*Neonatology Questions and Controversies*
# Neonatal Hemodynamics

# *Neonatology Questions and Controversies*
# Neonatal Hemodynamics
## Fourth Edition

### *Series Editor*

**Richard A. Polin, MD**
William T Speck Professor of Pediatrics
Executive Vice Chair Department of Pediatrics
Vagelos College of Physicians and Surgeons
Columbia University
New York, New York
United States

### *Other Volumes in the Neonatology Questions and Controversies Series*

GASTROENTEROLOGY AND NUTRITION

HEMATOLOGY AND TRANSFUSION MEDICINE

INFECTIOUS DISEASE, IMMUNOLOGY, AND PHARMACOLOGY

NEUROLOGY

RENAL, FLUID AND ELECTROLYTE DISORDERS

THE NEWBORN LUNG

**4th Edition**

## Neonatology Questions and Controversies

# Neonatal Hemodynamics

**Martin Kluckow, MBBS, FRACP, PhD, CCPU (Neonatal)**
University of Sydney and Royal North Shore
    Hospital
Sydney, NSW
Australia

**Patrick J. McNamara, MB, BCH, BAO, MSc, MRCP, MRCPCH, FASE**
University of Iowa Stead Family Children's
    Hospital
Iowa City, Iowa
United States

*Consulting Editor*
**Richard A. Polin, MD**
William T Speck Professor of Pediatrics
Executive Vice Chair Department of Pediatrics
Vagelos College of Physicians and Surgeons
Columbia University
New York, New York
United States

ELSEVIER

Elsevier
1600 John F. Kennedy Blvd.
Ste 1800
Philadelphia, PA 19103-2899

NEONATOLOGY QUESTIONS AND CONTROVERSIES:
NEONATAL HEMODYNAMICS, FOURTH EDITION

ISBN: 978-0-323-88073-2

---

**Notice**

Practitioners and researchers must always rely on their own experience and knowledge in evaluating and
using any information, methods, compounds or experiments described herein. Because of rapid
advances in the medical sciences, in particular, independent verification of diagnoses and drug dosages
should be made. To the fullest extent of the law, no responsibility is assumed by Elsevier, authors, editors
or contributors for any injury and/or damage to persons or property as a matter of products liability,
negligence or otherwise, or from any use or operation of any methods, products, instructions, or ideas
contained in the material herein.

---

Previous editions copyrighted 2019, 2012, and 2008.

Content Strategist: Sarah Barth
Senior Content Development Specialist: Vasowati Shome
Publishing Services Manager: Shereen Jameel
Project Manager: Nandhini Thanga Alagu
Design Direction: Margaret M. Reid

Printed in India

Last digit is the print number:    9   8   7   6   5   4   3   2   1

Working together
to grow libraries in
developing countries

www.elsevier.com • www.bookaid.org

*To my father, Padraic McNamara, whose passion for academia,*
*quest for new knowledge, and support of my career have been my lifelong*
*inspiration and major determinant in my desire for innovation and discovery;*
*I will be forever indebted.*

**Patrick J. McNamara**

**Regan Giesinger, MD**

*This book is also dedicated to an outstanding young investigator and contributor to two excellent chapters, Dr. Regan Giesinger, who passed away after an extensive battle with cancer on May 15, 2023. Dr. Giesinger was an exceptional young clinician-scientist who, at a very early stage of her career, achieved an international reputation in her field of neonatal hemodynamics and the application of targeted neonatal echocardiography (TnECHO) as a critical bedside tool to enhance clinical care and research through providing enhanced diagnostic and mechanistic insights. Her primary research work, which characterized the relationship between right ventricular dysfunction and neurodevelopmental outcomes in term neonates with hypoxic ischemic encephalopathy, was precedent setting and has laid the foundation for further investigation. She also published several original contributions related to novel therapies in pulmonary hypertension, and the use of nitric oxide in preterm infants. In addition, Regan showed outstanding strengths, integrity, and leadership in education, training, and administrative roles and represented the very best of academic medicine. She recognized that if we are to provide the "best" care, there was an urgent need to re-engage with physiology and in providing the "right" therapy, clinicians needed to recognize the importance of diagnostic precision and delineation of the specific phenotype. In teaching the importance of physiology and diagnostic precision in cardiovascular care, Regan has influenced a generation of trainees and young faculty. She is truly the "mother" of Neonatal Hemodynamics, and it has been an honor to have been her mentor, closest friend, and scientific collaborator.*

**Patrick J. McNamara**

# Contributors

**Carl Backes, MD**
**Professor of Pediatrics**
Departments of Neonatology and Cardiology
Nationwide Childrens Hospital
The Ohio State University Wexner Medical Center
Columbus, Ohio
United States

**Shazia Bhombal, MD**
**Clinical Associate Professor of Pediatrics**
Division of Neonatal and Developmental Medicine
Stanford University School of Medicine
Stanford, California
United States

**Adrianne Rahde Bischoff, MD**
**Clinical Assistant Professor**
Division of Neonatology
Department of Pediatrics
Univerity of Iowa
Iowa City, Iowa
United States

**Douglas A. Blank, MD, PhD**
**Research Fellow**
The Ritchie Centre, Hudson Institute of Medical
    Research and Department of Paediatrics
Monash University
**Neonatologist**
Monash Newborn
Monash Health
Clayton, Victoria
Australia

**TJ Boly, DO**
**Instructor of Pediatrics**
Division of Neonatology
Department of Pediatrics
University of Iowa
Iowa City, Iowa
United States

**Stephanie M. Boyd, MBBS (Hons), BSc (Med), MPHTM, FRACP, CCPU (Neonatal)**
**Staff Specialist Neonatologist**
Grace Centre for Newborn Intensive Care
The Children's Hospital at Westmead
Westmead, NSW
**Clinical Lecturer**
The University of Sydney
Sydney, NSW
Australia

**Neidin Bussmann, MB, BCh, BAO (NUI), LRCP, SI (Honours), MRCPI, PhD, PG Cert**
Department of Neonatology
NICU
Cork University Maternity Hospital
Cork
Ireland

**Trassanee Chatmethakul, MD**
**Assistant Professor**
Pediatrics, Section of Neonatal-Perinatal Medicine
University of Oklahoma Health Sciences Center
Oklahoma City, Oklahoma
United States

**David J. Cox, MBBS, PhD, MRCPCH**
**Consultant**
Department of Neonatal Medicine
Great Ormond Street Hospital for Children NHS
    Foundation Trust
London
United Kingdom

**Willem-Pieter de Boode, MD, PhD**
**Professor**
Department of Neonatology
Radboudumc Amalia Children's Hospital
Nijmegen
Netherlands

**Koert de Waal, PhD**
Associate Professor
Neonatology
John Hunter Children's Hospital
Newcastle, NSW
Australia

**Eugene Dempsey, FRCPI**
Professor
Paediatrics and Child Health
University College Cork, Cork
Principal Investigator
INFANT Centre
University College Cork,
Cork
Ireland

**Laura Dix, MD, PhD**
Department of Neonatology
Wilhelmina Children's Hospital, University Medical
    Centre Utrecht
Utrecht
Netherlands

**Adre J. du Plessis, MBChB, MPH**
Director
Prenatal Pediatrics Institute
Children's National Hospital
Chief
Division of Prenatal and Transitional Pediatrics
Children's National Hospital
Washington, District of Columbia
United States

**Afif Faisal El-Khuffash, MB, BCh, BAO, BA(Sci),
FRCPI, MD, DCE**
Professor
Department of Neonatology
The Rotunda Hospital
Dublin
Ireland

**Beate Horsberg Eriksen, MD, PhD**
Senior Consultant
Paediatric Department
Neonatal Intensive Care, Ålesund
Møra and Romsdal
Associate Professor
Clinical Research Unit
NTNU
Trondheim
Norway

**Nicholas Evans, DM, MRCPCH, CCPU
(Neonatal), OAM**
Clinical Associate Professor
Newborn Care
RPA Hospital and University of Sydney
Sydney, NSW
Australia

**Erika F. Fernandez, MD**
Neonatology Medical Director
Department of Pediatrics, Division of Neonatology
Dignity Health, Commonspirit
Santa Maria, California
United States

**Elizabeth Rachel Fisher, BMed, MMed(Clin Epi)**
Fellow
Neonatology
Royal North Shore Hospital
St Leonards, NSW
Clinical Associate Lecturer
Department of Obstetrics, Gynaecology and
    Neonatology, Northern Clinical School
University of Sydney
Sydney, NSW
Australia

**Drude Fugelseth, MD, PhD**
Professor
Institute of Clinical Medicine
University of Oslo
Consultant
Neonatal Intensive Care, Ullevål
Oslo University Hospital
Oslo
Norway

**Regan Giesinger (E), MD, FRCPC, FASE (Deceased)**
**Clinical Associate Professor**
Neonatology
University of Iowa
Iowa City, Iowa
United States

**Gorm Greisen, MD, DrMedSci**
**Honorary Consultant**
Neonatology
Rigshospitalet
**Emeritus Professor**
Institute of Clinical Medicine
University of Copenhagen
Copenhagen
Denmark

**Alan M. Groves, MBChB, MD, FRCPCH, BSc, FAAP**
**Associate Professor**
Pediatrics
Dell Medical School
The University of Texas at Austin
Austin, Texas
United States

**Samir Gupta, MD, MRCP, DM, FRCPCH, FRCPI**
**Professor of Neonatology**
Department of Engineering
Durham University
Durham
United Kingdom
**Division Chief of Neonatology**
Division of Neonatology
SIDRA Medicine
Doha
Qatar

**Audrey Hébert, MD, FRCPC**
**Assistant Professor**
Pediatrics
CHU de Québec, Laval University
Quebec City
Canada

**Stuart B. Hooper, BSc(Hons), PhD**
**Professor**
The Ritchie Centre
Hudson Institute for Medical Research
**Professor**
Obstetrics and Gynaecology
Monash University
Melbourne, Victoria
Australia

**Dr. Amish Jain, MBBS, MRCPCH, PhD, FASE**
**Professor**
Department of Paediatrics
University of Toronto
Toronto, Ontario
Canada

**Anup C. Katheria, MD, FAAP**
**Adjunct Associate Professor of Pediatrics**
Pediatrics
Loma Linda University
**Director**
Neonatal Research Institute
Sharp Mary Birch Hospital for Women and
    Newborns
San Diego, California
United States

**Martin Kluckow, MBBS, FRACP, PhD**
**Professor**
Division of Women's, Children's & Family Health
University of Sydney
**Senior Staff Specialist**
Department of Neonatology
Royal North Shore Hospital
Sydney, NSW
Australia

**Ganga Krishnamurthy, MBBS**
**Associate Professor**
Pediatrics
Columbia University Medical Center
New York, New York
United States

**David Van Laere, MD**
Neonatal Intensive Care
University Hospital Antwerp
Edegem
Life Sciences
University Antwerp
Antwerp
**Founder**
Innocens
Antwerp
Belgium

**Satyan Lakshminrusimha, MD, MBBS, FAAP**
**Dennis & Nancy Marks Professor and Chair**
Department of Pediatrics
UC Davis
**Pediatrician-in-Chief**
UC Davis Children's Hospital
Sacramento, California
United States

**Petra Lemmers, MD, PhD**
Department of Neonatology
Wilhelmina Children's Hospital and Brain Center
    Rudolph Magnus University Medical Center
Utrecht University
Utrecht
Netherlands

**Philip T. Levy, MD**
**Assistant Professor**
Neonatology
Division of Newborn Medicine
Boston Childrens Hospital
Brookline, Massachusetts
United States

**Patrick J. McNamara, MB, BCH, BAO, MRCPCH, DCh, MSc**
**Professor**
Pediatrics and Internal Medicine
University of Iowa
Iowa City, Iowa
United States

**Christopher McPherson, PharmD**
**Clinical Pharmacy Specialist**
Pharmacy
St. Louis Children's Hospital
**Associate Professor**
Pediatrics
Washington University School of Medicine
St. Louis, Missouri
United States

**Souvik Mitra, MD, MSc, PhD, FRCPC**
**Associate Professor**
Pediatrics, Community Health & Epidemiology
Dalhousie University
Halifax, Nova Scotia
Canada

**Bassel Mohammad Nijres, MD, MS**
**Assistant Professor**
Pediatric Cardiology
University of Iowa
Iowa City, Iowa
United States

**Sarah B. Mulkey, MD, PhD**
**Associate Professor**
Pediatrics and Neurology
George Washington University School of Medicine
    and Health Sciences
Washington, District of Columbia
United States

**Rema S. Nagpal, MD**
**Associate Professor**
Department of Pediatrics
B.J. Govt. Medical College & Sassoon General
    Hospitals
Pune, Maharashtra
India

**Gunnar Naulaers, MD,PhD**
**Professor**
Development and Regeneration
KU Leuven
Leuven
Belgium

**Elaine Neary, MD, PHD**
Consultant Neonatologist
Department of Family Health
Liverpool Neonatal Partnership
Liverpool
United Kingdom

**Eirik Nestaas, MD, PhD**
Associate Professor
Institute of Clinical Medicine
University of Oslo
Consultant
The Clinic of Paediatrics and Adolescence
Akershus University Hospital
Oslo
Norway

**Shahab Noori, MD, MS, CBTI**
Professor of Pediatrics
Fetal and Neonatal Institute, Division of
    Neonatology, Children's Hospital Los Angeles,
    Department of Pediatrics
Keck School of Medicine, University of Southern
    California
Los Angeles, California
United States

**Anthony N. Price, PhD**
Senior Research Fellow
School of Imaging Sciences & Biomedical
    Engineering
King's College London
London
United Kingdom

**Jay D. Pruetz, MD**
Associate Professor
Pediatrics
USC Keck School of Medicine
Associate Professor
Department of Clinical Obstetrics and Gynecology
USC Keck School of Medicine
Attending Cardiologist
Heart Institute
Children's Hospital Los Angeles
Los Angeles, California
United States

**Danielle R. Rios, MD, MS**
Associate Professor
Department of Pediatrics
University of Iowa
Iowa City, Iowa
United States

**Mohit Sahni, MBBS, DCH, DNB(peds), Fellowship
Neonatology**
Director
Neonatology
Nirmal hospital Pvt. Ltd
Surat, Gujarat
India

**Sarah D. Schlatterer, MD, PhD**
Assistant Professor
Neurology
George Washington University School of Medicine
    and Health Sciences
Assistant Professor
Pediatrics
George Washington University School of Medicine
    and Health Sciences
Prenatal/Neonatal Neurologist
Prenatal Pediatrics Institute
Children's National Hospital
Washington, District of Columbia
United States

**Istvan Seri, MD, PhD, HonD, HonP**
Professor
Pediatrics
Department of Pediatrics, Semmelweis University
Budapest
Hungary
Adjunct Professor
Pediatrics/Neonatology
Children's Hospital Los Angeles; USC Keck School of
    Medicine
Los Angeles, California
United States

**Prakesh S. Shah, MD, FRCPC, MSc**
Professor
Department of Pediatrics
University of Toronto
Toronto, Ontario
Canada

**Yogen Singh, MD, MA(Cantab), FRCPCH**
Professor
Department of Pediatrics, Division of Neonatology
Loma Linda University School of Medicine
Loma Linda, California
**Adjunct Clinical Professor of Pediatrics**
Department of Pediatrics
Stanford University School of Medicine
Stanford, California
United States

**Suresh Victor, FRCPCH, PhD**
Senior Lecturer
Perinatal Imaging and Health
King's College London
London
United Kingdom

**Pradeep Suryawanshi, MD, DCH, FNNF, FRCPCH**
Professor & Head
Department of Neonatology
Bharati Vidyapeeth University Medical College Pune
Pune, Maharashtra
India

**Frank van Bel, MD, PhD**
Professor
Neonatology
University Medical Center Utrecht
Utrecht
Netherlands

**Angelica Vasquez, MD**
Clinical Assistant Professor
Neonatal-Perinatal Medicine
Vagelos College of Physicians and Surgeons
Columbia University
New York, New York
United States

**Michael Weindling, BSc, MA, MD, FRCP, FRCPCH, HonFRCA**
Department of Women's and Children's Health
University of Liverpool, Liverpool Health Partners
Liverpool
United Kingdom

**Dany E. Weisz, MD, MSc, FRCP(C)**
Associate Professor
Pediatrics
University of Toronto
Toronto, Ontario
Canada

# Series Foreword

*"To study the phenomena of disease without books is to sail an uncharted sea, while to study books without patients is not to go to sea at all."*

*"Medicine is learned by the bedside and not in the classroom. Let not your conceptions of disease come from the words heard in the lecture room or read from the book. See and then reason and compare and control. But see first."*

William Osler

Before the invention of the movable type by Johannes Gutenberg in the 15th century, physicians learned medicine by serving an apprenticeship with individuals considered experienced. There were no printed textbooks, and medical journals were not published until the beginning of the 19th century. By apprenticing yourself to a physician over a period of years, one learned how to be a competent practitioner. Internships in the United States evolved from those apprenticeships in the 18th century. The term *residency* was chosen because the physicians in training had a "residence" at the hospital. Modern-day internships began at the Johns Hopkins Hospital in 1904. The Johns Hopkins Hospital was founded by Osler, Halstead, Welch, and Kelly. Halstead is credited with creating the first surgical residency and coined the phrase "see one, do one, teach one" (SODOTO). That educational philosophy has been adopted by nearly every specialty in medicine, including neonatology.

Modern-day trainees in neonatology still learn how to care for critically ill infants and how to perform procedures by watching, assisting, and listening to more experienced individuals at the bedside. The SODOTO approach is considered a fundamental educational tool. However, over a 3-year period, much of education occurs away from the bedside during teaching rounds and conferences. The teaching is often more theoretical, and by design, rounds in the nursery and conferences are passive learning exercises. In those settings, trainees listen but do not take an active role in the educational process. Learning is always more effective when the recipient takes an active role in their own education. Ideally, they should be questioning what they hear, reading pertinent literature and, when the opportunity arises, teaching others. Unfortunately, much of the information transmitted in those settings is not usually followed by an active phase of questioning and reading by the trainee.

Most graduates of fellowship programs turn out to be excellent practitioners, but once they leave the fellowship program, new information is acquired only intermittently either at conferences or from journals and textbooks. As a source of new information, journals provide access to the most up-to-date information. However, that information is unfiltered, and the conclusions of a study may not be appropriate (or perhaps risky) for a critically ill infant. Textbooks like the ones in the Neonatology Questions and Controversies series offer an opportunity to hear from experts in neonatal-perinatal medicine who have synthesized (and filtered) the existing literature and can provide up-to-date recommendations.

The fourth edition of the Questions and Controversies series will also have seven volumes. Each of them has been extensively revised, and we have added several new editors: Terri Inder has joined Jeffrey Perlman for the Neurology volume, James Wynn joined William Benitz and P. Brian Smith as a coeditor for the Infectious Disease, Immunology and Pharmacology volume, and Patrick J. McNamara is now a coeditor with Martin Kluckow for the Neonatal Hemodynamics volume. The reader will find many completely new chapters; however, like the last edition, each of them is focused on day-to day clinical decisions encountered by neonatologists. Nothing will replace the teaching that occurs at the bedside when confronted with a critically ill neonate, and the SODOTO educational approach still has an important role in education. Procedures are best learned by simulations and guidance from experienced practitioners at the bedside. However, expertise as a practitioner can only be enhanced by reading and incorporating new information into daily practice, once proven safe and effective. Perhaps SODOTO should be changed to LQRT (listen, question, read, and teach).

Questions and Controversies is a unique source to learn from experts in the field who have been through the LQRT process many times. Osler's quotes at the top of this foreword suggest that both bedside teaching and journals/textbooks have a synergistic role in physician education, and neither is sufficient by itself.

As with all prior editions, I am indebted to an exceptional group of volume editors who chose the content and authors and edited the manuscripts. I also want to thank Sarah Barth (Publisher) as well as Vasowati Shome and Vaishali Singh (Senior Content Development Specialists) at Elsevier, who have guided the development of this series.

Richard A. Polin, MD

# Preface

Hemodynamics represents the interaction between heart function, blood flow, and pressures in the systemic and pulmonary circulations and is by definition dynamic, varying with time and physiological conditions. Lessons learned over the past decade, by neonatologists who have studied neonatal hemodynamics using ultrasound and other noninvasive techniques, have demonstrated the complexity of the interaction between cardiovascular physiology and neonatal disease states. In particular, there is increasing recognition of the existence of multiple cardiovascular phenotypes in similar clinical situations. Therefore, neonatal hemodynamics continues to be an area of medicine ripe for study and trials as we remain at the infancy of our understanding of neonatal cardiovascular disease and the complexities of management.

The Hemodynamics and Cardiology volume of the book series Questions and Controversies in Neonatology continues to evolve as this relatively new specialty becomes more clinically relevant and important in neonatal care. The book has changed significantly from the combined Neonatal/Cardiac vision of the initial editors Charles Kleinman and Istvan Seri through to that of the current editors, Martin Kluckow and new co-editor Patrick J. McNamara. Patrick is one of the thought leaders in this new and evolving area and has been instrumental in expanding this specialty into an important component of acute neonatal care. Under the new editors we have focused the book primarily on the emerging specialty of neonatal hemodynamics, with a single overview chapter on cardiology/congenital heart disease.

The latest edition of the book covers everything from basic cardiovascular physiology through to advanced monitoring and hemodynamic assessment. It provides in-depth clinical overviews of the many hemodynamic conditions that are relevant for the neonatologist, including approach to blood pressure and blood flow, management of a patent ductus arteriosus (PDA) including percutaneous device closure, acute and chronic pulmonary hypertension, and congenital diaphragmatic hernia. The book contains a state-of-the-art review of advanced neonatal hemodynamic assessment methods including speckle echocardiography, novel methods of assessment of the right ventricle, and cardiac MRI.

Several chapters have been completely overhauled to focus on the novel concept of hemodynamic phenotypes and, from there, the concept of individualized assessment and management, according to the underlying physiology. Clinical controversies in management are discussed, and the expert opinion of our highly experienced and qualified authors is clearly set out. Several chapters are devoted to contemporary areas of hemodynamic controversy (e.g., PDA, hypotension, and pulmonary hypertension) but have been reimagined to focus on an individualistic approach to care based on the ambient physiology, enhanced diagnostic precision, and phenotypic profiling. Of note, the use of case-based examples in these chapters to emphasize areas of physiological variability and the dynamic nature of illness and response to treatment is a highlight of the new edition. A new chapter entitled Neonatal Hemodynamic Pharmacology brings together all commonly used cardiovascular pharmacological agents efficiently and summarizes their use. Other new chapters include hemodynamic management in special circumstances (twin-twin transfusion, infant of a diabetic mother, arteriovenous malformations), neonatal hemodynamic care written from the perspective of the resource-challenged country, and a more stream-lined review of the hemodynamics of umbilical cord clamping. We are immensely grateful to the contributing authors, all of whom we consider to be experts in their respective topics. We hope that this book will stimulate you to think more deeply about physiology when you are faced with hemodynamic pathology, and that this will lead to better, more focused care of your neonatal patients.

**Martin Kluckow, MBBS, FRACP,
PhD, CCPU (Neonatal)
Patrick J. McNamara, MB, BCH, BAO,
MSc, MRCP, MRCPCH, FASE**

# Contents

xvi

# Cardiovascular Physiology, Pathophysiology, and Pharmacology

# Chapter 1

# Principles of Developmental Cardiovascular Physiology and Pathophysiology

Shahab Noori and Istvan Seri

## Key Points

1. A successful hemodynamic transition from fetal to extrauterine life is a complex process and requires the interdependent sequential physiologic changes to take place in a timely manner
2. Immaturity- or pathophysiology-driven disturbances of the transitional process may have significant short- and long-term consequences
3. Timely diagnosis and pathophysiology-targeted management of neonatal shock pose difficult challenges for the clinician
4. Many questions remain unanswered, including, but not restricted to, the timely recognition of the subpopulation of neonates at high risk for the development of hemodynamic compromise in the transitional period, the definition of the individual patient-dependent blood pressure thresholds associated with inadequate tissue oxygen delivery, the role of physiologic cord clamping, and the recognition of the hemodynamic antecedents of peri-intraventricular hemorrhage

## Introduction

The last two decades have seen a growing controversy in the field of neonatal hemodynamics in general and over the diagnosis and treatment of neonatal cardiovascular insufficiency, especially in the very preterm infant. The complexities and difficulties associated with the design and execution of randomized controlled trials (RCTs) targeting clinically relevant outcome measures in very preterm neonates with cardiovascular compromise are the primary reason for the ongoing controversy. Indeed, essential questions such as the blood pressure (BP) threshold associated with inadequate tissue oxygen delivery (and thus necessitating treatment in a selected patient population) can only be answered by properly designed RCTs. In the absence of such information, applying the principles of developmental cardiovascular physiology and pathophysiology can aid the diagnosis and management of neonatal circulatory compromise. In addition, designing RCTs in this area also requires a thorough understanding of developmental cardiovascular physiology.

Therefore this chapter first reviews the principles of fetal, transitional, and post-transitional hemodynamics, with an emphasis on the principles of developmental cardiovascular physiology. The major goals of this chapter are to help the reader to appreciate the impact of immaturity and/or pathological events on the physiology of neonatal cardiovascular transition and understand the primary factors leading to cardiovascular compromise in the preterm and term neonate. Using this knowledge, along with carefully selected and relevant information from clinical trials, the clinician can best assess and manage hemodynamic disturbance in the immediate transitional period and beyond and potentially reduce the end-organ damage caused by decreased oxygen delivery to the organs, especially to the immature brain.

## Principles of Developmental Physiology

### FETAL CIRCULATION

The fetal circulation is characterized by low systemic vascular resistance (SVR) with high systemic blood flow and high pulmonary vascular resistance with low pulmonary blood flow. Given the low oxygen tension of the fetus, the fetal circulation allows for preferential flow of the most oxygenated blood to the heart and brain, two of the three "vital organs".[1,2]

With the placenta rather than the lungs being the organ of gas exchange, most of the right ventricular output is diverted through the patent ductus arteriosus (PDA) to the systemic circulation. In fact, the pulmonary blood flow only constitutes about 7–8% of the combined cardiac output in fetal lambs.[3] However, Doppler and magnetic resonance imaging studies have shown that the proportion of combined cardiac output that supplies the lungs is higher in the human fetus (11–25%), with some studies reporting an increase in this proportion with advancing gestational age to a peak around 30 weeks' gestation.[4-7] In fetal life both ventricles contribute to the systemic blood flow, and the circulation therefore depends on the persistence of shunts via the foramen ovale and PDA between the systemic and pulmonary circuits, with the two circulations functioning in "parallel". The right ventricle (RV) is the dominant pumping chamber, and its contribution to the combined cardiac output is about 60%. The combined cardiac output is in the range of 400–450 mL/kg/min in the fetus, which is much higher than the systemic flow after birth (about 200 mL/kg/min). Approximately one-third of the combined cardiac output (150 mL/kg/min) perfuses the placenta via the umbilical vessels. However, placental blood flow decreases to 21% of the combined cardiac output near term.[8] The umbilical vein carries the oxygenated blood from the placenta though the portal veins and the ductus venosus to the inferior vena cava (IVC) and eventually to the heart. About 50% of oxygenated blood in the umbilical vein is shunted through the ductus venosus and IVC to the right atrium, where the oxygenated blood is preferentially directed to the left atrium through the patent foramen ovale. This percentage decreases as gestation advances. One of the unique characteristics of the fetal circulation is that arterial oxygen saturation ($SaO_2$) is different between the upper and lower body. Having the most oxygenated blood in the left atrium ensures a supply of adequate oxygen to the heart and brain. Furthermore, in response to hypoxemia, most of the blood flow in the umbilical vein bypasses the portal circulation via the ductus venosus and again delivers the most oxygenated blood to the heart and brain.

## TRANSITIONAL PHYSIOLOGY

Transition from the fetal to the postnatal type of circulation is a complex process. In the past decade research interest has again focused on cardiovascular and pulmonary adaptation at birth. Amongst others, animal and human studies have investigated the impact of the timing of cord clamping on cardiovascular and pulmonary transitional physiology. The findings of these studies have highlighted the importance of allowing for placental transfusion to take place and suggested that lung aeration should be established prior to umbilical cord clamping to ensure that the source of left ventricular (LV) preload gradually changes over from the placenta to the lungs.[9] The maintenance of appropriate LV preload during the immediate hemodynamic transition from the fetal to the postnatal circulation has been shown to attenuate the abrupt decrease in preload and systemic blood flow seen with the practice of immediate cord clamping[10] and is associated with improved postnatal hemodynamic stability and clinical outcomes (Chapter 6). Among the clinical outcomes, improved postnatal transition, decreased need for blood transfusion, and lower incidence of intraventricular hemorrhage have been documented without significant untoward effects associated with delayed cord clamping in preterm infants.[11-15] In addition, a decreased need for blood transfusion has been observed in term neonates, albeit with higher rates of jaundice and polycythemia reported. As discussed in Chapter 6 in detail, these findings have led to a departure from the traditional approach of immediate cord clamping and a move to delayed clamping of the cord for all newborns who are vigorous at birth in the absence of conditions preventing placental transfusion.[16-18] Interestingly, cord milking seems to confer similar hemodynamic benefits to delayed cord clamping.[19,20] However, the finding of a higher rate of severe peri-/intraventricular hemorrhage (P/IVH) in the cord milking as compared to the delayed cord clamping group in preterm infants of <32 weeks' gestation is concerning.[21] The reason for the increased risk of P/IVH is unclear, although a rapid rise in cerebral blood flow (CBF) has been postulated as one of the possible etiological factors. In a subset of the patients in the trial by Katheria et al., cerebral oxygen saturation was also monitored in the delivery room and the findings were published in a separate paper.[22] Interestingly, arterial oxygen saturation was higher in the cord milking group, without a difference in cerebral tissue oxygen saturation between the groups. Therefore, as a group, subjects who underwent cord milking might not have had excessive CBF. However, it is possible that in selected vulnerable individuals, a rapid increase in the preload and thus CBF plays a role. Therefore, while cord milking could reduce the risk of cerebral ischemia by rapidly increasing circulating blood volume and thus preload and therefore improving systemic blood flow, it may increase the risk of P/IVH through yet unidentified mechanism(s), and its use is currently not recommended.

After birth, the circulation changes from parallel to series, and thus the left and RV outputs must become equal. However, this process, especially in very preterm infants, is not complete for days or even weeks after birth due to the inability of the fetal channels to close in a timely manner. The persistence of the PDA alters the hemodynamics during transition and beyond and has been associated with severe and even refractory hypotension.[23,24] The impact of the PDA on pulmonary and systemic blood flow in the preterm infant is discussed in Chapter 16. At birth, removal of the low-resistance placental circulation and the surge in catecholamines and other hormones increase the SVR. On the other hand, pulmonary vascular resistance (PVR) drops precipitously due to the act of breathing air and exposure of the pulmonary arteries to higher partial pressure of oxygen as compared to the very low level in utero. Organ blood flow also changes significantly. In the newborn lamb CBF drops in response to oxygen exposure.[25] A drop in CBF in the first few minutes after birth in normal-term neonates has also been reported.[26] This drop in CBF appears to be related, at least in part, to cerebral vasoconstriction in response to the increase in arterial blood oxygen content immediately after birth. In addition, the correlation between left-to-right PDA shunting and middle cerebral artery flow velocity (a surrogate for CBF) suggests a possible role of the ductus arteriosus in the observed reduction in CBF.[26] Finally, especially in some very preterm neonates,

the inability of the immature myocardium to pump against the suddenly increased SVR might lead to a transient decrease in systemic blood flow, which in turn could also contribute to the decrease in CBF (Chapters 2 and 20).

## POSTNATAL CIRCULATION

### Pressure, Flow, and Resistance

Poiseuille's equation ($Q = [\Delta P \times \pi\ r^4]/8\mu L$) describes the factors that determine the movement of fluid through a tube. This equation helps us understand how changes in cardiovascular parameters affect blood flow. Basically, flow (Q) is directly related to the pressure difference ($\Delta P$) across the vessel and the fourth power of the radius (r) and inversely related to the length (L) of the vessel and the viscosity of the fluid ($\mu$). Therefore, BP is the driving force behind moving blood through the vasculature. As there are several differences between laminar flow of water through a tube and blood flow through the body, the relationship between the above factors in the body does not exactly follow the equation. In addition, because we do not measure all components of this equation, in clinical practice the interaction among BP, flow, and SVR is described by using an analogy of Ohm's law (cardiac output = pressure gradient/SVR). Therefore blood flow is directly related to BP and inversely related to SVR. Regulation of and changes in cardiac output and SVR determine the BP. In other words, systemic BP is the dependent variable of the interaction between the two independent variables: cardiac output (flow) and SVR. Of note, since cardiac output is also partly affected by SVR, in theory, cardiac output cannot be considered a completely independent variable.

Cardiac output is determined by heart rate, preload, myocardial contractility, and afterload. Preload can be described in terms of pressure or volume: that is, central venous pressure or end-diastolic ventricular volume. Therefore preload is affected not only by the effective circulating blood volume but also by many other factors such as myocardial relaxation and compliance, contractility, and afterload. Increasing end-diastolic volume leads to an increase in stroke volume according to the Frank-Starling mechanism. The magnitude of increase in stroke volume depends on the Frank-Starling curve for the ventricle, which in turn is affected by the afterload and inotropic properties of the myocardium. The limited data available on diastolic function in the newborn in general and in preterm infants in particular suggests lower myocardial compliance and relaxation function. On the other hand, baseline myocardial contractility is high or comparable to older children, while the myocardial capacity to maintain contractility in the face of an increase in the afterload might be limited (see below). Afterload and SVR are related and usually change in the same direction. Yet, these two parameters are different and should not be used interchangeably. SVR is determined by the resistance of the vascular system and is regulated by changes in the diameter of the small resistance vessels, primarily the arterioles. In contrast, afterload is the force that the myocardium has to overcome to pump blood out of the ventricles during the ejection period. Wall tension can be used as a measure of afterload. Therefore, based on Laplace's law, LV afterload is directly related to the intraventricular pressure and the LV diameter at the end of systole and indirectly related to the myocardial wall thickness. Indeed, changes in SVR exert their effect on afterload indirectly by affecting BP.

## Organ Blood Flow Distribution

Under resting physiologic conditions, blood flow to each organ is regulated by a baseline vascular tone under the influence of the autonomic nervous system. Changes in the baseline vascular tone regulate organ blood flow. Vascular tone is regulated by local tissue (e.g., $H^+$, $CO_2$, and $O_2$), paracrine (e.g., nitric oxide [NO], prostacyclin and endothelin-1), and neurohormonal factors as well as by the myogenic properties of the blood vessel. Under pathologic conditions such as hypoxia-ischemia, the relative organ distribution of cardiac output favors the "vital" organs (the brain, heart, and adrenal glands). In principle, vital organ designation is operational even in fetal life. However, the vascular bed of the forebrain (cortex) might only achieve the characteristic "vital organ" vasodilatory response to a decrease in perfusion pressure late in the second trimester (see discussion below).

## Microcirculatory Physiology

Other than being the site of exchange of oxygen and nutrients and removal of metabolic byproducts, the microcirculation also plays a significant role in regulating systemic and local hemodynamics. The small arteries and arterioles are the main regulators of peripheral vascular resistance, and the venules and small veins play an important role as capacitance vessels. Coupling of oxygen supply and demand is one of the primary functions of the microcirculation. Oxygen delivery ($DO_2$) depends on blood flow and oxygen content. The total oxygen content of the blood (hemoglobin-bound and dissolved) can be calculated based on the hemoglobin concentration (Hb; g/dL), $SaO_2$, and partial pressure of oxygen ($PaO_2$; mmHg) in the arterial blood ($[1.36 \times Hb \times SaO_2] + [0.003 \times PaO_2]$). Tissue blood flow is adjusted based on the oxygen consumption ($VO_2$) determined by the metabolic requirements. When the blood flow cannot be increased beyond a certain point, oxygen extraction is increased to meet the demand for $VO_2$. Therefore $VO_2$ is not affected by decreases in blood flow until the tissue's capacity to extract more oxygen is exhausted. At this point, $VO_2$ becomes directly flow dependent.[27]

In healthy term infants localized peripheral (buccal) perfusion assessed by capillary-weighted saturation using visible light spectroscopy has only a weak correlation with central blood flow during the transitional period.[28] Therefore it is possible that under physiologic conditions, peripheral blood flow is not affected by the variability in the systemic blood flow. In other words, blood flow (cardiac output) is regulated to meet $VO_2$. In ventilated preterm infants limb blood flow assessed by near-infrared spectroscopy (NIRS) showed no correlation with BP.[29] Along with the poor correlation of buccal oxygen saturation with cardiac output in healthy term neonates, these findings suggest that regulation of the microcirculation and peripheral blood flow in relatively hemodynamically stable preterm and term neonates might be, at least to a certain point, independent from systemic blood flow.

Skin microcirculation has been more extensively studied in neonates. Orthogonal polarization spectral imaging studies of skin demonstrated that functional small vessel density, a measure of tissue perfusion and microcirculation, changes over the first postnatal month and directly correlates with hemoglobin concentration and environmental temperature in preterm infants.[30] In this study functional small vessel density was also inversely related to BP. This finding indicates that evaluation of skin microcirculation may be useful in the indirect assessment of SVR. Findings of laser Doppler flowmetry studies of the skin indicate that the relationship between peripheral microvascular blood flow and cardiovascular function evolves during the first few postnatal days and that it depends on the gestational age and sex of the patient.[31-33] Indeed, the inverse relationship between microvascular blood flow, calculated SVR, and mean BP immediately after delivery is no longer present by the fifth postnatal day.[31] Interestingly, male preterm infants are more likely to have peripheral vasodilation at 24 hours after birth and this may be related to the different maturational pattern of the autonomic nervous system in male compared to female neonates.[32,33] A recent study found a higher sympathetic output at 6 hours after birth in male preterm infants compared to females; however, sympathetic tone tends to decrease in males and increase in females over time during the first 3 postnatal days.[32] Gestational age has an inverse relationship with microvascular blood flow during the first few postnatal days.[32] Among the most immature neonates (≤28 weeks), those who died during the transitional period had higher baseline microvascular blood flow, that is, lower peripheral vascular resistance.[31] These findings suggest that developmental changes in the microcirculation also play a significant role in the regulation of transitional hemodynamics and that microcirculatory maladaptation is associated with and/or may increase the risk of mortality.

Given the limited data available and inconsistency of the findings, further studies of the regulation of microcirculation are needed to improve our understanding of the physiology and pathophysiology of the microcirculation during development and postnatal transition and to better characterize its role in the regulation of systemic hemodynamics in the preterm and term neonate.

## Myocardial Function – Developmental Aspects

There are important differences in myocardial structure and function between the immature myocardium of the neonate compared to that of the older child and adult.[34,35] The immature myocardium of the preterm and term neonate has less contractile elements, higher water content, greater surface-to-volume ratio, and an underdeveloped sarcoplasmic reticulum. The immature myocardium primarily relies on the function of L-type calcium channels and thus on extracellular calcium concentration for the calcium supply necessary for muscle contraction. In children and adults these channels only serve to trigger the release of calcium from its abundant intracellular sources in the sarcoplasmic reticulum. These characteristics of the immature myocardium explain the observed differences in myocardial compliance and contractility between preterm and term neonates and children and adults.

Echocardiography studies have shown that the immature myocardium has a higher baseline contractile state and that contractility rapidly decreases in the face of an increase in afterload.[36] The sensitivity of the immature myocardium to afterload means that for the same degree of rise in the afterload, the myocardium of the neonate has a more significant reduction in contractility compared to children or adults. With the rise in SVR after birth, LV afterload increases. This, in turn, may lead to a significant decrease in myocardial contractility with possible clinical implications (see discussion under myocardial dysfunction). Another difference between the immature myocardium of neonates and the mature heart of older children is the force-frequency relationship (FFR). FFR describes the relationship between the heart rate and contractile force. As heart rate increases, the contractility increases to a point beyond which contractility declines with further increases in heart rate. Therefore there is an optimal heart rate in relation to contractility. Little is known about the FFR in neonates. An in vivo pig model showed an adaptive response to tachycardia, with improved force generation at a greater heart rate in the newborn animals compared to a decreased force generation in adults.[37] This may explain, at least in part, the better tolerance of tachycardia in neonates compared to adults. Conversely, a study of ventricle muscle strips obtained during corrective cardiac surgery from subjects with congenital heart defects showed a flat FFR in newborns <2 weeks old, while the contractile force increased in response to increasing heart rate in 3- to 14-month-old infants.[38] Obviously, more data are needed to better define the FFR and its clinical implications in neonates.

## Impact of the Immature Autonomic Nervous System on Regulating Cardiac Function and Vascular Tone

Circulatory function is mediated at the central and local levels through neural, hormonal, and metabolic mechanisms and reflex pathways (Figure 1.1). Integral to the regulation of cardiac function and vascular tone is the central nervous system. The medulla generates complex patterns of sympathetic, parasympathetic, and cardiovascular responses that are essential for homeostasis, as well as behavioral patterning of autonomic activity.[39,40] The balance between sympathetic and parasympathetic outflow to the heart and blood vessels is regulated by peripheral baroreceptors and chemoreceptors in the aortic arch and carotid sinus, as well as by the mechanoreceptors in the heart and lungs.[41] Though many of these pathways have been identified, much work remains to delineate the adaptation of cardiovascular control in the immature infant, where the maturation of the many components of this complex system is at varying pace and has been shown to lead to instability in autonomic function and maintenance of adequate organ blood flow and BP. The effect of the dynamic nature of the developing system on cardiovascular function is unclear but it may have short- and long-term implications for neonates born premature or with growth restriction.[42,43]

Heart rate variability analysis is a non-invasive tool employed to assess the sympathetic and parasympathetic modulation of the cardiovascular system over a relatively short period of time.[44-46] This method has been found to be useful in conditions where cardiac output has been impacted, such as in patients with sepsis.[47,48] Heart rate variability analysis holds promise to further characterize the autonomic control of cardiovascular function since the relationship among heart rate variability, sympathovagal balance, and the modulation of the renin-angiotensin-aldosterone system in various pathophysiologic states can be explored.

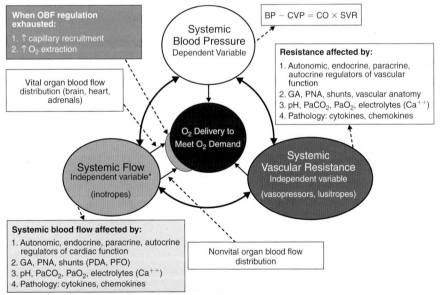

**Fig. 1.1  To meet cellular metabolic demand, a complex interaction among blood flow, vascular resistance, and blood pressure takes place.** Vascular resistance and blood flow are the independent variables and blood pressure is the dependent variable in this interaction characterized by the simplified equation using an analogy of Ohm's law: BP − CVP = CO × SVR. However, as cardiac output is also affected by SVR, it cannot be considered a completely independent variable. In addition to the interaction among the major determinants of cardiovascular function, complex regulation of blood flow distribution to vital and non-vital organs, recruitment of capillaries, and extraction of oxygen all play a fundamental role in the maintenance of hemodynamic homeostasis.[184] BP = blood pressure, CBF = cerebral blood flow; CO = cardiac output; CVP = central venous pressure; GA = gestational age; OBF = organ blood flow; PaCO$_2$ = partial pressure of carbon dioxide in the arteries; PaO$_2$ = partial pressure of oxygen in the arteries; PDA = patent ductus arteriosus; PFO = patent foramen ovale; PNA = postnatal age; SVR = systemic vascular resistance. See text for details.

## Developmental Cardiovascular Pathophysiology: Etiology and Pathophysiology of Neonatal Shock

To ensure normal cellular function and maintenance of structural integrity, delivery of oxygen must meet cellular oxygen demand. Oxygen delivery is determined by the oxygen content of the blood and cardiac output (see earlier). However, cardiac output can only deliver oxygen effectively to the organs if perfusion pressure (BP) is maintained in a range appropriate to the given conditions of the cardiovascular system. As BP is determined by the interaction between SVR and cardiac output (BP $\alpha$ SVR $\times$ systemic blood flow; Figure 1.1), the complex interdependence between perfusion pressure and systemic blood flow mandates that, if possible, both should be monitored in critically ill neonates (Chapter 14).

Indeed, if SVR is too low, BP (perfusion pressure) may drop below a critical level where cellular oxygen delivery becomes compromised despite normal or even high cardiac output. However, if SVR is too high, cardiac output and thus organ perfusion may decrease to a critical level such that cellular oxygen delivery becomes compromised despite maintenance of BP in the perceived normal range. Therefore the use of either BP or cardiac output *alone* for the assessment of the cardiovascular status is misleading, especially under certain critical circumstances in preterm and term neonates. Unfortunately, while BP can be continuously monitored, there are only a few recently developed and not yet fully validated invasive and non-invasive bedside techniques which continuously monitor systemic perfusion, in absolute numbers in the critically ill neonate (see Chapter 14). Therefore, in most intensive care units, the clinician has been left with monitoring the indirect and rather insensitive and non-specific measures of organ perfusion such as urine output and capillary refill time (CRT) (Chapter 20). Monitoring the time course of the development and cessation of lactic acidosis is the most specific indirect measure of the status of tissue perfusion and it has become available from small blood samples along with routine blood-gas analysis. However, this measure has its limitations as well, as elevated serum lactic acid levels may represent an ongoing impairment in tissue oxygenation or a previous event with improvement in tissue perfusion ("wash-out phenomenon"). Thus serum lactic acid concentration needs to be sequentially monitored and a single value may not provide appropriate information regarding tissue perfusion. Furthermore, when epinephrine is being administered, epinephrine induced-specific increases in lactic acid levels occur independent of the state of tissue perfusion.[49]

Because it is a common practice to routinely measure BP in neonates, population-based normative data are available for the statistically defined normal ranges of BP in preterm and term neonates.[50-52] It is very likely that the 5th or the 10th percentiles of these gestational- and postnatal-age-dependent normative data used to define hypotension do not represent BP values in every patient where autoregulation of organ blood flow or organ blood flow itself is necessarily compromised. Recent findings have described the possible lower limits of BP below which autoregulation of CBF, cerebral function, and, finally, cerebral perfusion are impaired in very-low-birth-weight (VLBW) preterm infants (Figure 1.2).[53-55] The true impact of gestational and postnatal age, and the individual patient's ability to compensate (with increased cardiac output and appropriate regulation of organ blood flow) on the dependency of CBF on BP in this population remains to be determined.[56-58] It is particularly interesting that two studies using different methods and patients with different gestational and postnatal age have found that the lower elbow of the CBF autoregulatory curve might be at 29 mmHg of mean BP.[53-55] However, there is not sufficient evidence to recommend that mean BP in preterm neonates during the first postnatal days be kept above this breakpoint. Several epidemiological studies have demonstrated that hypotension and/or low systemic perfusion are associated with increased mortality and morbidity in the neonatal patient population. Other studies found an increase in mortality and morbidity in preterm infants who received treatment for hypotension. Due to the retrospective and uncontrolled nature of these studies, it is hard to tease out the cause of adverse outcome associated with hypotension. It is possible that the poor outcome associated with hypotension is multifactorial; thus it may either be due to the direct effect of hypotension on organ perfusion, inappropriate use and titration of vasopressor-inotropes, inotropes or lusitropes,

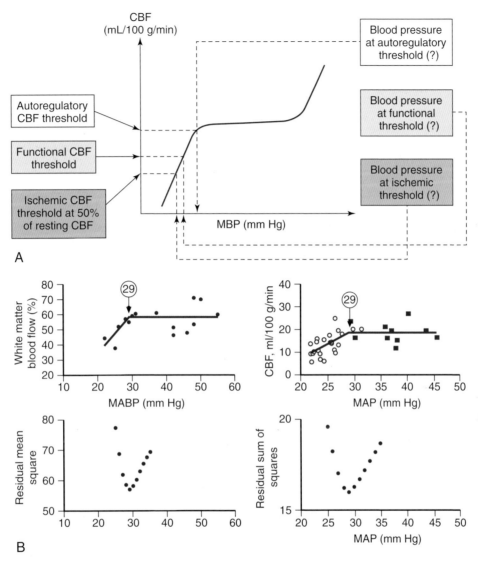

**Fig. 1.2** (A) Definition of hypotension by three pathophysiological phenomena of increasing severity: the "autoregulatory, functional, and ischemic thresholds" of hypotension. Cerebral blood flow (CBF) is compromised when blood pressure decreases to below autoregulatory threshold. With further decrease in blood pressure, first brain function is impaired, followed by tissue injury as ischemic threshold is crossed.[185] (B) Left panels: Upper panel shows the relationship between cerebral white matter blood flow (expressed as the percentage of total cerebral blood flow) and mean arterial blood pressure (MABP) in 13 preterm infants (16 measurements). A break point in the relationship was identified at 29 mm Hg mean blood pressure. Lower panel depicts the lowest residual mean square (best fit) with the breakpoint. Right panels: Serial measurements of cerebral blood flow (CBF) and mean arterial pressure (MAP) in normotensive and untreated hypotensive ELBW neonates at 13–40 hours after birth. Note the breakpoint at 29 mm Hg in the CBF-MAP autoregulation curve (the same value obtained in the study shown on the left-hand side). (Adapted with permission from references 53–55.)

coexistence of other pathologies with hypotension as a marker of disease severity, or a combination of all of these factors.[59]

## Definition and Phases of Shock

Shock is defined as a condition where supply of oxygen to the tissues does not meet oxygen demand. In the initial *"compensated" phase* of shock, neuroendocrine compensatory mechanisms and increased tissue oxygen extraction maintain perfusion pressure, blood flow, and oxygen supply to the vital organs (heart, brain and adrenal glands) at the expense of blood flow to the rest of the body. This is achieved by selective vasoconstriction of the resistance vessels in the non-vital organs leading to maintenance of BP in the normal range and redistribution of blood flow to the vital organs. Low normal to normal BP, increased heart rate, cold extremities, delayed CRT, and oliguria are the hallmarks of this phase. Unfortunately, while these clinical signs are useful in detecting early shock in pediatric and adult patients, they are of limited value in neonates, especially in preterm infants in the immediate postnatal period. Indeed, in preterm infants immediately after birth, shock is rarely diagnosed in this phase and is usually only recognized in the second, "uncompensated", phase. In the *uncompensated phase* of shock the neuroendocrine compensatory mechanisms fail and hypotension, decreased vital and non-vital organ perfusion, and oxygen delivery develop. These events first result in the loss of vital organ blood flow autoregulation and the development of lactic acidosis and, if the process progresses, cellular function and structural integrity become compromised. Even in the compensated phase, however, recognition of shock may be delayed because of the uncertainty about the definition of hypotension in preterm infants.[60,61] Finally, if treatment is delayed or ineffective, shock progresses to its final *"irreversible" phase*. In this phase irreparable cellular damage occurs in all organs and therapeutic interventions will fail to sustain life.

## Etiology of Neonatal Shock

Neonatal shock may develop because of volume loss (absolute hypovolemia), myocardial dysfunction, abnormal peripheral vasoregulation, or a combination of all of these factors.

## HYPOVOLEMIA

Adequate preload is essential for maintaining normal cardiac output and organ blood flow. Therefore pathological conditions associated with absolute or relative hypovolemia can lead to a decrease in cardiac output, poor tissue perfusion, and shock. Although absolute hypovolemia is a common cause of shock in the pediatric population, in neonates in the immediate postnatal period it is rarely the primary cause. Neonates are born with approximately 80–100 mL/kg of blood volume, and only a significant drop in blood volume leads to hypotension. Perinatal events that can cause hypovolemia include a tight nuchal cord, cord avulsion, cord prolapse, placental abruption, feto-maternal transfusion, and birth trauma such as subgaleal hemorrhage. Fortunately, either these perinatal events do not result in significant hypovolemia and shock in most instances (e.g., placental abruption) or their occurrence is very rare (e.g., cord avulsion). Another cause of absolute hypovolemia is transepidermal water loss in extremely-low-birth-weight (ELBW) infants in the immediate postnatal period. The potential role of early umbilical cord clamping in relative hypovolemia has recently been raised.

To explore the role of intravascular volume status in the occurrence of hypotension, several investigators have evaluated the relationship between blood volume and systemic arterial BP in normotensive and hypotensive preterm infants. Bauer et al. measured blood volume in 43 preterm neonates during the first 2 postnatal days and found a weak but statistically significant positive correlation between blood pressure and blood volume.[62] However, there was no correlation between blood volume and blood pressure until blood volume exceeded 100 mL/kg. Barr et al. found no relationship between arterial mean blood pressure and blood volume in preterm infants and no difference in blood volume between hypotensive and normotensive infants.[63] Similarly, Wright and Goodall reported no relationship between blood volume and blood pressure in preterm neonates in the immediate postnatal period.[64] Therefore absolute hypovolemia was for a long period thought to be an unlikely primary cause of hypotension in preterm infants in the immediate postnatal period. This notion was further supported by the fact that dopamine was shown to be more effective than volume administration in improving BP in preterm infants during the first days after delivery.[65,66] In addition, the response of hypotensive preterm infants to volume expanders has been absent, weak, or inconsistent.[67] However, the findings of improved cardiovascular status following delayed (physiologic) cord clamping indicate that the relationship between intravascular volume and hypotension depends on a number of factors, including but not restricted to the level of immaturity, postnatal age, the level of inflammatory response to noxious stimuli such as oxygen radicals, and/or infection affecting vascular tone.

On the other hand, delayed cord clamping and cord milking have been shown to confer short-term hemodynamic benefits and, in addition to the improved maintenance of LV preload during early hemodynamic transition, these beneficial hemodynamic effects are also thought to be the result of the associated increases in blood volume.[11,13,19,20,68] In summary, it is unclear at present to what extent and in which patient is the hypovolemic component a factor during hemodynamic transition.

## MYOCARDIAL DYSFUNCTION (SEE ALSO CHAPTER 20)

As discussed earlier, there are considerable differences in the structure and function of the myocardium among preterm and term infants and children. The significant immaturity of the myocardium of the preterm infant explains, at least in part, why these patients are prone to develop myocardial failure following delivery.[34,35]

The limited capacity to increase contractility above the baseline makes the immature myocardium prone to fail when SVR abruptly increases. This disadvantage associated with myocardial immaturity is especially important during the initial transitional period. As the low-resistance placental circulation is removed, SVR suddenly increases. This acute rise in the SVR and afterload may compromise left cardiac output and systemic blood flow. Indeed, superior vena cava (SVC) flow, used as a surrogate for systemic blood flow (LV output), is low in a proportion of VLBW infants during the first 6–12 postnatal hours.[69] The exaggerated decrease in myocardial contractility in response to increases in LV afterload may play a role in development of low SVC flow.[70] However, this low flow state appears to be transient as most patients recover by 24–36 hours after delivery. Similarly, findings of Doppler studies of CBF

suggest an increase in CBF shortly after delivery.[71] Therefore, although the myocardium of the preterm neonate undergoes structural and functional maturation over many months, it appears that after a transient dysfunction of varying severity immediately after delivery, it can relatively rapidly adapt to the postnatal changes in systemic hemodynamics.

In addition to the developmentally regulated susceptibility to dysfunction, a decrease in the oxygen supply associated with perinatal depression is a major cause of poor myocardial function and low cardiac output in preterm and term neonates immediately following delivery. During fetal life, despite being in a "hypoxic" environment by postnatal norms, neuroendocrine and other compensatory mechanisms and the unique fetal circulation enable the fetus to tolerate the "relative" hypoxemia and even brief episodes of true fetal hypoxemia. Indeed and as mentioned earlier, during fetal hypoxemia, the distribution of blood flow is altered to maintain perfusion and oxygen supply to the vital organs, including the heart.[72-74] However, a significant degree of hypoxemia, especially when associated with metabolic acidosis, can rapidly exhaust the compensatory mechanisms and result in myocardial dysfunction. The critical threshold of fetal arterial oxygen saturation below which metabolic acidosis develops varies depending on the cause of fetal hypoxia. In the animal model of maternal hypoxia-induced fetal hypoxia, fetal arterial oxygen saturations below 30% are associated with metabolic acidosis. In addition, it appears that the fetus is more or less susceptible to hypoxia if the cause of hypoxia is umbilical cord occlusion or decreased uterine blood flow, respectively. Human data obtained by fetal pulse oximetry are consistent with the results of animal studies and indicate that the oxygen saturation of 30% is indeed the threshold for the development of fetal metabolic acidosis.[75]

An increase in cardiac enzymes and cardiac troponin T and I are useful in the assessment of the degree of myocardial injury associated with perinatal asphyxia.[76-79] In addition, increases in cardiac troponin T and I have been shown to be helpful in diagnosing myocardial injury even in the mildly depressed neonate. While cardiac troponin T and I may be more sensitive than echocardiography findings in detecting myocardial injury,[80] the cardiovascular significance of elevated troponin in the absence of myocardial dysfunction remains unclear.

Modifications of the cardiac contractile protein myosin regulatory light chain 2 (MLC2) have also been implicated in the development of cardiac systolic dysfunction following newborn asphyxia. In a piglet model of perinatal asphyxia a decrease in MLC2 phosphorylation and an increase in MLC2 degradation via nitration were observed, suggesting that these are potential targets for therapeutic interventions to reduce myocardial damage in perinatal depression.[81] Nevertheless, documentation of clinical relevance of these findings is necessary in order to determine the future utility of such therapies.

Tricuspid regurgitation is the most common echocardiographic finding in neonates with perinatal depression and myocardial dysfunction. In cases with severe perinatal depression and myocardial injury, myocardial dysfunction frequently leads to decreases in cardiac output and the development of full-blown cardiogenic shock.[82,83] Finally, if the myocardium is not appropriately supported by inotropes, the ensuing low cardiac output will exacerbate the existing metabolic acidosis[84] (see Chapter 27).

Cardiogenic shock due to congenital heart defect, arrhythmia, cardiomyopathy, and PDA is discussed in other chapters of this book.

## VASODILATION

The regulation of vascular smooth muscle tone is complex and involves neuronal, endocrine, paracrine, and autocrine factors (Figure 1.3). Regardless of the regulatory stimuli, intracellular calcium availability plays the central role in regulating vascular smooth muscle tone. In the process of smooth muscle cell contraction, the regulatory protein calmodulin combines with calcium to activate myosin kinase. This enzyme phosphorylates the myosin light chain facilitating its binding with actin and thus resulting in contraction. As for vasodilation, in addition to the reduction in intracellular calcium availability, myosin phosphatase generates muscle relaxation by dephosphorylation of the myosin light chain.

Maintenance of the vascular tone depends on the balance between the opposing forces of vasodilation and vasoconstriction. The vasodilatory and vasoconstricting mediators exert their effects by inducing alteration in cytosolic calcium concentration and/or by

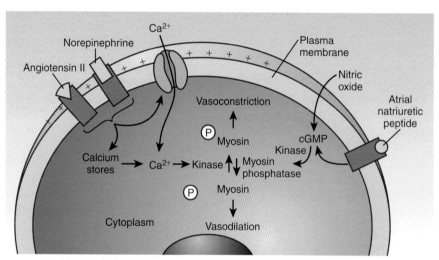

**Fig. 1.3 Regulation of vascular smooth muscle tone.** The steps involved in vasoconstriction and vasodilation are shown in blue and red, respectively. Phosphorylation (P) of myosin is the critical step in the contraction of vascular smooth muscle. The action of vasoconstrictors such as angiotensin II and norepinephrine result in an increase in cytosolic calcium concentration, which activates myosin kinase. Vasodilators such as atrial natriuretic peptide and nitric oxide activate myosin phosphatase and, by dephosphorylating myosin, cause vasorelaxation. The plasma membrane is shown at resting potential (plus signs). The abbreviation cGMP denotes cyclic guanosine monophosphate.[85]

direct activation of the enzymes involved in the process. Influx of calcium through cell membrane voltage-gated calcium channels and release of calcium from sarcoplasmic reticulum are the two sources responsible for the rise in cytosolic calcium required for muscle contraction.

Recently, the role of various potassium channels has been identified in the regulation of vascular tone. Among these, the adenosine triphosphate (ATP)–dependent potassium channel ($K_{ATP}$) emerged as the key channel through which many modulators exert their action on vascular smooth muscle tone. In addition, the $K_{ATP}$ channel has been implicated in pathogenesis of vasodilatory shock.[85] $K_{ATP}$ channels are located on the smooth muscle cell membrane and opening of these channels leads to $K^+$ efflux with resultant hyperpolarization of the cell membrane. Cell membrane hyperpolarization in turn causes the closure of the voltage-gated calcium channels in the cell membrane and thus a reduction in cytosolic calcium and a decreased vascular tone. Under normal conditions, the $K_{ATP}$ channels are closed for the most part. However, under pathological conditions, a number of stimuli may activate these channels and thus affect tissue perfusion. For instance, via the associated reduction in ATP and the increase in $H^+$ concentration and lactate levels, tissue hypoxia activates $K_{ATP}$ channels, resulting in vasodilation and a compensatory increase in tissue perfusion.[86]

As mentioned earlier, a number of vasodilators and vasoconstrictors exert their effects through the $K_{ATP}$ channels. For example, in septic shock several endocrine and paracrine factors such as atrial natriuretic peptide, adenosine, and NO are released, resulting in activation of $K_{ATP}$ channels.[87,88] Thus $K_{ATP}$ channels are thought to play an important role in pathogenesis of vasodilatory shock.[89] Indeed, animal studies have shown an improvement in BP following administration of $K_{ATP}$ channel blockers.[88,90] Inhibition of $K_{ATP}$ channels can improve vascular tone in vasodilatory shock; however, because $K_{ATP}$ channels are ubiquitously expressed and involved in a number of cellular and tissue functions, their inhibition can also lead to adverse effects.[91-93] Two human trials failed to show any benefit of administration of the $K_{ATP}$ channel inhibitor glibenclamide in adults with septic shock.[94,95] Although the sample size was small and several problems have been identified with the methodology,[96] the findings of these studies support the recent notion that the mechanism of vasodilation in septic shock is more complex than initially believed (see below).

Eicosanoids are derived from cell membrane phospholipids through metabolism of arachidonic acid by the cyclooxygenase or lipoxygenase enzymes and have a wide range of effects on vascular tone. For example, prostacyclin and prostaglandin $E_2$ are vasodilators, while thromboxane $A_2$ is a vasoconstrictor. Apart from their involvement in the physiological regulation of vascular tone, these eicosanoids also play a role in pathogenesis of shock. In addition, eicosanoids derived from the cytochrome P450 pathway of arachidonic acid metabolism such as hydroxyeicosatetraenoic acid and epoxyeicosatrienoic acid have also been shown to play a role in the inflammation associated with septic shock.[97] Animal studies and some human trials have shown a beneficial effect of cyclooxygenase inhibition in septic shock.[98-101] In addition, rats deficient in essential fatty acid and thus unable to produce significant amounts of eicosanoids are less susceptible to endotoxic shock than their wild-type counterparts. However, the role of eicosanoids in the pathogenesis of shock is also more complex, and some studies suggest that, under different conditions, they may actually have a beneficial role. For example, administration of prostaglandin $I_2$ ($PGI_2$), $PGE_1$, and $PGE_2$ improves the cardiovascular status in animals with hypovolemic shock.[102,103] Another layer of complexity is revealed by the observation that production of both the vasodilator and vasoconstrictor prostanoids is increased in shock.[104,105]

Nitric oxide (NO) is another paracrine substance that plays an important role in the regulation of vascular tone. Normally, NO is produced in vascular endothelial cells by the constitutive enzyme endothelial NO synthase (eNOS). NO then diffuses to the adjacent smooth muscle cells, where it activates guanylyl cyclase, resulting in increased cyclic guanosine monophosphate (cGMP) formation. cGMP then induces vasodilation by the activation of cGMP-dependent protein kinase and the different $K^+$ channels as well as by the inhibition of inositol triphosphate formation and calcium entry into the vascular smooth muscle cells. In septic shock (see also Chapter 21) endotoxin and cytokines, such as tumor necrosis factor-alpha, result in increased expression of inducible NO synthase (iNOS).[106-109] Studies in animals and humans have shown that the NO level significantly increases in various forms of shock, especially in septic shock.[110,111] This excessive and dysregulated production of NO then leads to severe vasodilation, hypotension, and vasopressor resistance (see below and Chapters 20 and 21). Because of the role of NO in the pathogenesis of vasodilatory shock, a number of studies have looked at the NO production pathway as a potential target of therapeutic interventions.[112,113]

Although initial studies using a non-selective NOS inhibitor in adult patients with septic shock have found improvement in vascular tone and resolution of shock,[114,115] subsequent studies showed significant side effects and increased mortality associated with this treatment modality.[116,117] The deleterious effects were likely due to inhibition of eNOS, the constitutive NOS that plays an important role in the physiologic regulation of vascular tone. In other words, while excessive NO production in septic shock adversely affects macro-circulatory and cellular function, reduced eNOS activity and NO availability may impair microcirculation.[89] Indeed, subsequent studies in animal models using a selective iNOS inhibitor found an improvement in BP and a reduction in lactic acidosis.[118-120] Despite the observation that the use of selective iNOS inhibitors might be promising, none of these agents has been approved for clinical use.[121]

Recently there has been a renewed interest in the cardiovascular effects of vasopressin.[122,123] Although in postnatal life and under physiologic conditions, this hormone is primarily involved in the regulation of osmolality, there is accumulating evidence suggesting a role of vasopressin in the pathogenesis of vasodilatory shock. Vasopressin exerts its vascular effects through the two isoforms of $V_1$ receptors. $V_{1a}$ receptor is expressed in all vessels, while $V_{1b}$ is only present in the pituitary gland. The renal epithelial effects of vasopressin are mediated through $V_2$ receptors.

Postnatally and under physiologic conditions, vasopressin contributes little, if any, to the maintenance of vascular smooth muscle tone. However, under pathologic conditions such as in shock, with the decrease in BP, vasopressin production increases, attenuating the further decline in BP. With progression of the circulatory compromise, however, vasopressin levels decline as pituitary vasopressin stores become depleted. The decline in vasopressin production leads to further losses of vascular tone and contributes to the development of refractory hypotension.[85] Findings on the effectiveness of vasopressin replacement therapy in reversing refractory hypotension further support the role of vasopressin in the pathogenesis of vasodilatory shock.[124,125] The vasoconstrictor effects of vasopressin appear to be dose dependent.[126] As mentioned earlier, excessive production of NO and activation of $K_{ATP}$ channels are some of the major mechanisms involved in the pathogenesis of vasodilatory shock. Under these circumstances, vasopressin inhibits NO-induced cGMP production and inactivates the $K_{ATP}$ channels, resulting in improvement in vascular tone. In addition, vasopressin releases calcium from sarcoplasmic reticulum and augments the vasoconstrictive effects of norepinephrine. As for its clinical use, vasopressin has been shown to improve cardiovascular function in neonates and children presenting with vasopressor-resistant vasodilatory shock after cardiac surgery.[127] However, the few published case series on preterm infants with refractory hypotension show variable effects of vasopressin treatment with improvement in BP and urine output only in some patients.[128,129] A recent pilot study showed similar efficacy of vasopressin to dopamine in improving BP and signs of shock in preterm infants.[130] Although vasopressin was associated with somewhat less tachycardia, the clinical significance of this finding is unclear. In adults, recent RCTs have demonstrated a reduction in mortality with the use of vasopressin in septic shock.[131,132] However, a recent metanalysis and trial sequential analysis concluded that vasopressin does not reduce mortality or intensive care unit stay in refractory shock and may increase risk of ischemic injury in the pediatric population.[133]

Given the systemic vasoconstrictor and potential pulmonary vasodilator effects of vasopressin, its use in selected cases of neonatal shock such as hypertrophic cardiomyopathy, where the use of medications with inotropic effects are contraindicated, and pulmonary hypertension, where low pulmonary blood flow, due to ventricular interdependence, resulting in low systemic blood flow have been reported.[134-136] However, as expression of vasopressin receptors is developmentally regulated, it is unclear to what extent vasopressin induces selective pulmonary vasodilation in the neonatal population.[137]

In general, vasodilation with or without decreased myocardial contractility is the dominant underlying cause of hemodynamic disturbances in septic shock. However, there are very limited data on changes in cardiovascular function in neonates with septic shock. A study in preterm infants with late-onset sepsis found that the high cardiac output characteristic for the earlier stages of septic shock diminished and SVR sharply increased before death in non-surviving patients, while there was only a mild increase in the SVR during the course of the cardiovascular disturbance in patients who survived. The authors also described a significant variability in hemodynamic response among the survivors.[138] In children two distinct presentations of shock are seen: one with vasodilation (warm shock) characterized by high CO and low SVR and the other with vasoconstriction (cold shock) characterized by high SVR and low CO. A study in children with fluid-resistant shock found different patterns of hemodynamic derangement in central venous catheter–related (CVCR) versus community-acquired (CA) infections. Low SVR and low cardiac output were the dominant pathophysiological findings in patients with CVCR and CA septic shock, respectively. These findings suggest that the hemodynamic response may be different depending on the type of bacterial pathogen and/or represent the fact that patients with CA septic shock are usually diagnosed at a later stage, and thus myocardial dysfunction might have already set in at the time of the diagnosis.[139] While vasodilatory shock is thought to be the main presentation of neonates with septic shock, a recent study in preterm infants provided some evidence suggestive of the prevalence of vasoconstrictive type shock.[140] In older children about 50% of patients with septic shock present with either systolic or diastolic dysfunction.[141] However, it is not known how common myocardial dysfunction is in the neonatal population with septic shock. The results of the above studies underscore the importance of direct assessment of cardiac function by echocardiography and tailoring the treatment strategy according to the hemodynamic finding in each individual patient.

The case study presented below underscores this point and illustrates that the population-based BP values defining hypotension must be viewed as guidelines only that do not necessarily apply to an individual patient. This is explained by the fact that a number of factors, including gestational and postnatal age, preexisting insults, $PaCO_2$ and $PaO_2$ levels, acidosis, and the underlying pathophysiology, all impact the critical BP value in any given patient at which perfusion pressure becomes progressively inadequate to first sustain vital organ (brain, heart, adrenal glands) perfusion and blood flow autoregulation, then brain function, and, finally structural integrity of the organs.

## Case Study

A preterm infant (twin A) was born at 31 + 1 weeks gestation (birth weight 1180 g, 8th percentile) via cesarean section due to abnormal umbilical cord Doppler findings. There was no evidence of chorioamnionitis, and Apgar scores were 4 and 7 at 1 and 5 minutes, respectively. The patient was not requiring any respiratory support and blood gases and capillary refill time had been normal during the first 3 postnatal hours in the NICU. However, the neonate's mean arterial BP had been low and, at 3 hours of age, it was 21 mmHg with systolic and diastolic blood pressures at 34 and 14 mmHg, respectively.

What would be the best course of action? Should one increase BP by increasing SVR and cardiac output using a vasopressor with inotropic property such as dopamine or epinephrine? Or, is increasing cardiac output using a primarily inotropic agent such as dobutamine more appropriate in hypotensive preterm neonates during the early postnatal transitional period? Or, should one attempt to further increase preload by giving additional boluses of physiologic saline? Or, should we ignore the MABP value as the clinical exam and laboratory findings were not suggestive of poor perfusion and there was no metabolic acidosis? Most neonatologists would choose one of the above-listed options and, in the absence of additional information on the hemodynamic status, it is indeed impossible to know what to do and whether the treatment choice chosen was the right one.

Therefore, before choosing a treatment option, we obtained additional information on the cardiovascular status by assessing cardiac function, systemic perfusion, and CBF

*Continued on following page*

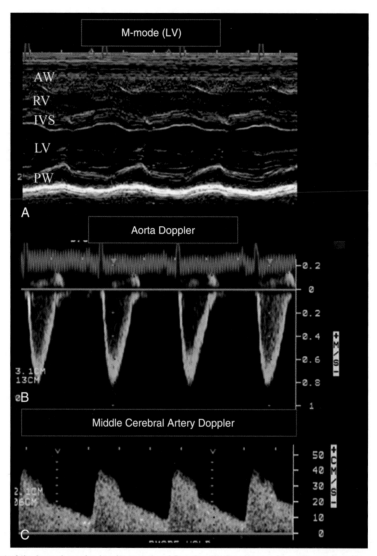

Fig. 1.4 Direct assessment of the hemodynamics by ultrasound and Doppler: (A) the changes in cardiac wall motions are shown in this M-mode image; note the normal motion of the IVS and PW resulting in normal shortening fraction; (B) the spectral Doppler at the aortic valve is shown here, along with the diameter of aorta, which is used to estimate the left ventricular output; (C) the middle cerebral artery flow Doppler depicts a normal pattern. AW = anterior wall; IVS = intraventricular septum; LV = left ventricle; PW = posterior wall; RV = right ventricle.

**Case Study** *(Continued)*

using point-of-care ultrasonography (Figure 1.4). Myocardial contractility, assessed by the shortening fraction, was 35% (normal 28–42%) and left ventricular output was 377 mL/kg/min (normal 150–300 mL/kg/min) in the presence of an equally bidirectional PDA flow. Middle cerebral artery (MCA) blood flow, assessed by MCA mean velocity and flow pattern, was normal. Using the additional hemodynamic information obtained by echocardiography and ultrasonography, it was clear that the cause of the low blood pressure was the low SVR with a compensatory increase in the cardiac output (BP α cardiac output × SVR). Given the normal myocardial contractility, the high cardiac

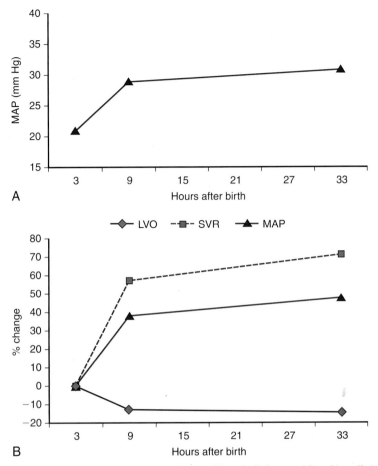

**Fig. 1.5** The changes in hemodynamics are shown in these graphs: (A) mean BP gradually increased from 21 mmHg to 31 mmHg over 30 hours; (B) the 38% increase in mean BP at 9 hours after birth was the result of an increase in SVR (57%) and a mild decrease in LVO (13%). SVR continued to rise without a significant change in LVO at 33 hours.

**Case Study** (*Continued*)

output, and the normal CBF along with the lack of clinical or laboratory signs of systemic hypoperfusion, we opted to closely monitor the patient without any intervention to attempt to increase the blood pressure. By 9 hours of age, mean blood pressure spontaneously increased to 29 mmHg and the repeat echocardiogram revealed a mild decrease in LVO. Accordingly, a significant increase in the calculated SVR occurred (Figure 1.5). After another 24 hours had passed, mean blood pressure increased to 31 mm Hg and, as cardiac output didn't change, calculated SVR continued to rise. The patient remained clinically stable during the entire hospital course and was discharged home without evidence of early brain morbidity.

This case study illustrates several important points. First, without appropriate assessment of systemic and organ blood flow and only relying on blood pressure and the indirect clinical and laboratory signs of tissue perfusion, it would have been impossible to ascertain the adequacy of systemic and brain perfusion *at the time of presentation*. Secondly, assessment of cardiac output and the calculation of the SVR did aid in choosing the most appropriate course of action. Thirdly, in addition to the evaluation of cardiac output and calculation of SVR, information on systemic blood flow distribution to the organs, especially the brain, may help in formulating a pathophysiology-based treatment strategy in neonates with suspected hemodynamic derangement.

*Continued on following page*

In this case we chose to closely monitor the infants rather than to treat the hypotension as we documented a compensatory increase in cardiac output and one of the surrogate measures of CBF (MCA Doppler and flow pattern) was normal. In this case it took 6 hours for the vascular tone to spontaneously improve to the degree where mean blood pressure reached the lower limit of the population-based normal value. One may argue for the careful titration of low-dose vasopressor support even in this situation so that normalization of SVR can be facilitated and hence mean blood pressure would have "normalized" faster. However, in a patient with evidence of adequate systemic and cerebral blood flow, the potential side effects of vasopressor use likely outweigh its benefits. This is especially true if vasopressors, when used, are not carefully titrated to achieve an appropriate hemodynamic target beyond the "normalization" of the blood pressure. As CBF autoregulation is impaired during hypotension, a significant and rapid rise in blood pressure results in an abrupt increase in CBF with a potential for cerebral injury, and possibly intracranial hemorrhage.[56] However, in patients in whom cardiac output does not compensate for the decreased SVR, hypotension will lead to decreased CBF with a potential for cerebral injury, possibly ischemic lesions especially in the white matter with or without a secondary hemorrhage.[56] In addition and as discussed earlier, as our ability to clinically assess the adequacy of the circulation is inaccurate,[142] it is very important that low blood pressure values are not disregarded without additional direct assessment of systemic hemodynamics and CBF and close and careful monitoring of the patient.

## ADRENAL INSUFFICIENCY (SEE ALSO CHAPTER 23)

The adrenal glands play a crucial role in cardiovascular homeostasis. *Mineralocorticoids* regulate intravascular volume through their effects on maintaining adequate extracellular sodium concentration. In addition, physiologic levels of mineralocorticoids play an important role in the regulation of cytosolic calcium availability in the myocardium and vascular smooth muscle cells.[143] *Glucocorticoids* exert their cardiovascular effects mainly by enhancing the sensitivity of the cardiovascular system to catecholamines. The rapid rise of BP in the early postnatal period has been attributed to maturation of glucocorticoid-regulated vascular smooth muscle cell response to central and local stimulatory mechanisms, changes in the expression of the vascular angiotensin II receptor subtypes, and accumulation of elastin and collagen in large arteries.[144-146] Glucocorticoids play a role in the latter mechanism via their stimulatory effect on collagen synthesis in the vascular wall.[147] Given the importance of corticosteroids in cardiovascular stability, it is not surprising that deficiency of these hormones plays a role in the pathogenesis of certain forms of neonatal shock.

Preterm infants are born with an immature hypothalamic-pituitary-adrenal axis. Several indirect pieces of evidence suggest that immature preterm infants are only capable of producing enough corticosteroids to meet their metabolic demand and support their growth during a healthy state (Chapter 23). When critically ill, a number of these patients cannot mount an adequate stress response. This condition has been referred to as relative adrenal insufficiency.

Relative adrenal insufficiency is defined as a low baseline total serum cortisol level considered inappropriate for the degree of severity of the patient's illness. However, there is no agreement on what this level might be.[151,152] For the purpose of replacement therapy in adults, a cortisol level below 15 mcg/dL is usually considered diagnostic for relative adrenal insufficiency.[153] To establish the presumptive diagnosis of relative adrenal insufficiency for the neonatal patient population, some authors have suggested the use of a total serum cortisol cutoff value of 5 mcg/dL, while others have used the cutoff value established for adults earlier (15 mcg/dL).[154,155] However, use of an arbitrary single serum cortisol level to define relative adrenal insufficiency may not be appropriate, especially in the neonatal period, primarily because there is a large variation in total serum cortisol levels in neonates.[148,150,156-162] In addition, during the first 3 months of postnatal life, total serum cortisol levels progressively decrease with advancing postnatal age.[163,164] Furthermore, most studies have shown an inverse relationship between total serum cortisol levels and gestational age.[163-166] The study by Ng et al. discussed earlier has also demonstrated a gestational age-independent correlation between serum cortisol level and the lowest BP registered in the immediate postnatal period in VLBW infants.[150] These authors also found that serum cortisol levels inversely correlate with the maximum and cumulative dose of vasopressor-inotropes. However, despite these correlations, they found an overlap of serum cortisol levels between normotensive and hypotensive VLBW infants, thus making it difficult to define a single serum cortisol level below which adrenal insufficiency can be diagnosed with certainty.

It has been demonstrated that more than half of the mechanically ventilated near-term and term infants receiving vasopressor-inotropes have total serum cortisol levels below 15 mcg/dL.[155] In more immature preterm infants an even larger proportion of patients have low serum cortisol levels. Korte et al have found that 76% of sick VLBW infants have serum cortisol levels <15 mcg/dL.[154] Recently, several studies investigated the role of adrenal insufficiency in the pathogenesis of hypotension in preterm neonates following PDA ligation. These studies found that random and post-stimulation cortisol levels prior to ligation do not predict hypotension.[167,168] However, after ligation, low cortisol levels in patients receiving vasopressor-inotrope therapy are associated with the development of vasopressor-resistant refractory hypotension

and need for hydrocortisone treatment.[169] Finally, studies demonstrating an improvement in the cardiovascular status in response to low-dose steroid administration in preterm and term neonates indirectly support the role of relative adrenal insufficiency in the pathogenesis of hypotension, especially in cases where the hypotension is resistant to vasopressor-inotrope treatment.[149,170-178]

## DOWNREGULATION OF ADRENERGIC RECEPTORS

Recently, downregulation of adrenergic receptors has been implicated in the pathogenesis of vasopressor-resistant hypotension. Improvement in the cardiovascular status in patients with refractory hypotension following administration of corticosteroids supports this notion as glucocorticoids upregulate adrenergic receptor gene function and result in enhanced expression of adrenergic receptors.[179,180] These *"genomic"* effects of corticosteroids may explain why vasopressor requirement decreases within 6–12 hours following corticosteroid administration (Figure 1.6).[173,174] However, it is important to point out that the beneficial steroidal effects on the cardiovascular system are not limited to adrenergic receptor upregulation. Other genomic mechanisms include inhibition of inducible

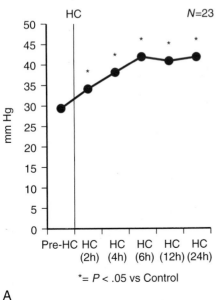

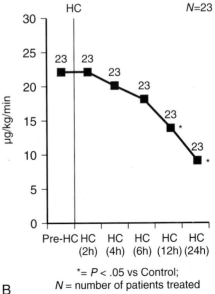

**Fig. 1.6** (A) The increase in mean blood pressure and (B) the decrease in dopamine requirement in response to low-dose hydrocortisone (HC) treatment in preterm infants with vasopressor-resistant hypotension.[177]

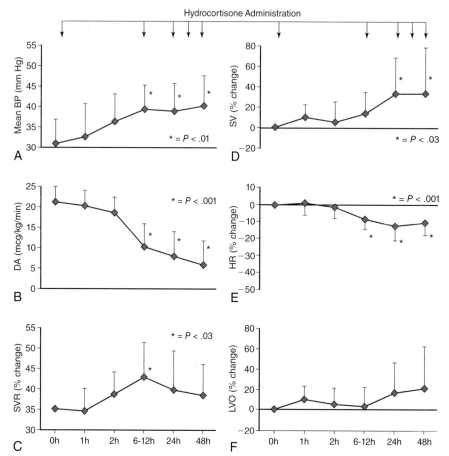

**Fig. 1.7** Changes in cardiovascular function in response to hydrocortisone (HC) in pressor-treated preterm neonates. Changes in mean BP (A) and dopamine dosage (DA) (B). Percentage changes relative to baseline (0 hours) in SVR (C), stroke volume (SV) (D), heart rate (HR) (E), and LVO (F).[179]

NO synthase and upregulation of myocardial angiotensin II receptors.[173,181-183] "*Non-genomic*" steroidal actions include the immediate increase in cytosolic calcium availability in vascular smooth muscle and myocardial cells, inhibition of degradation and reuptake of catecholamines, and inhibition of prostacyclin production.[173,182] The wide range of genomic and non-genomic effects of steroids explains the rapid and often sustained improvement in all components of the cardiovascular status (Figure 1.7) of the critically ill neonate treated with low-dose hydrocortisone.[173,175]

## Summary

This chapter has reviewed the principles of developmental hemodynamics during fetal life, postnatal transition, and the neonatal period, as well as the etiology and pathophysiology of neonatal cardiovascular compromise. Although significant advances have recently been made in these areas, much more needs to be understood before we can accurately diagnose and appropriately treat preterm and term neonates with cardiovascular compromise during transition and beyond.

## REFERENCES

1. Kiserud T. Physiology of the fetal circulation. *Semin Fetal Neonatal Med.* 2005;10:493-503.
2. Noori S, Friedlich P, Seri I. Pathophysiology of shock in the fetus and neonate. In: Polin R, Abman S, Benitz W, Rowitch D, eds. *Fetal and Neonatal Physiology.* Philadelphia: WB Saunders; 2022.
3. Rudolph AM. Distribution and regulation of blood flow in the fetal and neonatal lamb. *Circ Res.* 1985;57:811-821.
4. Sutton MS, Groves A, MacNeill A, Sharland G, Allan L. Assessment of changes in blood flow through the lungs and foramen ovale in the normal human fetus with gestational age: a prospective Doppler echocardiographic study. *Br Heart J.* 1994; 71:232-237.
5. Rasanen J, Wood DC, Weiner S, Ludomirski A, Huhta JC. Role of the pulmonary circulation in the distribution of human fetal cardiac output during the second half of pregnancy. *Circulation.* 1996;94:1068-1073.
6. Mielke G, Benda N. Cardiac output and central distribution of blood flow in the human fetus. *Circulation.* 2001;103: 1662-1668.
7. Prsa M, Sun L, van Ameron J, et al. Reference ranges of blood flow in the major vessels of the normal human fetal circulation at term by phase-contrast magnetic resonance imaging. *Circ Cardiovasc Imaging.* 2014;7:663-670.
8. Kiserud T, Ebbing C, Kessler J, Rasmussen S. Fetal cardiac output, distribution to the placenta and impact of placental compromise. *Ultrasound Obstet Gynecol.* 2006;28:126-136.
9. Bhatt S, Alison BJ, Wallace EM, et al. Delaying cord clamping until ventilation onset improves cardiovascular function at birth in preterm lambs. *J Physiol.* 2013;591:2113-2126.
10. Kluckow M, Hooper SB. Using physiology to guide time to cord clamping. *Semin Fetal Neonatal Med.* 2015;20:225-231.
11. Baenziger O, Stolkin F, Keel M, et al. The influence of the timing of cord clamping on postnatal cerebral oxygenation in preterm neonates: a randomized, controlled trial. *Pediatrics.* 2007;119:455-459.
12. Sommers R, Stonetreet BS, Oh William, et al. Hemodynamic effects of delayed cord clamping in premature infants. *Pediatrics.* 2012;129:e667-e672.
13. Rabe H, Reynolds G, Diaz-Rossello J. A systematic review and meta-analysis of a brief delay in clamping the umbilical cord of preterm infants. *Neonatology.* 2008;93:138-144.
14. Backes CH, Rivera BK, Haque U, et al. Placental transfusion strategies in very preterm neonates: a systematic review and meta-analysis. *Obstet Gynecol.* 2014;124:47-56.
15. Katheria AC, Lakshminrusimha S, Rabe H, McAdams R, Mercer JS. Placental transfusion: a review. *J Perinatol.* 2017; 37:105-111.
16. Wyckoff MH, Aziz K, Escobedo M, et al. Part 13: neonatal resuscitation: 2015 American Heart Association guidelines update for cardiopulmonary resuscitation and emergency cardiovascular care. *Circulation.* 2015;132:S543-S560.
17. Katheria AC, Lakshminrusimha S, Rabe H, McAdams R, Mercer JS. Placental transfusion: a review. *J Perinatol.* 2017;37:105-111. doi:10.1038/jp.2016.151.
18. Committee Opinion No. 684: delayed umbilical cord clamping after birth. *Obstet Gynecol.* 2017;129:e5-e10.
19. Hosono S, Mugishima H, Fujita H, et al. Blood pressure and urine output during the first 120 h of life in infants born at less than 29 weeks' gestation related to umbilical cord milking. *Arch Dis Child Fetal Neonatal Ed.* 2009;94:F328-F331.
20. Katheria AC, Truong G, Cousins L, Oshiro B, Finer NN. Umbilical cord milking versus delayed cord clamping in preterm infants. *Pediatrics.* 2015;136:61-69.
21. Katheria A, Reister F, Essers J, et al. Association of umbilical cord milking vs delayed umbilical cord clamping with death or severe intraventricular hemorrhage among preterm infants. *JAMA.* 2019;322:1877-1886.
22. Katheria AC, Szychowski JM, Essers J, et al. Early cardiac and cerebral hemodynamics with umbilical cord milking compared with delayed cord clamping in infants born preterm. *J Pediatr.* 2020;223:51-56.e1.
23. Liebowitz M, Koo J, Wickremasinghe A, Allen IE, Clyman RI. Effects of prophylactic indomethacin on vasopressor-dependent hypotension in extremely preterm infants. *J Pediatr.* 2017;182: 21-27.e2. doi:10.1016/j.jpeds.2016.11.008.
24. Sarkar S, Dechert R, Schumacher RE, Donn SM. Is refractory hypotension in preterm infants a manifestation of early ductal shunting? *J Perinatol.* 2007;27:353-358.
25. Iwamoto HS, Teitel D, Rudolph AM. Effects of birth-related events on blood flow distribution. *Pediatr Res.* 1987;22:634-640.
26. Noori S, Wlodaver A, Gottipati V, et al. Transitional changes in cardiac and cerebral hemodynamics in term neonates at birth. *J Pediatr.* 2012;160:943-948.
27. Weindling AM. Peripheral oxygenation and management in the perinatal period. *Semin Fetal Neonatal Med.* 2010;15:208-215.
28. Noori S, Drabu B, McCoy M, Sekar K. Non-invasive measurement of local tissue perfusion and its correlation with hemodynamic indices during the early postnatal period in term neonates. *J Perinatol.* 2011;31:785-788.
29. Kissack CM, Weindling AM. Peripheral blood flow and oxygen extraction in the sick, newborn very low birth weight infant shortly after birth. *Pediatr Res.* 2009;65:462-467.
30. Kroth J, Weidlich K, Hiedl S, et al. Functional vessel density in the first month of life in preterm neonates. *Pediatr Res.* 2008; 64:567-571.
31. Stark MJ, Clifton VL, Wright IMR. Microvascular flow, clinical illness severity and cardiovascular function in the preterm infant. *Arch Dis Child Fetal Neonatal Ed.* 2008;93:F271-F274.
32. de Meautsart CC, Dyson RM, Latter JL, et al. Influence of sympathetic activity in the control of peripheral microvascular tone in preterm infants. *Pediatr Res.* 2016;80:793-799.
33. Stark MJ, Clifton VL, Wright IMR. Sex-specific differences in peripheral microvascular blood flow in preterm infants. *Pediatr Res.* 2008;63:415-419.
34. Anderson PA. The heart and development. *Semin Perinatol.* 1996;20:482-509.
35. Noori S, Seri I. Pathophysiology of newborn hypotension outside the transitional period. *Early Hum Dev.* 2005;81:399-404.
36. Rowland DG, Gutgesell HP. Noninvasive assessment of myocardial contractility, preload, and afterload in healthy newborn infants. *Am J Cardiol.* 1995;75:818-821.
37. Schmidt MR, White PA, Khambadkone S, et al. The neonatal but not the mature heart adapts to acute tachycardia by beneficial modification of the force-frequency relationship. *Pediatr Cardiol.* 2011;32:562-567.
38. Wiegerinck RF, Cojoc A, Zeidenweber CM, et al. Force frequency relationship of the human ventricle increases during early postnatal development. *Pediatr Res.* 2009;65:414-419.
39. Gilbey MP, Spyer KM. Physiological aspects of autonomic nervous system function. *Curr Opin Neurol Neurosurg.* 1993;6:518-523.
40. Spyer KM. Annual review prize lecture. Central nervous mechanisms contributing to cardiovascular control. *J Physiol.* 1994; 474:1-19.

41. Segar J. Neural regulation of blood pressure during fetal and newborn life. In: Polin RA, Fox WW, Abman SH, eds. *Fetal and Neonatal Physiology*. Philadelphia: Elsevier; 2004:717-726.

42. Galland BC, Taylor BJ, Bolton DPG, Sayers RM. Heart rate variability and cardiac reflexes in small for gestational age infants. *J Appl Physiol (1985)*. 2006;100:933-939.

43. Patural H, et al. Autonomic cardiac control of very preterm newborns: a prolonged dysfunction. *Early Hum Dev*. 2008; 84:681-687.

44. Pomeranz B, et al. Assessment of autonomic function in humans by heart rate spectral analysis. *Am J Physiol*. 1985;248: H151-H153.

45. Heart rate variability: standards of measurement, physiological interpretation and clinical use. Task Force of the European Society of Cardiology and the North American Society of Pacing and Electrophysiology. *Circulation*. 1996;93:1043-1065.

46. Kleiger RE, Stein PK, Bigger JT. Heart rate variability: measurement and clinical utility. *Ann Noninvasive Electrocardiol*. 2005; 10:88-101.

47. Griffin MP, et al. Heart rate characteristics: novel physiomarkers to predict neonatal infection and death. *Pediatrics*. 2005;116: 1070-1074.

48. Fairchild KD, O'Shea TM. Heart rate characteristics: physiomarkers for detection of late-onset neonatal sepsis. *Clin Perinatol*. 2010;37:581-598.

49. Valverde E, et al. Dopamine versus epinephrine for cardiovascular support in low birth weight infants: analysis of systemic effects and neonatal clinical outcomes. *Pediatrics*. 2006;117: e1213-e1222.

50. Seri I. Circulatory support of the sick preterm infant. *Semin Neonatol*. 2001;6:85-95.

51. Nuntnarumit P, Yang W, Bada-Ellzey HS. Blood pressure measurements in the newborn. *Clin Perinatol*. 1999;26:981-996, x.

52. Zubrow AB, Hulman S, Kushner H, Falkner B. Determinants of blood pressure in infants admitted to neonatal intensive care units: a prospective multicenter study. Philadelphia Neonatal Blood Pressure Study Group. *J Perinatol*. 1995;15:470-479.

53. Munro MJ, Walker AM, Barfield CP. Hypotensive extremely low birth weight infants have reduced cerebral blood flow. *Pediatrics*. 2004;114:1591-1596.

54. Victor S, Marson AG, Appleton RE, Beirne M, Weindling AM. Relationship between blood pressure, cerebral electrical activity, cerebral fractional oxygen extraction, and peripheral blood flow in very low birth weight newborn infants. *Pediatr Res*. 2006;59:314-319.

55. Børch K, Lou HC, Greisen G. Cerebral white matter blood flow and arterial blood pressure in preterm infants. *Acta Paediatr*. 2010;99:1489-1492.

56. Tsuji M, et al. Cerebral intravascular oxygenation correlates with mean arterial pressure in critically ill premature infants. *Pediatrics*. 2000;106:625-632.

57. Tyszczuk L, Meek J, Elwell C, Wyatt JS. Cerebral blood flow is independent of mean arterial blood pressure in preterm infants undergoing intensive care. *Pediatrics*. 1998;102:337-341.

58. Kissack CM, Garr R, Wardle SP, Weindling AM. Cerebral fractional oxygen extraction in very low birth weight infants is high when there is low left ventricular output and hypocarbia but is unaffected by hypotension. *Pediatr Res*. 2004;55: 400-405.

59. Noori S, Stavroudis TA, Seri I. Systemic and cerebral hemodynamics during the transitional period after premature birth. *Clin Perinatol*. 2009;36:723-736, v.

60. Seri I, Evans J. Controversies in the diagnosis and management of hypotension in the newborn infant. *Curr Opin Pediatr*. 2001;13:116-123.

61. Al-Aweel I, et al. Variations in prevalence of hypotension, hypertension, and vasopressor use in NICUs. *J Perinatol*. 2001; 21:272-278.

62. Bauer K, Linderkamp O, Versmold HT. Systolic blood pressure and blood volume in preterm infants. *Arch Dis Child*. 1993; 69:521-522.

63. Barr PA, Bailey PE, Sumners J, Cassady G. Relation between arterial blood pressure and blood volume and effect of infused albumin in sick preterm infants. *Pediatrics*. 1977;60:282-289.

64. Wright IM, Goodall SR. Blood pressure and blood volume in preterm infants. *Arch Dis Child Fetal Neonatal Ed*. 1994;70: F230-F231.

65. Gill AB, Weindling AM. Echocardiographic assessment of cardiac function in shocked very low birthweight infants. *Arch Dis Child*. 1993;68:17-21.

66. Lundstrøm K, Pryds O, Greisen G. The haemodynamic effects of dopamine and volume expansion in sick preterm infants. *Early Hum Dev*. 2000;57:157-163.

67. Shalish W, Olivier F, Aly H, Sant'Anna G. Uses and misuses of albumin during resuscitation and in the neonatal intensive care unit. *Semin Fetal Neonatal Med*. 2017;22:328-335.

68. Zaramella P, et al. Early versus late cord clamping: effects on peripheral blood flow and cardiac function in term infants. *Early Hum Dev*. 2008;84:195-200.

69. Kluckow M, Evans N. Low superior vena cava flow and intraventricular haemorrhage in preterm infants. *Arch Dis Child Fetal Neonatal Ed*. 2000;82:F188-F194.

70. Osborn DA, Evans N, Kluckow M. Left ventricular contractility in extremely premature infants in the first day and response to inotropes. *Pediatr Res*. 2007;61:335-340.

71. Kehrer M, et al. Development of cerebral blood flow volume in preterm neonates during the first two weeks of life. *Pediatr Res*. 2005;58:927-930.

72. Noori S, Friedlich P, Seri I. Pathophysiology of neonatal shock. In: Polin RA, Fox WW, Abman SH, eds. *Fetal and Neonatal Physiology*. Philadelphia: Elsevier; 2004:772-778.

73. Reuss ML, Rudolph AM. Distribution and recirculation of umbilical and systemic venous blood flow in fetal lambs during hypoxia. *J Dev Physiol*. 1980;2:71-84.

74. Davies JM, Tweed WA. The regional distribution and determinants of myocardial blood flow during asphyxia in the fetal lamb. *Pediatr Res*. 1984;18:764-767.

75. Kühnert M, Seelbach-Göebel B, Butterwegge M. Predictive agreement between the fetal arterial oxygen saturation and fetal scalp pH: results of the German multicenter study. *Am J Obstet Gynecol*. 1998;178:330-335.

76. Güneş T, Öztürk MA, Köklü SM, Narin N, Köklü E. Troponin-T levels in perinatally asphyxiated infants during the first 15 days of life. *Acta Paediatr*. 2005;94:1638-1643.

77. Trevisanuto D, et al. Cardiac troponin I in asphyxiated neonates. *Biol Neonate*. 2006;89:190-193.

78. Gaze DC, Collinson PO. Interpretation of cardiac troponin measurements in neonates – The devil is in the details. Commentary to Trevisanuto et al.: cardiac troponin I in asphyxiated neonates (Biol Neonate 2006;89:190-193). *Biol Neonate*. 2006; 89:194-196.

79. El-Khuffash A, Davis PG, Walsh K, Molloy EJ. Cardiac troponin T and N-terminal-pro-B type natriuretic peptide reflect myocardial function in preterm infants. *J Perinatol*. 2008;28:482-486.

80. Szymankiewicz M, Matuszczak-Wleklak M, Hodgman JE, Gadzinowski J. Usefulness of cardiac troponin T and echocardiography in the diagnosis of hypoxic myocardial injury of full-term neonates. *Biol Neonate.* 2005;88:19-23.
81. Doroszko A, et al. Neonatal asphyxia induces the nitration of cardiac myosin light chain 2 that is associated with cardiac systolic dysfunction. *Shock Augusta Ga.* 2010;34:592-600.
82. Walther FJ, Siassi B, Ramadan NA, Wu PY. Cardiac output in newborn infants with transient myocardial dysfunction. *J Pediatr.* 1985;107:781-785.
83. Barberi I, et al. Myocardial ischaemia in neonates with perinatal asphyxia. Electrocardiographic, echocardiographic and enzymatic correlations. *Eur J Pediatr.* 1999;158:742-747.
84. Seri I, Noori S. Diagnosis and treatment of neonatal hypotension outside the transitional period. *Early Hum Dev.* 2005;81: 405-411.
85. Landry DW, Oliver JA. The pathogenesis of vasodilatory shock. *N Engl J Med.* 2001;345:588-595.
86. Quayle JM, Nelson MT, Standen NB. ATP-sensitive and inwardly rectifying potassium channels in smooth muscle. *Physiol Rev.* 1997;77:1165-1232.
87. Murphy ME, Brayden JE. Nitric oxide hyperpolarizes rabbit mesenteric arteries via ATP-sensitive potassium channels. *J Physiol.* 1995;486(Pt 1):47-58.
88. Vanelli G, Hussain SN, Dimori M, Aguggini G. Cardiovascular responses to glibenclamide during endotoxaemia in the pig. *Vet Res Commun.* 1997;21:187-200.
89. Lambden S. Bench to bedside review: therapeutic modulation of nitric oxide in sepsis-an update. *Intensive Care Med Exp.* 2019;7:64.
90. Gardiner SM, Kemp PA, March JE, Bennett T. Regional haemodynamic responses to infusion of lipopolysaccharide in conscious rats: effects of pre- or post-treatment with glibenclamide. *Br J Pharmacol.* 1999;128:1772-1778.
91. Foster MN, Coetzee WA. KATP channels in the cardiovascular system. *Physiol Rev.* 2016;96:177-252.
92. Sordi R, Fernandes D, Heckert BT, Assreuy J. Early potassium channel blockade improves sepsis-induced organ damage and cardiovascular dysfunction. *Br J Pharmacol.* 2011;163: 1289-1301.
93. Tinker A, Aziz Q, Thomas A. The role of ATP-sensitive potassium channels in cellular function and protection in the cardiovascular system. *Br J Pharmacol.* 2014;171:12-23.
94. Warrillow S, Egi M, Bellomo R. Randomized, double-blind, placebo-controlled crossover pilot study of a potassium channel blocker in patients with septic shock. *Crit Care Med.* 2006;34:980-985.
95. Morelli A, et al. Glibenclamide dose response in patients with septic shock: effects on norepinephrine requirements, cardiopulmonary performance, and global oxygen transport. *Shock Augusta Ga.* 2007;28:530-535.
96. Oliver JA, Landry DW. Potassium channels and septic shock. *Crit Care Med.* 2006;34:1255-1257.
97. Tunctan B, et al. Eicosanoids derived from cytochrome P450 pathway of arachidonic acid and inflammatory shock. *Prostaglandins Other Lipid Mediat.* 2019;145:106377.
98. Fink MP. Therapeutic options directed against platelet activating factor, eicosanoids and bradykinin in sepsis. *J Antimicrob Chemother.* 1998;41(suppl A):81-94.
99. Arons MM, et al. Effects of ibuprofen on the physiology and survival of hypothermic sepsis. Ibuprofen in Sepsis Study Group. *Crit Care Med.* 1999;27:699-707.
100. Memiş D, Karamanlioğlu B, Turan A, Koyuncu O, Pamukçu Z. Effects of lornoxicam on the physiology of severe sepsis. *Crit Care Lond Engl.* 2004;8:R474-R482.
101. Aronoff DM. Cyclooxygenase inhibition in sepsis: is there life after death? *Mediators Inflamm.* 2012;2012:696897.
102. Feuerstein G, Zerbe RL, Meyer DK, Kopin IJ. Alteration of cardiovascular, neurogenic, and humoral responses to acute hypovolemic hypotension by administered prostacyclin. *J Cardiovasc Pharmacol.* 1982;4:246-253.
103. Machiedo GW, Warden MJ, LoVerme PJ, Rush BF. Hemodynamic effects of prolonged infusion of prostaglandin E1 (PGE1) after hemorrhagic shock. *Adv Shock Res.* 1982;8:171-176.
104. Reines HD, Halushka PV, Cook JA, Wise WC, Rambo W. Plasma thromboxane concentrations are raised in patients dying with septic shock. *Lancet Lond Engl.* 1982;2:174-175.
105. Ball HA, Cook JA, Wise WC, Halushka PV. Role of thromboxane, prostaglandins and leukotrienes in endotoxic and septic shock. *Intensive Care Med.* 1986;12:116-126.
106. Rubanyi GM. Nitric oxide and circulatory shock. *Adv Exp Med Biol.* 1998;454:165-172.
107. Liu S, Adcock IM, Old RW, Barnes PJ, Evans TW. Lipopolysaccharide treatment in vivo induces widespread tissue expression of inducible nitric oxide synthase mRNA. *Biochem Biophys Res Commun.* 1993;196:1208-1213.
108. Taylor BS, Geller DA. Molecular regulation of the human inducible nitric oxide synthase (iNOS) gene. *Shock Augusta Ga.* 2000;13:413-424.
109. Titheradge MA. Nitric oxide in septic shock. *Biochim Biophys Acta.* 1999;1411:437-455.
110. Doughty L, Carcillo JA, Kaplan S, Janosky J. Plasma nitrite and nitrate concentrations and multiple organ failure in pediatric sepsis. *Crit Care Med.* 1998;26:157-162.
111. Carcillo JA. Nitric oxide production in neonatal and pediatric sepsis. *Crit Care Med.* 1999;27:1063-1065.
112. Barrington KJ, et al. The hemodynamic effects of inhaled nitric oxide and endogenous nitric oxide synthesis blockade in newborn piglets during infusion of heat-killed group B streptococci. *Crit Care Med.* 2000;28:800-808.
113. Mitaka C, et al. Effects of nitric oxide synthase inhibitor on hemodynamic change and O2 delivery in septic dogs. *Am J Physiol.* 1995;268:H2017-H2023.
114. Grover R, et al. An open-label dose escalation study of the nitric oxide synthase inhibitor, N(G)-methyl-L-arginine hydrochloride (546C88), in patients with septic shock. Glaxo Wellcome International Septic Shock Study Group. *Crit Care Med.* 1999;27:913-922.
115. Bakker J, et al. Administration of the nitric oxide synthase inhibitor NG-methyl-L-arginine hydrochloride (546C88) by intravenous infusion for up to 72 hours can promote the resolution of shock in patients with severe sepsis: results of a randomized, double-blind, placebo-controlled multicenter study (study no. 144-002). *Crit Care Med.* 2004;32:1-12.
116. López A, et al. Multiple-center, randomized, placebo-controlled, double-blind study of the nitric oxide synthase inhibitor 546C88: effect on survival in patients with septic shock. *Crit Care Med.* 2004;32:21-30.
117. Wong VWC, Lerner E. Nitric oxide inhibition strategies. *Future Sci OA.* 2015;1:FSO35.
118. Mitaka C, Hirata Y, Yokoyama K, Makita K, Imai T. A selective inhibitor for inducible nitric oxide synthase improves hypotension and lactic acidosis in canine endotoxic shock. *Crit Care Med.* 2001;29:2156-2161.

119. Pullamsetti SS, et al. Effect of nitric oxide synthase (NOS) inhibition on macro-and microcirculation in a model of rat endotoxic shock. *Thromb Haemost.* 2006;95:720-727.
120. Su F, et al. Effects of a selective iNOS inhibitor versus norepinephrine in the treatment of septic shock. *Shock Augusta Ga.* 2010;34:243-249.
121. Cinelli MA, Do HT, Miley GP, Silverman RB. Inducible nitric oxide synthase: regulation, structure, and inhibition. *Med Res Rev.* 2020;40:158-189.
122. Rozenfeld V, Cheng JW. The role of vasopressin in the treatment of vasodilation in shock states. *Ann Pharmacother.* 2000; 34:250-254.
123. Robin JK, Oliver JA, Landry DW. Vasopressin deficiency in the syndrome of irreversible shock. *J Trauma.* 2003;54:S149-S154.
124. Landry DW, et al. Vasopressin deficiency contributes to the vasodilation of septic shock. *Circulation.* 1997;95:1122-1125.
125. Liedel JL, Meadow W, Nachman J, Koogler T, Kahana MD. Use of vasopressin in refractory hypotension in children with vasodilatory shock: five cases and a review of the literature. *Pediatr Crit Care Med.* 2002;3:15-18.
126. Malay MB, et al. Heterogeneity of the vasoconstrictor effect of vasopressin in septic shock. *Crit Care Med.* 2004;32: 1327-1331.
127. Rosenzweig EB, et al. Intravenous arginine-vasopressin in children with vasodilatory shock after cardiac surgery. *Circulation.* 1999;100:II182-II186.
128. Meyer S, Gottschling S, Baghai A, Wurm D, Gortner L. Arginine-vasopressin in catecholamine-refractory septic versus non-septic shock in extremely low birth weight infants with acute renal injury. *Crit Care Lond Engl.* 2006;10:R71.
129. Bidegain M, et al. Vasopressin for refractory hypotension in extremely low birth weight infants. *J Pediatr.* 2010;157: 502-504.
130. Rios DR, Kaiser JR. Vasopressin versus dopamine for treatment of hypotension in extremely low birth weight infants: a randomized, blinded pilot study. *J Pediatr.* 2015;166:850-855.
131. Jiang L, Sheng Y, Feng X, Wu J. The effects and safety of vasopressin receptor agonists in patients with septic shock: a meta-analysis and trial sequential analysis. *Crit Care Lond Engl.* 2019;23:91.
132. Yao RQ, et al. Clinical efficiency of vasopressin or its analogs in comparison with catecholamines alone on patients with septic shock: a systematic review and meta-analysis. *Front Pharmacol.* 2020;11:563.
133. Masarwa R, et al. Role of vasopressin and terlipressin in refractory shock compared to conventional therapy in the neonatal and pediatric population: a systematic review, meta-analysis, and trial sequential analysis. *Crit Care Lond Engl.* 2017;21:1.
134. Boyd SM, Riley KL, Giesinger RE, McNamara PJ. Use of vasopressin in neonatal hypertrophic obstructive cardiomyopathy: case series. *J Perinatol.* 2021;41:126-133.
135. Acker SN, Kinsella JP, Abman SH, Gien J. Vasopressin improves hemodynamic status in infants with congenital diaphragmatic hernia. *J Pediatr.* 2014;165:53-58.e1.
136. Mohamed A, Nasef N, Shah V, McNamara PJ. Vasopressin as a rescue therapy for refractory pulmonary hypertension in neonates: case series. *Pediatr Crit Care Med.* 2014;15:148-154.
137. Enomoto M, Pan J, Shifrin Y, Belik J. Age dependency of vasopressin pulmonary vasodilatory effect in rats. *Pediatr Res.* 2014;75:315-321.
138. de Waal K, Evans N. Hemodynamics in preterm infants with late-onset sepsis. *J Pediatr.* 2010;156:918-922.e1.
139. Brierley J, Peters MJ. Distinct hemodynamic patterns of septic shock at presentation to pediatric intensive care. *Pediatrics.* 2008;122:752-759.
140. Saini SS, Kumar P, Kumar RM. Hemodynamic changes in preterm neonates with septic shock: a prospective observational study. *Pediatr Crit Care Med.* 2014;15:443-450.
141. Raj S, Killinger JS, Gonzalez JA, Lopez L. Myocardial dysfunction in pediatric septic shock. *J Pediatr.* 2014;164:72-77.e2.
142. de Boode WP. Clinical monitoring of systemic hemodynamics in critically ill newborns. *Early Hum Dev.* 2010;86:137-141.
143. Wehling M. Looking beyond the dogma of genomic steroid action: insights and facts of the 1990s. *J Mol Med Berl Ger.* 1995;73:439-447.
144. Cox BE, Rosenfeld CR. Ontogeny of vascular angiotensin II receptor subtype expression in ovine development. *Pediatr Res.* 1999;45:414-424.
145. Kaiser JR, Cox BE, Roy TA, Rosenfeld CR. Differential development of umbilical and systemic arteries. I. ANG II receptor subtype expression. *Am J Physiol.* 1998;274:R797-R807.
146. Bendeck MP, Langille BL. Rapid accumulation of elastin and collagen in the aortas of sheep in the immediate perinatal period. *Circ Res.* 1991;69:1165-1169.
147. Leitman DC, Benson SC, Johnson LK. Glucocorticoids stimulate collagen and noncollagen protein synthesis in cultured vascular smooth muscle cells. *J Cell Biol.* 1984;98:541-549.
148. Hanna CE, et al. Hypothalamic pituitary adrenal function in the extremely low birth weight infant. *J Clin Endocrinol Metab.* 1993;76:384-387.
149. Ng PC, et al. Refractory hypotension in preterm infants with adrenocortical insufficiency. *Arch Dis Child Fetal Neonatal Ed.* 2001;84:F122-F124.
150. Ng PC, et al. Transient adrenocortical insufficiency of prematurity and systemic hypotension in very low birthweight infants. *Arch Dis Child Fetal Neonatal Ed.* 2004;89:F119-F126.
151. Ng PC. Is there a "normal" range of serum cortisol concentration for preterm infants? *Pediatrics.* 2008;122:873-875.
152. Aucott SW. The challenge of defining relative adrenal insufficiency. *J Perinatol.* 2012;32:397-398.
153. Cooper MS, Stewart PM. Corticosteroid insufficiency in acutely ill patients. *N Engl J Med.* 2003;348:727-734.
154. Korte C, et al. Adrenocortical function in the very low birth weight infant: improved testing sensitivity and association with neonatal outcome. *J Pediatr.* 1996;128:257-263.
155. Fernandez E, Schrader R, Watterberg K. Prevalence of low cortisol values in term and near-term infants with vasopressor-resistant hypotension. *J Perinatol.* 2005;25:114-118.
156. Hingre RV, Gross SJ, Hingre KS, Mayes DM, Richman RA. Adrenal steroidogenesis in very low birth weight preterm infants. *J Clin Endocrinol Metab.* 1994;78:266-270.
157. Watterberg KL, Scott SM. Evidence of early adrenal insufficiency in babies who develop bronchopulmonary dysplasia. *Pediatrics.* 1995;95:120-125.
158. Jett PL, et al. Variability of plasma cortisol levels in extremely low birth weight infants. *J Clin Endocrinol Metab.* 1997;82: 2921-2925.
159. Hanna CE, et al. Corticosteroid binding globulin, total serum cortisol, and stress in extremely low-birth-weight infants. *Am J Perinatol.* 1997;14:201-204.
160. Ng PC, et al. The pituitary-adrenal responses to exogenous human corticotropin-releasing hormone in preterm, very low birth weight infants. *J Clin Endocrinol Metab.* 1997;82: 797-799.

161. Procianoy RS, Cecin SK, Pinheiro CE. Umbilical cord cortisol and prolactin levels in preterm infants. Relation to labor and delivery. *Acta Paediatr Scand.* 1983;72:713-716.

162. Terrone DA, et al. Neonatal effects and serum cortisol levels after multiple courses of maternal corticosteroids. *Obstet Gynecol.* 1997;90:819-823.

163. Rokicki W, Forest MG, Loras B, Bonnet H, Bertrand J. Free cortisol of human plasma in the first three months of life. *Biol Neonate.* 1990;57:21-29.

164. Wittekind CA, Arnold JD, Leslie GI, Luttrell B, Jones MP. Longitudinal study of plasma ACTH and cortisol in very low birth weight infants in the first 8 weeks of life. *Early Hum Dev.* 1993;33:191-200.

165. Goldkrand JW, Schulte RL, Messer RH. Maternal and fetal plasma cortisol levels at parturition. *Obstet Gynecol.* 1976;47:41-45.

166. Scott SM, Watterberg KL. Effect of gestational age, postnatal age, and illness on plasma cortisol concentrations in premature infants. *Pediatr Res.* 1995;37:112-116.

167. EL-Khuffash A, McNamara PJ, Lapointe A, Jain A. Adrenal function in preterm infants undergoing patent ductus arteriosus ligation. *Neonatology.* 2013;104:28-33.

168. Clyman RI, et al. Hypotension following patent ductus arteriosus ligation: the role of adrenal hormones. *J Pediatr.* 2014;164:1449-1455.e1.

169. Noori S, et al. Catecholamine-resistant hypotension and myocardial performance following patent ductus arteriosus ligation. *J Perinatol.* 2015;35:123-127.

170. Helbock HJ, Insoft RM, Conte FA. Glucocorticoid-responsive hypotension in extremely low birth weight newborns. *Pediatrics.* 1993;92:715-717.

171. Fauser A, Pohlandt F, Bartmann P, Gortner L. Rapid increase of blood pressure in extremely low birth weight infants after a single dose of dexamethasone. *Eur J Pediatr.* 1993;152:354-356.

172. Gaissmaier RE, Pohlandt F. Single-dose dexamethasone treatment of hypotension in preterm infants. *J Pediatr.* 1999;134:701-705.

173. Seri I, Tan R, Evans J. Cardiovascular effects of hydrocortisone in preterm infants with pressor-resistant hypotension. *Pediatrics.* 2001;107:1070-1074.

174. Noori S, et al. Cardiovascular effects of low-dose dexamethasone in very low birth weight neonates with refractory hypotension. *Biol Neonate.* 2006;89:82-87.

175. Noori S, et al. Hemodynamic changes after low-dosage hydrocortisone administration in vasopressor-treated preterm and term neonates. *Pediatrics.* 2006;118:1456-1466.

176. Ng PC, et al. A double-blind, randomized, controlled study of a "stress dose" of hydrocortisone for rescue treatment of refractory hypotension in preterm infants. *Pediatrics.* 2006;117:367-375.

177. Baker CFW. et al. Hydrocortisone administration for the treatment of refractory hypotension in critically ill newborns. *J. Perinatol.* 2008;28:412-419.

178. Higgins S, Friedlich P, Seri I. Hydrocortisone for hypotension and vasopressor dependence in preterm neonates: a meta-analysis. *J Perinatol.* 2010;30:373-378.

179. Davies AO, Lefkowitz RJ. Regulation of beta-adrenergic receptors by steroid hormones. *Annu Rev Physiol.* 1984;46:119-130.

180. Hadcock JR, Malbon CC. Regulation of beta-adrenergic receptors by "permissive" hormones: glucocorticoids increase steady-state levels of receptor mRNA. *Proc Natl Acad Sci U S A.* 1988;85:8415-8419.

181. Radomski MW, Palmer RM, Moncada S. Glucocorticoids inhibit the expression of an inducible, but not the constitutive, nitric oxide synthase in vascular endothelial cells. *Proc Natl Acad Sci U S A.* 1990;87:10043-10047.

182. Wehling M. Specific, nongenomic actions of steroid hormones. *Annu Rev Physiol.* 1997;59:365-393.

183. Segar JL, et al. Effect of cortisol on gene expression of the renin-angiotensin system in fetal sheep. *Pediatr Res.* 1995;37:741-746.

184. Soleymani S, Borzage M, Seri I. Hemodynamic monitoring in neonates: advances and challenges. *J Perinatol.* 2010;30(Suppl):S38-S45.

185. Noori S, McLean CW, Wu TW, Seri I. Cerebral circulation and hypotension in the premature infant: diagnosis and treatment. In: Perlman JM, Cilio MR, eds. *Neurology: Neonatology Questions and Controversies.* Philadelphia: Elsevier;2019:1-26.

# Chapter 2

# Vascular Regulation and Assessment of Blood Flow to Organs in the Neonatal Period

Gorm Greisen

## Key Points

- Multiple mechanisms operate to regulate blood flow to organs – these are also important in the newborn.
- Distribution of cardiac output is actively regulated.
- Autoregulation may best be described as a degree of capacity rather than an on-off phenomenon.
- Cerebral autoregulation, that is, the ability to buffer the effects of blood pressure on cerebral blood flow, is developed even at the limits of viability.
- Whereas the brain is relatively large in newborn infants, its blood flow is relatively low.
- A "diving" reflex–like response serves to prioritize vital organs during stress.
- The cerebral hemispheres may not be privileged, especially in the very preterm neonate.

## The Purposes of Blood Flow

In most organs the principal role of perfusion is to provide substrates for cellular energy metabolism, with the final purpose of maintaining normal intracellular concentrations of the high-energy phosphate metabolites adenosine triphosphate (ATP) and phosphocreatine. The critical substrate is usually oxygen. Accordingly, organ blood flow is regulated by the energy demand of the given tissue. For instance, during maximal activation by seizures in the brain, cerebral blood flow (CBF) increases threefold, while in the muscle during maximal exercise, blood flow increases up to eightfold. Some organs, such as the brain, heart, and liver, have higher baseline oxygen consumption and thus higher demand for blood flow than others.

Finally, in the kidney and skin, perfusion may be considerably above the metabolic needs to serve for glomerular filtration and thermoregulation, respectively. Indeed, during heating, skin blood flow may increase by as much as fourfold without any increase in energy demand.

In the developing organism, metabolic requirements are increased by as much as 40% due to the expenditures of growth. Since growth involves deposition of protein and fat, energy metabolism and oxygen requirements are not increased as much as are the requirements for protein and energy.

### TISSUE ISCHEMIA

When blood flow is failing, there are several lines of defense mechanisms at the tissue level before the tissue is damaged. First, more oxygen is extracted from the blood. Normal oxygen extraction is about 30%, resulting in a venous oxygen saturation ($SvO_2$) of 65–70%. Oxygen extraction can increase up to 50% to 60%, resulting in an $SvO_2$ of 40–50%, which corresponds to a venous (i.e., endcapillary) oxygen tension of 3–4 kPa. This is the critical value for oxygen tension for driving the diffusion of molecular oxygen from the capillary into the cell and to the mitochondria (Figure 2.1). Microvascular anatomy and the pathophysiology of the underlying disease process are both important for these final steps of oxygen delivery to tissue. When the cell senses oxygen insufficiency, its function is affected so that growth stops, organ function fails, and, finally, cellular function; thus, organ

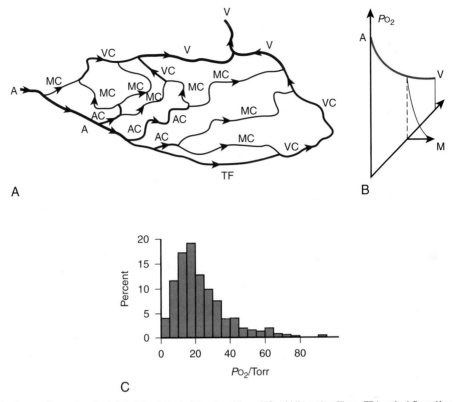

**Fig. 2.1** (A) Draft of a capillary network. *A,* Arteriole; *AC,* arterial endcapillary; *MC,* middle endcapillary; *TF,* terminal flow; *V,* venule; *VC,* venous endcapillary. (B) A three-dimensional graph illustrating the $Po_2$ gradients from the arterial *(A)* to the venous *(V)* end of the capillaries and the radial gradient of $Po_2$ in surrounding tissue to the mitochondrion *(M)*. Y-axis: $Po_2$; X-axis: distance along the capillary (typically 1000 μm); Z-axis: distance into tissue (typically 50 μm). (C) The wide distribution of tissue $Po_2$ as recorded by microelectrode. Y-axis: frequency of measurements; X-axis: $Po_2$. $Po_2$ values in tissue are typically 10–30 Torr (1.5–4.5 kPa), but range from near-arterial levels to near zero. The cells with the lowest $Po_2$ determine the ischemic threshold, that is, the most remote cells at the venous end of capillaries. Microvascular factors, such as capillary density, and distribution of blood flow among capillaries are very important for oxygen transport to the tissue.

survival is threatened (Figure 2.2). *Ischemia* is the term used for inadequate blood flow to maintain appropriate oxygen delivery and thus cellular function and integrity. Since there are several steps in the cellular reaction to oxygen insufficiency, more than one ischemic threshold may be defined. It is also possible that newborn infants can be, at least, partly protected against hypoxic-ischemic injury by mechanisms akin to hibernation by "hypoxic hypometabolism."[1]

## The Physics

Physically, blood simply flows toward the point of lowest resistance. While flow velocities in the heart

are high enough to allow the kinetic energy to thrust the blood forward, flow velocities are minimal in the peripheral circulation. Organs are perfused in parallel and the blood flow through a given tissue is the result of the pressure gradient between the arteries and the veins, the so-called perfusion pressure. Vascular resistance is composed of the limited diameter of blood vessels, particularly the smaller arteries and arterioles, their lengths, and blood viscosity. While veins also hold tone, their contribution to vascular resistance is very limited, so they will be disregarded here. Their importance lies in the regulation of blood return to the heart, which thus influences cardiac output (see Chapter 3).

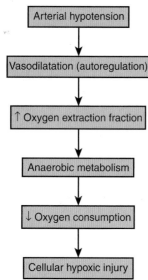

**Fig. 2.2 The lines of defense against oxygen insufficiency.** First, when blood pressure falls, autoregulation of organ blood flow will reduce vascular resistance and keep blood flow nearly unaffected. If the blood pressure falls below the lower limit of the autoregulatory elbow, or if autoregulation is impaired by vascular pathology, metabolic or respiratory acidosis, or immaturity, blood flow to the tissue falls. At this point, oxygen extraction increases from each milliliter of blood. The limit of this compensation is attained when the minimal $Svo_2$, or rather the minimal endcapillary oxygen tension, has been reached. This process is determined by microvascular factors as illustrated in Fig. 2.1. When the limits of oxygen extraction have been reached, the marginal cells resort to anaerobic metabolism (increase glucose consumption to produce lactate) to meet their metabolic needs. If this is insufficient, oxygen consumption decreases as metabolic functions related to growth and to organ function are shut down. However, in vital organs, such as the brain, heart, and adrenal glands, loss of function is life threatening. In nonvital organs normal development may be affected if this critical state is long lasting. Acute cellular death by necrosis occurs only when vital cellular functions break down and membrane potential and integrity cannot be maintained. In newborn mammals hypoxic hypometabolism is a mechanism that further reduces the sensitivity to hypoxic-ischemic injury.

## Regulation of Arterial Tone

The regulation of organ blood flow takes place by active modification of the arterial diameter, that is, by varying the tone of the smooth muscle cells of the arterial wall. Factors that influence vascular resistance are usually divided into four categories: blood pressure, chemical ($Pco_2$ and $Po_2$), metabolic (functional activation), and neurogenic. Most studies of vascular resistance have been done on cerebral vessels. Therefore the following account refers to cerebral vessels from mature animals, unless stated otherwise.

### THE ROLE OF CONDUIT ARTERIES IN REGULATING VASCULAR RESISTANCE

It is often assumed that the arteriole, the precapillary muscular artery with a diameter of 20–50 μm, is the primary determinant of vascular resistance, while the larger arteries are considered passive conduits. However, this is not the case. For instance, in the adult cat the pressure in the small cerebral arteries (150–200 μm) is only 50–60% of the aortic pressure. Thus nearly 50% of the total vascular resistance is "central" and the reactivity of the entire muscular arterial tree is of relevance in regulating organ blood flow and "distributing" cardiac output. The role of the prearteriolar arteries is likely to be even more important in the newborn than in the adult. *First*, the smaller body size translates to smaller conduit arteries (the resistance is proportional to length but is inversely proportional to the diameter to the power of 4). *Second*, conduit arteries are very reactive in the newborn. The diameter of the carotid artery increases by 75% during acute asphyxia in term lambs, whereas the diameter of the descending aorta decreases by 15% when blood pressure drops. For comparison, flow-induced vasodilatation in the forearm in adults is only in the order of 5%. These findings indicate a roughly 90% reduction of the arterial component of the cerebrovascular resistance coupled with a near doubling of the arterial component of vascular resistance to the lower body. Incidentally, they also suggest that blood flow velocity, as recorded from conduit arteries by Doppler ultrasound, may be potentially misleading and thus likely to be biased as a measure of perfusion in the neonates.

### ARTERIAL REACTION TO PRESSURE (AUTOREGULATION)

Smooth muscle cells of the arterial wall constrict in response to increased intravascular pressure in the local arterial segment to a degree that more than compensates for the passive stretching of the vessel wall by the increased pressure.[2] The net result is that arteries constrict when pressure increases and dilate when pressure drops.[3] This phenomenon is called the

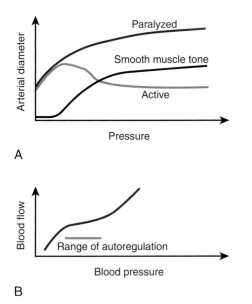

**Fig. 2.3 Increases in pressure lead to progressive dilatation of a paralyzed artery.** As pressure increases further, the elastic capacity is exhausted, and vasodilation decreases as collagen restricts further dilation, limiting the risk of rupture (A). A certain range of pressures is associated with a proportional variation in smooth muscle tone. The precise mechanism of this mechanochemical coupling is not known, but it is endogenous to all vascular smooth muscle cells. As a result, in an active artery, the diameter varies inversely with pressure over a certain range. This phenomenon constitutes the basis of arterial "autoregulation" (B).

autoregulation of blood flow (Figure 2.3). The response time in isolated, cannulated arterial segments is in the order of 10 seconds.[4] The cellular mechanisms of this process are now better understood. Vessel wall constriction constitutes an intrinsic myogenic reflex and is independent of endothelial function. Rather, pressure induces an increase in the smooth muscle cell membrane potential, which regulates vascular smooth muscle cell activity through the action of voltage-gated calcium channels. Although the precise mechanistic nature of the mechano-chemical coupling is unknown, several plasma membrane–bound receptors are involved, including G protein–coupled receptors and a class of transient potential receptors.[5] Furthermore, the calcium signal is modulated in many ways,[6] but a detailed discussion of this topic is beyond the scope of this chapter. Suffice to mention that phospholipases and activation of

protein kinase C are involved, and, at least in the rat middle cerebral artery, the arachidonic acid metabolite 20-HETE has also been implicated.[7] Furthermore, additional modulation of intracellular calcium concentration by alternative sources, such as the calcium-dependent $K^+$ channels, also exists. Local variations in the expression of these receptors and channels may, at least in part, explain the difference in responses to blood pressure in different vascular beds and the change in unique blood flow distribution between vital and non-vital organs during the diving reflex (see later).[8]

## INTERACTION OF AUTOREGULATION AND HYPOXIC VASODILATATION

As described earlier, arterial smooth muscle tone is affected by a number of factors, all contributing to determine the level of vascular resistance. Among the vasodilators, hypoxia is one of the most important, more potent, and physiologically relevant factors. Vascular reactivity to $O_2$ depends, in part, on intact endothelial function ensuring appropriate local nitric oxide (NO) production. Hypoxia also induces tissue lactic acidosis. The decreased pH constitutes a point of interaction between $O_2$ and $CO_2$ reactivity (see later). In addition, hypoxia decreases smooth muscle membrane potential by the direct and selective opening of both the calcium-activated and ATP-sensitive $K^+$ channels in the cell membrane.[9] In the immature brain adenosine is also an important regulator of the vascular response to hypoxia.[10] The membrane potential response to hypoxia is independent of the existing intravascular pressure.[11] However, at lower pressures, the decrease in membrane potential only leads to minimal further arterial dilation because, since at low vascular tone, the membrane potential-muscular tone relationship is already outside the steep part of the slope (Figure 2.4). In other words at low perfusion pressures, the dilator pathway has already been near maximally activated. Therefore in a hypotensive neonate, a superimposed hypoxic event cannot be appropriately compensated due to the low perfusion pressure. The end result is tissue hypoxia-ischemia with the potential of causing irreversible damage to organs, especially to the brain. This is a clinically highly relevant point when providing care for the hypotensive and hypoxic neonate.

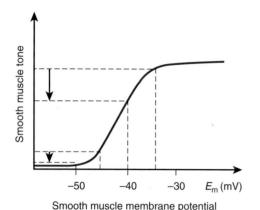

**Fig. 2.4 The relationship between smooth muscle cell membrane potential ($E_m$) and tone.** Pressure affects smooth muscle tone through membrane potential. Increased pressure increases membrane potential (i.e., makes it less negative), whereas decreased pressure induces hyperpolarization (i.e., membrane potential is more negative). Hyperpolarization induces relaxation and hence vasodilatation. The modifying effect of hypoxia is illustrated by the dashed lines and arrows. At high membrane potential ($-35$ mV), a decrease in membrane potential by 5 mV induces a marked reduction in muscular tone. Thus, at normal or high blood pressures, hypoxemia can be compensated by vasodilatation. However, at low membrane potential (hyperpolarization) a similar hypoxia-induced decrease in membrane potential has much less effect on muscular tone. This predicts that, at low blood pressure where there is a baseline low membrane potential to enable vasodilation keeping blood flow in the acceptable range, hypoxemia cannot be well compensated by further increases in blood flow. Many other factors may influence muscle tone by modifying membrane potential, and the magnitude of effects can be predicted to be interdependent.

## THE EFFECTS OF $P_{CO_2}$

Arteries and arterioles in the brain constrict with hypocapnia and dilate with hypercapnia. The principal part of this reaction is mediated through changes in pH, that is, $H^+$ concentration. Perivascular pH has a direct effect on the membrane potential of arterial smooth muscle cells since, mostly via activation of both the ATP-sensitive and calcium-activated $K^+$ channels, extracellular $H^+$ concentration is one of the main determinants of the potassium conductance of the plasma membrane in arterial smooth muscle cells regulating the outward $K^+$ current.[9] Therefore when the pH decreases, the $K^+$ outflow from the vascular smooth muscle cell increases, resulting in hyperpolarization of the cell membrane and, via the closure of

voltage-gated $Ca^{++}$ channels, it causes vasodilatation. Furthermore, increased extracellular and, to a lesser degree, intracellular $H^+$ concentrations reduce the conductance of the voltage-dependent calcium channels, further enhancing vascular smooth muscle cell relaxation.[12]

Hypercapnic vasodilatation is reduced by up to 50% when NO synthase (NOS) activity is blocked in the brain of the adult rat.[13] The hypercapnic response is restituted by the addition of an NO donor.[14] This finding suggests that unhindered local NO production is necessary for the pH to exert its vasoregulator effects. Indeed, it has been suggested that, although the calcium-activated and ATP-sensitive $K^+$ channels play the primary role in the vascular response to changes in $P_{CO_2}$, the function of these channels is regulated by local NO production.[15]

The role of prostanoids in mediating the vascular response to $P_{CO_2}$ is less clear.[16,17] The fact that indomethacin abolishes the normal CBF-$CO_2$ response in preterm infants is likely a direct effect of the drug independent of its inhibitory action on prostanoid synthesis.[18] This notion is supported by the finding that ibuprofen is devoid of such effects on the brain blood flow–$CO_2$ response.[19]

## FUNCTIONAL ACTIVATION (METABOLIC BLOOD FLOW CONTROL)

Several mechanisms operate to match local blood flow to metabolic requirements, including changes in pH, local production of adenosine, ATP and NO, and local neural mechanisms. It appears that, in the muscle, there is not a single factor dominating, since the robust and very fast coupling of activity and blood flow is almost unaffected by blocking any of these mechanisms one by one.[20] In the brain astrocytes may be the central sites of regulation of this response in the neurovascular unit via their perivascular end-feet and by using many of the aforementioned cellular mechanisms, such as changes in $K^+$ ion flux and the local production of prostanoids, ATP, and adenosine.[21] Among these cellular regulators, adenosine has been proposed to play a principal role.[22] Adenosine also works by regulating the activity of the calcium-activated and ATP-sensitive $K^+$ channels.

## FLOW-MEDIATED VASODILATATION

Endothelial cells sense flow by shear stress and produce NO in reaction to high shear stress at high flow velocities. NO diffuses freely and reaches the smooth muscle cell underneath the endothelium. NO acts on smooth muscle $K^+$ channels using cyclic guanosine monophosphate (GMP) as the secondary messenger and then a series of intermediate steps. Since NO is a vasodilator, the basic arterial reflex to high flow is vasodilation. Thus when a tissue is activated (e.g., a muscle contracts), the local vessels first dilate, as directed by the mechanisms of the metabolic flow control described earlier, and blood flow increases. This initial increase in blood flow is then sensed in the conduit arteries through the shear stress-induced increase in local NO production, and vascular resistance is further reduced, allowing flow to increase yet again. The action remains local as the generated NO diffusing into the bloodstream is largely inactivated by hemoglobin.

## SYMPATHETIC NERVOUS SYSTEM

Epinephrine in the blood originates from the adrenal glands, whereas norepinephrine is produced by sympathetic nerve endings and extra-adrenal chromaffin tissue. Sympathetic nerves are present in nearly all vessels, located in the adventitia and mixed in with the smooth muscle cells. Adrenoreceptors are widely distributed in the cardiovascular system located in the smooth muscle and endothelial cell membranes. Several different adrenoreceptors exist; alpha-1 receptors with at least three subtypes are present primarily in the arteries and the myocardium, while alpha-2, beta-1, and beta-2 receptors are expressed in all types of vessels and the myocardium. In the arteries and veins alpha-receptor stimulation causes vasoconstriction, and beta-receptor stimulation results in vasodilatation. Both alpha- and beta-adrenoreceptors are frequently expressed in the membrane of the same cell. Therefore the response of the given cell to epinephrine or norepinephrine depends on the relative abundance of the receptor types expressed.[23] Points of clinical importance are (1) the regulation of the expression of the cardiovascular adrenergic receptors are regulated by corticosteroids, (2) the high incidence of relative adrenal insufficiency in preterm neonates and critically ill term infants (see Chapter 23), and (3) the downregulation of the cardiovascular adrenergic receptors in response to the increased release of endogenous catecholamines or the administration of exogenous catecholamines given in critical illness.[24-26] Typically, arteries and arterioles of the skin, gut, and muscle constrict in response to increases in endogenous catecholamine production, whereas those of the heart and brain neither constrict nor even dilate (see later). The response also depends on the resting tone of the given vessel. Furthermore, circulating norepinephrine may be more effective than norepinephrine produced by sympathetic nerve activity, since alpha-1 receptors may be particularly abundant in the membrane regions close to where the nerve secretes the transmitter. Furthermore, the signaling pathways of the adrenoreceptors are complex and dependent on the receptor subtype. Activation of alpha-adrenoreceptors generally results in vasoconstriction mediated by increased release of calcium from intracellular stores as a first step, while beta-receptor-induced vasodilation is mediated by increased cyclic adenosine monophosphate (AMP) generation. However, the system is more complex and, among other mechanisms, receptor activation-associated changes in $K^+$ conductance and local NOS are also involved. Finally, the sympathetic nervous system is activated during hypoxia, hypotension, or hypovolemia via the stimulation of different chemoreceptors and baroreceptors in the vessel walls and the vasomotor centers in the medulla. Activation of the sympathetic nervous system plays a central role in the cardiovascular response to stress, and it is the mainstay of the diving reflex response during hypoxia-ischemia.

## HUMORAL FACTORS IN GENERAL CIRCULATION

Several endogenous vasoactive factors, other than those mentioned earlier, play a role in the processes of organ blood flow regulation, such as angiotensin II, arginine-vasopressin, vasointestinal peptide, neuropeptide gamma, and endothelin-1. However, none of these vasoactive factors has been shown to have any significant importance in themselves under normal conditions, except for the role of angiotensin II in regulating renal microhemodynamics.

## QUANTITATIVE PREDICTIONS OF LOCAL VASCULAR TONE ARE NOT POSSIBLE

In conclusion, many factors have an input and interact to define the degree of contraction of the local vascular smooth muscle cell to regulate local arterial and arteriolar tone (see Figure 2.4). Although many details are unknown, especially in the developing immature animal or human, the final common pathway appears to involve the smooth-cell membrane potential, cytoplasmic calcium concentration, and the calcium/calmodulin myosin light chain kinase–mediated phosphorylation of the regulatory light chains of myosin, resulting in the interaction of actin and myosin (Figure 2.5). The complexity of the known factors and their interplay, as well as the differences in the response among the different organs, are overwhelming, and no simple or unifying principle of vascular tone regulation has gained a foothold. Indeed, the complexity predicts that vascular tone and reactivity in a particular arterial segment in a particular tissue may differ markedly from that in other segments or other tissues. Practically, this means that the insights that are summarized above are as yet insufficient to allow any quantitative predictions for different organs or segments of the vascular tree.

## Blood Flow to the Brain

Brain injury is common in newborn infants. It can occur rapidly, is frequently irreversible, and rarely, in itself prevents survival. No other injury to other organs in the neonatal period has the same clinical importance, as the other organs have a better capacity to recover even from severe hypoxic-ischemic damage. Disturbances in blood flow and inflammation have been proposed as the major factors in the development of neonatal brain injury.

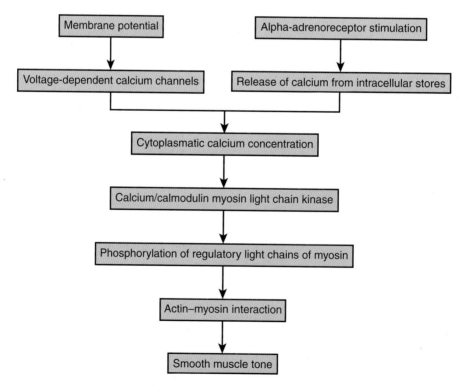

Fig. 2.5  A scheme of the pathway from smooth muscle cell membrane potential and alpha-adrenoreceptor stimulation to changes in smooth muscle tone.

## AUTOREGULATION OF CEREBRAL BLOOD FLOW IN THE IMMATURE BRAIN

Pressure-flow autoregulation has been widely investigated in the immature cerebral vasculature since the original observation of direct proportionality of CBF to systolic blood pressure in a group of neonates during stabilization after birth.[27]

An autoregulatory plateau, shifted to the left to match the lower perinatal blood pressure, has been demonstrated in several animal species shortly after birth, including dogs, lambs, and rats.[28-32] In fetal lambs autoregulation was weak or absent at 0.6 gestation but is functional at 0.9 gestation.[33] The lower autoregulation threshold appears developmentally regulated since it was closer to the normal resting systemic mean blood pressure at 0.75 gestation compared with 0.9 gestation.[34] Thus in the more immature subject there is less vasodilator reserve, which limits the effectiveness of CBF autoregulation at low blood pressures. In newborn lambs autoregulation could be completely abolished for 4–7 hours by 20 minutes of hypoxemia with arterial oxygen saturations of about 50%.[35]

Observational studies of global CBF in stable neonates without evidence of major brain injury suggest that autoregulation is well functioning.[36-44] In contrast, weak or absent autoregulation has been found under pathologic conditions, such as following severe birth asphyxia in term infants, and in preterm infants in association with brain injury or death.[39,41,45-49]

Imaging of CBF during arterial hypotension suggested that CBF to the periventricular white matter may be selectively reduced at blood pressures less than 30 mmHg,[50] supporting the notion that the periventricular white matter is a "watershed area." Another study also found some evidence for the lower threshold of the autoregulatory curve for the global CBF around 29 mmHg.[51]

In conclusion, the lower threshold for CBF autoregulation may be around 30 mmHg or somewhat below, and autoregulation can be assumed to operate in most well newborn infants, even the most immature. When blood pressure falls below the threshold, CBF will fall more than proportionally to blood pressure due to the elastic reduction in vascular diameter. However, significant blood flow is believed to be present until systemic mean blood pressure is less than 20 mmHg, and it may in general be more appropriate to consider arterial blood pressure-CBF reactivity (i.e., autoregulation) as a degree of capacity rather than an on-off phenomenon.[52] Finally, while poor clinical outcomes may be predicted by a weak autoregulation response, it remains to be demonstrated that it has clinical value.[53] One way could be to determine the level of arterial blood pressure, where the pressure-flow reactivity is lowest – the optimal blood pressure – and then to treat arterial hypotension using this individualized target.[54]

## EFFECT OF CARBON DIOXIDE ON CEREBRAL BLOOD FLOW

Changes in carbon dioxide tension ($Pco_2$) have more pronounced effects on CBF than on blood flow in other organs due to the presence of the blood-brain barrier. The blood-brain barrier is an endothelium with tight junctions, which does not allow $HCO_3^-$ to pass through readily. The restricted diffusion of $HCO_3^-$ means that pH in the perivascular space in the brain is decreased by hypercapnia and increased by hypocapnia more readily than in blood where buffering is more effective due to the presence of hemoglobin. This response to a change in $Pco_2$ continues until $HCO_3^-$ equilibrates over the course of hours.

In normocapnic adults small acute changes in arterial $Pco_2$ ($Paco_2$) result in a change in CBF by 30% per kPa (4% per mmHg $Paco_2$). Similar reactivity has been demonstrated in the normal human neonate.[38,55,56] However, $Paco_2$ reactivity was less than 30% per kPa during the first 24 hours.[39]

Contrary to the vasodilation induced by increases in the $Pco_2$, a hyperventilation-related decrease in $Paco_2$ causes hypocapnic cerebral vasoconstriction and has been found to be associated with brain injury in preterm but not in term infants or adults.[38,57-59] It is an open question whether hypocapnia alone can cause ischemia or if it works in combination with other factors, such as hypoxemia, hypoglycemia, the presence of high levels of cytokines, sympathetic activation, or seizures.

## METABOLIC CONTROL OF BLOOD FLOW TO THE BRAIN

CBF in term infants is higher during active sleep than during quiet sleep[60-62] and, in preterm infants of 32–35 weeks' postmenstrual age, in the wake state compared with sleep.[63] Thus there is flow-metabolism coupling even before term gestation in the brain. This finding is further supported by the increase in CBF seen during seizure activity and by the relation between CBF and blood hemoglobin concentration.[36,40]

The cerebrovascular response to functional activation by sensory stimulation was found to be variable by initial studies using magnetic resonance imaging and near-infrared spectroscopy (NIRS).[64-68] More recently, a clear coupling between increases in local metabolic rate and blood flow has been demonstrated in preterm infants[69] and also between burst activity and cerebral oxygenation in term infants with neonatal encephalopathy.[70]

Cerebrovenous oxygen saturation is entirely normal (65–70%) in normal, healthy, term infants in the first days after birth,[71,72] and in a simple way this finding indicates that there normally is a balance between blood flow and cerebral oxygen consumption in the newborn.

## ADRENERGIC MECHANISMS AFFECTING CEREBRAL BLOOD FLOW

Based on findings in animal studies, the sympathetic system appears to play a greater role affecting CBF and its autoregulation in the perinatal period than it does later in life.[73-77] This finding has been attributed to the relative immaturity of the NO-induced vasodilatory mechanisms during early development.[78] The adrenergic effect, at least in part, is due to constriction of conduit arteries.

A rare study of human neonatal arteries in vitro (obtained postmortem from preterm neonates of 23–34 weeks' gestation) showed basal tone and a pressure-diameter relation quite similar to those seen in the adult pial arteries.[79] However, the neonatal arteries were significantly more sensitive to exogenous norepinephrine and electrical field activation of adventitial sympathetic nerve fibers and had a much higher sympathetic nerve density compared with those in the adult pial arteries.[80,81]

## EFFECT OF MEDICATIONS ON CEREBRAL BLOOD FLOW

Indomethacin reduces CBF in experimental animals, adults, and preterm neonates.[82] The concern has been whether it reduces CBF to ischemic levels resulting in injury in the developing brain. Interestingly, although

indomethacin decreases the incidence of severe peri/intraventricular hemorrhage, this early effect does not seem to translate to better long-term neurodevelopmental outcomes.[83] Contrary to indomethacin, ibuprofen does not have significant cerebrovascular effects.[19,84]

Among the methylxanthines, aminophylline reduces CBF and $Paco_2$ in experimental animals, adults, and preterm infants, but caffeine has less of an effect on CBF.[85,86] Methylxanthines are potent adenosine receptor antagonists. However, it is not entirely clear whether the reduction of CBF is the direct effect of methylxanthines on the adenosine receptors, a result of the associated decrease in $Paco_2$, or a combination.

Dopamine does not appear to have a selective (dilatory) effect on brain vasculature,[87,88] and its administration has been found to be associated with impaired autoregulation.[49,89] Individual studies have varied regarding its effect on CBF,[87-91] but using a meta-analytic approach, dopamine administration results in increases in CBF in hypotensive neonates.[92] Surprisingly, perhaps, in newborn piglets dopamine infusion tended to improve rather than impair the ability to maintain CBF during hypovolemic hypotension.[93]

## ISCHEMIC THRESHOLDS IN THE BRAIN

In the newborn puppy $Svo_2$ may decrease from 75 to 40% without provoking significant lactate production.[94] The exact minimum value of "normal" $Svo_2$ depends on, among other factors, the oxygen dissociation curve. Therefore it may be affected by changes in pH and the proportion of fetal hemoglobin present in the blood.

In the cerebral cortex of the adult baboon and man the threshold of blood flow sufficient to maintain tissue integrity depends on the duration of the low flow. For instance, if the low flow lasts for a few hours, the limit of minimal CBF to maintain tissue integrity is around 10 mL/100 g/min.[95] In acute localized brain ischemia, blood flow may remain sufficient to maintain structural integrity but fail to sustain functional (electrical) activity, a phenomenon called "border zone" or "penumbra."[96] Indeed, in progressing ischemia electrical failure is a warning for the impending development of permanent tissue injury. In the adult human brain cortex electrical function ceases at about 20 mL/100 g/min of blood flow (40–50% normal resting values), while in the subcortical gray matter and brainstem of the adult baboon, the electrical threshold is 10–15 mL/100 g/min.[97]

In normal newborn infants at rest the global CBF is 15–20 mL/100 g/min.[98] The ischemic threshold values of CBF for neonates are not known. However, in view of the low resting levels of CBF and the comparatively longer survival in total ischemia or anoxia, neonatal CBF thresholds are likely to be considerably less than 10 mL/100 g/min. Indeed, in ventilated preterm infants visual evoked responses were unaffected at global CBF levels below 10 mL/100 g/min corresponding to a cerebral oxygen delivery of 50 μmol/100 g/min.[38,99] For comparison, normal oxygen consumption in normal preterm infants was estimated to be 32 μmol/100 g/min and in normal term infants to 48 μmol/100 g/min.[100]

Low CBF and cerebral oxygen delivery carry a risk of later death, cerebral atrophy, or neurodevelopmental deficit,[101-104] but it is unclear whether treatment aimed at increasing CBF (or its surrogate, cerebral oxygenation) can improve the outcome.[105]

## Blood Flow to Other Organs

Based on studies on the distribution of cardiac output in term fetal lambs and newborn piglets, the typical abdominal organ blood flow appears to be around 100–350 mL/100 g/min.[106,107] In the fetus abdominal organ blood flow is higher than in the newborn with the exception of the intestine.

### KIDNEY

The adult kidneys constitute 0.5% of body weight but represent 25% of resting cardiac output, making them the most richly perfused organ of the body. In the newborn, although the kidneys are relatively larger, they receive less blood flow, probably due to the immaturity of the renal function. Renal arteries display appropriate autoregulation with a lower threshold adjusted to the prevailing lower blood pressure.[108] In addition to structural immaturity, high levels of circulating vasoactive mediators, such as angiotensin II, vasopressin, and endogenous catecholamines, explain the relatively low renal blood flow in the immediate postnatal period. Indeed, after the alpha-adrenergic receptor blockade, renal nerve stimulation results in

increased blood flow. To counterbalance the renal vasoconstriction and increased sodium reabsorption caused by the aforementioned hormones, the neonatal kidney is more dependent on the local production of vasodilatory prostaglandins compared to later in life. This explains why indomethacin, a cyclooxygenase (COX) inhibitor, readily reduces renal blood flow and urinary output in the neonate but not in the euvolemic child or adult. Interestingly, the renal side effects of another COX inhibitor, ibuprofen, are less pronounced in the neonate.[109] Finally, dopamine may selectively increase renal blood flow at a low dose with minimal effect on blood pressure.[87]

### LIVER

The liver is a large organ that has a dual blood supply, with blood originating from the stomach and intestines through the portal system and also from the hepatic branch of the celiac artery through the hepatic artery. The proportion of blood flow from these sources in the normal adult is 3:1. Hepatic vessels are richly innervated with sympathetic and parasympathetic nerves. The hepatic artery constricts in response to sympathetic nerve stimulation and exogenous norepinephrine, while the response of the portal vein is less well characterized. Angiotensin II is a potent vasoconstrictor of the hepatic vascular beds. During the first days after birth, a portion of the portal blood flow continues to be shunted past the liver through the ductus venosus until it closes. Portal liver blood flow in lambs is 100–150 mL/100 g/min during the first postnatal day and increases to over 200 mL/100 g/min by the end of the first week.[110]

### STOMACH AND INTESTINES

The stomach and intestines are motile organs, and variation in intestinal wall tension influences vascular resistance.[111] For example, the stimulation of sympathetic nerves results in constriction of the intestinal arteries and arterioles and in the relaxation of the intestinal wall. Thus the sympathetic effects on vascular resistance and intestinal wall tension are opposite. Furthermore, several gastrointestinal hormones and paracrine substances, such as gastrin, glucagon, and cholecystokinin, dilate the intestinal vessels, which likely contributes to the increase in intestinal blood flow during digestion. Local metabolic coupling also contributes to the digestion-associated increase in intestinal blood flow. Intestinal blood flow also shows well-developed autoregulation, and responses to sympathetic nerve stimulation, exogenous catecholamines, and angiotensin II similar to that of the other abdominal organs in the immature animal.

## Distribution of Cardiac Output in the Healthy Human Neonate

If the heart fails to increase cardiac output to maintain systemic blood pressure, a selective and marked increase in the flow to one organ can, in principle, compromise blood flow to other organs (the "steal" phenomenon). No organ of critical importance is large at birth (Table 2.1).

### BLOOD FLOW TO THE UPPER PART OF THE BODY

Blood flow to various organs differs considerably at the resting state. The data from recent Doppler flow volumetric studies allow some comparisons for the organs in the upper part of the body in healthy term infants. Blood flow to the brain, defined as the sum of the blood flowing through the two internal carotids and two vertebral arteries, corresponds to 18 mL/100 g/min using a mean brain weight of 385 g for the term infant (Table 2.2). This blood flow is close to what is expected from the data using methods to measure perfusion directly as mL/100 g/min.

### BLOOD FLOW TO THE LOWER PART OF THE BODY

Lower body blood flows are less well studied in the human neonate. In a recent study in extremely low birth weight infants with no ductal shunt and a cardiac output of 200 mL/kg/min, aortic blood flow was found to be 90 mL/kg/min at the level of the diaphragm.[112] Although this finding is in agreement with the data by Kluckow and Evans showing that approximately 50% of left ventricular output returns through the superior vena cava (SVC) in preterm neonates, some caution is warranted because most preterm infants enrolled in the studies on SVC blood flow measurements had an open patent ductus arteriosus (PDA).[113]

The data on individual abdominal organ flow in neonates are less current but available with a renal blood flow (right + left) of 21 mL/kg/min body weight, a superior mesenteric artery blood flow of 43 mL/kg/min, and a celiac artery blood flow of 70 mL/kg/min.[114-116] In the study by Agata and colleagues the results were divided

| TABLE 2.1   Organ Weights in Term and Extremely Low Birth Weight Neonates | | |
|---|---|---|
| | Body and Organ Weight (g) | |
| Organ or Tissue | 3500 | 1000 |
| Brain | 411 (12%) | 143 (15%) |
| Heart | 23 (1%) | 8 (1%) |
| Liver | 153 (4%) | 47 (5%) |
| Kidney | 28 (1%) | 10 (1%) |
| Fat | 23%* | <5% |

Organ weight as a percentage of body weight (%).
Total body water is around 75% and 85% to 90% of body weight in term neonates and extremely low birth weight neonates, respectively.
*Data from Ref. 143. Other data from Ref. 144.

| TABLE 2.2   Volumetric Blood Flow by Doppler Ultrasound Measurement for the Upper Part of the Body in Healthy Term Infants | | | | | |
|---|---|---|---|---|---|
| Vessel | N | Age | Flow (mL/min) | Flow (mL/kg/min) | Reference |
| Vertebral arteries | 42 | 39–42* (weeks) | 22† | | Kehrer et al.[141] |
| Int. carotid arteries | | | 56† | | |
| Right com. carotid | 21 | Day 1–3 | 117** | | Sinha et al.[142] |
| Superior vena cava | 14 | Day 1 | 258 | 76 | Kluckow and Evans[128] |
| Ascending aorta | | | 500 | 147 | |

*Newborn infants born at term were mixed with former preterm infants reaching 39–40 postmenstrual weeks.[140]
†Values for sum of right and left.
**Value multiplied by 2 for comparison.

by 2 to account for the parabolic arterial flow profile.[116] However, since the sum of abdominal organ blood flow exceeds the blood flow in the descending aorta, and since blood flow from other organ systems in the lower body (e.g., bones, muscle, and skin) has not been taken into consideration, it is clear that blood flow to the abdominal organs has been overestimated in the neonate. The reasons for this discrepancy are unclear but they may, at least in part, be related to the use of less sophisticated Doppler equipment using lower ultrasound frequencies in the studies performed in the early 1990s. In terms of perfusion rate the renal blood flow of 21 mL/min/kg body weight transforms to 210 mL/100 g kidney weight/min. Again, this is higher than that expected from studies using hippuric acid clearance.[117] Taking all these findings into consideration, it is reasonable to conclude that normal abdominal organ flow in the human neonate is likely to be comparable to that in different animal species and is around 100–300 mL/100 g/min. For comparison, lower limb blood flow in the human infant has been estimated by NIRS and the venous occlusion technique to be around 3.5 mL/100 g/min only.[118]

In summary, cardiac output is distributed approximately equally to the upper and lower body in the normal healthy newborn infant at gestational ages from 28 to 40 weeks. It may come as a surprise to many readers that only 25–30% of the blood flow to the upper part of the body goes to the brain, whereas the abdominal organs can be assumed to account for the largest part of the blood flow to the lower part of the body. Although good estimates of abdominal organ perfusion rates are not available, they appear to be higher than the perfusion rate of the brain. Therefore a relative hyperperfusion of the abdominal organs could result in a significant "steal" of cardiac output from the brain.

## Mechanisms Governing the Redistribution of Cardiac Output in the Fetal "Diving" Reflex

The hypoxic "diving" reflex has similarities with but is not identical to the aerobic diving reflex.

### AEROBIC DIVING

The diving reflex of sea mammals occurs within the "aerobic diving limit," that is, without hypoxia severe

enough to lead to the production of lactic acid. The key components are reflex bradycardia mediated through the carotid chemoreceptors and the vagal nerve, reflex vasoconstriction of the vascular beds of "non-vital" organs, and recruitment of blood from the spleen. All of this results in a reduced cardiac output, a dramatically increased circulation time, and hence a lag before the $CO_2$ reaches the respiratory center.[119]

### FETAL REACTIONS TO HYPOXIA

Similarly, the immediate reaction to hypoxia in the perinatal mammal is bradycardia and peripheral vasoconstriction. Since the reaction to fetal distress is of great clinical interest, it has been extensively studied in the fetal lamb. The response to fetal distress is qualitatively similar but quantitatively different among the different modes of induction of fetal distress, such as maternal hypoxemia, graded reduction of umbilical blood flow, repeated or graded reduction or complete arrest of uterine blood flow, and reduction of fetal blood volume.[120] Among the vital organs, adrenal blood flow increases in all situations, whereas this is not the case for the heart when fetal distress is caused by the reduction of fetal blood volume or for the brain when uterine blood flow is arrested. The fetal circulation is different from the postnatal circulation, and its peculiar features may explain some of the differences between fetal and postnatal hemodynamic responses to stress.

## Methods to Assess Organ Blood Flow in the Neonate

This discussion focuses on CBF since this is where there is most experience. Blood flow may refer to an organ as a whole, to a specific region, or to a tissue compartment of a given organ, depending on the method of measurement.

It is important to emphasize that blood flow is a complex and dynamic variable. Aside from physiologic fluctuations in organ blood flow governed by the changes in functional activity and thus the metabolic demand of a given organ, blood flow may significantly change within seconds under pathologic conditions such as with abrupt changes in blood pressure or the onset of hypoxia. In addition, blood flow may vary from one part of an organ to the other as during functional activation, or during stress, the distribution may change markedly.

Unfortunately, measurement of blood flow has limited precision. For research purposes, a method of measurement is appropriate if it is unbiased. Even if it lacks precision, it is still possible to achieve meaningful and statistically significant results for groups of infants. For clinical use, however, it is necessary that measurements are sufficiently precise to be valuable for the individual infant.

## DOPPLER ULTRASOUND

Doppler ultrasound to assess changes in CBF was first used in neonates in 1979.[121] The use of Doppler ultrasound for functional echocardiography in the neonate is described in Chapters 9 and 10 in detail.

### Doppler Principle

According to the Doppler principle, the frequency shift of the reflected sound (the "echo") is proportional to the velocity of the reflector. Since erythrocytes in blood reflect ultrasound, blood flow velocity can be measured based on simple physics, there are several factors that need to be taken into consideration and corrected for with the use of the Doppler principle. *First*, the apparent velocity must be corrected for the angle between the blood vessel and the ultrasound beam. *Second*, it should be kept in mind that multiple frequencies are detected when performing an ultrasound study of a vessel, since the flow velocity decreases from the center of the bloodstream toward the vessel wall. In addition, even the vessel wall itself contributes to the signal. *Finally*, the velocity is pulsating in nature, as it is faster in systole than in diastole.

### Indices of Pulsatility

Indices of pulsatility reflect downstream resistance to flow. The pulsatility in the umbilical artery has achieved great clinical importance in fetal monitoring.[122] In newborn infants, however, the resistance index in the anterior cerebral artery was only weakly associated with CBF as measured by [133]Xe clearance.[123] In addition, more sophisticated modeling reveals that arterial blood pressure pulsatility and arterial wall compliance are just as important determinants of the indices of pulsatility as is the downstream resistance.[124] In summary, Doppler data on

resistance indices may be biased. In a seminal clinical study, however, the pulsatility index was shown to carry independent prognostic ability in term infants with neonatal hypoxic-ischemic encephalopathy.[125] With increased computational capacity, it has become possible to make full 2D Doppler images at full spatial resolution and a sufficient time resolution to track the cardiac cycle – called fast Doppler. This allows measurement of indices of resistance in all vessels in the field, and thereby will allow the study of functional activation and localized pathology.[126] Central hemodynamics will not bias local differences in pulsatility, but differences in local artery wall compliance may still be mistaken for local vaso-dilation or vaso-constriction.

### Blood Flow Velocity

Since the 1980s, duplex scanning combining imaging and Doppler, range-gating limiting flow detection to a small sample volume, and frequency analysis allowing proper estimation of maximum and mean frequency shift has been possible and all contributed to more reliable measurement of blood flow velocity. However, if arterial diameter is not measured, it is not straightforward to compare one infant to another, one organ to another, and even one physiological state to another in the same infant, since arterial diameter varies dynamically in the immature individual.[3,127]

### Volumetric Measurements

Absolute organ blood flow in mL/min equals flow velocity (cm/s) multiplied by arterial cross-sectional area (cm$^2$). To measure left and right ventricular output or SVC flow, the vessels are relatively large and the reproducibility is 10–15%.[128] With the advent of color-coded imaging and the use of higher ultrasound frequencies, volumetric measurement of distributary arteries have also become possible in the newborn. For instance, measurement of blood flow in the right common carotid artery with a diameter of 2–3 mm was reported to have a reproducibility of 10–15% using a 15-MHz transducer, while that in both internal carotid and both vertebral arteries with diameters of 1–2 mm was found to be 7% for the sum of the blood flows in the four arteries using a 10-MHz transducer.[129,130] Using table values of brain weights, the mean value 14 mL/100g/min for infants born at

32–33 weeks' gestation and 19 mL/100 g/min for infants born at term suggest that the bias is small.[130]

## MAGNETIC RESONANCE PHASE CONTRAST IMAGING

In the simplest way global CBF may be estimated by imaging the four arteries on the neck and multiplying their cross-sectional area with the blood flow velocity, estimated by the loss of magnetization caused by fresh blood (water) flowing into the plane of imaging, also called *phase contrast imaging*.[131] It is thus quite similar to volumetric Doppler ultrasound (see above) and is possible in newborns, although more complex and not a bedside method. The results are in mL/s, and can be related to body weight, or to brain weight as estimated from brain volume measured during the same procedure by MRI. An average global CBF of 15 mL/100g/min in 10 healthy term infants with a test-retest variability of 7% has been reported.[132]

## Methods for Measurement of Perfusion

These methods are based on measurements at the tissue level and the unit is always mL/100 g/min.

### MRI FLOW IMAGING

Arterial spin labeling is performed by applying the radio-frequency pulse to a thick slice (slab) at the base of the skull. This labels the blood in segments of the large arteries supplying the brain. After allowing for the arterial transit time (a little less than a second) to pass, imaging of as many slices as technically possible commences. Regions with higher flow will contain more labeled blood (the bolus distribution principle) and hence a higher signal. Flow is quantified by measuring the relative difference in signal intensity divided by the duration of the labeling pulse. This method also requires correcting for the blood-brain water partition coefficient, any incomplete arterial labeling, and the imaging delay compared to the relaxation time in the blood.[133] This method was first used in 25 neonates with congenital heart disease during normal ventilation and during inhalation of added $CO_2$.[134] All babies were mechanically ventilated and sedated. Mean slice CBF was 19.7 ± 9.2 mL/100 g/min and 40.1 ± 20.3 mL/100 g/min before and during $CO_2$ inhalation, respectively, giving an overall CBF-$CO_2$ reactivity of 1 mL/Torr or 35% change per

kPa suggesting little bias. In unsedated preterm infants near expected date of delivery and in normal term infants, and local CBF ranging from 39 mL/100 g/min in basal ganglia to 10 mL/100 g/min in white matter was found.[135] Improved computational capacity has allowed the development of multiple (pseudo-continuous) arterial spin labeling, and this is also possible in newborns and appears to provide better signal-to-noise and slightly higher values of CBF (25 mL/100 g/min).[136] The limits of agreement between the values of global CBF obtained by the two techniques, however, was as much as ±15 mL/100 g/min.

## METHODS USING X-RAYS OR RADIOACTIVE ISOTOPES

These are based on fewer assumptions than MRI and are by nature measures of perfusion in mL/100 g/min. The absolute values of the results have high credibility, but the radiation limits their application. Measurement of CBF by $^{133}$Xe clearance was used in the 1980s to demonstrate that global CBF in preterm infants is 15–20 mL/100 g/min, much lower than in adults.[137] Single photon emission computed tomography is also based on the bolus distribution principle and provided the first high-resolution tomographic flow images in preterm infants, suggesting that the white matter is particularly vulnerable to ischemia at low blood pressure.[51] Stable xenon-enhanced computed tomography uses repeated CT scans to detect the washout (clearance) of xenon and was able to detect very low levels of CBF that have been documented in young, brain-dead infants.[138] Positron emission tomography (PET) utilizes the fact that positron annihilation results in two photons emitted always at an angle of 180°, and therefore localization is achieved without collimation and loss of photons. Biologically relevant positron-emitting isotopes exist (e.g., $^{11}$C, $^{13}$N, and $^{15}$O) and many biochemical substances can be labeled. Furthermore, with the newest PET scanners, $^{15}$O-labeled water CBF imaging can be done with good spatial resolution[98,139] (Figure 2.6) and a dose of isotope that allows non-therapeutic research in children.[140]

## Conclusion

Multiple molecular mechanisms regulate the contraction of the vascular smooth muscle cell and thus the arterial vascular tone. The vascular muscle tone in the

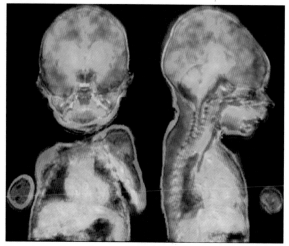

**Fig. 2.6  Flow image in normal infant born after 40 weeks' gestation with birth weight 3260 g, on the second day of life during natural sleep, using a hybrid PET/MR scanner. 14 MBq $^{15}$O-labeled water was used, resulting in a radiation dose of 0.3 mSv, which allows research for the purpose of "Increases in knowledge leading to health benefits."[140] The input function was taken from voxels in the left ventricle, imaged simultaneously. Coronal and sagittal sections. The global CBF was 22.2 mL/100 g/min. Due to the methodology, a value of high credibility. The blood flow to the liver is clearly higher – as predicted from ultrasound Doppler data but was not quantitated.** (Courtesy of Julie Bjerglund Andersen, Rigshospitalet, Copenhagen.)

various tissues and organs is central to the regulation of local blood flow and distribution of cardiac output. In the newborn infant the large distributary arteries take an active part. In the normal newborn infant cardiac output is distributed equally to the upper and lower parts of the body and the perfusion rate (in mL/100 g/min) is much higher in liver and kidneys, as compared to the brain.

Blood flow to the brain has been most studied due to the risks of hypoxic-ischemic brain injury and its potential life-long consequences. Cerebral autoregulation is developed already at the limit of viability, although autoregulation may be impaired and may best be described as a degree of capacity rather than an on-off phenomenon. Cerebral vascular reactivity to Pco$_2$ and to hypoxia is more robust. The sympathetic nervous system plays a particular role in newborn infants and may be responsible for the decrease in blood flow to the cerebral hemispheres during the diving reflex, as elicited by hypoxia and in states of low cardiac output.

These complexities – as well as the limitations of the methods to measure organ blood flow and oxygenation – are likely reasons for the lack of strong evidence behind the management of circulatory compromise in newborn infants.

## REFERENCES

1. Mortola JP. Implications of hypoxic hypometabolism during mammalian ontogenesis. *Respir Physiol Neurobiol.* 2004;141: 345-356.
2. Heistad DD. What is new in cerebral microcirculation. Landis award lecture. *Microcirculation.* 2001;8:365-375.
3. Malcus P, Kjellmer I, Lingman G, et al. Diameters of the common carotid artery and aorta change in different directions during acute asphyxia in the fetal lamb. *J Perinat Med.* 1991;19:259-267.
4. Lagaud G, Gaudreault N, Moore ED, et al. Pressure-dependent myogenic constriction of cerebral arteries occurs independently of voltage-dependent activation. *Am J Physiol Heart Circ Physiol.* 2002;283:H2187-H2195.
5. Li Y, Baylie RL, Tavares MJ, et al. TRPM4 channels couple purinergic receptor mechanoactivation and myogenic tone development in cerebral parenchymal arterioles. *J Cereb Blood Flow Metab.* 2014;34(10):1706-1714.
6. Hill MA, Zou H, Potocnik SJ, et al. Invited review. Arteriolar smooth muscle mechanotransduction. Ca2+ signaling pathways underlying myogenic reactivity. *J Appl Physiol.* 2001;91:973-983.
7. Gebremedin A, Lange AR, Lowry TF, et al. Production of 20-HETE and its role in autoregulation of cerebral blood flow. *Circ Res.* 2000;87:60-65.
8. Dora KA. Does arterial myogenic tone determine blood distribution in vivo? *Am J Physiol Heart Circ Physiol.* 2005;289:1323-1325.
9. Pearce WJ, Harder DR. Cerebrovascular smooth muscle and endothelium. In: Mraovitch S, Sercombe R, eds. *Neurophysiological Basis of Cerebral Blood Flow Control. An Introduction.* London: John Libbey; 1996:153-158.
10. Pearce WJ. Hypoxic regulation of the fetal cerebral circulation. *J Appl Physiol.* 2006;100:731-738.
11. Liu Y, Harder DR, Lombard JH. Interaction of myogenic mechanisms and hypoxic dilation in rat middle cerebral arteries. *Am J Physiol Heart Circ Physiol.* 2002;283:H2276-H2281.
12. Aalkjær C, Poston L. Effects of pH on vascular tension. Which are the important mechanisms? *J Vasc Res.* 1996;33:347-359.
13. Wang Q, Pelligrino DA, Baughman VL, et al. The role of neuronal nitric oxide synthetase in regulation of cerebral blood flow in normocapnia and hypercapnia in rats. *J Cereb Blood Flow Metab.* 1995;15:774-778.
14. Iadecola C, Zhang F. Permissive and obligatory roles of NO in cerebrovascular responses to hypercapnia and acetylcholine. *Am J Physiol.* 1996;271:R990-R1001.
15. Lindauer U, Vogt J, Schuh-Hofer S, et al. Cerebrovascular vasodilation to extraluminal acidosis occurs via combined activation of ATP-sensitive and Ca2+-activated potassium channels. *J Cereb Blood Flow Metab.* 2003;23:1227-1238.
16. Wagerle LC, Mishra OP. Mechanism of CO2 response in cerebral arteries of the newborn pig: role of phospholipase, cyclooxygenase, and lipooxygenase pathways. *Circ Res.* 1988; 62:1019-1026.

17. Rama GP, Parfenova H, Leffler CW. Protein kinase Cs and tyrosine kinases in permissive action of prostacyclin on cerebrovascular regulation in newborn pigs. *Pediatr Res.* 1996; 41:83-89.

18. Edwards AD, Wyatt JS, Ricardsson C, et al. Effects of indomethacin on cerebral haemodynamics in very preterm infants. *Lancet.* 1990;23:1491-1495.

19. Patel J, Roberts I, Azzopardi D, et al. Randomized double-blind controlled trial comparing the effects of ibuprofen with indomethacin on cerebral hemodynamics in preterm infants with patent ductus arteriosus. *Pediatr Res.* 2000;47:36-42.

20. Clifford PS, Hellsten Y. Vasodilatory mechanisms in contracting skeletal muscle. *J Appl Physiol.* 2004;97:393-403.

21. Koehler RC, Gebremedhin D, Harder DR. Role of astrocytes in cerebrovascular regulation. *J Appl Physiol.* 2006;100:307-317.

22. Phillis JW. Adenosine and adenine nucleotides as regulators of cerebral blood flow: roles of acidosis, cell swelling, and KATP channels. *Crit Rev Neurobiol.* 2004;16:237-270.

23. Guimaraes S, Moura D. Vascular adrenoreceptors. An update. *Pharm Rev.* 2001;53:319-356.

24. Seri I, Tan R, Evans J. The effect of hydrocortisone on blood pressure in preterm neonates with vasopressor-resistant hypotension. *Pediatrics.* 2001;107:1070-1074.

25. Watterberg KL. Adrenal insufficiency and cardiac dysfunction in the preterm infant. *Pediatr Res.* 2002;51:422-424.

26. Noori S, Seri I. Pathophysiology of newborn hypotension outside the transitional period. *Early Hum Dev.* 2005;81:399-404.

27. Lou HC, Lassen NA, Friis-Hansen B. Low cerebral blood flow in hypotensive perinatal distress. *Acta Neurol Scand.* 1977;56: 343-352.

28. Hernandez MJ, Brennan RW, Bowman GS. Autoregulation of cerebral blood flow in the newborn dog. *Brain Res.* 1980; 184:199-201.

29. Pasternak JF, Groothuis DR. Autoregulation of cerebral blood flow in the newborn beagle puppy. *Biol Neonate.* 1985;48: 100-109.

30. Tweed WA, Cote J, Pash M, et al. Arterial oxygenation determines autoregulation of cerebral blood flow in the fetal lamb. *Pediatr Res.* 1983;17:246-249.

31. Papile LA, Rudolph AM, Heyman MA. Autoregulation of cerebral blood flow in the preterm fetal lamb. *Pediatr Res.* 1985; 19:59-161.

32. Pryds A, Pryds O, Greisen G. Cerebral pressure autoregulation and vasoreactivity in the newborn rat. *Pediatr Res.* 2005;57: 294-298.

33. Helau S, Koehler RC, Gleason CA, et al. Cerebrovascular autoregulation during fetal development in sheep. *Am J Physiol Heart Circ Physiol.* 1994;266:H1069-H1074.

34. Müller T, Löhle M, Schubert H, et al. Developmental changes in cerebral autoregulatory capacity in the fetal sheep parietal cortex. *J Physiol.* 2002;539:957-967.

35. Tweed WA, Cote J, Lou H, et al. Impairment of cerebral blood flow autoregulation in the newborn lamb by hypoxia. *Pediatr Res.* 1986;20:516-519.

36. Younkin DP, Reivich M, Jaggi JL, et al. The effect of haematocrit and systolic blood pressure on cerebral blood flow in newborn infants. *J Cereb Blood Flow Metab.* 1987;7:295-299.

37. Greisen G. Cerebral blood flow in preterm infants during the first week of life. *Acta Paediatr Scand.* 1986;75:43-51.

38. Greisen G, Trojaborg W. Cerebral blood flow, PaCO2 changes, and visual evoked potentials in mechanically ventilated, preterm infants. *Acta Paediatr Scand.* 1987;76:394-400.

39. Pryds O, Greisen G, Lou H, et al. Heterogeneity of cerebral vasoreactivity in preterm infants supported by mechanical ventilation. *J Pediatr.* 1989;115:638-645.

40. Pryds O, Andersen GE, Friis-Hansen B. Cerebral blood flow reactivity in spontaneously breathing, preterm infants shortly after birth. *Acta Paediatr Scand.* 1990;79:391-396.

41. Pryds O, Greisen G, Lou H, et al. Vasoparalysis is associated with brain damage in asphyxiated term infants. *J Pediatr.* 1990;117:119-125.

42. Tyszczuk L, Meek J, Elwell C, et al. Cerebral blood flow is independent of mean arterial blood pressure in preterm infants undergoing intensive care. *Pediatrics.* 1998;102:337-341.

43. Noone MA, Sellwood M, Meek JH, et al. Postnatal adaptation of cerebral blood flow using near infrared spectroscopy in extremely preterm infants undergoing high-frequency oscillatory ventilation. *Acta Paediatr.* 2003;92:1079-1084.

44. Wardle SP, Yoxall CW, Weindling AM. Determinants of cerebral fractional oxygen extraction using near-infrared spectroscopy in preterm neonates. *J Cereb Blood Flow Metab.* 2000;20:272-279.

45. Milligan DWA. Failure of autoregulation and intraventricular haemorrhage in preterm infants. *Lancet.* 1980;1:896-899.

46. Tsuji M, Saul JP, du Plessis A, et al. Cerebral intravascular oxygenation correlates with mean arterial pressure in critically ill premature infants. *Pediatrics.* 2000;106:625-632.

47. Wong FY, Leung TS, Austin T, et al. Impaired autoregulation in preterm infants identified by using spatially resolved spectroscopy. *Pediatrics.* 2008;121:e604-e611.

48. O'Leary H, Gregas MC, Limperopoulos C, et al. Elevated cerebral pressure passivity is associated with prematurity-related intracranial hemorrhage. *Pediatrics.* 2009;124:302-309.

49. Howlett JA, Northington FJ, Gilmore MM, et al. Cerebrovascular autoregulation and neurologic injury in neonatal hypoxic-ischemic encephalopathy. *Pediatr Res.* 2013;74(5):525-535.

50. Børch K, Lou HC, Greisen G. Cerebral white matter flow and arterial blood pressure in preterm infants. *Acta Paediatr.* 2010;99:1489-1492.

51. Munro MJ, Walker AM, Barfield CP. Hypotensive extremely low birth weight infants have reduced cerebral blood flow. *Pediatrics.* 2004;114:1591-1596.

52. Greisen G. To autoregulate or not to autoregulate–that is no longer the question. *Semin Pediatr Neurol.* 2009;16(4):207-215.

53. Greisen G. Cerebral autoregulation in preterm infants. How to measure it–and why care? *J Pediatr.* 2014;165(5):885-886.

54. da Costa CS, Greisen G, Austin T. Is near-infrared spectroscopy clinically useful in the preterm infant? *Arch Dis Child Fetal Neonatal Ed.* 2015;100(6):F558-F561.

55. Leahy FAN, Cates D, MacCallum M, et al. Effect of CO2 and 100% O2 on cerebral blood flow in preterm infants. *J Appl Physiol.* 1980;48:468-472.

56. Rahilly PM. Effects of 2% carbon dioxide, 0.5% carbon dioxide, and 100% oxygen on cranial blood flow of the human neonate. *Pediatrics.* 1980;66:685-689.

57. Calvert SA, Hoskins EM, Fong KW, et al. Atiological factors associated with the development of periventricular leucomalacia. *Acta Paediatr Scand.* 1987;76:254-259.

58. Graziani LJ, Spitzer AR, Mitchell DG, et al. Mechanical ventilation in preterm infants. Neurosonographic and developmental studies. *Pediatrics.* 1992;90:515-522.

59. Ferrara B, Johnson DE, Chang PN, et al. Efficacy and neurologic outcome of profound hypocapneic alkalosis for the treatment of persistent pulmonary hypertension in infancy. *J Pediatr.* 1984;105:457-461.

60. Milligan DWA. Cerebral blood flow and sleep state in the normal newborn infant. *Early Hum Develop.* 1979;3:321-328.
61. Rahilly PM. Effects of sleep state and feeding on cranial blood flow of the human neonate. *Arch Dis Child.* 1980;55:265-270.
62. Mukhtar AI, Cowan FM, Stothers JK. Cranial blood flow and blood pressure changes during sleep in the human neonate. *Early Hum Develop.* 1982;6:59-64.
63. Greisen G, Hellstrom-Westas L, Lou H, et al. Sleep-waking shifts and cerebral blood flow in stable preterm infants. *Pediatr Res.* 1985;19:1156-1159.
64. Born P, Leth H, Miranda MJ, et al. Visual activation in infants and young children studied by functional magnetic resonance imaging. *Pediatr Res.* 1998;44:578-583.
65. Martin E, Joeri P, Loenneker T, et al. Visual processing in infants and children studied using functional MRI. *Pediatr Res.* 1999;46:135-140.
66. Meek JH, Firbank M, Elwell CE, et al. Regional hemodynamic responses to visual stimulation in awake infants. *Pediatr Res.* 1998;43:840-843.
67. Erberich GS, Friedlich P, Seri I, et al. Brain activation detected by functional MRI in preterm neonates using an integrated radiofrequency neonatal head coil and MR compatible incubator. *Neuroimage.* 2003;20:683-692.
68. Erberich SG, Panigrahy A, Friedlich P, et al. Somatosensory lateralization in the newborn brain. *Neuroimage.* 2006;29:155-161.
69. Roche-Labarbe N, Fenoglio A, Radhakrishnan H, et al. Somatosensory evoked changes in cerebral oxygen consumption measured non-invasively in premature neonates. *Neuroimage.* 2014;85(Pt 1):279-286.
70. Chalia M, Lee CW, Dempsey LA, et al. Hemodynamic response to burst-suppressed and discontinuous electroencephalography activity in infants with hypoxic ischemic encephalopathy. *Neurophotonics.* 2016;3(3):031408.
71. Buchvald FF, Keshe K, Greisen G. Measurement of cerebral oxyhaemoglobin saturation and jugular blood flow in term healthy newborn infants by near-infrared spectroscopy and jugular venous occlusion. *Biol Neonate.* 1999;75:97-103.
72. Jiang D, Lu H, Parkinson C, et al. Vessel specific quantification of neonatal cerebral venous oxygenation. *Magn Res Med.* 2019;82:1129-1139.
73. Hernandez MJ, Hawkins RA, Brennan RW. Sympathetic control of regional cerebral blood flow in the asphyxiated newborn dog. In: Heistad DD, Marcus ML, eds. *Cerebral Blood Flow, Effects of Nerves and Neurotransmitters.* New York: Elsevier; 1982:359-366.
74. Hayashi S, Park MK, Kuelh TJ. Higher sensitivity of cerebral arteries isolated from premature and newborn baboons to adrenergic and cholinergic stimulation. *Life Sciences.* 1984;35:253-260.
75. Wagerle LC, Kumar SP, Delivoria-Papadopoulos M. Effect of sympathetic nerve stimulation on cerebral blood flow in newborn piglets. *Pediatr Res.* 1986;20:131-135.
76. Kurth CD, Wagerle LC, Delivoria-Papadopoulos M. Sympathetic regulation of cerebral blood flow during seizures in newborn lambs. *Am J Physiol.* 1988;255:H563-H568.
77. Goplerud JM, Wagerle LC, Delivoria-Papadopoulos M. Sympathetic nerve modulation of regional cerebral blood flow during asphyxia in newborn piglets. *Am J Physiol.* 1991;260:H1575-H1580.
78. Wagerle LC, Moliken W, Russo P. Nitric oxide and alpha-adrenergic mechanisms modify contractile responses to norepinephrine in ovine fetal and newborn cerebral arteries. *Pediatr Res.* 1995;38:237-242.
79. Bevan RD, Vijayakumaran E, Gentry A, et al. Intrinsic tone of cerebral artery segments of human infants between 23 weeks of gestation and term. *Pediatr Res.* 1998;43:20-27.
80. Bevan R, Dodge J, Nichols P, et al. Responsiveness of human infant cerebral arteries to sympathetic nerve stimulation and vasoactive agents. *Pediatr Res.* 1998;44:730-739.
81. Bevan RD, Dodge J, Nichols P, et al. Weakness of sympathetic neural control of human pial compared with superficial temporal arteries reflects low innervation density and poor sympathetic responsiveness. *Stroke.* 1998;29:212-221.
82. Pryds O, Greisen G, Johansen K. Indomethacin and cerebral blood flow in preterm infants treated for patent ductus arteriosus. *Eur J Pediatr.* 1988;147:315-316.
83. Schmidt B, Davis P, Moddemann D, et al. Trial of Indomethacin Prophylaxis in Preterms Investigators. Long-term effects of indomethacin prophylaxis in extremely-low-birth-weight infants. *N Engl J Med.* 2001;344:1966-1972.
84. Mosca F, Bray M, Lattanzio M, et al. Comparative evaluation of the effects of indomethacin and ibuprofen on cerebral perfusion and oxygenation in preterm infants with patent ductus arteriosus. *J Pediatr.* 1997;131:549-554.
85. Pryds O, Schneider S. Aminophylline induces cerebral vasoconstriction in stable, preterm infants without affecting the visual evoked potential. *Eur J Pediatr.* 1991;150:366-369.
86. Lundström KE, Larsen PB, Brendstrup L, et al. Cerebral blood flow and left ventricular output in spontaneously breathing, newborn preterm infants treated with caffeine or aminophylline. *Acta Paediatr.* 1995;84:6-9.
87. Seri I, Abbasi S, Wood DC, et al. Regional hemodynamic effects of dopamine in the sick preterm neonate. *J Pediatr.* 1998;133:728-734.
88. Zhang J, Penny DJ, Kim NS, et al. Mechanisms of blood pressure increase induced by dopamine in hypotensive preterm neonates. *Arch Dis Child.* 1999;81:F99-F104.
89. Eriksen VR, Hahn GH, Greisen G. Dopamine therapy is associated with impaired cerebral autoregulation in preterm infants. *Acta Paediatr.* 2014;103(12):1221-1226.
90. Lundström KE, Pryds O, Greisen G. The haemodynamic effect of dopamine and volume expansion in sick preterm infants. *Early Hum Develop.* 2000;57:157-163.
91. Jayasinghe D, Gill AB, Levene MI. CBF reactivity in hypotensive and normotensive preterm infants. *Pediatr Res.* 2003;54:848-853.
92. Sassano-Higgins S, Friedlich P, Seri I. A meta-analysis of dopamine use in hypotensive preterm infants: blood pressure and cerebral hemodynamics. *J Perinatol.* 2011;31(10):647-655.
93. Eriksen VR, Rasmussen MB, Hahn GH, et al. Dopamine therapy does not affect cerebral autoregulation during hypotension in newborn piglets. *PLoS One.* 2017;12:e0170738.
94. Reuter JH, Disney TA. Regional cerebral blood flow and cerebral metabolic rate of oxygen during hyperventilation in the newborn dog. *Pediatr Res.* 1986;20:1102-1106.
93. Jones TH, Morawetz RB, Crowell RM, et al. Thresholds of focal cerebral ischaemia in awake monkeys. *J Neurosurg.* 1981;54:773-782.
96. Astrup J. Energy-requiring cell functions in the ischaemic brain. *J Neurosurg.* 1982;56:482-497.
97. Branston NM, Ladds A, Symon L, et al. Comparison of the effects of ischaemia on early components of somatosensory evoked potentials in brainstem, thalamus, and cerebral cortex. *J Cereb Blood Flow Metab.* 1984;4:68-81.

98. Andersen JB, Lindberg U, Olesen OV, et al. Hybrid PET/MRI imaging in healthy unsedated newborn infants with quantitative rCBF measurements using 15O-water PET. *J Cereb Blood Flow Metab.* 2019;39:782-793.
99. Pryds O, Greisen G. Preservation of single flash visual evoked potentials at very low cerebral oxygen delivery in sick, newborn, preterm infants. *Pediatr Neurol.* 1990;6:151-158.
100. Qi Y, He J. Neurophysiologic profiling of at-risk low and very low birth weight infants using magnetic resonance imaging. *Front Physiol.* 2021;12:638868.
101. Lou HC, Skov H. Low cerebral blood flow: a risk factor in the neonate. *J Pediatr.* 1979;95:606-609.
102. Ment RL, Scott DT, Lange RC, et al. Postpartum perfusion of the preterm brain: relationship to neurodevelopmental outcome. *Childs Brain.* 1983;10:266-272.
103. Pryds O. Low neonatal cerebral oxygen delivery is associated with brain injury in preterm infants. *Acta Paediatr.* 1994;83:1233-1236.
104. Krageloh-Mann I, Toft P, Lunding J, et al. Brain lesions in preterms: origin, consequences and compensation. *Acta Paediatr.* 1999;88:897-908.
105. Hyttel-Sorensen S, Pellicer A, Alderliesten T, et al. Cerebral near infrared spectroscopy oximetry in extremely preterm infants: phase II randomised clinical trial. *BMJ.* 2015;350:g7635.
106. Fujimori K, Honda S, Sanpei M, et al. Effects of exogenous big endothelin-1 on regional blood flow in fetal lambs. *Obstet Gynecol.* 2005;106:818-823.
107. Powell RW, Dyess DL, Collins JN, et al. Regional blood flow response to hypothermia in premature, newborn, and neonatal piglets. *J Pediatr Surg.* 1999;34:193-198.
108. Jose PA, Haramati A, Fildes RD. Postnatal maturation of renal blood flow. In: Polin RA, Fox WW, eds. *Fetal and Neonatal Physiology.* Philadelphia: WB Saunders; 1998:1573-1578.
109. Pezzati M, Vangi V, Biagiotti R, et al. Effects of indomethacin and ibuprofen on mesenteric and renal blood flow in preterm infants with patent ductus arteriosus. *J Pediatr.* 1999;135:733-738.
110. Rudolph CD, Rudolph AM. Fetal and postnatal hepatic vasculature and blood flow. In: Polin RA, Fox WW, eds. *Fetal and Neonatal Physiology.* Philadelphia: WB Saunders; 1998:1442-1449.
111. Clark DA, Miller MJS. Development of the gastrointestinal circulation in the fetus and newborn. In: Polin RA, Fox WW, eds. *Fetal and Neonatal Physiology.* Philadelphia: WB Saunders; 1998:929-933.
112. Shimada S, Kasai T, Hoshi A, et al. Cardiocirculatory effects of patent ductus arteriosus in extremely low-birth-weight infants with respiratory distress syndrome. *Pediatr Int.* 2003;45:255-262.
113. Kluckow M, Evans N. Superior vena cava flow. A novel marker of systemic blood flow. *Arch Dis Child.* 2000;82:F182-F187.
114. Visser MO, Leighton JO, van de Bor M, et al. Renal blood flow in the neonate: quantitation with color and pulsed Doppler ultrasound. *Radiology.* 1992;183:441-444.
115. Van Bel F, van Zwieten PH, Guit GL, et al. Superior mesenteric artery blood flow velocity and estimated volume flow. Duplex Doppler US study of preterm and term neonates. *Radiology.* 1990;174:165-169.
116. Agata Y, Hiraishi S, Misawa H, et al. Regional blood flow distribution and left ventricular output during early neonatal life: a quantitative ultrasonographic assessment. *Pediatr Res.* 1994;36:805-810.
117. Yao LP, Jose PA. Developmental renal hemodynamics. *Pediatr Nephrol.* 1995;9:632-637.
118. Bay-Hansen R, Elfving B, Greisen G. Use of near infrared spectroscopy for estimation of peripheral venous saturation in newborns; comparison with co-oximetry of central venous blood. *Biol Neonate.* 2002;82:1-8.
119. Stephenson R. Physiological control of diving behaviour in the Weddell seal Leptonychotes weddelli; a model based on cardiorespiratory control theory. *J Exp Biol.* 2005;208:1971-1991.
120. Jensen A, Garnier Y, Berger R. Dynamics of fetal circulatory responses to hypoxia and asphyxia. *Eur J Obstet Gynecol Reprod Biol.* 1999;84:155-172.
121. Bada HS, Hajjar W, Chua C, et al. Noninvasive diagnosis of neonatal asphyxia and intraventricular hemorrhage by Doppler ultrasound. *J Pediatr.* 1979;95:775-779.
122. Neilson JP, Alfirevic Z. Doppler ultrasound for fetal assessment in high risk pregnancies. *Cochrane Database Syst Rev.* 2000;(2):CD000073.
123. Greisen G, Johansen K, Ellison PH, et al. Cerebral blood flow in the newborn infant: comparison of Doppler ultrasound and 133-Xenon clearance. *J Pediatr.* 1984;104:411-418.
124. Greisen G. Analysis of cerebroarterial Doppler flow velocity waveforms in newborn infants: towards an index of cerebrovascular resistance. *J Perinat Med.* 1986;4:181-187.
125. Levene MI, Sands C, Grindulis H, et al. Comparison of two methods of predicting outcome in perinatal asphyxia. *Lancet.* 1985;8472:67-69.
126. Demené C, Pernot M, Biran V, et al. Ultrafast Doppler reveals the mapping of cerebral vascular resistivity in neonates. *J Cereb Blood Flow Metab.* 2014;34:1009-1017.
127. Drayton MR, Skidmore R. Vasoactivity of the major intracranial arteries in newborn infants. *Arch Dis Child.* 1987;62:236-240.
128. Kluckow M, Evans N. Superior vena cava flow in newborn infants: a novel marker of systemic blood flow. *Arch Dis Child.* 2000;82:F182-F187.
129. Ehehalt S, Kehrer M, Goelz R, et al. Cerebral blood flow volume measurement with ultrasound: interobserver reproducibility in preterm and term neonates. *Ultrasound Med Biol.* 2005;31:191-196.
130. Kehrer M, Krägeloh-Mann-I, Goeltz M, et al. The development of cerebral perfusion in healthy preterm and term neonates. *Neuropediatrics.* 2003;34:281-286.
131. Benders MJ, Hendrikse J, de Vries LS, et al. Phase contrast magnetic resonance angiography measurements of global cerebral blood flow in the neonate. *Pediatr Res.* 2011;69(6):544-547.
132. Liu P, Huang H, Rollins N, et al. Quantitative assessment of global cerebral metabolic rate of oxygen (CMRO2) in neonates using MRI. *NMR Biomed.* 2014;27:332-340.
133. Wang J, Licht DJ, Jahng GH, et al. Pediatric perfusion imaging using arterial spin labelling. *J Magn Res Imag.* 2003;18:404-413.
134. Licht DJ, Wang J, Silvestre DW, et al. Preoperative cerebral blood flow is diminished in neonates with severe congenital heart defects. *J Thorac Cardiovasc Surg.* 2004;128:841-849.
135. Miranda MJ, Olofsson K, Sidaros K. Noninvasive measurements of regional cerebral perfusion in preterm and term neonates by magnetic resonance arterial spin labeling. *Pediatr Res.* 2006;60:359-363.
136. Boudes E, Gilbert G, Leppert IR, et al. Measurement of brain perfusion in newborns: pulsed arterial spin labeling (PASL)

versus pseudo-continuous arterial spin labeling (pCASL). *Neuroimage Clin.* 2014;6:126-133.

137. Greisen G, Pryds O. Intravenous 133Xe clearance in preterm neonates with respiratory distress. Internal validation of CBF-infinity as a measure of global cerebral blood flow. *Scand J Clin Lab Invest.* 1988;48:673-678.

138. Ashwal S, Schneider S, Thompson J. Xenon computed tomography measuring blood flow in the determination of brain death in children. *Ann Neurol.* 1989;25:539-546.

139. Andersen JB, Henning WS, Lindberg U, et al. Positron emission tomography/magnetic resonance hybrid scanner imaging of cerebral blood flow using 15O-water positron emission tomography and arterial spin labeling magnetic resonance imaging in newborn piglets. *J Cereb Blood Flow Metab.* 2015;35(11):1703-1710.

140. European Commission. Guidance on medical exposures in medical and biomedical research. 1998. Available at: https://energy.ec.europa.eu/system/files/2014-11/099_en_1.pdf, 1998.

141. Kehrer M, Krägeloh-Mann L, Goelz R, et al. The development of cerebral perfusion in healthy preterm and term neonates. *Neuropediatrics.* 2003;34:281-286.

142. Sinha AK, Cane C, Kempley ST. Blood flow in the common carotid artery in term and preterm infants: reproducibility and relation to cardiac output. *Arch Dis Child.* 2006;91:31-35.

143. Uthaya S, Bell J, Modi N. Adipose tissue magnetic resonance imaging in the newborn. *Horm Res.* 2004;62(suppl 3):1430-1438.

144. Charles AD, Smith NM. Perinatal postmortem. In: Rennie JM, ed. *Roberton's Textbook of Neonatology.* Beijing: Elsevier; 2005:1207-1215.

# Chapter 3

# Blood Pressure and Cardiovascular Physiology

Eugene Dempsey, Neidin Bussmann, and Istvan Seri

## Key Points

- In the context of neonatal care, invasive or noninvasive measurement of blood pressure can be accomplished with acceptable precision across all gestational age categories.
- Gestational and postnatal-age-dependent population-based normative blood pressure ranges are available. However, their usefulness in the assessment of adequacy of circulatory status remains limited.
- Interrogation of the individual components of the patient's blood pressure may provide a greater understanding of the underlying physiology. This includes systolic, diastolic, mean blood pressure and pulse pressure.
- Clinical, biochemical, and echocardiographic hemodynamic information in addition to individual BP components will provide a more complete assessment of cardiovascular well-being as we await more objective comprehensive hemodynamic monitoring and data acquisition systems to permit an individualized approach to care.

## Introduction

Historically blood pressure, in particular mean blood pressure, was the main determinant of circulatory well-being in the neonatal intensive care unit. Typically, it was the sole criterion used to initiate intervention, especially in preterm infants.[1] The primary reason was the assumption that low blood pressure, however defined, was directly and strongly correlated with cardiac output and end-organ blood flow. While this practice remains commonplace, we now understand that as hemodynamic monitoring

tools become more accessible and utilized at the bedside, the many shortcomings of our overreliance on blood pressure measurements to guide intervention is highlighted. However, rather than neglecting this measurement, we contend that it remains a critically important hemodynamic value and one of several other important measurements to be considered in the assessment of circulatory well-being.

In this chapter we have set out to address several factors: What is meant by blood pressure, how it is regulated, how it should be measured, what factors determine blood pressure, and how blood pressure should be factored into decision-making in commonly encountered conditions in the neonatal intensive care unit.

## What Is Blood Pressure?

When the term blood pressure is used, it typically refers to the systemic arterial pressure. This is derived from the pumping action of the left ventricle (LV), and a characteristic aortic pressure waveform is generated with each contraction. This is the standard blood pressure waveform that we visualize in the neonatal unit every day, transduced from the aorta, displayed at the patient bedside. The peak pressure generated refers to the *systolic* pressure. The pressure subsequently falls to its lowest level in the cardiac cycle prior to the next contraction and is termed the *diastolic* pressure. The numerical difference between systolic and diastolic pressure is the *pulse* pressure (PP). An understanding of the individual components of the arterial pressure waveform can provide greater insights into cardiovascular status.

The pressure waveform can be separated into upstroke (anacrotic) and downstroke (dicrotic) limbs. The elements of the waveform consist of the systolic up-stroke, the peak systolic pressure, the systolic decline, dicrotic notch, diastolic run-off, and end-diastolic pressure (Figure 3.1). The area under the curve represents the mean arterial pressure and historically was calculated as the mean arterial pressure equal to the diastolic pressure plus one-third of the PP. However, this is a simplification of the calculation. In two patients the systolic and diastolic components can measure the same, but the area under the curve might be substantially different, resulting in significantly different mean arterial blood pressure measurements.

The systolic upstroke is a direct reflection of left ventricular (LV) ejection and corresponds to the peak aortic blood flow acceleration across the aortic valve. Thus factors that influence these will result in alterations of the upstroke. A prime example may be a slurred upstroke in the setting of aortic stenosis. The peak systolic pressure represents the maximum pressure in the central arteries and is directly related to LV contraction, the compliance of the arterial system, and

reflected waves. Reflected waveforms refer to backward wave reflection as the resistance increases in the distal arteries. The effect of reflected waves is to increase the systolic blood pressure and alter the shape of the waveform. This phenomenon in the aorta is not typically seen in the neonate. As one moves further distally from the aorta, the phenomenon of distal systolic pulse amplification occurs as the systolic pressure increases due to augmentation of the reflected waves. However, the overall area of the waveform tends to decrease, resulting in a reduction in the overall mean blood pressure.

The systolic decline represents the drop in blood pressure as the ventricular contraction ceases and blood moves from the central arterial compartment faster than the influx from the later phase of ventricular contraction. Conditions such as LV outflow tract obstruction in the setting of hypertrophic obstructive cardiomyopathy result in a very rapid decline in this phase.

The dicrotic notch seen on the systolic decline represents a sudden small increase in blood pressure.

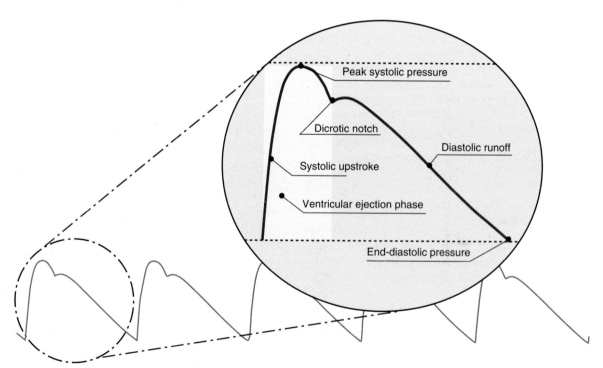

**Fig. 3.1  The arterial pressure waveform characterized by the upstroke (anacrotic) and downstroke (dicrotic) limbs.** The elements consist of the systolic upstroke, the peak systolic pressure, the systolic decline, dicrotic notch, diastolic run-off, and end-diastolic pressure.

This notch when measured in the aorta is referred to as the incisura because it "cuts into" the descending waveform. This increase in blood pressure represents aortic valve closure. As one moves further into the distal circulation, the dicrotic notch is more likely a reflection of the peripheral vascular resistance rather than aortic valve closure. Also, the latency between the peak systolic pressure and the dicrotic notch increases. Loss of the incisura/dicrotic notch on central invasive blood pressure monitoring may reflect transducer damping (discussed later).

Diastolic run-off is related to the cushioning effect of the elastic recoil of the large vessels and is often referred to as the Windkessel effect. In essence the large vessels act as reservoirs that distend during systole and recoil during diastole, permitting movement of blood throughout the cardiac cycle. The cushioning effect enables conversion of highly pulsatile flow from LV ejection into steady, non-pulsatile flow in downstream capillaries while also limiting large fluctuations in PP. Distal vessel structure contains a greater proportion of elastin. Otto Frank (of the Frank-Starling Law) pioneered work in this area. The end-diastolic pressure represents the pressure exerted primarily by the terminal resistance arterioles and is a very important factor in determining coronary blood flow.

Mean arterial BP (MAP) is the product of cardiac output and systemic vascular resistance. Accordingly, it is the dependent variable determined by the two independent variables in the circulation. It is in essence the hydrodynamic form of Ohm's law (voltage difference is equal to current times resistance), where pressure difference is equal to flow times resistance.

$$\text{Mean arterial Pressure} = \text{Cardiac output} \times \text{systemic vascular resistance}$$

Changes in cardiac output and systemic vascular resistance can result in significant alterations in blood pressure values. An understanding of each of these factors and their interrelatedness is essential to interpreting blood pressure, particularly in the first postnatal hours and days when significant changes in each may occur. The problem to date has been the fact that measuring cardiac output was previously challenging; however, with the use of echocardiography and non-invasive cardiac output monitoring, this has become feasible. Chapters 9, 10, and 12 deal with these assessments in much greater detail.

Briefly, cardiac output is the amount of blood pumped with each contraction and is the product of heart rate and stroke volume (SV). SV is influenced by several factors including preload, afterload, inotropy, ventricular compliance, and chronotropy. Preload represents the sarcomere length just prior to contraction (at the end of diastole) and as this cannot be measured, we rely on indirect measures such as end-diastolic volume. This in turn is dependent on ventricular compliance and pressure. An increase in venous return will result in an increase in ventricular filling, end-diastolic volume, and thus in preload. This increase in preload results in an increase in the force of the contraction and thus an increase in SV. This is the Frank-Starling mechanism described by Otto Frank and Ernest Starling. In newborns the curve is relatively flat across a range of normal filling pressures. A typical example might be an increase in cardiac output following a bolus of fluid.

Afterload is the load against which the heart must contract to eject blood. An increase in afterload (for whatever reason) will typically result in a decrease and shift to the right in the Frank-Starling curve and ultimately a decrease in SV and cardiac output. Both ventricles are particularly sensitive to increases in afterload. However, a sudden increase in afterload may result in an increase in preload and thus a Frank-Starling response resulting in short-term increased SV (Anrep effect), highlighting the interdependency of preload and afterload.

Inotropy (activation of the contractile proteins) occurs independent of sarcomere length. Changes in inotropy will result in changes in the Frank-Starling relationship such that an increase in inotropy effects an increase in SV. An increase in heart rate may also result in an increase in inotropy termed the Bowditch effect or force frequency relationship. This refers to the increase in inotropy that occurs with an increase in heart rate. This effect is most likely due to an increase in intracellular calcium. This phenomenon has not been investigated to any great extent in the newborn. However, an increase in heart rate may have a negative effect on diastolic filling time and thus negatively impact preload. These factors are one example of the interdependency of preload, afterload, and inotropy that need to be considered in the newborn, especially where medications which may have differing effects on each are utilized in preterm or term infants with low blood pressure.

An understanding of the vascular system and its function is essential to understanding blood pressure and blood pressure regulation. The vascular system is essentially made up of three types of vessels: distributive, exchange, and capacitance vessels. The distributive vessels include the aorta, large, and small arteries. The primary function of the aorta is to distribute blood into the arterial system and dampen the pulsatile flow. The small arteries and arterioles are the primary resistance vessels and account for approximately 70% of the systemic vascular resistance. These vessels are innervated by the autonomic nervous system and constrict and dilate depending on the underlying situation. The pressure within the arterial system is greatest in the aorta and large arteries. The greatest drop in pressure occurs in the small arterioles due to the increased resistance to flow.

The exchange vessels include the capillaries and small venules. These have a very large surface area and therefore flow across these vessels is low; hence these vessels are the primary sites for exchange to occur. To a lesser extent, they also contribute to the systemic vascular resistance. The capacitance vessels include the large venules, large veins, and venae cavae. Approximately 70–80% of the blood volume at any given point is in the venous system. These vessels have smooth muscle and therefore also contribute to the total systemic vascular resistance by approximately 15%. Venous constriction will result in an increase in venous return and ultimately an increase in SV.

Vascular tone is determined by the interaction between extrinsic and intrinsic factors acting on the smooth muscle of the blood vessel. Extrinsic factors include autonomic nervous system innervation and circulating hormones such as catecholamines, angiotensin, and vasopressin. The intrinsic factors include various endothelial factors, local metabolites, and local hormones among others (see Chapter 2 for a more detailed discussion). Systemic vascular resistance is expressed in mmHg/mL/min or dyn/s/cm$^{-5}$, where 1 dyn is 1330 mmHg. While somewhat of an oversimplification, vasoconstrictor elements can be thought of as maintaining SVR and MAP, whereas vasodilator elements are more related to organ blood flow.

## Regulation of Systemic Arterial Blood Pressure

Blood pressure regulation is a complex process involving input from multiple sources, including baroreceptors, volume receptors, and chemoreceptors located either peripherally or centrally. Each of these feedbacks to the cardiovascular center is located in the region of the pons and medulla (nucleus tractus solitarius [NTS]). These regions also receive input from the hypothalamus (e.g., temperature regulation), the cortex, and the limbic system (e.g., stress). Efferents from the cardiovascular center act primarily on the myocardium and peripheral vasculature to alter blood pressure as necessary. Sympathetic effects include increased inotropy, increased heart rate, increased conduction velocity (dromotropy) within the heart, and increased vascular smooth muscle activation resulting in vasoconstriction. Vagal activation has the opposite effect.

Arterial baroreceptors are located in the carotid sinus and the aortic arch. When systemic arterial blood pressure drops, there is a decrease in the stretch in the vessel resulting in a reduction in baroreceptor firing to the NTS. As a result, sympathetic activity increases and basal vagal activity decreases. This typically results in an increase in cardiac output and systemic vascular resistance to increase the arterial blood pressure.

Cardiopulmonary baroreceptors are located primarily in the atria or venoatrial area and are often referred to as low pressure receptors or volume receptors. A drop in venous return may result in a reduction in signals from the receptors and thus an increase in sympathetic activity, similar to the arterial baroreceptors response.

Chemoreceptors (central and peripheral) influence cardiovascular function. Hypoxia typically results in an increase in sympathetic activity leading to an increase in arterial blood pressure. Pulmonary stretch receptor activation can result in an inhibition in sympathetic activity and a drop in arterial blood pressure. This is something that should be considered in the setting of mechanical ventilation and overdistension. Humoral factors also have a very important role to play in blood pressure regulation, either directly affecting cardiovascular function or indirectly via alterations in blood volume. These include circulating catecholamines, atrial natriuretic peptide, vasopressin, and renin-angiotensin system (RAS). Some result in relatively quick changes in blood pressure such as circulating catecholamines, whereas others result in gradual increases or decreases in blood pressure over time such as occurs with the RAS via hormonal-mediated mechanisms.

It is not too difficult to appreciate that maturation of these systems will vary with many factors such as in utero environment, gender, gestational age, and postnatal age.[2,3] One measure of autonomic function is baroreceptor sensitivity (BRS). BRS can be calculated from spontaneous oscillations of systolic BP and pulse intervals by the cross-correlation sequence method. Javorka et al. studied this among preterm infants matched for postconceptual age (approximately 34 weeks) but who differed in gestational age at birth. Those born more preterm had markedly decreased values of BRS despite having similar postconceptional age. The more mature the infant, the higher the BRS and diastolic and mean blood pressure.[4] This would suggest that in very preterm infants, cardiovascular maturation occurs faster in utero, or alternatively that neonatal interventions may negatively impact on this expected maturation. Other studies have confirmed that BRS in preterm infants is lower than term matched controls. One of these evaluated BRS weekly, and while they did find a significant increase in BRS with postnatal age, this was reduced compared to term controls.[5]

Golder et al. studied autonomic control in the setting of hypotension during the first postnatal days in preterm infants.[6] They evaluated heart rate variability (HRV), blood pressure variability (BPV), and BRS. The assumption was that reduced BRS could potentially be harmful. The study was limited by relatively small numbers of subjects (23 preterm infants). The authors found that gestational age correlated with all measures of HRV but not with BPV and BRS. In the group who received inotropes BRS was lower ($3.8 \pm 0.9$ vs $6.9 \pm 1.6$ ms/mmHg), and the low-frequency/high-frequency HRV ratio was also lower ($5.7 \pm 1.3$ vs $13.6 \pm 2.8$, $P < 0.05$). This ratio may reflect decreased sympathetic activity in those infants who receive inotropes.

Vesoulis assessed BPV in preterm infants (40 in total) who were either normotensive or hypotensive as a method to assess vasomotor function.[7] Hypotensive infants (9 in total) who received inotropes had decreased low-frequency variability at baseline compared with normotensive infants, which did increase after inotrope initiation. However, low-frequency power did not change for those with treatment failure. This points to the fact that vasomotor dysregulation is associated with cardiovascular instability and that vasomotor dysregulation is a potential measure of treatment failure.

## How to Measure Blood Pressure?

There are two main methods of obtaining BP measurements in newborn infants, noninvasively or invasively. Both methods have their own inherent advantages and potential problems, but the standard of care for any critically ill newborn infant should be invasive BP monitoring where feasible. Detailed recent reviews of BP measurement and monitoring in the neonate are available.[8]

The noninvasive method is based on oscillometry. Marey first described this method in 1876. When a limb was placed in a pressure chamber, the pressure in the chamber would fluctuate, and the magnitude of these fluctuations was dependent on the pressure contained within the chamber. The oscillometric method is based on the principle that blood moving through an artery creates oscillations/vibrations of the arterial vessel wall. Thus application of external pressure via an inflated cuff placed on the limb will allow determination of "arterial" BP parameters. These oscillations are transmitted to the cuff, converted into an electrical signal by the transducer, and ultimately display systolic, mean, and diastolic noninvasive BP measurements. Prior to the development of automated devices, values were obtained clinically by either palpation or auscultation. The palpation method relies on feeling a pulse, the auscultation method on listening for sounds of turbulence generated by flow in the partially compressed vessel. Korotkoff first described indirect measurements of BP by auscultation in 1905.[9]

The systolic component of the BP measurement is just less than the systolic pressure at which the oscillations begin. The pressure at which the oscillations are at their maximum amplitude is the mean arterial pressure (MAP). The pressure in the cuff when blood first starts to flow continuously without vibration is an estimate of diastolic BP component. Various devices incorporate different algorithms to estimate the systolic and diastolic measurements.

There are several important factors to be considered when noninvasively measuring BP. Incorrect cuff size is the principal factor that will cause inaccurate measurements. The location of measurement, either an upper limb or a lower limb, may result in an overestimation or underestimation of the true value, respectively. Also, different devices may result in slightly different readings related to the algorithm used. These will be discussed later.

The invasive method uses a fluid-filled transducer directly attached to an indwelling arterial catheter placed either in the aorta or a peripheral artery. The pressure transducer converts the energy into an electrical signal that is then processed, amplified, and converted by a microprocessor into a visual display on the bedside monitor. There are a number of technical challenges that can result in inaccurate measurements due to either overdamping or underdamping of the signal.[10] One possible source of inaccuracy is the presence of small air bubbles introduced into the system. These can cause excessive damping of the PP waveform, causing an underreading of systolic BP and overreading of diastolic BP, although the mean BP is relatively unaffected. The absence or distortion of the dicrotic notch of the downward slope of the arterial waveform suggests the presence of overdamping. Further sources of overdamping may occur if blood contaminates the tubing, if the tubing is too long or too compliant, or if the initial calibration process is inaccurate. Underdamping can occur with stiff noncompliant tubing or when there is hypothermia, characterized by excessively high systolic BP and low diastolic BP, as in a resonant signal.

A number of groups have compared different noninvasive devices and observed how they compare with invasive measurements.[11-14] One of the authors (ED) previously evaluated noninvasive measurements compared to invasive measurements with three different automated oscillometric devices: (1) Procare 300 Compact (Criticon Inc., Tampa, Florida), (2) GE Marquette Solar 8000 Patient Monitor (General Electric, Fairfield,

Connecticut), and (3) GE Dash 4000 Patient Monitor with DINAMAP technology (General Electric, Fairfield, Conneticut). Measurement of the mid-arm and mid-calf circumference was obtained for each baby prior to placement of the appropriate-sized cuff (mid-arm and mid-calf circumference 0.45–0.55), consistent with the American Heart Association's recommendation that the cuff bladder width and length be 40% and 80%, respectively, of the mid-arm circumference.[15] Invasive measurements were recorded using a fluid-coupled pressure transducer (Transtar R 19 Neonatal Monitoring Kit with Kids Kit Blood Sampling System; Medex Inc., Carlsbad, California). No difference between the noninvasive recordings simultaneously obtained from the upper or lower limbs was found. However, all three noninvasive recorders consistently overestimated invasive BP values. The average difference between mean invasive and noninvasive BP was 5.1 mmHg overall and was device specific: 2.4, 4.5, and 8.4 mmHg for Dash, Dinamap, and Marquette monitors, respectively. Several other studies highlighted similar findings. Dannevig et al. found that Dinamap overreads mean BP by approximately 7.6 mmHg, particularly in smaller infants.[16] Diprose et al. also reported that Dinamap tends to overread mean BP in hypotensive infants.[17] These are important points to consider in low flow states, where noninvasive BP measurements may be falsely reassuring.

The site at which the noninvasive recording is obtained may be one reason for this difference. Several other studies comparing BP measurements from upper versus lower limbs have produced conflicting results. In term neonates Park and Lee observed no difference in BP measurements between arm and calf measurements.[18] Piazza and colleagues compared upper and lower limb systolic BP in term neonates in the first 24 hours and found that higher readings were generally present in the upper versus lower limb.[19] However, higher readings in the lower limb were also common (28%). Cowan and colleagues determined arm and calf BP in term neonates in active and quiet sleep in the first 5 postnatal days.[20] The increase in BP was greater in the arm than in the calf during these periods. In summary, noninvasive BP measurements are device specific, and upper and lower limb mean BP values are similar, whereas noninvasive BP measurements tend to overestimate invasive BP values, particularly in immature hypotensive preterm infants.[21] Perhaps the greatest challenges persist for the most immature infants (22–23 weeks) and those of <500 g where appropriate cuff size and optimization of measurement techniques remain challenging.

The International Neonatal Committee Hemodynamics Working Group recently published a systematic review addressing methods of BP measurement in neonates <3 months of age, including proper cuff size, optimal location, and measurement method performed. This review highlighted some of the challenges in obtaining reliable noninvasive BP measurements and lists the recommendations around standardizing these measurements.[22]

## Blood Pressure Ranges

Defining these BP ranges in the newborn population is both challenging and contentious. When we investigate BP standards or normative ranges, the striking findings are first, the lack of consistency across these numerous ranges and second, the absolute number of ranges that exist. Ranges are often based on birth weight, gestational age, and postnatal age criteria.[23-26] Similar populations of babies with different reference ranges suggest methodologic differences or problems. These statistically determined values vary considerably, which is not surprising considering how many of these ranges were derived. The following limitations need consideration: retrospective data collection; inclusion of small numbers of patients; collection of only a few data points and summation over wide time ranges; the combination of invasive and noninvasive measurements; and the inclusion of small for dates and appropriate for gestational age infants. In some instances newborns who received volume or vasopressor-inotrope or inotrope infusions are included in normative range development. Thus it makes interpretation of these values challenging, as they are very unlikely to constitute population-based "normative ranges."

One of the first reference ranges developed was by Versmold et al. in 1981.[26] Data were obtained invasively on 16 infants less than 1000 g and were subsequently combined with data from 45 larger infants to develop new nomograms for BP values during the first 12 postnatal hours in infants weighing 610–4220 g.

The authors concluded that they "hope that the new, extended nomograms for mean, systolic, and diastolic blood pressures will lead to more accurate assessment of the cardiovascular state in newborn infants, particularly in those born very prematurely." It is now more than 30 years since this statement was written. Other reference ranges were developed in the 1980s and 1990s, including those from Watkins et al.,[25] Spinazzola et al.,[24] and Hegyi et al.[27] While each study has some limitations, each provides important information. For example, Hegyi et al.[27] highlight lower BP values in preterm infants receiving mechanical ventilation.

Kent et al. measured BP values in 406 healthy term infants on the postnatal ward over the first 4 postnatal days.[28] The median systolic, diastolic, and mean BP values on the first postnatal day were 65, 45, and 48 mmHg, respectively. On day 4, these values had increased to 70, 46, and 54 mmHg. These are useful reference guides when evaluating term newborns. Kent and colleagues also evaluated noninvasive BP measurements in a group of stable preterm infants 28–36 weeks' gestation.[29] They measured BP on days 1, 2, 3, 4, 7, 14, 21, and 28 in a group of 147 infants. They found that premature neonates stabilize their mean BP after postnatal day 14, and at this time, they have a BP similar to that of term infants. Others have also shown an increase in BP over the first postnatal days.[30-32] Watkins et al. document the mean and 10th percentile BP over the first days based on birth weight alone (Table 3.1). These weight-based values are often used to guide therapy. Zubrow and colleagues reported the findings of a large multicenter study conducted by the Philadelphia Neonatal Blood Pressure Study Group.[31] In this study systolic and diastolic BP was significantly correlated with birth weight, gestational age, and postconceptional age. In each of four gestational age groups systolic and diastolic BP was significantly correlated with postnatal age over the first 5 postnatal days.

Batton and colleagues recently evaluated the change in BP over the first 24 postnatal hours in a population of extreme preterm infants.[33] A drop in BP values characterized the first 4 postnatal hours. For the 164 untreated infants in this cohort, the systolic, diastolic, and mean arterial BP increased ($P < .001$) by an estimated mean ± SD rate of 0.3 ± 0.5 (range: −2.15 to 1.50), 0.2 ± 0.4 (range: −1.10 to 1.10), and 0.2 ± 0.4

## TABLE 3.1   Variation of Mean Blood Pressure* With Birth Weight at 3–96 Hours of Postnatal Age

| Birth Weight (g) | Time (h) Postnatal Age | | | | | | | | |
|---|---|---|---|---|---|---|---|---|---|
| | 3 | 12 | 24 | 36 | 48 | 60 | 72 | 84 | 96 |
| 500 | 35/23 | 36/24 | 37/25 | 38/26 | 39/28 | 41/29 | 42/30 | 43/31 | 44/33 |
| 600 | 35/24 | 36/25 | 37/26 | 39/27 | 40/28 | 41/29 | 42/31 | 44/32 | 45/33 |
| 700 | 36/24 | 37/25 | 38/26 | 39/28 | 42/29 | 42/30 | 43/31 | 44/32 | 45/34 |
| 800 | 36/25 | 37/26 | 39/27 | 40/28 | 41/29 | 42/31 | 44/32 | 45/33 | 46/34 |
| 900 | 37/25 | 38/26 | 39/27 | 40/29 | 42/30 | 43/31 | 44/32 | 45/34 | 47/35 |
| 1000 | 38/26 | 39/27 | 40/28 | 41/29 | 42/31 | 43/32 | 45/33 | 46/34 | 47/35 |
| 1100 | 38/27 | 39/27 | 40/29 | 42/30 | 43/31 | 44/32 | 45/34 | 46/35 | 48/36 |
| 1200 | 39/27 | 40/28 | 41/29 | 42/30 | 43/32 | 45/33 | 46/34 | 47/35 | 48/37 |
| 1300 | 39/28 | 40/29 | 41/30 | 43/31 | 44/32 | 45/33 | 46/35 | 48/36 | 49/37 |
| 1400 | 40/28 | 41/29 | 42/30 | 43/32 | 44/33 | 46/34 | 47/35 | 48/36 | 49/38 |
| 1500 | 40/29 | 42/30 | 43/31 | 44/32 | 45/33 | 46/35 | 48/36 | 49/37 | 50/38 |

*Numbers refer to average mean BP/10th percentile for mean blood pressure.
From Watkins AM, West CR, Cooke RW Blood pressure and cerebral haemorrhage and ischaemia in very low birthweight infants. Early Hum Dev. 1989;19(2):103-110.). Used with permission from Elsevier Ltd.

(range: −0.90 to 1.25) mmHg/h, respectively, thereafter. This equates to an approximately 5 mmHg increase in mean BP over the first 24 postnatal hours in preterm infants born less than 26 weeks' gestation. Utilizing a large number of data points in a cohort of 35 extremely preterm infants, Vesoulis documented a greater increase in systolic compared to diastolic blood pressure over the first 72 postnatal hours.[34]

Another "normative range" often used to warrant intervention is a single absolute mean BP value chosen over a wide range of gestational ages. The most common is a mean BP less than 30 mmHg.[35] This approach is based on findings suggesting that the lower limit of the BP autoregulatory curve for cerebral blood flow is around 28–30 mmHg in neonatal animal models as well as preterm neonates.[36,37] Munro and colleagues studied the relationship between mean arterial BP and cerebral blood flow assessed by near-infrared spectroscopy (NIRS) in 17 extremely preterm infants, 12 of whom were hypotensive and 5 were normotensive. Patients who were hypotensive had lower cerebral blood flow compared with normotensive infants. When dopamine was commenced in the hypotensive infants, the mean BP and cerebral blood flow increased. Cerebral blood flow correlated with mean arterial BP in hypotensive infants before ($R = 0.62$) and during ($R = 0.67$) dopamine administration but not in normotensive infants. Using

complex statistical analysis, the authors suggested a "breakpoint" of mean arterial BP of 29 mmHg in the untreated cohort of infants. These findings need to be interpreted cautiously considering the small number of patients included and the lack of inclusion of potential confounders, including the effect of gestational age and the partial pressure of carbon dioxide. An interesting finding was that once dopamine therapy was commenced, cerebral blood flow seemed to continue along a pressure-passive curve, suggesting a loss of autoregulatory capacity even when BP increased beyond the lower autoregulatory elbow of 29 mmHg. Greisen and colleagues explored the relationship between white matter injury and blood flow in 13 preterm infants, using single-photon emission computed tomography with [99]Tc labeled hexamethylpropylenamide oxime as the tracer.[37] They found no relationship between white matter blood flow percentage (WMBF%) and any of the variables studied, including mean arterial BP. However, using nonlinear regression assuming a plateau over a certain BP threshold and a positive slope below this threshold, the relation to WMBF% was statistically significant ($P = .02$) with a threshold identified at 29 mmHg (95% confidence interval 26–33 mmHg). They concluded that periventricular white matter is selectively vulnerable to ischemia during episodes of low BP. There were several limitations to this study, including the small number of infants studied; two imaging studies were performed in only 3 of the 13 infants, while the relation between BP and WMBF% was statistically significant, two-thirds of the variance of WM% was still unexplained. Interestingly, these values approximate to data published almost 30 years ago by Miall-Allen et al.,[38] showing that in 33 infants of less than 31 weeks' gestation, a mean BP of less than 30 mmHg for over an hour was *associated with* severe intracranial hemorrhage, ischemic cerebral lesions, or death within 48 hours. No severe lesions were developed in infants with a mean BP of 30mm Hg or greater. Accordingly, this value (30 mmHg) is considered by some as a threshold to start intervention.[2] However, again these findings need to be interpreted cautiously when applying this principle to those at greatest risk of brain injury, that is, the most immature preterm infants. Applying this principle to infants less than 26 weeks' gestation would essentially mean intervening for a significant majority in the first postnatal hours. Indeed Greisen and colleagues state that their "result should not be used for clinical decision-making."[37] Therefore routine intervention based solely on maintaining a BP greater than 30 mmHg for extreme preterm infants should be avoided as the risks associated with vasopressor-inotrope administration may be significant in this population of infants,[39] especially if the medications are not carefully titrated. Again, these are very important considerations when caring for babies delivered at 22–24 weeks and <500 g, where very limited normative data exists.

Another "range" commonly used is that of the Joint Working Group of the British Association of Perinatal Medicine. They recommended that the mean arterial BP in mmHg should be maintained at or greater than the mean gestational age in weeks.[40] Again, there is little published evidence to support this "rule," but it remains the most common criteria used to define hypotension.[41] Lee and colleagues identified that the lower limits of mean arterial BP for infants between 26 and 32 weeks' gestation were numerically similar to the gestational age.[23] The German Neonatal Network presented data on a very large cohort of preterm infants[42] and identified that the lowest mean arterial BP recorded on postnatal day 1 was similar to the gestational age in weeks (Table 3.2). However, there is growing evidence highlighting the inadequacy of this guideline. Cunningham et al. have shown a poor

**TABLE 3.2 Lowest Mean arterial BP During the First 24 Hours and Gestational Age (Completed Weeks)**

| Gestational Age Weeks | Number of Infants With Data | Lowest Mean Arterial BP (mmHg; Median [IQR]) |
|---|---|---|
| 22 | 25 | 21 (18–25) |
| 23 | 178 | 21 (19–24) |
| 24 | 339 | 22 (20–25) |
| 25 | 431 | 24 (21–26) |
| 26 | 583 | 24 (21–28) |
| 27 | 666 | 26 (22–29) |
| 28 | 725 | 27 (24–31) |
| 29 | 725 | 29 (25–32) |
| 30 | 709 | 30 (27–34) |
| 31 | 526 | 31 (27–35) |
| All | 4907 | 27 (23–31) |

*IQR,* Interquartile range.
From Faust K, Hartel C, Preuss M, et al. Short-term outcome of very-low-birthweight infants with arterial hypotension in the first 24 h of life. Arch Dis Child Fetal Neonatal Ed. 2015;100(5):F388-F392. doi:10.1136/archdischild-2014-306483..

relationship between this rule and the incidence of intraventricular hemorrhage.[32] Data collected by the Canadian Neonatal Network (CNN) show that over 52% of preterm infants less than 28 weeks' gestation are "hypotensive" by this rule alone in the first postnatal day and, as such, may warrant intervention.[43] This simple rule also needs to be interpreted cautiously in light of the normal increase in BP over the first days, especially during the first 3 days after delivery. What is clear is that this rule is very easy to remember and is consistently used by many to guide intervention.[1,41] While intervention is dealt with in other chapters, what is clear is that dopamine remains one of the most common drugs used in the neonatal intensive care unit, especially in infants at 22–23weeks' gestation.[44]

In summary numerous reference ranges exist. Many of these are problematic, especially because of the lack of a consistent relationship between low BP values and clinically relevant short- and long-term outcomes and because there are very few data on the effectiveness of the commonly used treatment modalities to decrease the incidence of peri-/intraventricular hemorrhage (P/IVH) and white matter injury. However, consistent observations demonstrate that the BP in the first postnatal days is gestation specific, typically characterized by a drop in the first hours after birth followed by an increase thereafter over the first 3 days. This is critical to our understanding of cardiovascular support in preterm infants as the timing of intervention for low BP in preterm infants occurs on day 1 in over 90% of cases, regardless of gestational age.[45] There is no evidence that treating normal transitional changes in BP is beneficial and therefore is not recommended. In addition, the complexity of cardiovascular instability and adaptive physiologic changes is such that picking a single value to initiate therapy is somewhat naïve and illogical. What is important for clinicians to consider are as follows: a range of blood pressure values that might trigger further evaluation, the normal evolution of blood pressure over time, review the individual components of blood pressure, and understand that blood pressure values alone are likely a poor marker of end-organ blood flow.

## Blood Pressure, Cardiac Output, and Clinical Assessment

End-organ blood flow through a vessel is ultimately dependent on resistance. Three factors influence resistance (R) to blood flow: the length (L) of the vessel, the viscosity of the blood, and the radius of the vessel (Poiseuille law). The longer the vessel and the more viscous the blood, the lower the flow with a constant pressure. The greater the radius, the greater the flow as resistance to flow decreases to the power of four. These factors need to be considered when addressing end-organ blood flow and are dealt with in greater detail in Chapter 2. From a practical viewpoint at the bedside, it is easy to appreciate that blood flow and blood pressure are not interchangeable. Several studies have highlighted the discrepancy between cardiac output measurements and blood pressure measurements.[46-51] Kharrat et al. found that MBP and DBP demonstrated no correlation with LVO, whereas SBP and PP positively correlated with low LVO. The best predictor of low LVO (<150 mL/kg/min) was a narrower PP.

Recent surveys of practice highlight the use of other relevant parameters including clinical, biochemical, and echocardiographic measures, not just blood pressure values alone, to aid in decision-making.[41,52] Three recent studies suggest that this is occurring in clinical practice.[42,53,54] Detail is lacking on the individual parameters leading to intervention, but one can assume that many babies in these studies had clinical signs consistent with good perfusion and were not treated, and the contrary may also hold true. There is no validated clinical scoring system available to diagnose shock in newborns. The assessment of capillary refill time (CRT), color, heart rate, BP, and urine output are readily made at the bedside but none of these parameters in isolation is specific in identifying poor perfusion. CRT values exist for the term neonate,[55,56] but there are limited data available for the preterm infant,[46,57] with some asking whether it is a useful parameter to be evaluated at all.[58] Osborn and colleagues studied the ability of CRT, central-peripheral temperature difference (CPTd) ≥2°C, and BP to detect low SVC flow in neonates less than 30 weeks' gestation. Results for CPTd and CRT are listed in Table 3.3. The authors showed a statistically significant but weak association between CRT and systemic blood flow.[57] The sensitivity improved when mean BP values and central CRT ≥3 seconds were combined. Wodey and colleagues have shown a significant relationship between cardiac index (cardiac output/body surface area) and CRT in preterm neonates in a study using echocardiography in 100 preterm infants.[59] We previously also identified a weak relationship between CRT and simultaneously obtained SVC flow measurements in a preterm population.[46]

The relationship between skin color and illness severity in the newborn has been evaluated using a tristimulus colorimeter, an objective measurement tool for skin color.[60] Colorimeter values were found to be different in the high illness severity group, particularly in the blue-yellow axis. However, no data on BP or cardiac function were provided. Heart rates are extremely variable; they vary with gestational and postnatal age and correlate with oxygen consumption. However, neither absolute heart rate nor trend analysis of heart rate has been validated to assess cardiac function in term or preterm infants. In the first postnatal day, urine output is not a particularly useful parameter due to the perinatal surge of vasoconstrictive hormones and the complex transitional process of postnatal hemodynamics. Urine output is typically low and variable in the immediate postnatal period; however, an acceptable urine output (>1.5–2.0 mL/kg/h) is somewhat reassuring to the clinician at the

**TABLE 3.3  Relationship Between Central-Peripheral Temperature Difference and Capillary Refill Time and Other Parameters at 3- and 10-Hours Postnatal Age**

| CPTd or CRT | Sn | Sp | PPV | NPV | LR+ | LR− |
|---|---|---|---|---|---|---|
| **CPTd ≥2°C** | | | | | | |
| 3 h | 29 (15–42) | 78 (65–90) | 20 (8–32) | 85 (74–96) | 1.29 | 0.92 |
| 10 h | 41 (27–55) | 66 (52–79) | 41 (27–55) | 66 (52–79) | 1.19 | 0.90 |
| All observations | 40 (32–48) | 69 (61–77) | 23 (16–30) | 83 (77–90) | 1.30 | 0.87 |
| **CRT ≥3 s** | | | | | | |
| 3 h | 54 (45–63) | 79 (72–86) | 23 (16–31) | 93 (89–98) | 2.55 | 0.58 |
| 10 h | 59 (50–68) | 75 (67–82) | 51 (42–60) | 80 (73–87) | 2.33 | 0.55 |
| All observations | 55 (50–60) | 80 (76–84) | 33 (29–38) | 91 (88–94) | 2.78 | 0.56 |
| **CRT ≥4 s** | | | | | | |
| 3 h | 38 (30–47) | 93 (88–97) | 38 (30–47) | 93 (88–97) | 5.24 | 0.66 |
| 10 h | 26 (18–33) | 97 (93–100) | 77 (70–84) | 74 (67–82) | 7.44 | 0.77 |
| All observations | 29 (24–33) | 96 (94–98) | 55 (50–60) | 88 (85–91) | 6.84 | 0.75 |

Values in parentheses are 95% confidence intervals.

*CPTd*, Central-peripheral temperature difference; *CRT*, capillary refill time; *LR−*, negative likelihood ratio; *LR+*, positive likelihood ratio; *NPV*, negative predictive value; *PPV*, positive predictive value; *Sn*, sensitivity; *Sp*, specificity.

From Osborn DA, Evans N, Kluckow M Clinical detection of low upper body blood flow in very premature infants using blood pressure, capillary refill time, and central-peripheral temperature difference. Arch Dis Child Fetal Neonatal Ed. 2004;89(2): F168-F173. Used with permission from BMJ Publishing Group.

bedside when deciding if one needs to initiate therapy. While the positive predictive value of each of these individual parameters identifying poor perfusion is unknown and likely to be low, it does appear that clinical assessment using a combination of signs allows one to better identify patients with poor outcomes.[61] Combining clinical parameters along with BP values is clearly more logical than intervening based solely on BP values alone, unless the mean arterial BP is very low. We previously suggested using a BP value of at least 5 mmHg below the lower gestational age rule as the lowest acceptable BP during the first postnatal day.[61] This would equate to somewhere in the region of 18–20 mmHg for babies delivered at 23–25 weeks' gestation, and this value is numerically similar to the critical closing pressure for cerebral blood flow in animal models (see Chapter 2) and preterm neonates during the first postnatal days.[62] In this study critical closing pressure was studied in preterm neonates from 23 to 31 weeks' gestation and found to increase with increasing gestational age. Evidence in preterm neonates less than 28 weeks is not available as to whether this BP cutoff value is safe and effective to use when initiation of treatment is considered. Data

from the EPIPAGE-2 study would suggest that a mean BP of at least 5 mmHg less than gestational age is associated with adverse outcome.[63] The recent HIP Trial attempted to determine if intervening with a vasopressor-inotrope based on this rule was associated with worse outcome.[64] The study stopped early due to poor enrollment rates. Some key findings were that approximately 25% of all extremely low gestational age infants have a mean BP less than their gestational age at some point in the first postnatal days, the majority occurring on the first day. For those enrolled in the trial and randomized to the placebo arm, half had a spontaneous increase in blood pressure without treatment, the other half received a vasopressor-inotrope based on a combination of clinical and biochemical factors. The group who did not receive treatment thus had signs of good perfusion and a spontaneous increase in blood pressure over the ensuing hours.

There are some potential objective parameters readily available at the bedside, but their usefulness in term and preterm newborns is debatable. These include central venous pressure (CVP) monitoring, mixed venous oxygen saturation, and plasma lactate levels. CVP monitoring is commonly performed in adult and pediatric intensive care where it is often used to guide fluid management, less so in neonatal intensive care units.[65] Rudolph and colleagues recorded CVP in six babies with respiratory distress syndrome and found values between −6.5 and 0 mmHg.[66] These patients were not ventilated and generated large negative intrathoracic pressures, hence the negative values. Siassi and colleagues reported a mean CVP of +1.6 mmHg in healthy preterm neonates and negative values in babies with respiratory distress (−16 to +3 mmHg).[67] A more recent study suggests normal values for CVP in preterm infants have a very wide range (2.8–13.9 mmHg),[68] but there were numerous technical difficulties obtaining CVP measurements. It is unclear whether CVP correlates with circulating blood volume in the preterm infant[69] and, in any case, most preterm infants with lower BP in the first few days are not significantly hypovolemic.[70] Thus CVP monitoring is probably of limited value in the NICU setting. Others have suggested noninvasive methods of assessing CVP, with subcostal estimates of the maximum and minimum diameter of the inferior vena cava (IVC) obtained by echocardiography.[71] The ratio of minimum to maximum diameter correlated with CVP in this study of 14 newborns. However, a previous study showed a poor correlation between similar noninvasive echocardiographic assessments of IVC diameter and CVP, especially in mechanically ventilated infants.[72] A recent meta-analysis of 37 studies concluded that the evidence does not support the measurement of IVC diameter by ultrasonography as an acceptable surrogate to determine CVP in critically ill patients.[73]

Mixed venous saturation monitoring is frequently used in adult and pediatric intensive care, but interatrial shunting and technical difficulties in obtaining a value have limited its role, especially in the preterm neonate. There have been few studies in newborns incorporating mixed venous saturation, outside the setting of postoperative cardiac surgery. O'Connor and colleagues studied 18 newborns in the first 3 postnatal days and obtained 100 paired values of arterial saturation and mixed venous saturation. They found that the mean mixed venous oxygen saturation was 83.3% and that there was a strong correlation with fractionated oxygen extraction.[74] Van der Hoeven and colleagues measured venous oxygen saturation continuously with a fiberoptic catheter placed in the right atrium via the IVC.[75] They found a central venous

oxygen saturation ranging from 65 to 82% (5th and 95th percentile) during the first days after delivery in 10 stable preterm infants. More recently, Yapakci et al. measured IVC oxygen saturation in preterm infants as an indicator of mixed venous oxygenation in the first 3 postnatal days.[76] They identified a progressive decrease in venous oxygen saturation over the first few days, with the highest mean IVC oxygen saturation of 79.9% on initial measurement and the lowest value of 64.8% for the final measurement performed at 72 hours postnatally. However, the usefulness of mixed venous saturation monitoring in assessing cardiovascular well-being, especially for the preterm infant, remains unanswered.

Lactate values have been analyzed in a number of clinical situations in the preterm infant, including the need for erythrocyte transfusion,[77] sepsis,[78] and necrotizing enterocolitis.[79] Lactate values obtained in the first postnatal day have been used to predict outcome. Groenendaal and colleagues estimated the positive (PPV) and negative predictive value (NPV) of arterial lactate values obtained within 3 hours after birth and found that with a cutoff value of 5.7 mmol/L, the PPV was 0.47 and NPV 0.92 for a combined adverse outcome (death or poor neurodevelopmental outcome) in a cohort of preterm babies.[80] We have previously identified an association with an increased risk of adverse outcome, defined as death or severe P/IVH with a single lactate value greater than 5.6 mmol/L obtained during the first postnatal day.[81] Deshpande and Paltt showed a worse outcome when plasma lactate concentrations remained persistently elevated in sick ventilated newborns of 23–40 weeks' gestation.[82] Mortality was 57% if two lactate values were above 5.6 mmol/L, highlighting the importance of serial lactate assessments. However, these measurements were obtained beyond the transitional period. Data are limited on the utilization of plasma lactate values specifically in hypotensive newborns. Yoxall and Weindling found no difference in lactate levels between normotensive and hypotensive preterm infants.[83] In a cohort of VLBW infants we previously identified a weak negative correlation between lactate values and SVC flow.[46] A combined lactate value of greater than 4 mmol/L and prolonged CRT greater than 4 seconds resulted in a PPV of 80% and an NPV of 88% for identifying low SVC flow, which highlights the value of combining clinical and biochemical parameters in the overall assessment.[46]

de Boode provides an excellent overview of the predictive value of the most commonly used indicators of circulatory failure, including BP, heart rate, urine output, CRT, and plasma lactate concentration.[84] In summary, combining different clinical hemodynamic and biochemical parameters enhances the predictive value in the overall detection of circulatory failure, but the accuracy is still limited.

## Interpretation of Blood Pressure Values in Clinical Scenarios

An understanding of the individual (systolic and diastolic blood pressure) and combined components of blood pressure values may permit a better understanding of the complexity of "normal/abnormal"

blood pressure values in the context of end-organ blood flow. Theoretically, this should permit enhanced management of reduced blood pressure states and thus an approach based more on the physiological principles of the newborn circulation.[85] The elephant in the room remains defining "normative" systolic and diastolic blood pressure values, and deciding that a definition based on the 3rd, 5th, or 10th percentile represents the value at which intervention is required. We would contend that these individual components obtained from a population of preterm neonates provide a greater insight and understanding, but that clinical decision-making for the individual patient is much more complex and requires inclusion of a multitude of factors as highlighted in Figure 3.2. This algorithm includes several of the subjective and

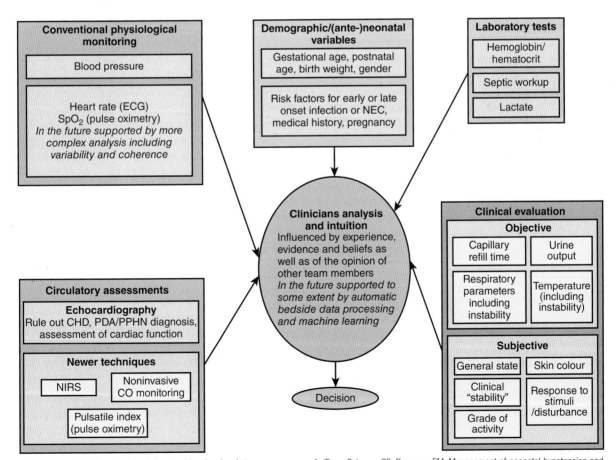

**Fig. 3.2 The complexity of decision-making in circulatory management.** (From Schwarz CE, Dempsey EM. Management of neonatal hypotension and shock. *Semin Fetal Neonatal Med.* Oct 2020;25(5):101121.)

objective parameters addressed previously. The combination of each of these, along with clinical intuition utilized humbly at the bedside should permit a more rational approach to management.

In general terms, systolic blood pressure largely reflects the force of the blood expelled into the arterial vessel walls during systole and therefore effective LV contractility. Diastolic blood pressure is more a measure of the resting vascular tone and as such reflects the systemic vascular resistance/tone and the intravascular blood volume. Systolic hypotension may be caused by any of the following: increase in LV afterload, a reduction in contractility, and decrease in preload. The increased afterload has a negative effect on the force-velocity relationship. The force (or stress) velocity relationship describes the myocardium's ability to increase contractility in the face of increased afterload but uncoupling of this relationship can occur if the LV cannot maintain this level of increased contractility, subsequently resulting in a reduction in cardiac output.[86] This can be caused by clinical conditions such as necrotizing enterocolitis, severe pulmonary hypertension, early septic (cold) shock, cardiogenic shock (e.g., hypoxic-ischemic injury, secondary to therapeutic hypothermia), during the state of transitional circulation and in patients with an early pneumothorax or pericardial effusion. Specific therapeutic options are discussed in greater detail in other chapters. The various medications, the rationale behind their use, and their effectiveness are discussed in Chapter 5. The overall focus in managing systolic hypotension should be to consider inodilator agents that reduce SVR and improve LV function while also providing appropriate volume resuscitation and treating the underlying cause of systolic hypotension.[85,87] The pathophysiology behind diastolic hypotension may include reduced preload and/or decreased SVR, thus negatively impacting the Frank-Starling relationship (length-tension relationship). In a normal physiological environment an increase in preload causes improved contractility due to stretching of the sarcomeres in the myocardium and normal or increased cardiac output.[86] Causes of diastolic hypotension include systemic hypovolemia and blood loss, severe pulmonary hemorrhage, mechanical ventilation impairing venous return, warm vasoactive septic shock, a hemodynamically significant patent

ductus arteriosus, and reduced systemic vascular resistance in the setting of transitional hypotension in the first postnatal day.[88] The treatment options may include no intervention, vasopressor, or vasopressor-inotrope agents that increase SVR and improve LV filling while also supporting volume replacement and treating a hemodynamically significant PDA.[85,87]

Combined systolic and diastolic hypotension reflects circulatory failure with progression of the underlying disease, potential adrenal insufficiency, and/or LV failure. Initial systolic hypotension that has progressed to combined hypotension is seen in the setting of a tension pneumothorax or cardiac tamponade and evolving cardiogenic shock. Conditions that initially presented as diastolic hypotension but progress to combined hypotension include severe NEC or sepsis, severe pulmonary hypertension refractory to treatment, an HsPDA with underlying LV diastolic dysfunction, and severe volume loss. In these scenarios aggressive inotropic and vasopressor support may be required, while considering steroid therapy for adrenal insufficiency and ensuring adequate volume resuscitation has been performed.[85,87] Some conditions can present with either diastolic or systolic hypotension initially with a progression to combined hypotension depending on their hemodynamic profile at presentation. We will briefly discuss specific disease profiles in further detail below but each of these is dealt with in greater detail in Chapters 19, 21, 22, and 27.

## PATENT DUCTUS ARTERIOSUS AND BLOOD PRESSURE

The ductus arteriosus plays an important role in the transition from fetal circulation to the ex utero state. However, in the premature infant patency of the ductus is the most common congenital heart condition and can lead to deleterious outcomes. Echocardiography is the mainstay of diagnosis and monitoring of response to therapy. How does a PDA affect the individual and combined components of blood pressure? Although pulmonary overcirculation from a large left-to-right shunt causes an increase in LV preload, SVR is reduced due to an overall enlarged vascular bed capacity. This is reflected in reduced diastolic blood pressure in the setting of maintained SV with normal (or high) systolic blood pressure, thus causing the typical widened PP seen on invasive monitoring. It is not clear if there is a difference between location of measurement when performed noninvasively.

Progression of the disease process sees an evolution to reduced combined blood pressure. The myocardium becomes overstretched due to the persistently high LV preload, causing sarcomere dysfunction. This negatively impacts the Frank-Starling curve, causing a reduced cardiac output and a reduced diastolic blood pressure. In conjunction with pulmonary overcirculation secondary to the large left-to-right shunt, the "ductal steal" condition, due to systemic hypoperfusion, takes effect. This has potential for end-organ damage, increased afterload, and causing systolic hypotension.[89] Boldt and colleagues used a data-driven approach assessing mean blood pressure values in the first 24 hours in a cohort of >800 VLBW infants.[90] They identified infants whose mean MAP was lower at 18–24 hours than at 4–10 hours after birth and found that they were more likely to undergo surgical ligation of the PDA and to develop P/IVH.[90] Weisz et al. in a case-control study of 14 preterm infants with hypotension but clinically well otherwise identified that a large PDA, driven by reduced systemic afterload, was the most likely underlying physiology with no evidence of LV dysfunction. Echocardiography thus has the potential to optimize targeted interventions in this population of preterm infants. Post-ligation cardiac syndrome (PLCS) can occur in up to 45% of babies undergoing surgical closure and typically presents with problems of ventilation and oxygenation, as well as systemic hypotension within approximately 6–12 hours of surgery.[91] This is discussed in greater detail in Chapter 12.

## PULMONARY HYPERTENSION (PH) AND BLOOD PRESSURE

Pulmonary hypertension (PH) affects both the term and preterm neonate and is defined as "the presence of increased pulmonary vascular resistance (PVR) associated with shunting of deoxygenated blood from the pulmonary to the systemic circulation causing severe hypoxemia."[92] The hemodynamic profile in pulmonary hypertension can vary between patients depending on the underlying cause or severity of disease, thus leading to significant variability in blood pressure profiles. Systemic hypotension is very common in the setting of PH. Through greater knowledge of the disease process and using bedside tools such as echocardiography one can develop an individualized approach to managing and monitoring systemic blood pressure in the setting of PH.

Right ventricular failure secondary to increased afterload causes a reduction in right ventricle (RV) SV and reduced pulmonary blood flow, leading to a reduction in left sided venous return and a reduction in LV preload. This is often exacerbated by the reduced venous return secondary to higher mechanical ventilation requirements, all resulting in diastolic hypotension. The impact of marked RV dilatation may include interference with LV preload (ventriculoventricular interaction) manifesting as diastolic hypotension and if profound LV outflow tract obstruction manifesting as systolic hypotension. LV hypoplasia in the context of congenital diaphragmatic hernia may cause reduced contractility and cardiac output, primarily manifesting as systolic hypotension. RV and LV failure in disease refractory to treatment often will present as combined hypotension and, unless provision of ECMO support is available, it is a poor prognostic sign.[87,92,93]

## SEPSIS AND BLOOD PRESSURE

Typically, BP is maintained in the early stages of sepsis. The clinical presentation can vary between "warm" and "cold" shock, necessitating a differential approach to therapeutic intervention. Warm shock is typically secondary to endotoxin release resulting in peripheral vasodilation, decreased SVR, and diastolic hypotension. Systemic vasodilation and reduced systemic vascular resistance in the setting of severe sepsis in combination with myocardial dysfunction can cause reduced contractility manifesting as both systolic and diastolic hypotension.[87,93] In cold shock an increase primarily in circulating endothelin levels results in peripheral vasoconstriction and elevated SVR resulting in a reduction in systolic blood pressure due to an increase in afterload and reduced cardiac output.[85,87] Targeted neonatal echocardiography can aid in guiding the management. Dual therapy (inodilator and vasopressor) is often used, and treatment requires a thorough understanding of cardiovascular physiology and neonatal pharmacodynamics along with close monitoring and appropriate antibiotic administration and use of supportive therapy.[85,87]

## HYPOXIC-ISCHEMIC ENCEPHALOPATHY AND BLOOD PRESSURE

Hypoxic-ischemic injury during the perinatal period can lead to multiorgan injury, and the myocardium can be affected in up to two-thirds of patients. Myocardial contractility is directly affected by the ischemic event but concomitant pulmonary hypertension also plays a role in the development of systemic hypotension often seen in HIE.[94] Furthermore, therapeutic hypothermia itself can place additional stress on the myocardium by causing peripheral vasoconstriction and increasing SVR, thus reducing LV cardiac output, as well as increasing pulmonary pressures and thus reducing LV preload.[87,95] These infants tend to present with systolic hypotension but can progress to combined systolic and diastolic hypotension if there is advanced myocardial injury or coinciding pulmonary hypertension.[85,87] Adrenal injury may occur in the setting of HIE, resulting in refractory hypotension, and corticosteroid administration may be considered in these cases.

## Conclusion

Understanding the complexities of the cardiovascular system remains a key challenge in neonatal care, especially over the first days after delivery when so many changes are occurring in the same time frame. Many new novel bedside techniques are on the horizon and are covered in other chapters (see Chapters 10, 12, and 14). These include the use of data-driven solutions and augmented intelligence incorporating multiple bedside signals. Techniques to continuously measure cardiac output are on the horizon, but many challenges need to be overcome before these are used routinely in neonatal intensive care units. No continuous measures of systemic vascular resistance are currently available. As for BP, the mainstay of continuous assessment remains invasive BP monitoring. While this has many shortcomings, it remains the primary reason for initiating intervention in most centers. However, a greater understanding of the individual components of blood pressure assessment (MBP, SBP, DBP, PP) and their trend over time are of great importance to the clinician. In addition, obtaining relevant clinical, biochemical, and echocardiography-derived hemodynamic profiling to enhance diagnostic precision may provide a more complete assessment while we await more objective, comprehensive monitoring systems. Using this approach, an individualized care plan can be initiated, continuously evaluated, and updated over time.

## REFERENCES

1. Dempsey EM, Barrington KJ. Diagnostic criteria and therapeutic interventions for the hypotensive very low birth weight infant. *J Perinatol.* 2006;26(11):677-681.
2. Haskova K, Javorka M, Czippelova B, Zibolen M, Javorka K. Baroreflex sensitivity in premature infants – relation to the parameters characterizing intrauterine and postnatal condition. *Physiol Res.* 2017;66(suppl 2):S257-S264. doi:10.33549/physiolres.933681.
3. Fyfe KL, Yiallourou SR, Wong FY, Odoi A, Walker AM, Horne RS. Gestational age at birth affects maturation of baroreflex control. *J Pediatr.* 2015;166(3):559-565. doi:10.1016/j.jpeds.2014.11.026.
4. Javorka K, Haskova K, Czippelova B, Zibolen M, Javorka M. Baroreflex sensitivity and blood pressure in premature infants – dependence on gestational age, postnatal age and sex. *Physiol Res.* 2021;70(suppl 3):S349-S356. doi:10.33549/physiolres.934829.
5. Gournay V, Drouin E, Roze JC. Development of baroreflex control of heart rate in preterm and full term infants. *Arch Dis Child Fetal Neonatal Ed.* 2002;86(3):F151-F154. doi:10.1136/fn.86.3.f151.
6. Golder V, Hepponstall M, Yiallourou SR, Odoi A, Horne RS. Autonomic cardiovascular control in hypotensive critically ill preterm infants is impaired during the first days of life. *Early Hum Dev.* 2013;89(6):419-423. doi:10.1016/j.earlhumdev.2012.12.010.
7. Vesoulis ZA, Hao J, McPherson C, El Ters NM, Mathur AM. Low-frequency blood pressure oscillations and inotrope treatment failure in premature infants. *J Appl Physiol.* 2017;123(1):55-61. doi:10.1152/japplphysiol.00205.2017.
8. Darnall R. Blood-pressure monitoring. In: Brans YW, Hay Jr WW, eds. *Physiological monitoring and instrument diagnosis in perinatal and neonatal medicine.* UK Cambridge University Press; 1995:246-266.
9. Korotkoff N. On methods of studying blood pressure [in Russian]. *Bull Imperial Mil Med Acad.* 1905;11:365-367.
10. Cunningham S, Symon AG, McIntosh N. Changes in mean blood pressure caused by damping of the arterial pressure waveform. *Early Hum Dev.* 1994;36(1):27-30.
11. Shimokaze T, Akaba K, Saito E. Oscillometric and intra-arterial blood pressure in preterm and term infants: extent of discrepancy and factors associated with inaccuracy. *Am J Perinatol.* 2015;32(3):277-282. doi:10.1055/s-0034-1383851.
12. Lalan S, Blowey D. Comparison between oscillometric and intra-arterial blood pressure measurements in ill preterm and full-term neonates. *J Am Soc Hypertens.* 2014;8(1):36-44. doi:10.1016/j.jash.2013.10.003.
13. Holt TR, Withington DE, Mitchell E. Which pressure to believe? A comparison of direct arterial with indirect blood pressure measurement techniques in the pediatric intensive care unit. *Pediatr Crit Care Med.* 2011;12(6):e391-e394. doi:10.1097/PCC.0b013e3182230f43.

14. O'Shea J, Dempsey EM. A comparison of blood pressure measurements in newborns. *Am J Perinatol.* 2009;26(2):113-116. doi:10.1055/s-0028-1091391.

15. Pickering TG, Hall JE, Appel LJ, et al. Recommendations for blood pressure measurement in humans: an AHA scientific statement from the Council on High Blood Pressure Research Professional and Public Education Subcommittee. *J Clin Hypertens (Greenwich).* 2005;7(2):102-109.

16. Dannevig I, Dale HC, Liestol K, Lindemann R. Blood pressure in the neonate: three non-invasive oscillometric pressure monitors compared with invasively measured blood pressure. *Acta Paediatr.* 2005;94(2):191-196.

17. Diprose GK, Evans DH, Archer LN, Levene MI. Dinamap fails to detect hypotension in very low birthweight infants. *Arch Dis Child.* 1986;61(8):771-773.

18. Park MK, Lee DH. Normative arm and calf blood pressure values in the newborn. *Pediatrics.* 1989;83(2):240-243.

19. Piazza SF, Chandra M, Harper RG, Sia CG, McVicar M, Huang H. Upper- vs lower-limb systolic blood pressure in full-term normal newborns. *Am J Dis Child.* 1985;139(8):797-799.

20. Cowan F, Thoresen M, Walloe L. Arm and leg blood pressures – are they really so different in newborns? *Early Hum Dev.* 1991; 26(3):203-211.

21. Dasnadi S, Aliaga S, Laughon M, Warner DD, Price WA. Factors influencing the accuracy of noninvasive blood pressure measurements in NICU infants. *Am J Perinatol.* 2015;32(7): 639-644. doi:10.1055/s-0034-1390345.

22. Dionne JM, Bremner SA, Baygani SK, et al. Method of blood pressure measurement in neonates and infants: a systematic review and analysis. *J Pediatr.* 2020;221:23-31.e5. doi:10.1016/j.jpeds.2020.02.072.

23. Lee J, Rajadurai VS, Tan KW. Blood pressure standards for very low birthweight infants during the first day of life. *Arch Dis Child Fetal Neonatal Ed.* 1999;81(3):F168-F170.

24. Spinazzola RM, Harper RG, de Soler M, Lesser M. Blood pressure values in 500- to 750-gram birthweight infants in the first week of life. *J Perinatol.* 1991;11(2):147-151.

25. Watkins AM, West CR, Cooke RW. Blood pressure and cerebral haemorrhage and ischaemia in very low birthweight infants. *Early Hum Dev.* 1989;19(2):103-110.

26. Versmold HT, Kitterman JA, Phibbs RH, Gregory GA, Tooley WH. Aortic blood pressure during the first 12 hours of life in infants with birth weight 610 to 4,220 grams. *Pediatrics.* 1981; 67(5):607-613.

27. Hegyi T, Carbone MT, Anwar M, et al. Blood pressure ranges in premature infants. I. The first hours of life. *J Pediatr.* 1994; 124(4):627-633.

28. Kent AL, Kecskes Z, Shadbolt B, Falk MC. Normative blood pressure data in the early neonatal period. *Pediatr Nephrol.* 2007;22(9):1335-1341. doi:10.1007/s00467-007-0480-8.

29. Kent AL, Kecskes Z, Shadbolt B, Falk MC. Blood pressure in the first year of life in healthy infants born at term. *Pediatr Nephrol.* 2007;22(10):1743-1749. doi:10.1007/s00467-007-0561-8.

30. Batton B, Batton D, Riggs T. Blood pressure during the first 7 days in premature infants born at postmenstrual age 23 to 25 weeks. *Am J Perinatol.* 2007;24(2):107-115. doi:10.1055/s-2007-970178.

31. Zubrow AB, Hulman S, Kushner H, Falkner B. Determinants of blood pressure in infants admitted to neonatal intensive care units: a prospective multicenter study. Philadelphia Neonatal Blood Pressure Study Group. *J Perinatol.* 1995;15(6): 470-479.

32. Cunningham S, Symon AG, Elton RA, Zhu C, McIntosh N. Intra-arterial blood pressure reference ranges, death and morbidity in very low birthweight infants during the first seven days of life. *Early Hum Dev.* 1999;56(2–3):151-165.

33. Batton B, Li L, Newman NS, et al. Evolving blood pressure dynamics for extremely preterm infants. *J Perinatol.* 2014;34(4): 301-305. doi:10.1038/jp.2014.6.

34. Vesoulis ZA, El Ters NM, Wallendorf M, Mathur AM. Empirical estimation of the normative blood pressure in infants <28 weeks gestation using a massive data approach. *J Perinatol.* 2016;36(4): 291-295. doi:10.1038/jp.2015.185.

35. Bada HS, Korones SB, Perry EH, et al. Mean arterial BP changes in premature infants and those at risk for intraventricular hemorrhage. *J Pediatr.* 1990;117(4):607-614.

36. Munro MJ, Walker AM, Barfield CP. Hypotensive extremely low birth weight infants have reduced cerebral blood flow. *Pediatrics.* 2004;114(6):1591-1596. doi:10.1542/peds.2004-1073.

37. Borch K, Lou HC, Greisen G. Cerebral white matter blood flow and arterial blood pressure in preterm infants. *Acta Paediatr.* 2010;99(10):1489-1492. doi:10.1111/j.1651-2227.2010.01856.x.

38. Miall-Allen VM, de Vries LS, Whitelaw AG. Mean arterial BP and neonatal cerebral lesions. *Arch Dis Child.* 1987;62(10): 1068-1069.

39. Batton B, Li L, Newman NS, et al. Early blood pressure, antihypotensive therapy and outcomes at 18–22 months' corrected age in extremely preterm infants. *Arch Dis Child Fetal Neonatal Ed.* 2016;101(3):F201-F206. doi:10.1136/archdischild-2015-308899.

40. Development of audit measures and guidelines for good practice in the management of neonatal respiratory distress syndrome. Report of a Joint Working Group of the British Association of Perinatal Medicine and the Research Unit of the Royal College of Physicians. *Arch Dis Child.* 1992;67(10 Spec No):1221-1227.

41. Stranak Z, Semberova J, Barrington K, et al. International survey on diagnosis and management of hypotension in extremely preterm babies. *Eur J Pediatr.* 2014;173(6):793-798. doi:10.1007/s00431-013-2251-9.

42. Faust K, Hartel C, Preuss M, et al. Short-term outcome of very-low-birthweight infants with arterial hypotension in the first 24 h of life. *Arch Dis Child Fetal Neonatal Ed.* 2015;100(5): F388-F392. doi:10.1136/archdischild-2014-306483.

43. Barrington KJ, Stewart S, Lee S. Differing blood pressure thresholds in preterm infants, effects on frequency of diagnosis of hypotension and intraventricular haemorrhage. *Pediatr Res.* 2002;51:455A.

44. Miller LE, Laughon MM, Clark RH, et al. Vasoactive medications in extremely low gestational age neonates during the first postnatal week. *J Perinatol.* 2021;41(9):2330-2336. doi:10.1038/s41372-021-01031-8.

45. Laughon M, Bose C, Allred E, et al. Factors associated with treatment for hypotension in extremely low gestational age newborns during the first postnatal week. *Pediatrics.* 2007; 119(2):273-280. doi:10.1542/peds.2006-1138.

46. Miletin J, Pichova K, Dempsey EM. Bedside detection of low systemic flow in the very low birth weight infant on day 1 of life. *Eur J Pediatr.* 2009;168(7):809-813. doi:10.1007/s00431-008-0840-9.

47. Groves AM, Kuschel CA, Knight DB, Skinner JR. Relationship between blood pressure and blood flow in newborn preterm infants. *Arch Dis Child Fetal Neonatal Ed.* 2008;93(1):F29-F32. doi:10.1136/adc.2006.109520.

48. Kluckow M, Evans N. Relationship between blood pressure and cardiac output in preterm infants requiring mechanical ventilation. *J Pediatr.* 1996;129(4):506-512.

49. Groves AM, Kuschel CA, Knight DB, Skinner JR. Echocardiographic assessment of blood flow volume in the superior vena cava and descending aorta in the newborn infant. *Arch Dis Child Fetal Neonatal Ed.* 2008;93(1):F24-F28. doi:10.1136/adc.2006.109512.

50. Pladys P, Wodey E, Beuchee A, Branger B, Betremieux P. Left ventricle output and mean arterial BP in preterm infants during the 1st day of life. *Eur J Pediatr.* 1999;158(10):817-824.

51. Kharrat A, Rios DI, Weisz DE, et al. The relationship between blood pressure parameters and left ventricular output in neonates. *J Perinatol.* 2019;39(5):619-625. doi:10.1038/s41372-019-0337-6.

52. Sehgal A, Osborn D, McNamara PJ. Cardiovascular support in preterm infants: a survey of practices in Australia and New Zealand. *J Paediatr Child Health.* 2012;48(4):317-323. doi:10.1111/j.1440-1754.2011.02246.x.

53. Popat H, Robledo KP, Sebastian L, et al. Effect of delayed cord clamping on systemic blood flow: a randomized controlled trial. *J Pediatr.* 2016;178:81-86.e2. doi:10.1016/j.jpeds.2016.08.004.

54. Batton B, Li L, Newman NS, et al. Use of antihypotensive therapies in extremely preterm infants. *Pediatrics.* 2013;131(6):e1865-e1873. doi:10.1542/peds.2012-2779.

55. Raju NV, Maisels MJ, Kring E, Schwarz-Warner L. Capillary refill time in the hands and feet of normal newborn infants. *Clin Pediatr (Phila).* 1999;38(3):139-144.

56. Strozik KS, Pieper CH, Roller J. Capillary refilling time in newborn babies: normal values. *Arch Dis Child Fetal Neonatal Ed.* 1997;76(3):F193-F196.

57. Osborn DA, Evans N, Kluckow M. Clinical detection of low upper body blood flow in very premature infants using blood pressure, capillary refill time, and central-peripheral temperature difference. *Arch Dis Child Fetal Neonatal Ed.* 2004;89(2):F168-F173.

58. LeFlore JL, Engle WD. Capillary refill time is an unreliable indicator of cardiovascular status in term neonates. *Adv Neonatal Care.* 2005;5(3):147-154.

59. Wodey E, Pladys P, Betremieux P, Kerebel C, Ecoffey C. Capillary refilling time and hemodynamics in neonates: a Doppler echocardiographic evaluation. *Crit Care Med.* 1998;26(8):1437-1440.

60. De Felice C, Flori ML, Pellegrino M, et al. Predictive value of skin color for illness severity in the high-risk newborn. *Pediatr Res.* 2002;51(1):100-105.

61. Dempsey EM, Al Hazzani F, Barrington KJ. Permissive hypotension in the extremely low birthweight infant with signs of good perfusion. *Arch Dis Child Fetal Neonatal Ed.* 2009;94(4):F241-F244. doi:10.1136/adc.2007.124263.

62. Rhee CJ, Fraser CD III, Kibler K, et al. Ontogeny of cerebrovascular critical closing pressure. *Pediatr Res.* 2015;78(1):71-75. doi:10.1038/pr.2015.67.

63. Durrmeyer X, Marchand-Martin L, Porcher R, et al. Abstention or intervention for isolated hypotension in the first 3 days of life in extremely preterm infants: association with short-term outcomes in the EPIPAGE 2 cohort study. *Arch Dis Child Fetal Neonatal Ed.* 2017;102(6):490-496. doi:10.1136/archdischild-2016-312104.

64. Dempsey EM, Barrington KJ, Marlow N, et al. Hypotension in preterm infants (HIP) randomised trial. *Arch Dis Child Fetal Neonatal Ed.* 2021;106(4):398-403. doi:10.1136/archdischild-2020-320241.

65. Sivarajan VB, Bohn D. Monitoring of standard hemodynamic parameters: heart rate, systemic blood pressure, atrial pressure, pulse oximetry, and end-tidal $CO_2$. *Pediatr Crit Care Med.* 2011;12(suppl 4):S2-S11. doi:10.1097/PCC.0b013e318220e7ea.

66. Rudolph AM, Drorbaugh JE, Auld PA, et al. Studies on the circulation in the neonatal period. The circulation in the respiratory distress syndrome. *Pediatrics.* 1961;27:551-566.

67. Siassi B, Wu PY, Li RK, Mondanlou H. Central venous pressure in preterm infants. *Biol Neonate.* 1980;37(5-6):285-290.

68. Trevor Inglis GD, Dunster KR, Davies MW. Establishing normal values of central venous pressure in very low birth weight infants. *Physiol Meas.* 2007;28(10):1283-1291. doi:10.1088/0967-3334/28/10/012.

69. Choi YS, Lee BS, Chung SH, Kim JH, Kim EA, Kim KS. Central venous pressure and renal function in very low birth weight infants during the early neonatal period. *J Matern Fetal Neonatal Med.* 2016;29(3):430-434. doi:10.3109/14767058.2014.1002766.

70. Bauer K, Linderkamp O, Versmold HT. Systolic blood pressure and blood volume in preterm infants. *Arch Dis Child.* 1993;69(5 Spec No):521-522.

71. Sato Y, Kawataki M, Hirakawa A, et al. The diameter of the inferior vena cava provides a noninvasive way of calculating central venous pressure in neonates. *Acta Paediatr.* 2013;102(6):e241-e246. doi:10.1111/apa.12247.

72. Hruda J, Rothuis EG, van Elburg RM, Sobotka-Plojhar MA, Fetter WP. Echocardiographic assessment of preload conditions does not help at the neonatal intensive care unit. *Am J Perinatol.* 2003;20(6):297-303. doi:10.1055/s-2003-42771.

73. Alavi-Moghaddam M, Kabir A, Shojaee M, Manouchehrifar M, Moghimi M. Ultrasonography of inferior vena cava to determine central venous pressure: a meta-analysis and meta-regression. *Acta Radiol.* 2017;58(5):537-541. doi:10.1177/0284185116663045.

74. O'Connor TA, Hall RT. Mixed venous oxygenation in critically ill neonates. *Crit Care Med.* 1994;22(2):343-346.

75. van der Hoeven MA, Maertzdorf WJ, Blanco CE. Continuous central venous oxygen saturation (ScvO2) measurement using a fibre optic catheter in newborn infants. *Arch Dis Child Fetal Neonatal Ed.* 1996;74(3):F177-F181.

76. Yapakci E, Ecevit A, Ince DA, et al. Inferior vena cava oxygen saturation during the first three postnatal days in preterm newborns with and without patent ductus arteriosus. *Balkan Med J.* 2014;31(3):230-234. doi:10.5152/balkanmedj.2014.13197.

77. Moller JC, Schwarz U, Schaible TF, Artlich A, Tegtmeyer FK, Gortner L. Do cardiac output and serum lactate levels indicate blood transfusion requirements in anemia of prematurity? *Intensive Care Med.* 1996;22(5):472-476.

78. Nguyen HB, Rivers EP, Knoblich BP, et al. Early lactate clearance is associated with improved outcome in severe sepsis and septic shock. *Crit Care Med.* 2004;32(8):1637-1642. doi is: 10.1097/01.CCM.0000132904.35713.A7

79. Abubacker M, Yoxall CW, Lamont G. Peri-operative blood lactate concentrations in pre-term babies with necrotising enterocolitis. *Eur J Pediatr Surg.* 2003;13(1):35-39. doi:10.1055/s-2003-38298.

80. Groenendaal F, Lindemans C, Uiterwaal CS, de Vries LS. Early arterial lactate and prediction of outcome in preterm neonates admitted to a neonatal intensive care unit. *Biol Neonate.* 2003;83(3):171-176.

81. Nadeem M, Clarke A, Dempsey EM. Day 1 serum lactate values in preterm infants less than 32 weeks gestation. *Eur J Pediatr.* 2010;169(6):667-670. doi:10.1007/s00431-009-1085-y.

82. Deshpande SA, Platt MP. Association between blood lactate and acid-base status and mortality in ventilated babies. *Arch Dis Child Fetal Neonatal Ed.* 1997;76(1):F15-F20.

83. Yoxall CW, Weindling AM. Blood lactate concentrations in sick neonates: normal range and prognostic significance of hyper-lactataemia. *Pediatr Res.* 1996;40:557.

84. de Boode WP. Clinical monitoring of systemic hemodynamics in critically ill newborns. *Early Hum Dev.* 2010;86(3):137-141. doi:10.1016/j.earlhumdev.2010.01.031.

85. El-Khuffash A, McNamara PJ Hemodynamic assessment and monitoring of premature infants. *Clin Perinatol.* 2017;44(2): 377–393. doi:10.1016/j.clp.2017.02.001.

86. Bussmann N, El-Khuffash A Future perspectives on the use of deformation analysis to identify the underlying pathophysio-logical basis for cardiovascular compromise in neonates. *Pediatr Res.* 2019;85:591–595. doi:10.1038/s41390-019-0293-z.

87. Giesinger RE, McNamara PJ Hemodynamic instability in the critically ill neonate: an approach to cardiovascular support based on disease pathophysiology. Semin Perinatol. 2016;40(3): 174–188.

88. Aldana-Aguirre JC, Deshpande P, Jain A, Weisz DE. Physiology of low blood pressure during the first day after birth among extremely preterm neonates. *J Pediatr.* 2021;236:40-46.e3. doi:10.1016/j.jpeds.2021.05.026.

89. Rios DR, Bhattacharya S, Levy PT, McNamara PJ Circulatory insufficiency and hypotension related to the ductus arteriosus in neonates. Front Pediatr. 2018;6:62. doi:10.3389/fped.2018. 00062.

90. Boldt R, Makela PM, Immeli L, et al. Blood pressure changes during the first 24 hours of life and the association with the persistence of a patent ductus arteriosus and occurrence of in-traventricular haemorrhage. *PLoS One.* 2021;16(11):e0260377. doi:10.1371/journal.pone.0260377. doi:10.1371/journal.pone. 0260377.

91. Jain A, Sahni M, El-Khuffash A, et al. Use of targeted neonatal echocardiography to prevent postoperative cardiorespiratory instability after patent ductus arteriosus ligation. J Pediatr. 2012;160(4):584–589.e1. doi:10.1016/j.jpeds.2011.09.027.

92. de Boode WP, Singh Y, Molnar Z, et al. Application of neona-tologist performed echocardiography in the assessment and management of persistent pulmonary hypertension of the newborn. Paediatr Res. 2018;84(Suppl 1):68–77. doi:10.1038/ s41390-018-0082-0.

93. Singh Y, Katheria AC, Vora F Advances in diagnosis and man-agement of hemodynamic instability in neonatal shock. Front Pediatr. 2018;6:2. doi:10.3389/fped.2018.00002.

94. Armstrong K, Franklin O, Sweetman D, Molloy EJ Cardiovas-cular dysfunction in infants with neonatal encephalopathy. Arch Dis Child. 2012;97(4):372–375. doi:10.1136/adc.2011. 214205.

95. Breatnach CR, Forman E, Foran A, et al. Left ventricular rotational mechanics in infants with hypoxic ischemic encephalopathy and preterm infants at 36 weeks postmenstrual age: a comparison with healthy term controls. Echocardiography. 2017;34(2):232–239. doi:10.1111/echo.13421.

# Chapter 4

# Cardiopulmonary Interactions in the Mechanically Ventilated Neonate

Dany E. Weisz

## Introduction

Cardiopulmonary interactions are crucial considerations in the intensive care management of critically ill neonates. The understanding of the impact of mechanical ventilation on the heart and lungs permits the prediction of a neonate's response to the initiation or modification of positive pressure ventilation, or the effect of cardiovascular therapeutics. These interactions are guided by the laws of hydrodynamics as applied to a distensible or compressible structure. The thoracic cavity limits the space available for the heart and lungs. With this external constraint, changes in intrathoracic pressure (ITP) throughout the respiratory cycle may have varying effects on cardiac and respiratory function. Conversely, the serial nature of the pulmonary and systemic circulations implies that cardiac dysfunction may adversely impact vascular pressures in the lung and thereby deleteriously affect gas exchange. This chapter will illustrate core principles of cardiopulmonary interactions and their importance in the clinical management of critically ill neonates.

## Physiological Principles of Cardiorespiratory Interactions in Neonates

### POSITIVE PRESSURE VENTILATION AND THE RIGHT HEART

#### Systemic Venous Return

Systemic venous return occurs due to a pressure gradient between the systemic venous reservoirs ($P_{venous}$, upstream pressure) and the right atrium ($P_{RA}$, downstream pressure) such that

$$\text{Systemic venous return} = \frac{P_{venous} - P_{RA}}{Venous\ Resistance}$$

The venous system pressure ($P_{venous}$) is influenced by both intravascular volume and venous compliance. Low-pressure venous reservoirs in the hepatic, splanchnic, and splenic circulations contain most of the circulating blood volume, and healthy neonates have sufficient capacity to receive substantial increases in intravascular volume without appreciable increases in venous pressure. Venous compliance is dependent upon both capacitance and venomotor tone. Increased skeletal muscle contraction and systemic vascular resistance augment the venous tone.

Right atrial pressure is the major resistor to systemic venous return and is, under normal conditions, typically low.[1] The $P_{venous} - P_{RA}$ pressure gradient is augmented, facilitating improvement in systemic venous return, in the setting of higher peripheral venous pressure (e.g., intravascular volume administration or increased skeletal muscle activity) and lower right atrial pressure. Catecholamines mediate acute compensatory increases in systemic venous return by facilitating vascular smooth muscle contraction (which reduces venous capacitance and increases $P_{venous}$), and this may be induced by neurosympathetic activation or through exogenous catecholamine administration[2] (Table 4.1).

### Spontaneous Respiration and Right Ventricular Preload

During normal, spontaneous respiration, ventilation occurs through the generation of negative ITP. Diaphragm descent and rib cage expansion increase the chest cavity volume, creating negative pleural pressure and reducing ITP. The lungs expand to fill the chest cavity and the negative ITP is transmitted to the vena cava and right atrium,

| TABLE 4.1 Factors and Conditions That Affect Systemic Venous Return | |
|---|---|
| **Increase Systemic Venous Return** | **Decrease Systemic Venous Return** |
| • Increase system venous pressure<br>↑ venous tone: catecholamines, skeletal muscle activity, supine, or Trendelenburg position<br>↑ intravascular volume: exogenous fluid administration for volume expansion<br>• Decrease right atrial pressure<br>Removal of mechanical ventilation (i.e., endotracheal extubation) | • Decrease system venous pressure<br>↓ venous tone: venodilators, skeletal muscle paralysis, anti-gravity positioning<br>↓ intravascular volume: fluid losses, hemorrhage<br>Skeletal muscle paralysis<br>• Increase right atrial (or downstream); pressure<br>↑ pressure from adjacent structures: pericardial effusion/tamponade; tension pneumothorax or hydrothorax; excessive lung volumes |

resulting in increased transmural RA pressure, RA expansion, and reduced $P_{RA}$. Simultaneously, intraabdominal pressure increases due to diaphragm descent, resulting in decreased venous reservoir capacitance and an increase in $P_{venous}$.[3,4] The combined increase in $P_{venous}$ and reduction in $P_{RA}$ increase the $P_{venous} - P_{RA}$ pressure gradient, increasing systemic venous return, right heart preload, and right ventricular stroke volume.

The augmentation in systemic venous return and right heart preload associated with the reduction in $P_{RA}$ associated with negative pressure inspiration is limited by the collapsibility of the vena cava. While negative ITP and lung expansion result in reduced $P_{RA}$, there is an associated reduction in transmural pressure ($P_{TM}$) of the intrathoracic great veins. Increasingly, negative ITP and consequently reduced $P_{RA}$ will result in increasing systemic venous return up until vena cava $P_{TM}$ becomes negative at the thoracic inlet.[5] At this point, vena cava collapse occurs at the thoracic inlet, and further systemic venous return is determined by the difference between $P_{venous}$ and vena cava pressures at the thoracic inlet (intraabdominal pressure for inferior vena cava; atmospheric pressure for superior vena cava).

Altogether, under normal physiological conditions of spontaneous respirations, these cardiopulmonary interactions culminate in small but detectable and cyclical variations in ventricular stroke volume and systolic blood pressure during the respiratory cycle. During inspiration, the increase in RV preload alters the interventricular septal configuration and increases LV elastance, resulting in reduced LV preload and stroke volume and reduced systolic blood pressure.[6]

During expiration, this process is reversed and is associated with an increase in systolic blood pressure.

### Mechanical Ventilation and Right Ventricular Preload

The administration of positive pressure ventilation, through increases in ITP, reverses the cardiopulmonary interactions that occur with spontaneous ventilation. Inspiration is associated with a reduction in right ventricular preload and an increase in systolic blood pressure[7] (Figure 4.1). While these breath-to-breath hemodynamic fluctuations that occur over the respiratory cycle illustrate the dynamic cardiopulmonary interactions that exist, they have limited clinical importance in the administration and titration of intensive care.

In contrast, sustained influences of positive pressure ventilation on the circulation have the potential to have a significant impact on cardiorespiratory stability, which necessitates consideration in clinical decision making. In contemporary practice, mechanical ventilation is universally administered with positive end-expiratory pressure (PEEP), resulting in an ITP that is higher than atmospheric pressure throughout the respiratory cycle. For mechanically ventilated neonates, the effect of ITP on systemic and pulmonary hemodynamics is mediated by lung volumes. During the administration of positive pressure ventilation, lung compliance is the predominant determinant of the lung volume attained for the given pressure administered. In the setting of excessive lung volumes ("overdistention"), the lungs exert positive pressure on adjacent structures, including the pleura and pericardium, resulting in an increase in intrapleural, pericardial, and ultimately intracardiac pressure. The transmission of

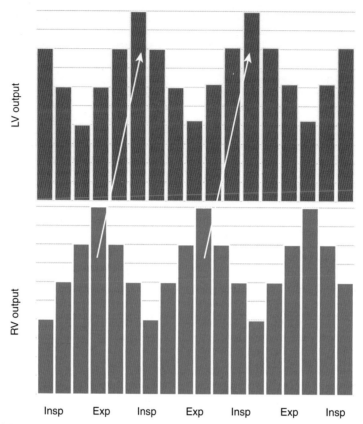

**Fig. 4.1  Cyclic changes in right and left ventricular output (RVO and LVO) with respiration.** During spontaneous ventilation (not shown), inspiration results in an increase in RVO due to increased systemic venous return and a decrease in LVO as interventricular septal deviation limits LV end-diastolic volume. During positive pressure ventilation, the process is reversed. During mechanical ventilation, rise of pleural pressure to supra-atmospheric level during inspiration impedes venous return to the right atrium. Right ventricular outflow during lung inflation is further diminished due to an increase in pulmonary vascular resistance (observed as a slight increase in pulmonary artery diastolic pressure) when lung volume increases above functional residual capacity. The inspiratory reduction in pulmonary arterial flow is followed, after a phase lag of 2 beats, by a reduction in LVO, beginning at the end of inhalation and most pronounced during expiration. *Exp*, Expiration; *Insp*, inspiration; *LV*, left ventricular; *RV*, right ventricular. (Based on data from Jardin et al.[7])

positive pressure from the lungs to the heart results in increased pressure within the cardiac chambers, including $P_{RA}$. Increased $P_{RA}$ decreases the $P_{venous} - P_{RA}$ pressure gradient, thereby reducing systemic venous return. The reduction in systemic venous return reduces both right ventricular preload and stroke volume and, ultimately, left ventricular (LV) output.[8] If $P_{RA}$ rises to the level of $P_{venous}$, then systemic venous return ceases and both RV stroke volume and pulmonary blood flow fall precipitously, representing tamponade physiology. Mean airway pressure–induced reductions in cardiac output have been confirmed in preterm neonates.[9]

However, compensatory mechanisms exist that mitigate the reduction in systemic venous return associated with increased ITP and $P_{RA}$. Although increased ITP may increase $P_{RA}$ and reduce systemic venous return, the associated reduction in cardiac output elicits arterial baroreceptor–mediated neurosympathetic activation, which results in decreased venous capacitance and increased $P_{venous}$ through increased venomotor tone. The potential reduction in systemic venous return associated with an increase in ITP is thus partially mitigated (Figure 4.2).

Among ventilated patients where higher ITP and increased lung volumes are deemed to be necessary,

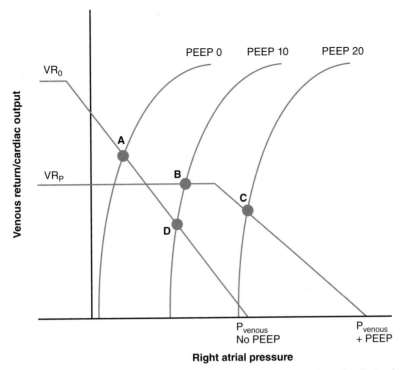

**Fig. 4.2 Relationship between cardiac function and venous return curves illustrating the hemodynamic effects of positive end-expiratory pressure (PEEP).** As lung volume increases with PEEP, intrathoracic pressure increases by an amount influenced by chest wall and pulmonary compliance and lung volume. Positive intrathoracic pressure is transmitted to the right atrium, resulting in decreased systemic venous return. Under conditions of zero PEEP, venous return would theoretically decrease from point A to point D ($VR_0$ is the venous return curve under conditions of zero PEEP). However, as PEEP increases from 0 to 20, a rightward shift in the cardiac function curve occurs (PEEP 10 and PEEP 20 are the cardiac function curves with 10 and 20 cm $H_2O$ of PEEP, respectively). There is also an increase in venous system pressure mediated by arterial baroreceptor–mediated neurosympathetic activation. Hence the intersection of the venous return and cardiac function curves shifts from A to B to C, representing a mitigation of the decline in systemic venous return and cardiac output with mechanical ventilation.

or for whom there is uncertainty regarding the magnitude of the $P_{Venous} - P_{RA}$ pressure gradient, the administration of intravenous fluid may transiently augment systemic venous return. Among mechanically ventilated patients who have sustained reductions in ventricular preload associated with progressive increases in mean airway and ITP, a bolus of 0.9% saline restores end-diastolic volume to pre-ventilation levels.[10]

### Mechanical Ventilation, Lung Volumes, and Right Ventricular Afterload

The impact of mechanical ventilation on right ventricular afterload is mediated through the relationship of PVR and lung volumes. PVR is the net resistance

across alveolar vessels (contributing to gas exchange and exposed to alveolar pressure) and extra-alveolar vessels (larger vessels, located in the interstitium and exposed to intrapleural pressures). Alveolar and extra-alveolar vessels lie in series, and thus the net PVR is the sum of their total resistances.

At low lung volumes, alveoli are atelectatic, resulting in more tortuous extra-alveolar vessels (high resistance), while alveolar vessels have low resistance owing to low intra-alveolar pressure. Atelectasis also promotes V/Q mismatch and intra-pulmonary shunting, leading to hypoxia, which increases PVR. At high lung volumes, alveolar overdistention compresses alveolar vessels (resulting in high resistance), while extra-alveolar vessels assume a straighter configuration and develop lower resistance. Overdistention also results in V/Q mismatch by increasing ventilatory dead space, leading to hypercarbia, which increases PVR. As net PVR is the sum of the alveolar and extra-alveolar vascular resistance, PVR is minimized and pulmonary blood flow maximized, when lung volumes are at functional residual capacity (FRC) (Figure 4.3).

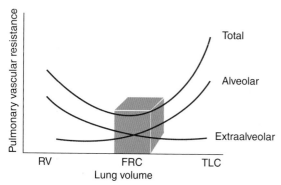

**Fig. 4.3 Schematic representation of the relationship between pulmonary vascular resistance (PVR) and lung volume.** As lung volume increases from residual volume (RV) to total lung capacity (TLC), the alveolar vessels become increasingly compressed by the distending alveoli, resulting in increased resistance in the intra-alveolar vessels. The resistance of extra-alveolar vessels decreases with increasing lung volumes because they become less tortuous. The net effect of increasing lung volumes on the pulmonary vasculature produces a "U-shaped" curve, with its nadir (representing optimal PVR) at functional residual capacity (FRC). (Reproduced from Weisz et al.[63] with permission.)

## POSITIVE PRESSURE VENTILATION AND THE LEFT VENTRICLE: INTRATHORACIC PRESSURE AND LEFT VENTRICULAR AFTERLOAD

LV afterload ($\sigma$) is the resistance that must be overcome for the LV to eject blood into the aorta and is represented by wall stress ($\sigma$).

$$\sigma = \frac{Pressure \times Radius}{Wall\ thickness}$$

During normal spontaneous respiration ("quiet breathing"), the left ventricular transmural pressure (P-LV$_{TM}$) is equal to the aortic pressure because the ITP is negligible. However, during periods of severe respiratory distress due to obstructive lung disease (e.g., neonate with severe bronchopulmonary dysplasia or subglottic stenosis), increased inspiratory effort leads to exaggerated negative ITP and an increase in P-LV$_{TM}$[11] (Figure 4.4). In the presence of large negative ITP swings, increased LV afterload may precipitate LV systolic dysfunction and pulmonary edema.[11] Sustained increases in respiratory effort also result in increased endogenous catecholamine release, leading to increased systemic vascular resistance and arterial blood pressure and further increases in LV afterload.

The administration of positive pressure ventilation may improve LV loading conditions, resulting in improved cardiac output. LV afterload is altered by changes in ITP through its effects on both LV end-diastolic

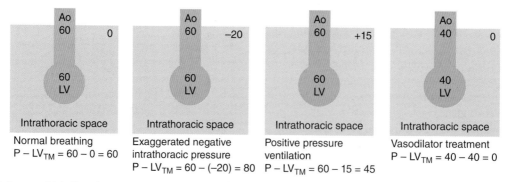

**Fig. 4.4 Influence of intrathoracic pressure on left ventricular afterload.** Changes in aortic pressure or intrathoracic pressure affect the left ventricular transmural pressure (P-LV$_{TM}$), which is the pressure generated by LV myocardial contraction to generate stroke volume. During normal quiet breathing, intrathoracic pressure is minimal and therefore P-LV$_{TM}$ is equal to the aortic pressure (first panel). During exaggerated spontaneous respirations, such as a neonate with severe respiratory distress syndrome, the P-LV$_{TM}$ will increase, resulting in increased LV afterload (second panel). During mechanical ventilation, positive intrathoracic pressure results in a reduced P-LV$_{TM}$, reducing LV afterload (third panel). Treatment with a systemic vasodilator reduces P-LV$_{TM}$ and LV afterload, but through a reduction in aortic pressure, as intrathoracic pressure is unchanged (fourth panel).

volume and ejection pressure. LV ejection pressure is aortic pressure relative to ITP. The thoracic aorta is subject to changes in pleural pressure, due to its position within the thorax. If arterial pressure remains constant as ITP increases (e.g., with initiation of mechanical ventilation), then $P\text{-}LV_{TM}$ will decrease, and LV stroke volume will increase. Conversely, decreases in ITP would result in increased $P\text{-}LV_{TM}$ (and LV afterload) and LV stroke volume would decrease, assuming arterial pressure remains constant.[12,13] Thus increases in ITP decrease LV afterload and decreases in ITP increase LV afterload.

However, studies in adults have suggested that ITP-mediated decreases in LV afterload may be preload dependent and may therefore mitigate associated improvements in LV stroke volume.[13,14] The initiation of mechanical ventilation, and associated increase in ITP, results in a reduction in LV afterload, augmentation of LV stroke volume, and increase in systemic blood pressure.[15] Overall, $P\text{-}LV_{TM}$ decreases owing to a greater rise in ITP than in LV and thoracic arterial pressures; however, associated improvements in LV performance may be self-limited because venous return also decreases, due to the effect of increased ITP in reducing intrathoracic blood volume. Nonetheless, positive pressure ventilatory support probably still effectively reduces $P\text{-}LV_{TM}$ by reducing inspiratory effort and preventing the adverse effect of large negative swings of ITP on LV performance, which would reduce LV afterload regardless of (and uninfluenced by) venous return.[16] Positive pressure ventilatory support also improves the oxygen supply-demand relationship by promoting alveolar patency and reducing respiratory muscle oxygen consumption, which will dampen systemic catecholamine release and further reduce LV afterload.[17]

## PHYSIOLOGICAL IMPACT OF CARDIOVASCULAR ANOMALIES AND DYSFUNCTION ON THE RESPIRATORY SYSTEM

Postnatally, the existence of the pulmonary and systemic circulations in series implies that alterations in atrial and/or ventricular pressures may adversely impact the pulmonary circulation. Blood flows through a vessel in the circulation only when there exists a pressure gradient between the inflow (Pi) and outflow (Po) pressures. Friction between the vessel walls and the moving blood creates an intrinsic vascular resistance. This relationship is described by a variation of Ohm's law:

$$Q\ (Flow) = \frac{Pressure\ Gradient\ (Pi-Po)}{Vascular\ resistane}$$

When applied to the pulmonary circulation:

$$\begin{array}{l} Pulmonary \\ Blood\ Flow \\ (PBF) \end{array} = \frac{\begin{array}{c} Mean\ Pulmonary\ Artery \\ Pressure\ (mPAp) - Pulmonary \\ Copillary\ [Wedge]\ Pressure\ (PCWP) \end{array}}{Pulmonary\ Vascular\ Resistance\ (PVR)}$$

This may be further rearranged as: $mPAp = (PBF \times PVR) + PCWP$. Pulmonary vascular resistance represents the net resistance to pulmonary blood flow and is influenced primarily by the number and diameter of pulmonary arterioles and blood viscosity. Pulmonary vascular resistance may remain elevated in infants with impaired transition and congenital or acquired lesions, which may be pulmonary or extra-pulmonary in origin. Pulmonary capillary wedge pressure is the "back-pressure" mitigating pulmonary venous return and is analogous to left atrial pressure in the setting of anatomically and functionally normal pulmonary venous drainage.

### Acute Pulmonary Hypertension

For neonates with hypoxic respiratory failure (HRF) and a clinical phenotype of acute pulmonary hypertension, clinicians should consider etiologies associated not only with increased PVR but also PBF or PCWP, especially among neonates with an incomplete response to inhaled nitric oxide (Figure 4.5). Increased pulmonary blood flow may result in increased PAp[18] and occurs in the setting of systemic-to-pulmonary shunt lesions, which may be cardiac (ventricular or atrial septal defect, patent ductus arteriosus) or extra-cardiac (arteriovenous malformation, twin-to-twin transfusion) in origin. PVR (and PAp) increases linearly with increasing PCWP,[19] which occurs with left heart obstructive lesions (e.g., pulmonary vein obstruction or mitral valve stenosis) or impairment in LV filling (e.g., LV systolic dysfunction, which may be due, for example, to hypoxic ischemic encephalopathy).

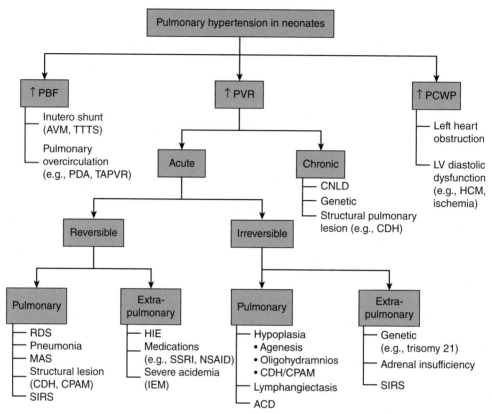

**Fig. 4.5  Causes of pulmonary hypertension in neonate.** Pulmonary hypertension in neonates may be due to increased pulmonary blood flow (PBF), pulmonary vascular resistance (PVR), or pulmonary capillary wedge pressure (PCWP). Increased PVR may be classified as acute or chronic and may arise from a variety of underlying disorders. *AVM,* Arteriovenous malformation; *CDH,* congenital diaphragmatic hernia; *CNLD,* chronic neonatal lung disease of prematurity; *CPAM,* cystic pulmonary adenomatoid malformation; *HCM,* hypertrophic cardiomyopathy; *IEM,* inborn error of metabolism; *LV,* left ventricle; *MAS,* meconium aspiration syndrome; *NSAID,* non-steroidal anti-inflammatory drug; *PDA,* patent ductus arteriosus; *SIRS,* systemic inflammatory response syndrome; *SSRI,* selective serotonin reuptake inhibitor; *TAPVR,* total anomalous pulmonary venous return; *TTTS,* twin-to-twin transfusion. (Reproduced with permission from Weisz and McNamara.[64])

## Patent Ductus Arteriosus

The relationship between the PDA and the lung is extensively reviewed in Chapters 16 and 19. The effect of a PDA on the lung occurs at multiple levels and at differing time points. The magnitude of the PDA shunt and its associated cardiopulmonary interactions dictate the pathophysiologic features of this lesion in clinical care. Specific features of cardiovascular mechanics associated with prematurity particularly predispose neonates to greater PDA-associated adverse cardiopulmonary effects. A left-to-right ductal shunt results in increased PBF and left heart dilatation, resulting in higher left-ventricular end-diastolic pressures, upstream pulmonary venous pressure and pulmonary congestion, a pathophysiology exacerbated among preterm neonates owing to decreased compliance of the immature ventricle.[20] Unlike in adults where increased pulmonary vascular distention and recruitment of the capillary bed assist in managing higher PBF without associated changes in capillary hydrostatic pressure, the pulmonary vascular bed in neonates is poorly compliant and already nearly fully recruited.[21] PDA-associated increases in PBF therefore result in increased PAp and a shift in the pulmonary pressure head to downstream capillary filtration sites, leading to pulmonary interstitial edema, reduced lung compliance, and impaired oxygenation.[22,23] Additional increases in left atrial and volume and pressure overload associated with larger ductal shunts may further worsen pulmonary venous pressure and culminate in alveolar edema and further deterioration in respiratory mechanics and function. Preterm neonates with respiratory distress syndrome are more sensitive to increases in microvascular perfusion pressure and demonstrate exaggerated increases in interstitial and alveolar lung fluid accumulation, resulting in secondary surfactant dysfunction.[24,25]

## Management of the Critically Ill Neonate: Implications of Cardiorespiratory Interactions in Clinical Decisions

Among neonates, the cardiopulmonary interactions of positive pressure support, ITP, lung volumes, and cardiac preload and afterload carry potentially significant implications for clinical management. Overall, the association of airway pressure and lung volumes is determined by lung and chest wall compliance and airway resistance. Commonly encountered clinical scenarios in neonates involve rapid changes in these physiological indices, with the potential for clinicians to either improve or iatrogenically induce hemodynamic derangement. Conversely, abnormal cardiac anatomy or function may primarily lead, or contribute to, severe HRF in neonates. Titration of mechanical ventilation alone may be insufficient in achieving respiratory stability.

### CARDIORESPIRATORY INTERACTIONS DURING PERINATAL TRANSITION

The initial, and likely most critical, cardiorespiratory interactions in neonates occur at birth, at the time of respiratory and circulatory transition to extra-uterine life. Pulmonary pathology, such as respiratory distress syndrome or pulmonary hypoplasia, may result in impairment in the normal and programmed drop in PVR and/or necessitate therapeutic interventions such as positive pressure ventilation, both of which may adversely affect cardiovascular function. Similarly, abnormal cardiac anatomy or function may be the primary derangement(s) that result in pulmonary venous congestion or impaired pulmonary blood flow,

and adversely impact respiratory function. Cardiorespiratory interactions associated with the transitional period are described in detail in Chapter 6.

### SURFACTANT ADMINISTRATION

Respiratory distress syndrome of the newborn is caused by surfactant deficiency, often in the context of immature lungs. Surfactant deficiency increases the surface tension within the alveoli and small airways, resulting in reduced lung compliance. Atelectasis occurs throughout the lung in the setting of surfactant deficiency, resulting in impairment in gas exchange. The therapeutic administration of exogenous surfactant induces a rapid increase in pulmonary compliance among preterm neonates with respiratory distress syndrome.[26] After the administration of surfactant, the provision of an unchanged mean airway pressure results in an increase in lung distention, with the potential to cause an increase in $P_{RA}$, reducing systemic venous return and right heart preload. If unrecognized, obstructive shock can ensue with impairment in ventricular preload and output, characterized by severe HRF (due to reduced pulmonary blood flow) and simultaneous systemic hypotension (due to low LV output or increased left-right flow across the PDA when PVR falls). Such a critical scenario, albeit iatrogenic in nature, may be further aggravated by an unsuspecting clinician who empirically administers systemic vasopressors (further reducing LV output) or inhaled nitric oxide (ineffective at improving oxygenation in the setting of impaired pulmonary blood flow). However, hemodynamic instability may be entirely avoided if clinicians anticipate such rapid changes in pulmonary compliance and take steps to prevent pulmonary overdistention, such as regularly considering weaning the mean airway pressure or employing a volume-targeted, pressure-limited mode of ventilation.[27] Echocardiographic evaluation is diagnostic and assists in differentiating from acute pulmonary hypertension, often demonstrating reduced biventricular preload, normal systolic function, and sub-systemic pulmonary artery pressure.

### ACUTE PULMONARY HYPERTENSION OF THE NEWBORN

The syndrome of acute pulmonary hypertension (aPH) at birth, previously termed persistent pulmonary hypertension of the newborn (PPHN), presents clinically as an infant with HRF out of proportion to the degree of lung abnormality and is associated with significant interaction between the lungs and cardiovascular system. This syndrome is often not simply a uniform entity of raised pulmonary vascular resistance but rather is potentially a conglomerate of clinical conditions, of which the clinical response to therapeutic agents is dependent on the relative effect of each of the components. The effect of each component on the respiratory system is also variable. The underlying components of aPH include lung pathology and VQ mismatch (meconium aspiration, pneumonia), the effect on ventricular systolic dysfunction (potentiated by conditions such as asphyxia), patency of the ductus arteriosus, the relative pressures across the PDA guiding the direction of the transductal shunt, the pulmonary vascular resistance, and the systemic vascular resistance. Each of these components has some influence on the respiratory system – some more directly than others.

The adverse effect of pulmonary parenchymal disease, which results in VQ mismatch, is reduced gas exchange with poor oxygenation and carbon dioxide retention, both of which in turn may result in increased pulmonary vascular resistance. Increased PVR and associated increased PAp may both reduce pulmonary blood flow and facilitate a pulmonary-to-systemic shunt across the PDA (depending on the relative systemic blood pressure). Pulmonary blood flow may be reduced due to poor RV function, increased afterload from both pulmonary vascular resistance and lung air space changes that directly impinge on the patency of pulmonary blood vessels. The iatrogenic effect of mechanical ventilation or increased positive pressure also contributes to this impingement on the pulmonary blood vessels. The effect of reduced pulmonary blood flow due to multiple underlying causes flows onto the systemic side of the heart with reduced filling of the left atrium and subsequently decreased LV output. The reduced LV output may be exacerbated by asphyxial myocardial injury – with up to 70% of asphyxiated infants demonstrating evidence of abnormal cardiac function when cardiac output is measured.[28,29] The reduction in systemic blood flow may then in turn result in reduced systemic blood flow and blood pressure, which results in more right-to-left shunting through the PDA. Finally, the ventricular interdependence of the right and left

ventricles, which share a septum and fibers and are constrained by the pericardium, can result in further reductions in the LV output due to decreased cavity size and preload from septal bowing away from the right ventricle in the setting of high pulmonary vascular pressures.[30]

The titration of mechanical ventilatory support to modulate PVR may be clinically important for conditions, such as hydrops fetalis or aPH, where RV systolic dysfunction and associated decreased pulmonary blood flow, are common contributors to HRF and circulatory instability. Among most neonates with normal cardiac anatomy, PVR is the main contributor to pulmonary artery pressure (and RV afterload). Hence the titration of mechanical ventilation to target lung volumes at FRC and minimize PVR (and RV afterload) is a core tenet of clinical management to improve RV performance and pulmonary blood flow, in part because the RV is intolerant of increased afterload. In contrast to the ellipse-shaped and thicker-walled left ventricle that is well-equipped to function under conditions of increased afterload, the RV is thin walled and crescent shaped, designed to function as a flow generator accommodating the entire systemic venous return to the heart.[31] In response to high PVR (and increased pulmonary artery pressure), the RV may adapt by increasing myocardial contractility (known as a homeometric adaptation),[32] but if this adaptation fails, RV dilatation occurs, damaging the RV contractile apparatus by lengthening the individual sarcomeres beyond their optimal interactive capacity.

Among term and near-term neonates with severe HRF after birth, inhaled nitric oxide improves oxygenation and reduces the risk of death or treatment with extracorporeal membrane oxygenation.[33] However, a minority of neonates exhibit no improvement in oxygenation with iNO, which is associated with increased mortality/ECMO[34] and may be due to ongoing reduced pulmonary blood flow potentiated by RV systolic dysfunction.[35] The combination of high PAp, low PBF, and worsening RV systolic dysfunction may potentiate a vicious cycle of severe systemic hypoxemia and cardiogenic shock, owing to "right-to-left" shunts at the level of the patent foramen ovale and ductus arteriosus, declining biventricular outputs and worsening lactic acidosis. Among neonates with severe HRF and PH who are iNO non-responders, urgent echocardiography evaluation is important to identify the underlying pathophysiology of elevated PAp to guide appropriate treatment. For example, neonates with persistent fetal circulation ("right-to-left" shunts at the level of the PFO and ductus arteriosus) with severe RV dysfunction should be treated with inotropic agents aimed at augmenting RVO (e.g., epinephrine, dobutamine). Clinicians performing echocardiography on neonates with suspected PPHN should also remember to rule out obstructed total anomalous pulmonary venous connections, as the elevated pulmonary venous pressure and ensuing low left atrial pressure (combined with elevated right heart pressures) may present as otherwise "classic" persistent fetal circulation.

## ATYPICAL ACUTE PULMONARY HYPERTENSION

Among neonates with severe HRF who do not experience improved oxygenation with administration of inhaled nitric oxide, echocardiography evaluation is critical to identify the relative contributory effects of "pre-capillary" vs. "post-capillary" disease (Figure 4.6). In contrast to "classic PPHN", which is characterized by persistent fetal circulation and often complicated by severe right heart dysfunction, severe HRF and acute pulmonary hypertension may be associated with

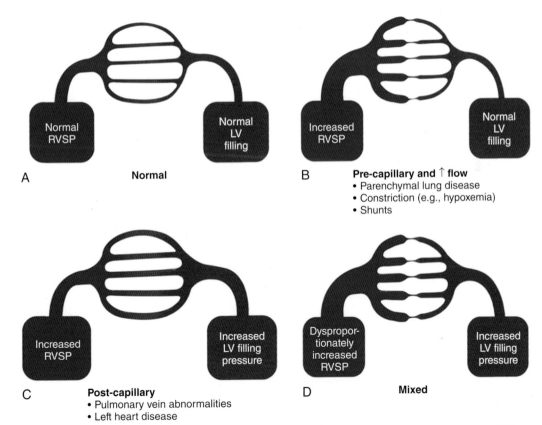

**Fig. 4.6 Range of abnormalities in pulmonary hypertension.** Panel A shows a normal scenario with normal PVR and normal LV filling pressures. Panel B shows normal LV filling pressures but increased PVR resulting in elevated pulmonary artery pressure. Panel C demonstrates increased LV filling pressures with normal PVR, resulting in pulmonary hypertension due to left heart disease. Panel D shows a mixed picture, with increased LV filling pressure but a disproportionate increase in pulmonary artery pressure caused by increased PVR. *LV*, Left ventricle; *PVR*, pulmonary vascular resistance; *RVSP*, right ventricular systolic pressure. (Reproduced with permission from Naing et al.[65])

increased PCWP. Recognition of a potentially dominant contributory role of increased PCWP typically occurs after a lack of improvement in oxygenation with the administration of iNO, prompting echocardiography evaluation, which may demonstrate severely reduced LV systolic function, often with relatively spared RV systolic function. Chest radiography may demonstrate pulmonary edema, but often an absence of radiographic evidence of pulmonary parenchymal disease. Such pathophysiology may be encountered among a minority of neonates with hypoxic-ischemic encephalopathy undergoing therapeutic hypothermia and is associated with increased mortality.[20]

Neonates whose pathophysiology of severe HRF is dominated by increased PCWP require intensive care management with different hemodynamic goals compared with neonates with classic PPHN. Specifically, these neonates may derive greater benefit from mechanical ventilatory support and pharmacological therapies aimed at optimizing LV loading conditions, augmenting LV stroke volume, and reducing LV filling pressures rather than the administration of pulmonary arterial vasodilators.[21] Positive pressure ventilatory support may have a beneficial effect by both reducing LV afterload and facilitating alveolar recruitment and patency in the setting of pulmonary edema from pulmonary venous hypertension. Improvement in LV stroke volume may be facilitated through the administration of inotropic (e.g., low-dose epinephrine [0.01–0.1 μg/kg/min], dobutamine) or inodilator agents (e.g., milrinone), the selection should be influenced by systemic blood pressure and the presence or absence of tachycardia. Cardiovascular therapeutic agents with a predominantly vasopressor effect, such as vasopressin, phenylephrine or high-dose epinephrine (≥0.3 μg/kg/min) are contraindicated, as LV stroke volume would be further compromised.

### PATENT DUCTUS ARTERIOSUS

The effect of a PDA on the lung occurs at multiple levels and at differing time points. The initial effect occurs with increasing left-to-right shunt through a PDA that has failed to constrict fully, usually in the setting of a premature birth. Failure of full constriction in the first few hours in the setting of an infant who has rapidly improving lung compliance results in

an increasing left-to-right shunt through the PDA. The resultant increased pulmonary blood flow has several effects. The first is the physical effect of stiffer lungs, which are more difficult for the infant to inflate or require a higher positive pressure. Premature infants may develop carbon dioxide retention or have increasing apnoea and need for respiratory support. Secondly, the increased blood flow through lung blood vessels and capillaries results in fluid leakage into the interstitial tissues, predisposing infants to lung damage and the need for increased respiratory support.

The association between PDA and BPD is clear but the causal pathways leading to this are less so. This area is further confused by the apparent lack of effect in reducing BPD in clinical trials of early treatment to close the PDA. These trials however are problematic in that there were large variations in patient clinical features, limited echocardiography standardization, and a high incidence of open-label treatment confounding the results. Recent studies have implicated a minimum duration of mechanical ventilation in concert with a large PDA shunt in the pathophysiology of BPD.[36,37]

## Cardiopulmonary Interactions Associated With Modes of Positive Pressure Ventilation

### CONVENTIONAL VS. HIGH-FREQUENCY VENTILATION: WHICH MODE OF MECHANICAL VENTILATION OPTIMIZES CARDIOPULMONARY INTERACTIONS IN NEONATES?

The hemodynamic impact of mechanical ventilation appears to be dependent on the mean airway pressure administered rather than being affected by the mode of ventilation (conventional vs. high-frequency ventilation). In an animal model of the preterm neonate with respiratory distress syndrome during the first day after birth, both conventional and high-frequency ventilation had similar effects on LV output and effective systemic blood flow for an equivalent mean airway pressure.[38,39] Similarly, no adverse effects on the systemic, cerebral, or splanchnic circulations were identified among human preterm neonates with RDS or pulmonary interstitial emphysema who required rescue high-frequency oscillatory ventilation (HFOV).[40,41]

Over the past decade, volume-targeted, pressure-limited modes of high-frequency ventilation have become available with the aim of achieving stable tidal volume and minute ventilation, though the hemodynamic impact of this change has only recently been evaluated. In a randomized trial involving late-preterm piglets with induced RDS, HFOV using a volume-targeted, pressure-limited mode ("volume guarantee", HFOV-VG) resulted in similar LV output and brain, lung, and heart markers of oxidative stress, ischemia, and inflammation compared with pressure-targeted HFOV.[26] However, HFOV-VG resulted in reduced cerebral blood flow and oxygenation, a finding whose clinical significance and impact on outcomes requires further study.[42]

In contrast, no neonatal studies have evaluated the hemodynamic impact of high-frequency jet ventilation (HFJV) in neonates. Adult animal models of heart failure have reported an overall neutral hemodynamic effect of HFJV compared with CMV, with HFJV causing a reduction in LV transmural systolic pressure (reduced afterload) but no improvement in stroke volume due to a simultaneous increase in LV end-diastolic pressure (reduced preload).[43]

## NEURALLY ADJUSTED VENTILATORY ASSIST

Neurally adjusted ventilatory assist (NAVA) is increasingly being applied during ventilatory support for neonates treated with both invasive and non-invasive ventilation (NIV). Clinical trials among preterm neonates have demonstrated lower diaphragmatic electrical activity and improved ventilator synchrony and respiratory efforts and extubation success with NIV-NAVA, compared with nasal continuous positive airway pressure (nCPAP) or non-invasive positive pressure ventilation (NIPPV).[44-46] While the cardiopulmonary effects of NAVA among preterm neonates have not been investigated, studies in adults with heart failure and children with congenital heart disease have reported favorable hemodynamic effects. Compared with conventional mechanical ventilation, invasive NAVA facilitates improved cerebral blood flow after cardiac surgery.[47] In addition, use of NAVA results in less RV dysfunction, possibly due to preservation of cyclic ITP changes characteristic of spontaneous ventilation and/or limitation of RV outflow impedance during inspiration.[48] Additional investigations are required to identify specific hemodynamic conditions, beyond undifferentiated respiratory failure, where adjunct support with NAVA may be beneficial in neonates.

## SYSTEMIC AND CEREBRAL HEMODYNAMIC IMPACT OF NON-INVASIVE RESPIRATORY SUPPORT IN NEONATES

High-quality evidence supports avoiding delivery room mechanical ventilation among extremely preterm neonates, to improve neonatal mortality and morbidity,[49-51] including employing minimally invasive methods for the administration of exogenous surfactant for respiratory distress syndrome.[52] Although primary non-invasive positive pressure support is now the preferred initial method of ventilatory support after birth, the optimal mode of non-invasive respiratory support among preterm neonates is controversial. Moreover, the systemic and cerebral hemodynamic impact of less invasive surfactant administration and the various modes of non-invasive respiratory support have only recently been evaluated.

Although there remains uncertainty regarding the relative effectiveness of nasal continuous positive airway pressure (nCPAP) versus NIPPV for respiratory support among preterm neonates, they appear to have similar impacts on the systemic, pulmonary, and cerebral circulations. Prospective, randomized, cross-over, clinical trials in stable moderately and extremely preterm neonates have identified similar left and right ventricular outputs, superior vena cava flow and cerebral artery flow velocities among these two common modes of respiratory support.[53,54] These studies suggest that among stable preterm neonates requiring non-invasive respiratory support, clinicians may select either nCPAP or NIPPV without an appreciable hemodynamic impact. Additional studies enrolling neonates with hemodynamic disturbance are needed to determine whether a particular mode of non-invasive respiratory support may be beneficial in the critical management of neonates with disease.

The administration of surfactant via endotracheal tube is known to result in rapid changes in systemic and pulmonary hemodynamics.[55] Less invasive surfactant administration has recently been demonstrated to have a similar hemodynamic impact, including rapid reduction in PVR and improvement in echocardiography indices of RV systolic performance.[56] However, fetal growth restriction (FGR) appears to modulate the hemodynamic impact of surfactant administration. Compared with appropriate for gestational age (AGA) preterm neonates, FGR preterm neonates experience smaller increases in indices of right ventricular systolic performance, and cerebral blood flow, which may reflect the lasting effects of altered cardiac maldevelopment from an *in utero* maladaptive state.[57,58] The clinical implications of these circulatory differences among preterm neonates with FGR require further study.

## Cardiopulmonary Interactions in the Management of Structural Heart Disease

The impact of positive pressure ventilation on hemodynamics among neonates with structural heart disease depends on the underlying physiology, with the potential for both beneficial and deleterious effects. Among neonates with single-ventricle physiology (e.g., hypoplastic left heart syndrome), modulation of PVR is a primary mechanism of balancing systemic and pulmonary blood flow and can be influenced by titrating lung volumes, $FiO_2$, serum pH, and minute ventilation ($PaCO_2$).[59,60]

In addition, neonates with severe ventricular hypertrophy (e.g., among neonates born to mothers with poorly controlled diabetes mellitus) and obstruction to LV outflow may experience hemodynamic instability with the initiation or escalation of mechanical ventilation. Increased LV filling pressures (diastolic dysfunction) in these neonates necessitate close attention to loading conditions, including preservation of both preload and afterload to maintain LV output. However, positive pressure support will decrease both LV preload and afterload, which may exacerbate outflow tract obstruction and compromise LV stroke volume.[61] Hemodynamic support of neonates with LV outflow obstruction who are supported with mechanical ventilation may be optimized with sufficient administration of volume expanders and systemic vasopressors (e.g., vasopressin), and avoidance of therapies with positive β1-adrenergic effects (which reduce time for LV filling, e.g., dopamine, dobutamine, epinephrine) or systemic vasodilators (which reduce LV end-diastolic volume, as well as coronary perfusion pressure; e.g., milrinone, sodium nitroprusside).[62]

## Conclusion

Understanding the interaction between the respiratory and cardiovascular systems is important in the management of neonates in the intensive care unit. The impact of respiration on circulatory function and vice versa is prominent throughout the period of critical illness. There is an optimal balance between the use of positive pressure ventilation to improve alveolar ventilation and the effects that higher MAP will have on systemic, and particularly pulmonary, blood flow. As both alveolar oxygenation and systemic blood flow are required for oxygen delivery, this balance must be carefully considered. The nature of the pulmonary and systemic circulations in series implies that alterations in atrial and/or ventricular pressures may adversely impact the pulmonary circulation. While the clinical phenotype of HRF associated with aPH is common in the NICU, cardiorespiratory interactions are key considerations in intensive care decisions, depending on the underlying pathophysiology. Both the selection of cardiovascular therapeutics and titration of mechanical ventilation depend on the nature of pulmonary parenchymal disease and contributory effects of left and/or right heart disease. Finally, although a multitude of modes of invasive and non-invasive ventilation support are now available in the NICU, their relative effects on the cardiovascular system appear similar for a given mean airway pressure.

## REFERENCES

1. Drees JA, Rothe CF. Reflex venoconstriction and capacity vessel pressure-volume relationships in dogs. *Circ Res.* 1974;34(3):360-373.
2. Guyton AC, Lindsey AW, Abernathy B, Langston JB. Mechanism of the increased venous return and cardiac output caused by epinephrine. *Am J Physiol.* 1958;192(1):126-130.
3. Takata M, Robotham JL. Effects of inspiratory diaphragmatic descent on inferior vena caval venous return. *J Appl Physiol (1985).* 1992;72(2):597-607.
4. Takata M, Wise RA, Robotham JL. Effects of abdominal pressure on venous return: abdominal vascular zone conditions. *J Appl Physiol (1985).* 1990;69(6):1961-1972.
5. Guyton AC, Adkins LH. Quantitative aspects of the collapse factor in relation to venous return. *Am J Physiol.* 1954;177(3):523-527.
6. Peters J, Kindred MK, Robotham JL. Transient analysis of cardiopulmonary interactions. II. Systolic events. *J Appl Physiol (1985).* 1988;64(4):1518-1526.

7. Jardin F, Farcot JC, Gueret P, Prost JF, Ozier Y, Bourdarias JP. Cyclic changes in arterial pulse during respiratory support. *Circulation*. 1983;68(2):266-274.

8. Haldén E, Jakobson S, Janerås L. The effect of positive end-expiratory pressure on central haemodynamics in the pig. *Acta Anaesthesiol Scand*. 1981;25(6):538-542.

9. Tana M, Polglase GR, Cota F, et al. Determination of lung volume and hemodynamic changes during high-frequency ventilation recruitment in preterm neonates with respiratory distress syndrome. *Crit Care Med*. 2015;43(8):1685-1691.

10. Dhainaut JF, Devaux JY, Monsallier JF, Brunet F, Villemant D, Huyghebaert MF. Mechanisms of decreased left ventricular preload during continuous positive pressure ventilation in ARDS. *Chest*. 1986;90(1):74-80.

11. Stalcup SA, Mellins RB. Mechanical forces producing pulmonary edema in acute asthma. *N Engl J Med*. 1977;297(11):592-596.

12. Pinsky MR, Summer WR. Cardiac augmentation by phasic high intrathoracic pressure support in man. *Chest*. 1983;84(4):370-375.

13. Pinsky MR, Summer WR, Wise RA, Permutt S, Bromberger-Barnea B. Augmentation of cardiac function by elevation of intrathoracic pressure. *J Appl Physiol Respir Environ Exerc Physiol*. 1983;54(4):950-955.

14. Denault AY, Gorcsan J III, Pinsky MR. Dynamic effects of positive-pressure ventilation on canine left ventricular pressure-volume relations. *J Appl Physiol (1985)*. 2001;91(1):298-308.

15. Fessler HE, Brower RG, Wise RA, Permutt S. Mechanism of reduced LV afterload by systolic and diastolic positive pleural pressure. *J Appl Physiol (1985)*. 1988;65(3):1244-1250.

16. Rasanen J, Heikkila J, Downs J, Nikki P, Vaisanen I, Viitanen A. Continuous positive airway pressure by face mask in acute cardiogenic pulmonary edema. *Am J Cardiol*. 1985;55(4):296-300.

17. Kennedy SK, Weintraub RM, Skillman JJ. Cardiorespiratory and sympathoadrenal responses during weaning from controlled ventilation. *Surgery*. 1977;82(2):233-240.

18. Kulik TJ. Pulmonary blood flow and pulmonary hypertension: is the pulmonary circulation flowophobic or flowophilic? *Pulm Circ*. 2012;2(3):327-339.

19. Wood P, Besterman EM, Towers MK, McIlroy MB. The effect of acetylcholine on pulmonary vascular resistance and left atrial pressure in mitral stenosis. *Br Heart J*. 1957;19(2):279-286.

20. Friedman WF. The intrinsic physiologic properties of the developing heart. In: Friedman WF, Lesch M, Sonnenblick EH, eds. *Neonatal Heart Disease*. New York: Grune and Stratton; 1972:21-49.

21. Nelin LD, Wearden ME, Welty SE, Hansen TN. The effect of blood flow and left atrial pressure on the DLCO in lambs and sheep. *Respir Physiol*. 1992;88(3):333-342.

22. Pérez Fontán JJ, Clyman RI, Mauray F, Heymann MA, Roman C. Respiratory effects of a patent ductus arteriosus in premature newborn lambs. *J Appl Physiol (1985)*. 1987;63(6):2315-2324.

23. Alpan G, Scheerer R, Bland R, Clyman R. Patent ductus arteriosus increases lung fluid filtration in preterm lambs. *Pediatr Res*. 1991;30(6):616-621.

24. Matsuda T, Anderson-Morris J, Raj JU. Microvascular pressures in isolated perfused immature lamb lungs: effects of flow rate, left atrial pressure and surfactant therapy. *Biol Neonate*. 1996;70(6):349-358.

25. Ikegami M, Jacobs H, Jobe A. Surfactant function in respiratory distress syndrome. *J Pediatr*. 1983;102(3):443-447.

26. Baraldi E, Pettenazzo A, Filippone M, Magagnin GP, Saia OS, Zacchello F. Rapid improvement of static compliance after surfactant treatment in preterm infants with respiratory distress syndrome. *Pediatr Pulmonol*. 1993;15(3):157-162.

27. Klingenberg C, Wheeler KI, McCallion N, Morley CJ, Davis PG. Volume-targeted versus pressure-limited ventilation in neonates. *Cochrane Database Syst Rev*. 2017;10(10):CD003666.

28. Altit G, Bonifacio SL, Guimaraes CV, et al. Cardiac dysfunction in neonatal HIE is associated with increased mortality and brain injury by MRI [published online ahead of print, 2021 Sep 7]. *Am J Perinatol*. 2021. doi:10.1055/s-0041-1735618.

29. Sehgal A, Wong F, Menahem S. Speckle tracking derived strain in infants with severe perinatal asphyxia: a comparative case control study. *Cardiovasc Ultrasound*. 2013;11:34.

30. Jain A, El-Khuffash AF, van Herpen CH, et al. Cardiac function and ventricular interactions in persistent pulmonary hypertension of the newborn. *Pediatr Crit Care Med*. 2021;22(2):e145-e157.

31. Haddad F, Hunt SA, Rosenthal DN, Murphy DJ. Right ventricular function in cardiovascular disease, part I: anatomy, physiology, aging, and functional assessment of the right ventricle. *Circulation*. 2008;117(11):1436-1448.

32. Sarnoff SJ, Mitchell JH, Gilmore JP, Remensnyder JP. Homeometric autoregulation in the heart. *Circ Res*. 1960;8:1077-1091.

33. Barrington KJ, Finer N, Pennaforte T, Altit G. Nitric oxide for respiratory failure in infants born at or near term. *Cochrane Database Syst Rev*. 2017;1(1):CD000399.

34. Dillard J, Pavlek LR, Korada S, Chen B. Worsened short-term clinical outcomes in a cohort of patients with iNO-unresponsive PPHN: a case for improving iNO responsiveness. *J Perinatol*. 2022;42(1):37-44.

35. Bischoff AR, Giesinger RE, Neary E, Weisz DE, Belik J, McNamara PJ. Clinical and echocardiography predictors of response to inhaled nitric oxide in hypoxemic term and near-term neonates. *Pediatr Pulmonol*. 2021;56(5):982-991.

36. Clyman RI, Kaempf J, Liebowitz M, et al. Prolonged tracheal intubation and the association between patent ductus arteriosus and bronchopulmonary dysplasia: a secondary analysis of the PDA-TOLERATE trial. *J Pediatr*. 2021;229:283-288.e2.

37. Clyman RI, Hills NK, Cambonie G, et al. Patent ductus arteriosus, tracheal ventilation, and the risk of bronchopulmonary dysplasia. *Pediatr Res*. 2022;91:652-658.

38. Kinsella JP, Gerstmann DR, Clark RH, et al. High-frequency oscillatory ventilation versus intermittent mandatory ventilation: early hemodynamic effects in the premature baboon with hyaline membrane disease. *Pediatr Res*. 1991;29(2):160-166.

39. Oguchi K, Baylen BG, Ikegami M, et al. Hemodynamic effects of high frequency ventilation in surfactant-treated preterm lambs. *Biol Neonate*. 1986;49(1):21-28.

40. Nelle M, Zilow EP, Linderkamp O. Effects of high-frequency oscillatory ventilation on circulation in neonates with pulmonary interstitial emphysema or RDS. *Intensive Care Med*. 1997;23(6):671-676.

41. Ayoub D, Elmashad A, Rowisha M, Eltomey M, El Amrousy D. Hemodynamic effects of high-frequency oscillatory ventilation in preterm neonates with respiratory distress syndrome. *Pediatr Pulmonol*. 2021;56(2):424-432.

42. Bhogal J, Solevåg AL, O'Reilly M, et al. Hemodynamic effects of high frequency oscillatory ventilation with volume guarantee in a piglet model of respiratory distress syndrome. *PLoS One*. 2021;16(2):e0246996.

43. Weber A, Mathru M, Rooney MW. Effect of jet ventilation on heart failure: decreased afterload but negative response in left ventricular end-systolic pressure-volume function. *Crit Care Med.* 1996;24(4):647-657.

44. Treussart C, Decobert F, Tauzin M, et al. Patient-ventilator synchrony in extremely premature neonates during non-invasive neurally adjusted ventilatory assist or synchronized intermittent positive airway pressure: a randomized crossover pilot trial. *Neonatology.* 2022;119(3):386-393.

45. Shin SH, Shin SH, Kim SH, et al. Noninvasive neurally adjusted ventilation in postextubation stabilization of preterm infants: a randomized controlled study. *J Pediatr.* 2022;247:53-59.e1.

46. Latremouille S, Bhuller M, Shalish W, Sant'Anna G. Cardiorespiratory effects of NIV-NAVA, NIPPV, and NCPAP shortly after extubation in extremely preterm infants: a randomized crossover trial. *Pediatr Pulmonol.* 2021;56(10):3273-3282.

47. Zhu L, Xu Z, Gong X, et al. Mechanical ventilation after bidirectional superior cavopulmonary anastomosis for single-ventricle physiology: a comparison of pressure support ventilation and neurally adjusted ventilatory assist. *Pediatr Cardiol.* 2016; 37(6):1064-1071.

48. Berger D, Bloechlinger S, Takala J, Sinderby C, Brander L. Heart-lung interactions during neurally adjusted ventilatory assist. *Crit Care.* 2014;18(5):499.

49. Stevens TP, Finer NN, Carlo WA, et al. Respiratory outcomes of the surfactant positive pressure and oximetry randomized trial (SUPPORT). *J Pediatr.* 2014;165(2):240-249.e4.

50. Vaucher YE, Peralta-Carcelen M, Finer NN, et al. Neurodevelopmental outcomes in the early CPAP and pulse oximetry trial. *N Engl J Med.* 2012;367(26):2495-2504.

51. Finer NN, Carlo WA, Walsh MC, et al. Early CPAP versus surfactant in extremely preterm infants. *N Engl J Med.* 2010;362(21): 1970-1979.

52. Abdel-Latif ME, Davis PG, Wheeler KI, De Paoli AG, Dargaville PA. Surfactant therapy via thin catheter in preterm infants with or at risk of respiratory distress syndrome. *Cochrane Database Syst Rev.* 2021;5(5):CD011672.

53. Mukerji A, Abdul Wahab MG, Razak A, et al. High CPAP vs. NIPPV in preterm neonates – A physiological cross-over study. *J Perinatol.* 2021;41(7):1690-1696.

54. Chang HY, Cheng KS, Lung HL, et al. Hemodynamic effects of nasal intermittent positive pressure ventilation in preterm infants. *Medicine (Baltimore).* 2016;95(6):e2780.

55. Sehgal A, Mak W, Dunn M, et al. Haemodynamic changes after delivery room surfactant administration to very low birth weight infants. *Arch Dis Child Fetal Neonatal Ed.* 2010;95(5): F345-F351.

56. Sehgal A, Bhatia R, Roberts CT. Cardiorespiratory physiology following minimally invasive surfactant therapy in preterm infants. *Neonatology.* 2019;116(3):278-285.

57. Sehgal A, Bhatia R, Roberts CT. Cardiovascular response and sequelae after minimally invasive surfactant therapy in growth-restricted preterm infants. *J Perinatol.* 2020;40(8):1178-1184.

58. Malhotra A, Miller SL, Jenkin G, et al. Fetal growth restriction is associated with an altered cardiopulmonary and cerebral hemodynamic response to surfactant therapy in preterm lambs. *Pediatr Res.* 2019;86(1):47-54.

59. Triantaris A, Aidonidis I, Hatziefthimiou A, Gourgoulianis K, Zakynthinos G, Makris D. Elevated $PaCO_2$ levels increase pulmonary artery pressure. *Sci Prog.* 2022;105(2):368504221094161.

60. Magoon R, Makhija N, Jangid SK. Balancing a single-ventricle circulation: "physiology to therapy". *Indian J Thorac Cardiovasc Surg.* 2020;36(2):159-162.

61. Braunwald E, Oldham Jr HN, Ross Jr J, Linhart JW, Mason DT, Fort L III. The circulatory response of patients with idiopathic hypertrophic subaortic stenosis to nitroglycerin and to the Valsalva maneuver. *Circulation.* 1964;29:422-431.

62. Boyd SM, Riley KL, Giesinger RE, McNamara PJ. Use of vasopressin in neonatal hypertrophic obstructive cardiomyopathy: case series. *J Perinatol.* 2021;41(1):126-133.

63. Weisz DE, Jain A, McNamara PJ *Patent Ductus Arteriosus.* Buenos Aires: Ediciones Journal S.A; 2016. https://www.amazon.com/Patent-Ductus-Arteriosus-Dany-Weisz-ebook/dp/B01EVTIIG8.

64. Weisz DE, McNamara PJ. Cardiovascular assessment. In: Goldsmith J, Karotkin E, Suresh G, Keszler M, eds. *Assisted Ventilation of the Neonate.* 6th ed. Philadelphia: Elsevier; 2016.

65. Naing P, Kuppusamy H, Scalia G, Hillis GS, Playford D. Non-invasive assessment of pulmonary vascular resistance in pulmonary hypertension: current knowledge and future direction. *Heart Lung Circ.* 2017;26(4):323-330.

# Chapter 5

# Neonatal Cardiovascular Drugs

Danielle R. Rios, Angelica Vasquez, and Christopher McPherson

## Key Points

- Highlighting the importance of understanding physiology prior to prescribing medications will enable the provider to choose the preferred regimen for each particular patient.

- Extrapolating data from older pediatric populations and adults must be done with caution, considering the unique physiology and differences in pharmacokinetics and pharmacodynamics in critically ill neonates and infants.

- Understanding the mechanism of action and therapeutic effects (both desired and side effects) will enable the provider to better anticipate changes to be seen and monitor effects.

## Introduction

There are a number of cardiovascular medications that are used in neonatology on a regular basis. An understanding of physiology can guide the clinician toward the selection of a specific medication based on mechanism of action that is necessary to manage the patient-specific disease state. Each medication will have a range of side effects that should be considered when choosing a medication therapy regimen, and even more so when utilizing this class of medications in critically ill neonates. Extrapolating data from older pediatric or adult patients must be done with caution considering the unique physiology of critically ill neonates. For example, the premature neonatal heart contains only 30% contractile tissue, in contrast to 60% in the adult heart.[1] Additionally, expression of sarcoplasmic reticulum and t-tubules is low, while mitochondria are abundant, resulting in disorganized myocyte activity. These maturational differences are tolerated in the intrauterine environment dominated by low placental resistance. However, with exposure to ex utero systemic vascular resistance, the stress of illness, and inotropes or vasopressors, cardiovascular function may be impaired.

The adrenergic system and myocardial innervation both mature throughout gestation.[2] This maturation is driven to some extent by stimulation, and fetal adrenoreceptors have a low threshold for provocation. In preterm neonates this manifests as "denervation hypersensitivity," in which myocardial adrenoreceptors demonstrate maximal response to even small concentrations of catecholamine.[3] Importantly, maturation is not uniform, as active alpha-1-receptors outnumber beta-1-receptors in early gestation.[4] Consequently, agents with non-specific activity like dopamine have a different dose-response profile in premature neonates, term neonates, and older patients. Critical illness further complicates dose-response. Renal maldevelopment or maladaptation has implications on drug elimination with lower albumin binding leading to increased drug available for metabolism in the setting of less efficient renal clearance of active drug and metabolites. Hypoxic-ischemic encephalopathy complicates the consequences of bradycardia (induced by therapeutic hypothermia or medications like dexmedetomidine in the setting of existing cardiac dysfunction induced by hypoxia-ischemia) and tachycardia (induced by exogenous catecholamines in the setting of metabolic insufficiency and/or hypocalcemia compromising right ventricular performance).[5] Additionally, decreased renal clearance in this population may exacerbate the therapeutic or adverse effects of pharmacologic interventions.[6] In confluence, this complex milieu highlights the vital nature of optimizing diagnostic techniques and understanding the specific impacts of available pharmacotherapies.

This chapter will discuss the mechanism of action and therapeutic effects of cardiovascular medications used most commonly in critically ill neonates and infants based on predominant pathology grouping (Tables 5.1 and 5.2). We will not be discussing medication regimens for treatment of a hemodynamically significant patent ductus arteriosus (PDA), as these are discussed in detail in Chapter 17. Critical evaluation of available pharmacologic studies and randomized controlled trials was vital to generation of the content of this chapter. However, this evaluation highlighted the profound limitations of the available data. Therefore the information in this chapter should be interpreted in the context of emerging evidence.

## Cardiovascular Support of Heart Function

When attempting to support heart function, a combination of inotropes and vasodilators may be utilized. Inotropes are medications that act primarily on the cardiac myocyte (Figure 5.1) to increase contractility, whereas vasodilators decrease wall tension leading to an improvement in stroke volume and cardiac output. In this section we will discuss two predominant inotropes, dobutamine and epinephrine; two inotropes with vasodilator effects, milrinone and levosimendan; and sodium nitroprusside, a primary vasodilator.

### PREDOMINANT INOTROPE

#### Dobutamine

1. **Mechanism of action:** Dobutamine is a synthetic catecholamine that is a racemic mixture of two parts (negative and positive isomers) and promotes direct stimulation of adrenergic receptors in the myocardium.[7] The negative isomer is an alpha-1-receptor agonist and increases systemic vascular resistance (SVR) and myocardial contractility. The positive isomer is a beta-1- and beta-2-receptor agonist, which increases myocardial contractility and heart rate while decreasing SVR. It is also a potent alpha-1-receptor antagonist that blocks the effects of the negative isomer. The resulting effects of dobutamine are increased inotropy and chronotropy, with no effect on, or a decrease in, SVR.[8,9]
2. **Dosing** is via continuous infusion; the usual dosing range is 2–20 mcg/kg/min. Improved left ventricular (LV) performance in preterm infants is achieved at doses of 5–10 mcg/kg/min[10-12]

with changes in cardiac output within 20 minutes and improvement in systemic markers after 8–10 hours.[13]
3. **Pharmacokinetics:** Dobutamine is metabolized by the liver and excreted in the urine. The half-life is 3–36 minutes in preterm neonates.[14]
4. **Examples of clinical use:** Right ventricular (RV) dysfunction in the setting of pulmonary hypertension (PH) or hypoxic-ischemic encephalopathy, LV dysfunction following interventional closure of PDA, myocarditis, or asphyxia.
5. **Adverse effects** include tachycardia, arrhythmias, hypertension, and hypotension.[12,15]
6. **Special considerations:** Expression of α-adrenergic receptors is upregulated in preterm infants as compared to β-adrenergic expression, which may result in attenuated decreases in SVR when compared to term infants.[8] Dobutamine has been shown to improve superior vena cava flow in preterm neonates when compared to dopamine.[16]

### Epinephrine

1. **Mechanism of action:** Epinephrine is an endogenous hormone secreted by the adrenal medulla. It is a potent stimulator of both α- and β-adrenergic receptors and its effects on body organ systems are expressed in a dose-dependent manner. The cardiac and vascular beta-1- and beta-2-adrenoreceptors are primarily stimulated at low doses (0.01–0.1 mcg/kg/min), which leads to increased inotropy, chronotropy, and conduction velocity and peripheral vasodilation (primarily in the muscles).[8] Doses >0.1 mcg/kg/min stimulate vascular and cardiac alpha-1-receptors leading to vasoconstriction and increased inotropy, while the alpha-2-receptor effects are less prominent.[8] Epinephrine has been shown to increase coronary artery blood flow,[17,18] cerebral perfusion,[19] and SVR and pulmonary vascular resistance (PVR) in a 1:1 ratio[20] or less[21] with some dose-dependent variability. However, it has also been shown in high doses to irreversibly disrupt the myocardial sarcolemma and swell the mitochondria with calcium deposition in a neonatal animal model.[22]

## TABLE 5.1  Overview of Cardiovascular Medications Used for Heart Function or Pulmonary Hypertension

| CARDIOVASCULAR SUPPORT OF HEART FUNCTION | | | | | |
|---|---|---|---|---|---|
| | Receptors/ Action | Predominant Effects | Dosing Range | Common Clinical Use | Comments |
| **Predominant Inotropes** | | | | | |
| 1. Dobutamine | Alpha-1-agonist Alpha-1-antagonist Beta-1, beta-2-agonist | ↑ HR, inotropy ↓/↔ SVR | 2–20 mcg/kg/min | RV dysfunction in PH or HIE, cardiac dysfunction in premature infants | Improvement seen in premature infants at doses limited to 5–10 mcg/kg/min |
| 2. Epinephrine | Alpha-1-agonist Alpha-2 effects less prominent beta-1, beta-2-agonist | ↑ HR, inotropy Vasodilation (muscle) Vasoconstriction ↑ PVR = SVR | 0.01–0.5 mcg/kg/min | Septic shock with cardiac dysfunction, severe cardiac dysfunction | Avoid in patients with hypertrophic cardiomyopathy |
| **Inotropes With Vasodilator Effects** | | | | | |
| 1. Milrinone | PDE-3 inhibitor | ↓ SVR, PVR, inotropy, and lusitropy | 0.25–1 mcg/kg/min | Low cardiac output syndrome after cardiac surgery, PLCS, PH, CDH | Caution in poor renal function or decreased renal clearance |
| 2. Levosimendan | PDE-3 inhibitor | ↓ SVR, PVR, inotropy | 0.05–0.2 mcg/kg/min | Patients requiring afterload reduction and inotropy | Not available in United States or Canada |
| **Primary Vasodilator** | | | | | |
| 1. Sodium nitroprusside | Arterial and venous vasodilator | Vasodilation ↓ SVR | 0.5–2 mcg/kg/min | Hypertensive crisis | Close monitoring needed to avoid severe hypotension and hypoperfusion |
| CARDIOVASCULAR SUPPORT FOR ACUTE AND/OR CHRONIC PULMONARY HYPERTENSION | | | | | |
| **Pulmonary Vasodilator** | | | | | |
| 1. Inhaled nitric oxide | Selective pulmonary vasodilator | ↓ PVR | 1–20 ppm | Acute and chronic PH | Should be avoided in left-sided outflow tract obstruction and increased PCWP |
| **Phosphodiesterase Inhibitor** | | | | | |
| 1. Sildenafil | PDE-5 inhibitor | ↓ PVR ↓/↔ SVR | Continuous IV: 0.4 mg/kg over 3 hours, then 1.6 mg/kg/day IV: 0.4 mg/kg q6 PO: 0.5–3 mg/kg q6–8 | Chronic and occasionally acute PH | Could contribute to worsened V:Q mismatch |

*Continued on following page*

**TABLE 5.1 Overview of Cardiovascular Medications Used for Heart Function or Pulmonary Hypertension (Continued)**

| | Receptors/ Action | Predominant Effects | Dosing Range | Common Clinical Use | Comments |
|---|---|---|---|---|---|
| **Endothelin Receptor Antagonist** | | | | | |
| 1. Bosentan | $ET_A$ and $ET_B$ blocker | ↓ PVR | 1–2 mg/kg BID | Chronic PH | Liver enzymes need to be followed closely |
| **Prostacyclin Analogues** | | | | | |
| 1. Epoprostenol | Pulmonary and systemic vasodilator | ↓ PVR, SVR | Continuous IV: 50–80 ng/kg/min Inhalation: 20–50 ng/kg/min | Chronic PH and elevated PVR | Abrupt discontinuation results in rebound PH |
| 2. Treprostinil | Analogue of epoprostenol | ↓ PVR, SVR | IV or subcutaneous infusion 2–20 ng/kg/min | Chronic PH | Optimal for prolonged subcutaneous infusion due to stability in solution and relatively long half-life |
| 3. Iloprost | Analogue of epoprostenol | ↓ PVR, SVR | Inhalation: 0.25–2.5 mcg/kg q2–6 Nebulization: 0.8 mcg/kg/h | Chronic and occasionally acute PH | Less basic pH compared to epoprostenol facilitates nebulized delivery; however, data limited in neonates |
| **Prostaglandin E1** | | | | | |
| 1. Alprostadil | Vasodilation of vascular and PDA smooth muscle | ↓ PVR ↓/↔ SVR | 0.01–0.1 mcg/kg/min | CHD, PH with failing RV, acute PH | Apnea seen more often in <2 kg BW, higher starting doses, and during the first hour of infusion |
| **Soluble Guanylate Cyclase Stimulators** | | | | | |
| 1. Riociguat | sGC stimulation | ↓ PVR | 0.5–2 mg up to TID | Chronic PH | Should not be used within 24 hours of sildenafil |

*BID*, twice daily; *CDH*, congenital diaphragmatic hernia; *ET*, endothelin; *HIE*, hypoxic-ischemic encephalopathy; *HR*, heart rate; *IV*, intravenous; *PCWP*, pulmonary capillary wedge pressure; *PDA*, patent ductus arteriosus; *PDE*, phosphodiesterase; *PH*, pulmonary hypertension; *PLCS*, post-ligation cardiac syndrome; *PO*, per oral route; *PVR*, pulmonary vascular resistance; *RV*, right ventricle; *sGC*, soluble guanylate cyclase; *SVR*, systemic vascular resistance; *TID*, three times daily.

2. **Dosing** is via continuous infusion with a usual dosing range of 0.01–0.5 mcg/kg/min.[19,23]
3. **Pharmacokinetics:** Epinephrine is metabolized in the liver and excreted in the urine as inactivated compound. Data characterizing the pharmacokinetics of epinephrine in neonates are limited; the half-life in adults is less than 5 minutes.

4. **Examples of clinical use:** Septic shock with cardiac dysfunction and diseases associated with severe cardiac dysfunction.
5. **Adverse effects** include tachycardia, lactic acidosis independent of improvement in hemodynamic status, and hyperglycemia requiring insulin seen in premature infants.[19,23]

## TABLE 5.2 Overview of Cardiovascular Medications Used for Blood Pressure Support

### SUPPORT FOR SYSTEMIC HYPOTENSION

| | Receptors/Action | Predominant Effects | Dosing Range | Common Clinical Use | Comments |
|---|---|---|---|---|---|
| **Predominant Vasoconstrictors** | | | | | |
| 1. Vasopressin | Arginine vasopressin, oxytocin, and purinergic receptors | ↑ SVR<br>↓/↔ PVR<br>↓/↔ HR | 0.1–1.2 mU/kg/min<br>(0.006–0.072 U/kg/h) | Vasodilatory shock, PH with preserved LV function, hypotension, hypertrophic cardiomyopathy | Sodium levels must be monitored during use, prolonged therapy may result in polyuria and fluid imbalance upon discontinuation |
| 2. Norepinephrine | Alpha-1, alpha-2, beta-1 > beta-2 | ↑ SVR<br>Minor inotropy, chronotropy | 0.02–1 mcg/kg/min | Sepsis and shock | In presence of high oxygen concentrations, can induce pulmonary vasoconstriction |
| 3. Dopamine | CNS and peripheral dopaminergic, adrenergic (alpha-1, beta-1, beta-2), and serotonergic receptors | ↑ HR<br>↑ PVR > SVR | 2–20 mcg/kg/min | Sepsis in setting of no PH | Should be used with caution in premature infants due to the unpredictable nature of its effects |
| 4. Phenylephrine | Alpha-agonist | ↑ SVR | 0.1–0.5 mcg/kg/min | "Tet spells" | May cause severe bradycardia |
| **Glucocorticoids** | | | | | |
| 1. Hydrocortisone | Genomic and non-genomic effects | Variable | LD: 1–2 mg/kg<br>0.5–1 mg/kg q6–12 | Adjunctive therapy for relative or absolute adrenal insufficiency and pressor-resistant hypotension when increased cell surface receptors required (e.g., adrenergic receptors) | Concurrent use with indomethacin should be avoided |

### SUPPORT FOR SYSTEMIC HYPERTENSION

| | Receptors/Action | Predominant Effects | Dosing Range | Common Clinical Use | Comments |
|---|---|---|---|---|---|
| **Dihydropyridine** | | | | | |
| 1. Isradipine | CCB | ↓ SVR | 0.05–0.15 mg/kg QID | Acute hypertension | Rapid onset of action |
| 2. Amlodipine | CCB | ↓ SVR | 0.05–0.3 mg/kg 1–2 times daily | Chronic hypertension | Slower onset of action and longer duration of effect |
| **Angiotensin-Converting Enzyme (ACE) Inhibitors** | | | | | |
| 1. Enalapril(at) | Competitive inhibitor of ACE | ↓ SVR | PO: 0.04–0.3 mg/kg/day div 1–2 times daily<br>IV: 5–10 mcg/kg q8–24 | Hypertension, LV diastolic dysfunction, congestive heart failure | Use with caution in patients with impaired renal function or hypovolemia |

*ACE*, angiotensin-converting enzyme; *CCB*, calcium channel blocker; *HR*, heart rate; *IV*, intravenous; *LD*, loading dose; *PH*, pulmonary hypertension; *PO*, per oral route; *PVR*, pulmonary vascular resistance; *SVR*, systemic vascular resistance.

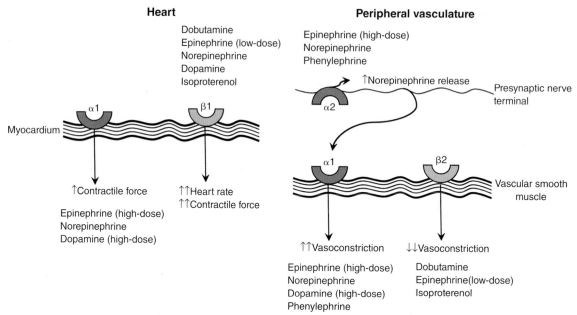

**Fig. 5.1** Effects of medications on adrenergic receptors in the heart and peripheral vasculature. (Adapted from Giesinger RE, McNamara PJ. Hemodynamic instability in the critically ill neonate: an approach to cardiovascular support based on disease pathophysiology. *Semin Perinatol.* 2016;40(3):174-188.)

6. **Special considerations:** In patients with acute PH caution is advised due to the potential increase in PVR and pulmonary artery pressure seen in animal studies.[20] Epinephrine, as is true with all drugs with β-adrenergic activity and chronotropic effects, should be avoided in patients with hypertrophic cardiomyopathy.

## INOTROPES WITH VASODILATOR EFFECTS

### Milrinone

1. **Mechanism of action:** Milrinone is a selective phosphodiesterase-3 (PDE-3) inhibitor that inhibits the degradation of cyclic adenosine monophosphate (cAMP).[8] The increased concentration of cAMP leads to the multiple cardiovascular effects of milrinone, including vasodilation in the systemic and pulmonary vascular beds, inotropy through activation of contractile proteins, and a lusitropic effect by prolonging the relaxation period of the cardiac cycle.[8]

2. **Dosing** is via continuous infusion, with the usual dosing range being 0.25–1 mcg/kg/min. Loading doses ranging from 25 to 75 mcg/kg have been described in the literature[24-26] but have been

associated with hypotension, with some recommending avoidance.[27] A normal saline bolus of 10–15 mL/kg administered during the first hour of infusion may assist in the prevention of low diastolic blood pressure (BP) due to vasodilation.[28]

3. **Pharmacokinetics:** Most of the circulating milrinone is not metabolized and is excreted unchanged in the urine. The mean half-life is approximately 4 hours in term neonates and 10 hours in preterm neonates.[26,29]

4. **Examples of clinical use:** Milrinone has been shown to improve hemodynamics in low cardiac output syndrome after cardiac surgery,[30] post-ligation cardiac syndrome,[28] PH,[27,31] and congenital diaphragmatic hernia.[32]

5. **Adverse effects** include hypotension and arrhythmias; less commonly seen are thrombocytopenia, hypokalemia, and other laboratory value changes.[24]

6. **Special considerations:** Caution is advised in therapeutic situations associated with poor renal function or decreased renal clearance of medications. Patients with hypoxic-ischemic encephalopathy undergoing therapeutic hypothermia

have been shown to exhibit profound hypotension with milrinone administration,[6] likely due to vasodilation after accumulation from poor excretion. Clearance will vary based on gestational and chronological age.[26,29] Additionally, it has been postulated in an animal model that PDE-4 is the predominant enzyme in fetal life leading to a potential delay in the inotropic effect for the first several days.[33,34]

### Levosimendan

1. **Mechanism of action:** While levosimendan has not been approved for use in the United States or Canada, it is used in over 60 countries, including many in the European Union and Latin America. It enhances myocardial contractility by binding to troponin C, a cytosolic calcium-dependent interaction, thereby also improving LV diastolic function without promoting arrhythmogenesis or altering myocardial oxygen demand.[8,35] Levosimendan also inhibits cardiac PDE-3 at higher doses[8,35] and promotes vasodilation by activation of adenosine triphosphate (ATP)–sensitive potassium channels.[8,35] Affected vasculatures include coronary, pulmonary, renal, splanchnic, cerebral, and systemic arteries as well as saphenous, portal, and systemic veins.[35]

2. **Dosing:** More studies are required to establish a safe dosing range in neonates and premature infants. Reported dosing range for continuous infusion is 0.05–0.2 mcg/kg/min with variable use of loading doses.

3. **Pharmacokinetics:** The metabolism of levosimendan results in active metabolites that are likely responsible for prolonged hemodynamic effects after discontinuation of continuous infusion.[35] These metabolites are excreted in the feces and urine. Pharmacokinetic data on its use in neonates are not available; in adults the half-life of the parent drug is approximately 1 hour, while the active metabolite has a prolonged elimination half-life of 70–80 hours.

4. **Examples of clinical use:** Since the hemodynamic profile is similar to milrinone, levosimendan may be beneficial in patients requiring afterload reduction and inotropy (e.g., post-ligation cardiac syndrome).

5. **Adverse effects** include, as with any medications that cause vasodilation, hypotension. Further studies in neonates and infants are needed to delineate other potential adverse effects.

6. **Special considerations:** More data on its use in neonates and infants are required to evaluate potential effects and associations with clinical procedures (e.g., therapeutic hypothermia) and diagnoses (e.g., renal failure).

## PRIMARY VASODILATOR

### Sodium Nitroprusside

1. **Mechanism of action:** Sodium nitroprusside is a non-specific vasodilator (arterial and venous) with no direct effect on myocardial contractility or heart rate.[36] It functions as a prodrug, reacting with sulfhydryl groups on erythrocytes, albumin, and other proteins to release nitric oxide (NO), which activates guanylate cyclase stimulating production of cyclic guanosine monophosphate (cGMP).[36] Its main hemodynamic effect is reducing SVR, resulting in decreased afterload. The vasodilator properties lead to decreased ventricular filling pressures, reduced wall stress, and lower myocardial oxygen demand. Together, these result in increased cardiac output and systemic tissue oxygenation as long as coronary perfusion pressure is adequate.[36]

2. **Dosing** is via continuous infusion, with a usual dosing range of 0.5–2 mcg/kg/min, though maximum dosing as high as 10 mcg/kg/min has been reported for control of hypertensive emergencies.[37] Doses higher than 1.8 mcg/kg/min and/or prolonged therapy have been associated with elevated cyanide levels.[36,38]

3. **Pharmacokinetics:** Sodium nitroprusside combines with hemoglobin, forming cyanide and cyanmethemoglobin. This process is rapid, with a half-life of approximately 2 minutes. Cyanide is then converted to thiocyanate in the liver and kidney, a process with limited capacity which can be overwhelmed in high doses, resulting in toxicity. Sodium nitroprusside is excreted in the urine as thiocyanate. The half-life of thiocyanate is approximately 3 days in adults with normal renal function.

4. **Examples of clinical use:** Hypertensive crisis (e.g., paradoxical hypertension following correction of coarctation of the aorta).[39]

5. **Adverse effects** include cyanide toxicity (especially in those who have hypoalbuminemia and hepatic impairment and those undergoing cardiopulmonary bypass or therapeutic hypothermia),[40] hypotension, increased intracranial pressure,[41] and methemoglobinemia.

6. **Special considerations:** Upon initiation of sodium nitroprusside, it is important to maintain close monitoring to avoid life-threatening hypotension and hypoperfusion, especially in populations at increased risk, such as premature infants.

## Cardiovascular Support for Acute and/or Chronic Pulmonary Hypertension (Figure 5.2)

The major goal of medication therapy in PH in the *acute setting* is to improve pulmonary blood flow, and, more often than not, fast-acting medications are utilized first-line (e.g., pulmonary vasodilator). In addition, there are likely to be secondary beneficial effects to RV function and cardiac output. In the *chronic setting*, while fast-acting agents may be utilized initially, more often than not, chronic medication therapy is required to affect pulmonary pressures. In both cases, evaluation, and support, when decreased, of both RV and LV heart function is still required.

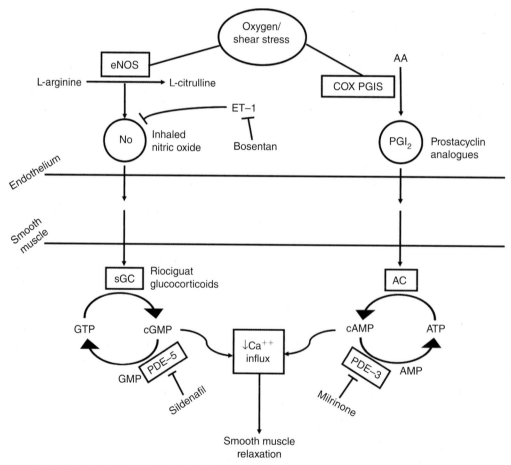

Fig. 5.2 Pathways for medication effect and therapeutic benefit in acute and chronic pulmonary hypertension.

## PULMONARY VASODILATOR

### Inhaled Nitric Oxide

1. **Mechanism of action:** Inhaled nitric oxide (iNO) acts as a selective pulmonary vasodilator that relaxes vascular smooth muscle by binding to the heme moiety of guanylate cyclase, which leads to its activation and increased levels of cGMP.[42] It improves oxygenation via reduction of PVR, improved ventilation/perfusion matching, and decreased right to left extrapulmonary shunting.[43] These actions together improve pulmonary blood flow, which leads to improved pulmonary venous return and LV output.

2. **Dosing** is via inhalation, with a usual dosing range of 1–20 ppm, with starting doses ranging from 5 to 20 ppm. Doses >20 ppm are not recommended due to increased risk of methemoglobinemia and pulmonary injury from elevated nitrogen dioxide.[43]

3. **Pharmacokinetics:** iNO combines with oxyhemoglobin to produce methemoglobin and nitrate.[42] The half-life of NO is 2–6 seconds in neonates.[44] Nitrate is excreted in the urine.

4. **Examples of clinical use:** Acute or chronic PH.

5. **Adverse effects** include methemoglobinemia, which should be measured within 4–8 hours of initiation and periodically throughout administration, inflammation and lung tissue injury caused by nitrogen dioxide, and possible decreased platelet aggregation without increased bleeding time.[42] In the presence of high concentrations of oxygen, it is possible that iNO may react with reactive oxygen species to form reactive nitrogen species (e.g., peroxynitrite) that can lead to cytotoxicity.[42] Use in patients with LV systolic or diastolic dysfunction may increase pulmonary capillary pressure resulting in pulmonary edema. iNO should be avoided in patients with left-sided outflow tract obstruction (e.g., hypoplastic left heart syndrome) or those with excessive pulmonary blood flow (e.g., anomalous pulmonary venous return or vein stenosis, PDA).[43]

6. **Special considerations:** Echocardiography, prior to iNO use, should be considered to confirm features of PH (especially in premature infants),[45] to determine RV and LV function, and to establish normal cardiac anatomy.[43] Abrupt discontinuation of iNO may lead to worsening of oxygenation and/or rebound pulmonary hypertension; weaning is recommended.[43,44]

## PHOSPHODIESTERASE INHIBITORS

### Sildenafil

1. **Mechanism of action:** Sildenafil is a selective PDE-5 inhibitor in the smooth muscle of the pulmonary vasculature, which promotes increased cGMP and pulmonary vasculature relaxation.[46] While sildenafil is more selective for the pulmonary vasculature, both pulmonary and systemic vasodilation may occur.

2. **Dosing** may be via intravenous (IV less commonly) or oral route. Recommended dosing for continuous infusion is 0.4 mg/kg load over 3 hours followed by 1.6 mg/kg/day.[47,48] IV intermittent dosing is 0.4 mg/kg given over 1–3 hours every 6 hours.[49] Oral dosing in neonatal case series of acute PH ranges from 0.5 to 3 mg/kg/dose q 6–8 hours.[47,50,51] Chronic oral therapy is typically limited to a maximum dose of 2 mg/kg/dose, or 10 mg, orally every 8 hours.[52]

3. **Pharmacokinetics:** Sildenafil is metabolized in the liver by CYP3A4 (major) and CYP2C9 (minor) forming a major metabolite (desmethyl-sildenafil), which retains 50% of the activity of sildenafil. Elimination increases with increasing postmenstrual age (half-life of the parent compound ~56 hours in term newborns with maturation to ~48 hours by week 1 of age).[53] Excretion is mainly as metabolites via feces and some urine. Clearance may be decreased in patients with hepatic or renal impairment.[50]

4. **Examples of clinical use:** Chronic and, less frequently, acute PH.

5. **Adverse effects** include hypotension and flushing. Due to risk of severe hypotension, concurrent use of riociguat (a soluble guanylate cyclase stimulator) is contraindicated and should not be given less than 24 hours apart. Caution is required with other vasodilators.

6. **Special considerations:** Pulmonary vasodilatory effects are not confined to well-ventilated portions of the lung, as is the case with iNO,

which could contribute to worsened V:Q (ventilation:perfusion) mismatch.

## ENDOTHELIN RECEPTOR ANTAGONISTS

### Bosentan

1. **Mechanism of action:** Bosentan blocks endothelin (ET) receptors, which induce vasoconstriction, on the endothelium and in vascular smooth muscle. While it blocks both $ET_A$ and $ET_B$ receptors, it has a slightly higher affinity for the A subtype receptor.[54]
2. **Dosing** is via the oral route with an initial dose of 1 mg/kg/dose twice daily, which may be increased to 2 mg/kg/dose twice daily if necessary.[55,56]
3. **Pharmacokinetics:** Bosentan is metabolized in the liver via CYP2C9 and CYP3A4 to one active and two inactive metabolites.[54] Bosentan also induces both enzymes. The maximum concentration occurs at a median of 12 hours after administration of initial doses but this time decreases to a median of 7.5 hours by day 5 of therapy.[55] It is mostly excreted in the feces as metabolites, with a small amount excreted in the urine as unchanged drug.[54]
4. **Examples of clinical use:** Chronic PH.
5. **Adverse effects** include hepatotoxicity and anemia requiring close monitoring of liver enzymes (baseline, then monthly) and hemoglobin (baseline, 1 and 3 months, then every 3 months).[54]
6. **Special considerations:** Bosentan is only available in the United States through a Risk Evaluation and Mitigation Strategy (REMS) program. It has been classified as a hazardous substance due to its associated risk of birth defects.[54] Single gloving is recommended for administration of intact tablets or capsules. Double gloving, a protective gown, and eye/face protection are recommended for manipulating tablets and administration of oral suspension to neonates and infants. A suspension recipe has been shown to be stable for up to 1 month.[57] Bosentan was shown to rapidly improve oxygenation index in the absence of iNO[56] but was shown to have limited acute efficacy as an adjunct to iNO.[55]

## PROSTACYCLIN (ANALOGUES)

### Epoprostenol

1. **Mechanism of action:** Epoprostenol is a potent pulmonary and systemic vasodilator and inhibitor of platelet aggregation by increasing cAMP levels.[58] It has also been shown to have vascular remodeling and anti-inflammatory properties.[58]
2. **Dosing** is via continuous infusion or inhalation. Initial dosage for continuous infusion is 1–2 ng/kg/min, titrated to effect with usual dosing range of 50–80 ng/kg/min.[47] Dosing range for inhalation is 20–50 ng/kg/min.[59,60]
3. **Pharmacokinetics:** Epoprostenol is rapidly hydrolyzed with a half-life of approximately 6 minutes to form two active (though with minimal activity) and multiple inactive metabolites.[61] It is predominantly excreted in the urine.
4. **Examples of clinical use:** Chronic PH and/or elevated PVR.
5. **Adverse effects** include flushing and hypotension when used systemically.[47,61]
6. **Special considerations:** In patients with LV systolic or diastolic dysfunction or increased pulmonary capillary wedge pressure, caution is advised with use due to the potential for pulmonary edema.[61] Abrupt discontinuation of the IV formulation can result in rebound PH or pulmonary hypertensive crisis.[47] The intravenous formulation has been associated with a higher incidence of gram-negative rod bloodstream infections, though more data is required.[62]

### Treprostinil

1. **Mechanism of action:** Synthetic analogue of epoprostenol with superior stability in solution (facilitating subcutaneous infusion) and a longer half-life.[63]
2. **Dosing** is typically initiated as an IV or subcutaneous continuous infusion through dedicated access at 2–5 ng/kg/min, titrated to effect with a usual maximum dose of 20 ng/kg/min, but reported maximum of 52 ng/kg/min.[64-68]
3. **Pharmacokinetics:** Treprostinil is metabolized in the liver to inactive metabolites, primarily by CYP2C8, before renal elimination. The half-life is approximately 4 hours in adults.[69]

4. **Examples of clinical use:** Chronic PH.
5. **Adverse effects** are similar to epoprostenol with the addition of mild-to-moderate infusion site pain when administered subcutaneously.[63]
6. **Special considerations:** Treprostinil has a lower risk of rebound PH, compared to epoprostenol, due to a longer half-life. Multidisciplinary planning is required prior to initiation and during titration and stabilization to ensure optimization of the delivered concentration, maintain line patency, and avoid volume overload. IV formulation has been associated with higher incidence of gram-negative rod bloodstream infections than IV epoprostenol, though more data is required.[62]

## Iloprost

1. **Mechanism of action:** Synthetic analogue of epoprostenol with superior stability in solution (along with more neutral pH facilitating nebulization) and a slightly longer half-life.[70]
2. **Dosing** is via inhalation and may be delivered intermittently as 0.25–2.5 mcg/kg every 2–6 hours or via continuous nebulization at 0.8 mcg/kg/h or 5–10 mcg/h.[71-74]
3. **Pharmacokinetics:** Iloprost is metabolized by beta oxidation of a carboxyl side chain in the liver prior to renal elimination, thereby prolonging the effective half-life to 20–30 minutes.
4. **Examples of clinical use:** Chronic and, less frequently, acute PH.
5. **Adverse effects** including flushing and cough are common. Patients should be monitored carefully for hypotension, although this adverse effect is mitigated to some extent when administered directly to the lungs. Acute desaturations have been observed during administration of nebulized therapy.
6. **Special considerations:** Although iloprost inhalation has been extensively described in adults, descriptions in neonates are limited. Delivery of nebulized solution to distal airways may be challenging, especially during high-frequency ventilation.[75] Multidisciplinary planning is required to ensure optimal preparation and procedures for nebulized administration.

## PROSTAGLANDIN E1
### Alprostadil

1. **Mechanism of action:** Alprostadil causes vasodilation by direct effect on vascular and ductus arteriosus smooth muscle.[76]
2. **Dosing** is via continuous infusion, with a usual dosing range of 0.01–0.1 mcg/kg/min.[76] Higher initial doses (0.05–0.1 mcg/kg/min) may be required for patients with restrictive ductal flow, and once response is seen, the dose should be reduced to lowest effective dose (may be as low as 0.01 mcg/kg/min).
3. **Pharmacokinetics:** Alprostadil is mostly oxidized during a single pass through the lungs into an active metabolite, resulting in a half-life of less than 1 minute in neonates. Elimination occurs predominately as metabolites in the urine, with a small amount in feces.[76]
4. **Examples of clinical use:** Ductal-dependent congenital heart defects and acute PH in the setting of RV failure to offload the right heart.
5. **Adverse effects** include apnea, fever, flushing, and, less commonly, hypotension.[76] Reversible cortical proliferation of the long bones is seen with prolonged treatment courses.[77] Apnea is seen more often in neonates <2 kg at birth, with higher starting doses, and usually within the first hour of infusion.
6. **Special considerations:** Though alprostadil is most commonly used for maintenance of ductal patency in cases of congenital heart disease, it may play a role in disease states where a restrictive or closed ductus arteriosus is detrimental (e.g., acute PH with failing RV).[78] Its pulmonary vasodilator effects may also be beneficial in acute PH and other disease states.[79]

## SOLUBLE GUANYLATE CYCLASE STIMULATORS
### Riociguat

1. **Mechanism of action:** Riociguat sensitizes soluble guanylate cyclase (sGC) to endogenous NO and directly stimulates sGC independent of NO. This leads to increased cGMP levels and subsequently vasodilation.[80]
2. **Dosing** is via the oral route; pharmacological dose range studies in the neonatal and infant

populations are not available; however, preliminary data is emerging.[81] Suggested dosing range in adults is 0.5–2 mg/dose three times daily. Dosing should be titrated gradually to monitor for adverse effects; for instance, starting at 0.5 mg daily for 48 hours, then to twice daily for 48 hours. If tolerated, it can be increased to 0.5 mg three times daily, then to 1 mg three times daily, if necessary.

3. **Pharmacokinetics:** Riociguat is metabolized in the liver by CYP1A1, CYP3A, CYP2C8, and CYP2J2 into one active and other inactive metabolites. It is excreted in both urine and feces.[80] The half-life in adults with PH is ~12 hours.
4. **Examples of clinical use:** Chronic PH refractory to sildenafil.
5. **Adverse effects** include hypotension and bleeding.[82] Use is contraindicated with specific PDE-5 inhibitors (e.g., sildenafil) and caution advised with non-specific PDE inhibitors (e.g., caffeine, theophylline). Riociguat should not be administered within 24 hours of a dose of sildenafil.
6. **Special considerations:** Riociguat is only available in the United States for neonates and infants through a REMS program. There is a paucity of data on its use in neonates and infants. Caution is advised in transitioning from sildenafil to riociguat, as clinical deterioration may be seen upon discontinuation of sildenafil even in non-responders. Up-titration of iNO or use of other pulmonary vasodilators (e.g., milrinone) may be of benefit during the wash-out period.

## Support for Systemic Hypotension

Systemic hypotension is a common diagnosis in the neonatal intensive care unit (NICU), though its frequency varies considerably between institutions. The choice of medication will vary based on the presence or absence and degree of systemic perfusion, cerebral blood flow, heart function, pulmonary or systemic vascular resistance, and intra- or extra-cardiac shunt flow and direction. Commonly used medications in this setting include predominant systemic vasoconstrictors (i.e., dopamine, norepinephrine, vasopressin, and phenylephrine) and glucocorticoids.

## PREDOMINANT VASOCONSTRICTORS

### Dopamine

1. **Mechanism of action:** Dopamine is an endogenous catecholamine and a precursor of norepinephrine and epinephrine. It stimulates both central and peripheral nervous system dopaminergic and adrenergic (both alpha-1 and beta) receptors (Figure 5.1) while also having serotonergic effects.[83] Approximately half of the cardiovascular effects are thought to be due to released norepinephrine, but low stores can lead to tachyphylaxis.[83]
2. **Dosing** is via continuous infusion into a large vein, reported dosing range of 2–20 mcg/kg/min, though in critically ill infants, receptor saturation is often seen by 8 mcg/kg/min.[84,85] Low doses stimulate predominantly dopaminergic receptors (0.5–4 mcg/kg/min), medium doses additionally stimulate beta-receptors (beta-1 > beta-2; 2–10 mcg/min), and high doses additionally stimulate alpha-1-receptors (5–20 mcg/kg/min). Preterm neonates typically experience receptor effects at lower doses than term neonates, although high interpatient variability exists in the dose-response relationship regardless of gestational age; therefore, due to the unpredictable nature of its effects, dopamine should be used with caution in preterm infants.
3. **Pharmacokinetics:** Dopamine is irreversibly metabolized in the liver, kidney, and pulmonary endothelium and reversibly metabolized in the plasma. It is excreted in the urine as metabolites or unchanged drug.[83] The mean half-life in critically ill newborns is 7 minutes.[86]
4. **Examples of clinical use:** Disease states with low SVR (e.g., septic shock) and no evidence of PH given potential risk of increased PVR.
5. **Adverse effects** include tachycardia, tachyarrhythmias, natriuresis, which may result in hyponatremia,[85] increased oxygen consumption,[87] increased pulmonary artery pressure and PVR,[20] neutrophil apoptosis,[88] and inhibition of thyrotropin.[83] Dopamine is also associated with severe vasoconstriction after extravasation.[83]
6. **Special considerations:** Dopamine, as is true with all drugs with marked chronotropic effects

due to β-adrenergic activity, should be avoided in patients with hypertrophic cardiomyopathy. Dopamine may be preferred over epinephrine, as a predominant vasoconstrictor in neonates, due to a lower incidence of transient tachycardia, lactic acidosis, and hyperglycemia.[23]

## Norepinephrine

1. **Mechanism of action:** Norepinephrine is a nonselective α-adrenergic receptor agonist with more beta-1 than beta-2 activity[89] (Figure 5.1). Stimulation of these receptors results in a primary vasoconstriction effect with minor inotropic and chronotropic properties, which leads to increased systemic BP and coronary blood flow.
2. **Dosing** is via continuous infusion into a large vein, with a usual dosing range of 0.02–1 mcg/kg/min,[89] although doses as high as 2 mcg/kg/min have been published.[90] The initial dose is usually 0.02–0.05 mcg/kg/min, with subsequent titration to effect.
3. **Pharmacokinetics:** Norepinephrine is metabolized via catechol-o-methyltransferase and monoamine oxidase and excreted as mostly inactive metabolites and some unchanged drug in the urine. The half-life is approximately 1 minute in critically ill infants and young children.[90]
4. **Examples of clinical use:** Disease states with low SVR (e.g., septic shock).
5. **Adverse effects** include reflex bradycardia in the setting of a sudden increase in SVR,[90] tachycardia and/or cardiac arrhythmias, peripheral ischemia, and extravasation injury.
6. **Special considerations:** Caution is advised in patients with LV dysfunction as increased afterload may be poorly tolerated. Norepinephrine, as is true with all drugs with marked chronotropic effects due to β-adrenergic activity, should be avoided in patients with hypertrophic cardiomyopathy. Additionally, norepinephrine in the presence of 100% oxygen concentrations has been shown to induce vasoconstriction in pulmonary arteries[91]; however, norepinephrine has also been shown to increase pulmonary blood flow and improve oxygenation in hypotensive neonates with acute PH.[92,93] Additionally, norepinephrine may be preferred over dopamine in hypotensive patients with underlying cardiogenic shock, based predominantly on adult data.[94]

## Vasopressin

1. **Mechanism of action:** Vasopressin stimulates arginine vasopressin, oxytocin, and purinergic receptors.[95] V1 receptors are expressed on vascular smooth muscle, hepatocytes, and platelets. They are responsible for vasoconstriction via a phosphatidyl-inositol-calcium signaling pathway and vasodilation in the coronary and pulmonary vessels via NO production. V2 receptors are expressed in the renal collecting duct, where they have an antidiuretic effect and mediate vasodilation via NO. V3 receptors are expressed in the anterior pituitary and hippocampus, where they release adrenocorticotropic hormone (ACTH) when stimulated. Stimulation of oxytocin receptors causes vasodilation via increased NO. The vasodilatory effect of low-dose vasopressin on purinergic receptors is reversed in higher doses by stimulation of the V1 receptors.
2. **Dosing** is via continuous infusion. Extreme caution must be taken as dosing units of measure vary by institution; the most common units of measure in the neonatal population are mU/kg/min and U/kg/h. Usual dosing range is 0.1–1.2 mU/kg/min (0.006–0.072 U/kg/h) though higher ranges have been reported.[96] Suggested starting dose is 0.3 mU/kg/min (0.018 U/kg/h) and titrating to effect. Once goals have been achieved, vasopressin can be weaned in increments of 0.1–0.2 mU/kg/min (0.006–0.012 U/kg/h) as tolerated.
3. **Pharmacokinetics:** Vasopressin is metabolized in the liver and kidney into inactive metabolites, which are excreted in the urine with a small amount of unchanged drug. The half-life in adults is 10–20 minutes; limited neonatal data exist.
4. **Examples of clinical use:** Data on vasopressin in the neonatal and premature population are limited,[97] though it has been used in hypotension,[96,98,99] pulmonary hypertension,[100,101] shock,[102] and low cardiac output syndrome following surgery for congenital heart disease.[103] Vasopressin is the vasoactive medication of choice in patients with hypotension

and/or low cardiac output state in the setting of hypertrophic cardiomyopathy due to its lack of chronotropic effects.[78,104]

5. **Adverse effects** mostly include natriuresis, which may result in hyponatremia. There have been reports of peripheral ischemic changes infrequently associated with higher dosing ranges than recommended and/or with terlipressin use (a longer-acting vasopressin analogue).[102]

6. **Special considerations:** Caution is advised in patients with LV dysfunction as increased afterload may be poorly tolerated. Prolonged therapy may result in decreased endogenous production of vasopressin, which may lead to polyuria and fluid imbalance upon discontinuation. Urine output and electrolytes should be monitored carefully. During administration, sodium replacement at or above the amount excreted in the urine should be sufficient to avoid hyponatremia. After discontinuation, hyponatremia will resolve, and rapid adjustment of supplementation may be required to avoid iatrogenic hypernatremia.

### Phenylephrine

1. **Mechanism of action:** Phenylephrine is a pure α-adrenergic receptor agonist (Figure 5.1) and, as such, results in vasoconstriction without inotropy or chronotropy.[105]

2. **Dosing** is via continuous infusion, with a usual dosing range of 0.1–0.5 mcg/kg/min titrated to response.[106] Doses up to 2 mcg/kg/min have been reported.[107]

3. **Pharmacokinetics:** Phenylephrine is metabolized in the liver via oxidative deamination, sulfation, or glucuronidation to form inactive metabolites that are excreted in the urine.[105] Phenylephrine rapidly distributes but has a relatively prolonged elimination half-life of ~3 hours in adults.

4. **Examples of clinical use:** Phenylephrine has utility in neonates with tetralogy of Fallot during "Tet spells" as it increases systemic BP, and therefore pulmonary blood flow is augmented through reversal of excessive right-left flow across the ventricular septal defect.[106,107]

5. **Adverse effects** include severe bradycardia, likely baroreflex mediated, and reduced cardiac output caused by increased afterload especially in patients with heart dysfunction.[108]

6. **Special considerations:** If extravasation occurs, phentolamine may be used as an antidote.

## GLUCOCORTICOIDS

### Hydrocortisone

1. **Mechanism of action:** Hydrocortisone has both genomic and non-genomic effects that differ in timing of onset of effect, with genomic actions taking longer. The variable and complex actions include inducing the final enzyme in the transformation of norepinephrine to epinephrine, increasing adrenergic receptor expression, upregulation of angiotensin II receptors, inhibition of inducible NO synthase expression, inhibition of vasodilatory prostaglandin action, suppressing migration of polymorphonuclear leukocytes, and decreasing capillary permeability.[109]

2. **Dosing** is via intermittent IV or oral route, with a loading dose range of 1–2 mg/kg/dose followed by 0.5–1 mg/kg/dose every 6–12 hours. For neonates >35 weeks' gestation, dosing interval is usually 6–8 hours. In premature infants <35 weeks' gestation, dosing interval is usually 8–12 hours.[110]

3. **Pharmacokinetics:** Hydrocortisone is metabolized in the liver via glucuronidation or sulphation to inactive metabolites, and a small amount of unchanged drug is excreted in addition to the inactive metabolites in the urine.[109] The mean half-life in neonates is approximately 3 hours, with slower clearance observed in extremely preterm neonates and with a rapid maturation after term age.[111]

4. **Examples of clinical use:** Adjunctive therapy for relative or absolute adrenal insufficiency and pressor-resistant hypotension.

5. **Adverse effects** include hyperglycemia, hypertension, thrombus formation, development of hypertrophic cardiomyopathy, and increased risk of infection.[112] Hydrocortisone has not been associated with neurodevelopmental impairment.[113,114]

6. **Special considerations:** Concurrent use of hydrocortisone and indomethacin should be avoided due to increased risk of intestinal perforation.[115]

## Support for Systemic Hypertension

Systemic hypertension is, perhaps, a less recognized but equally important entity in the NICU. More often associated with bronchopulmonary dysplasia (BPD) in former premature infants, systemic hypertension may result in LV systolic or diastolic dysfunction if left untreated. Common medications used in the NICU are calcium channel blockers and, in infants >36 weeks' gestation, angiotensin-converting enzyme (ACE) inhibitors.

### CALCIUM CHANNEL BLOCKER

#### Isradipine

1. **Mechanism of action:** Isradipine is a dihydropyridine calcium antagonist with a high affinity for L-type calcium channels on vascular smooth muscles, which gives it a fairly specific and potent antihypertensive effect.[116]
2. **Dosing** is via the oral route with recommended dosing of 0.05–0.15 mg/kg/dose four times daily and a maximum dose of 0.8 mg/kg/day (total dose no more than 10 mg/day).[117,118]
3. **Pharmacokinetics:** Isradipine has a rapid onset after oral administration (~1–2 hours) and undergoes hepatic metabolism via cytochrome P450 isoenzyme CYP3A4, with a relatively long terminal half-life (~8 hours).[119,120]
4. **Examples of clinical use:** Treatment of acute systemic hypertension.
5. **Adverse effects** include flushing, dizziness, and tachycardia.[116]
6. **Special considerations:** Isradipine is used for treatment of acute hypertension in pediatric patients.[116,120-122] Dihydropyridines have little to no negative effect upon cardiac contractility or conduction.

#### Amlodipine

1. **Mechanism of action:** Amlodipine is a dihydropyridine calcium channel antagonist that acts on vascular smooth muscle to produce peripheral arterial vasodilation resulting in an antihypertensive effect.[120,123-125]
2. **Dosing** is via the oral route; usual dosing is 0.05–0.3 mg/kg/dose one to two times daily, with a maximum dose of 0.6 mg/kg/day.[117]

3. **Pharmacokinetics:** Limited data on its use in neonates are available. Amlodipine undergoes metabolism in the liver and, unlike other calcium channel blockers, has high oral bioavailability (60–65%) and a long half-life (30–50 hours), resulting in prolonged duration of effect.[120,123-125]
4. **Examples of clinical use:** Treatment of chronic systemic hypertension.
5. **Adverse effects** include peripheral edema, flushing,[126] and reflex tachycardia.[117]
6. **Special considerations:** Slower onset of action and prolonged duration of effect make it a good option for management of less severe or chronic systemic hypertension rather than acute hypertension.[120,127] Dihydropyridines have little to no negative effect on cardiac contractility or conduction.

### ACE INHIBITORS

#### Enalapril(at)

1. **Mechanism of action:** Enalapril is a competitive inhibitor of ACE, which is responsible for conversion of angiotensin I to angiotensin II (a potent vasoconstrictor). Inhibition of ACE thus results in reduced angiotensin II and aldosterone, with subsequent decrease in peripheral vascular resistance resulting in an anti-hypertensive effect.[119,128,129]
2. **Dosing** is via the oral route, with a usual dosing range of 0.04–0.3 mg/kg/day divided one to two times daily.[117,130,131] Dosing should be initiated at the low end of the dosing range and titrated to effect due to the potential of a potent hypotensive effect in some neonates.[132]
   a. **Enalaprilat** is the IV formulation of enalapril. Limited data on its use in neonates are available. Current recommended IV dose is 5–10 mcg/kg/dose every 8–24 hours.[133]
3. **Pharmacokinetics:** Limited data on its pharmacokinetics in neonates are available. Enalapril undergoes hepatic biotransformation into the active compound enalaprilat and is excreted primarily in the urine.[119,128,134] The onset of action occurs after approximately 1 hour, with peak activity at 4–6 hours and an elimination half-life of 10–12 hours in neonates.[135] Enalapril is less bioavailable and has a shorter duration of

action in infants with congestive heart failure than in adults.[136]

4. **Examples of clinical use:** Treatment of systemic hypertension and congestive heart failure in neonates.[117,127,137-140] ACE inhibitors have anti-remodeling effects and decrease peripheral vascular resistance leading to decreased afterload.[141-147] There is emerging evidence that ACE inhibitors may have a modulatory effect on LV diastolic dysfunction in neonates with BPD.[148,149]

5. **Adverse effects** include hyperkalemia, oliguria, acute kidney injury (AKI),[138,150] reflex tachycardia,[117] and hypotension.[138] Cough has been reported in adults.[151]

6. **Special considerations:** Treatment should be used with caution in patients with impaired renal function or hypovolemia. There is a potential for nephrotoxicity in premature infants still undergoing nephrogenesis,[127,152,153] so avoidance or caution should be taken in patients <36 weeks postmenstrual age.

## Fluid Modulation

### LOOP DIURETICS

#### Furosemide

1. **Mechanism of action:** Furosemide is a loop diuretic that inhibits active reabsorption of sodium, chloride, and potassium in the ascending limb of the loop of Henle by blocking the $Na^+$-$K^+$-$Cl^-$ cotransporter.[154-160] Thus furosemide has a potent natriuretic effect.

2. **Dosing** may be via the IV (intermittent or continuous infusion), intramuscular (IM), or oral route. Doses are NOT interchangeable, due to decreased bioavailability orally.
   a. Recommended *oral* dose: 2 mg/kg/dose (range 0.5–4 mg/kg/dose) with a frequency that varies with postnatal maturation in premature infants: Postmenstrual age (PMA) < 31 weeks – every 24 hours; PMA ≥ 31 weeks – every 12 hours.[161-164] There is evidence of drug accumulation and increased risk of toxicity with doses >2 mg/kg/dose administered more frequently than every 24 hours.[162]

   b. Recommended *IM* and *intermittent IV* dose: 1 mg/kg/dose (range 0.5–2 mg/kg/dose); PMA < 31 weeks – every 24 hours; PMA ≥ 31 weeks – every 12–24 hours.[133,161-163,165] There is evidence of drug accumulation and increased risk of toxicity with doses >1 mg/kg/dose administered more frequently than every 24 hours.[162]

   c. Recommended dosing for *continuous IV infusion* (term neonates): Optional initial IV bolus dose 1–2 mg/kg followed by continuous IV infusion (range 0.1–0.4 mg/kg/h). In existing trials, infusions were initiated at 0.1–0.2 mg/kg/h and titrated based on urine output every 12–24 hours in 0.1 mg/kg/h increments up to a max dose of 0.4 mg/kg/h.[166,167]

3. **Pharmacokinetics:** Furosemide metabolism occurs mainly in the kidneys and to a lesser extent in the liver.[159,168,169] In newborn infants furosemide has a prolonged half-life (12–24 hours at <31 weeks PMA compared to ~2 hours near term age) and reduced clearance in the setting of immature renal function, reducing metabolic elimination.[160-162,170-174] This slow elimination is associated with prolonged diuretic effects and can increase the risk of drug accumulation and toxicity.[157,175] There can be substantial pharmacokinetic alterations in loop diuretics when neonates are on extracorporeal membrane oxygenation (ECMO).[157,159,161,176]

4. **Examples of clinical use:** Loop diuretics are used for management of both acute and chronic fluid overload, most commonly in the setting of congenital heart disease, congestive heart failure, and renal dysfunction.[177-179] A trial of loop diuretics can be useful in neonates with oliguric AKI to improve diuresis and avoid volume overload.[159,180-183] There is strong evidence supporting the efficacy of furosemide in critically ill and postoperative cardiac patients.[167,184,185] Loop diuretics, thiazides, and aldosterone antagonists are not first-line for fast onset hypertension, but may be used to treat slow onset neonatal hypertension secondary to sodium or water retention.[159]

5. **Adverse effects** include AKI due to fluid loss.[159,186] Electrolyte imbalances including hyponatremia,[156] hypokalemia,[156,160] hypomagnesemia,[156,160,187,188]

metabolic alkalosis,[156,189] and hypocalcemia due to hypercalciuria[160,188] are also common. Chronic hypercalciuria has been associated with nephrocalcinosis and nephrolithiasis secondary to high urinary calcium excretion.[190-194] Increased cumulative furosemide exposure is associated with bone demineralization and metabolic bone disease, as bone is demineralized to maintain normal serum calcium levels.[160,195,196] There are many reports of loop diuretic–induced ototoxicity; however, currently existing data are of low quality in assessing for an association between furosemide and sensorineural hearing loss in premature infants.[197-199]

6. **Special considerations:** Loop diuretic resistance can be overcome by adding thiazide diuretics.[160,163,200,201] In addition to diuretic effects, loop modulators can have a variety of extrarenal effects.[202] Furosemide can induce transient improvement in pulmonary mechanics,[203-205] but there are limited data supporting substantial and long-lasting improvement in respiratory status.[159,206,207] Loop diuretics decrease pulmonary edema, resulting in improved PVR and lung compliance. These effects may be beneficial for symptomatic improvement of acute pulmonary edema in certain patients.[208] Furosemide also appears to have a direct relaxant effect on airway smooth muscle unrelated to its diuretic effects.[202,203,209,210] Furosemide is not recommended for routine management of respiratory distress syndrome or early or late phases of BPD.[159,208,211,212] There is evidence that loop diuretics can induce non-diuretic mediated relaxation of the vascular smooth muscle; however, the dose required for therapeutic effect exceeds the threshold for renal injury and recommended dosing ranges in neonates treated in the NICU.[202,213-215] Furosemide is known to stimulate renal synthesis of prostaglandin E2 and can subsequently function as a potent vasodilator of the ductus arteriosus.[202,216-220] Therefore furosemide is not recommended as the primary therapy for pulmonary overcirculation in the setting of PDA or in combination with cyclo-oxygenase inhibitors. Furosemide is a potent displacer of bilirubin and should be used with caution in neonates with hyperbilirubinemia.[221]

## Bumetanide

1. **Mechanism of action:** Bumetanide, like furosemide, is a loop diuretic that inhibits active reabsorption of sodium, chloride, and potassium in the ascending limb of the loop of Henle by blocking the $Na^+$-$K^+$-$Cl^-$ cotransporter,[154-160] resulting in a potent natriuresis.

2. **Dosing** may be via the IV or oral route. Limited data on its use in neonates are available (based on small trials and one retrospective study). In preterm infants the recommended oral, IM, and IV dosing is 0.01–0.06 mg/kg/dose every 12–24 hours[222,223]; IV doses as high as 0.1 mg/kg/dose have been reported.[222] In term neonates the recommended oral, IM, and IV dosing is 0.01–0.05 mg/kg/dose every 12–24 hours, with doses as high as 0.1 mg/kg/dose reported.[224,225]

3. **Pharmacokinetics:** Bumetanide is partially metabolized in the liver and excreted in the urine as unchanged drug and inactive metabolites.[160,222,226] Bumetanide is 40 times more potent than furosemide[157,227-229] and has a shorter half-life than furosemide.[157,230] Infants have significantly lower clearance (mean half-life of 6 hours).[160,230] Renal clearance of bumetanide increases about threefold from birth to 6 months of age.[157,231] There are no data currently available on the pharmacokinetics of continuous bumetanide infusions in critically ill neonates.[157,159] There can be substantial pharmacokinetic alterations in bumetanide when neonates are on ECMO.[157,232]

4. **Examples of clinical use:** Bumetanide can be useful in the treatment of severe oliguria, renal insufficiency, congestive heart failure, or edema refractory to furosemide treatment.[202]

5. **Adverse effects** include electrolyte imbalances such as hyponatremia,[156] hypokalemia,[156,160] hypomagnesemia,[156,160,187,188] metabolic alkalosis,[156,189] and hypocalcemia due to hypercalciuria.[160,188] In premature neonates, when compared to furosemide, bumetanide has lower sodium losses, higher urine calcium losses,[233] and less ototoxicity.[229]

6. **Special considerations:** There are very few studies on the use of bumetanide in preterm infants with AKI.[159,223] The limited available literature

suggests that bumetanide has no significant effect on ductal diameter.[202] Use in combination with thiazide diuretics can enhance the clinical response to bumetanide.[229] It is a potent displacer of bilirubin and caution should be used in neonates with hyperbilirubinemia.[234]

## THIAZIDE DIURETICS

1. **Mechanism of action:** Thiazide diuretics work by inhibiting NaCl reabsorption in the distal convoluted tubule, resulting in increased excretion of sodium and water, as well as potassium and bicarbonate.[155,156,159,235-237] They also act as a calcium-activated potassium channel blocker in smooth muscle cells,[238-240] resulting in vasodilation and a possible anti-hypertensive effect.[239] Thiazide diuretics also have a weak inhibitory effect on carbonic anhydrase, which contributes to the excretion of bicarbonate and its vasodilatory effect.[165,239,241] They are also known to have a calcium sparing effect by stimulating calcium reabsorption in the proximal and distal nephron.[156,242] Chlorothiazide and hydrochlorothiazide are structurally similar, but hydrochlorothiazide is more potent.

2. **Dosing of chlorothiazide** may be via the IV or oral route. Recommended oral dosing for diuresis (edema), heart failure, and hypertension is 10–40 mg/kg/day in divided doses once or twice daily.[137,243,244] Recommended IV dosing is 5–10 mg/kg/day in divided doses once or twice daily[245]; however, doses up to 12 mg/kg/day have been reported.[246]

3. **Dosing of hydrochlorothiazide** is via the oral route; usual dosing is 1–2 mg/kg/dose every 12 hours.[159,247]

4. **Pharmacokinetics:** There are limited data available on its pharmacokinetics in neonates. Chlorothiazide is not metabolized but is eliminated as unchanged drug by the kidney.[248] Hydrochlorothiazide is not metabolized but is rapidly excreted by tubular secretion in the kidney.[249-251] Organic anion transporter 1 (OAT1) and OAT3 transporters in the kidney are responsible for clearance of hydrochlorothiazide; however, there is very little data about maturation of these transporters in humans.[251,252]

5. **Examples of clinical use:** Thiazides can be used to treat neonates with nephrogenic diabetes insipidus.[159,253,254] Limited data suggest that thiazide diuretics can improve pulmonary mechanics in infants with BPD.[255] Loop diuretics, thiazides, and aldosterone antagonists are not first-line for rapid-onset hypertension but may be used to treat slow-onset neonatal hypertension secondary to sodium or water retention.[159]

6. **Adverse effects include hyponatremia,[156,256] hypokalemia,[156] hypomagnesemia,[156,257] and hypercalcemia.[156]** Thiazide diuretics can also result in metabolic alkalosis, but to a lesser degree than loop diuretics.[156] Hyperglycemia can occur secondary to inhibition of pancreatic release of insulin.[156,239] Hyperuricemia[156,258] and dyslipidemia (by unclear mechanism) have also been reported.[156]

7. **Special considerations:** Thiazide diuretics are less potent than loop diuretics. Thiazides may help inhibit bone demineralization by improving calcium retention.[160] These medications should be used with caution in patients with significant impairment of renal or hepatic function. Thiazide diuretics can displace bilirubin from albumin and should be used with caution in infants with hyperbilirubinemia.[259]

## MINERALOCORTICOID RECEPTOR ANTAGONIST

### Spironolactone

1. **Mechanism of action:** Spironolactone is a potassium sparing diuretic that is a competitive antagonist of the aldosterone receptor in the principal cells of the collecting duct.[159] Spironolactone also has an antiandrogen effect via peripheral antagonism of androgens.[260]

2. **Dosing** is via the oral route and the usual dosing is 1–3 mg/kg/day divided every 12–24 hours.[133,261]

3. **Pharmacokinetics:** Spironolactone is rapidly metabolized by the liver, and excretion occurs primarily in the urine and secondarily in the bile.[262]

4. **Examples of clinical use:** There is emerging evidence that spironolactone can be effective in treating select cases of neonatal hypertension

related to phthalate exposure.[127,263,264] Potassium sparing diuretics can be used to counteract the effects of loop or thiazide diuretic-induced hyperaldosteronism, hypokalemia, hypomagnesemia, and metabolic alkalosis.[156] Loop diuretics, thiazides, and aldosterone antagonists are not first-line for rapid-onset neonatal hypertension but may be used to treat slow-onset hypertension secondary to sodium or water retention.[159]

5. **Adverse effects** include hyperkalemia.[156,235,265] There are also some reports of nephrocalcinosis in preterm infants.[192]

6. **Special considerations:** Spironolactone must be used with caution in patients with renal impairment and serum potassium levels should be monitored closely.[156,159]

## Modulators of Heart Rate

### BETA-BLOCKERS

#### Propranolol

1. **Mechanism of action:** Propranolol is a non-selective β-adrenergic blocker.[266]

2. **Dosing** may be via the IV or oral route. Recommended starting oral dose for treatment of hypertension and tachyarrhythmias is 0.25–1 mg/kg/dose orally every 6–8 hours,[267-269] with a maximum dose of 5–10 mg/kg/day. Recommended starting IV dose is 0.01 mg/kg/dose every 6 hours, with a maximum dose of 0.15 mg/kg/dose every 6 hours.[269]

3. **Pharmacokinetics:** Limited pharmacokinetic data available in neonates suggest a prolonged half-life compared to adults (mean 15 hours compared to 3–6 hours).[270] Propranolol is metabolized in the liver, and elimination is by renal excretion of metabolites.[266]

4. **Examples of clinical use:** Propranolol has been shown to treat supraventricular arrythmias, selective arrythmias, and long QT syndrome.[226,267,271] It can also be used to treat hypertension. Rate control with propranolol also helps improve filling in patients with hypertrophic cardiomyopathy.[272,273]

5. **Adverse effects** include hypoglycemia and bronchospasm.[274,275]

6. **Special considerations:** Caution should be taken in neonates with chronic lung disease given the risk of bronchoconstriction. Serum half-life is prolonged in patients with liver disease.

### Esmolol

1. **Mechanism of action:** Esmolol is a potent rapid-onset cardio selective beta-1-specific antagonist with a short duration of action. beta-1 specific antagonism results in reduced heart rate, AV-nodal conduction, and BP.[276]

2. **Dosing** is via continuous IV infusion. The starting dose for term neonates (PNA 0–7 days) is 50 mcg/kg/min and should be titrated up by 25–50 mcg/kg/min every 20 minutes to response. The starting dose for term neonates (PNA 8–28 days) is 75 mcg/kg/min and dose should be titrated up by 50 mcg/kg/min every 20 minutes to response. Maximum dose: 1000 mcg/kg/min.[277]

3. **Pharmacokinetics:** Esmolol is rapidly metabolized in blood by esterases in red blood cells.[278] Pharmacokinetic data in newborns/infants suggest a faster elimination than in adults (half-life of 2–5 minutes in infants compared to mean of 9 minutes in adults).[276,277,279,280] It is excreted predominantly as inactive metabolites in urine.

4. **Examples of clinical use:** Esmolol has been shown to control hypertension in children after repair of coarctation of aorta.[277,279,281,282] Esmolol can be used to increase ventricular filling time and augment cardiac output in patients with hypertrophic obstructive cardiomyopathy.[283,284] It can also be used to treat hypercyanotic spells in tetralogy of Fallot.[285]

5. **Adverse effects** include severe bradycardia, hypotension, and reaction at injection site.[279]

6. **Special considerations:** Esmolol should be used with caution in patients with heart block.

### BETA-AGONIST

#### Isoproterenol

1. **Mechanism of action:** Isoproterenol is a non-specific beta-agonist with very low affinity for α-adrenergic receptors (Figure 5.1). Stimulation of these receptors results in inotropic, chronotropic, and systemic and pulmonary vasodilatory effects.[286] In vitro studies have demonstrated a

greater inotropic effect in newborns compared to adults.[287]

2. **Dosing** is via continuous infusion. There is very limited data on dosing for neonates; however, the usual dosing range is 0.05–1 mcg/kg/min.[288,289] Initial dose is usually 0.05 mcg/kg/min titrated to effect.

3. **Pharmacokinetics:** Isoproterenol is metabolized in the liver and lungs via catechol-o-methyltransferase and excreted as both inactive metabolites and some unchanged drug in the urine.[286] The elimination half-life is 2.5–5 minutes. Postoperative cardiac patients have lower clearance rates.[286]

4. **Examples of clinical use:** Isoproterenol is indicated for mild or transient episodes of heart block that do not require elective shock or pacemaker therapy.

5. **Adverse effects:** Patients may exhibit dose-dependent vasodilation, resulting in hypotension due to unopposed beta-2 agonism. Additionally, there is a potential risk for myocardial ischemia.[290] Atrial and ventricular arrythmias can also occur.

6. **Special considerations:** Isoproterenol, as is true with all drugs with β-adrenergic activity, should be avoided in patients with hypertrophic cardiomyopathy. Caution should also be utilized in patients with fixed outflow obstructions and compromised coronary blood flow given increased oxygen consumption.

## Conclusion

Understanding the mechanism of action, clinical utility, and potential unwanted side effects is important in choosing medication regimens for critically ill neonates and infants in the NICU. While care was taken to ensure accurate dosing recommendations in this chapter, local prescribing guidelines may differ and should always be referred to when treating patients. There are still limited data on pharmacokinetics in premature infants and neonates in general. For this reason, as evidence emerges or new studies are conducted, the dosing strategies for any of the listed medications may change. Additionally, new therapeutics not listed may be discovered. The information in this chapter should be combined with emerging data to complement current and future practice.

## REFERENCES

1. Xu A, Hawkins C, Narayanan N. Ontogeny of sarcoplasmic reticulum protein phosphorylation by Ca2+-calmodulin-dependent protein kinase. *J Mol Cell Cardiol*. 1997;29(1):405-418.
2. Kojima M, Ishima T, Taniguchi N, Kimura K, Sada H, Sperelakis N. Developmental changes in beta-adrenoceptors, muscarinic cholinoceptors, and Ca2+ channels in rat ventricular muscles. *Br J Pharmacol*. 1990;99(2):334-339.
3. Friedman WF. The intrinsic physiologic properties of the developing heart. *Prog Cardiovasc Dis*. 1972;15(1):87-111.
4. Chemtob S, Guest I, Potvin W, Varma DR. Ontogeny of responses of rabbit aorta to atrial natriuretic factor and isoproterenol. *Dev Pharmacol Ther*. 1991;16(2):108-115.
5. Wiegerinck RF, Cojoc A, Zeidenweber CM, et al. Force frequency relationship of the human ventricle increases during early postnatal development. *Pediatr Res*. 2009;65(4):414-419.
6. Bischoff AR, Habib S, McNamara PJ, Giesinger RE. Hemodynamic response to milrinone for refractory hypoxemia during therapeutic hypothermia for neonatal hypoxic ischemic encephalopathy. *J Perinatol*. 2021;41(9):2345-2354.
7. Ruffolo Jr RR. The pharmacology of dobutamine. *Am J Med Sci*. 1987;294(4):244-248.
8. Noori S, Seri I. Neonatal blood pressure support: the use of inotropes, lusitropes, and other vasopressor agents. *Clin Perinatol*. 2012;39(1):221-238.
9. Seri I. Management of hypotension and low systemic blood flow in the very low birth weight neonate during the first postnatal week. *J Perinatol*. 2006;26(suppl 1):S8-S13.
10. Stopfkuchen H, Queisser-Luft A, Vogel K. Cardiovascular responses to dobutamine determined by systolic time intervals in preterm infants. *Crit Care Med*. 1990;18(7):722-724.
11. Stopfkuchen H, Schranz D, Huth R, Jüngst BK. Effects of dobutamine on left ventricular performance in newborns as determined by systolic time intervals. *Eur J Pediatr*. 1987;146(2):135-139.
12. Martinez AM, Padbury JF, Thio S. Dobutamine pharmacokinetics and cardiovascular responses in critically ill neonates. *Pediatrics*. 1992;89(1):47-51.
13. Robel-Tillig E, Knüpfer M, Pulzer F, Vogtmann C. Cardiovascular impact of dobutamine in neonates with myocardial dysfunction. *Early Hum Dev*. 2007;83(5):307-312.
14. Pellicer A, Fernández R, Jullien V, et al. Pharmacokinetic study (phase I–II) of a new dobutamine formulation in preterm infants immediately after birth. *Pediatr Res*. 2021;89(4):981-986.
15. Mahoney L, Shah G, Crook D, Rojas-Anaya H, Rabe H. A literature review of the pharmacokinetics and pharmacodynamics of dobutamine in neonates. *Pediatr Cardiol*. 2016;37(1):14-23.
16. Osborn D, Evans N, Kluckow M. Randomized trial of dobutamine versus dopamine in preterm infants with low systemic blood flow. *J Pediatr*. 2002;140(2):183-191.
17. Barrington K, Chan W. The circulatory effects of epinephrine infusion in the anesthetized piglet. *Pediatr Res*. 1993;33(2):190-194.
18. Hardin RA, Scott JB, Haddy FJ. Effect of epinephrine and norepinephrine on coronary vascular resistance in dogs. *Am J Physiol*. 1961;201:276-280.
19. Pellicer A, Valverde E, Elorza MD, et al. Cardiovascular support for low birth weight infants and cerebral hemodynamics: a randomized, blinded, clinical trial. *Pediatrics*. 2005;115(6):1501-1512.

20. Cheung PY, Barrington KJ. The effects of dopamine and epinephrine on hemodynamics and oxygen metabolism in hypoxic anesthetized piglets. *Crit Care.* 2001;5(3):158-166.
21. Barrington KJ, Finer NN, Chan WK. A blind, randomized comparison of the circulatory effects of dopamine and epinephrine infusions in the newborn piglet during normoxia and hypoxia. *Crit Care Med.* 1995;23(4):740-748.
22. Caspi J, Coles JG, Benson LN, et al. Age-related response to epinephrine-induced myocardial stress. A functional and ultrastructural study. *Circulation.* 1991;84(suppl 5):III394-III399.
23. Valverde E, Pellicer A, Madero R, Elorza D, Quero J, Cabañas F. Dopamine versus epinephrine for cardiovascular support in low birth weight infants: analysis of systemic effects and neonatal clinical outcomes. *Pediatrics.* 2006;117(6):e1213-e1222.
24. Samiee-Zafarghandy S, Raman SR, van den Anker JN, et al. Safety of milrinone use in neonatal intensive care units. *Early Hum Dev.* 2015;91(1):31-35.
25. Chang AC, Atz AM, Wernovsky G, Burke RP, Wessel DL. Milrinone: systemic and pulmonary hemodynamic effects in neonates after cardiac surgery. *Crit Care Med.* 1995;23(11):1907-1914.
26. Paradisis M, Jiang X, McLachlan AJ, Evans N, Kluckow M, Osborn D. Population pharmacokinetics and dosing regimen design of milrinone in preterm infants. *Arch Dis Child Fetal Neonatal Ed.* 2007;92(3):F204-F209.
27. McNamara PJ, Laique F, Muang-In S, Whyte HE. Milrinone improves oxygenation in neonates with severe persistent pulmonary hypertension of the newborn. *J Crit Care.* 2006;21(2):217-222.
28. El-Khuffash AF, Jain A, Weisz D, Mertens L, McNamara PJ. Assessment and treatment of post patent ductus arteriosus ligation syndrome. *J Pediatr.* 2014;165(1):46-52.e1.
29. Bailey JM, Hoffman TM, Wessel DL, et al. A population pharmacokinetic analysis of milrinone in pediatric patients after cardiac surgery. *J Pharmacokinet Pharmacodyn.* 2004;31(1):43-59.
30. Ferrer-Barba A, Gonzalez-Rivera I, Bautista-Hernandez V. Inodilators in the management of low cardiac output syndrome after pediatric cardiac surgery. *Curr Vasc Pharmacol.* 2016;14(1):48-57.
31. James AT, Bee C, Corcoran JD, McNamara PJ, Franklin O, El-Khuffash AF. Treatment of premature infants with pulmonary hypertension and right ventricular dysfunction with milrinone: a case series. *J Perinatol.* 2015;35(4):268-273.
32. Patel N. Use of milrinone to treat cardiac dysfunction in infants with pulmonary hypertension secondary to congenital diaphragmatic hernia: a review of six patients. *Neonatology.* 2012;102(2):130-136.
33. Akita T, Joyner RW, Lu C, Kumar R, Hartzell HC. Developmental changes in modulation of calcium currents of rabbit ventricular cells by phosphodiesterase inhibitors. *Circulation.* 1994;90(1):469-478.
34. Artman M, Kithas PA, Wike JS, Strada SJ. Inotropic responses change during postnatal maturation in rabbit. *Am J Physiol.* 1988;255(2 Pt 2):H335-H342.
35. Toller WG, Stranz C. Levosimendan, a new inotropic and vasodilator agent. *Anesthesiology.* 2006;104(3):556-569.
36. Hottinger DG, Beebe DS, Kozhimannil T, Prielipp RC, Belani KG. Sodium nitroprusside in 2014: a clinical concepts review. *J Anaesthesiol Clin Pharmacol.* 2014;30(4):462-471.
37. Flynn JT. Neonatal hypertension: diagnosis and management. *Pediatr Nephrol.* 2000;14(4):332-341.
38. Moffett BS, Price JF. Evaluation of sodium nitroprusside toxicity in pediatric cardiac surgical patients. *Ann Pharmacother.* 2008;42(11):1600-1604.
39. Roeleveld PP, Zwijsen EG. Treatment strategies for paradoxical hypertension following surgical correction of coarctation of the aorta in children. *World J Pediatr Congenit Heart Surg.* 2017;8(3):321-331.
40. Rindone JP, Sloane EP. Cyanide toxicity from sodium nitroprusside: risks and management. *Ann Pharmacother.* 1992;26(4):515-519.
41. Turner JM, Powell D, Gibson RM, McDowall DG. Intracranial pressure changes in neurosurgical patients during hypotension induced with sodium nitroprusside or trimetaphan. *Br J Anaesth.* 1977;49(5):419-425.
42. Griffiths MJ, Evans TW. Inhaled nitric oxide therapy in adults. *N Engl J Med.* 2005;353(25):2683-2695.
43. Kinsella JP. Inhaled nitric oxide in the term newborn. *Early Hum Dev.* 2008;84(11):709-716.
44. Peliowski A. Inhaled nitric oxide use in newborns. *Paediatr Child Health.* 2012;17(2):95-100.
45. Ahmed MS, Giesinger RE, Ibrahim M, et al. Clinical and echocardiography predictors of response to inhaled nitric oxide in hypoxic preterm neonates. *J Paediatr Child Health.* 2019;55(7):753-761.
46. Porta NFM, Steinhorn RH. Pulmonary vasodilator therapy in the NICU: inhaled nitric oxide, sildenafil, and other pulmonary vasodilating agents. *Clin Perinatol.* 2012;39(1):149-164.
47. Abman SH, Hansmann G, Archer SL, et al. Pediatric pulmonary hypertension: guidelines from the American Heart Association and American Thoracic Society. *Circulation.* 2015;132(21):2037-2099.
48. Steinhorn RH, Kinsella JP, Pierce C, et al. Intravenous sildenafil in the treatment of neonates with persistent pulmonary hypertension. *J Pediatr.* 2009;155(6):841-847.e1.
49. Stultz JS, Puthoff T, Backes Jr C, Nahata MC. Intermittent intravenous sildenafil for pulmonary hypertension management in neonates and infants. *Am J Health Syst Pharm.* 2013;70(5):407-413.
50. Lakshminrusimha S, Mathew B, Leach CL. Pharmacologic strategies in neonatal pulmonary hypertension other than nitric oxide. *Semin Perinatol.* 2016;40(3):160-173.
51. Vargas-Origel A, Gómez-Rodríguez G, Aldana-Valenzuela C, Vela-Huerta MM, Alarcón-Santos SB, Amador-Licona N. The use of sildenafil in persistent pulmonary hypertension of the newborn. *Am J Perinatol.* 2010;27(3):225-230.
52. Barst RJ, Beghetti M, Pulido T, et al. STARTS-2: long-term survival with oral sildenafil monotherapy in treatment-naive pediatric pulmonary arterial hypertension. *Circulation.* 2014;129(19):1914-1923.
53. Mukherjee A, Dombi T, Wittke B, Lalonde R. Population pharmacokinetics of sildenafil in term neonates: evidence of rapid maturation of metabolic clearance in the early postnatal period. *Clin Pharmacol Ther.* 2009;85(1):56-63.
54. Rubin LJ, Roux S. Bosentan: a dual endothelin receptor antagonist. *Expert Opin Investig Drugs.* 2002;11(7):991-1002.
55. Steinhorn RH, Fineman J, Kusic-Pajic A, et al. Bosentan as adjunctive therapy for persistent pulmonary hypertension of the newborn: results of the randomized multicenter placebo-controlled exploratory trial. *J Pediatr.* 2016;177:90-96.e3.
56. Mohamed WA, Ismail M. A randomized, double-blind, placebo-controlled, prospective study of bosentan for the treatment of persistent pulmonary hypertension of the newborn. *J Perinatol.* 2012;32(8):608-613.
57. Malik A, Gorman G, Coward L, Arnold JJ. Stability of an extemporaneously compounded oral suspension of bosentan. *Hosp Pharm.* 2016;51(5):389-395.

58. Vane JR. Prostacyclin. *J R Soc Med.* 1983;76(4):245-249.

59. Kelly LK, Porta NF, Goodman DM, Carroll CL, Steinhorn RH. Inhaled prostacyclin for term infants with persistent pulmonary hypertension refractory to inhaled nitric oxide. *J Pediatr.* 2002; 141(6):830-832.

60. Bindl L, Fahnenstich H, Peukert U. Aerosolised prostacyclin for pulmonary hypertension in neonates. *Arch Dis Child Fetal Neonatal Ed.* 1994;71(3):F214-F216.

61. Ivy DD. Prostacyclin in the intensive care setting. *Pediatr Crit Care Med.* 2010;11(suppl 2):S41-S45.

62. Kaye KM, Evans S, Choi Y, Barritt K, Engel J. Bloodstream infections among patients treated with intravenous epoprostenol or intravenous treprostinil for pulmonary arterial hypertension – seven sites, United States, 2003–2006. *MMWR Morb Mortal Wkly Rep.* 2007;56(8):170-172. Available at: https://www.cdc.gov/mmwr/preview/mmwrhtml/mm5608a5.htm.

63. Vachiéry JL, Hill N, Zwicke D, Barst R, Blackburn S, Naeije R. Transitioning from IV epoprostenol to subcutaneous treprostinil in pulmonary arterial hypertension. *Chest.* 2002;121(5):1561-1565.

64. Olson E, Lusk LA, Fineman JR, Robertson L, Keller RL. Short-term treprostinil use in infants with congenital diaphragmatic hernia following repair. *J Pediatr.* 2015;167(3):762-764.

65. Park BY, Chung SH. Treprostinil for persistent pulmonary hypertension of the newborn, with early onset sepsis in preterm infant: 2 case reports. *Medicine (Baltimore).* 2017;96(26):e7303.

66. Carpentier E, Mur S, Aubry E, et al. Safety and tolerability of subcutaneous treprostinil in newborns with congenital diaphragmatic hernia and life-threatening pulmonary hypertension. *J Pediatr Surg.* 2017;52(9):1480-1483.

67. Lawrence KM, Hedrick HL, Monk HM, et al. Treprostinil improves persistent pulmonary hypertension associated with congenital diaphragmatic hernia. *J Pediatr.* 2018;200:44-49.

68. Jozefkowicz M, Haag DF, Mazzucchelli MT, Salgado G, Fariña D. Neonates effects and tolerability of treprostinil in hypertension with persistent pulmonary. *Am J Perinatol.* 2020;37(9):939-946.

69. Wade M, Baker FJ, Roscigno R, et al. Pharmacokinetics of treprostinil sodium administered by 28-day chronic continuous subcutaneous infusion. *J Clin Pharmacol.* 2004;44(5):503-539.

70. Hoeper MM, Olschewski H, Ghofrani HA, et al. A comparison of the acute hemodynamic effects of inhaled nitric oxide and aerosolized iloprost in primary pulmonary hypertension. German PPH study group. *J Am Coll Cardiol.* 2000;35(1):176-182.

71. Mulligan C, Beghetti M. Inhaled iloprost for the control of acute pulmonary hypertension in children: a systematic review. *Pediatr Crit Care Med.* 2012;13(4):472-480.

72. Kahveci H, Yilmaz O, Avsar UZ, et al. Oral sildenafil and inhaled iloprost in the treatment of pulmonary hypertension of the newborn. *Pediatr Pulmonol.* 2014;49(12):1205-1213.

73. Dykes JC, Torres M, Alexander PJ. Continuous inhaled iloprost in a neonate with d-transposition of the great arteries and severe pulmonary arterial hypertension. *Cardiol Young.* 2016; 26(3):571-573.

74. Kim SH, Lee HJ, Kim NS, Park HK. Inhaled iloprost as a first-line therapy for persistent pulmonary hypertension of the newborn. *Neonatal Med.* 2019;26(4):191-197.

75. DiBlasi RM, Crotwell DN, Shen S, Zheng J, Fink JB, Yung D. Iloprost drug delivery during infant conventional and high-frequency oscillatory ventilation. *Pulm Circ.* 2016;6(1):63-69.

76. Heymann MA, Clyman RI. Evaluation of alprostadil (prostaglandin E1) in the management of congenital heart disease in infancy. *Pharmacotherapy.* 1982;2(3):148-155.

77. Kaufman MB, El-Chaar GM. Bone and tissue changes following prostaglandin therapy in neonates. *Ann Pharmacother.* 1996;30(3):269-274, 277.

78. Giesinger RE, McNamara PJ. Hemodynamic instability in the critically ill neonate: an approach to cardiovascular support based on disease pathophysiology. *Semin Perinatol.* 2016;40(3):174-188.

79. Weesner KM. Hemodynamic effects of prostaglandin E1 in patients with congenital heart disease and pulmonary hypertension. *Cathet Cardiovasc Diagn.* 1991;24(1):10-15.

80. Kenny M, Clarke MM, Pogue KT. Overview of riociguat and its role in the treatment of pulmonary hypertension. *J Pharm Pract.* 2022;35(3):437-444.

81. Giesinger RE, Stanford AH, Thomas B, Abman SH, McNamara PJ. Safety and feasibility of riociguat therapy for the treatment of chronic pulmonary arterial hypertension in infancy. *J Pediatr.* 2022;255:224-229.e1.

82. Hoeper MM, Gomez Sanchez MA, Humbert M, et al. Riociguat treatment in patients with pulmonary arterial hypertension: final safety data from the EXPERT registry. *Respir Med.* 2020;177:106241.

83. Seri I. Cardiovascular, renal, and endocrine actions of dopamine in neonates and children. *J Pediatr.* 1995;126(3):333-344.

84. Padbury JF, Agata Y, Baylen BG, et al. Dopamine pharmacokinetics in critically ill newborn infants. *J Pediatr.* 1987;110(2):293-298.

85. Seri I, Tulassay T, Kiszel J, Machay T, Csömör S. Cardiovascular response to dopamine in hypotensive preterm neonates with severe hyaline membrane disease. *Eur J Pediatr.* 1984;142(1):3-9.

86. Bhatt-Mehta V, Nahata MC, McClead RE, Menke JA. Dopamine pharmacokinetics in critically ill newborn infants. *Eur J Clin Pharmacol.* 1991;40(6):593-597.

87. Li J, Zhang G, Holtby H, et al. Adverse effects of dopamine on systemic hemodynamic status and oxygen transport in neonates after the Norwood procedure. *J Am Coll Cardiol.* 2006;48(9):1859-1864.

88. Aslan Y, Koca L, Mutlu M, Tekelioglu Y, Erduran E. Apoptotic effects of dopamine and dobutamine on neutrophils of premature neonates. *J Mater Fetal Neonatal Med.* 2011;24(9):1155-1158.

89. Dempsey E, Rabe H. The use of cardiotonic drugs in neonates. *Clin Perinatol.* 2019;46(2):273-290.

90. Oualha M, Tréluyer JM, Lesage F, et al. Population pharmacokinetics and haemodynamic effects of norepinephrine in hypotensive critically ill children. *Br J Clin Pharmacol.* 2014;78(4):886-897.

91. Lakshminrusimha S, Russell JA, Wedgwood S, et al. Superoxide dismutase improves oxygenation and reduces oxidation in neonatal pulmonary hypertension. *Am J Respir Crit Care Med.* 2006;174(12):1370-1377.

92. Magnenant E, Jaillard S, Deruelle P, et al. Role of the alpha2-adrenoceptors on the pulmonary circulation in the ovine fetus. *Pediatr Res.* 2003;54(1):44-51.

93. Tourneux P, Rakza T, Bouissou A, Krim G, Storme L. Pulmonary circulatory effects of norepinephrine in newborn infants with persistent pulmonary hypertension. *J Pediatr.* 2008;153(3):345-349.

94. De Backer D, Biston P, Devriendt J, et al. Comparison of dopamine and norepinephrine in the treatment of shock. *N Engl J Med.* 2010;362(9):779-789.

95. Russell JA. Bench-to-bedside review: vasopressin in the management of septic shock. *Crit Care*. 2011;15(4):226.
96. Ikegami H, Funato M, Tamai H, Wada H, Nabetani M, Nishihara M. Low-dose vasopressin infusion therapy for refractory hypotension in ELBW infants. *Pediatr Int*. 2010;52(3):368-373.
97. Rios DR, Moffett BS, Kaiser JR. Trends in pharmacotherapy for neonatal hypotension. *J Pediatr*. 2014;165(4):697-701.
98. Rios DR, Kaiser JR. Vasopressin vs dopamine for treatment of hypotension in ELBW infants: a randomized, blinded pilot study. *J Pediatr*. 2015;166(4):850-855.
99. Ni M, Kaiser JR, Moffett BS, et al. Use of vasopressin in neonatal intensive care unit patients with hypotension. *J Pediatr Pharmacol Ther*. 2017;22(6):430-435.
100. Mohamed A, Nasef N, Shah V, McNamara PJ. Vasopressin as a rescue therapy for refractory pulmonary hypertension in neonates: case series. *Pediatr Crit Care Med*. 2014;15(2):148-154.
101. Acker SN, Kinsella JP, Abman SH, Gien J. Vasopressin improves hemodynamic status in infants with congenital diaphragmatic hernia. *J Pediatr*. 2014;165(1):53-58.e1.
102. Meyer S, Gortner L, McGuire W, Baghai A, Gottschling S. Vasopressin in catecholamine-refractory shock in children. *Anaesthesia*. 2008;63(3):228-234.
103. Chandler HK, Kirsch R. Management of the low cardiac output syndrome following surgery for congenital heart disease. *Curr Cardiol Rev*. 2016;12(2):107-111.
104. Boyd SM, Riley KL, Giesinger RE, McNamara PJ. Use of vasopressin in neonatal hypertrophic obstructive cardiomyopathy: case series. *J Perinatol*. 2021;41(1):126-133.
105. Hengstmann JH, Goronzy J. Pharmacokinetics of 3H-phenylephrine in man. *Eur J Clin Pharmacol*. 1982;21(4):335-341.
106. Wessel DL. Managing low cardiac output syndrome after congenital heart surgery. *Crit Care Med*. 2001;29(suppl 10):S220-S230.
107. Shaddy RE, Viney J, Judd VE, McGough EC. Continuous intravenous phenylephrine infusion for treatment of hypoxemic spells in tetralogy of Fallot. *J Pediatr*. 1989;114(3):468-470.
108. Goertz AW, Lindner KH, Seefelder C, Schirmer U, Beyer M, Georgieff M. Effect of phenylephrine bolus administration on global left ventricular function in patients with coronary artery disease and patients with valvular aortic stenosis. *Anesthesiology*. 1993;78(5):834-841.
109. Czock D, Keller F, Rasche FM, Häussler U. Pharmacokinetics and pharmacodynamics of systemically administered glucocorticoids. *Clin Pharmacokinet*. 2005;44(1):61-98.
110. Watterberg KL. Hydrocortisone dosing for hypotension in newborn infants: less is more. *J Pediatr*. 2016;174:23-26.e1.
111. Vezina HE, Ng CM, Vazquez DM, Barks JD, Bhatt-Mehta V. Population pharmacokinetics of unbound hydrocortisone in critically ill neonates and infants with vasopressor-resistant hypotension. *Pediatr Crit Care Med*. 2014;15(6):546-553.
112. Röhr SB, Sauer H, Gortner L, Gräber S, Meyer S. Cardiovascular and metabolic side effects associated with hydrocortisone and dexamethasone use in VLBW infants: a single-centre experience. *Acta Paediatr*. 2013;102(10):e436.
113. Baud O, Trousson C, Biran V, et al. Association between early low-dose hydrocortisone therapy in extremely preterm neonates and neurodevelopmental outcomes at 2 years of age. *JAMA*. 2017;317(13):1329-1337.
114. Halbmeijer NM, Onland W, Cools F, et al. Effect of systemic hydrocortisone initiated 7 to 14 days after birth in ventilated preterm infants on mortality and neurodevelopment at 2 years'

corrected age: follow-up of a randomized clinical trial. *JAMA*. 2021;326(4):355-357.
115. Watterberg KL, Gerdes JS, Cole CH, et al. Prophylaxis of early adrenal insufficiency to prevent bronchopulmonary dysplasia: a multicenter trial. *Pediatrics*. 2004;114(6):1649-1657.
116. Flynn JT, Warnick SJ. Isradipine treatment of hypertension in children: a single-center experience. *Pediatr Nephrol*. 2002;17(9):748-753.
117. Starr MC, Flynn JT. Neonatal hypertension: cases, causes, and clinical approach. *Pediatr Nephrol*. 2019;34(5):787-799.
118. Fuhrman B. *Pediatric Critical Care*. Philadelphia Elsevier Saunders; 2011.
119. Yu ASL. *Brenner & Rector's the Kidney*. Philadelphia, PA: Elsevier; 2020.
120. Flynn JT, Pasko DA. Calcium channel blockers: pharmacology and place in therapy of pediatric hypertension. *Pediatr Nephrol*. 2000;15(3-4):302-316.
121. Miyashita Y, Peterson D, Rees JM, Flynn JT. Isradipine for treatment of acute hypertension in hospitalized children and adolescents. *J Clin Hypertens (Greenwich)*. 2010;12(11):850-855.
122. Johnson CE, Jacobson PA, Song MH. Isradipine therapy in hypertensive pediatric patients. *Ann Pharmacother*. 1997;31(6):704-707.
123. Meredith PA, Elliott HL. Clinical pharmacokinetics of amlodipine. *Clin Pharmacokinet*. 1992;22(1):22-31.
124. Abernethy DR. Pharmacokinetics and pharmacodynamics of amlodipine. *Cardiology*. 1992;80(suppl 1):31-36.
125. Elliott HL, Meredith PA. The clinical consequences of the absorption, distribution, metabolism and excretion of amlodipine. *Postgrad Med J*. 1991;67(suppl 3):S20-S23.
126. Pedrinelli R, Dell'Omo G, Mariani M. Calcium channel blockers, postural vasoconstriction and dependent oedema in essential hypertension. *J Hum Hypertens*. 2001;15(7):455-461.
127. Flynn JT. The hypertensive neonate. *Semin Fetal Neonatal Med*. 2020;25(5):101138.
128. Davies RO, Gomez HJ, Irvin JD, Walker JF. An overview of the clinical pharmacology of enalapril. *Br J Clin Pharmacol*. 1984;18(suppl 2):215S-229S.
129. Goodman LS, Brunton LL, Chabner B, Knollmann BrC. *Goodman & Gilman's Pharmacological Basis of Therapeutics*. New York: McGraw-Hill; 2011.
130. Artman M, Graham Jr TP. Guidelines for vasodilator therapy of congestive heart failure in infants and children. *Am Heart J*. 1987;113(4):994-1005.
131. Leversha AM, Wilson NJ, Clarkson PM, Calder AL, Ramage MC, Neutze JM. Efficacy and dosage of enalapril in congenital and acquired heart disease. *Arch Dis Child*. 1994;70(1):35-39.
132. Lindle KA, Dinh K, Moffett BS, et al. Angiotensin-converting enzyme inhibitor nephrotoxicity in neonates with cardiac disease. *Pediatr Cardiol*. 2014;35(3):499-506.
133. Eichenwald EC, Hansen AR, Martin C, Stark AR, eBook Nursing Collection W. *Cloherty and Stark's Manual of Neonatal Care*. Philadelphia: Wolters Kluwer; 2017.
134. MacFadyen RJ, Meredith PA, Elliott HL. Enalapril clinical pharmacokinetic-pharmacodynamic relationships. An overview. *Clin Pharmacokinet*. 1993;25(4):274-282.
135. Nakamura H, Ishii M, Sugimura T, Chiba K, Kato H, Ishizaki T. The kinetic profiles of enalapril and enalaprilat and their possible developmental changes in pediatric patients with congestive heart failure. *Clin Pharmacol Ther*. 1994;56(2):160-168.
136. Lloyd TR, Mahoney LT, Knoedel D, Marvin Jr WJ, Robillard JE, Lauer RM. Orally administered enalapril for infants with

congestive heart failure: a dose-finding study. *J Pediatr.* 1989;114(4 Pt 1):650-654.

137. Flynn JT, Kaelber DC, Baker-Smith CM, et al. Clinical practice guideline for screening and management of high blood pressure in children and adolescents. *Pediatrics.* 2017;140(3): e20181739.

138. Ku LC, Zimmerman K, Benjamin DK, et al. Safety of enalapril in infants admitted to the neonatal intensive care unit. *Pediatr Cardiol.* 2017;38(1):155-161.

139. Dutertre JP, Billaud EM, Autret E, Chantepie A, Oliver I, Laugier J. Inhibition of angiotensin converting enzyme with enalapril maleate in infants with congestive heart failure. *Br J Clin Pharmacol.* 1993;35(5):528-530.

140. Mason T, Polak MJ, Pyles L, Mullett M, Swanke C. Treatment of neonatal renovascular hypertension with intravenous enalapril. *Am J Perinatol.* 1992;9(4):254-257.

141. Onodera H, Matsunaga T, Tamura Y, et al. Enalapril suppresses ventricular remodeling more effectively than losartan in patients with acute myocardial infarction. *Am Heart J.* 2005;150(4):689.

142. Marijianowski MM, Teeling P, Becker AE. Remodeling after myocardial infarction in humans is not associated with interstitial fibrosis of noninfarcted myocardium. *J Am Coll Cardiol.* 1997;30(1):76-82.

143. Investigators S, Yusuf S, Pitt B, Davis CE, Hood WB, Cohn JN. Effect of enalapril on survival in patients with reduced left ventricular ejection fractions and congestive heart failure. *N Engl J Med.* 1991;325(5):293-302.

144. Pfeffer MA, Braunwald E, Moye LA, et al. Effect of captopril on mortality and morbidity in patients with left ventricular dysfunction after myocardial infarction. Results of the survival and ventricular enlargement trial. The SAVE Investigators. *N Engl J Med.* 1992;327(10):669-677.

145. Konstam MA, Kronenberg MW, Rousseau MF, et al. Effects of the angiotensin converting enzyme inhibitor enalapril on the long-term progression of left ventricular dilatation in patients with asymptomatic systolic dysfunction. SOLVD (Studies of Left Ventricular Dysfunction) Investigators. *Circulation.* 1993; 88(5 Pt 1):2277-2283.

146. Jugdutt BI. Effects of amlodipine versus enalapril on left ventricular remodelling after reperfused anterior myocardial canine infarction. *Can J Cardiol.* 1997;13(10):945-954.

147. Frenneaux M, Stewart RA, Newman CM, Hallidie-Smith KA. Enalapril for severe heart failure in infancy. *Arch Dis Child.* 1989;64(2):219-223.

148. Stanford AH, Reyes M, Rios DR, et al. Safety, feasibility, and impact of enalapril on cardiorespiratory physiology and health in preterm infants with systemic hypertension and left ventricular diastolic dysfunction. *J Clin Med.* 2021; 10(19):4519.

149. Sehgal A, Krishnamurthy MB, Clark M, Menahem S. ACE inhibition for severe bronchopulmonary dysplasia – an approach based on physiology. *Physiol Rep.* 2018;6(17):e13821.

150. Pandey R, Koshy RG, Dako J. Angiotensin converting enzyme inhibitors induced acute kidney injury in newborn. *J Matern Fetal Neonatal Med.* 2017;30(6):748-750.

151. Song WJ, Niimi A. Angiotensin-converting enzyme inhibitors, asthma, and cough: relighting the torch. *J Allergy Clin Immunol Pract.* 2021;9(9):3440-3441.

152. Gubhaju L, Sutherland MR, Black MJ. Preterm birth and the kidney: implications for long-term renal health. *Reprod Sci.* 2011;18(4):322-333.

153. Frolich S, Slattery P, Thomas D, et al. Angiotensin II-AT1-receptor signaling is necessary for cyclooxygenase-2-dependent postnatal nephron generation. *Kidney Int.* 2017;91(4): 818-829.

154. Brater DC. Diuretic therapy. *N Engl J Med.* 1998;339(6): 387-395.

155. Rose BD. Diuretics. *Kidney Int.* 1991;39(2):336-352.

156. Palmer BF. Metabolic complications associated with use of diuretics. *Semin Nephrol.* 2011;31(6):542-552.

157. Pacifici GM. Clinical pharmacology of the loop diuretics furosemide and bumetanide in neonates and infants. *Paediatr Drugs.* 2012;14(4):233-246.

158. Kokko JP. Site and mechanism of action of diuretics. *Am J Med.* 1984;77(5A):11-17.

159. Guignard JP, Iacobelli S. Use of diuretics in the neonatal period. *Pediatr Nephrol.* 2021;36(9):2687-2695.

160. Eades SK, Christensen ML. The clinical pharmacology of loop diuretics in the pediatric patient. *Pediatr Nephrol.* 1998; 12(7):603-616.

161. Pacifici GM. Clinical pharmacology of furosemide in neonates: a review. *Pharmaceuticals (Basel).* 2013;6(9):1094-1129.

162. Mirochnick MH, Miceli JJ, Kramer PA, Chapron DJ, Raye JR. Furosemide pharmacokinetics in very low birth weight infants. *J Pediatr.* 1988;112(4):653-657.

163. van der Vorst MM, Kist JE, van der Heijden AJ, Burggraaf J. Diuretics in pediatrics: current knowledge and future prospects. *Paediatr Drugs.* 2006;8(4):245-264.

164. MacDonald MG, Seshia MMK. *Avery's Neonatology: Pathophysiology & Management of the Newborn.* Philadelphia: Wolters Kluwer; 2016.

165. Chemtob S, Kaplan BS, Sherbotie JR, Aranda JV. Pharmacology of diuretics in the newborn. *Pediatr Clin North Am.* 1989;36(5):1231-1250.

166. Schoemaker RC, van der Vorst MM, van Heel IR, Cohen AF, Burggraaf J, Pediatric Pharmacology Network. Development of an optimal furosemide infusion strategy in infants with modeling and simulation. *Clin Pharmacol Ther.* 2002;72(4): 383-390.

167. van der Vorst MM, Ruys-Dudok van Heel I, Kist-van Holthe JE, et al. Continuous intravenous furosemide in haemodynamically unstable children after cardiac surgery. *Intensive Care Med.* 2001;27(4):711-715.

168. Kerdpin O, Knights KM, Elliot DJ, Miners JO. In vitro characterisation of human renal and hepatic frusemide glucuronidation and identification of the UDP-glucuronosyltransferase enzymes involved in this pathway. *Biochem Pharmacol.* 2008; 76(2):249-257.

169. Pichette V, du Souich P. Role of the kidneys in the metabolism of furosemide: its inhibition by probenecid. *J Am Soc Nephrol.* 1996;7(2):345-349.

170. Tuck S, Morselli P, Broquaire M, Vert P. Plasma and urinary kinetics of furosemide in newborn infants. *J Pediatr.* 1983; 103(3):481-485.

171. Vert P, Broquaire M, Legagneur M, Morselli PL. Pharmacokinetics of furosemide in neonates. *Eur J Clin Pharmacol.* 1982;22(1):39-45.

172. Peterson RG, Simmons MA, Rumack BH, Levine RL, Brooks JG. Pharmacology of furosemide in the premature newborn infant. *J Pediatr.* 1980;97(1):139-143.

173. Aranda JV, Perez J, Sitar DS, et al. Pharmacokinetic disposition and protein binding of furosemide in newborn infants. *J Pediatr.* 1978;93(3):507-511.

174. Aranda JV, Lambert C, Perez J, Turmen T, Sitar DS. Metabolism and renal elimination of furosemide in the newborn infant. *J Pediatr.* 1982;101(5):777-781.

175. Ross BS, Pollak A, Oh W. The pharmacologic effects of furosemide therapy in the low-birth-weight infant. *J Pediatr.* 1978;92(1):149-152.

176. Sutiman N, Koh JC, Watt K, et al. Pharmacokinetics alterations in critically Ill pediatric patients on extracorporeal membrane oxygenation: a systematic review. *Front Pediatr.* 2020; 8:260.

177. Holtta T, Jalanko H. Congenital nephrotic syndrome: is early aggressive treatment needed? Yes. *Pediatr Nephrol.* 2020; 35(10):1985-1990.

178. Richardson H. Frusemide in heart failure of infancy. *Arch Dis Child.* 1971;46(248):520-524.

179. Witte MK, Stork JE, Blumer JL. Diuretic therapeutics in the pediatric patient. *Am J Cardiol.* 1986;57(2):44A-53A.

180. Gouyon JB, Guignard JP. Management of acute renal failure in newborns. *Pediatr Nephrol.* 2000;14(10-11):1037-1044.

181. Guignard JP, Ali US. Acute renal failure in the neonate. *J Pediatr Intensive Care.* 2016;5(2):42-49.

182. Nada A, Bonachea EM, Askenazi DJ. Acute kidney injury in the fetus and neonate. *Semin Fetal Neonatal Med.* 2017;22(2): 90-97.

183. Pandey V, Kumar D, Vijayaraghavan P, Chaturvedi T, Raina R. Non-dialytic management of acute kidney injury in newborns. *J Renal Inj Prev.* 2017;6(1):1-11.

184. van der Vorst MM, Kist-van Holthe JE, den Hartigh J, van der Heijden AJ, Cohen AF, Burggraaf J. Absence of tolerance and toxicity to high-dose continuous intravenous furosemide in haemodynamically unstable infants after cardiac surgery. *Br J Clin Pharmacol.* 2007;64(6):796-803.

185. Klinge JM, Scharf J, Hofbeck M, Gerling S, Bonakdar S, Singer H. Intermittent administration of furosemide versus continuous infusion in the postoperative management of children following open heart surgery. *Intensive Care Med.* 1997;23(6): 693-697.

186. Liu C, Yan S, Wang Y, et al. Drug-induced hospital-acquired acute kidney injury in China: a multicenter cross-sectional survey. *Kidney Dis (Basel).* 2021;7(2):143-155.

187. Ryan MP, Devane J, Ryan MF, Counihan TB. Effects of diuretics on the renal handling of magnesium. *Drugs.* 1984;28(suppl 1):167-181.

188. Reyes AJ. Renal excretory profiles of loop diuretics: consequences for therapeutic application. *J Cardiovasc Pharmacol.* 1993;22(suppl 3):S11-S23.

189. Palmer BF, Alpern RJ. Metabolic alkalosis. *J Am Soc Nephrol.* 1997;8(9):1462-1469.

190. Gimpel C, Krause A, Franck P, Krueger M, von Schnakenburg C. Exposure to furosemide as the strongest risk factor for nephrocalcinosis in preterm infants. *Pediatr Int.* 2010;52(1):51-56.

191. Adams ND, Rowe JC. Nephrocalcinosis. *Clin Perinatol.* 1992;19(1):179-195.

192. Atkinson SA, Shah JK, McGee C, Steele BT. Mineral excretion in premature infants receiving various diuretic therapies. *J Pediatr.* 1988;113(3):540-545.

193. Myracle MR, McGahan JP, Goetzman BW, Adelman RD. Ultrasound diagnosis of renal calcification in infants on chronic furosemide therapy. *J Clin Ultrasound.* 1986;14(4):281-287.

194. Schell-Feith EA, Kist-van Holthe JE, van der Heijden AJ. Nephrocalcinosis in preterm neonates. *Pediatr Nephrol.* 2010; 25(2):221-230.

195. Orth LE, O'Mara KL. Impact of early versus late diuretic exposure on metabolic bone disease and growth in premature neonates. *J Pediatr Pharmacol Ther.* 2018;23(1):26-33.

196. Jensen EA, White AM, Liu P, et al. Determinants of severe metabolic bone disease in very low-birth-weight infants with severe bronchopulmonary dysplasia admitted to a tertiary referral center. *Am J Perinatol.* 2016;33(1):107-113.

197. Ding D, Liu H, Qi W, et al. Ototoxic effects and mechanisms of loop diuretics. *J Otol.* 2016;11(4):145-156.

198. Rybak LP. Furosemide ototoxicity: clinical and experimental aspects. *Laryngoscope.* 1985;95(9 Pt 2 Suppl 38):1-14.

199. Jackson W, Taylor G, Selewski D, Smith PB, Tolleson-Rinehart S, Laughon MM. Association between furosemide in premature infants and sensorineural hearing loss and nephrocalcinosis: a systematic review. *Matern Health Neonatol Perinatol.* 2018;4:23.

200. Lunau HE, Bak M, Petersen JS, Shalmi M, Marcussen N, Christensen S. Renal adaptations to continuous administration of furosemide and bendroflumethiazide in rats. *Pharmacol Toxicol.* 1994;74(4-5):216-222.

201. Huang X, Dorhout Mees E, Vos P, Hamza S, Braam B. Everything we always wanted to know about furosemide but were afraid to ask. *Am J Physiol Renal Physiol.* 2016;310(10):F958-F971.

202. Cotton R, Suarez S, Reese J. Unexpected extra-renal effects of loop diuretics in the preterm neonate. *Acta Paediatr.* 2012;101(8):835-845.

203. Rush MG, Engelhardt B, Parker RA, Hazinski TA. Double-blind, placebo-controlled trial of alternate-day furosemide therapy in infants with chronic bronchopulmonary dysplasia. *J Pediatr.* 1990;117(1 Pt 1):112-118.

204. Stewart A, Brion LP. Intravenous or enteral loop diuretics for preterm infants with (or developing) chronic lung disease. *Cochrane Database Syst Rev.* 2011;(9):CD001453.

205. Stewart A, Brion LP, Soll R. Diuretics for respiratory distress syndrome in preterm infants. *Cochrane Database Syst Rev.* 2011;(12):CD001454.

206. Blaisdell CJ, Troendle J, Zajicek A, Prematurity and Respiratory Outcomes Program. Acute responses to diuretic therapy in extremely low gestational age newborns: results from the prematurity and respiratory outcomes program cohort study. *J Pediatr.* 2018;197:42-47.e1.

207. Brion LP, Primhak RA, Yong W. Aerosolized diuretics for preterm infants with (or developing) chronic lung disease. *Cochrane Database Syst Rev.* 2006;(3):CD001694.

208. Michael Z, Spyropoulos F, Ghanta S, Christou H. Bronchopulmonary dysplasia: an update of current pharmacologic therapies and new approaches. *Clin Med Insights Pediatr.* 2018; 12:1179556518817322.

209. Prabhu VG, Keszler M, Dhanireddy R. Dose-dependent evaluation of the effects of nebulized furosemide on pulmonary function in ventilated preterm infants. *J Perinatol.* 1998; 18(5):357-360.

210. Stevens EL, Uyehara CF, Southgate WM, Nakamura KT. Furosemide differentially relaxes airway and vascular smooth muscle in fetal, newborn, and adult guinea pigs. *Am Rev Respir Dis.* 1992;146(5 Pt 1):1192-1197.

211. Greenberg RG, Gayam S, Savage D, et al. Furosemide exposure and prevention of bronchopulmonary dysplasia in premature infants. *J Pediatr.* 2019;208:134-140.e2.

212. Bamat NA, Nelin TD, Eichenwald ECK, et al. Loop diuretics in severe bronchopulmonary dysplasia: cumulative use and associations with mortality and age at discharge. *J Pediatr.* 2021;231:43-49.e3.

213. Barthelmebs M, Stephan D, Fontaine C, Grima M, Imbs JL. Vascular effects of loop diuretics: an in vivo and in vitro study in the rat. *Naunyn Schmiedebergs Arch Pharmacol.* 1994;349(2): 209-216.

214. de Berrazueta JR, Gonzalez JP, de Mier I, Poveda JJ, Garcia-Unzueta MT. Vasodilatory action of loop diuretics: a plethysmography study of endothelial function in forearm arteries and dorsal hand veins in hypertensive patients and controls. *J Cardiovasc Pharmacol.* 2007;49(2):90-95.

215. Mackay IG, Muir AL, Watson ML. Contribution of prostaglandins to the systemic and renal vascular response to frusemide in normal man. *Br J Clin Pharmacol.* 1984;17(5):513-519.

216. Sulyok E, Varga F, Nemeth M, et al. Furosemide-induced alterations in the electrolyte status, the function of renin-angiotensin-aldosterone system, and the urinary excretion of prostaglandins in newborn infants. *Pediatr Res.* 1980;14(5): 765-768.

217. Wiemer G, Fink E, Linz W, Hropot M, Scholkens BE, Wohlfart P. Furosemide enhances the release of endothelial kinins, nitric oxide and prostacyclin. *J Pharmacol Exp Ther.* 1994; 271(3):1611-1615.

218. Green TP, Thompson TR, Johnson DE, Lock JE. Furosemide promotes patent ductus arteriosus in premature infants with the respiratory-distress syndrome. *N Engl J Med.* 1983;308(13): 743-748.

219. Friedman Z, Demers LM, Marks KH, Uhrmann S, Maisels MJ. Urinary excretion of prostaglandin E following the administration of furosemide and indomethacin to sick low-birth-weight infants. *J Pediatr.* 1978;93(3):512-515.

220. Toyoshima K, Momma K, Nakanishi T. In vivo dilatation of the ductus arteriosus induced by furosemide in the rat. *Pediatr Res.* 2010;67(2):173-176.

221. Shankaran S, Poland RL. The displacement of bilirubin from albumin by furosemide. *J Pediatr.* 1977;90(4):642-646.

222. Lopez-Samblas AM, Adams JA, Goldberg RN, Modi MW. The pharmacokinetics of bumetanide in the newborn infant. *Biol Neonate.* 1997;72(5):265-272.

223. Oliveros M, Pham JT, John E, Resheidat A, Bhat R. The use of bumetanide for oliguric acute renal failure in preterm infants. *Pediatr Crit Care Med.* 2011;12(2):210-214.

224. Sullivan JE, Witte MK, Yamashita TS, Myers CM, Blumer JL. Dose-ranging evaluation of bumetanide pharmacodynamics in critically ill infants. *Clin Pharmacol Ther.* 1996;60(4):424-434.

225. Ward OC, Lam LK. Bumetanide in heart failure in infancy. *Arch Dis Child.* 1977;52(11):877-882.

226. Vetter VL. *Pediatric Cardiology: The Requisites in Pediatrics.* Philadelphia, PA: Mosby Elsevier; 2006.

227. Ramsay LE, McInnes GT, Hettiarachchi J, Shelton J, Scott P. Bumetanide and frusemide: a comparison of dose-response curves in healthy men. *Br J Clin Pharmacol.* 1978;5(3): 243-247.

228. Asbury MJ, Gatenby PB, O'Sullivan S, Bourke E. Bumetanide: potent new "loop" diuretic. *Br Med J.* 1972;1(5794):211-213.

229. Ward A, Heel RC. Bumetanide. A review of its pharmacodynamic and pharmacokinetic properties and therapeutic use. *Drugs.* 1984;28(5):426-464.

230. Sullivan JE, Witte MK, Yamashita TS, Myers CM, Blumer JL. Pharmacokinetics of bumetanide in critically ill infants. *Clin Pharmacol Ther.* 1996;60(4):405-413.

231. Sullivan JE, Witte MK, Yamashita TS, Myers CM, Blumer JL. Analysis of the variability in the pharmacokinetics and pharmacodynamics of bumetanide in critically ill infants. *Clin Pharmacol Ther.* 1996;60(4):414-423.

232. Wells TG, Fasules JW, Taylor BJ, Kearns GL. Pharmacokinetics and pharmacodynamics of bumetanide in neonates treated with extracorporeal membrane oxygenation. *J Pediatr.* 1992; 121(6):974-980.

233. Shankaran S, Liang KC, Ilagan N, Fleischmann L. Mineral excretion following furosemide compared with bumetanide therapy in premature infants. *Pediatr Nephrol.* 1995;9(2):159-162.

234. Walker PC, Shankaran S. The bilirubin-displacing capacity of bumetanide in critically ill neonates. *Dev Pharmacol Ther.* 1988;11(5):265-272.

235. Wells TG. The pharmacology and therapeutics of diuretics in the pediatric patient. *Pediatr Clin North Am.* 1990;37(2): 463-504.

236. Haas M. The Na-K-Cl cotransporters. *Am J Physiol.* 1994;267 (4 Pt 1):C869-C885.

237. Stanton BA. Cellular actions of thiazide diuretics in the distal tubule. *J Am Soc Nephrol.* 1990;1(5):832-836.

238. Calder JA, Schachter M, Sever PS. Potassium channel opening properties of thiazide diuretics in isolated guinea pig resistance arteries. *J Cardiovasc Pharmacol.* 1994;24(1):158-164.

239. Duarte JD, Cooper-DeHoff RM. Mechanisms for blood pressure lowering and metabolic effects of thiazide and thiazide-like diuretics. *Expert Rev Cardiovasc Ther.* 2010; 8(6):793-802.

240. Pickkers P, Hughes AD, Russel FG, Thien T, Smits P. Thiazide-induced vasodilation in humans is mediated by potassium channel activation. *Hypertension.* 1998;32(6):1071-1076.

241. Pickkers P, Russel FG, Hughes AD, Thien T, Smits P. Hydrochlorothiazide exerts no direct vasoactivity in the human forearm. *J Hypertens.* 1995;13(12 Pt 2):1833-1836.

242. Friedman PA. Codependence of renal calcium and sodium transport. *Annu Rev Physiol.* 1998;60:179-197.

243. Kliegman RM. *Nelson Textbook of Pediatrics.* Philadelphia, MO: Elsevier; 2019.

244. Hobbins SM, Fowler RS, Rowe RD, Korey AG. Spironolactone therapy in infants with congestive heart failure secondary to congenital heart disease. *Arch Dis Child.* 1981;56(12): 934-938.

245. Costello J, Almodovar M. Emergency care for infants and children with acute cardiac disease. *Clin Pediatr Emerg Med.* 2007;8(3):145-155.

246. Moffett BS, Tsang R, Kennedy C, Bronicki RA, Akcan-Arikan A, Checchia PA. Efficacy of sequential nephron blockade with intravenous chlorothiazide to promote diuresis in cardiac intensive care infants. *Cardiol Young.* 2017;27(6):1104-1109.

247. Kearns GL, Abdel-Rahman SM, Alander SW, Blowey DL, Leeder JS, Kauffman RE. Developmental pharmacology – drug disposition, action, and therapy in infants and children. *N Eng J Med.* 2003;349(12):1157-1167.

248. Welling PG. Pharmacokinetics of the thiazide diuretics. *Biopharm Drug Dispos.* 1986;7(6):501-535.

249. Niemeyer C, Hasenfuss G, Wais U, Knauf H, Schafer-Korting M, Mutschler E. Pharmacokinetics of hydrochlorothiazide in relation to renal function. *Eur J Clin Pharmacol.* 1983;24(5): 661-665.

250. Fernandez E, Perez R, Hernandez A, Tejada P, Arteta M, Ramos JT. Factors and mechanisms for pharmacokinetic differences between pediatric population and adults. *Pharmaceutics.* 2011;3(1):53-72.

251. Commander SJ, Wu H, Boakye-Agyeman F, et al. Pharmacokinetics of hydrochlorothiazide in children: a potential surrogate for renal secretion maturation. *J Clin Pharmacol.* 2021; 61(3):368-377.

252. Sweeney DE, Vallon V, Rieg T, Wu W, Gallegos TF, Nigam SK. Functional maturation of drug transporters in the developing, neonatal, and postnatal kidney. *Mol Pharmacol.* 2011;80(1):147-154.

253. Kirchlechner V, Koller DY, Seidl R, Waldhauser F. Treatment of nephrogenic diabetes insipidus with hydrochlorothiazide and amiloride. *Arch Dis Child.* 1999;80(6):548-552.

254. Duicu C, Pitea AM, Sasaran OM, Cozea I, Man L, Banescu C. Nephrogenic diabetes insipidus in children (Review). *Exp Ther Med.* 2021;22(1):746.

255. Brion LP, Primhak RA, Ambrosio-Perez I. Diuretics acting on the distal renal tubule for preterm infants with (or developing) chronic lung disease. *Cochrane Database Syst Rev.* 2000;(2):CD001817.

256. Leung AA, Wright A, Pazo V, Karson A, Bates DW. Risk of thiazide-induced hyponatremia in patients with hypertension. *Am J Med.* 2011;124(11):1064-1072.

257. Nijenhuis T, Vallon V, van der Kemp AW, Loffing J, Hoenderop JG, Bindels RJ. Enhanced passive Ca2+ reabsorption and reduced Mg2+ channel abundance explains thiazide-induced hypocalciuria and hypomagnesemia. *J Clin Invest.* 2005;115(6):1651-1658.

258. Reyes AJ. Cardiovascular drugs and serum uric acid. *Cardiovasc Drugs Ther.* 2003;17(5-6):397-414.

259. Wennberg RP, Rasmussen F, Ahlfors CE. Displacement of bilirubin from human albumin by three diuretics. *J Pediatr.* 1977;90(4):647-650.

260. Corvol P, Michaud A, Menard J, Freifeld M, Mahoudeau J. Antiandrogenic effect of spirolactones: mechanism of action. *Endocrinology.* 1975;97(1):52-58.

261. Fanaroff AA, Fanaroff AA, Fanaroff JM, Klaus MH. *Klaus & Fanaroff's Care of the High-Risk Neonate.* Philadelphia, PA: Elsevier/Saunders; 2013.

262. Los LE, Pitzenberger SM, Ramjit HG, Coddington AB, Colby HD. Hepatic metabolism of spironolactone. Production of 3-hydroxy-thiomethyl metabolites. *Drug Metab Dispos.* 1994;22(6):903-908.

263. Jenkins R, Tackitt S, Gievers L, et al. Phthalate-associated hypertension in premature infants: a prospective mechanistic cohort study. *Pediatr Nephrol.* 2019;34(8):1413-1424.

264. Jenkins RD, Aziz JK, Gievers LL, Mooers HM, Fino N, Rozansky DJ. Characteristics of hypertension in premature infants with and without chronic lung disease: a long-term multicenter study. *Pediatr Nephrol.* 2017;32(11):2115-2124.

265. Buck ML. Clinical experience with spironolactone in pediatrics. *Ann Pharmacother.* 2005;39(5):823-828.

266. Al-Majed AA, Bakheit AHH, Abdel Aziz HA, Alajmi FM, AlRabiah H. Propranolol. *Profiles Drug Subst Excip Relat Methodol.* Elsevier; 2017;42:287-338.

267. Barton AL, Moffett BS, Valdes SO, Miyake C, Kim JJ. Efficacy and safety of high-dose propranolol for the management of infant supraventricular tachyarrhythmias. *J Pediatr.* 2015;166(1):115-118.

268. Pfammatter JP, Bauersfeld U. Safety issues in the treatment of paediatric supraventricular tachycardias. *Drug Saf.* 1998;18(5):345-356.

269. Luedtke SA, Kuhn RJ, McCaffrey FM. Pharmacologic management of supraventricular tachycardias in children. Part 2: atrial flutter, atrial fibrillation, and junctional and atrial ectopic tachycardia. *Ann Pharmacother.* 1997;31(11):1347-1359.

270. Filippi L, Cavallaro G, Fiorini P, et al. Propranolol concentrations after oral administration in term and preterm neonates. *J Matern Fetal Neonatal Med.* 2013;26(8):833-840.

271. Gillette P, Garson A, Jr., Eterovic E, Neches W, Mullins C, McNamara DG. Oral propranolol treatment in infants and children. *J Pediatr.* 1978;92(1):141-144.

272. Seggewiss H, Rigopoulos A. Management of hypertrophic cardiomyopathy in children. *Paediatr Drugs.* 2003;5(10):663-672.

273. Ostman-Smith I, Wettrell G, Riesenfeld T. A cohort study of childhood hypertrophic cardiomyopathy: improved survival following high-dose beta-adrenoceptor antagonist treatment. *J Am Coll Cardiol.* 1999;34(6):1813-1822.

274. McBride JT, McBride MC, Viles PH. Hypoglycemia associated with propranolol. *Pediatrics.* 1973;51(6):1085-1087.

275. Holland KE, Frieden IJ, Frommelt PC, Mancini AJ, Wyatt D, Drolet BA. Hypoglycemia in children taking propranolol for the treatment of infantile hemangioma. *Arch Dermatol.* 2010;146(7):775-778.

276. Cuneo BF, Zales VR, Blahunka PC, Benson Jr DW. Pharmacodynamics and pharmacokinetics of esmolol, a short-acting beta-blocking agent, in children. *Pediatr Cardiol.* 1994;15(6):296-301.

277. Wiest DB, Garner SS, Uber WE, Sade RM. Esmolol for the management of pediatric hypertension after cardiac operations. *J Thorac Cardiovasc Surg.* 1998;115(4):890-897.

278. Reynolds RD, Gorczynski RJ, Quon CY. Pharmacology and pharmacokinetics of esmolol. *J Clin Pharmacol.* 1986;26(suppl 1):A3-A14.

279. Tabbutt S, Nicolson SC, Adamson PC, et al. The safety, efficacy, and pharmacokinetics of esmolol for blood pressure control immediately after repair of coarctation of the aorta in infants and children: a multicenter, double-blind, randomized trial. *J Thorac Cardiovasc Surg.* 2008;136(2):321-328.

280. Wiest DB, Trippel DL, Gillette PC, Garner SS. Pharmacokinetics of esmolol in children. *Clin Pharmacol Ther.* 1991;49(6):618-623.

281. Smerling A, Gersony WM. Esmolol for severe hypertension following repair of aortic coarctation. *Crit Care Med.* 1990;18(11):1288-1290.

282. Vincent RN, Click LA, Williams HM, Plauth WH, Williams WH. Esmolol as an adjunct in the treatment of systemic hypertension after operative repair of coarctation of the aorta. *Am J Cardiol.* 1990;65(13):941-943.

283. Östman-Smith I. Beta-blockers in pediatric hypertrophic cardiomyopathies. *Rev Recent Clin Trials.* 2014;9(2):82-85.

284. Ross M, Ungerleider, Nelson K, Cooper D. *Critical Heart Disease in Infants and Children.* Philadelphia, PA: Elsevier; 2019.

285. Nussbaum J, Zane EA, Thys DM. Esmolol for the treatment of hypercyanotic spells in infants with tetralogy of Fallot. *J Cardiothorac Anesth.* 1989;3(2):200-202.

286. Reyes G, Schwartz PH, Newth CJ, Eldadah MK. The pharmacokinetics of isoproterenol in critically ill pediatric patients. *J Clin Pharmacol.* 1993;33(1):29-34.

287. Nishioka K, Nakanishi T, George BL, Jarmakani JM. The effect of calcium on the inotropy of catecholamine and paired electrical stimulation in the newborn and adult myocardium. *J Mol Cell Cardiol.* 1981;13(5):511-520.

288. Matsubara S, Morimatsu Y, Shiraishi H, et al. Fetus with heart failure due to congenital atrioventricular block treated by maternally administered ritodrine. *Arch Gynecol Obstet.* 2008;278(1):85-88.

289. Castilla M, Jerez M, Llacer M, Martinez S. Anaesthetic management in a neonate with congenital complete heart block. *Paediatr Anaesth.* 2004;14(2):172-175.

290. Mikhail MS, Hunsinger SY, Goodwin SR, Loughlin GM. Myocardial ischemia complicating therapy of status asthmaticus. *Clin Pediatr (Phila).* 1987;26(8):419-421.

# Hemodynamics of Postnatal Transition

# Chapter 6

# Hemodynamic Significance and Clinical Relevance of Deferred Cord Clamping and Umbilical Cord Milking

Douglas A. Blank, Stuart B. Hooper, Anup C. Katheria, and Martin Kluckow

## Key Points

- Cardiorespiratory transition at birth is a complex series of changes in which the lungs replace the placenta as the organ of gas exchange and the main source of preload to the left side of the heart.
- Lung aeration, driven by spontaneous inhalations or mechanical inflation, is the key stimulus leading to pulmonary vascular relaxation.
- Umbilical cord clamping, prior to lung aeration, reduces cardiac output by up to 50% and increases the risk of hypoxia. Cardiac output after umbilical cord clamping is restored with an increase in pulmonary blood flow.
- Deferred cord clamping after birth is currently recommended for vigorous preterm and term newborns, leading to improved preterm survival, increased hemoglobin, and increased iron stores.
- Physiologically based cord clamping is an emerging strategy for non-vigorous newborns requiring respiratory support at birth in which umbilical cord clamping is deferred until the lungs are aerated and exchanging gases.
- Umbilical cord milking (UCM) has been the subject of numerous clinical trials, mostly in near-term infants not requiring resuscitation, suggesting that UCM is safe, appears to confer the same benefits of deferred cord clamping, and may be more effective in infants delivered by cesarean section. However, the recent finding of a fourfold increase in severe IVH rates in extremely preterm infants receiving UCM has led to the recommendation against UCM in extremely preterm infants.

## The Transition to Newborn Life and Lung Liquid Clearance

The transition from intra- to extra-uterine life involves a remarkable sequence of physiological events that allow the fetus to survive after birth independent of placental support and in a gaseous environment.[1,2] Before birth, the developing lungs are liquid filled and gas exchange occurs across the placenta.[3] Cardiopulmonary adaption at birth is triggered by the one event that cannot occur in utero, lung aeration. At birth, the airways must be cleared of liquid to allow the entry of air and the onset of pulmonary ventilation so that gas exchange can transfer from the placenta to the lungs.[3] To facilitate the onset of pulmonary gas exchange, lung aeration also triggers a large decrease in pulmonary vascular resistance (PVR). As a result, right ventricular output is redirected through the lungs rather than flowing through the ductus arteriosus (DA), causing a large increase in pulmonary blood flow (PBF).[4,5] Before birth, as PBF is low, most venous return and ventricular preload for the left ventricle is supplied by umbilical venous return, which flows via the ductus venosus and foramen ovale directly into the left atrium.[6] The increase in PBF plays a vital role in sustaining the infant's cardiac output by replacing umbilical venous flow as the primary source of left ventricular preload after umbilical venous return is lost due to umbilical cord clamping (UCC). Therefore UCC, before pulmonary ventilation has commenced and PBF has increased, is potentially problematic and causes a large reduction (up to 50%) in cardiac output and increased risk of hypoxemia and ischemia.[4,7-9] Thus it is important to understand the physiological changes that occur at birth, as well as be able to recognize the stage within this transitional process that the infant has reached, in order to choose the correct timing for UCC after birth.

## AIRWAY LIQUID CLEARANCE

In utero, the fetus grows and develops in a liquid environment, with gas exchange occurring across the placenta. The future airways are filled with a liquid that is produced by the lung and plays a vital role in stimulating fetal lung growth and development.[10] This liquid is actively retained within the airways by the fetus and keeps the lungs under a constant state of distension, resulting in a resting lung volume that is larger than the functional residual capacity of the newborn lung.[10] This constant state of distension provides a mechanical stimulus for lung growth, which, if absent, results in severe lung hypoplasia that is either lethal or causes significant morbidity in the newborn.[10,11] However, while airway liquid is essential for fetal lung growth, its presence prevents the entry of air and the onset of pulmonary gas exchange after birth. As such, it is important that the airways are cleared as rapidly as possible during the birth process to ensure that air can enter the terminal gas exchange regions of the lung and facilitate the onset of gas exchange.

Much interest has focused on the mechanisms of airway liquid clearance at birth, as reduced or variable airway liquid clearance is a major cause of perinatal morbidity, particularly in premature infants or term infants born by cesarean section. There are potentially three mechanisms that can contribute to airway liquid clearance at birth, which depend upon the timing and mode of birth: (i) expulsion of liquid with uterine contractions after rupture of membranes, (ii) increased circulating adrenaline levels during labor which activate amiloride-sensitive $Na^+$ channels and stimulate liquid reabsorption, and (iii) trans-epithelial hydrostatic pressures generated during initial inspirations or mechanical inflations after birth.[12]

As the fetal respiratory system is highly compliant, small increases in transthoracic pressure, for example, due to postural changes, can greatly reduce the volume of airway liquid. It is well established that the loss of amniotic fluid and uterine contractions increase fetal spinal flexion, which in turn increases both abdominal and intrathoracic pressures, resulting in lung liquid loss.[13,14] While this mechanism can account for large reductions in airway liquid at birth, it does not explain how residual volumes of liquid are cleared from the airways after birth. It has been proposed that increased circulating adrenaline levels during labor activate amiloride-sensitive $Na^+$ channels located on the apical surface of pulmonary epithelial cells.[15,16] The resulting uptake of $Na^+$ from the lung lumen and its transport across the epithelium into the pulmonary interstitium also increases the electropotential gradient for $Cl^-$ ion flux in the same direction.[16] This reverses the osmotic gradient driving fetal lung liquid secretion, leading to liquid reabsorption from the airway lumen.[16] While this mechanism has been extensively studied and described, it only develops late in gestation and requires very high levels of circulating adrenaline, and at maximally stimulated rates (30 mL/h), it would take hours to clear all airway liquid.[12,17,18] As a result, this mechanism likely accounts for only a small proportion (<5%) of airway liquid clearance at birth.[19,20]

Phase contrast X-ray imaging has allowed researchers to visualize the entry of air onto the lungs at birth in both spontaneously breathing and mechanically ventilated term and preterm rabbits.[21-25] These studies clearly show that the air-liquid interface only moves distally during inspiration or during positive pressure inflations (Figure 6.1). Between breaths or inflations,

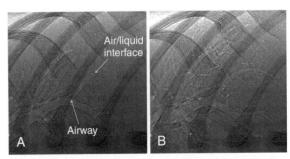

**Fig. 6.1 High-resolution phase contrast X-ray images of a non-dependent region of the lung shortly after the beginning of lung aeration.** Images were acquired before (A) and after (B) a single breath in a spontaneously breathing near-term rabbit, demonstrating the amount of aeration that occurs with a single inspiration. Using this technique, liquid-filled airways are not visible and only become visible after they aerate. The air-liquid interface is clearly visible in (Panel A) After one breath at least another two generations of airways become visible (Panel B).

the air-liquid interface either remains stationary or moves proximally, indicating that some airway liquid re-entry may occur between breaths.[19,20,25] Based on these results, it was concluded that after birth, airway liquid clearance primarily results from trans-epithelial hydrostatic pressures generated during inspiration/inflation.[12,20] That is, inspiration-induced hydrostatic pressure gradients between the airways and surrounding tissue drive the movement of liquid out of the airways across the pulmonary epithelium. This process was found to be extraordinarily rapid, with some newborn rabbits completely aerating their lungs in 3–5 breaths, generating an FRC of 15–20 mL/kg in that time (~30 seconds).[19,20] Similarly, in spontaneously breathing term newborns delivered via cesarean section without labor, 90% had aerated lungs (measured by ultrasound), and 100% had detectable exhaled carbon dioxide within 7 breaths after birth. This confirms a dominant role for inspirations in airway liquid clearance as a single mechanism.[26,27]

## INCREASE IN PULMONARY BLOOD FLOW AT BIRTH IN RESPONSE TO LUNG AERATION

At birth, lung aeration increases PBF 20- to 30-fold,[6] which not only enhances pulmonary gas exchange capacity but also plays a critical role in taking over the supply of preload for the left ventricle from umbilical venous return.[1,3] Numerous mechanisms are believed to mediate the pulmonary vasodilation in response to lung aeration, including increased oxygenation leading to the release of vasodilators such as nitric oxide, a reduction in lung distension caused by the formation of surface tension, and a vagal-mediated vasodilation caused by the movement of liquid out of the airways into the surrounding tissue.[28] The latter mechanism was identified using simultaneous phase contrast X-ray imaging and angiography, designed to examine the spatial relationship between ventilation and perfusion during transition.[29] While the imaging was expected to show that partial lung aeration would increase PBF in only aerated lung regions, unexpectedly, the imaging unequivocally demonstrated that partial lung aeration caused a global increase in PBF (Figure 6.2). As ventilation with 100% nitrogen was able to produce a similar response as well as an increase in heart rate,[30] it appears that increased oxygenation is not a prerequisite for pulmonary vasodilation at birth, which is a consistently reported finding.[31,32] Nevertheless, ventilation with 100% oxygen enhanced the increase in PBF, but only in ventilated lung regions, indicating that the increase in PBF in response to lung aeration is multifactorial, with different mechanisms working independently.[30] As vagal nerve section abolished the increase in PBF induced by partial lung ventilation with 100% nitrogen, it was suggested that the movement of airway liquid into lung tissue activated receptors (possibly J receptors), which signaled via the vagus to stimulate a global increase in PBF.[33]

While the global increase in PBF that is stimulated by partial lung aeration causes a large ventilation/perfusion mismatch after birth, this is not necessarily problematic.[29] Indeed, as lung aeration is usually quite heterogeneous,[34] restricting the overall increase in PBF by only increasing PBF in aerated lung regions will reduce pulmonary venous return and may affect cardiac output. This is because, following UCC, pulmonary venous return becomes the primary source of preload for the left ventricle and restricting the increase in PBF restricts cardiac output.[4] As a result, the importance of clamping the umbilical cord at the appropriate time within this physiological sequence (lung aeration followed by PBF increase) becomes self-evident.[3]

## The Cardiovascular Transition at Birth: Effect of Umbilical Cord Clamping

The fetal circulatory system is very different than that of the newborn and must undergo substantial and rapid changes to transform from a fetal into a newborn phenotype.[3,6] Before birth PBF is low, and most of right ventricular output bypasses the lung and enters the descending thoracic aorta via the DA.[6] As a result, the left and right fetal ventricles pump in parallel, with both providing output for the systemic circulation. Of note, this circulation also includes perfusing an organ (the placenta) which at times during pregnancy is as big, if not bigger, than the fetus.

As the placenta receives a high percentage (30–50%) of fetal cardiac output, umbilical venous return must also provide a large proportion of venous return to the heart, which flows via both the ductus venous and the liver via the IVC.[6] Of the umbilical venous return flowing through the ductus venosus, most of this blood bypasses the right atrium, right ventricle,

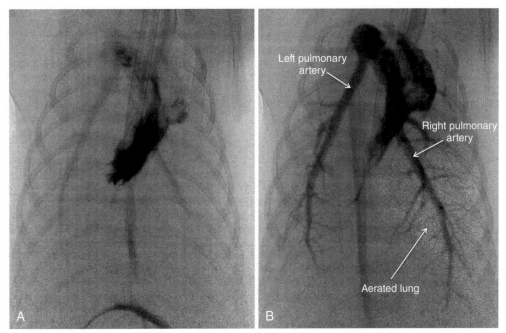

**Fig. 6.2 Simultaneous phase contrast X-ray images and angiogram of a near-term newborn rabbit before (A) and after partial lung aeration of the right lung (B).** An iodine solution is used as a contrast agent to highlight the blood vessels. Before lung aeration (A), pulmonary blood flow (PBF) is low and so very little iodine solution penetrates into the pulmonary arteries. However, after partial aeration of the right lung (B), PBF into both lungs is greatly increased, irrespective of whether partial lung aeration occurs on the left or right side. This indicates that the increase in PBF at birth is not dependent upon total lung aeration and is not spatially related to aerated lung regions.

and the lungs by flowing through the foramen ovale into the left atrium.[6] This has two important consequences. The first is that highly oxygenated umbilical venous blood can pass directly into the left side of the heart, resulting in higher blood oxygen levels in preductal arteries perfusing the head and upper body.[6] The second, often overlooked consequence, is that umbilical venous blood provides a large percentage of the left ventricular preload in the fetus, particularly as PBF is low.[1,3]

The consequences of umbilical cord clamping at birth are multifactorial. The healthy placenta has a low-resistance, highly compliant vascular bed that receives a large percentage of fetal cardiac output. As a result, clamping the umbilical cord at birth not only separates the infant from its site of gas exchange but also greatly increases systemic vascular resistance and therefore increases afterloads on both the left and right ventricles.[4] This causes an instantaneous (within

4 heartbeats) increase in arterial blood pressure (by ~30%), which results in an equally rapid increase in cerebral blood flow.[4] In addition, upon clamping the umbilical cord, umbilical venous return is lost, which reduces left ventricular preload and, combined with the increase in afterload, greatly reduces cardiac output. The loss in cardiac output persists until the lung aerates and PBF increases to restore ventricular preload.[35] As such, if this period of reduced cardiac output at birth coincides with even a mild level of birth asphyxia, then the infant is at risk of further hypoxic/ischemic injury. This is because the fetus's primary defense against periods of hypoxia is to increase and redistribute cardiac output to increase blood flow to vital organs such as the brain.[36] However, if cardiac output is reduced, as occurs after cord clamping and before the onset of pulmonary ventilation, then the capacity of the fetus to defend itself from hypoxia is severely limited.

## NEONATAL CARDIOVASCULAR RESPONSES TO UMBILICAL CORD CLAMPING

Realization that the supply of left ventricular preload must switch from umbilical venous return to pulmonary venous return after birth underpins the rationale for deferring umbilical cord clamping until after the onset of pulmonary ventilation.[1,3,4] That is, if PBF increases before the umbilical cord is clamped, pulmonary venous return can immediately replace umbilical venous return as the primary source of preload for the left ventricle without any diminution in supply (Figure 6.3).[4] Under these circumstances, umbilical cord clamping does not result in a reduction in cardiac output. It is also important to recognize that the increase in pulmonary venous return following ventilation onset also increases right ventricular output, which increases rapidly with the increase in PBF.[4] For this to occur, blood flow through the foramen ovale (FO) must reverse to allow blood to flow from the left into the right atrium and contribute to right ventricular preload. While it has long been considered that the FO is a one-way valve, only flowing from right to left,[37] both experimental evidence and clinical observations indicate that this is not entirely accurate.[38]

Ventilating the lung and reducing PVR before clamping the umbilical cord also greatly mitigates the increase in arterial pressure caused by UCC, because the vasodilated lungs provide an additional low-resistance pathway for blood flow.[4,7,9] This initiates a competitive interplay between the pulmonary and placental circulations, whereby flow into either circulation depends upon the downstream resistance (or, more precisely, impedance) in each vascular bed.[1,3] As such, following the reduction in PVR, the proportion of right ventricular output passing through the DA into the descending aorta is reduced and redirected into the pulmonary circulation. The result is a substantial reduction in umbilical blood flow entering and leaving the placenta (Figure 6.4).[9,39] It is interesting to speculate whether the decrease in PVR contributes to reduced flow and gradual closure of the umbilical vessels after birth. Indeed, anything that alters resistances in either vascular bed will alter the distribution of cardiac output between the two vascular beds and may contribute to umbilical vessel closure when flow into the pulmonary circulation is favored.[3] For instance, as uterine contractions increase placental vascular resistance and reduce umbilical blood

flow, they increase the distribution of cardiac output into the pulmonary circulation. Similarly, the effect of gravity, caused by positioning the newborn above or below the placenta, induces the same response. That is, following ventilation onset, while umbilical artery flow is reduced as PBF increases, the reduction is much greater if the newborn is placed above the placenta compared with below the placenta.[39]

UCC following ventilation onset markedly alters the distribution of cardiac output within the newborn.[4] The loss of the low resistance placental vascular bed causes a large increase in PBF, due to (1) the redirection of the entire right ventricular output into the lungs and (2) the very rapid reversal of blood flow through the DA, leading to a large left-to-right DA shunt.[4,5] As a result, both left and right ventricles contribute to PBF after birth, with the contribution of the left gradually diminishing as the DA closes.[5] It has been suggested that this ensures that pulmonary venous return and left ventricular preload is sufficient to maintain or increase (as needed) left ventricular output in the newborn period. It also allows the output of the two ventricles to gradually (over a few hours) come into balance before the two circulations separate, as at that time, the outputs of the two ventricles must be equal.[3] Indeed, a continuing but gradually diminishing communication between the two atria (via the FO) and between the two arterial circulations (via the DA) should theoretically facilitate the balancing of the two ventricular outputs.

## NEONATAL CARDIOVASCULAR CONSEQUENCES OF UMBILICAL CORD MILKING

Umbilical cord milking (UCM) is a procedure in which the clinician milks or pushes the blood in the UC from the placenta to the infant. There are two established techniques of UCM that have been described in the literature. One method is "intact umbilical cord milking" (I-UCM). In this technique the clinician milks 20 cm of the UC over 1–2 seconds and releases the umbilical cord after each milk to allow the cord to refill with blood. This process is repeated 2–4 times prior to umbilical cord clamping.[40-45] Another UCM technique, called "cut-umbilical cord milking" (cut-UCM), is clamping the UC close to the placenta and milking the residual volume in the UC after cord clamping.[46-49] Currently international recommendations discourage

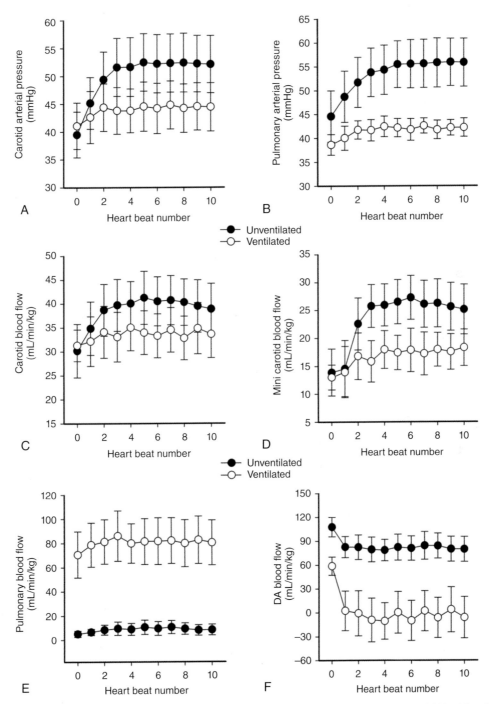

**Fig. 6.3** Changes in mean (± SEM) carotid arterial blood pressure (A), pulmonary arterial pressure (B), carotid arterial blood flow (C), minimum carotid arterial blood flow (D), pulmonary blood flow (E), and ductus arteriosus (DA) blood flow (F) in ventilated (*open circles*) and unventilated lambs (*filled circles*) for the first 10 heartbeats after umbilical cord occlusion (indicated by *dotted line*). '0' represents the heartbeat immediately before cord clamping. (From Bhatt et al.[4])

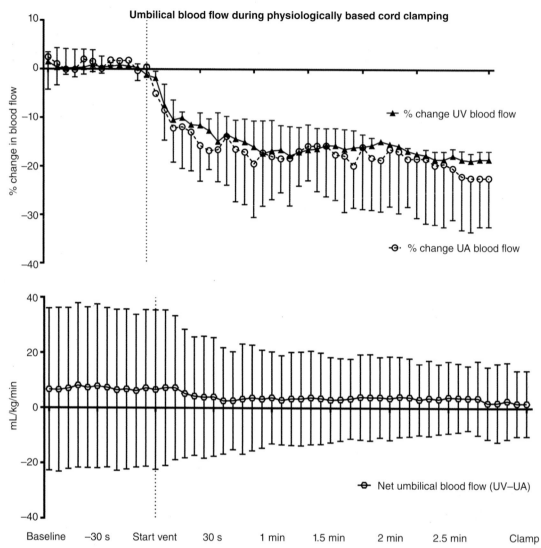

**Fig. 6.4 Umbilical blood flow measured during ventilation prior to umbilical cord clamping in anesthetized preterm lambs.** Umbilical venous and umbilical arterial blood flow was significantly reduced after the initiation of ventilation ($P < 0.001$). However, net umbilical blood flow did not change during this time ($P = 0.99$), resulting in no placental transfusion. *UA,* umbilical artery; *UV,* umbilical vein. (From Blank et al.[9])

the use of UCM outside of clinical studies.[50-54] The primary advantage of UCM over deferred UCC is the rapid blood transfer from the placenta to the infant immediately after birth without interfering with evaluation and resuscitation of the newborn. In several small trials authors concluded that UCM conferred the same benefits of deferred UCC.[41-43,55-57] In addition, UCM maybe a more effective method to transfer blood during cesarean deliveries because the uterus is not

vigorously contracting.[43] However, this assumes that the only benefit of deferred UCC is placental transfusion (see below), which it clearly is not, and also neglects the effect that total or intermittent occlusions of the umbilical cord have on the newborn's circulation.

Recent studies have clarified the physiological consequences of UCM procedures.[9,58] As expected, UCM necessitates that the cord is occluded during the milking procedure, which causes both a rapid increase in

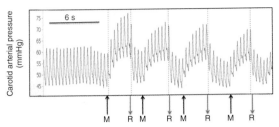

**Fig. 6.5 Changes in Carotid Arterial Pressure in Response to Four Consecutive Umbilical Cord Milkings.** Each cord milk is indicated by "M," whereas the cord release that occurred at the end of each milk is indicated by "R". Note the large increases in arterial pressure that occurred with each milk.

arterial pressure and cerebral blood flow and presumably a decrease in cardiac output, similar to that seen after actual cord clamping.[4,9] As arterial pressures are quickly restored following release of the cord to allow it to refill, the resulting changes in arterial blood pressure and cerebral flow in subsequent "milks" are precisely replicated. The net result is a concerning picture of several rapid increases and decreases in arterial pressure and cerebral blood flow, which resemble a "saw tooth" and are in stark contrast to the very stable pressures and flows that occur during deferred UCC. In a newborn infant with either an immature or inflamed cerebral vascular bed, these large "see-sawing" changes in arterial pressures and flows may be of even more concern (Figure 6.5). UCM has been the subject of numerous clinical trials, mostly in near-term infants not requiring resuscitation, and involves milking a 20 cm length of cord over 2–3 seconds, 3–4 times. These trials have suggested that UCM is safe, appears to confer the same benefits of DCC,[41,42,55-57,59] and may be more effective in infants delivered by cesarean section.[43,60] However, the recent finding of a fourfold increase in severe IVH rates in extremely preterm infants receiving UCM has led to the recommendation against UCM in extremely preterm infants.[58,61] There are no published results on the physiologic effects of cut-UCM.

## Placental Transfusion During Delayed Umbilical Cord Clamping

The concept that blood volume will automatically shift from the placenta to the infant in a time-dependent manner after birth if UCC is delayed is complex and

difficult to explain physiologically. This assumes that throughout deferred UCC, umbilical venous flow will exceed umbilical artery flow, despite the vein being much more susceptible to reduced flow in response to external influences than the artery.[1] However, the fundamental principles of circulatory physiology dictate that flow into an organ will always equal flow out of an organ unless there is a major change in vascular compliance (Figure 6.4).[9] While a large change in compliance will cause an imbalance in flow, the flow difference will always be transient. As such, blood volume will not automatically shift from the placenta to the infant unless the compliance of the vascular beds within either the infant or the placenta changes.[3,35] This is consistent with the fact that fetuses spend ~9 months in utero perfusing the placenta, and during this time, the distribution of blood volume between the fetus and placenta must be balanced to avoid a continuing net shift of blood from one compartment to the other.

## POTENTIAL MECHANISMS FOR PLACENTAL BLOOD TRANSFUSION

Numerous mechanisms have been suggested to enhance placental-to-infant blood transfusion after birth, including gravity, uterine contractions, the increase in PBF, and thoracic pressure changes arising during inspiration.[3] On the other hand, an increase in thoracic and abdominal pressures arising from crying or grunting may lead to fetal-to-placental blood transfusion, as would peripheral vasoconstriction possibly caused by birth asphyxia.[62] Doppler ultrasound measurements in the umbilical cords of human infants have revealed that breathing, particularly inspiration, and crying have a profound impact on blood flow in both the umbilical arteries and veins.[62] Large inspiratory efforts increase umbilical venous flow, leading to an increase in flow through the ductus venosus (and presumably across the foramen ovale), whereas vigorous crying caused flow to cease in both vessels.[62,63] In contrast to humans, large inspiratory efforts decrease umbilical venous flow in lambs.[64] This discrepancy is most probably anatomical in nature because the ductus venosus enters the IVC before it passes through the diaphragm in sheep, but the ductus venosus does not enter the IVC in humans. As such, it appears that breathing has a major influence on umbilical blood flows that differ between species and more research is required to determine whether this mechanism could drive placental-to-infant blood transfusion in humans.

**Gravity and Uterine Contractions:** While placing newborns below the placenta after birth reduces umbilical artery flow, it does not result in significant placental-to-newborn blood transfusion because umbilical venous flow is reduced by the same amount. On the other hand, placing the newborn above the placenta doesn't result in infant-to-placental blood transfusion as flows in both umbilical vessels are changed by this procedure.[39] These findings are consistent with a clinical trial showing no effect on placental transfusion when placing infants at the vaginal introitus versus on the maternal abdomen.[65]

Blood volume measurements in human infants suggest that uterine contractions facilitate blood transfusion into the infant after birth.[66] However, during labor, uterine contractions are known to increase placental vascular resistance and decrease umbilical blood flow, having differential effects on umbilical arteries and veins.[67,68] That is, as the veins are highly compliant low-pressure vessels, during contractions, the veins close earlier than arteries and then reopen after the arteries when the uterus relaxes.[67,68] This reasoning explains the bradycardic fetal heart rate response to uterine contractions during labor, causing a transient increase in placental blood volume, which is released back into the infant following the contraction.[67] Consequently uterine contractions do not readily explain placental-to-infant blood transfusion, and in particular, they do not "squeeze" blood out of the placenta and into the infant (Figure 6.6).[68]

**Increase in Pulmonary Blood Flow at Birth:** A common explanation for placental-to-infant blood transfusion is the increase in PBF at birth, which results in an increase in blood volume to accommodate the increased blood volume residing in the lung at any moment in time. However, while the increase in PBF after birth leads to a 40% increase in pulmonary blood volume, as the lung's blood volume is so small, this increase only accounts for a 2% overall increase in total blood volume (i.e., 2 mL/kg).[69] The mathematical explanation for this is simple. Dilation of a blood vessel increases its volume by the square of the radius change ($r^2$), whereas the resistance decreases by the change in radius to the fourth power ($r^4$). As such, the

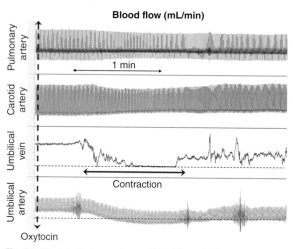

**Fig. 6.6** Physiological recordings of blood flows in the left pulmonary artery (PA), carotid artery, umbilical vein (UV), and umbilical artery (UA) before and immediately after oxytocin administration (IV) to the ewe in a newborn lamb prior to UCC and before ventilation onset. Note that during the contraction, UV flow decreases to 0, UA flow decreases and reverses during diastole (indicated by diastolic flows below zero), and CA flow increases. (From Stenning et al.[68])

increase in PBF resulting from vasodilation is two orders of magnitude greater than the volume change, which explains why a large increase in organ blood flow does not necessarily translate into a large increase in organ blood volume.

**Vaginal Birth:** The early observations demonstrating a time-dependent increase in infant blood volume during deferred cord clamping only provide measurements made after birth in vaginally born infants.[66,70-72] The question therefore arises: what happens to an infant's blood volume during labor before birth? It is possible that during labor, the forces imposed on the infant increase abdominal and thoracic pressures, causing a net shift of blood from the infant into the placenta, which is then restored or "rebalanced" following delivery. As measurements have only been made after birth, this could appear as a placental transfusion. This concept explains why deferred UCC is less effective at promoting a placental transfusion in infants delivered by cesarean section[43] and why in multiple sheep experiments in which the lambs are delivered by cesarean section, researchers have not been able to detect any placental transfusion.[39]

Recent studies in twins have shown that hemoglobin levels are higher in the second-born twin for the first 48 hours after birth if the infants are delivered vaginally but not if the twins were delivered by cesarean section.[73,74] This effect was first observed in monochorionic twins, leading to the theory that labor induced the net movement of blood from the first-born twin into the second-born twin via anastomoses in the placenta.[74] However, as this effect was also present in dichorionic twins, it was suggested that earlier UCC in the first-born twin resulted in less placental blood transfusion compared with the second-born twin.[73] However, it is also possible that second-born twins are exposed to less compression than the first-born twin during delivery, resulting in less blood loss into the placenta during labor. Whatever the explanation, these studies indicate that the effects of labor and vaginal delivery are major determinants of whether increased hemoglobin content is observed postnatally. In any event the term "placental transfusion" during delayed UCC is likely to be misleading and the concept of "blood volume restoration" or "rebalancing of the circulation" is probably more accurate.

## Clinical Effects of Deferred Umbilical Cord Clamping

Until recently, early UCC was performed on nearly every newborn baby in the developed world. The clinical reasons for introducing early UCC as one of the "three pillars" of the active management of the third stage of labor are unclear, although reducing the length of the third stage may have been the goal. Nevertheless, while the active management of the third stage of labor has reduced the risk of maternal postpartum hemorrhage, it appears that early cord clamping plays little to no role in this benefit. Indeed, systematic reviews have clearly shown that the rates of postpartum hemorrhage are similar between early and late cord clamping, thus supporting the concept that early UCC has no role in reducing the risk of PPH.[57]

### POTENTIAL MECHANISMS OF BENEFIT: TRANSFUSION VERSUS TIMING

There are several possible mechanisms that may explain the apparent benefits of a deferral of cord clamping time in the preterm infant. The first and most accepted

mechanism is that of allowing a placental transfusion – or a net flow of blood from the placenta to the infant.[72] However, as explained above, the physiology of this is complex and there is little physiological rationale for it. An important principle is the fetal ability to maintain euvolemia and the physics of blood supply to an organ, such that what goes in should come out again. The concept of a restoration of blood volume lost to the placenta during labor discussed earlier also affects the way we understand placental transfusion. There are a number of suggested determinants of placental transfusion beyond that of time, including relative position/gravity, uterine contractions and the role of oxytocin, mode of delivery, the role of breathing/crying, and the patency of the umbilical vessels with differential flow cessation times.[62] Another mechanism of benefit might include prevention of hypotension and low systemic blood flow,[75,76] both known associations with acute IVH[77] and longer-term neurological injury.[78] The benefits of allowing some time for the infant to commence breathing and aerate their lungs while still receiving warm oxygenated blood from the placenta increases the likelihood that PBF will have increased prior to cord clamping. The physiological benefits of this approach have been described above, which is now termed *physiologically based cord clamping*.[2] Leading on from this benefit is the further development of a more hands-off, non-interventionist approach to preterm infant delivery – the concept of supporting the transition rather than "resuscitating" every infant. Supporting the transition while still attached to the placenta takes the pressure off the team to intervene with suction, occlusive masks, and attempted endotracheal intubation all of which can be associated with vagal responses, hypoxia, and delay in establishing normal breathing. The subsequent reduced need for mechanical ventilation and higher pressure/oxygen may partially explain the benefit seen in preterm infants who have a deferral in cord clamping time.

### DETERMINANTS OF THE PLACENTAL TRANSFUSION

**Time:** This is the most well-understood and most commonly cited determinant of the placental transfusion and is the basis of most of the recommendations for delay. However, there is little consistency between studies as to what the optimum time to UCC should be, with times ranging from 30 seconds to 3 minutes and more. Again, this most likely reflects our lack of understanding of the physiology and hemodynamics, as well as our inability to accurately measure placental transfusion. The concept that placental transfusion was time dependent was originally described by Yao et al. in the late 1960s,[72] but the observations have been repeated by others with similar results.[79] While there are some methodological concerns regarding these studies, the large systematic reviews of both active versus expectant management of the third stage of labor[80] and deferred versus early UCC have clearly shown a significant difference in birthweight.[81] While this is the most conclusive evidence for "placental transfusion", the physiology underpinning this transfusion is still not clear.

**Position/Gravity:** Intuitively, placing the infant below the level of the placenta should induce a gravity-based placental transfusion; however, there are a number of important caveats to this hypothesis. The physiological rationale for this is discussed earlier, but from a clinical viewpoint, there has only been a single study addressing the relative position of the baby to the placenta and the effect on placental transfusion.[65] In this multicenter randomized controlled trial of 546 term healthy infants born vaginally, infants were weighed immediately at birth, then randomized to be held for 2 minutes at the level of the vaginal introitus or on the mother's abdomen or chest. The umbilical cord was then clamped and the infant reweighed. The main finding was that *both* groups of infants had significant weight gain (56 vs 53 g), equivalent to about a 50-mL transfusion. A difference in birthweight between early (60 seconds) and delayed cord clamp groups has been noted previously – with an average weight gain of about 100 g in the delayed group.[81] The implication from this large clinical study is that gravity is not the main driving factor for placental transfusion and that other factors (including lung inflation and breathing) may be more important. A recent study in preterm lambs, born by cesarean section, where a 10-cm change in height above/below the placenta was combined with the effect of initiation of ventilation prior to UCC, demonstrated that changing the body position had minimal and only transient effects on umbilical and cerebral blood flow, with no change in net blood volume recorded.[39]

**Contractions/Oxytocics:** The role of uterine contraction and the timing of oxytocic administration in relation to cord clamping time is surprisingly poorly studied.[65] In an animal model early oxytocin administration prior to clamping the cord resulted in a rapid decline in umbilical arterial and venous blood flow and partly negated the benefits of deferred umbilical cord clamping seen in this model.[68] No published trials to date investigating deferred UCC with placental transfusion as a primary outcome have considered the timing of uterotonic administration.

**Mode of Delivery:** Several clinical studies have noted a difference between the amount of placental transfusion and change in hemoglobin level seen in a cesarean delivery versus vaginal delivery.[43,79] The fundamental difference between these modes of delivery is that the uterus is incised to deliver the infant and so the consequences of uterine contractions on the infant and placenta during delivery are absent. While the role of uterine contractions enhancing placental transfusion is a convenient explanation, it is not supported by the science/physiology (see above). The novel concept that placental transfusion may actually be a homeostatic restoration of blood volume following fetal blood loss into the placenta during labor/delivery may also explain differences in mode of delivery. That is, the volume of placental transfusion is consistently greater following vaginal birth (i.e., following labor) than delivery via cesarean section without labor.[43,79] This may simply reflect the fact that vaginally delivered infants, who have all experienced labor and uterine contractions, lose more blood into the placenta during the labor and delivery process. Consequently, active transfer of blood via UCM may be more efficient at improving hemodynamic outcomes in infants born by cesarean section, although at the expense of other potential complications.[43,58]

**Umbilical Blood Vessel Patency:** The equal flow of blood from fetus to placenta relies on both the umbilical artery and veins being patent. A cessation of flow in one of these vessels may result in differential transfer of blood from one side to the other. Studies examining blood flow in umbilical vessels during the third stage are few, although an early study has assessed flow indirectly,[71] whereas a more recent study[62] has measured flow in real time. A clinical study of 62 normal term deliveries[71] measured placental residual volume as the index of placental transfusion and compared clamping all blood vessels versus clamping arteries or veins differentially to estimate flow. They concluded that arterial flow was maintained for about 40 seconds after birth, while umbilical venous flow continued for about 3 minutes and was influenced by uterine contractions. However, there are serious limitations with this study as they did not measure actual flow, but measured placental residual volumes, and compared these to expected volumes (from previous studies) to determine if there had been umbilical artery or venous flow. Published animal experiments using preterm fetal lambs and observations from fetal surgery and the ex utero intrapartum treatment (EXIT) procedure demonstrate that changes in umbilical blood flow are matched between venous and arterial vessels.[9] Other physiological events such as breathing and crying, as well as differential constriction of umbilical arteries and veins during uterine contractions, may affect the volume of blood transfused. Boere et al. used Doppler ultrasound to measure umbilical blood flow and direction of flow in normally transitioning term infants who had their cord clamped at a time point determined by the midwife.[62] This study demonstrated that up to one-third of babies still had umbilical venous flow when the cord was clamped (mean 05:13 mins Range 02:56–09:15) and 43% of infants had umbilical arterial flow at cord clamp time (mean 05:16 mins Range 03:32–10:10). Most importantly they found that flow ceased in the umbilical vein before the umbilical artery in over 50% of infants. Significant perturbations of blood flow were seen with breathing and crying; in particular, stopping or reversal of flow was often observed with crying and forced expirations.

**Breathing/Crying:** The effects of breathing and/or crying on the transitional circulation were reviewed earlier in this chapter. In addition to the direct effects on umbilical blood flow of crying and breathing seen in the study described earlier,[62] there is also a study from the 1960s that demonstrated the relationship of the onset of breathing to a change in residual placental volume.[82] In this study normal-term infants who established respirations 10 seconds or more before UCC had less placental residual volume and by implication received more blood back from the placenta. The authors concluded that: "During delivery, cord-clamping should be delayed until spontaneous or induced breathing has begun".

## PREVENTION OF HYPOTENSION/LOW SYSTEMIC BLOOD FLOW

An important beneficial mechanism strongly associated with delayed cord clamping is the prevention of low systemic blood flow and/or hypotension. The transitional circulation, particularly in very-low-birth-weight (VLBW) infants, is vulnerable to impairment, which can arise for several reasons (see Chapter 1). For instance, (i) the preterm myocardium is poorly adapted to respond to the postnatal increase in systemic vascular resistance, (ii) the transitional circulation is affected by systemic to pulmonary shunts that move blood out of the systemic circulation, (iii) preload is affected by positive pressure respiratory support, and (iv) the infant may be relatively hypovolemic due to a failure to restore blood volume following labor and delivery. All of these variables lead to a low cardiac output state that is associated with adverse outcomes such as cerebral injury, including periventricular or intraventricular hemorrhage (P/IVH) and periventricular leukomalacia (PVL)[77] (see Chapters 7 and 20). An accurate diagnosis of low cardiac output is not possible by simply measuring blood pressure,[83] and other measures of cardiovascular adequacy such as capillary refill time or lactic acidosis are nonspecific in these patients.[84] The measure of superior vena cava (SVC) flow was first described over 20 years ago and has been correlated with both short- and long-term adverse events (see Chapter 10).[77,78] It is utilized as a measurement in the transitional setting, where other cardiac output measures such as the ventricular outputs are likely to be affected by the fetal shunts. It is therefore a useful measure to assess adequacy of systemic blood flow in a transitioning preterm infant. As such, SVC flow has been utilized as an outcome in a number of cord clamping time studies. Initially these were small observational or practice change studies, but more recently, results of larger randomized control studies have been published (Table 6.1).

Low SVC flow has been associated with an increased incidence of P/IVH,[77] so prevention of low SVC flow by delayed cord clamping may be at least a partial reason as to why the systematic reviews of the outcomes of delayed cord clamping in preterm infants show a reduction in severe grade P/IVH.[57] Meyer et al. were the first to recognize an association between later clamping of the cord (30–45 seconds) and improved

**TABLE 6.1    Summary of Studies of Systemic Blood Flow Changes After Different Types of Umbilical Cord Management**

| Study | N | Mean GA Weeks | Intervention | ICC SVC Flow (mL/kg/min) | DCC/UCM SVC Flow (mL/kg/min) | Age (h) |
|---|---|---|---|---|---|---|
| Meyer, 2012[75] | 30 | 26 | DCC 30–40 s | 52 (42–100) | 91 (81–101)* | 16 |
| Sommers, 2012[76] | 51 | 28 | DCC 41 s vs. 5 s | 89 ± 24 | 112 ± 30* | 6 |
| Katheria, 2014[42] | 28 | <29 | Intact UCM | 66 ± 18 | 98 ± 27* | 5 |
| Popat, 2016[85] | 266 | 28 | DCC 60 s | 92 ± 35 | 95 ± 41 | 3–6 |
| Katheria 2016[94] | 125 | 28 | DCC vs. VDCC | 86 ± 32$ | 83 ± 26# | <12 |

*$P < 0.05$ compared to ICC.

#, Values for LSCS/DCC and ventilation.

$, values for LSCS/DCC of 60 seconds.

*DCC,* delayed cord clamping; *ICC,* immediate cord clamping; *SVC Flow,* superior vena cava flow; *UCM,* umbilical cord milking; *VDCC,* ventilated DCC.

SVC flow in a small retrospective cohort study.[75] Subsequently, similar findings with improved SVC flow in the delayed clamping arm of a randomized control trial of immediate versus delayed (45 seconds) cord clamping in a group of less than 32 weeks' gestation infants were demonstrated.[76] More recently, UCM has also been shown to improve SVC flow.[41,55] The largest study to date of SVC flow in the setting of immediate versus delayed (60 seconds) cord clamping has recently been published.[85] This trial demonstrated that there was no difference in SVC flow in a group of 266 infants less than 30 weeks' gestation randomized into the two arms, even though there was an increase in the hematocrit in the delayed arm group. Additionally, right ventricular output was found to be lower in the delayed arm, which may have reflected a higher hematocrit or an increase in left-to-right shunting across the ductus arteriosus due to a higher resistance in the systemic versus pulmonary vascular bed. The causes of the discrepancy between the findings of the previous smaller studies and those of this study are unclear. Reassuringly, the recently published 2-year follow-up of the Australian Placental Transfusion Study confirmed improved neurodevelopmental outcomes in extremely preterm babies who were managed with deferred UCC.[86] Further research is needed to better understand the mechanisms that lead to the benefit of deferred UCC.

## LONG-TERM OUTCOMES AND MORTALITY AFTER DEFERRED UMBILICAL CORD CLAMPING

Recent evidence has established deferred umbilical cord clamping as the standard of care for spontaneously breathing preterm and term newborns.[87,88] Studies of >2800 preterm infants have shown that deferred UCC confers important benefits for preterm newborns, which include a reduction in mortality, fewer blood transfusions, lower risk of intraventricular hemorrhage (IVH) and necrotizing enterocolitis, improved hemodynamics, and improved motor function at 18–22 months of age.[4,57,89] This benefit also appears to hold true for extremely preterm infants,[90] who, as the science predicts, would benefit to a greater extent than term infants as they take longer to aerate their lungs and are more vulnerable to hemodynamic instability.

Deferral of cord clamping in the term infant has long been practiced by midwives in low-risk settings, resulting in both improved short-term[81] and longer-term outcomes, including improved iron stores at 6 months of age.[91] In a cohort of over 12,000 spontaneously breathing term and late preterm infants, delaying umbilical cord clamping until after the initiation of spontaneous respirations reduced the risk of death and the combined risk of death or ICU admission within 24 hours after birth.[92] However, the number of infants who died in this cohort was small, representing only 0.2% of the total number of infants studied.

A randomized trial of over 380 healthy term infants born in Sweden compared DCC for ≥180 seconds to ICC (≤10 seconds).[93] Although neonatal hemoglobin and IgG levels and iron stores at 4 months were higher in the DCC group, no differences in iron status and neurodevelopment development, assessed by the Ages and Stages Questionnaire (ASQ), were seen at 12 months.

Neurodevelopmental scores were higher in female infants and infants receiving early breastfeeding. Male infants who received DCC had higher ASQ scores than male infants who received ICC, whereas female infants who received DCC had lower ASQ scores than female infants who received ICC. These potential gender differences are puzzling and unexpected but have not been further evaluated.

## Less Intervention at Birth: Resuscitation Versus Transitioning

A largely unrecognized benefit of deferred cord clamping is the observation that many babies, including the smallest and most immature, have the opportunity to establish spontaneous breathing while still supported by the placental circulation. A randomized trial of resuscitation with an intact cord[94] demonstrated that up to 90% of infants less than 32 weeks were able to establish breathing prior to clamping the cord at 60 seconds. Other trials have also shown that up to 80% of extremely preterm infants commence breathing at birth if left to transition spontaneously.[95] Spontaneous breathing has many advantages, including making resuscitation easier, opening the glottis, and allowing transition to commence while the infant is still attached to the placenta. Indeed, closure of the vocal cords during apnea, including apnea induced unintentionally by trigeminal nerve stimulation during facemask ventilation, impedes resuscitation efforts until the hypoxic and bradycardic neonate can no longer maintain tonic constriction of the vocal cords and they passively relax or are bypassed with an endotracheal tube.[96,97] Other potential hemodynamic advantages include avoiding significant mechanical ventilation, which has been closely associated with lung injury and impairment of the cardiovascular system.[98] Many neonatologists have begun to reconsider the role of resuscitation – which often entails intervention with subsequent regression in the transition process (suction, masks, positive pressure breaths) versus that of waiting and supporting the infant's transition. The fact that the newborn is still attached to the placenta and (assuming placental blood flow is still intact) receiving warmed, oxygenated blood makes waiting for transition to happen spontaneously a more acceptable option.

## PHYSIOLOGICALLY BASED CORD CLAMPING

Polglase et al. coined the term *physiologically based cord clamping* (PBCC) to underscore the importance of taking into account the stages in the cardiorespiratory transition and timing of cord clamping to fit with the transition of an individual infant.[7] As with many things in medicine, the concept of arbitrarily picking a time interval to apply to a physiological process such as time of cord clamping (45 seconds, 60 seconds, 3 minutes) is problematic. As discussed in this review, there are many factors to consider – immaturity, degree of lung aeration and level of asphyxia, distribution of the fetal-placental blood, position of the infant relative to the placenta, uterine contractions, and mode of delivery and facilitating the transition (breathing first, clamp later) or inhibiting the transition by intervention. There will not be a single time interval that suits all of these situations and maximizes the cardiorespiratory outcomes of the infant, particularly infants needing respiratory support after birth.

Research is underway to discover the best signal or signals to let the clinician know the newborn is ready for umbilical cord clamping, including evidence of lung aeration and umbilical blood flow using ultrasound and pulmonary gas exchange using exhaled carbon dioxide.[26,27,62,99,100] The results of these studies have been incorporated into a series of pilot trials demonstrating feasibility and safety of PBCC that have led to larger RCTs investigating the benefits of PBCC in both preterm and term infants, including term infants with congenital diaphragmatic hernia.[101-107] However, there is accumulating evidence that heart rates and oxygen levels of newborns receiving deferred UCC are higher in newborns who had early UCC (Figure 6.7), thus requiring a change in established thinking and protocols.[101,102,108-110]

## Conclusions

The act of early clamping of the umbilical cord (usually within 15–20 seconds) is probably the most frequently performed medical procedure since the 1950s. The procedure was introduced into obstetric care as part of a bigger "package of care", with little understanding of the physiological effects that it might have in term and particularly preterm infants. It is only in the past 5–10 years that the physiologic rationale and an understanding of

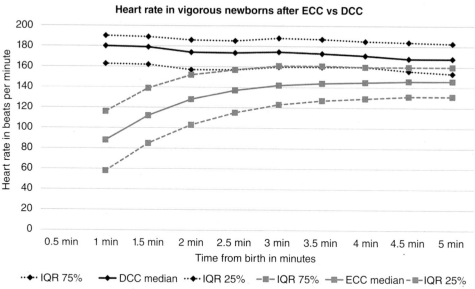

**Fig. 6.7** Heart rate (median and interquartile range) from *N* = 295 newborns, ≥35 weeks receiving deferred cord clamping (DCC) for 2 or more minutes (with deferred postpartum uterotonic administration until after umbilical cord clamping, shown in *black*)[102] versus *N* = 306 newborns, ≥37 receiving early cord clamping (ECC, shown in *gray*).[109] The median heart rate in the first 3 minutes after birth is higher in newborns in whom deferred cord clamping was performed. *M,* Minutes from birth.

the potential benefits of waiting before cord clamping has emerged. This has been led by a group of clinicians and midwives documenting the clinical benefits of deferral of clamping and by a group of scientists using physiology and animal models to understand the physiological consequences of early clamping (similar to the backgrounds of the authors of this chapter – one a physiologist and the other three neonatologists). Understanding the complex cardiorespiratory physiology of the transition has been key to this discussion. The findings of the largest RCT of early versus late cord clamping to date and an updated systematic review support the notion that a deferral in clamping of the umbilical cord can reduce mortality in preterm infants without harm to either mother or baby.[89,90] The importance of the respiratory transition (airway liquid absorption, lung aeration, and increase in PBF) and its very close relationship to the cardiovascular transition (left ventricular preload, maintenance of cardiac output, and stabilization of a potentially labile circulation) has been increasingly understood. New concepts discussed here include that of fetal blood volume restoration rather than placental transfusion and the importance of a physiological endpoint to determine when to

clamp the umbilical cord rather than an arbitrary time point. Along the way, much has been learned about very preterm infants and what they are capable of, if left to transition on their own, while still supported by a placental circulation. The iatrogenic insults of suction, inadvertent airway occlusion by mask in a spontaneously breathing infant and mechanical ventilation with the significant change in physiology that it entails have been put increasingly under the spotlight as we understand the normal transition and what is required to support even our tiniest babies through this process. Although there are neonates, especially among the very preterm, that will still require resuscitation in the traditional sense, most neonates appear to do better if supported in commencing the transition to extrauterine life with the umbilical cord unclamped. There are some specific situations where it is unclear if there is a benefit in later cord clamping and where there may be possibility of harm. These clinical situations include infants at higher risk of polycythemia (IUGR, recipient twin in twin-twin transfusion), infants with high-risk cardiovascular states such as congenital diaphragmatic hernia and congenital heart disease, and the asphyxiated infant.

# REFERENCES

1. Hooper SB, Polglase GR, te Pas AB. A physiological approach to the timing of umbilical cord clamping at birth. *Arch Dis Child Fetal Neonatal Ed.* 2015;100(4):F355-F360.
2. Hooper SB, Binder-Heschl C, Polglase GR, et al. The timing of umbilical cord clamping at birth: physiological considerations. *Matern Health Neonatol Perinatol.* 2016;2:4.
3. Hooper SB, Te Pas AB, Lang J, et al. Cardiovascular transition at birth: a physiological sequence. *Pediatr Res.* 2015;77(5):608-614.
4. Bhatt S, Alison BJ, Wallace EM, et al. Delaying cord clamping until ventilation onset improves cardiovascular function at birth in preterm lambs. *J Physiol.* 2013;591(8):2113-2126.
5. Crossley KJ, Allison BJ, Polglase GR, Morley CJ, Davis PG, Hooper SB. Dynamic changes in the direction of blood flow through the ductus arteriosus at birth. *J Physiol.* 2009;587 (Pt 19):4695-4704.
6. Rudolph AM. Fetal and neonatal pulmonary circulation. *Annual Review of Physiology.* 1979;41:383-395.
7. Polglase GR, Dawson JA, Kluckow M, et al. Ventilation onset prior to umbilical cord clamping (physiological-based cord clamping) improves systemic and cerebral oxygenation in preterm lambs. *PLoS One.* 2015;10(2):e0117504.
8. Polglase GR, Blank DA, Barton SK, et al. Physiologically based cord clamping stabilises cardiac output and reduces cerebrovascular injury in asphyxiated near-term lambs. *Arch Dis Child Fetal Neonatal Ed.* 2018;103(6):F530-F538.
9. Blank DA, Polglase GR, Kluckow M, et al. Haemodynamic effects of umbilical cord milking in premature sheep during the neonatal transition. *Arch Dis Child Fetal Neonatal Ed.* 2018;103(6):F539-F546.
10. Harding R, Hooper SB. Regulation of lung expansion and lung growth before birth. *J Appl Physiol (1985).* 1996;81(1):209-224.
11. Hooper SB, Harding R. Fetal lung liquid: a major determinant of the growth and functional development of the fetal lung. *Clin Exp Pharmacol Physiol.* 1995;22:235-247.
12. Hooper SB, Te Pas AB, Kitchen MJ. Respiratory transition in the newborn: a three-phase process. *Arch Dis Child Fetal Neonatal Ed.* 2016;101(3):F266-F271.
13. Harding R, Hooper SB, Dickson KA. A mechanism leading to reduced lung expansion and lung hypoplasia in fetal sheep during oligohydramnios. *Am J Obstet Gynecol.* 1990;163(6 Pt 1): 1904-1913.
14. Albuquerque CA, Smith KR, Saywers TE, Johnson C, Cock ML, Harding R. Relation between oligohydramnios and spinal flexion in the human fetus. *Early Hum Dev.* 2002;68(2):119-126.
15. Olver RE, Walters DV, S MW. Developmental regulation of lung liquid transport. *Annu Rev Physiol.* 2004;66:77-101.
16. Olver RE, Ramsden CA, Strang LB, Walters DV. The role of amiloride-blockable sodium transport in adrenaline-induced lung liquid reabsorption in the fetal lamb. *J Physiol.* 1986;376:3 21-340.
17. Jain L, Dudell GG. Respiratory transition in infants delivered by cesarean section. *Semin Perinatol.* 2006;30(5):296-304.
18. Jobe AH. The new bronchopulmonary dysplasia. *Curr Opin Pediatr.* 2011;23(2):167-172.
19. Hooper SB, Kitchen MJ, Wallace MJ, et al. Imaging lung aeration and lung liquid clearance at birth. *FASEB J.* 2007;21:3329-3337.
20. Siew ML, Wallace MJ, Kitchen MJ, et al. Inspiration regulates the rate and temporal pattern of lung liquid clearance and lung aeration at birth. *J Appl Physiol.* 2009;106(6):1888-1895.
21. Kitchen MJ, Siew ML, Wallace MJ, et al. Changes in positive end-expiratory pressure alter the distribution of ventilation within the lung immediately after birth in newborn rabbits. *PLoS One.* 2014;9(4):e93391.
22. te Pas AB, Siew M, Wallace MJ, et al. Effect of sustained inflation length on establishing functional residual capacity at birth in ventilated premature rabbits. *Pediatr Res.* 2009;66(3):295-300.
23. Siew ML, Te Pas AB, Wallace MJ, et al. Positive end-expiratory pressure enhances development of a functional residual capacity in preterm rabbits ventilated from birth. *J Appl Physiol (1985).* 2009;106(5):1487-1493.
24. te Pas AB, Siew M, Wallace MJ, et al. Establishing functional residual capacity at birth: the effect of sustained inflation and positive end-expiratory pressure in a preterm rabbit model. *Pediatr Res.* 2009;65(5):537-541.
25. Siew ML, Wallace MJ, Allison BJ, et al. The role of lung inflation and sodium transport in airway liquid clearance during lung aeration in newborn rabbits. *Pediatr Res.* 2013;73(4 Pt 1):443-449.
26. Blank DA, Rogerson SR, Kamlin COF, et al. Lung ultrasound during the initiation of breathing in healthy term and late preterm infants immediately after birth, a prospective, observational study. *Resuscitation.* 2017;114:59-65.
27. Blank DA, Gaertner VD, Kamlin COF, et al. Respiratory changes in term infants immediately after birth. *Resuscitation.* 2018;130: 105-110.
28. Gao Y, Raj JU. Regulation of the pulmonary circulation in the fetus and newborn. *Physiol Rev.* 2010;90(4):1291-1335.
29. Lang JA, Pearson JT, Te Pas AB, et al. Ventilation/perfusion mismatch during lung aeration at birth. *J Appl Physiol.* 2014;117(5): 535-543.
30. Lang JA, Pearson JT, Binder-Heschl C, et al. Increase in pulmonary blood flow at birth: role of oxygen and lung aeration. *J Physiol.* 2016;594(5):1389-1398.
31. Teitel DF, Iwamoto HS, Rudolph AM. Changes in the pulmonary circulation during birth-related events. *Pediatr Res.* 1990;27(4):372-378.
32. Sobotka KS, Hooper SB, Allison BJ, et al. An initial sustained inflation improves the respiratory and cardiovascular transition at birth in preterm lambs. *Pediatr Res.* 2011;70(1):56-60.
33. Lang JA, Pearson JT, Binder-Heschl C, et al. Vagal denervation inhibits the increase in pulmonary blood flow during partial lung aeration at birth. *J Physiol.* 2017;595(5):1593-1606.
34. Siew ML, Te Pas AB, Wallace MJ, et al. Surfactant increases the uniformity of lung aeration at birth in ventilated preterm rabbits. *Pediatr Res.* 2011;70(1):50-55.
35. Bhatt S, Polglase GR, Wallace EM, Te Pas AB, Hooper SB. Ventilation before umbilical cord clamping improves the physiological transition at birth. *Front Pediatr.* 2014;2:113.
36. Cohn HE, Sacks EJ, Heymann MA, Rudolph AM. Cardiovascular responses to hypoxemia and acidemia in fetal lambs. *Am J Obstet Gynecol.* 1974;120(6):817-824.
37. Dawes GS, Mott JC, Widdicombe JG. Closure of the foramen ovale in newborn lambs. *J Physiol.* 1955;128(2):384-395.
38. Evans N, Iyer P. Incompetence of the foramen ovale in preterm infants supported by mechanical ventilation. *J Pediatr.* 1994; 125(5 Pt 1):786-792.
39. Hooper SB, Crossley KJ, Zahra VA, et al. Effect of body position and ventilation on umbilical artery and venous blood flows during delayed umbilical cord clamping in preterm lambs. *Arch Dis Child Fetal Neonatal Ed.* 2017;102(4):F312-F319.
40. March MI, Hacker MR, Parson AW, Modest AM, de Veciana M. The effects of umbilical cord milking in extremely preterm infants: a randomized controlled trial. *J Perinatol.* 2013;33(10): 763-767.

41. Katheria A, Blank D, Rich W, Finer N. Umbilical cord milking improves transition in premature infants at birth. *PLoS One.* 2014;9(4):e94085.

42. Katheria AC, Leone TA, Woelkers D, Garey DM, Rich W, Finer NN. The effects of umbilical cord milking on hemodynamics and neonatal outcomes in premature neonates. *J Pediatr.* 2014;164(5):1045-1050.

43. Katheria AC, Truong G, Cousins L, Oshiro B, Finer NN. Umbilical cord milking versus delayed cord clamping in preterm infants. *Pediatrics.* 2015;136(1):61-69.

44. Rabe H, Jewison A, Alvarez RF, et al. Milking compared with delayed cord clamping to increase placental transfusion in preterm neonates: a randomized controlled trial. *Obstet Gynecol.* 2011;117(2 Pt 1):205-211.

45. Rabe H, Sawyer A, Amess P, Ayers S, Brighton Perinatal Study Group. Neurodevelopmental outcomes at 2 and 3.5 years for very preterm babies enrolled in a randomized trial of milking the umbilical cord versus delayed cord clamping. *Neonatology.* 2016;109(2):113-119.

46. Hosono S, Mugishima H, Fujita H, et al. Umbilical cord milking reduces the need for red cell transfusions and improves neonatal adaptation in infants born at less than 29 weeks' gestation: a randomised controlled trial. *Arch Dis Child Fetal Neonatal Ed.* 2008;93(1):F14-F19.

47. Hosono S, Mugishima H, Takahashi S, et al. One-time umbilical cord milking after cord cutting has same effectiveness as multiple-time umbilical cord milking in infants born at <29 weeks of gestation: a retrospective study. *J Perinatol.* 2015;35(8):590-594.

48. Hosono S, Hine K, Nagano N, et al. Residual blood volume in the umbilical cord of extremely premature infants. *Pediatr Int.* 2015;57(1):68-71.

49. Katheria AC, Lakshminrusimha S, Rabe H, McAdams R, Mercer JS. Placental transfusion: a review. *J Perinatol.* 2017;37(2):105-111.

50. WHO. *Guideline: Delayed umbilical cord clamping for improved maternal and infant health and nutrition outcomes.* Geneva: World Health Organization; 2014.

51. Committee on Obstetric Practice ACoO, Gynecologists. Committee Opinion No. 543: timing of umbilical cord clamping after birth. *Obstet Gynecol.* 2012;120(6):1522-1526.

52. Perlman JM, Wyllie J, Kattwinkel J, et al. Part 7: Neonatal resuscitation: 2015 International consensus on cardiopulmonary resuscitation and emergency cardiovascular care science with treatment recommendations. *Circulation.* 2015;132(16 Suppl 1):S204-S241.

53. Wyckoff MH, Aziz K, Escobedo MB, et al. Part 13: Neonatal resuscitation: 2015 American Heart Association guidelines update for cardiopulmonary resuscitation and emergency cardiovascular care. *Circulation.* 2015;132(18 Suppl 2):S543-S560.

54. American Academy of Pediatrics. Timing of umbilical cord clamping after birth. *Pediatrics.* 2013;131(4):e1323-e1323.

55. Takami T, Suganami Y, Sunohara D, et al. Umbilical cord milking stabilizes cerebral oxygenation and perfusion in infants born before 29 weeks of gestation. *J Pediatr.* 2012;161(4):742-747.

56. Upadhyay A, Gothwal S, Parihar R, et al. Effect of umbilical cord milking in term and near term infants: randomized control trial. *Am J Obstet Gynecol.* 2013;208(2):120.e1-e6.

57. Rabe H, Gyte GML, Díaz-Rossello JL, Duley L. Effect of timing of umbilical cord clamping and other strategies to influence placental transfusion at preterm birth on maternal and infant outcomes. *Cochrane Database Syst Rev.* 2019;9(9):CD003248.

58. Katheria A, Reister F, Essers J, et al. Association of umbilical cord milking vs delayed umbilical cord clamping with death or severe intraventricular hemorrhage among preterm infants. *JAMA.* 2019;322(19):1877-1886.

59. Patel S, Clark EA, Rodriguez CE, Metz TD, Abbaszadeh M, Yoder BA. Effect of umbilical cord milking on morbidity and survival in extremely low gestational age neonates. *Am J Obstet Gynecol.* 2014;211(5):519.e1-e7.

60. Safarulla A. A review of benefits of cord milking over delayed cord clamping in the preterm infant and future directions of research. *J Matern Fetal Neonatal Med.* 2017;30(24):2966-2973.

61. Balasubramanian H, Ananthan A, Jain V, Rao SC, Kabra N. Umbilical cord milking in preterm infants: a systematic review and meta-analysis. *Arch Dis Child Fetal Neonatal Ed.* 2020; 105(6):572-580.

62. Boere I, Roest AA, Wallace E, et al. Umbilical blood flow patterns directly after birth before delayed cord clamping. *Arch Dis Child Fetal Neonatal Ed.* 2015;100(2):F121-F125.

63. Brouwer E, Knol R, Kroushev A, et al. Effect of breathing on venous return during delayed cord clamping: an observational study. *Arch Dis Child Fetal Neonatal Ed.* 2022;107(1):65-69.

64. Brouwer E, Te Pas AB, Polglase GR, et al. Effect of spontaneous breathing on umbilical venous blood flow and during delayed cord clamping in preterm lambs. *Arch Dis Child Fetal Neonatal Ed.* 2020;105(1):26-32.

65. Vain NE, Satragno DS, Gorenstein AN, et al. Effect of gravity on volume of placental transfusion: a multicentre, randomised, non-inferiority trial. *Lancet.* 2014;384(9939):235-240.

66. Yao AC, Hirvensalo M, Lind J. Placental transfusion-rate and uterine contraction. *Lancet.* 1968;1(7539):380-383.

67. Westgate JA, Wibbens B, Bennet L, Wassink G, Parer JT, Gunn AJ. The intrapartum deceleration in center stage: a physiologic approach to the interpretation of fetal heart rate changes in labor. *Am J Obstet Gynecol.* 2007;197(3):236.e1-236.e11.

68. Stenning FJ, Polglase GR, Te Pas AB, et al. Effect of maternal oxytocin on umbilical venous and arterial blood flows during physiological-based cord clamping in preterm lambs. *PLoS One.* 2021;16(6):e0253306.

69. Walker AM, Alcorn DG, Cannata JC, Maloney JE, Ritchie BC. Effect of ventilation on pulmonary blood volume of the fetal lamb. *J Appl Physiol.* 1975;39(6):969-975.

70. Yao AC, Lind J. Effect of gravity on placental transfusion. *Lancet.* 1969;2(7619):505-508.

71. Yao AC, Lind J. Blood flow in the umbilical vessels during the third stage of labor. *Biol Neonate.* 1974;25(3-4):186-193.

72. Yao AC, Moinian M, Lind J. Distribution of blood between infant and placenta after birth. *Lancet.* 1969;2(7626):871-873.

73. Verbeek L, Zhao DP, Middeldorp JM, et al. Haemoglobin discordances in twins: due to differences in timing of cord clamping? *Arch Dis Child Fetal Neonatal Ed.* 2017;102(4):F324-F328.

74. Verbeek L, Zhao DP, Te Pas AB, et al. Hemoglobin differences in uncomplicated monochorionic twins in relation to birth order and mode of delivery. *Twin Res Hum Genet.* 2016;19(3):241-245.

75. Meyer MP, Mildenhall L. Delayed cord clamping and blood flow in the superior vena cava in preterm infants: an observational study. *Arch Dis Child Fetal Neonatal Ed.* 2012;97(6):F484-F486.

76. Sommers R, Stonestreet BS, Oh W, et al. Hemodynamic effects of delayed cord clamping in premature infants. *Pediatrics.* 2012;129(3):e667-e672.

77. Kluckow M, Evans N. Low superior vena cava flow and intraventricular haemorrhage in preterm infants. *Arch Dis Child Fetal Neonat Ed.* 2000;82:188-194.

78. Hunt RW, Evans N, Rieger I, Kluckow M. Low superior vena cava flow and neurodevelopment at 3 years in very preterm infants. *J Pediatr.* 2004;145(5):588-592.

79. Aladangady N, McHugh S, Aitchison TC, Wardrop CA, Holland BM. Infants' blood volume in a controlled trial of placental transfusion at preterm delivery. *Pediatrics.* 2006;117(1):93-98.

80. Begley CM, Gyte GML, Devane D, McGuire W, Weeks A. Active versus expectant management for women in the third stage of labour. *Cochrane Database Syst Rev.* 2011;11:CD007412.

81. McDonald SJ, Middleton P, Dowswell T, Morris PS. Effect of timing of umbilical cord clamping of term infants on maternal and neonatal outcomes. *Cochrane Database Syst Rev.* 2013;7: CD004074.

82. Redmond A, Isana S, Ingall D. Relation of onset of respiration to placental transfusion. *Lancet.* 1965;1(7380):283-285.

83. Kluckow M, Evans N. Relationship between blood pressure and cardiac output in preterm infants requiring mechanical ventilation. *J Pediatr.* 1996;129(4):506-512.

84. Osborn DA, Evans N, Kluckow M. Clinical detection of low upper body blood flow in very premature infants using blood pressure, capillary refill time, and central-peripheral temperature difference. *Arch Dis Child Fetal Neonatal Ed.* 2004;89(2): F168-F173.

85. Popat H, Robledo KP, Sebastian L, et al. Effect of delayed cord clamping on systemic blood flow: a randomized controlled trial. *J Pediatr.* 2016;178:81-86.e2.

86. Robledo KP, Tarnow-Mordi WO, Rieger I, et al. Effects of delayed versus immediate umbilical cord clamping in reducing death or major disability at 2 years corrected age among very preterm infants (APTS): a multicentre, randomised clinical trial. *Lancet Child Adolesc Health.* 2022;6(3):150-157.

87. Wyckoff MH, Wyllie J, Aziz K, et al. Neonatal life support: 2020 International consensus on cardiopulmonary resuscitation and emergency cardiovascular care science with treatment recommendations. *Circulation.* 2020;142(16_suppl_1):S185-S221.

88. Kamath-Rayne BD, Thukral A, Visick MK, et al. Helping Babies Breathe, Second Edition: a model for strengthening educational programs to increase global newborn survival. *Glob Health Sci Pract.* 2018;6(3):538-551.

89. Fogarty M, Osborn DA, Askie L, et al. Delayed vs early umbilical cord clamping for preterm infants: a systematic review and meta-analysis. *Am J Obstet Gynecol.* 2018;218(1):1-18.

90. Tarnow-Mordi W, Morris J, Kirby A, et al. Delayed versus immediate cord clamping in preterm infants. *N Engl J Med.* 2017;377(25):2445-2455.

91. Gupta R, Ramji S. Effect of delayed cord clamping on iron stores in infants born to anemic mothers: a randomized controlled trial. *Indian Pediatrics.* 2002;39(2):130-135.

92. Ersdal HL, Linde J, Mduma E, Auestad B, Perlman J. Neonatal outcome following cord clamping after onset of spontaneous respiration. *Pediatrics.* 2014;134(2):265-272.

93. Andersson O, Domellof M, Andersson D, Hellstrom-Westas L. Effect of delayed vs early umbilical cord clamping on iron status and neurodevelopment at age 12 months: a randomized clinical trial. *JAMA Pediatr.* 2014;168(6):547-554.

94. Katheria A, Poeltler D, Durham J, et al. Neonatal resuscitation with an intact cord: a randomized clinical trial. *J Pediatr.* 2016;178:75-80.e3.

95. O'Donnell CP, Kamlin CO, Davis PG, Morley CJ. Crying and breathing by extremely preterm infants immediately after birth. *J Pediatr.* 2010;156(5):846-847.

96. Crawshaw JR, Kitchen MJ, Binder-Heschl C, et al. Laryngeal closure impedes non-invasive ventilation at birth. *Arch Dis Child Fetal Neonatal Ed.* 2018;103(2):F112-F119.

97. Gaertner VD, Ruegger CM, O'Currain E, et al. Physiological responses to facemask application in newborns immediately after birth. *Arch Dis Child Fetal Neonatal Ed.* 2021;106(4): 381-385.

98. Evans N, Kluckow M. Early determinants of right and left ventricular output in ventilated preterm infants. *Arch Dis Child Fetal Neonatal Ed.* 1996;74(2):F88-F94.

99. Blank D, Rich W, Leone T, Garey D, Finer N. Pedi-cap color change precedes a significant increase in heart rate during neonatal resuscitation. *Resuscitation.* 2014;85(11):1568-1572.

100. Hooper SB, Fouras A, Siew ML, et al. Expired $CO_2$ levels indicate degree of lung aeration at birth. *PLoS One.* 2013; 8(8):e70895.

101. Blank DA, Badurdeen S, Omar FKC, et al. Baby-directed umbilical cord clamping: a feasibility study. *Resuscitation.* 2018; 131:1-7.

102. Badurdeen S, Davis PG, Hooper SB, et al. Physiologically based cord clamping for infants $\geq 32^{+0}$ weeks gestation: a randomised clinical trial and reference percentiles for heart rate and oxygen saturation for infants $\geq 35^{+0}$ weeks gestation. *PLoS Med.* 2022;19(6):e1004029.

103. Winter J, Kattwinkel J, Chisholm C, Blackman A, Wilson S, Fairchild K. Ventilation of preterm infants during delayed cord clamping (VentFirst): a pilot study of feasibility and safety. *Am J Perinatol.* 2017;34(2):111-116.

104. Brouwer E, Knol R, Vernooij ASN, et al. Physiological-based cord clamping in preterm infants using a new purpose-built resuscitation table: a feasibility study. *Arch Dis Child Fetal Neonatal Ed.* 2019;104(4):F396-F402.

105. Foglia EE, Ades A, Hedrick HL, et al. Initiating resuscitation before umbilical cord clamping in infants with congenital diaphragmatic hernia: a pilot feasibility trial. *Arch Dis Child Fetal Neonatal Ed.* 2020;105(3):322-326.

106. Knol R, Brouwer E, Klumper F, et al. Effectiveness of stabilization of preterm infants with intact umbilical cord using a purpose-built resuscitation table-study protocol for a randomized controlled trial. *Front Pediatr.* 2019;7:134.

107. Knol R, Brouwer E, van den Akker T, et al. Physiological-based cord clamping in very preterm infants – randomised controlled trial on effectiveness of stabilisation. *Resuscitation.* 2020;147:26-33.

108. Dawson JA, Kamlin CO, Vento M, et al. Defining the reference range for oxygen saturation for infants after birth. *Pediatrics.* 2010;125(6):e1340-e1347.

109. Dawson JA, Kamlin CO, Wong C, et al. Changes in heart rate in the first minutes after birth. *Arch Dis Child Fetal Neonatal Ed.* 2010;95(3):F177-F181.

110. Padilla-Sanchez C, Baixauli-Alacreu S, Canada-Martinez AJ, Solaz-Garcia A, Alemany-Anchel MJ, Vento M. Delayed vs immediate cord clamping changes oxygen saturation and heart rate patterns in the first minutes after birth. *J Pediatr.* 2020; 227:149-156.e1.

# Chapter 7

# Transitional Hemodynamics and Pathophysiology of Peri-/Intraventricular Hemorrhage

Shahab Noori and Istvan Seri

## Key Points

- A period of systemic and cerebral hypoperfusion in the immediate postnatal period predisposes the extremely preterm infant to peri-/intraventricular hemorrhage (P/IVH).
- Cardiovascular immaturity and maladaptation after birth contribute to postnatal hypoperfusion.
- Ventilatory support, especially inappropriately high mean airway pressure, can accentuate the early postnatal hypoperfusion.
- Following the initial hypoperfusion, a period of improvement in systemic and cerebral perfusion precedes occurrence of P/IVH on the second or third postnatal days. Therefore ischemia-reperfusion is a major hemodynamic contributor to the pathogenesis of P/IVH.
- Hypercapnia, especially $PaCO_2$ above low 50s, may increase the risk of P/IVH by potentiating the reperfusion phase via increasing the cerebral blood flow and attenuating autoregulation.
- Delayed cord clamping is associated with hemodynamic stability and appears to be beneficial in preventing P/IVH by mitigating the risk of hypoperfusion.
- Cord milking is associated with decreased need for cardiovascular support during the transitional period. However, this procedure is not recommended due to the increased rate of P/IVH found in a recent randomized control trial. Although the mechanism(s) of the development of P/IVH with cord milking is unclear, a rapid change in cerebral blood flow has been postulated.

## Introduction

Peri-/intraventricular hemorrhage (P/IVH) is a devastating complication of prematurity that affects about a third of extremely preterm infants (<28 weeks' gestation).[1] P/IVH is a major risk factor for poor neurodevelopmental outcome, hydrocephalus, and mortality amongst these patients.[2] Although the pathogenesis of P/IVH is complex and likely involves multiple different mechanisms, alteration in cerebral hemodynamics is thought to play a major role. Recent advances in noninvasive monitoring have highlighted the hemodynamic antecedents of P/IVH. This chapter reviews the inherent vulnerabilities of preterm infants during the transitional period and how the interaction between transitional hemodynamics and interventions aimed at supporting respiratory and cardiovascular function can increase the risk of P/IVH.

## Fetal and Transitional Circulation

As the physiology of fetal circulation is discussed in Chapter 1, we only provide a brief review of its main characteristics pertinent to the topic of this chapter. In utero, the most oxygenated blood, with oxygen saturation of around 75–85%, flows from the umbilical vein through the ductus venosus to the inferior vena cava (IVC). Due to mixing with venous blood from the portal and hepatic circulations in the liver and to some mixing with the venous blood flowing from the lower body in the IVC, the oxygen saturation of blood entering the heart is only about 70%. Of note, blood flowing in from the ductus venosus into the IVC is primarily diverted by the Eustachian valve toward the foramen ovale and into the left atrium.[3-5] The low flow of poorly oxygenated pulmonary venous return to the left atrium admixing with this flow via the foramen ovale still ensures supply of relatively well-oxygenated blood to the heart and brain with an oxygen saturation around 60%. On the other hand, blood returning from superior vena cava (SVC) and the stream in the IVC, representing blood returning from the lower parts of the body, are preferentially directed to right ventricle. As most of right ventricular output is diverted through the patent ductus arteriosus (PDA) to the systemic circulation, both ventricles contribute to the systemic circulation. Given the low blood flow to the lungs, due to high pulmonary vascular resistance, left ventricular preload is relatively small. As such, during fetal life, the contribution of the right ventricle to systemic blood flow is greater than that of the left ventricle. In the fetus the combined cardiac output is about 400–450 mL/kg/min, with only about 11–25% constituting the pulmonary circulation.[3,6-9] This is in contrast to postnatal circulation, where the left and right cardiac outputs are equal and average about 200 mL/kg/min. The low-resistance placental circulation facilitates the high cardiac output in the fetus by reducing the afterload. At birth, pulmonary vascular resistance drops precipitously as the newborn starts breathing and the lungs become the organ of gas exchange. This increases pulmonary blood flow and changes the ductal flow pattern in a way that progressively directs blood from the right ventricle to the pulmonary circulation.[10] The increased pulmonary blood flow in turn increases left-sided preload and promotes functional closure of the foramen ovale. This, along with the closure of the ductus arteriosus over the following 2–3 days, transforms the circulation to the adult-type (postnatal) circulation, in which the pulmonary and systemic circuits are not functioning as parallel circulations anymore but as circulations in series. Despite its complexity, this transformation occurs smoothly in most term infants. However, in preterm infants, especially those born before 28 weeks' gestation, this process is hindered by immaturity of the organ systems and is more likely to represent an abnormal cardiorespiratory transition. Accordingly, it is likely to be associated with circulatory compromise, as discussed in detail in this chapter.

## Cerebral Blood Flow

Understanding the evolution of cerebral hemodynamics from fetal circulation through the postnatal transition is critical in understanding the role of abnormal transition in pathogenesis of P/IVH. However, measurement of cerebral blood flow (CBF) is challenging in neonates, especially in preterm infants and during the immediate postnatal period. CBF has been assessed using radioactive xenon clearance, positron emission tomography, Doppler ultrasonography, magnetic resonance imaging, and near-infrared spectroscopy (NIRS). Each of these methods has its own intrinsic limitations. Due to their noninvasive nature and bedside availability, Doppler and NIRS are the most commonly used methods for the assessment of CBF. With Doppler ultrasonography, various surrogates of CBF, such as SVC blood flow and a major cerebral artery blood flow velocity, have been used to characterize intermittent changes in cerebral hemodynamics. On the other hand, NIRS allows for the continuous assessment of regional tissue oxygen saturation (rSO$_2$) or tissue oxygenation index (TOI). Although NIRS does not measure blood flow directly, by considering *cerebral* regional oxygen saturation (CrSO$_2$), clinical information, and certain other parameters, changes in CBF can be deduced. Considering arterial oxygen saturation (SPO$_2$), the index of cerebral fractional oxygen extraction (CFOE) can be calculated according to the following formula: (SPO$_2$ – CrSO$_2$)/SPO$_2$. CrSO$_2$ has a direct and CFOE an inverse relationship with changes in CBF. In other words, a reduction in CrSO$_2$ or an increase in CFOE indicates a decrease in CBF provided certain assumptions hold true. These assumptions include no significant changes in SPO$_2$ (with CrSO$_2$), organ metabolism, hemoglobin, and/or the distribution of blood in tissue among arteries, veins, and capillaries.

### NORMAL CHANGES IN CBF

During fetal development, brain blood flow increases both as an absolute value and per gram of tissue.[11,12] Animal and human studies have shown a decrease in CBF at and immediately after birth.[13,14] The cause of this reduction is unclear but in part may be related to an increase in tissue oxygenation at birth compared to the fetal life.[10,13] Interestingly, the progressive change of PDA flow pattern from right to left to left to right during the first few minutes after birth strongly and inversely correlates with middle cerebral artery mean blood flow velocity (MCA-MV), a surrogate of CBF.[10] This suggests a possible role of PDA immediately after birth in reduction of CBF. Alternatively, the changes in PDA flow pattern and reduction in CBF may be independent, and both reflective of the increasing oxygen tension following delivery. More data are needed to elucidate the normal changes in cardiovascular function and cerebral hemodynamics at and immediately after birth, especially in preterm infants.

After the immediate postnatal period, CBF increases rather significantly over the following days and more gradually afterward in both preterm and term infants.[15-18] Despite the rise in CBF, it remains at only a fraction of the adult value.[19,20] Moreover, sick preterm infants have even lower CBF.[19] The low CBF in neonates may be explained by lower brain metabolism; however, cardiovascular maladaptation in preterm infants may also contribute to the observed low CBF.

## CBF AND P/IVH

Preterm infants who develop P/IVH have lower CBF after birth. Studies using NIRS found higher CFOE on the first postnatal day in preterm infants who later develop P/IVH.[21] Serial measurements of SVC flow, a surrogate for CBF, also found that low SVC blood flow in the first few hours after birth is a risk factor for P/IVH.[22] However, caution needs to be exercised when using SVC flow as a surrogate of CBF since, in the preterm neonate, it is estimated that only around 30% of the blood flow in the SVC represents blood coming back from the brain (Chapter 2). The last two decades have seen an increased use of ultrasonography by neonatologists to elucidate the cardiovascular adaptation during the transitional period. In addition, advances in monitoring technology have brought NIRS to a more widespread use in research and also have facilitated its introduction into clinical care. The newer NIRS sensors have allowed for more continuous and prolonged monitoring of regional tissue oxygen saturation and for quick applications of the sensors in situations when time is of the essence, for example, in the delivery room. Therefore, despite the limitations mentioned earlier, increased application of the newer

NIRS technology and ultrasonography have provided valuable insights into the cerebral hemodynamic changes that precede P/IVH.

A recent nested case-control study compared $CrSO_2$ and CFOE between preterm infants with and without P/IVH during the first 15 days after birth.[23] Measurements were done daily for 2 hours for 8 days and then on day 15.[23] The authors found lower $CrSO_2$ and higher CFOE in the P/IVH group, suggestive of lower CBF throughout the first 8 days. While low CBF in the first postnatal day has consistently been reported, its persistence for a week has not.[17,21,22,24] In contrast, another nested case-control study monitoring cerebral oxygenation during the first few postnatal days found higher $CrSO_2$ and lower CFOE during the 24 hours prior to detection of severe P/IVH.[25] In other words, this study suggests that higher rather than lower CBF precedes brain hemorrhage. This discrepancy may be explained by the differences in the timing and duration of monitoring between the two studies.[26] In a recent study, in addition to performing frequent and regularly timed head ultrasounds and echocardiography, we prospectively and continuously monitored NIRS indices in extremely preterm infants (<28 weeks) during the first 3 postnatal days. The study found a unique pattern with identifiable phases of changes, among others, in the indices of CBF in patients who developed P/IVH (Figure 7.1).[27] The $CrSO_2$ and CFOE were indicative of low CBF in the earlier hours of the first postnatal day, followed by a period of an increase in CBF before detection of P/IVH around 48 hours after birth and, thereafter, a subsequent decrease in CBF. These findings suggest that there are two distinct hemodynamic phases in the pathogenesis of P/IVH: an early hypoperfusion and a later reperfusion phase. The prospective, comprehensive, and continuous design of the study allowed for detection of the two phases. Given the dynamic changes in CBF over the first few days, intermittent or a short period of monitoring will miss either the hypoperfusion or reperfusion phase.[26]

In the remainder of this chapter we will discuss the vulnerabilities of preterm infants during the transitional period that increase the risk of P/IVH and focus on the causes and risk factors that lead to or potentiate the hypoperfusion and/or reperfusion phases.

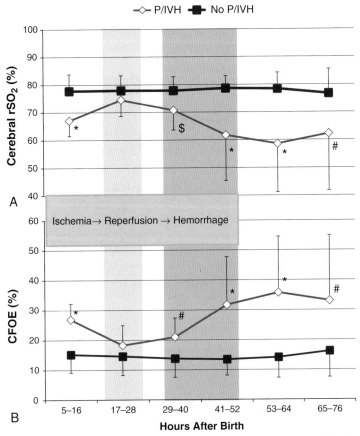

**Fig. 7.1** Changes in cerebral regional oxygen saturation ($rSO_2$) and cerebral fractional oxygen extraction (CFOE) in two groups of very preterm neonates presenting with (*white diamonds*) and without (*red squares*) peri-/intraventricular hemorrhage (PIVH) during first 3 postnatal days. The No-P/IVH group exhibited stable cerebral $rSO_2$ (a) and CFOE (b) values, while the P/IVH group presented with a characteristic pattern of changes. The P/IVH group had lower cerebral $rSO_2$ and higher CFOE during the first 12 hours of the study, followed by normalization of these parameters (highlighted in *light pink*) just before the two study periods when P/IVH was detected (highlighted in *pink*). These findings suggest that initial cerebral hypoperfusion is followed by a period of reperfusion before the occurrence of the P/IVH. After the second study period, cerebral $rSO_2$ decreased and CFOE increased, suggesting a decrease in CBF during and after the development of P/IVH. Statistically significant differences between the two groups: $*P < 0.005$, $\#P < 0.04$, and $\$P < 0.05$. The values represent the mean ± SD of the data obtained in each 12-hour data collection period.[27]

## Vulnerabilities of Preterm Infants During Transition

### INHERENT VULNERABILITY OF THE IMMATURE BRAIN

The brain of a preterm infant is vulnerable to development of P/IVH due to both structural and functional immaturity. The germinal matrix is the site of active proliferation of future neuronal and glial cells and, as such, is a highly vascularized and metabolically active tissue.[28] Its capillary network consisting of thin-walled fragile vessels is susceptible to rupture.[29] The germinal

matrix involutes between 28 and 34 weeks.[28,30] Therefore, until its final involution, the germinal matrix is susceptible to bleeding, especially in preterm infants <28 weeks' gestation. In addition, the germinal matrix lies within an arterial end zone, which makes it particularly vulnerable to hypoperfusion-reperfusion injury.[31] The immature venous system is prone to congestion, which further increases the risk of hemorrhage in this population.[28,30]

The ability to maintain CBF relatively constant despite fluctuations in blood pressure (i.e., CBF autoregulation) is an important protective mechanism against ischemia and hyperperfusion (Chapter 2). The correlation between mean blood pressure and tissue oxygenation index or regional tissue oxygen saturation using NIRS allows for continuous assessment of CBF autoregulation by analyzing coherence and transfer function gain. Coherence is a measure of linear correlation between blood pressure and an index of CBF (i.e., cerebral oxygenation), and therefore an arbitrary cutoff, usually 0.5, is used to define presence or absence of autoregulation. On the other hand, transfer function gain assesses the degree of impairment by measuring the effects of changes in the amplitude of the blood pressure waveform on the amplitude of changes in cerebral tissue oxygenation. Both methods have their strengths and limitations and are not routinely used in clinical settings (Chapter 2).[32]

The brain of preterm infants has immature CBF autoregulation.[33-35] In addition, most very preterm neonates have mean blood pressures very close to the lower elbow of the blood pressure autoregulatory curve during the first 24 hours after delivery (Chapter 2). Although CBF autoregulation is present even in the most immature preterm infant, the autoregulatory plateau is quite narrow. Moreover, immaturity per se and/or the interventions aiming to support these patients can result in systemic changes that alter CBF autoregulation (see hypotension and permissive hypercapnia). Given the role of CBF autoregulation in ensuring maintenance of adequate CBF and prevention of hyperperfusion, immature and impaired autoregulation has long been considered a risk factor for P/IVH. Indeed most, but not all, studies of CBF autoregulation in preterm infants have shown an association between impaired autoregulation and the occurrence P/IVH.[33-38]

Another vulnerability of the brain of the very preterm neonate ($\leq$28 weeks' gestation) is the immaturity of the forebrain (including cortex, thalamus, hypothalamus, basal ganglia) vasculature displaying characteristics of the blood flow regulation of a non-vital organ during the first postnatal days. In other words, the vessels of the forebrain respond with vasoconstriction to decreasing perfusion pressure or hypoxia rather than with vasodilation as expected for the vessels of a vital organ (brain, heart, and adrenal gland).[39] Several lines of evidence support this notion.[40-42] For example, beagle pups exposed to hypoxia exhibit vasodilation of the hindbrain (medulla, pons, cerebellum) but vasoconstriction of the forebrain.[40] In humans CBF autoregulation appears in the brainstem first and in the forebrain only later in gestation.[41] Therefore vital organ assignment appears to be developmentally regulated, with the forebrain lagging behind the hindbrain in acquiring the properties of a high-priority vascular bed.

## IMMATURE MYOCARDIUM

The myocardium of a neonate, even at term, is immature and quite different than that of older children and adults. It has more water content and less contractile elements. In addition, the immature sarcoplasmic reticulum makes cytosolic calcium the primary source of second messenger, calcium for myocardial function. These differences affect both systolic and diastolic functions. Indeed, the neonatal myocardium is more sensitive to afterload; specifically, its lower compliance adversely affects ventricular filling and is dependent on extracellular calcium for its function. Preterm infants, especially during the transition, exhibit a cardiovascular response to acidosis that is different from that of adults. A recent study in hemodynamically stable very preterm infants during the transitional period showed that, while acidic pH was not associated with a decrease in myocardial contractility, cardiac output failed to increase, presumably because the expected acidosis-associated decrease in systemic vascular resistance didn't take place.[43] It has been postulated that immaturity of the myocardium predisposes preterm infants to a low systemic flow state[22,44] and therefore contributes to the low CBF observed in a subset of very preterm neonates who later develop P/IVH. If we consider SVC flow as a surrogate for systemic flow, the finding of low SVC flow in the P/IVH group represents low cardiac output in the immediate postnatal period, with the fetal channels open.[22] Indeed, low left (LVO) and right ventricular output (RVO) have been shown to be prevalent in those who later develop P/IVH (Figure 7.2).[27] However, the underlying causes of this low cardiac output are unclear. Among others, a suddenly increased *high afterload* following removal of low-resistance placental circulation in the setting of an immature myocardium has been postulated to be one of the underlying causes of this finding. Indeed, there is a difference in the inverse linear relationship of contractility and afterload among

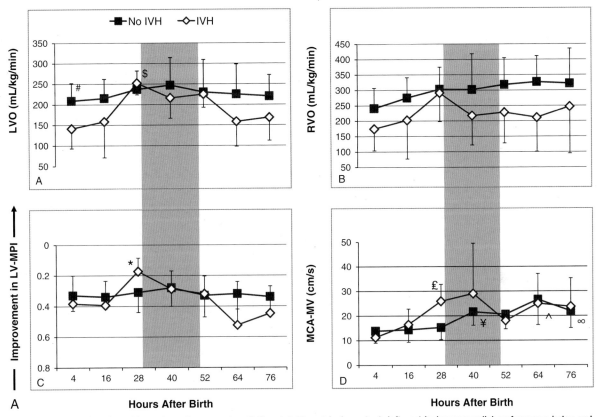

**Fig. 7.2a** Changes in selected hemodynamic parameters (left and right ventricular output, left ventricular myocardial performance index and middle cerebral artery mean flow velocity) during the first 76 hours in very preterm neonates with (*white diamonds*) and without (*red squares*) P/IVH. The changes in LVO (a), RVO (b), left ventricular myocardial performance index (LV-MPI) (c), and MCA-MV (d) in the two groups during the study are shown. There was a trend for a lower LVO in the P/IVH group at baseline, with a trend for improvement before the occurrence of P/IVH (highlighted in *pink*). Lower MPI (i.e., better function) and higher MCA-MV in the P/IVH group also preceded occurrence of P/IVH. The pattern of changes in LVO between the two groups tended to be statistically significant ($P = 0.068$), while that in RVO, MPI, and MCA-MV did not reach statistical significance.[27] Statistically significant differences between groups: $*P = 0.04$ and $£P = 0.016$. No-P/IVH group; compared to baseline: $¥P = 0.02$, $^P < 0.0001$, and $\infty P = 0.044$. Differences approaching statistical significance and suggesting a difference between the groups: $\#P < 0.055$; and within the P/IVH group compared to baseline: $\$P = 0.07$. The values represent the mean ± SD of the data obtained upon entry into the study and every 12 hours thereafter. *LVO*, left ventricular output; *MCA*, middle cerebral artery mean flow velocity; *MPI*, myocardial performance index; *RVO*, right ventricular output.

preterm infants with normal and low SVC flow, with patients having low SVC flow as a group exhibiting a steeper regression line suggestive of lower contractility in this group.[44] However, this is not a consistent finding and a recent study found no difference in afterload or load-dependent and load-independent indices of contractility between patients who develop P/IVH and those who don't.[27] Whether *low preload* could explain the observed low cardiac output is not known, in part because of the difficulty in assessing preload using noninvasive techniques. However, recent studies of delayed cord clamping and cord milking suggest a possible role for low preload in the observed low cardiac output state (see below). Thus it is likely that the low cardiac output is multifactorial, with abnormalities in preload, contractility, and afterload and other factors such as ductal shunting contributing to a varying degree in different patients. Following the initial low flow state, cardiovascular function improves, and cardiac output normalizes. This improvement in systemic flow is also associated with reperfusion of the brain and precedes occurrence of P/IVH (Figure 7.2).[27]

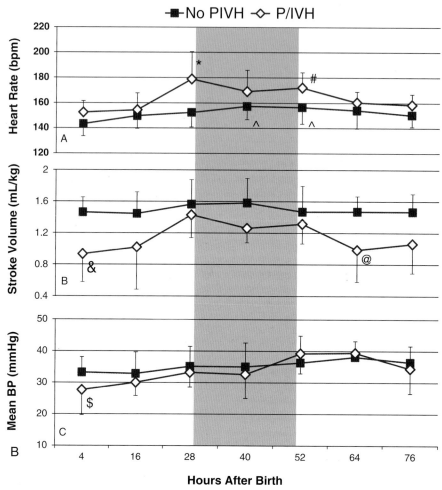

**Fig. 7.2b** Changes in selected hemodynamic parameters (heart rate, left ventricular stroke volume, and mean blood pressure) during the first 76 hours in very preterm neonates with and without P/IVH. Changes in heart rate (a), left ventricular stroke volume (b), and mean blood pressure (c) in the two groups during the study are shown. Heart rate significantly increased in the No-P/IVH group (ANOVA $P = 0.004$), while there was a trend for an increase in the P/IVH group (ANOVA $P = 0.051$) during the study. Compared to the No-P/IVH group, left ventricular stroke volume in patients of the P/IVH group was lower at the baseline but similar before the occurrence of the P/IVH. Mean blood pressure (c) tended to increase in the P/IVH group (ANOVA $P = 0.052$), while it remained unchanged and relatively stable in the No-P/IVH group (ANOVA $P = 0.2$). In addition, mean blood pressure at baseline also tended to be lower in patients in the P/IVH group. The pattern of changes in heart rate and stroke volume, but not in mean blood pressure, was different between the two groups.[27] No-P/IVH group; compared to baseline: ^$P = 0.007$ Between groups: *$P = 0.004$, #$P = 0.03$, &$P = 0.007$, @$P = 0.048$, $$P = 0.085$. *bpm*, beats per minute. The values represent the mean ± SD of the data obtained upon entry into the study and every 12 hours thereafter. Area highlighted in pink represents the period when P/IVH occurred.

## HYPOVOLEMIA AND TIMING OF CORD CLAMPING

Recent studies of timing of cord clamping show enhanced hemodynamic status and possible lower rate of P/IVH when clamping of the umbilical cord is delayed for 30–60 seconds, although in more recent studies there is less association seen with cord clamping and P/IVH.[45-48] These data suggest a better postnatal transition with delayed cord clamping. A more gradual separation from the low-resistance placental circulation might facilitate the adaptation of the left ventricle to the postnatal increase in afterload. Prolonging the time of cord clamping also promotes placental transfusion. In the term neonate it is estimated that 16–23 mL/kg of blood is transfused from the placenta to the neonate, with a 1- and 3-minute delay in the timing of cord clamping, respectively.[49] Importantly, the onset of breathing before cord clamping promotes earlier establishment of pulmonary blood flow, and thus better maintains left ventricular preload, and increases placental transfusion to the newborn.[50] Although all of the above mechanisms are likely contributory, increased intravascular volume due to placental transfusion has been speculated as the most important cause for the better transition in preterm infants with delayed or physiologic cord clamping. This speculation is based on the finding that similar cardiovascular benefits are seen with milking of the cord.[51-53] Preterm infants receiving placental transfusion by milking of the cord have higher cerebral oxygenation and SVC flow, cardiac output and urine output, and a decreased incidence of hypotension and are less likely to receive vasopressor-inotropes or inotropes compared to those with immediate cord clamping.[51-53] However, the finding of a higher rate of P/IVH among the extremely preterm infants randomized to cord milking in a recent RCT has raised significant concerns about the safety of this procedure intended to be used to facilitate placental transfusion.[54] The underlying mechanisms for the increase in P/IVH are unknown. Although there was no indirect evidence of an increase in CBF with cord milking in patients monitored with NIRS in the delivery room,[55] it is possible that in vulnerable individuals, a rapid increase in the preload, and thus CBF, may play a role.

Historically, hypovolemia was thought not to be prevalent in the newborn, given the absent or weak relationship between measured blood volume and blood pressure. However, the finding of a more stable cardiovascular status in preterm infants with placental transfusion, either from delayed cord clamping or cord milking, indicates that hypovolemia may indeed play a role in hemodynamic instability during the immediate transition period and, as such, might contribute to pathogenesis of P/IVH. Indeed, the recent report of an association between lower initial hematocrit used as a surrogate for intravascular volume and the occurrence of P/IVH supports the role of hypovolemia in the pathogenesis of P/IVH.[56] As mentioned earlier,

preterm infants who develop P/IVH have lower CBF in the first hours after birth, as suggested by lower $CrSO_2$ and SVC flow. The findings of a higher $CrSO_2$ and SVC flow in patients with delayed cord clamping or cord milking suggest that the incidence of low CBF occurring immediately after delivery can be reduced. Thus enhancing placental transfusion may, at least in theory, be associated with a lower incidence of P/IVH. While reduction in cerebral hypoperfusion with placental transfusion appears to decrease the predisposition to P/IVH, cord milking likely increases the risk of P/IVH.[54] Although the mechanism(s) leading to the increased occurrence of P/IVH with cord milking are unclear, the use of this intervention is currently not recommended.[57] Furthermore, the importance of the onset of breathing in delayed/physiological cord clamping also suggests that a gradual, smoother shift from placental blood flow to pulmonary blood as the source of left ventricular preload immediately after birth is among the key contributors associated with an improved hemodynamic status in the very preterm neonates during early transition.

## PATENT DUCTUS ARTERIOSUS

Although a large PDA with *and* without hypotension during early transition has been associated with P/IVH,[22,58,59] the extent of the contribution, if any, of the PDA to the pathogenesis of P/IVH is unclear. As discussed in Chapter 2, the pattern of CBF is affected by a PDA. Moreover, with an inadequately compensated cardiac output for the degree of the left-to-right PDA shunt, CBF is also reduced. Most studies assessing cerebral oxygenation using NIRS have shown a lower $CrSO_2$, with a PDA and improvement after closure of the ductus arteriosus.[60-62] The increased stroke volume and, as a result, the left ventricular output represent a compensatory mechanism to attenuate the effect of the shunt on systemic perfusion, especially pre-ductally. This adaptive process may be limited in a subset of patients, especially during first few hours after birth. As discussed earlier, this is the period when cerebral ischemia is prevalent in patients who later develop P/IVH. Indeed, there is a temporal relationship between a hemodynamically significant PDA and low indices of CBF during this critical period.[10,22] Authors of earlier studies showing a reduction of the incidence of P/IVH with indomethacin prophylaxis suggested that early PDA might have a role in development of P/IVH. However, lack of any effect of prophylactic ibuprofen on the incidence of P/IVH, despite a significant reduction in PDA rate, leads to the casting of doubt on the role of early PDA in the development of P/IVH and suggests a more direct effect of indomethacin on cerebral hemodynamics. Nevertheless, the strong relationship between a significant PDA and low CBF and $CrSO_2$ does suggest that PDA may be a contributing factor to the ischemic phase preceding the development of P/IVH.

## HYPOTENSION

Hypotension is common in preterm infants during transition. Hypotension is discussed in detail in Chapter 3; suffice to say that there are many reasons for a preterm infant to be hypotensive during the transitional period. These include postnatal maladaptation superimposed on immaturity of the cardiovascular system, inadequate compensation for the PDA shunt, prevalence of relative adrenal insufficiency, increased rate of sepsis, acidosis, and the detrimental impact of inappropriate ventilatory support on neonatal hemodynamics. Hypotension has long been recognized as a risk factor for P/IVH.[63-66] Given the fact that hypotension is a hallmark of uncompensated shock, the association between hypotension and P/IVH is not surprising. However, the uncertainty about the definition of hypotension and the influence of other coexisting variables (see Chapter 3) make it difficult to propose a "safe" blood pressure range.

Over the past decade, there has been an increasing concern about the possible role of treatment of hypotension in the occurrence of P/IVH and poor neurodevelopmental outcome associated with hypotension.[67-69] This is indeed a possibility, at least theoretically. By definition, hypotensive preterm infants are outside the CBF autoregulatory range, where cerebral perfusion is pressure passive.[70,71] Therefore inappropriate titration of vasopressor-inotropes can increase blood pressure and brain blood flow[70,72] and thus, in theory, increase the risk of P/IVH (Chapter 3). However, of note is that, although careful, stepwise titration of vasopressor-inotropes for hypotension

restores brain blood flow along with the blood pressure, CBF autoregulation does not regain its functionality for a period of time.[70,72] Yet, there are data, although not conclusive, on the potential beneficial effects of careful titration of cardiovascular medications.[64,73,74] A retrospective study of dopamine-treated preterm infants <28 weeks' gestation found that failure to respond to dopamine was associated with almost a sixfold greater likelihood of developing P/IVH. On the other hand, a strong response to dopamine was associated with a reduction in risk of P/IVH.[74] In contrast, the secondary analysis of a recent RCT of peripheral perfusion–based approach versus blood pressure–based approach to circulatory management of the preterm infants during the transitional period found a higher incidence of P/IVH in the subset of the blood pressure–based management group who had responded to the treatment (volume, pressors, and/or inotropes).[75] Although the reasons for these findings are unclear, differences in the choice of medication and the approach to drug titration to avoid significant and rapid fluctuations in blood pressure may have played a role.[70,76]

During the last decade, the trend toward less aggressive treatment of hypotension[77] has provided a glimpse into the potential effects of sustained hypotension in patients without clinical evidence of poor perfusion ("isolated hypotension"). For example, the analysis of the French national prospective population-based cohort study allowed for the matching of 119 extremely preterm infants with untreated, "isolated hypotension" to 119 neonates who received treatment despite also having no clinical evidence of poor perfusion.[78] Accordingly, none of the patients included in this study had any clinical sign of inadequate cardiovascular function other than hypotension. Hypotension was defined as a mean blood pressure less than gestational age in weeks during the first 3 postnatal days. The findings revealed that the group treated for the "isolated hypotension" had a higher rate of survival without severe morbidity and a lower rate of severe P/IVH and cerebral injury. Interestingly, the association between treatment and better outcome was even stronger when hypotension was defined as a mean blood pressure in mmHg less than gestational age in weeks by more than 5 points. Although this dose-effect relationship strengthens the possibility of causality, further studies are clearly needed to verify the impact of hypotension on P/IVH and long-term outcome.

It is likely that the underlying pathophysiology of brain injury associated with hypotension is multifactorial and that low CBF due to low perfusion pressure, inappropriate treatment, and titration of vasopressor-inotropes resulting in intermittent cerebral hypo- and hyperperfusion and other coexisting factors independent of hypotension all contribute to varying degrees to the development of P/IVH. The fact that hypotension is almost always treated,[79] albeit at different thresholds, makes establishing causality for adverse outcomes and defining the extent of contribution of various aspects of clinical care to the development of P/IVH in response to hypotension nearly impossible. There are many challenges in designing a study to ascertain the impact of each of these factors in the pathogenesis of P/IVH and poor neurodevelopmental outcome. These include the inability to utilize a physiology-based and individualized definition of hypotension for each patient, the heterogeneous etiology and pathophysiology of hypotension (i.e., abnormality in preload, contractility, afterload and/or vascular tone dysregulation), and complexity of selecting the appropriate treatment for the given pathophysiology and clinical presentation. In addition, given the strong belief among neonatologists of harmful effect of hypotension and difficulties in recruitment, conducting randomized control trials with a no-treatment arm does not appear feasible.[79,80]

## CARDIORESPIRATORY INTERACTION

The close anatomic and physiologic relationship between the respiratory and cardiovascular systems results in the notion that changes in the two systems mutually affect one another. Due to the vulnerability of the preterm infant, these interactions are particularly important during the early postnatal transitional period. Most very preterm infants require some level of respiratory support for immaturity of the lungs and the respiratory center.

The impact of positive airway pressure and invasive or noninvasive ventilation have been studied in animals and to a lesser extent in humans. Animal studies demonstrate that with increasing positive end-expiratory pressure, pulmonary vascular resistance increases, thereby raising right ventricular afterload, resulting in reductions in RVO.[81,82] In addition, the increased intrathoracic pressure-driven decrease in systemic venous return further reduces RVO and, as a result, systemic blood flow also decreases. Studies in human neonates have reported inconsistent results, with some findings being similar to those obtained in animal models, albeit with a milder impact, while others show no effect.[83-86] The reason for this discrepancy is unclear but likely involves limitations of assessment tools and differences in lung compliance among the patients in the different studies. The latter reason could explain the significant hemodynamic alteration observed in animal models where lung compliance is normal and therefore intrathoracic pressure is more readily transmitted to the vasculature and the heart. Although the effect of positive airway pressure in the range commonly used in clinical practice appears to be relatively small, inappropriately high pressure for the degree of lung disease can reduce systemic blood flow and also lead to increased cerebral venous pressure, both of which may contribute to pathogenesis of P/IVH. Indeed, a recent study showed that an altered internal cerebral venous flow pattern is associated with an increased rate of P/IVH.[87] This increase in P/IVH is presumably due to the effect of elevated intrathoracic and right atrial pressures on cerebral venous pressure. However, other variables, including high blood pressure and a PDA, have also been associated with altered internal cerebral venous flow.[88] Given the prevalence of less effective or impaired CBF autoregulation in sick, extremely preterm infants, decreases in systemic perfusion can relatively easily lead to a drop in CBF. In addition, the fluctuation of CBF associated with mechanical ventilation, perhaps due to asynchrony, increases the risk of P/IVH.[89] While positive pressure ventilation increases central and cerebral venous pressure, tension pneumothorax can result in a significant, abrupt rise in these pressures and increases the risk of P/IVH.[90,91] Surfactant administration can also impact CBF initially by altering carbon dioxide levels and subsequently by the hemodynamic consequences of potential lung hyperinflation following improvement in lung compliance, provided that ventilator support has not been weaned in a timely fashion.[92-94] Tracheal suction can also alter cerebral hemodynamics by increasing both arterial and venous blood pressure. In addition to the direct effects of ventilatory support, treatment strategies such as permissive hypercapnia with the resultant acidosis can impact cardiovascular function and CBF (see below).

## HYPOCAPNIA AND HYPERCAPNIA

Carbon dioxide has a potent effect on the vascular system in general and brain in particular. Increases and decreases in partial pressure of $CO_2$ ($PaCO_2$) cause cerebral vasodilation and vasoconstriction, respectively. In fact, changes in $PaCO_2$ are more potent regulators of CBF than are changes in blood pressure, even outside the autoregulatory blood pressure range (Chapter 2). Therefore hypocapnia and hypercapnia may impact the hypoperfusion and reperfusion phases preceding P/IVH, respectively. Although hypocapnia is associated with ischemic brain injury and periventricular leukomalacia,[95,96] it does not appear to play a significant role in pathogenesis of P/IVH.[97] This could be due to absent or low reactivity of CBF to changes in $PaCO_2$ during the first postnatal day, a period when hypoperfusion is commonly reported in this population. Indeed, there is an evolution of the CBF-$CO_2$ reactivity in preterm infants with higher responsiveness of the cerebral vasculature to changes in $PaCO_2$ with each passing day during the first few postnatal days.[98,99] In one study the CBF reactivity per kPa (7.5 mmHg) change in $PaCO_2$ was about 11% on the first postnatal day compared to 32% on the second day.[100] A weak relationship between $PaCO_2$ and CBF on the first postnatal day has also been shown using NIRS.[101] We found no relationship between MCA-MV, a surrogate for CBF, and $PaCO_2$ on the first postnatal day and a progressively stronger positive linear relationship on postnatal days 2 and 3 in preterm infants.[99]

On the other hand, hypercapnia has consistently been shown to be associated with P/IVH.[97,102-104] The highest $PaCO_2$ during the first 3 postnatal days has a dose-dependent relationship with odds of developing P/IVH.[102] Although cause-and-effect relationship has not been established, the increase in CBF with hypercapnia can accentuate the reperfusion phase preceding the occurrence of P/IVH.[27] In addition, hypercapnia attenuates CBF autoregulation. A study of the correlation between blood pressure and MCA-MV demonstrated a steeper coefficient line with higher $PaCO_2$ values suggesting a progressive impairment of CBF autoregulation with rising $PaCO_2$ above normal.[105] Similarly, we found no relationship between MCA-MV and blood pressure in normotensive preterm infants but, when adjusted for $PaCO_2$ levels, a significant positive relationship emerged, suggesting that higher $PaCO_2$ is associated with impairment of CBF autoregulation.[99] Furthermore, we found a breakpoint in the relationship between $PaCO_2$ and MCA-MV with no relationship below $PaCO_2$ values of 52–53 mmHg and a strong positive linear relationship above this cutoff (Figure 7.3).

Despite being used as a common treatment strategy during the first postnatal days and weeks, permissive hypercapnia is poorly defined and the safe cutoff for a given gestational and chronological age is unknown. Several randomized controlled trials (RCTs) were unable to show any reduction in rate of BPD with this strategy and some have also raised the possibility of harm.[106-108] A recent RCT in Europe comparing mild permissive hypercapnia to a higher $PaCO_2$ strategy among extremely preterm infants on mechanical ventilation during the first postnatal day found no effect on the primary outcome of death or moderate to severe BPD but an increase in necrotizing enterocolitis in the higher $PaCO_2$ group.[108] Yet, the 2-year follow-up of this study showed no difference in neurodevelopmental outcome, contrary to an earlier study finding worse outcomes in the permissive hypercapnia group.[107,109]

## Conclusions

Pathogenesis of P/IVH is complex and involves different mechanisms. Most agree that disturbances in CBF play a major role in development of P/IVH. Improved understanding of the physiology of the transitional circulation, especially in preterm infants, during the past decade has shed some light on the role of cardiovascular compromise and altered cerebral hemodynamics in the pathogenesis of P/IVH. The increased availability of more sophisticated, comprehensive monitoring technology and the more widespread application of these tools provide us with an opportunity to identify the subpopulation at greatest risk for circulatory compromise and development of P/IVH. This in

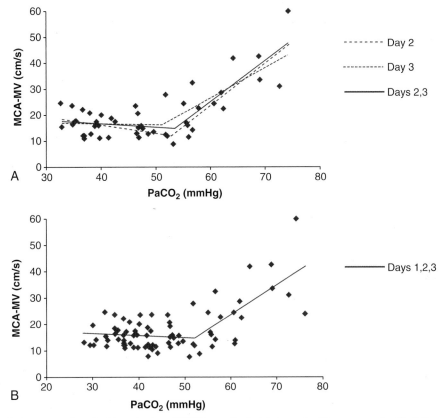

**Fig. 7.3 Relationship between carbon dioxide and index of CBF.** The graphs depict piece-wise bilinear regression identifying a breakpoint in the MCA-MV–PaCO$_2$ relationship. "Graph A" shows the breakpoints at a PaCO$_2$ value of 52.7 mmHg for day 2 (*broken line*, $R^2 = 0.74$, $P < 0.0001$), 51.0 mmHg for day 3 (*dotted line*, $R^2 = 0.60$, $P < 0.034$), and 53.2 mmHg for days 2 and 3 combined (*solid line*, $R^2 = 0.66$, $P < 0.0001$). "Graph B" shows the breakpoint at PaCO$_2$ of 51.7 mmHg ($R^2 = 0.49$, $P < 0.0001$) for all data points, including postnatal "day 1".[99] *MCA-MV*, middle cerebral artery mean flow velocity; *PaCO$_2$*, partial pressure of arterial carbon dioxide.

turn could prove useful in designing appropriate RCTs targeting the high-risk population and the underlying pathophysiology rather than enrolling all patients in the same gestational age range and unnecessarily exposing many patients to intervention who are at minimal or no risk for the development of P/IVH.

## REFERENCES

1. Stoll BJ, Stoll BJ, Hansen NI, Bell EF, et al. Neonatal outcomes of extremely preterm infants from the NICHD Neonatal Research Network. *Pediatrics*. 2010;126:443-456.
2. Mukerji A, Shah V, Shah PS. Periventricular/intraventricular hemorrhage and neurodevelopmental outcomes: a meta-analysis. *Pediatrics*. 2015;136:1132-1143.
3. Rudolph AM. Distribution and regulation of blood flow in the fetal and neonatal lamb. *Circ Res*. 1985;57:811-821.
4. Rothstein R, Longo L. Respiration in the fetal-placental unit. In: Cowett R, ed. *Principles of Perinatal-Neonatal Metabolism*. New York: Springer-Verlag; 1998:451.
5. Kiserud T, Acharya, G. The fetal circulation. *Prenat Diagn*. 2004;24:1049-1059.
6. Sutton MS, Groves A, MacNeill A, Sharland, G, Allan, L. Assessment of changes in blood flow through the lungs and foramen ovale in the normal human fetus with gestational age: a prospective Doppler echocardiographic study. *Br Heart J*. 1994;71:232-237.
7. Rasanen, J, Wood DC, Weiner S, Ludomirski A, Huhta JC. Role of the pulmonary circulation in the distribution of human fetal cardiac output during the second half of pregnancy. *Circulation*. 1996;94:1068-1073.
8. Mielke G, Benda N. Cardiac output and central distribution of blood flow in the human fetus. *Circulation*. 2001;103:1662-1668.
9. Prsa M, Sun L, van Amerom J, et al. Reference ranges of blood flow in the major vessels of the normal human fetal circulation at term by phase-contrast magnetic resonance imaging. *Circ Cardiovasc Imaging*. 2014;7:663-670.

10. Noori S, Wlodaver A, Gottipati V, et al. Transitional changes in cardiac and cerebral hemodynamics in term neonates at birth. *J Pediatr.* 2012;160:943-948.

11. Rudolph AM, Heymann, MA. Circulatory changes during growth in the fetal lamb. *Circ Res.* 1970;26:289-299.

12. Meerman RJ, van Bel F, van Zwieten PH, Oepkes D, den Ouden L. Fetal and neonatal cerebral blood flow velocity in the normal fetus and neonate: a longitudinal Doppler ultrasound study. *Early Hum Dev.* 1990;24:209-217.

13. Iwamoto HS, Teitel D, Rudolph AM. Effects of birth-related events on blood flow distribution. *Pediatr Res.* 1987;22:634-640.

14. Kempley ST, Vyas S, Bower S, Nicolaides KH, Gamsu, H. Cerebral and renal artery blood flow velocity before and after birth. *Early Hum Dev.* 1996;46:165-174.

15. Meek JH, Tyszczuk L, Elwell CE, Wyatt JS. Cerebral blood flow increases over the first three days of life in extremely preterm neonates. *Arch Dis Child Fetal Neonatal Ed.* 1998;78:F33-F37.

16. Kluckow M, Evans N. Superior vena cava flow in newborn infants: a novel marker of systemic blood flow. *Arch Dis Child Fetal Neonatal Ed.* 2000;82:F182-F187.

17. Kissack CM, Garr R, Wardle SP, Weindling AM. Postnatal changes in cerebral oxygen extraction in the preterm infant are associated with intraventricular hemorrhage and hemorrhagic parenchymal infarction but not periventricular leukomalacia. *Pediatr Res.* 2004;56:111-116.

18. Kehrer M, Blumenstock G, Ehehalt S, Goelz R, Poets C, Schöning M. Development of cerebral blood flow volume in preterm neonates during the first two weeks of life. *Pediatr Res.* 2005;58:927-930.

19. Greisen G. Cerebral blood flow in preterm infants during the first week of life. *Acta Paediatr Scand.* 1986;75:43-51.

20. Altman DI, Powers WJ, Perlman JM, Herscovitch P, Volpe SL, Volpe JJ. Cerebral blood flow requirement for brain viability in newborn infants is lower than in adults. *Ann Neurol.* 1988; 24:218-226.

21. Meek JH, Tyszczuk L, Elwell CE, Wyatt JS. Low cerebral blood flow is a risk factor for severe intraventricular haemorrhage. *Arch Dis Child Fetal Neonatal Ed.* 1999;81:F15-F18.

22. Kluckow M, Evans N. Low superior vena cava flow and intraventricular haemorrhage in preterm infants. *Arch Dis Child Fetal Neonatal Ed.* 2000;82:F188-F194.

23. Verhagen EA, Ter Horst HJ, Keating P, Martijn A, Van Braeckel KN, Bos AF. Cerebral oxygenation in preterm infants with germinal matrix-intraventricular hemorrhages. *Stroke J Cereb Circ.* 2010;41:2901-2907.

24. Sorensen LC, Maroun LL, Borch K, Lou HC, Greisen G. Neonatal cerebral oxygenation is not linked to foetal vasculitis and predicts intraventricular haemorrhage in preterm infants. *Acta Paediatr Oslo Nor.* 2008;97:1529-1534.

25. Alderliesten T, Lemmers PM, Smarius JJ, van de Vosse RE, Baerts W, van Bel F. Cerebral oxygenation, extraction, and autoregulation in very preterm infants who develop peri-intraventricular hemorrhage. *J Pediatr.* 2013;162:698-704.e2.

26. Noori S, Seri I. Hemodynamic antecedents of peri/intraventricular hemorrhage in very preterm neonates. *Semin Fetal Neonatal Med.* 2015;20:232-237.

27. Noori S, McCoy M, Anderson MP, Ramji F, Seri I. Changes in cardiac function and cerebral blood flow in relation to peri/intraventricular hemorrhage in extremely preterm infants. *J Pediatr.* 2014;164:264-270.e1-3.

28. Bassan H. Intracranial hemorrhage in the preterm infant: understanding it, preventing it. *Clin Perinatol.* 2009;36:737-762, v.

29. Ballabh P. Intraventricular hemorrhage in premature infants: mechanism of disease. *Pediatr Res.* 2010;67:1-8.

30. Hambleton G, Wigglesworth JS. Origin of intraventricular haemorrhage in the preterm infant. *Arch Dis Child.* 1976;51: 651-659.

31. du Plessis AJ. Cerebrovascular injury in premature infants: current understanding and challenges for future prevention. *Clin Perinatol.* 2008;35:609-641, v.

32. Greisen G. Cerebral autoregulation in preterm infants. How to measure it – and why care? *J Pediatr.* 2014;165:885-886.

33. Soul JS, Hammer PE, Tsuji M, et al. Fluctuating pressure-passivity is common in the cerebral circulation of sick premature infants. *Pediatr Res.* 2007;61:467-473.

34. Wong FY, Leung TS, Austin T, et al. Impaired autoregulation in preterm infants identified by using spatially resolved spectroscopy. *Pediatrics.* 2008;121:e604-e611.

35. Vesoulis ZA, Liao SM, Trivedi SB, Ters NE, Mathur AM. A novel method for assessing cerebral autoregulation in preterm infants using transfer function analysis. *Pediatr Res.* 2016;79:453-459.

36. Tsuji M, Saul JP, du Plessis A, et al. Cerebral intravascular oxygenation correlates with mean arterial pressure in critically ill premature infants. *Pediatrics.* 2000;106:625-632.

37. O'Leary H, Gregas MC, Limperopoulos C, et al. Elevated cerebral pressure passivity is associated with prematurity-related intracranial hemorrhage. *Pediatrics.* 2009;124:302-309.

38. Riera J, Cabañas F, Serrano JJ, et al. New time-frequency method for cerebral autoregulation in newborns: predictive capacity for clinical outcomes. *J Pediatr.* 2014;165:897-902.e1.

39. Noori S, Stavroudis TA, Seri I. Systemic and cerebral hemodynamics during the transitional period after premature birth. *Clin Perinatol.* 2009;36:723-736, v.

40. Hernandez M, Hawkins R, Brennan R. Sympathetic control of regional cerebral blood flow in the asphyxiated newborn dog. In: Heistad D, Marcus M, eds. *Cerebral Blood Flow, Effects of Nerves and Neurotransmitters.* North Holland: Elsevier; 1982:359-366.

41. Ashwal S, Dale PS, Longo LD. Regional cerebral blood flow: studies in the fetal lamb during hypoxia, hypercapnia, acidosis, and hypotension. *Pediatr Res.* 1984;18:1309-1316.

42. Victor S, Appleton RE, Beirne M, Marson AG, Weindling AM. The relationship between cardiac output, cerebral electrical activity, cerebral fractional oxygen extraction and peripheral blood flow in premature newborn infants. *Pediatr Res.* 2006;60:456-460.

43. Noori S, Wu TW, Seri I. pH effects on cardiac function and systemic vascular resistance in preterm infants. *J Pediatr.* 2013;162:958-963.e1.

44. Osborn DA, Evans N, Kluckow M. Left ventricular contractility in extremely premature infants in the first day and response to inotropes. *Pediatr Res.* 2007;61:335-340.

45. Baenziger O, Stolkin F, Keel M, et al. The influence of the timing of cord clamping on postnatal cerebral oxygenation in preterm neonates: a randomized, controlled trial. *Pediatrics.* 2007;119:455-459.

46. Sommers R, Stonestreet BS, Oh W, et al. Hemodynamic effects of delayed cord clamping in premature infants. *Pediatrics.* 2012;129:e667-e672.

47. Rabe H, Reynolds, G, Diaz-Rossello, J. A systematic review and meta-analysis of a brief delay in clamping the umbilical cord of preterm infants. *Neonatology.* 2008;93:138-144.

48. Ghavam S, Batra D, Mercer J, et al. Effects of placental transfusion in extremely low birthweight infants: meta-analysis of long- and short-term outcomes. *Transfusion (Paris).* 2014;54: 1192-1198.

49. Yao AC, Moinian M, Lind J. Distribution of blood between infant and placenta after birth. *Lancet.* 1969;2:871-873.
50. Bhatt S, Alison BJ, Wallace EM, et al. Delaying cord clamping until ventilation onset improves cardiovascular function at birth in preterm lambs. *J Physiol.* 2013;591:2113-2126.
51. Hosono S, Mugishima H, Fujita H, et al. Blood pressure and urine output during the first 120 h of life in infants born at less than 29 weeks' gestation related to umbilical cord milking. *Arch Dis Child Fetal Neonatal Ed.* 2009;94:F328-F331.
52. Takami T, Suganami Y, Sunohara D, et al. Umbilical cord milking stabilizes cerebral oxygenation and perfusion in infants born before 29 weeks of gestation. *J Pediatr.* 2012;161:742-747.
53. Katheria AC, Truong G, Cousins L, Oshiro B, Finer NN. Umbilical cord milking versus delayed cord clamping in preterm infants. *Pediatrics.* 2015;136:61-69.
54. Katheria A, Reister F, Essers J, et al. Association of umbilical cord milking vs delayed cord clamping with death or severe intraventricular hemorrhage among preterm infants. *JAMA.* 2019;322:1877-1886.
55. Katheria AC, Szychowski JM, Essers J, et al. Early cardiac and cerebral hemodynamics with umbilical cord milking compared with delayed cord clamping in infants born preterm. *J Pediatr.* 2020;223:51-56.e1.
56. Dekom S, Vachhani A, Patel K, Barton L, Ramanathan R, Noori S. Initial hematocrit values after birth and peri/intraventricular hemorrhage in extremely low birth weight infants. *J Perinatol.* 2018;38:1471-1475.
57. American College of Obstetricians and Gynecologists' Committee on Obstetric Practice. Delayed umbilical cord clamping after birth: ACOG committee opinion, number 814. *Obstet Gynecol.* 2020;136:e100-e106.
58. Aldana-Aguirre JC, Deshpande P, Jain A, Weisz DE. Physiology of low blood pressure during the first day after birth among extremely preterm neonates. *J Pediatr.* 2021;236:40-46.e3. doi:10.1016/j.jpeds.2021.05.026.
59. Noori S, Seri I. Hypotension and significant patent ductus arteriosus in infants born extremely preterm during the postnatal transitional period: normal adaptation? *J Pediatr.* 2022;240:314-315.
60. Lemmers PMA, Toet MC, van Bel F. Impact of patent ductus arteriosus and subsequent therapy with indomethacin on cerebral oxygenation in preterm infants. *Pediatrics.* 2008;121:142-147.
61. Lemmers PMA, Benders MJ, D'Ascenzo R, et al. Patent ductus arteriosus and brain volume. *Pediatrics.* 2016;137:e20153090.
62. Chock VY, Rose LA, Mante JV, Punn R. Near-infrared spectroscopy for detection of a significant patent ductus arteriosus. *Pediatr Res.* 2016;80:675-680.
63. Watkins AM, West CR, Cooke RW. Blood pressure and cerebral haemorrhage and ischaemia in very low birthweight infants. *Early Hum Dev.* 1989;19:103-110.
64. Pellicer A, Bravo MC, Madero R, Salas S, Quero J, Cabañas F. Early systemic hypotension and vasopressor support in low birth weight infants: impact on neurodevelopment. *Pediatrics.* 2009;123:1369-1376.
65. Thewissen L, Naulaers G, Hendrikx D, et al. Cerebral oxygen saturation and autoregulation during hypotension in extremely preterm infants. *Pediatr Res.* 2021;90:373-380. doi:10.1038/s41390-021-01483-w.
66. da Costa CS, Czosnyka M, Smielewski P, Austin T. Optimal mean arterial blood pressure in extremely preterm infants within the first 24 hours of life. *J Pediatr.* 2018;203:242-248.
67. Batton B, Batton D, Riggs T. Blood pressure during the first 7 days in premature infants born at postmenstrual age 23 to 25 weeks. *Am J Perinatol.* 2007;24:107-115.
68. Dempsey EM, Al Hazzani F, Barrington KJ. Permissive hypotension in the extremely low birthweight infant with signs of good perfusion. *Arch Dis Child Fetal Neonatal Ed.* 2009;94:F241-F244.
69. Batton B, Zhu X, Fanaroff J, et al. Blood pressure, anti-hypotensive therapy, and neurodevelopment in extremely preterm infants. *J Pediatr.* 2009;154:351-357.e1.
70. Munro MJ, Walker AM, Barfield CP. Hypotensive extremely low birth weight infants have reduced cerebral blood flow. *Pediatrics.* 2004;114:1591-1596.
71. Lightburn MH, Gauss CH, Williams DK, Kaiser JR. Observational study of cerebral hemodynamics during dopamine treatment in hypotensive ELBW infants on the first day of life. *J Perinatol.* 2013;33:698-702.
72. Seri I, Rudas G, Bors Z, Kanyicska B, Tulassay T. Effects of low-dose dopamine infusion on cardiovascular and renal functions, cerebral blood flow, and plasma catecholamine levels in sick preterm neonates. *Pediatr Res.* 1993;34:742-749.
73. Pellicer A, Valverde E, Elorza MD, et al. Cardiovascular support for low birth weight infants and cerebral hemodynamics: a randomized, blinded, clinical trial. *Pediatrics.* 2005;115:1501-1512.
74. Vesoulis ZA, Ters NE, Foster A, Trivedi SB, Liao SM, Mathur AM. Response to dopamine in prematurity: a biomarker for brain injury? *J Perinatol.* 2016;36:453-458. doi:10.1038/jp.2016.5.
75. Ishiguro A, Sasaki A, Motojima Y, et al. Randomized trial of perfusion-based circulatory management in infants of very low birth weight. *J Pediatr.* 2022;243:27-32.e2. doi:10.1016/j.jpeds.2021.12.020.
76. Vesoulis ZA, Flower AA, Zanelli S, et al. Blood pressure extremes and severe IVH in preterm infants. *Pediatr Res.* 2020;87:69-73.
77. Miller LE, Laughon MM, Clark RH, et al. Vasoactive medications in extremely low gestational age neonates during the first postnatal week. *J Perinatol.* 2021;41:2330-2336.
78. Durrmeyer X, Marchand-Martin L, Porcher R, et al. Abstention or intervention for isolated hypotension in the first 3 days of life in extremely preterm infants: association with short-term outcomes in the EPIPAGE 2 cohort study. *Arch Dis Child Fetal Neonatal Ed.* 2017;102:490-496.
79. Batton BJ, Li L, Newman NS, et al. Feasibility study of early blood pressure management in extremely preterm infants. *J Pediatr.* 2012;161:65-69.e1.
80. Dempsey EM, Barrington KJ, Marlow N, et al. Hypotension in Preterm Infants (HIP) randomised trial. *Arch Dis Child Fetal Neonatal Ed.* 2021;106:398-403.
81. Cheifetz IM, Craig DM, Quick G, et al. Increasing tidal volumes and pulmonary overdistention adversely affect pulmonary vascular mechanics and cardiac output in a pediatric swine model. *Crit Care Med.* 1998;26:710-716.
82. Polglase GR, Morley CJ, Crossley KJ, et al. Positive end-expiratory pressure differentially alters pulmonary hemodynamics and oxygenation in ventilated, very premature lambs. *J Appl Physiol (1985).* 2005;99:1453-1461.
83. Hausdorf G, Hellwege HH. Influence of positive end-expiratory pressure on cardiac performance in premature infants: a Doppler-echocardiographic study. *Crit Care Med.* 1987;15:661-664.
84. de Waal KA, Evans N, Osborn DA, Kluckow M. Cardiorespiratory effects of changes in end expiratory pressure in ventilated newborns. *Arch Dis Child Fetal Neonatal Ed.* 2007;92:F444-F448.

85. Abdel-Hady H, Matter M, Hammad A, El-Refaay A, Aly H. Hemodynamic changes during weaning from nasal continuous positive airway pressure. *Pediatrics.* 2008;122:e1086-e1090.

86. Beker F, Rogerson SR, Hooper SB, Wong C, Davis PG. The effects of nasal continuous positive airway pressure on cardiac function in premature infants with minimal lung disease: a crossover randomized trial. *J Pediatr.* 2014;164:726-729.

87. Ikeda T, Amizuka T, Ito Y, et al. Changes in the perfusion waveform of the internal cerebral vein and intraventricular hemorrhage in the acute management of extremely low-birth-weight infants. *Eur J Pediatr.* 2015;174:331-338.

88. Ikeda T, Ito Y, Mikami R, Matsuo K, Kawamura N, Yamoto A. Hemodynamics of infants with strong fluctuations of internal cerebral vein. *Pediatr Int.* 2019;61:475-481.

89. Perlman JM, McMenamin JB, Volpe JJ. Fluctuating cerebral blood-flow velocity in respiratory-distress syndrome. Relation to the development of intraventricular hemorrhage. *N Engl J Med.* 1983;309:204-209.

90. Cowan F, Thoresen M. The effects of intermittent positive pressure ventilation on cerebral arterial and venous blood velocities in the newborn infant. *Acta Paediatr Scand.* 1987;76:239-247.

91. Skinner JR, Milligan DW, Hunter S, Hey EN. Central venous pressure in the ventilated neonate. *Arch Dis Child.* 1992;67: 374-377.

92. Kaiser JR, Gauss CH, Williams DK. Surfactant administration acutely affects cerebral and systemic hemodynamics and gas exchange in very-low-birth-weight infants. *J Pediatr.* 2004;144: 809-814.

93. Saliba E, Nashashibi M, Vaillant MC, Nasr C, Laugier J. Instillation rate effects of Exosurf on cerebral and cardiovascular haemodynamics in preterm neonates. *Arch Dis Child Fetal Neonatal Ed.* 1994;71:F174-F178.

94. Roll C, Knief J, Horsch S, Hanssler L. Effect of surfactant administration on cerebral haemodynamics and oxygenation in premature infants – a near infrared spectroscopy study. *Neuropediatrics.* 2000;31:16-23.

95. Wiswell TE, Graziani LJ, Kornhauser MS, et al. Effects of hypocarbia on the development of cystic periventricular leukomalacia in premature infants treated with high-frequency jet ventilation. *Pediatrics.* 1996;98:918-924.

96. Shankaran S, Langer JC, Kazzi SN, et al. Cumulative index of exposure to hypocarbia and hyperoxia as risk factors for periventricular leukomalacia in low birth weight infants. *Pediatrics.* 2006;118:1654-1659.

97. Ambalavanan N, Carlo WA, Wrage LA, et al. PaCO$_2$ in surfactant, positive pressure, and oxygenation randomised trial (SUPPORT). *Arch Dis Child Fetal Neonatal Ed.* 2015;100:F145-F149.

98. Levene MI, Shortland D, Gibson N, Evans DH. Carbon dioxide reactivity of the cerebral circulation in extremely premature infants: effects of postnatal age and indomethacin. *Pediatr Res.* 1988;24:175-179.

99. Noori S, Anderson M, Soleymani S, Seri I. Effect of carbon dioxide on cerebral blood flow velocity in preterm infants during postnatal transition. *Acta Paediatr Oslo Nor.* 2014; 103:e334-e339.

100. Pryds O, Greisen G, Lou H, Friis-Hansen B. Heterogeneity of cerebral vasoreactivity in preterm infants supported by mechanical ventilation. *J Pediatr.* 1989;115:638-645.

101. Tyszczuk L, Meek J, Elwell C, Wyatt JS. Cerebral blood flow is independent of mean arterial blood pressure in preterm infants undergoing intensive care. *Pediatrics.* 1998;102:337-341.

102. Kaiser JR, Gauss CH, Pont MM, Williams DK. Hypercapnia during the first 3 days of life is associated with severe intraventricular hemorrhage in very low birth weight infants. *J Perinatol.* 2006;26:279-285.

103. Fabres J, Carlo WA, Phillips V, Howard G, Ambalavanan N. Both extremes of arterial carbon dioxide pressure and the magnitude of fluctuations in arterial carbon dioxide pressure are associated with severe intraventricular hemorrhage in preterm infants. *Pediatrics.* 2007;119:299-305.

104. McKee LA, Fabres J, Howard G, Peralta-Carcelen M, Carlo WA, Ambalavanan N. PaCO$_2$ and neurodevelopment in extremely low birth weight infants. *J Pediatr.* 2009;155:217-221.e1.

105. Kaiser JR, Gauss CH, Williams DK. The effects of hypercapnia on cerebral autoregulation in ventilated very low birth weight infants. *Pediatr Res.* 2005;58:931-935.

106. Carlo WA, Stark AR, Wright LL, et al. Minimal ventilation to prevent bronchopulmonary dysplasia in extremely-low-birth-weight infants. *J Pediatr.* 2002;141:370-374.

107. Thome UH, Carroll W, Wu TJ, et al. Outcome of extremely preterm infants randomized at birth to different PaCO$_2$ targets during the first seven days of life. *Biol Neonate.* 2006;90:218-225.

108. Thome UH, Genzel-Boroviczeny O, Bohnhorst B, et al. Permissive hypercapnia in extremely low birthweight infants (PHELBI): a randomised controlled multicentre trial. *Lancet Respir Med.* 2015;3:534-543.

109. Thome UH, Genzel-Boroviczeny O, Bohnhorst B, et al. Neurodevelopmental outcomes of extremely low birthweight infants randomised to different PCO$_2$ targets: the PHELBI follow-up study. *Arch Dis Child Fetal Neonatal Ed.* 2017;102(5): F376-F382. doi:10.1136/archdischild-2016-311581.

# Chapter 8

# The Immature Autonomic Nervous System, Hemodynamic Regulation, and Brain Injury in the Early Developing Brain

Sarah D. Schlatterer, Sarah B. Mulkey, and Adre J. du Plessis

## Key Points

- The autonomic nervous system (ANS) plays a key role in maintaining homeostasis in the critically ill preterm or term infant.
- Prematurity, an adverse intrauterine environment, and intrinsic fetal factors, such as congenital heart disease (CHD), may impact the development and function of the ANS.
- Autonomic dysfunction may have long-term health (e.g., adult hypertension) and psycho-affective consequences and can be associated with brain injury.
- Knowledge about cerebral hemodynamics in critically ill infants is limited by the lack of bedside continuous monitoring techniques.
- Further understanding of ANS development and cerebral autoregulation and factors that support or impede that maturation is critical.
- Development of novel neuromonitoring techniques is required to better understand the relationship between ANS function, cerebral autoregulation, and brain injury in the fragile newborn.
- Simple techniques such as skin-to-skin contact or pacifier use may support ANS development in the at-risk newborn.

## Introduction

Regulation of brain perfusion and oxygen/substrate delivery is, broadly speaking, dependent upon two partially overlapping systems. These are cardiovascular-respiratory regulation by the brainstem, autonomic nervous system (ANS) centers, and intrinsic cerebral autoregulatory systems. The period of transition from the relatively protected intrauterine environment to the complexities of the external world requires the coordination of the newborn's cardiovascular and respiratory systems.

The ANS plays a central role in maintaining homeostasis for the infant under fluctuating external conditions. ANS maturation begins in the fetal period and continues after birth. Therefore intrauterine conditions that do not provide a supportive environment for ANS development, including certain maternal medical conditions or illnesses, placental insufficiency, and intrinsic fetal conditions (e.g., congenital heart disease [CHD]), and preterm birth, may significantly affect ANS development and function. ANS immaturity or abnormal maturation may leave vulnerable infants unprepared for ex utero respiratory and hemodynamic demands, exposing the infant to the risks of respiratory, cardiovascular, and hemodynamic instability. Importantly, immature ANS regulation and impaired hemodynamics may not only lead to brain injury but also result in a spectrum of more subtle neurodevelopmental changes whose effects may not become evident until later in childhood.

Significant advances in obstetrical, neonatal, and cardiovascular intensive care, ventilation strategies, and management of neonatal hemodynamics have led to a decline in the earlier, often devastating, forms of brain injury seen in the preterm newborn, for example, cystic periventricular leukomalacia (PVL) and periventricular hemorrhagic infarction (grade IV intraventricular hemorrhage, [P/IVH]) and improved survival for other at-risk newborns, including those with CHD. Although survival of at-risk newborns has greatly improved and, in certain groups, there is a reduced prevalence of severe neuromotor disability and epilepsy among survivors, neuropsychologic disorders continue to manifest in ex-preterm children, former fetal growth-restricted children, and survivors of CHD. Thus neurologic morbidity remains prevalent in survivors of premature birth, high-risk near-term and term births, and cases of complicated fetal-neonatal transition. In this chapter we explore the immature ANS and its relation to brain injury and seek to understand the influence of the developing ANS on brainstem responses and higher cortical functions and outcome.

## Why Focus on the Developing ANS?

There is a complex, potentially bidirectional relationship between immaturity and dysfunction at the brainstem level ANS centers and injury/developmental dysfunction in higher cerebral structures. The link between ANS maturation and brain injury has been most widely studied in the preterm population. Preterm infants with poor neurologic outcomes often have abnormal ANS maturation.[1] ANS dysfunction and brain injury are also prevalent in other at-risk neonatal populations. For example, in infants with CHD, certain forms of which are known to cause delayed brain development, lower ANS function is associated with higher preoperative brain injury scores.[2] In term neonates with neonatal encephalopathy from hypoxia-ischemia (hypoxic ischemic encephalopathy [HIE]) specific patterns of cortical injury were associated with ANS dysfunction.[3] Similarly, neonatal stroke severity is inversely correlated with sympathetic tone.[1,2,4] The causal pathway is not always clear in these cases, and further studies are needed to clarify these relationships. Whether ANS dysfunction causes brain injury or whether brain injury leads to ANS dysfunction remains debatable, and the interaction is likely reciprocal.

The ANS regulates functions of the respiratory, cerebrovascular, and cardiovascular systems, and any abnormal function in these inter-related systems puts the immature brain at risk for injury or maldevelopment. Immature ANS responses likely contribute to hemodynamic and cardiovascular instability in at-risk infants, with impact on the cerebrovascular system.[5,6]

The prevailing paradigm for hemodynamically mediated brain injury in the premature infant is centered on a confluence of insults emanating from the unstable immature cardiovascular system and dysfunctional intrinsic cerebral autoregulation in the context of fragile cerebral vasculature. The brain's cellular elements are also vulnerable to hypoxemia and inflammation, in particular, the immature oligodendrocytes, enhancing risk for brain injury from periods of hemodynamic instability.

## ANS Development and Metrics

The ANS consists of the sympathetic and parasympathetic divisions and has integral control functions on many physiologic aspects of the human body. In addition, the ANS might also provide key inputs to the development of higher cortical and limbic structures involved in emotion, behavior, and thought processing. This important component of our nervous system matures during fetal development and into infancy.[7,8] Key ANS centers within the brainstem, namely the nucleus tractus solitarius, receive sensory input from peripheral receptors and respond through ANS efferent systems, including the dorsal motor nucleus of the vagus. In addition, supratentorial ANS centers including the anterior thalamus, anterior cingulate gyrus, and the amygdala integrate the more primitive functions of the ANS with higher cortical processes, a major evolutionary advantage for humans. The influence of the impaired developmental ANS on these higher-order cortical structures may contribute to the high rate of psycho-affective disorders in survivors of an abnormal third-trimester environment in utero or ex utero.[9]

The central ANS develops in a "bottom-up" manner, beginning with brainstem and hypothalamic centers early in gestation. Cerebral ANS structures develop later in gestation and during early infancy. Functional maturation of the ANS begins with the sympathetic system, which develops structurally and functionally early in gestation and continues to develop progressively throughout the fetal period. While the unmyelinated vagal (parasympathetic) system is earliest to develop, it remains functionally quiescent until the third trimester when its function becomes integrated with higher cortical centers.[10] The remainder of the parasympathetic system begins to develop after the sympathetic system and does not begin to exert functional influence until the third trimester, when parasympathetic tone increases significantly.[5,10-13]

Development in an unsupportive intrauterine or extrauterine environment (as may occur in preterm infants) can have significant effects on ANS function, resulting in alterations in hemodynamic control and risk for brain injury. Early delivery, even late preterm or early term, may be associated with ANS dysfunction.[14] The premature engagement of the ANS in responding to postnatal cardiorespiratory changes may result in "*dysmaturation*", or a shift in the temporal program of ANS maturation, and aberrant programming of the ANS.[15] Prematurity and ANS development ex utero has been associated with impaired ANS function in several studies,[16-19] and preterm infants with higher levels of prematurity-related complications appear to have more impaired autonomic function than preterm infants with low levels of complications.[17-21] This association holds true for neurologic outcomes as well, as preterm infants with adverse neurologic outcomes have lower autonomic tone (measured by heart rate variability [HRV]) compared to age-matched infants with favorable neurologic outcomes.[1]

Measurement of ANS function is challenging in the fetus and fragile newborn. HRV, the fluctuation in the length of time between heart beats (R-R intervals), can be analyzed noninvasively to assess sympathetic and parasympathetic tone, providing a window on the developing ANS.[7,22] High-frequency variability reflects parasympathetic function and is influenced by the respiratory rate (respiratory sinus arrhythmia), while low-frequency variability results from a combination of sympathetic and parasympathetic inputs and reflects baroreflex-induced changes in HR.[23] HRV is also influenced by the newborns' sleep state, with active sleep having higher sympathetic tone (low-frequency variability) compared to quiet sleep.[7]

For premature or critically ill term newborns, there are a multitude of "unexpected" stimuli in the ex utero environment, which the immature ANS may be unprepared to experience and process. The neonatal intensive care unit (NICU) or cardiovascular intensive care unit (CICU) environments are harsher than the muted intrauterine milieu for the developing neurosensory systems. Depending on the gestational age (GA) and

morbidity of the infant, the extraordinary experiences may include oxygenation disturbances and positive pressure ventilation forces on the lungs, hemodynamic instability increased by a patent ductus arteriosus, infections, painful procedures, light, and air and temperature changes on the delicate skin, among others. These stimuli can create a challenging environment for maturation of the ANS, resulting in delayed or abnormal maturation. ANS dysmaturation may then increase the risk for certain adverse events, including IVH,[24] sudden infant death syndrome, and brief resolved unexplained events (BRUEs, formerly "apparent life-threatening events" [ALTEs]),[25-27] among others.

In addition to prematurity, development in an unsupportive intrauterine environment, whether secondary to placental insufficiency or intrinsic fetal factors, may have consequences for ANS function. Growth-restricted fetuses (FGR) exhibit delayed/immature ANS function,[28-30] as evidenced by depressed HRV[28] and suppressed baroreflex and chemoreflex responses.[19] Similarly, fetuses with specific types of critical CHD, including hypoplastic left heart syndrome (HLHS) and transposition of the great arteries (TGA), also have abnormal ANS function.[11,31] Mechanisms underlying aberrant ANS development under the aforementioned conditions are not well understood. However, both FGR and critical CHD fetuses exhibit delayed brain growth and development.[32-34] Poor growth and development of the fetus overall and of the central nervous system, specifically, likely contribute.

## Cerebral Hemodynamic Control in the Developing Brain

The hemodynamic physiology of the developing brain increases its vulnerability to injury. Unlike the mature brain, where cerebral blood flow (CBF) exceeds the ischemic injury threshold by fivefold,[35] the developing brain has significantly lower global and regional CBF,[36] (see Chapter 2). These changes are most evident in the white matter, where there is a much lower ischemic injury threshold.[37,38] This suggests a reduced margin of safety for cerebral perfusion but has to be considered in the context of reduced oxygen metabolism in the developing brain. Monitoring of cerebral tissue oxygenation during transition of the premature newborn during the first few hours after birth is an emerging and important approach to help protect the immature brain (Chapter 15).[39]

Under normal conditions, cerebral perfusion is maintained by a background perfusion pressure provided by the cardiovascular system, which is then "fine-tuned" within the cerebral vasculature by complex intrinsic autoregulatory mechanisms (Chapter 2). However, during sustained physiologic instability and after brain insults, these responses eventually fail, leading to brain injury.[9,40] Cerebral pressure autoregulation maintains a relatively constant CBF across a range of cerebral perfusion pressures called the autoregulatory plateau.[41] In addition to these upper and lower pressure bounds, cerebral pressure autoregulation also has a limited impulse-response time, of the order of 5–15 seconds.[42] Outside these pressure and temporal bounds, CBF is pressure passive, with an increased risk of cerebrovascular injury.

Cerebral pressure-flow autoregulation emerges during fetal life but is underdeveloped in the immature brain. With decreasing GA, the autoregulatory plateau is narrower and lower,[43-45] and normal resting blood pressure (BP) is closer to the lower threshold of autoregulation.[45] Although cerebral pressure-flow autoregulation is well characterized in children and adults, this is not the case for the newborn,[45] least of all the sick premature infant.[46-53] Some studies in stable preterm infants have suggested a lower autoregulatory limit of around 25–30 mmHg[48,54,55]; however, in the sick premature infant the existence and limits of cerebral pressure autoregulation remain controversial.[46,47,52,56-60]

## Autonomic Function and Hemodynamics in Labor

The integrity of the fetal ANS is tested during the events of parturition. The sympathetic and parasympathetic nervous systems work to support and maintain the fetal HR and BP during periods of increased stress and uterine contractions, and then transition of the fetus at birth to extrauterine life. However, fetal-neonatal transition, especially for a fetus that has endured a suboptimal intrauterine environment for development of the ANS, or when preterm, presents a complicated and critical time for hemodynamic regulation. During most labors, fetal HR is monitored via

Doppler ultrasound (US) cardiotocography (CTG), which is typically combined with a monitor for maternal HR and a tocogram to detect uterine contractions. CTG-measured fetal HR produces an average of fetal heartbeats and so does not provide the data of high enough temporal resolution necessary for quantitative fetal HRV analysis but can display changing HRV via the fluctuation in the fetal HR. Fetal ECG devices can provide a true measure of the R-R interval and allow for quantitative fetal HRV analysis, although they are not often used clinically at this time.[61]

The fetal HR is influenced by the current state of the ANS, both its maturational level and the intrinsic intrauterine environment. In a study of fetal lambs developing in a hypoxic environment over 12 days, ANS maturation was slower than that of normoxic fetuses over the same gestational interval.[62] Thus chronic hypoxia may impair maturation of the fetal ANS and impact its function at the time of parturition. Fetal stress from acute hypoxia can manifest as a reduction in HRV and as a change in the baseline fetal HR. Fetuses may have a bradycardic or tachycardic response to hypoxia, depending upon the fetus's compensatory mechanisms available and on the duration and level of the hypoxia-stress exposure.[63] The Fetal Stress Index is measured by fetal HRV analysis and reflects parasympathetic tone, which correlates with arterial pH in a fetal lamb model.[64,65] During parturition in low-risk human labors, there is a reduction in the parasympathetic tone, seen as lower fetal HRV.[66] In this same study sympathetic tone in the fetal HR was higher during parturition than prior to the onset of labor, although the actual baseline fetal HR was not different between the pre-labor and labor periods.[66] Fetal HRV is therefore dynamic and responds to chronic and acute hypoxia states and during parturition.

Much has been learned regarding the effects of acute fetal hypoxemia in near-term or term labors from fetal lamb models. Fetal bradycardia can develop from the parasympathetic nervous system response to developing hypoxemia.[63] The degree of fetal HR lowering relates to the severity and duration of the hypoxemic exposure in an effort for the fetus to lower myocardial metabolic demand and to increase stroke volume.[63] Meanwhile, the fetus maintains BP by peripheral vasoconstriction, which is mediated by sympathetic activation. In a fetal lamb model exposed to repeated fetal umbilical cord occlusions causing fetal hypoxemia for 1 minute, every 5 minutes, the fetal lamb is able to maintain baseline fetal HR and BP between occlusions for an extended period of time.[67,68] This experiment simulates the repetitive uterine contractions in a human labor and shows the importance of the ANS in supporting the fetal cardiovascular response. In the same experiment a shorter duration between umbilical cord occlusions (1-minute exposure every 2.5 minutes) resulted in the fetal lamb responding to the more significant fetal hypoxemia with an initial tachycardia, followed by bradycardia and falling of mean arterial pressure.[67,68] The fetal lamb showed reduced cardiovascular compensation when exposed to more frequent hypoxemic events, with the ANS not able to adequately maintain the fetus in a normal range of HR and BP as time progressed. Another effect of shorter interval hypoxemia exposure is fetal tachycardia following the decelerations. This may be due to beta-adrenergic myocardial stimulation from adrenal activation to increase HR following the period of umbilical cord occlusion.[69] Thus the fetal ANS helps to support the complicated process of parturition and, under most circumstances, to enable birth of an infant with normal cardiovascular function in the first minutes of postnatal life.

## Prematurity, Brain Injury, and Systemic Hemodynamic Disturbances

Prematurity-related brain injury remains a major public health concern.[70,71] Survivors of prematurity are at risk for long-term motor, cognitive, and psycho-affective disorders (Figure 8.1).[72-74] Both the incidence and severity of brain injury in premature infants are inversely related to GA.[74] Because advances in survival have been greatest among the sickest, smallest, most immature infants, that is, those at greatest risk for cerebral circulatory instability and brain injury,[75] it is perhaps not surprising that survivors of extreme prematurity have the highest risk for the development of cerebral palsy.[76] Of major concern are the 25 to 50% of ex-preterm children who demonstrate potentially debilitating behavioral or learning problems by school age,[72,73,77,78] with moderate to severe impairment in academic achievement,[79] and increased risk of autism spectrum disorder.[74,80]

The principal forms of prematurity-related brain injury are germinal matrix–intraventricular hemorrhage (GM-IVH) and injury to the parenchyma, particularly to the immature white matter. The germinal matrices in the periventricular regions of the developing brain are supported by a profuse but transient vascular system of fragile thin-walled vessels with a deficient basal lamina, no muscularis layer,[81,82] and a predisposition to hypoxia-ischemia/reperfusion injury, increasing their vulnerability to rupture.[83] These germinal matrices are also vulnerable to rupture during fluctuations in perfusion pressure, the so-called "water-hammer" effect.[84] The most serious complications of GM-IVH are periventricular hemorrhagic infarction, with an adverse long-term outcome rate exceeding 85%,[85,86] and post-hemorrhagic hydrocephalus,[87] which has an adverse long-term outcome in up to 75% of patients.[88,89] Fortunately, the incidence of this type of white matter injury has also declined.[75]

Under-vascularized end-zones in the premature cerebral white matter are susceptible to hypoxic-ischemic injury during periods of decreased perfusion pressure due to incomplete arterial in-growth during prematurity.[90-96] White matter injury increases the risk of long-term neurologic impairment.[97] The severe form of white matter injury, termed cystic PVL, that can be easily appreciated on US, now has a very low prevalence, but magnetic resonance imaging (MRI) studies[98] describe a high prevalence of diffuse non-cystic white matter injury[99,100] to which cranial US is insensitive.[101] This diffuse form of white matter injury is detected by MRI in more than 50% of very premature infants.[98,100]

Cerebrovascular insults leading to both hemorrhagic and hypoxic-ischemic injury have long been considered a leading cause of acute and long-term neurologic morbidity in premature infants.[102-106] Systemic hemodynamic impairment is commonly diagnosed and treated in the premature infant and is related inversely to GA at birth. This maturational association between disturbed systemic hemodynamics and cerebrovascular injury has led to the notion that the relationship is causative. However, despite plausible extrapolations from human adult and supporting animal studies,[107-110] establishing a causal link between unstable hemodynamics and brain injury in the premature infant has many challenges.

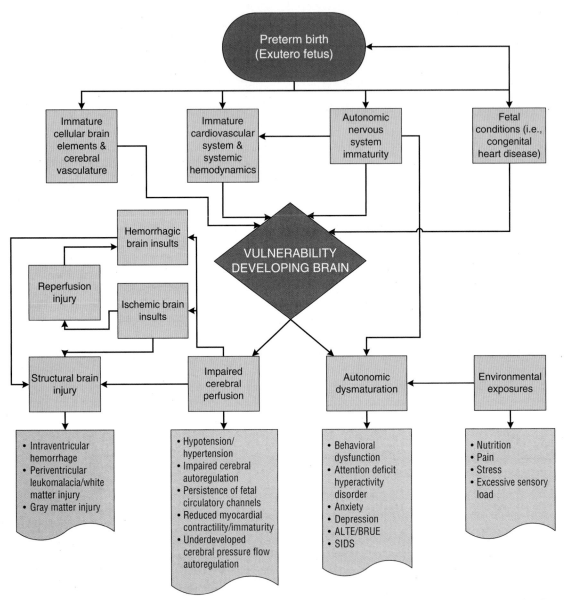

**Fig. 8.1 Developing brain vulnerability.** There is a complex interplay of multiple factors that affect the developing brain. The immature cardiovascular, hemodynamic, and autonomic nervous systems, as well as fetal and maternal conditions and environmental exposures, contribute to vulnerability of the developing brain. Structural brain injury and autonomic dysmaturation may occur, which can impact long-term neurologic, cognitive, and behavioral outcomes. Apparent life-threatening events (ALTEs); brief resolved unexplained events (BRUEs); sudden infant death syndrome (SIDS).

A variety of BP-associated disturbances have been implicated in prematurity-related brain injury, including arterial hypotension,[111-118] hypertension,[119,120] cerebral venous hypertension,[121-123] and/or fluctuating BP.[84,124,125] Different mechanisms have been proposed for the role of "hypotension" in GM-IVH. With intact pressure autoregulation, hypotension triggers cerebral vasodilation, with the increased cerebral blood volume potentially leading to the rupture of fragile vessels. With disrupted cerebral pressure autoregulation, or with BPs below the autoregulatory plateau, there is greater variability in CBF. During hypotension, hypoxic-ischemic injury to the vessel walls may further disrupt cerebral pressure autoregulation,[126-133] and vessels may rupture during reperfusion. In addition to GM-IVH, systemic hypotension has also been implicated in the development of white matter injury in premature infants.[111,112,134-136] However, other studies have shown no such relationship.[116,120,137,138] The diastolic closing margin, the difference between the diastolic arterial BP and the critical closing pressure (the arterial BP at which CBF stops), is higher in premature infants that develop GM-IVH.[139,140] However, critical closing pressure increases during the second and third trimesters, which may be why some premature newborns tolerate hypotension without resulting brain injury.[141] Sustained hypertension is not commonly diagnosed in premature infants, although it may also result in the development of GM-IVH.[119,120] Fluctuating BP in premature infants, particularly during positive pressure ventilation, has been associated with GM-IVH in a number of reports.[51,112,114,119,124,125,142-144] However, the role of fluctuating cerebral perfusion in prematurity-related brain injury remains controversial, since several studies found no such association.[47,125] The role of systemic BP disturbances and impaired cerebral pressure-flow autoregulation in prematurity-related brain injury is unclear, and further studies are needed to more appropriately address this important question.

Doppler US and functional echocardiography studies have identified periods of low cardiac output and low "cerebral" perfusion in premature infants during the early hours after birth. These low-flow states are not reliably detected by systemic BP measurements[145-149] and do not always respond to vasopressor-inotropes.[148] These low cardiac output states are associated with low superior vena cava (SVC) flow, suggesting decreased cerebral perfusion.[145,149-153] Periods of low SVC flow are associated with disturbed cerebral oxygenation by near-infrared spectroscopy (NIRS).[154,155] Both the nadir and duration of low SVC flow are associated with severe GM-IVH,[151,155,156] and later adverse neurologic outcome.[145,149] The association between systemic BP disturbances, as currently measured and interpreted, and prematurity-related brain injury remains controversial (Chapter 7).

## Congenital Heart Disease, Autonomic Function, and Cerebral Hemodynamics

Neonates with critical CHD are vulnerable to brain injury and are known to be at high risk for neurologic disability.[157-161] There are multiple and cumulative influences beginning in the fetal period and extending through the postoperative phase that may contribute to these outcomes.[162-165] Structural brain development and cerebral metabolism are impaired in critical CHD.[159,160,166] White matter injury, including PVL, is commonly found both pre- and postoperatively.[167,168] Preoperative brain injury in CHD appears to be strongly related to microstructural and metabolic brain development[166] and may be related to differences in cerebral circulation.[169] Fetuses and neonates may have impaired brain perfusion and oxygenation that likely contribute to delayed cerebral maturation and brain injury in this population.[170,171]

In the early transitional/neonatal period autonomic tone is depressed in infants with HLHS or TGA (both critical forms of CHD) when compared with healthy controls, supporting the notion that ANS development is delayed in the CHD population.[11] Mechanisms underlying aberrant ANS function in neonatal CHD remain poorly understood. Delayed brain growth and development is known to occur in infants with critical CHD[34,172,173] and may contribute to delayed development of the ANS. However, this remains to be proven.

There appears to be a link between autonomic dysfunction and preoperative brain injury in neonates with CHD. HRV metrics correlate with preoperative brain injury scores in neonates with CHD, suggesting interplay between autonomic function and brain injury in this population.[2] Depressed HRV precedes cardiac arrest in CHD infants,[174] again supporting the role of the ANS in maintaining hemodynamic stability.

Alterations in autonomic development in CHD may begin in the fetal period. Third-trimester fetal HRV is lower in fetuses with HLHS than in controls.[31] A trend toward lower autonomic tone in fetuses with tetralogy of Fallot (ToF) and TGA has also been shown.[31] Interestingly, fetal HRV correlates with 18-month developmental outcomes in survivors of CHD, supporting the association between ANS and neurocognitive function in this population.[175]

Several studies have found abnormal patterns of cerebral blood flow, including lower cerebrovascular resistance, in fetuses with CHD.[176-178] This suggests that cerebral autoregulation in these fetuses is actively redirecting blood flow toward the brain. The timing of alterations in cerebral blood flow appears to correlate with the associated neurocognitive outcomes. Abnormal cerebro-placental ratios (CPR < 1) early in pregnancy (≤26 weeks' GA), suggesting early cerebral hypoxia, correlate with lower 18-month cognitive development scores in CHD fetuses with HLHS, TGA, and ToF.[179] However, lower cerebrovascular resistance later in pregnancy seems to correlate with better neurocognitive outcomes, indicating a need for more investigation into the role of cerebrovascular resistance in neurodevelopment in this population.[180]

Studies using frequency-domain near-infrared spectroscopy (FDNIRS) and diffuse correlation spectroscopy (DCS)[181] and arterial spin-labeling techniques[182] have shown that neonates with single-ventricle CHD have impaired CBF compared to controls. Votava-Smith et al. found fluctuating pressure-passive cerebral perfusion in full-term neonates with CHD,[183] similar to what has been described in premature infants without CHD[47] and in preterm infants with hemodynamically significant PDA.[184] While several studies have shown decreased CBF in CHD, others have associated an increased CBF, in addition to other factors, including longer time to surgery and delayed sternal closure, with white matter injury in neonates with HLHS.[185] Interestingly, fluctuating cerebral pressure-passivity can occur in the term preoperative infant with CHD despite systemic normotension.[183] Cerebral pressure autoregulation also may be disturbed in the early postoperative period, particularly in the context of fluctuating systemic BP and higher $CO_2$ tension.[186]

## Resolving the Relationship Between Systemic Hemodynamics and Brain Injury: Obstacles to Progress

Several fundamental and inter-related challenges continue to impede our understanding of the relationship between changes in systemic hemodynamics, the immature response of the ANS, and brain injury in the developing brain. Advancing the field will require greater insight into the interaction between the immature systemic and cerebral hemodynamic systems, the ANS, and how this mediates injury in the immature brain.

## Measurement of Relevant Hemodynamic and Metabolic Indices

Currently, there are no established techniques for making continuous, *quantitative* measurements of systemic or CBF in the fragile newborn infant (Chapter 14). Arterial BP, the only continuous systemic hemodynamic signal available in the critically ill infant, has several limitations. First, there are no widely accepted noninvasive techniques for acquiring continuous BP in the critically ill infant.[26,187-189] Second, the relationship between BP and systemic blood flow is not constant, particularly during periods of critical physiological instability. Arterial BP is often used as a surrogate for cerebral perfusion pressure because the effect of venous pressure is disregarded in many clinical situations. However, in critically ill infants requiring positive pressure ventilatory support, the effect of increased intra-thoracic pressure may have a significant impact on cerebral perfusion, and ventilator-related cerebral venous volume fluctuations have been shown to predispose to cerebral pressure passivity in a cohort that included preterm infants, infants with CHD, and term infants with HIE.[190] At present, noninvasive techniques for monitoring cerebral perfusion pressure are not readily available for clinical use.

There are currently no well-accepted techniques for the measurement of continuous volumetric CBF. Transcranial Doppler US measures CBF velocity,[42,58,124,191-194] but not volumetric CBF. In the absence of reliable techniques for *continuous* CBF measurement, a number of intermittent ("static") approaches have been used to measure quantitative CBF.[57,145,149-151,195-199] These techniques are largely based on the Fick principle, using tracers ranging from $Xe^{133}$ to oxyhemoglobin measured by NIRS. Another approach has been the use of intermittent measurement of SVC flow by Doppler US as a surrogate for CBF. These studies have demonstrated the association between abnormally low SVC flow and neurologic morbidity.[145,149,150,152,153] However, these measurements of SVC flow are not continuous and, in the very preterm infant, less than 50% of the blood in the SVC represents the blood coming from the brain (Chapter 2).[200] Thus all of the so-called "static" measurements of CBF suffer from the inability to capture the dynamic nature of cerebral hemodynamics during the period of major physiologic change associated with transition to premature postnatal life.

The ability to measure the relationship between cerebral oxygen demand and supply would provide major insights into the mechanisms of brain injury in premature infants. This is important because it is clear that not only cerebral oxygen deficiency but also excessive cerebral oxygenation may be harmful to the immature brain.[201,202] Even in stable infants, the premature brain might be "hyper-oxygenated" at room air compared with the mature brain.[203] NIRS devices in current clinical use measure continuous cerebral tissue hemoglobin saturation as a surrogate measure of the adequacy of cerebral oxygen delivery (Chapter 15). The rationale behind this approach is that normal autoregulatory mechanisms maintain appropriate cerebral oxygen delivery and cerebral oxygen extraction[9,140]; conversely, increasing cerebral oxygen extraction is interpreted as a decrease in the cerebral oxygen delivery to demand ratio due to either decreasing CBF or increased cerebral activation. However, measures of cerebral tissue hemoglobin oxygenation may be misleading when considered in isolation because this approach assumes that neurovascular coupling is intact and because cerebral oxygen extraction may actually decrease after significant brain insults.

Understanding CBF in the medically fragile infant has been limited by the lack of bedside techniques capable of measuring *regional* blood flow within the brain. Not only is global CBF lower in these infants, but blood flow is also particularly low in the most vulnerable white matter regions.[204,205] Arterial spin labeling (ASL) perfusion MRI at 3 Tesla can measure regional cerebral perfusion noninvasively and without contrast.[169,206] In a study using pseudo-continuous ASL, frontal lobe perfusion increased more rapidly with increasing GA compared to the occipital regions.[204] In another study using ASL, neonates born prematurely had higher perfusion at term GA equivalence compared to term newborns, indicating a potential effect of ex utero development on brain perfusion.[207] The ASL technique does have some technical challenges in the high-risk preterm neonate, and

similar to many other imaging techniques, it is not portable to the bedside. Near-infrared spectroscopy in its various formats provides greater temporal resolution and is discussed in Chapter 15.

## Characterizing "Significant" Systemic Hemodynamic Insults and Establishing a Temporal Relationship Between Hemodynamic Changes and Brain Insults Difficult in Neonates

Understanding the role of systemic hemodynamic factors in brain injury in medically fragile infants has been impeded by a fundamental lack of understanding of the "dose" of hemodynamic insult required to injure the immature brain. Insults capable of causing injury to the developing brain may be distinctly different from those injuring the mature brain. In the extremely premature infant the risk period for hypoxic-ischemic brain insults may extend for weeks or months during the prolonged NICU stay. In the infant with CHD exposure to (often multiple) bypass procedures and a persistently altered cardiovascular physiology results in prolonged, often life-long, risk for brain injury. Presumably, injury thresholds exist for brief but severe, mild but prolonged, and repetitive hemodynamic insults, as well as for the cumulative impact of these insults. It is difficult to design appropriate experimental models or to monitor the human premature brain due to the prolonged period of risk for brain injury and the variety of hemodynamic insults that may occur.

Establishing a temporal association between systemic hemodynamic disturbances and brain insult is challenging in the medically fragile infant because the exact onset of brain injury is often unknown and brain injury may be cumulative.[208] Furthermore, neurodevelopmental deficits may only become evident months to years after the initial injury, sometimes as late as school age,[74,209] or beyond. During this interval, multiple factors, such as socioeconomic status and maternal education that are unrelated to the initial insult, may significantly influence long-term outcomes.[210] In the premature infant brain injury precedes critical normal third-trimester events in brain development.[211] Normal third-trimester developmental events may be derailed by acute injury resulting in acquired brain malformations (developmental disruptions).[212] Conversely, the ameliorating effect of brain plasticity may play a beneficial role in outcome.[213] Other potentially injurious mechanisms may operate before (e.g., fetal inflammation, altered fetal oxygen delivery), during (e.g., blood gas disturbances), and after (e.g., apnea and bradycardia, altered circulation, infection and inflammation[214-216]) the immediate period of postnatal hemodynamic instability and may act in concert with hemodynamic insults.

Establishing a causal link between early hemodynamic insults and brain injury is also challenging; specifically, the identification of *acute structural injury* during periods of critical illness has been limited by the lack of sensitive portable neuroimaging. Infants are usually too ill to be transported to MRI scanners, especially early in their hospitalization. Cranial US, although sensitive to hemorrhage, is insensitive to and delayed in its detection of diffuse white matter injury. This has been confirmed at autopsy[216,217] but also in MRI studies that indicate that most white matter injury is undetected by neonatal cranial US.[98,218] MRI-compatible incubators allow for safer transport of critically ill infants to MRI scanners and may advance detection of hyperacute brain injury.

Because the onset of cerebral pressure autoregulatory failure heralds an elevated risk for cerebrovascular injury at a point prior to irreversible injury, detection of cerebral pressure passivity might provide a sensitive cerebrovascular biomarker to relate to systemic BP changes. However, the presence and characteristics of pressure autoregulation in the sick premature infant remain controversial, in part due to the ongoing lack of established techniques for detecting cerebral pressure passivity. In a neonatal piglet model of hypotension cerebral autoregulation assessed by the linear correlation between arterial BP and $rSO_2$ (measured by NIRS) was as accurate as cerebral autoregulation assessed by the linear correlation between invasively monitored cerebral perfusion pressure.[219] The NIRS hemoglobin difference (HbD) signal, which can be measured continuously, can be time-locked to measurements of systemic BP and applied to the study of cerebral pressure-flow autoregulation in premature infants.[46,186,220] This approach can identify periods of pressure passivity using coherence function analysis to identify significant concordance between systemic BP and cerebral HbD changes.[186] The magnitude of pressure passivity during these periods can then be measured using transfer gain analysis.[47] Using this approach, an association between cerebral pressure-passivity and brain injury has been described,[46] as well as between the magnitude of pressure passivity and GM-IVH,[220] and in the term newborn with HIE.[221] This approach highlighted the prevalence and dynamic nature of cerebral pressure flow autoregulation, with periods of pressure passivity interspersed with apparent autoregulation in most extremely premature infants.[47]

Pressure autoregulation is affected not only by changes in arterial pressure but also by other influences, including reactivity to vasodilators such as carbon dioxide and the regulation of arterial pressure itself.[47,222] Brain injury such as hemorrhage or stroke may affect cerebral autoregulation, as well as conditions that alter intracranial pressure (i.e., hydrocephalus).[222] A continuous, robust cerebral circulation monitor that allows for both regional and global CBF assessment at the bedside is needed in this vulnerable population.[222] Predictable gestational/postnatal age–related BP bounds remain difficult to determine and multiple, simultaneous influences are likely at play in the critically ill neonate.

## Future Directions

Because the ANS plays a key role in maintaining hemodynamic stability during transition and during critical periods for the fetus and vulnerable neonate, strategies to support ANS development and function are critical. To date, the focus has been on providing support in the ex utero environment, and studies have concentrated on the preterm infant who may need weeks to months of neonatal intensive care.

Kangaroo care, the practice of placing the preterm infant skin-to-skin on the chest of its mother, has been studied in this context. Kangaroo care has been shown to support appropriate ANS development and neurobehavioral maturation (as measured by habituation and orientation scores on the Neonatal Behavioral Assessment Scale) in preterm neonates, as evidenced by increased sympathetic tone at 28 weeks' GA[223] and increased parasympathetic tone at 37 weeks' GA.[224] Kangaroo care combined with maternal singing had the added benefit of reducing maternal anxiety.[225] Other simple interventions, such as pacifier use, may improve sympathetic tone in former preterm infants.[226]

The Family Nurture Intervention (FNI), developed by Welch and colleagues, also shows promise in supporting appropriate ANS development in preterm infants. Preterm infants who underwent FNI had more rapid increases in parasympathetic function in HR data collected between ~35 weeks' and ~40 weeks' GA compared with standard-of-care controls, although there was no group difference in HR at term age.[227] In a follow-up study of the same cohort at 5 years, children and mothers who participated in the FNI had higher vagal tone than the standard-of-care control group.[228] Even when an infant is exposed to non-optimal conditions during critical periods of development (i.e., prematurity), non-pharmacologic interventions including skin-to-skin contact, pacifier use, and FNI may promote healthier ANS development.

Maternal stress and mood disorders are some of the most common complications of pregnancy,[229-231] and studies have shown an association between maternal depression, stress, and delayed ANS development during the fetal period,[232-235] although these are not always straightforward. An association between maternal and fetal HR and infant HRV at 1 year of age has been reported by DiPietro and colleagues.[236] Lower parasympathetic tone was found in infants of mothers with depressive symptoms in the third trimester[237] and in infants of mothers with high anxiety in the second trimester.[238] Conversely, other studies found no correlation between maternal negative trait emotionality and infant parasympathetic tone in pregnant adolescents, suggesting that the effect of maternal depression and anxiety during pregnancy on the brainstem ANS may be transient.[239,240] The type and degree of maternal stress or mental distress experienced as well as underlying genetic and epigenetic factors may impact the influence of maternal mental state on fetal and neonatal autonomic function. There is a need for future studies to better understand relationships between maternal mental health and the developing ANS.

## Conclusion

Successful transition of the fetus to the extrauterine environment is mediated by the most complex physiological changes anywhere across the lifespan. For premature and critically ill newborns, transition may be suboptimal due to, among others, immaturity of the systems necessary for the effective regulation of HR, BP, and CBF. Brain injury may result due to impaired regulation of these systems and may translate into a long-term neurologic burden of neurodevelopmental delay, cerebral palsy, and psycho-affective disorders that may persist across the lifespan. In this chapter we have outlined evidence for the key role the ANS plays in hemodynamic stability and neuroprotection and have explored the fundamental challenges in our understanding of systemic and cerebral hemodynamics and the immature ANS, as well as the limitations of current techniques for addressing these complex but critically important questions. The etiology of brain injury in premature and at-risk term newborns is multifactorial and the insult may be chronic and cumulative (Figure 8.1). The ANS is an integral driver in brainstem control of HR and BP, but more importantly, at least for the long-term neurologic health of infants, it is emerging as an important brain system for promoting affect, mood, stress responses, and behavior through its linkages to higher order cortical centers.[62,200] Much remains to be learned, and in order to support ANS development and maturation in at-risk neonates, further understanding of ANS development and factors that support or impede that maturation is critical. Innovative techniques and novel tools for monitoring and measuring autonomic function will be required to better understand the interplay between the ANS and its higher cortical and subcortical systems as they relate to brain injury and long-term neurodevelopmental and neuropsychological dysfunction in vulnerable populations.

## REFERENCES

1. Thiriez G, Mougey C, Vermeylen D, et al. Altered autonomic control in preterm newborns with impaired neurological outcomes. *Clin Auton Res.* 2015;25(4):233-242.
2. Schlatterer SD, Govindan RB, Murnick J, et al. In infants with congenital heart disease autonomic dysfunction is associated with pre-operative brain injury. *Pediatr Res.* 2022;91(7):1723-1729.
3. Schneebaum Sender N, Govindan RB, Sulemanji M, et al. Effects of regional brain injury on the newborn autonomic nervous system. *Early Hum Dev.* 2014;90(12):893-896.
4. Reich DA, Govindan RB, Whitehead MT, et al. The effect of unilateral stroke on autonomic function in the term newborn. *Pediatr Res.* 2019;85(6):830-834.

5. Longin E, Gerstner T, Schaible T, Lenz T, Konig S. Maturation of the autonomic nervous system: differences in heart rate variability in premature vs. term infants. *J Perinat Med.* 2006;34(4): 303-308.

6. Patural H, Barthelemy JC, Pichot V, et al. Birth prematurity determines prolonged autonomic nervous system immaturity. *Clin Auton Res.* 2004;14:391-395.

7. Fyfe KL, Yiallourou SR, Wong FY, Odoi A, Walker AM, Horne RS. The effect of gestational age at birth on post-term maturation of heart rate variability. *Sleep.* 2015;38(10):1635-1644.

8. Karin J, Hirsch M, Akselrod S. An estimate of fetal autonomic state by spectral analysis of fetal heart rate fluctuations. *Pediatr Res.* 1993;34(2):134-138.

9. Porges SW, Furman SA. The early development of the autonomic nervous system provides a neural platform for social behavior: a polyvagal perspective. *Infant Child Dev.* 2011;20(1): 106-118.

10. Porges SW. *The Polyvagal Theory.* New York: WW Norton & Company; 2011.

11. Mulkey SB, Govindan R, Metzler M, et al. Heart rate variability is depressed in the early transitional period for newborns with complex congenital heart disease. *Clin Auton Res.* 2020;30(2): 165-172.

12. Mulkey SB, du Plessis AJ. Autonomic nervous system development and its impact on neuropsychiatric outcome. *Pediatr Res.* 2019;85(2):120-126.

13. Clairambault J, Curzi-Dascalova L, Kauffmann F, Medigue C, Leffler C. Heart rate variability in normal sleeping full-term and preterm neonates. *Early Hum Dev.* 1992;28(2):169-183.

14. Burtchen N, Myers MM, Lucchini M, Ordonez Retamar M, Rodriguez D, Fifer WP. Autonomic signatures of late preterm, early term, and full term neonates during early postnatal life. *Early Hum Dev.* 2019;137:104817.

15. Zouikr I, Bartholomeusz MD, Hodgson DM. Early life programming of pain: focus on neuroimmune to endocrine communication. *J Transl Med.* 2016;14(1):123.

16. Mulkey SB, Plessis AD. The critical role of the central autonomic nervous system in fetal-neonatal transition. *Semin Pediatr Neurol.* 2018;28:29-37.

17. Mulkey SB, Kota S, Swisher CB, et al. Autonomic nervous system depression at term in neurologically normal premature infants. *Early Hum Dev.* 2018;123:11-16.

18. Yiallourou SR, Witcombe NB, Sands SA, Walker AM, Horne RS. The development of autonomic cardiovascular control is altered by preterm birth. *Early Hum Dev.* 2013;89(3):145-152.

19. Patural H, Pichot V, Jaziri F, et al. Autonomic cardiac control of very preterm newborns: a prolonged dysfunction. *Early Hum Dev.* 2008;84(10):681-687.

20. Mulkey SB, Govindan RB, Hitchings L, et al. Autonomic nervous system maturation in the premature extrauterine milieu. *Pediatr Res.* 2021;89(4):863-868.

21. Schlatterer SD, Govindan RB, Barnett SD, et al. Autonomic development in preterm infants is associated with morbidity of prematurity. *Pediatr Res.* 2022;91(1):171-177.

22. Task Force of the European Society of Cardiology and the North American Society of Pacing and Electrophysiology. Heart rate variability. Standards of measurement, physiological interpretation, and clinical use. *Circulation.* 1996;93(5):1043-1065.

23. Malliani A, Lombardi F, Pagani M. Power spectrum analysis of heart rate variability: a tool to explore neural regulatory mechanisms. *Br Heart J.* 1994;71(1):1-2.

24. Tuzcu V, Nas S, Ulusar U, Ugur A, Kaiser JR. Altered heart rhythm dynamics in very low birth weight infants with impending intraventricular hemorrhage. *Pediatrics.* 2009;123(3):810-815.

25. Tieder JS, Bonkowsky JL, Etzel RA, et al. Brief resolved unexplained events (formerly apparent life-threatening events) and evaluation of lower-risk infants: executive summary. *Pediatrics.* 2016;137(5):e20160591.

26. Fyfe KL, Odoi A, Yiallourou SR, Wong FY, Walker AM, Horne RS. Preterm infants exhibit greater variability in cerebrovascular control than term infants. *Sleep.* 2015;38(9):1411-1421.

27. Nino G, Govindan RB, Al-Shargabi T, et al. Premature infants rehospitalized because of an apparent life-threatening event had distinctive autonomic developmental trajectories. *Am J Respir Crit Care Med.* 2016;194(3):379-381.

28. Stampalija T, Casati D, Montico M, et al. Parameters influence on acceleration and deceleration capacity based on trans-abdominal ECG in early fetal growth restriction at different gestational age epochs. *Eur J Obstet Gynecol Reprod Biol.* 2015;188:104-112.

29. Stampalija T, Casati D, Monasta L, et al. Brain sparing effect in growth-restricted fetuses is associated with decreased cardiac acceleration and deceleration capacities: a case-control study. *BJOG.* 2016;123(12):1947-1954.

30. DiPietro JA, Costigan KA, Voegtline KM. Studies in fetal behavior: revisited, renewed, and reimagined. *Monogr Soc Res Child Dev.* 2015;80(3):vii;1-94.

31. Siddiqui S, Wilpers A, Myers M, Nugent JD, Fifer WP, Williams IA. Autonomic regulation in fetuses with congenital heart disease. *Early Hum Dev.* 2015;91(3):195-198.

32. Andescavage N, duPlessis A, Metzler M, et al. In vivo assessment of placental and brain volumes in growth-restricted fetuses with and without fetal Doppler changes using quantitative 3D MRI. *J Perinatol.* 2017;37(12):1278-1284.

33. Miller SL, Huppi PS, Mallard C. The consequences of fetal growth restriction on brain structure and neurodevelopmental outcome. *J Physiol.* 2016;594(4):807-823.

34. Limperopoulos C, Tworetzky W, McElhinney DB, et al. Brain volume and metabolism in fetuses with congenital heart disease: evaluation with quantitative magnetic resonance imaging and spectroscopy. *Circulation.* 2010;121(1):26-33.

35. Powers WJ, Grubb Jr RL, Darriet D, Raichle ME. Cerebral blood flow and cerebral metabolic rate of oxygen requirements for cerebral function and viability in humans. *J Cereb Blood Flow Metab.* 1985;5(4):600-608.

36. Ouyang M, Liu P, Jeon T, et al. Heterogeneous increases of regional cerebral blood flow during preterm brain development: preliminary assessment with pseudo-continuous arterial spin labeled perfusion MRI. *Neuroimage.* 2017;147:233-242.

37. Altman DI, Powers WJ, Perlman JM, Herscovitch P, Volpe SL, Volpe JJ. Cerebral blood flow requirement for brain viability in newborn infants is lower than in adults. *Ann Neurol.* 1988; 24(2):218-226.

38. Borch K, Greisen G. Blood flow distribution in the normal human preterm brain. *Pediatr Res.* 1998;43(1):28-33.

39. Pichler G, Binder C, Avian A, Beckenbach E, Schmolzer GM, Urlesberger B. Reference ranges for regional cerebral tissue oxygen saturation and fractional oxygen extraction in neonates during immediate transition after birth. *J Pediatr.* 2013;163(6): 1558-1563.

40. du Plessis AJ. Cerebrovascular injury in premature infants: current understanding and challenges for future prevention. *Clin Perinatol.* 2008;35(4):609-641.

41. Lassen NA, Christensen MS. Physiology of cerebral blood flow. *Br J Anaesth.* 1976;48(8):719-734.
42. Panerai RB, Kelsall AW, Rennie JM, Evans DH. Cerebral autoregulation dynamics in premature newborns. *Stroke.* 1995;26(1): 74-80.
43. van Os S, Liem D, Hopman J, Klaessens J, van de Bor M. Cerebral O2 supply thresholds for the preservation of electrocortical brain activity during hypotension in near-term-born lambs. *Pediatr Res.* 2005;57(3):358-362.
44. Van Os S, Klaessens J, Hopman J, Liem D, Van De Bor M. Cerebral oxygen supply during hypotension in near-term lambs: a near-infrared spectroscopy study. *Brain Dev.* 2006;28(2): 115-121.
45. Szymonowicz W, Walker AM, Yu VY, Stewart ML, Cannata J, Cussen L. Regional cerebral blood flow after hemorrhagic hypotension in the preterm, near-term, and newborn lamb. *Pediatr Res.* 1990;28(4):361-366.
46. Tsuji M, Saul JP, du Plessis A, et al. Cerebral intravascular oxygenation correlates with mean arterial pressure in critically ill premature infants. *Pediatrics.* 2000;106(4):625-632.
47. Soul JS, Hammer PE, Tsuji M, et al. Fluctuating pressure-passivity is common in the cerebral circulation of sick premature infants. *Pediatr Res.* 2007;61(4):467-473.
48. Pryds O, Andersen GE, Friis-Hansen B. Cerebral blood flow reactivity in spontaneously breathing, preterm infants shortly after birth. *Acta Paediatr Scand.* 1990;79(4):391-396.
49. Pryds O. Control of cerebral circulation in the high-risk neonate. *Ann Neurol.* 1991;30(3):321-329.
50. Milligan DW. Failure of autoregulation and intraventricular haemorrhage in preterm infants. *Lancet.* 1980;1(8174):896-898.
51. Miall-Allen VM, de Vries LS, Dubowitz LM, Whitelaw AG. Blood pressure fluctuation and intraventricular hemorrhage in the preterm infant of less than 31 weeks' gestation. *Pediatrics.* 1989;83(5):657-661.
52. Ramaekers VT, Casaer P, Daniels H, Marchal G. Upper limits of brain blood flow autoregulation in stable infants of various conceptional age. *Early Hum Dev.* 1990;24(3):249-258.
53. Verma PK, Panerai RB, Rennie JM, Evans DH. Grading of cerebral autoregulation in preterm and term neonates. *Pediatr Neurol.* 2000;23(3):236-242.
54. Van Bel F, Van de Bor M, Walther FJ. Cerebral blood flow velocity and cardiac output in infants of insulin-dependent diabetic mothers. *Acta Paediatr Scand.* 1991;80(10):905-910.
55. Munro MJ, Walker AM, Barfield CP. Hypotensive extremely low birth weight infants have reduced cerebral blood flow. *Pediatrics.* 2004;114(6):1591-1596.
56. Lou HC, Skov H, Pedersen H. Low cerebral blood flow: a risk factor in the neonate. *J Pediatr.* 1979;95(4):606-609.
57. Younkin DP, Reivich M, Jaggi J, Obrist W, Delivoria-Papadopoulos M. Noninvasive method of estimating human newborn regional cerebral blood flow. *J Cereb Blood Flow Metab.* 1982; 2(4):415-420.
58. Boylan GB, Young K, Panerai RB, Rennie JM, Evans DH. Dynamic cerebral autoregulation in sick newborn infants. *Pediatr Res.* 2000;48(1):12-17.
59. Anthony MY, Evans DH, Levene MI. Neonatal cerebral blood flow velocity responses to changes in posture. *Arch Dis Child.* 1993;69(3 Spec No):304-308.
60. Lou HC, Lassen NA, Friis-Hansen B. Low cerebral blood flow in the hypotensive distressed newborn. *Acta Neurol Scand Suppl.* 1977;64:428-429.
61. Mannella P, Billeci L, Giannini A, et al. A feasibility study on noninvasive fetal ECG to evaluate prenatal autonomic nervous system activity. *Eur J Obstet Gynecol Reprod Biol.* 2020;246:60-66.
62. Shaw CJ, Allison BJ, Itani N, et al. Altered autonomic control of heart rate variability in the chronically hypoxic fetus. *J Physiol.* 2018;596(23):6105-6119.
63. Bennet L, Gunn AJ. The fetal heart rate response to hypoxia: insights from animal models. *Clin Perinatol.* 2009;36(3):655-672.
64. Garabedian C, Clermont-Hama Y, Sharma D, et al. Correlation of a new index reflecting the fluctuation of parasympathetic tone and fetal acidosis in an experimental study in a sheep model. *PLoS One.* 2018;13(1):e0190463.
65. Jonckheere J, Garabedian C, Charlier P, Storme L, Debarge V, Logier R. Influence of averaged fetal heart rate in heart rate variability analysis. *Annu Int Conf IEEE Eng Med Biol Soc.* 2019; 2019:5979-5982.
66. Montalvo-Jaramillo CI, Pliego-Carrillo AC, Pena-Castillo MA, et al. Comparison of fetal heart rate variability by symbolic dynamics at the third trimester of pregnancy and low-risk parturition. *Heliyon.* 2020;6(3):e03485.
67. de Haan HH, Gunn AJ, Gluckman PD. Fetal heart rate changes do not reflect cardiovascular deterioration during brief repeated umbilical cord occlusions in near-term fetal lambs. *Am J Obstet Gynecol.* 1997;176(1 Pt 1):8-17.
68. Westgate JA, Bennet L, Gunn AJ. Fetal heart rate variability changes during brief repeated umbilical cord occlusion in near term fetal sheep. *Br J Obstet Gynaecol.* 1999;106(7):664-671.
69. Schifrin BS, Hamilton-Rubinstein T, Shields JR. Fetal heart rate patterns and the timing of fetal injury. *J Perinatol.* 1994; 14(3):174-181.
70. Behrman R, Stith Butler A. *Institute of Medicine Committee on Understanding Premature Birth and Assuring Healthy Outcomes Board on Health Sciences Outcomes: Preterm Birth: Causes,* Consequences, and Prevention. Washington DC: The National Academies Press; 2007.
71. Martin JA, Kung HC, Mathews TJ, et al. Annual summary of vital statistics: 2006. *Pediatrics.* 2008;121(4):788-801.
72. Schendel DE, Stockbauer JW, Hoffman HJ, Herman AA, Berg CJ, Schramm WF. Relation between very low birth weight and developmental delay among preschool children without disabilities. *Am J Epidemiol.* 1997;146(9):740-749.
73. Piecuch RE, Leonard CH, Cooper BA, Sehring SA. Outcome of extremely low birth weight infants (500 to 999 grams) over a 12-year period. *Pediatrics.* 1997;100(4):633-639.
74. Bhutta AT, Cleves MA, Casey PH, Cradock MM, Anand KJ. Cognitive and behavioral outcomes of school-aged children who were born preterm: a meta-analysis. *JAMA.* 2002;288(6): 728-737.
75. Stoll BJ, Hansen NI, Bell EF, et al. Trends in care practices, morbidity, and mortality of extremely preterm neonates, 1993-2012. *JAMA.* 2015;314(10):1039-1051.
76. Hagberg B, Hagberg G, Beckung E, Uvebrant P. Changing panorama of cerebral palsy in Sweden. VIII. Prevalence and origin in the birth year period 1991-1994. *Acta Paediatr.* 2001;90(3): 271-277.
77. Leonard CH, Piecuch RE. School age outcome in low birth weight preterm infants. *Semin Perinatol.* 1997;21(3):240-253.
78. O'Shea TM, Klinepeter KL, Goldstein DJ, Jackson BW, Dillard RG. Survival and developmental disability in infants with birth weights of 501 to 800 grams, born between 1979 and 1994. *Pediatrics.* 1997;100(6):982-986.

79. Aarnoudse-Moens CS, Weisglas-Kuperus N, van Goudoever JB, Oosterlaan J. Meta-analysis of neurobehavioral outcomes in very preterm and/or very low birth weight children. *Pediatrics*. 2009;124(2):717-728.

80. Limperopoulos C, Bassan H, Sullivan NR, et al. Positive screening for autism in ex-preterm infants: prevalence and risk factors. *Pediatrics*. 2008;121(4):758-765.

81. Anstrom JA, Brown WR, Moody DM, Thore CR, Challa VR, Block SM. Subependymal veins in premature neonates: implications for hemorrhage. *Pediatr Neurol*. 2004;30(1):46-53.

82. Ghazi-Birry HS, Brown WR, Moody DM, Challa VR, Block SM, Reboussin DM. Human germinal matrix: venous origin of hemorrhage and vascular characteristics. *Am J Neuroradiol*. 1997;18(2):219-229.

83. Grunnet ML. Morphometry of blood vessels in the cortex and germinal plate of premature neonates. *Pediatr Neurol*. 1989;5(1):12-16.

84. Hambleton G, Wigglesworth JS. Origin of intraventricular haemorrhage in the preterm infant. *Arch Dis Child*. 1976;51(9):651-659.

85. Bassan H, Benson CB, Limperopoulos C, et al. Ultrasonographic features and severity scoring of periventricular hemorrhagic infarction in relation to risk factors and outcome. *Pediatrics*. 2006;117(6):2111-2118.

86. Bassan H, Feldman HA, Limperopoulos C, et al. Periventricular hemorrhagic infarction: risk factors and neonatal outcome. *Pediatr Neurol*. 2006;35(2):85-92.

87. Volpe JJ, ed. Intracranial hemorrhage: germinal matrix-intraventricular hemorrhage of the premature infant. In: *Neurology of the Newborn*. 5th ed. Philadelphia, PA: Saunders Elsevier; 2008:517-588.

88. du Plessis AJ. Posthemorrhagic hydrocephalus and brain injury in the preterm infant: dilemmas in diagnosis and management. *Semin Pediatr Neurol*. 1998;5(3):161-179.

89. Ventriculomegaly Trial Group. Randomised trial of early tapping in neonatal posthaemorrhagic ventricular dilatation: results at 30 months. *Arch Dis Child Fetal Neonatal Ed*. 1994;70(2):F129-F136.

90. De Reuck JL. Cerebral angioarchitecture and perinatal brain lesions in premature and full-term infants. *Acta Neurol Scand*. 1984;70(6):391-395.

91. Takashima S, Armstrong DL, Becker LE. Subcortical leukomalacia. Relationship to development of the cerebral sulcus and its vascular supply. *Arch Neurol*. 1978;35(7):470-472.

92. De Reuck J. The human periventricular arterial blood supply and the anatomy of cerebral infarctions. *Eur Neurol*. 1971;5(6):321-334.

93. De Reuck J. The cortico-subcortical arterial angio-architecture in the human brain. *Acta Neurol Belg*. 1972;72(5):323-329.

94. Rorke LB. Anatomical features of the developing brain implicated in pathogenesis of hypoxic-ischemic injury. *Brain Pathol*. 1992;2(3):211-221.

95. Takashima S, Tanaka K. Development of cerebrovascular architecture and its relationship to periventricular leukomalacia. *Arch Neurol*. 1978;35(1):11-16.

96. Nakamura Y, Okudera T, Hashimoto T. Vascular architecture in white matter of neonates: its relationship to periventricular leukomalacia. *J Neuropathol Exp Neurol*. 1994;53(6):582-589.

97. O'Shea TM, Allred EN, Kuban KC, et al. Intraventricular hemorrhage and developmental outcomes at 24 months of age in extremely preterm infants. *J Child Neurol*. 2012;27(1):22-29.

98. Maalouf EF, Duggan PJ, Counsell SJ, et al. Comparison of findings on cranial ultrasound and magnetic resonance imaging in preterm infants. *Pediatrics*. 2001;107(4):719-727.

99. Volpe JJ. Cerebral white matter injury of the premature infant-more common than you think. *Pediatrics*. 2003;112(1 Pt 1):176-180.

100. Dyet LE, Kennea N, Counsell SJ, et al. Natural history of brain lesions in extremely preterm infants studied with serial magnetic resonance imaging from birth and neurodevelopmental assessment. *Pediatrics*. 2006;118(2):536-548.

101. De Vries LS, Wigglesworth JS, Regev R, Dubowitz LM. Evolution of periventricular leukomalacia during the neonatal period and infancy: correlation of imaging and postmortem findings. *Early Hum Dev*. 1988;17(2-3):205-219.

102. Shalak L, Perlman JM. Hemorrhagic-ischemic cerebral injury in the preterm infant: current concepts. *Clin Perinatol*. 2002;29(4):745-763.

103. Khwaja O, Volpe JJ. Pathogenesis of cerebral white matter injury of prematurity. *Arch Dis Child Fetal Neonatal Ed*. 2008;93(2):F153-F161.

104. Volpe JJ. Brain injury in the premature infant – current concepts. *Preven Med*. 1994;23:638-645.

105. Volpe JJ. Brain injury in the premature infant: overview of clinical aspects, neuropathology, and pathogenesis. *Semin Pediatr Neurol*. 1998;5(3):135-151.

106. du Plessis AJ, Volpe JJ. Intracranial hemorrhage in the newborn infant. In: Burg FD, Ingelfinger JR, Wald ER, Polin RA, Fletcher J, eds. *Gellis & Kagan's Current Pediatric Therapy 16*. Philadelphia, PA: W. B. Saunders Company; 1999:304-308.

107. Back SA, Riddle A, Hohimer AR. Role of instrumented fetal sheep preparations in defining the pathogenesis of human periventricular white-matter injury. *J Child Neurol*. 2006;21(7):582-589.

108. Ment LR, Stewart WB, Duncan CC, Lambrecht R. Beagle puppy model of intraventricular hemorrhage. *J Neurosurg*. 1982;57(2):219-223.

109. Goddard J, Lewis RM, Alcala H, Zeller RS. Intraventricular hemorrhage – an animal model. *Biol Neonate*. 1980;37(1):39-52.

110. Goddard-Finegold J, Michael LH. Cerebral blood flow and experimental intraventricular hemorrhage. *Pediatr Res*. 1984;18(1):7-11.

111. Watkins AM, West CR, Cooke RW. Blood pressure and cerebral haemorrhage and ischaemia in very low birthweight infants. *Early Hum Dev*. 1989;19(2):103-110.

112. Miall-Allen VM, de Vries LS, Whitelaw AG. Mean arterial blood pressure and neonatal cerebral lesions. *Arch Dis Child*. 1987;62(10):1068-1069.

113. Bada HS, Korones SB, Perry EH, et al. Frequent handling in the neonatal intensive care unit and intraventricular hemorrhage. *J Pediatr*. 1990;117(1 Pt 1):126-131.

114. Bada HS, Korones SB, Perry EH, et al. Mean arterial blood pressure changes in premature infants and those at risk for intraventricular hemorrhage. *J Pediatr*. 1990;117(4):607-614.

115. Low JA, Froese AB, Smith JT, Galbraith RS, Sauerbrei EE, Karchmar EJ. Hypotension and hypoxemia in the preterm newborn during the four days following delivery identify infants at risk of echosonographically demonstrable cerebral lesions. *Clin Invest Med*. 1992;15(1):60-65.

116. Perlman JM, Risser R, Broyles RS. Bilateral cystic periventricular leukomalacia in the premature infant: associated risk factors. *Pediatrics*. 1996;97(6 Pt 1):822-827.

117. Murphy DJ, Hope PL, Johnson A. Neonatal risk factors for cerebral palsy in very preterm babies: case-control study. *BMJ.* 1997;314(7078):404-408.

118. Fanaroff JM, Wilson-Costello DE, Newman NS, Montpetite MM, Fanaroff AA. Treated hypotension is associated with neonatal morbidity and hearing loss in extremely low birth weight infants. *Pediatrics.* 2006;117(4):1131-1135.

119. Gronlund JU, Korvenranta H, Kero P, Jalonen J, Valimaki IA. Elevated arterial blood pressure is associated with peri-intraventricular haemorrhage. *Eur J Pediatr.* 1994;153(11): 836-841.

120. Trounce JQ, Shaw DE, Levene MI, Rutter N. Clinical risk factors and periventricular leucomalacia. *Arch Dis Child.* 1988; 63(1):17-22.

121. Cowan F, Thoresen M. The effects of intermittent positive pressure ventilation on cerebral arterial and venous blood velocities in the newborn infant. *Acta Paediatr Scand.* 1987; 76(2):239-247.

122. Svenningsen L, Lindemann R, Eidal K. Measurements of fetal head compression pressure during bearing down and their relationship to the condition of the newborn. *Acta Obstet Gynecol Scand.* 1988;67(2):129-133.

123. Skinner JR, Milligan DW, Hunter S, Hey EN. Central venous pressure in the ventilated neonate. *Arch Dis Child.* 1992;67(4 Spec No):374-377.

124. Perlman JM, McMenamin JB, Volpe JJ. Fluctuating cerebral blood-flow velocity in respiratory-distress syndrome. Relation to the development of intraventricular hemorrhage. *N Engl J Med.* 1983;309(4):204-209.

125. Van Bel F, Van de Bor M, Stijnen T, Baan J, Ruys JH. Aetiological role of cerebral blood-flow alterations in development and extension of peri-intraventricular haemorrhage. *Dev Med Child Neurol.* 1987;29(5):601-614.

126. Lou HC. The "lost autoregulation hypothesis" and brain lesions in the newborn – an update. *Brain Dev.* 1988;10(3):143-146.

127. Pryds O, Christensen NJ, Friis-Hansen B. Increased cerebral blood flow and plasma epinephrine in hypoglycemic, preterm neonates. *Pediatrics.* 1990;85(2):172-176.

128. Leffler CW, Busija DW, Mirro R, Armstead WM, Beasley DG. Effects of ischemia on brain blood flow and oxygen consumption of newborn pigs. *Am J Physiol.* 1989;257(6 Pt 2):H1917-H1926.

129. Leffler CW, Busija DW, Beasley DG, Armstead WM, Mirro R. Postischemic cerebral microvascular responses to norepinephrine and hypotension in newborn pigs. *Stroke.* 1989;20(4): 541-546.

130. Laptook AR, Corbett RJ, Ruley J, Olivares E. Blood flow and metabolism during and after repeated partial brain ischemia in neonatal piglets. *Stroke.* 1992;23(3):380-387.

131. Conger JD, Weil JV. Abnormal vascular function following ischemia-reperfusion injury. *J Investig Med.* 1995;43(5):431-442.

132. Blankenberg FG, Loh NN, Norbash AM, et al. Impaired cerebrovascular autoregulation after hypoxic-ischemic injury in extremely low-birth-weight neonates: detection with power and pulsed wave Doppler US. *Radiology.* 1997;205(2): 563-568.

133. Lou HC, Lassen NA, Friis-Hansen B. Impaired autoregulation of cerebral blood flow in the distressed newborn infant. *J Pediatr.* 1979;94(1):118-121.

134. Low JA, Froese AB, Galbraith RS, Smith JT, Sauerbrei EE, Derrick EJ. The association between preterm newborn hypotension and hypoxemia and outcome during the first year. *Acta Paediatr.* 1993;82(5):433-437.

135. de Vries LS, Regev R, Dubowitz LM, Whitelaw A, Aber VR. Perinatal risk factors for the development of extensive cystic leukomalacia. *Am J Dis Child.* 1988;142(7):732-735.

136. Weindling AM, Wilkinson AR, Cook J, Calvert SA, Fok TF, Rochefort MJ. Perinatal events which precede periventricular haemorrhage and leukomalacia in the newborn. *Br J Obstet Gynaecol.* 1985;92(12):1218-1223.

137. Dammann O, Allred EN, Kuban KC, et al. Systemic hypotension and white-matter damage in preterm infants. *Dev Med Child Neurol.* 2002;44(2):82-90.

138. Bejar RF, Vaucher YE, Benirschke K, Berry CC. Postnatal white matter necrosis in preterm infants. *J Perinatol.* 1992;12(1):3-8.

139. Rhee CJ, Kaiser JR, Rios DR, et al. Elevated diastolic closing margin is associated with intraventricular hemorrhage in premature infants. *J Pediatr.* 2016;174:52-56.

140. Rhee CJ, Kibler KK, Easley RB, et al. The diastolic closing margin is associated with intraventricular hemorrhage in premature infants. *Acta Neurochir Suppl.* 2016;122:147-150.

141. Rhee CJ, Fraser CD, III, Kibler K, et al. The ontogeny of cerebrovascular critical closing pressure. *Acta Neurochir Suppl.* 2016;122:249-253.

142. Fujimura M, Salisbury DM, Robinson RO, et al. Clinical events relating to intraventricular haemorrhage in the newborn. *Arch Dis Child.* 1979;54(6):409-414.

143. McDonald MM, Koops BL, Johnson ML, et al. Timing and antecedents of intracranial hemorrhage in the newborn. *Pediatrics.* 1984;74(1):32-36.

144. Perlman J, Thach B. Respiratory origin of fluctuations in arterial blood pressure in premature infants with respiratory distress syndrome. *Pediatrics.* 1988;81(3):399-403.

145. Kluckow M, Evans N. Low superior vena cava flow and intraventricular haemorrhage in preterm infants. *Arch Dis Child Fetal Neonatal Ed.* 2000;82(3):F188-F194.

146. Kluckow M, Evans N. Low systemic blood flow and hyperkalemia in preterm infants. *J Pediatr.* 2001;139(2):227-232.

147. Kluckow M, Evans N. Relationship between blood pressure and cardiac output in preterm infants requiring mechanical ventilation. *J Pediatr.* 1996;129(4):506-512.

148. Osborn D, Evans N, Kluckow M. Randomized trial of dobutamine versus dopamine in preterm infants with low systemic blood flow. *J Pediatr.* 2002;140(2):183-191.

149. Hunt RW, Evans N, Rieger I, Kluckow M. Low superior vena cava flow and neurodevelopment at 3 years in very preterm infants. *J Pediatr.* 2004;145(5):588-592.

150. Miletin J, Dempsey EM. Low superior vena cava flow on day 1 and adverse outcome in the very low birthweight infant. *Arch Dis Child Fetal Neonatal Ed.* 2008;93(5):F368-F371.

151. Evans N, Kluckow M, Simmons M, Osborn D. Which to measure, systemic or organ blood flow? Middle cerebral artery and superior vena cava flow in very preterm infants. *Arch Dis Child Fetal Neonatal Ed.* 2002;87(3):F181-F184.

152. Kluckow M, Evans N. Superior vena cava flow in newborn infants: a novel marker of systemic blood flow. *Arch Dis Child Fetal Neonatal Ed.* 2000;82(3):F182-F187.

153. Kluckow M, Evans N. Low systemic blood flow in the preterm infant. *Semin Neonatol.* 2001;6(1):75-84.

154. Moran M, Miletin J, Pichova K, Dempsey EM. Cerebral tissue oxygenation index and superior vena cava blood flow in the very low birth weight infant. *Acta Paediatr.* 2009;98(1):43-46.

155. Kissack CM, Garr R, Wardle SP, Weindling AM. Cerebral fractional oxygen extraction in very low birth weight infants is high when there is low left ventricular output and hypocarbia

but is unaffected by hypotension. *Pediatr Res.* 2004;55(3): 400-405.

156. Osborn DA, Evans N, Kluckow M. Hemodynamic and antecedent risk factors of early and late periventricular/intraventricular hemorrhage in premature infants. *Pediatrics.* 2003; 112(1 Pt 1):33-39.

157. Donofrio MT, Duplessis AJ, Limperopoulos C. Impact of congenital heart disease on fetal brain development and injury. *Curr Opin Pediatr.* 2011;23(5):502-511.

158. Shillingford AJ, Ittenbach RF, Marino BS, et al. Aortic morphometry and microcephaly in hypoplastic left heart syndrome. *Cardiol Young.* 2007;17(2):189-195.

159. Licht DJ, Shera DM, Clancy RR, et al. Brain maturation is delayed in infants with complex congenital heart defects. *J Thorac Cardiovasc Surg.* 2009;137(3):529-537.

160. Miller SP, McQuillen PS, Hamrick S, et al. Abnormal brain development in newborns with congenital heart disease. *N Engl J Med.* 2007;357(19):1928-1938.

161. Sarajuuri A, Jokinen E, Mildh L, et al. Neurodevelopmental burden at age 5 years in patients with univentricular heart. *Pediatrics.* 2012;130(6):e1636-e1646.

162. Mulkey SB, Swearingen CJ, Melguizo MS, et al. Multi-tiered analysis of brain injury in neonates with congenital heart disease. *Pediatr Cardiol.* 2013;34(8):1772-1784.

163. Limperopoulos C, Majnemer A, Shevell MI, Rosenblatt B, Rohlicek C, Tchervenkov C. Neurodevelopmental status of newborns and infants with congenital heart defects before and after open heart surgery. *J Pediatr.* 2000;137(5):638-645.

164. Limperopoulos C, Majnemer A, Shevell MI, Rosenblatt B, Rohlicek C, Tchervenkov C. Neurologic status of newborns with congenital heart defects before open heart surgery. *Pediatrics.* 1999;103(2):402-408.

165. Donofrio MT, Massaro AN. Impact of congenital heart disease on brain development and neurodevelopmental outcome. *Int J Pediatr.* 2010;2010:359390.

166. Dimitropoulos A, McQuillen PS, Sethi V, et al. Brain injury and development in newborns with critical congenital heart disease. *Neurology.* 2013;81(3):241-248.

167. Mahle WT, Tavani F, Zimmerman RA, et al. An MRI study of neurological injury before and after congenital heart surgery. *Circulation.* 2002;106(12 Suppl 1):I109-I114.

168. Beca J, Gunn JK, Coleman L, et al. New white matter brain injury after infant heart surgery is associated with diagnostic group and the use of circulatory arrest. *Circulation.* 2013; 127(9):971-979.

169. Ortinau C, Beca J, Lambeth J, et al. Regional alterations in cerebral growth exist preoperatively in infants with congenital heart disease. *J Thorac Cardiovasc Surg.* 2012;143(6):1264-1270.

170. Sethi V, Tabbutt S, Dimitropoulos A, et al. Single-ventricle anatomy predicts delayed microstructural brain development. *Pediatr Res.* 2013;73(5):661-667.

171. Petit CJ, Rome JJ, Wernovsky G, et al. Preoperative brain injury in transposition of the great arteries is associated with oxygenation and time to surgery, not balloon atrial septostomy. *Circulation.* 2009;119(5):709-716.

172. Clouchoux C, du Plessis AJ, Bouyssi-Kobar M, et al. Delayed cortical development in fetuses with complex congenital heart disease. *Cereb Cortex.* 2013;23(12):2932-2943.

173. McQuillen PS, Goff DA, Licht DJ. Effects of congenital heart disease on brain development. *Prog Pediatr Cardiol.* 2010;29(2):79-85.

174. Bose SN, Verigan A, Hanson J, et al. Early identification of impending cardiac arrest in neonates and infants in the cardiovascular ICU: a statistical modelling approach using physiologic monitoring data – CORRIGENDUM. *Cardiol Young.* 2019;29(11):1349.

175. Siddiqui S, Fifer WP, Ordonez-Retamar M, Nugent JD, Williams IA. An antenatal marker of neurodevelopmental outcomes in infants with congenital heart disease. *J Perinatol.* 2017;37(8):953-957.

176. Donofrio MT, Bremer YA, Schieken RM, et al. Autoregulation of cerebral blood flow in fetuses with congenital heart disease: the brain sparing effect. *Pediatr Cardiol.* 2003;24(5):436-443.

177. Kaltman JR, Di H, Tian Z, Rychik J. Impact of congenital heart disease on cerebrovascular blood flow dynamics in the fetus. *Ultrasound Obstet Gynecol.* 2005;25(1):32-36.

178. Modena A, Horan C, Visintine J, Chanthasenanont A, Wood D, Weiner S. Fetuses with congenital heart disease demonstrate signs of decreased cerebral impedance. *Am J Obstet Gynecol.* 2006;195(3):706-710.

179. Williams IA, Tarullo AR, Grieve PG, et al. Fetal cerebrovascular resistance and neonatal EEG predict 18-month neurodevelopmental outcome in infants with congenital heart disease. *Ultrasound Obstet Gynecol.* 2012;40(3):304-309.

180. Williams IA, Fifer C, Jaeggi E, Levine JC, Michelfelder EC, Szwast AL. The association of fetal cerebrovascular resistance with early neurodevelopment in single ventricle congenital heart disease. *Am Heart J.* 2013;165(4):544-550.e1.

181. Dehaes M, Cheng HH, Buckley EM, et al. Perioperative cerebral hemodynamics and oxygen metabolism in neonates with single-ventricle physiology. *Biomed Opt Express.* 2015;6(12): 4749-4767.

182. Nagaraj UD, Evangelou IE, Donofrio MT, et al. Impaired global and regional cerebral perfusion in newborns with complex congenital heart disease. *J Pediatr.* 2015;167(5):1018-1024.

183. Votava-Smith JK, Statile CJ, Taylor MD, et al. Impaired cerebral autoregulation in preoperative newborn infants with congenital heart disease. *J Thorac Cardiovasc Surg.* 2017; 154(3):1038-1044.

184. Chock VY, Ramamoorthy C, Van Meurs KP. Cerebral autoregulation in neonates with a hemodynamically significant patent ductus arteriosus. *J Pediatr.* 2012;160(6):936-942.

185. Lynch JM, Buckley EM, Schwab PJ, et al. Time to surgery and preoperative cerebral hemodynamics predict postoperative white matter injury in neonates with hypoplastic left heart syndrome. *J Thorac Cardiovasc Surg.* 2014;148(5):2181-2188.

186. Bassan H, Gauvreau K, Newburger JW, et al. Identification of pressure passive cerebral perfusion and its mediators after infant cardiac surgery. *Pediatr Res.* 2005;57(1):35-41.

187. Fyfe KL, Yiallourou SR, Wong FY, Odoi A, Walker AM, Horne RS. Gestational age at birth affects maturation of baroreflex control. *J Pediatr.* 2015;166(3):559-565.

188. Witcombe NB, Yiallourou SR, Sands SA, Walker AM, Horne RS. Preterm birth alters the maturation of baroreflex sensitivity in sleeping infants. *Pediatrics.* 2012;129(1):e89-e96.

189. Andriessen P, Schoffelen RL, Berendsen RC, et al. Noninvasive assessment of blood pressure variability in preterm infants. *Pediatr Res.* 2004;55(2):220-223.

190. Govindan V, Govindan R, Massaro AN, et al. Cerebral venous volume changes and pressure autoregulation in critically ill infants. *J Perinatol.* 2020;40(5):806-811.

191. van Bel F, de Winter PJ, Wijnands HB, van de Bor M, Egberts J. Cerebral and aortic blood flow velocity patterns in preterm

infants receiving prophylactic surfactant treatment. *Acta Paediatr.* 1992;81(6-7):504-510.

192. Perlman JM, Volpe JJ. Cerebral blood flow velocity in relation to intraventricular hemorrhage in the premature newborn infant. *J Pediatr.* 1982;100(6):956-959.

193. O'Brien NF. Reference values for cerebral blood flow velocities in critically ill, sedated children. *Childs Nerv Syst.* 2015; 31(12):2269-2276.

194. Rennie JM, South M, Morley CJ. Cerebral blood flow velocity variability in infants receiving assisted ventilation. *Arch Dis Child.* 1987;62(12):1247-1251.

195. Edwards AD, Wyatt JS, Richardson C, Delpy DT, Cope M, Reynolds EO. Cotside measurement of cerebral blood flow in ill newborn infants by near infrared spectroscopy. *Lancet.* 1988;2(8614):770-771.

196. Tyszczuk L, Meek J, Elwell C, Wyatt JS. Cerebral blood flow is independent of mean arterial blood pressure in preterm infants undergoing intensive care. *Pediatrics.* 1998;102(2 Pt 1):337-341.

197. Meek JH, Tyszczuk L, Elwell CE, Wyatt JS. Cerebral blood flow increases over the first three days of life in extremely preterm neonates. *Arch Dis Child Fetal Neonatal Ed.* 1998; 78(1):F33-F37.

198. Lassen NA. Control of cerebral circulation in health and disease. *Circ Res.* 1974;34(6):749-760.

199. Greisen G, Pryds O. Intravenous 133Xe clearance in preterm neonates with respiratory distress. Internal validation of CBF infinity as a measure of global cerebral blood flow. *Scand J Clin Lab Invest.* 1988;48(7):673-678.

200. Drayton MR, Skidmore R. Vasoactivity of the major intracranial arteries in newborn infants. *Arch Dis Child.* 1987;62(3): 236-240.

201. Cerbo RM, Scudeller L, Maragliano R, et al. Cerebral oxygenation, superior vena cava flow, severe intraventricular hemorrhage and mortality in 60 very low birth weight infants. *Neonatology.* 2015;108(4):246-252.

202. Verhagen EA, Van Braeckel KN, van der Veere CN, et al. Cerebral oxygenation is associated with neurodevelopmental outcome of preterm children at age 2 to 3 years. *Dev Med Child Neurol.* 2015;57(5):449-455.

203. Sorensen LC, Greisen G. The brains of very preterm newborns in clinically stable condition may be hyperoxygenated. *Pediatrics.* 2009;124(5):e958-e963.

204. Ouyang M, Liu P, Jeon T, et al. Heterogeneous increases of regional cerebral blood flow during preterm brain development: preliminary assessment with pseudo-continuous arterial spin labeled perfusion MRI. *Neuroimage.* 2016;147:233-242.

205. Borch K, Lou HC, Greisen G. Cerebral white matter blood flow and arterial blood pressure in preterm infants. *Acta Paediatr.* 2010;99(10):1489-1492.

206. Goff DA, Buckley EM, Durduran T, Wang J, Licht DJ. Noninvasive cerebral perfusion imaging in high-risk neonates. *Semin Perinatol.* 2010;34(1):46-56.

207. Miranda MJ, Olofsson K, Sidaros K. Noninvasive measurements of regional cerebral perfusion in preterm and term neonates by magnetic resonance arterial spin labeling. *Pediatr Res.* 2006;60(3):359-363.

208. Noori S, McCoy M, Anderson MP, Ramji F, Seri I. Changes in cardiac function and cerebral blood flow in relation to peri/intraventricular hemorrhage in extremely preterm infants. *J Pediatr.* 2014;164(2):264-270.e1-3.

209. Msall ME. Measuring functional skills in preschool children at risk for neurodevelopmental disabilities. *Ment Retard Dev Disabil Res Rev.* 2005;11(3):263-273.

210. Gross SJ, Mettelman BB, Dye TD, Slagle TA. Impact of family structure and stability on academic outcome in preterm children at 10 years of age. *J Pediatr.* 2001;138(2):169-175.

211. Paredes MF, James D, Gil-Perotin S, et al. Extensive migration of young neurons into the infant human frontal lobe. *Science.* 2016;354(6308):aaf7073.

212. Messerschmidt A, Brugger PC, Boltshauser E, et al. Disruption of cerebellar development: potential complication of extreme prematurity. *AJNR Am J Neuroradiol.* 2005;26(7):1659-1667.

213. Karolis VR, Froudist-Walsh S, Brittain PJ, et al. Reinforcement of the brain's rich-club architecture following early neurodevelopmental disruption caused by very preterm birth. *Cereb Cortex.* 2016;26(3):1322-1335.

214. Kadhim H, Tabarki B, Verellen G, De Prez C, Rona AM, Sebire G. Inflammatory cytokines in the pathogenesis of periventricular leukomalacia. *Neurology.* 2001;56(10):1278-1284.

215. Volpe JJ. Neurobiology of periventricular leukomalacia in the premature infant. *Pediatr Res.* 2001;50(5):553-562.

216. Yoon BH, Romero R, Yang SH, et al. Interleukin-6 concentrations in umbilical cord plasma are elevated in neonates with white matter lesions associated with periventricular leukomalacia. *Am J Obstet Gynecol.* 1996;174(5):1433-1440.

217. Hope PL, Gould SJ, Howard S, Hamilton PA, Costello AM, Reynolds EO. Precision of ultrasound diagnosis of pathologically verified lesions in the brains of very preterm infants. *Dev Med Child Neurol.* 1988;30(4):457-471.

218. Ou X, Glasier CM, Ramakrishnaiah RH, et al. Impaired white matter development in extremely low-birth-weight infants with previous brain hemorrhage. *AJNR Am J Neuroradiol.* 2014;35(10):1983-1989.

219. Brady KM, Mytar JO, Kibler KK, et al. Noninvasive autoregulation monitoring with and without intracranial pressure in the naive piglet brain. *Anesth Analg.* 2010;111(1):191-195.

220. O'Leary H, Gregas MC, Limperopoulos C, et al. Elevated cerebral pressure passivity is associated with prematurity-related intracranial hemorrhage. *Pediatrics.* 2009;124(1):302-309.

221. Massaro AN, Govindan RB, Vezina G, et al. Impaired cerebral autoregulation and brain injury in newborns with hypoxic-ischemic encephalopathy treated with hypothermia. *J Neurophysiol.* 2015;114(2):818-824.

222. Donnelly J, Budohoski KP, Smielewski P, Czosnyka M. Regulation of the cerebral circulation: bedside assessment and clinical implications. *Crit Care.* 2016;20(1):129.

223. Kommers DR, Joshi R, van Pul C, et al. Features of heart rate variability capture regulatory changes during kangaroo care in preterm infants. *J Pediatr.* 2017;182:92-98.e1.

224. Feldman R, Eidelman AI. Skin-to-skin contact (Kangaroo Care) accelerates autonomic and neurobehavioural maturation in preterm infants. *Dev Med Child Neurol.* 2003;45(4): 274-281.

225. Arnon S, Diamant C, Bauer S, Regev R, Sirota G, Litmanovitz I. Maternal singing during kangaroo care led to autonomic stability in preterm infants and reduced maternal anxiety. *Acta Paediatr.* 2014;103(10):1039-1044.

226. Horne RS, Fyfe KL, Odoi A, Athukoralage A, Yiallourou SR, Wong FY. Dummy/pacifier use in preterm infants increases blood pressure and improves heart rate control. *Pediatr Res.* 2016;79(2):325-332.

227. Porges SW, Davila MI, Lewis GF, et al. Autonomic regulation of preterm infants is enhanced by Family Nurture Intervention. *Dev Psychobiol.* 2019;61(6):942-952.

228. Welch MG, Barone JL, Porges SW, et al. Family nurture intervention in the NICU increases autonomic regulation in mothers and children at 4–5 years of age: follow-up results from a randomized controlled trial. *PLoS One.* 2020;15(8):e0236930.

229. Fisher J, Cabral de Mello M, Patel V, et al. Prevalence and determinants of common perinatal mental disorders in women in low- and lower-middle-income countries: a systematic review. *Bull World Health Organ.* 2012;90(2):139G-149G.

230. Howard LM, Molyneaux E, Dennis CL, Rochat T, Stein A, Milgrom J. Non-psychotic mental disorders in the perinatal period. *Lancet.* 2014;384(9956):1775-1788.

231. Loomans EM, van Dijk AE, Vrijkotte TG, et al. Psychosocial stress during pregnancy is related to adverse birth outcomes: results from a large multi-ethnic community-based birth cohort. *Eur J Public Health.* 2013;23(3):485-491.

232. DiPietro JA, Costigan KA, Shupe AK, Pressman EK, Johnson TR. Fetal neurobehavioral development: associations with socioeconomic class and fetal sex. *Dev Psychobiol.* 1998;33(1):79-91.

233. Allister L, Lester BM, Carr S, Liu J. The effects of maternal depression on fetal heart rate response to vibroacoustic stimulation. *Dev Neuropsychol.* 2001;20(3):639-651.

234. Dieter JNI, Emory EK, Johnson KC, Raynor BD. Maternal depression and anxiety effects on the human fetus: preliminary findings and clinical implications. *Infant Ment Health J.* 2008;29(5):420-441.

235. Ghiasi S, Greco A, Barbieri R, Scilingo EP, Valenza G. Assessing autonomic function from electrodermal activity and heart rate variability during cold-pressor test and emotional challenge. *Sci Rep.* 2020;10(1):5406.

236. DiPietro JA, Costigan KA, Pressman EK, Doussard-Roosevelt JA. Antenatal origins of individual differences in heart rate. *Dev Psychobiol.* 2000;37(4):221-228.

237. Jones NA, Field T, Fox NA, Davalos M, Lundy B, Hart S. Newborns of mothers with depressive symptoms are physiologically less developed. *Infant Behav Dev.* 1998;21(3):537-541.

238. Field T, Diego M, Hernandez-Reif M, et al. Pregnancy anxiety and comorbid depression and anger: effects on the fetus and neonate. *Depress Anxiety.* 2003;17(3):140-151.

239. Ponirakis A, Susman EJ, Stifter CA. Negative emotionality and cortisol during adolescent pregnancy and its effects on infant health and autonomic nervous system reactivity. *Dev Psychobiol.* 1998;33(2):163-174.

240. van Dijk AE, van Eijsden M, Stronks K, Gemke RJ, Vrijkotte TG. Prenatal stress and balance of the child's cardiac autonomic nervous system at age 5–6 years. *PLoS One.* 2012;7(1):e30413.

# Diagnosis of Neonatal Cardiovascular Compromise: Methods and Clinical Applications

# ASSESSMENT OF HEMODYNAMICS AND CARDIAC FUNCTION: ULTRASOUND

# Chapter 9

# Ultrasound-Guided Hemodynamic Management

Nicholas Evans, Martin Kluckow, and Audrey Hébert

## Key Points

- The use of Clinician Performed Ultrasound (CPU) in the care of sick and preterm neonates is rapidly expanding.
- The benefits of a portable, bedside technique that provides real-time, longitudinal data regarding the physiology of individual patients and allows more targeted treatment are being progressively recognized as important.
- CPU has an important role in managing the transitioning term or preterm infant, the septic/asphyxiated infant, the shocked or hypotensive infant, and infants with suspected PPHN or congenital heart disease.
- CPU is usually a predominantly "rule-in" diagnostic modality and does not aim to "rule out" all diagnoses, whereas consultative ultrasound should also be used as a "rule-out" diagnostic modality.
- With the acceptance of the usefulness of ultrasound in the clinical setting, the need for appropriate training programs and accreditation increases.
- Approaches to training and accreditation vary across different countries.

## Introduction

It is a limitation in the intensive care of the newborn infant that we have few tools with which to monitor cardiovascular and hemodynamic function. The mainstay has been to continuously monitor invasive blood pressure and heart rate. Beyond that, reliance is placed on rather inaccurate measures of contemporaneous hemodynamic well-being such as skin capillary refill time and urine output and measures that do not reflect the changes in the hemodynamic status in real time such as the acid-base status. Near-infrared spectroscopy (NIRS) is evolving as a potentially useful monitoring tool[1] for the real-time assessment of tissue oxygenation of the organ interrogated (brain, kidney, muscle, or intestines). As for measuring cardiac output, there is little outcome-based validation for tools designed to measure cardiac output (Chapters 14 and 21). The difficulties of small patient size and a smaller commercial market, limit neonatology's access to a range of tools for monitoring cardiac output that are available for the intensive care of the older subject. These tools include thermodilution, electrical impedance velocimetry, continuous Doppler methodologies, and derivations from blood pressure waveforms.

Doppler cardiac ultrasound provides a noninvasive, albeit non-continuous, technique from which it is possible to derive estimates of a wide range of hemodynamic parameters as well as information on structure and function of the organ that drives the circulation, the heart. Integration of cardiac ultrasound into routine neonatal intensive care has been limited by the concentration of the necessary skills in specialist groups who work predominantly outside the NICU. This results in information that is often neither timely nor particularly well focused on hemodynamics. From a research perspective, it meant that there were assumptions derived from a limited number of snapshots rather than serial studies to document natural history.

Neonatology, like many acute care specialties, has recognized the limitations of an external consultative ultrasound model and neonatologists are increasingly developing cardiac ultrasound skills themselves so that it can be applied at the acute point of care.[2] This has allowed more systematic serial studies, which in turn is facilitating the development of the research agenda and the clinical monitoring potential of these methodologies. It should be emphasized that acute CPU does not replace the need for consultative ultrasound. Rather it addresses different questions and complements consultative ultrasound. The best outcomes are achieved when the two models work collaboratively alongside each other.

This chapter will provide an overview of the use of cardiac ultrasound to assess the neonatal circulation (details of the individual techniques will be outlined in other chapters) as well as discuss issues of training, accreditation, and interaction with other imaging specialists.

## Politics of Ultrasound

The evolution of ultrasound into the area of acute care has resulted in political controversies, and this has not been confined to neonatology. On one side of the argument, acute care specialists have recognized the rapid diagnostic potential of ultrasound, a potential that is difficult to fulfill within a consultative model of ultrasound.[3] The improvement in quality of imaging and portability of equipment has made ultrasound accessible to anyone with a good understanding of anatomy and access to training. On the other side of the argument, some consultative imaging specialists have resisted this on the basis of concerns about lack of accredited training and about the risk of diagnostic error.[4] Importantly, a review of medicolegal cases involving neonatal/pediatric CPU in the United States found no evidence of this risk[5] and several more recent case series show excellent anatomical concordance between cardiologists and appropriately trained CPU practitioners. Like all political divides, there are merits to both arguments. Consultative ultrasound specialists have neither the ability (nor often the desire) to be available 24/7 for the rapid diagnostic situations facing acute care specialists. CPU, particularly in neonatology, has often evolved with a lack of good training and accreditation

structures. Many of the early adopters of CPU were largely self-taught or taught by a cardiologist with a balanced perspective of the usefulness of functional ultrasound in the NICU. While this is changing, as will be described later, there is risk that this may lead to diagnostic error. As always, the answer lies in the middle, with a system that takes advantage of the strengths of both systems and minimizes the risks. Clinician-performed ultrasound (CPU) is usually a predominantly "rule-in" diagnostic modality and does not aim to "rule out" all diagnoses, whereas consultative ultrasound should also be viewed as a "rule-out" diagnostic modality.

From our experience, much of the resistance to establishing a CPU program is based on a lack of understanding of the goals. Resolution comes from reassurance about training and quality issues and education about purpose, most importantly, that the intent is to complement, not replace, the role of those consultative specialties.

## Training and Accreditation in Australia/New Zealand

It is the nature of the evolution of any procedure or technology that the early adopters are often self-taught. Development of training and accreditation structures follows when the need is identified and there is enough of a critical mass of early adopters to provide the necessary support. There are good examples of training structures in CPU such as that developed by the American College of Emergency Physicians[6,7]; however, there is a long way to go in neonatal CPU. Internationally, there is difference of opinion in the relative weight that should be given to training provided by those outside neonatology compared to those within. In Australia and New Zealand, we have developed a training program that is based on the philosophy that training for CPU in the NICU is best undertaken in the NICU under supervision of appropriately trained and accredited neonatologists, while also recognizing the need for support from the consultative imaging specialists.[3] The program was developed in 2007 under the auspices of the Australasian Society of Ultrasound in Medicine (ASUM), who, having recognized the inevitable evolution of ultrasound into acute care areas, had developed a qualification called the Certificate in Clinician Performed Ultrasound (CCPU). There were already modules for several acute care specialties and neonatology was developed as another module. The program was developed by a steering committee consisting of mainly neonatologists from around Australia and New Zealand but included a radiologist and a pediatric cardiologist. The qualification is based on course attendance and supervised logbooks of ultrasound scans. The trainees have to complete an online physics course, following which the ultrasound training is in two stages, basic and advanced. Basic training is aimed at normal image acquisition of the heart and brain, while advanced training is aimed at interpretation of abnormal hemodynamic and cerebral findings, as well as learning some other aspects of neonatal CPU such as basic abdominal organ imaging and central line localization. The core part of training is undertaken within the neonatal unit under the supervision of a qualified CPU clinician who can also teach the skills of integration of the ultrasound and clinical findings. The advanced module includes training in recognition of common congenital heart disease with the understanding that the ability to exclude congenital heart disease will require further training under the supervision of pediatric cardiology. The expectation is that only a few neonatologists undertake this extra training and others will continue to consult with pediatric cardiology colleagues to exclude structural cardiac abnormalities. This program has been running since 2007; there are more than 60 graduates with the CCPU (neonatal) and approximately 40 trainees currently undertaking training.[8]

Consensus statements on neonatal cardiac ultrasound training have been published in North America, Europe, and the UK.[9,10] Both these statements take a different focus, with an emphasis on training within pediatric cardiology. Neither of these statements addresses the wider role for neonatal CPU beyond the heart. The development of national or regional administered structured training programs under these guidelines is still in progress.

It is our view that to achieve the goal of quality assurance in standards of neonatal CPU, a training program needs to be both relevant and workable. For this to happen, the practical component of the training needs to occur mainly within the NICU and the training needs to be mainly provided by neonatologists. A core component of training is understanding how to integrate imaging skills into the other clinical information available for a particular patient. Further, the training program needs to embrace the fact that CPU in any acute care specialty embraces more than one organ.

## Training and Accreditation in North America

The concept of neonatal hemodynamics has received broad adoption with the establishment of new programs across North America and in many parts of the world.[11] The impetus for the growth of these programs is the need for rapid evaluation, an individualized approach to neonates with hemodynamic disturbances, and the call for standardization through research. Program structure and quality assurance are an integral part of the hemodynamic consultation process. In addition, access to dedicated echocardiography equipment, systems for study archiving and report generation, safety, quality assurance, and infection control practices are essential components of successful programs. In centers with Pediatric Cardiology services, close collaboration on operational, training, and research matters is encouraged. The field has grown exponentially in the past decade, particularly in North America, with the establishment of neonatal hemodynamics programs in more than 20 centers. Importantly, the concept of Targeted Neonatal Echocardiography (TNE) and neonatal hemodynamics has been positively embraced by major societies such as the American Echocardiography Society (ASE); specifically the establishment of the Neonatal Hemodynamics and TNE Specialty Interest Group (NHTS SIG) provides an avenue for cultivation of knowledge and scientific discovery and a path for collaboration between disciplines. Finally, the creation of academic consortia, such as the Pan American Hemodynamics Collaborative, and the establishment of a Neonatal Hemodynamics Research Center (https://neonatalhemodynamics.com) enable clinical, educational, and academic oversight of the field and the development of formal mentorship processes.

The implementation of neonatal hemodynamics programs has also influenced the development of training programs. The training model for neonatal hemodynamics requires exposure to a broad range of illnesses in both term (e.g., pulmonary hypertension, hypoxic-ischemic encephalopathy, surgical disease) and preterm infants. The curriculum should include extensive "hands-on" training (image acquisition and measurement analyses) and "cognitive" (advanced cardiovascular physiology, core pharmacology, and pathophysiology) components as they apply to common neonatal cardiovascular health problems. Although training in the echo lab, as suggested in the ASE 2011 guidelines,[12] can provide additional exposure to congenital cardiac malformations that trainees should recognize, the lack of access to pediatric echocardiography laboratories in many regions may represent an obstacle to establishing training programs. It is important to highlight, however, that the primary goal of the neonatologist with hemodynamics expertise is to recognize deviations from normal anatomy and appropriately refer to a cardiologist. Therefore most training may take place within the NICU and be supervised by neonatologists with expertise in neonatal hemodynamics. Trainees gain image acquisition skills within the NICU through graded exposure to a variety of neonatal cardiovascular health problems, and time in the echo lab is often integrated into the training program. Review sessions, collaborative discussions with pediatric cardiology, participation in special interest groups in neonatal hemodynamics, and research are all fundamental components of training. A singular approach to training may not be achievable and regional or international variance must be allowed for developing training guidelines. The development of echocardiography simulators and web-based APPs provides a novel opportunity to modernize learning. Standardized imaging protocols for the diagnosis and longitudinal evaluation of common neonatal problems are desirable. These protocols may include evaluation of the hemodynamic significance of patent ductus arteriosus (PDA), evaluation of pulmonary hemodynamics and right heart function (e.g., acute or chronic pulmonary

hypertension), and evaluation of left heart function and systemic hypoperfusion (e.g., post-PDA ligation, septic shock). The incorporation of advanced echocardiography techniques (e.g., tissue Doppler imaging, strain analysis) into standardized imaging protocols based on new knowledge requires thoughtful consideration.

## Moving Toward the Hemodynamic Consultation

The growth of the field of Neonatal Hemodynamics represents a natural evolution to further optimize clinical care and scientific knowledge in a subpopulation of critically ill preterm and term infants with intrinsic developmental vulnerability, which places them at increased risk of disease-dependent hemodynamic instability and cardiopulmonary maldevelopment. The publication of the American Society of Echocardiography (ASE) Guidelines for TNE in 2011[12] was a pivotal step in cultivating the growth of this expert model of hemodynamic care. The subsequent 10 years have witnessed major expansion in North America in terms of new clinical programs, scientific advancement, and innovation. Importantly, a key component of TNE and one of the primary differences compared with traditional echocardiography is that performance of the imaging and study interpretation by the neonatologist enables enhanced integration within the intensive care context. Appraisal of physiology-based echocardiography requires detailed knowledge of the modifiers of neonatal physiology, such as ventilation, fluid balance, and other important variables. The concept of a "hemodynamic consultation" was proposed to encompass the comprehensive, integrated assessment by a neonatologist with advanced echocardiography skills and a strong foundation in neonatal pathophysiology and neonatal cardiovascular pharmacotherapeutics.[13] Indications for hemodynamic consultation may include "disease-specific" evaluation such as hemodynamic significance of patent ductus arteriosus (PDA), assessment of pulmonary hemodynamics and right heart function (e.g., acute or chronic pulmonary hypertension), assessment of left heart function and systemic hypoperfusion (e.g., post-PDA ligation, septic shock), or "symptom-based" evaluation such as systemic hypotension or hypoxemia. As such, the assessment is dependent on the knowledge of cardiovascular physiology and pharmacotherapeutics, and the ability to integrate this information.

The hemodynamics consultation process may be summarized into three major phases:

(1) *Clinical evaluation*, including review of medical history, relevant investigations (laboratory, radiological), and current treatments (mechanical ventilation, fluid, and cardiovascular therapy).

(2) *Comprehensive TNE*, if indicated, including (a) recognizing abnormal cardiac anatomy and the need for pediatric cardiology appraisal if anomalies are suspected; (b) acquiring images in a systematic manner to comprehensively assess hemodynamics relevant to the specific clinical indication; (c) completing measurements in a standardized manner; (d) completing a formal report that includes information regarding anatomic surveillance and relevant hemodynamic measurements; and (e) archiving all relevant images in a format that aligns with the diagnostic report and is suitable for future audit and quality assurance.

(3) *Integration and medical recommendation*, including (a) completing a diagnostic impression based on integration of the relevant clinical and echocardiography information and (b) providing a medical recommendation and plan for longitudinal follow-up, if needed, in consultation with the clinical team.

## Integrating Clinical and Physiological Information to Target Treatment

A key use of CPU in the clinical setting is to help understand the underlying physiology and subsequently to decide on what treatment is most useful for the individual patient. An illustration of the process of identifying individual physiology in a focused ultrasound, applying this information, and assessing the outcome of treatment choices is shown in Figure 9.1. This targeting of treatment with the ability to longitudinally monitor response is the way we most often use CPU and is best demonstrated by some case presentations.

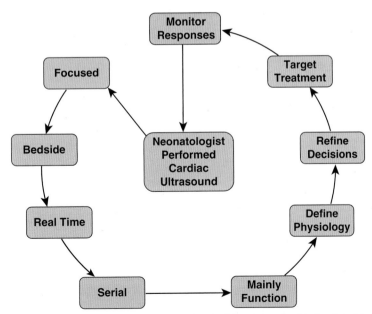

**Fig. 9.1** Diagrammatic representation of the process of use of CPU, diagnosing physiology, integrating into the clinical decision-making, and obtaining longitudinal feedback to validate treatment decisions made. (Adapted from Kluckow M. Use of ultrasound in the haemodynamic assessment of the sick neonate. Arch Dis Child Fetal Neonatal Ed. 2014;99:F332–F337. doi:10.1136/archdischild-2013-304926.)

## Case Presentation 1

Baby A was born at 38 weeks' gestation following an emergency Cesarean section for maternal pre-eclampsia. The amniotic fluid was clear. Respiratory distress began immediately after birth, requiring CPAP at 7–8 cm $H_2O$ and increased oxygen. By 6 hours of age, requiring 0.75 $FiO_2$ to maintain arterial $O_2$ saturation of >85%. At 6.5 hours, there was a sudden deterioration with arterial $O_2$ saturations below 80% requiring $FiO_2$ 1.0. Chest X-ray (CXR) showed some opacification in both lung fields and a small right-sided pneumothorax. Options considered include mechanical ventilation, needle drainage of pneumothorax, and use of inhaled nitric oxide (iNO). The oxygen requirements were out of proportion to CXR with a labile clinical state, so iNO was the favored clinical option. Prior to commencement of iNO, a CPU was performed.

Findings: See Figure 9.2.

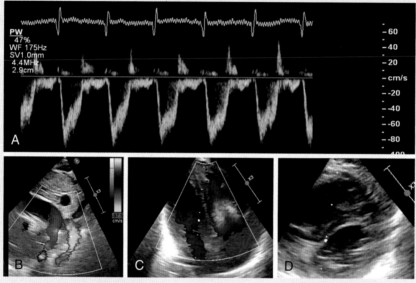

**Fig. 9.2 Findings for Case Presentation 1.** (A) Parasternal view – normal right ventricular output. (B) Ductal view – no patent ductus arteriosus. (C) Subcostal view – good contractility and no evidence of tricuspid incompetence. (D) Parasternal short axis view – normal right ventricle. Normal cardiac anatomy – later confirmed by cardiology team.

### OUTCOME CASE 1

Cardiac CPU showed no evidence of raised pulmonary pressures with normal cardiovascular function. Consequently, no iNO was administered. There was an attempted needle aspiration of the pneumothorax – no air recovered. Mechanical ventilation was transitioned to high-frequency ventilation, surfactant was administered, and a lung recruitment strategy was utilized. The $FiO_2$ requirements gradually improved. There was rapid recovery in 12–18 hours. This case illustrates that sometimes CPU supports a clinical decision to not introduce specific therapies – such as iNO.

## Case Presentation 2

Baby B was delivered at 25 weeks' gestation with incomplete antenatal steroid coverage. The infant was initially placed on CPAP at 6 cm $H_2O$ but then was intubated and given surfactant because of increasing oxygen requirements (0.35 $FiO_2$). Intravenous antibiotics were administered. The infant was rapidly extubated back to CPAP 6 cm $H_2O$ in room air. At 10 hours of age, the $FiO_2$ increased to >0.40 with borderline blood pressure (mean BP = 25 mmHg). The CPAP was increased to 7 cm $H_2O$ with transient improvement. The chest X-ray showed well-expanded lungs. Options considered were to re-ventilate and give further surfactant, wait for further improvement, or gain more clinical information from a CPU.

Findings: See Figure 9.3.

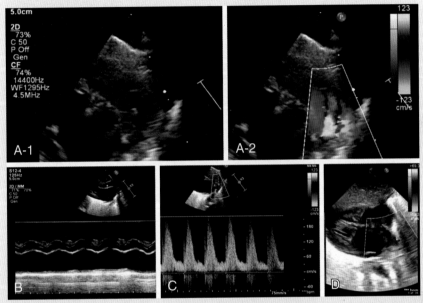

**Fig. 9.3 Findings for Case Presentation 2. (A-1) 2D Ductal view. (A-2) Color Doppler ductal view – large PDA measuring 2.5 mm, unconstricted. Left to right shunt. (B) Dilated left atrium (left atrial:aortic ratio = 1:2.2). (C) Ductal view Doppler – high-velocity pulsatile pattern. (D) Parasternal views – large left-to-right shunt at patent foramen ovale. In addition, there was reverse flow in diastole in the descending aorta and increased diastolic flow in the left pulmonary artery.**

### OUTCOME CASE 2

Cardiac CPU showed evidence of an unconstricted large left-to-right ductal shunt, with added left-to-right shunt at the patent foramen ovale (PFO). There were also signs of increased pulmonary blood flow and impairment of systemic blood flow. Early targeted treatment with indomethacin at 0.2 mg/kg was started to attempt PDA closure. Cardiac CPU 24 hours later showed a closed PDA and return of the hemodynamic state to normal. There was concurrent improvement in ventilation requirements, with decreasing $FiO_2$ and CPAP pressure requirements. This case illustrates that a small number of infants (particularly <26 weeks with incomplete steroid coverage) may have an early symptomatic PDA that has the potential to respond well to early treatment.

## Case Presentation 3

Baby C was born at term gestation by elective cesarean section. The infant was admitted to the NICU at 2 hours with persisting mild tachypnea. The cardiovascular examination was normal and CXR showed normal heart size and changes consistent with transient tachypnea of the newborn. The infant was commenced on antibiotics and nursed in FiO$_2$ 0.25. At 48 hours, the infant was still tachypneic, with increased work of breathing. The chest X-ray was unchanged and the cardiac examination was normal. A CPU was performed.

Findings: See Figure 9.4.

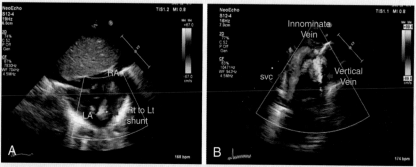

**Fig. 9.4 Findings for Case Presentation 3.** (A) Subcostal four-chamber view – pure right-to-left atrial shunt. (B) Suprasternal coronal posterior view – ascending vertical vein to innominate vein consistent with supra-diaphragmatic total anomalous pulmonary venous drainage (unobstructed) confirmed by a cardiologist.

### OUTCOME CASE 3

The CPU confirmed a structurally normal heart but there was uncertainty about the pulmonary veins. There was a pure right-to-left shunt across the PFO. Knowing the latter could be a marker of congenital heart disease (CHD), the clinicians requested early review by a pediatric cardiologist who confirmed total anomalous pulmonary venous drainage (TAPVD). This case highlights the importance of non-specific ultrasound markers in recognizing CHD and potential of CPU in early diagnosis of clinically unsuspected CHD.

## Case Presentation 4

This pregnancy was complicated by a prolonged period of oligohydramnios due to premature rupture of membranes at 20 weeks' gestation. A cesarean section was performed at 30 weeks' gestation. Baby D was born with limb contractures and stiff lungs that required high pressures during resuscitation. Adequate oxygenation was achieved with surfactant, FiO$_2$ 1.0, and high-pressure conventional ventilation. After transfer to the NICU, a rapid CPU of the lungs (to exclude pneumothorax) and heart was performed by the neonatologist while awaiting a chest X-ray.

## Case Presentation 4 *(Continued)*

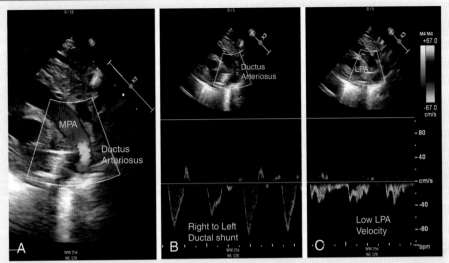

**Fig. 9.5** Findings for Case Presentation 4. (A) Ductal view color Doppler – showed right-to-left ductal shunt. (B) Ductal view pulsed Doppler – showed right-to-left ductal shunt. (C) Ductal view left pulmonary artery (LPA) – showed very low velocity consistent with low pulmonary blood flow.

### OUTCOME CASE 4

Ultrasound of the lungs confirmed no pneumothorax. A cardiac ultrasound showed low pulmonary blood flow and pulmonary hypertension with pure right-to-left shunt at ductal level and a right-to-left atrial shunt. Findings: See Figure 9.5 inhaled NO was started at 45 minutes of age. Ventilator pressures fell over the next 30 minutes and oxygen requirements decreased to FiO$_2$ 0.25. A repeat cardiac ultrasound showed bidirectional ductal shunt and increased left pulmonary artery (LPA) velocities. The baby was extubated to CPAP by 48 hours of life. This case highlights that CPU is useful to exclude lung pathology and the use of CPU to define acute pulmonary hypertension (aPH), as the primary problem allows very early treatment targeted at actual rather than presumed physiology.

## Case Presentation 5

Baby E was born at 41 weeks' gestational age and was diagnosed with meconium aspiration syndrome. She was intubated at 2 hours of life for hypoxemic respiratory failure. The baby remained in FiO$_2$ 1.0 despite starting iNO at 20 ppm. The referring center gave two saline boluses of (10 mL/kg) and started on dopamine up to 15 mcg/kg/min for low systolic BP (48/32 mmHg). The infant was transferred to a quaternary NICU for evaluation to receive ECMO. On arrival, there was a significant pre-/post-ductal saturation difference and a high lactate level.

Targeted echocardiography was performed to assess pulmonary pressure, left and right ventricular function,

and guide management. The ultrasound demonstrated severe RV dysfunction and dilatation with low right ventricular output, elevated pulmonary pressure (92 mmHg estimated by the tricuspid incompetence jet [Figure 6A] and bowing of the interventricular septum into the left ventricle [Figure 6B]). There was mild left ventricular dysfunction (ejection fraction by the Simpson method was 50%) with low left ventricular output (LVO 80 mL/kg/min – normal 200–300 mL/kg/min) with a small restrictive 1 mm PDA with pure right to left shunt and right to left shunting at atrial level.

Findings: See Figure 9.6.

*Continued on following page*

## Case Presentation 5 (Continued)

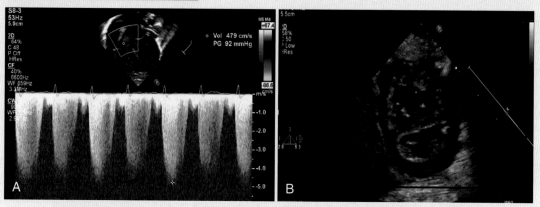

Fig. 9.6 Findings for Case Presentation 5. (A) Tricuspid incompetence jet. (B) Right ventricular septal bowing.

### OUTCOME CASE 5

Based on the assessment of RV systolic dysfunction with acute pulmonary hypertension, the hemodynamic team recommended weaning dopamine, which may have increased pulmonary vascular resistance and worsened hypoxemic respiratory failure. Dobutamine was begun to enhance myocardial performance. Vasopressin was commenced to lower pulmonary vascular resistance and improve atrial filling pressure while supporting the blood pressure. A prostaglandin infusion was begun to maintain ductal patency. A follow-up TnECHO 4 hours later showed improvement in RV function (tricuspid annular plane extension increased from 3 to 7 mm and right ventricular fractional area change increased from 18 to 35%) and decreased estimated pulmonary pressures with a large 2.5 mm PDA with bidirectional flow and bidirectional flow at atrial level.

## Case Presentation 6

Baby F was born at 24 weeks' gestation baby to a mother with chorioamnionitis. Antenatal steroids were given. The baby was intubated and given surfactant at 4 hours of life. There was rapid improvement in the respiratory distress; however, at 12 hours of life, the blood pressure declined to 32/11 (23) mmHg. The baby received one saline bolus of 10 mL/kg normal saline and was started on intravenous antibiotics. The diastolic blood pressure remained below the third percentile for gestational age despite fluid resuscitation. The team requested a hemodynamic consultation to assist with patient management.

### OUTCOME CASE 6

Hemodynamic consultation: The baby had an HR of 180 bpm and BP 32/11 mmHg in the right upper arm and was receiving 0.25 FiO$_2$ on conventional ventilation with an SpO$_2$ of 90% on the right upper arm. On cardiovascular examination, there was rapid capillary refill and bounding peripheral pulses and no heart murmurs.

Arterial blood gas showed metabolic acidosis with a lactate of 4.2. There had been no urine output since birth. Targeted echocardiography was performed to assess function and guide management. The ultrasound showed normal left ventricular function (ejection fraction by Simpson: 60%), high left ventricular output of 300 mL/kg/min, normal right ventricular function, and a small non-hemodynamically significant PDA of 1 mm. The hemodynamic team suggested a vasopressor agent such as norepinephrine to increase systemic vascular resistance and to consider early use of hydrocortisone.

## Uses of CPU in the NICU

While the focus of this book (and so this chapter) is on the cardiovascular system, it must be emphasized that the value of CPU extends well beyond the heart to include many organ systems, as well as procedural uses such as long-line placement.

M-mode and two-dimensional imaging results from ultrasound waves reflecting off solid or liquid interfaces of different densities to allow definition of structure. In the heart this is the interface between muscle, fiber, and blood. Projection of these structures against time allows definition of movement within the cardiac cycle, both of the structures themselves, and also relative to other structures. The Doppler principle can be applied to ultrasound waves because they change frequency as they reflect off moving objects; in the case of the heart and blood vessels, these are the red blood cells. From this change of frequency, both the direction and the velocity of the blood can be derived. Color Doppler maps this direction and the velocity of blood onto the 2D image. Measurement of movement from 2D and M-mode is the basis of most myocardial function tests. Doppler allows identification of the presence of shunts as well as the direction and velocity of shunt flow. Measurement of velocity also allows estimation of pressure gradient (dp) using the modified Bernoulli equation ($dp = 4V^2$); that is, the pressure gradient is equal to 4 times the velocity (V) squared. Measuring these pressure gradients across the tricuspid valve or a patent ductus arteriosus allows estimation of pulmonary artery pressure. Flow measurements, such as ventricular outputs, can be derived by integrating vessel cross-sectional area (using 2D or M-mode), mean velocity, and heart rate. By putting all this together, cardiac ultrasound allows understanding of the complete hemodynamic presentation and allows treatment targeted at that hemodynamic pattern.

In general terms, the traditional clinical pointers to circulatory failure are limited in their accuracy and often only become reliably abnormal when the hemodynamic pathology is well established.[14] In other words, the problem will often be identified late. Because of this, the best use of cardiac ultrasound is proactively in defined high-risk clinical situations.

## THE IMMEDIATE POSTNATAL PERIOD

Babies with signs of circulatory failure in the immediate post-resuscitation period are usually asphyxiated, hypovolemic, or, occasionally, both. This is often, but not exclusively seen, in term babies. These two main pathologies can be difficult to differentiate on clinical grounds.

Asphyxia is diagnosed on the basis of the usual markers: fetal distress, low Apgar scores, need for resuscitation, and lactic acidosis seen in measurement of the umbilical cord arterial blood. Such babies will appear pale and poorly perfused in the immediate post-resuscitation period. In many infants this will

improve with time with resolution of the acidosis. However, some of these babies remain at risk of circulatory failure due to compromised myocardial function and abnormal peripheral vasoregulation.[15] While recognizing the importance of initially addressing respiratory, metabolic, and neurological abnormalities and neuroprotection, an early cardiac ultrasound to assess myocardial function and systemic blood flow with measurement of superior vena cava (SVC) flow and right ventricular (RV) output may allow early direction of appropriate circulatory support (see Chapters 22 and 24). This post-resuscitation pallor needs to be differentiated from hypovolemia, which is rare, but the immediate postnatal period is the most likely time when there can be life-threatening hypovolemia. The causes of perinatal hypovolemia are often clinically occult at the time of resuscitation and include vasa previa, feto-placental hemorrhage, and acute feto-fetal and feto-maternal hemorrhage. All these occult hemorrhages can be acute or chronic but, when chronic, the problem is anemia, not hypovolemia. Cardiac ultrasound allows immediate differentiation of the well-filled, poorly contractile asphyxiated heart from the poorly filled hypovolemic heart, which, in turn, can be differentiated from the dilated hyperdynamic heart, which results from chronic fetal anemia. Appropriate treatment can then be provided.

## CIRCULATORY TRANSITION IN THE VERY PRETERM BABY

The early transitional period is one of exquisite circulatory vulnerability for the very preterm infant and 10–20% of babies born before 30 weeks' gestation will have a period of low systemic blood flow (SBF).[16] The causes of this are complex and relate to many factors, including immaturity, positive pressure ventilation, and shunts through the fetal channels, mainly the ductus arteriosus (also see Chapters 1, 7, and 20). Low SBF is predictive of mortality and a range of morbidities.[17] Low SBF develops during the first 12 hours and then improves spontaneously in almost all babies by 24 hours. Early detection depends on prospective measures of SBF (most frequently by cardiac ultrasound) during the high-risk period of the first 12 hours because low SBF is poorly predicted by clinical parameters including blood pressure (Chapter 20). In our own services we perform prospective cardiac ultrasound from 3 to 6 hours of age with a focus on measures of systemic blood flow using SVC flow and RV output in all preterm neonates born before 28 weeks' gestation. In addition, we screen preterm neonates born after 27 weeks' gestation who are at higher risk for low SBF, for example, limited exposure to antenatal steroids and/or with RDS requiring significant ventilator support. We also use cardiac ultrasound in any baby with severely or persistently low blood pressure or other clinical signs of circulatory compromise. With the latter group, it's important to highlight that low SBF is uncommon in preterm babies after 24 hours unless critically unwell and most hypotension after this time is vasodilatory, for example, low blood pressure in association with normal or high systemic blood flow. This highlights the illogicality of a single standard treatment for all preterm infants with hypotension as the correct treatment for pump failure will often be the wrong treatment for loss of vascular tone, and vice versa (see Chapter 24).

These cardiac ultrasound examinations should also include the common assessments used for pulmonary hypertension (described below). Severe pulmonary hypertension is uncommon as a primary pathology in preterm babies but can occur in certain subgroups; in particular, it is almost universal in babies born after premature prolonged rupture of membranes and oligohydramnios.[18,19]

## ASSESSMENT FOR PATENT DUCTUS ARTERIOSUS (PDA)

Assessment of the ductus arteriosus should be a part of all preterm neonatal cardiac ultrasounds, whether it be proactive during circulatory transition or reactive in response to clinical signs. Ultrasound allows estimation of the two main factors determining the significance of a PDA, that is, the diameter (or degree of constriction) using color Doppler and/or 2D imaging, as well as the pressure gradient across the ductus from the Doppler-derived flow direction and velocity. Additional information on shunt significance can be derived from the change in diastolic flow at either side of the ductus in the descending aorta and the left pulmonary artery. A significant left-to-right ductal shunt causes reversed diastolic flow in the former and exaggerated forward diastolic flow in the latter. How to use this information to determine whether to treat a PDA is addressed in Chapters 16 and 19. However, it is important to highlight here that early postnatal constriction of the ductus arteriosus predicts early spontaneous closure and may be a useful guide to the need for early treatment.[20]

## THE SEPTIC BABY

Cardiac ultrasound is useful for determining the hemodynamics in suspected or proven sepsis with measures of systemic blood flow and assessment for pulmonary hypertension. The hemodynamic compromise of late-onset sepsis is almost always vasodilatory (low BP but normal or high SBF) in the newborn.[21,22] In advanced septic shock evidence of tissue ischemia can persist despite normalization of systemic hemodynamics. Although less well studied in the newborn, this may be due to microvascular dysfunction described in older subjects with sepsis. The hemodynamics of early-onset sepsis is more variable. It can be vasodilatory but pulmonary hypertension can be a significant factor, particularly in early-onset group B streptococcal pneumonia. Assessment and management of neonatal sepsis and shock is discussed in Chapter 21.

## SUSPECTED PERSISTENT PULMONARY HYPERTENSION OF THE NEWBORN

This is usually a term or late preterm baby with high ventilator/oxygen requirements. Not all babies with high ventilator/oxygen requirements have pulmonary hypertension. The hemodynamics are as varied as the underlying pathologies and need to be assessed individually with cardiac ultrasound. It is particularly important that congenital heart disease is excluded immediately upon presentation in these babies. Transposition of the great arteries and total anomalous pulmonary venous drainage can both masquerade as pulmonary hypertension. Pulmonary artery pressure can be estimated from the pressure gradient across the tricuspid valve or, if patent, the ductus arteriosus. The direction and degree of shunting across the ductus arteriosus and foramen ovale can be assessed. These babies are at high risk for low SBF, particularly during the first 24 hours.[23] In some babies the low SBF probably results, at least in part, from the negative circulatory effect of high positive intrathoracic pressure during the period of circulatory transition. In most babies with low pulmonary blood flow PPHN the systemic compromise is the consequence of the restricted pulmonary blood flow and will improve if the pulmonary vascular resistance can be reduced with iNO or other vasodilators. Pulmonary blood flow can be estimated using Doppler velocity in the left pulmonary artery (LPA). Babies with primary PPHN often have low LPA velocities, indicating that blood is bypassing the lung. This low pulmonary blood flow hemodynamic predicts the oxygenation response to iNO.[24,25] Assessment and management of the infant with PPHN is discussed in more detail in Chapters 25 and 27.

## BABIES PRESENTING WITH COLLAPSE/SHOCK

Babies with primary cardiac problems can also present with circulatory failure. This presentation is not common but must be considered in any baby presenting with shock. Because the neonatologist using cardiac CPU spends most of their time examining structurally normal hearts, the ability to spot a heart that is not structurally normal and which needs an expert opinion comes quite early in the learning process. Therefore the reality is that in a hospital without an on-site pediatric cardiology service, cardiac CPU can be useful for rapid/early diagnosis of primary cardiac conditions such as ductal-dependent congenital heart disease, cardiomyopathies, or myocarditis. It can be life-saving in patients without CHD e.g., babies have died from central venous long-line tips misplaced in the heart, perforating the atrial wall and causing tamponade.[26] These babies die because this is a clinically occult diagnosis, often made at autopsy. With ultrasound, it is an obvious diagnosis, even to an inexpert eye, and needs an immediate pericardiocentesis and line removal or repositioning.

## IN NEWBORN TRANSPORT

Many of the above issues are brought into focus in babies who need retrieval from smaller hospitals to a center with a NICU. These are a particularly high-risk group. Preterm babies needing ex utero transfer tend to be born after precipitate delivery, without full antenatal steroid cover, and may have received inexperienced resuscitation and early management. Their high risk results in worse outcomes. More mature babies often present with unexpected respiratory failure/PPHN or asphyxia, or both. Sometimes these babies have acute presentations, which may be cardiac in origin. Increasing portability of ultrasound equipment creates the opportunity to take imaging equipment on transport. Our group has recently completed a prospective observational study of point-of-care cardiac and cerebral ultrasound in the transport of about 100 sick newborns across New South Wales, Australia.[27] We showed that CPU in newborn transport is feasible and, in the late preterm/term group of babies, we confirmed a high incidence of clinically unsuspected hemodynamic compromise, as well as several patients with congenital heart disease who had been diagnosed clinically as PPHN and in whom transport was redirected to a cardiac center. In preterm neonates there was a high risk of hemodynamic abnormalities, particularly low SBF, and subsequent IVH.[28] There are clearly challenges to implementing this practice on a wider basis, most specifically with having equipment and skills available for the transport. The portability of ultrasound equipment continues to improve with tablet-sized machines available with adequate resolution, and more neonatologists are learning ultrasound skills, particularly those now in training. It is now unusual for neonatologists in Australia and New Zealand to qualify without appropriate ultrasound skills. It would seem inevitable that neonatal retrieval is another area where CPU will become commonplace in the not-too-distant future.

## Avoiding Inappropriate Therapy and Weaning

Much research time and energy has been spent on developing guidelines for commencing extra therapy in response to hemodynamic complications and abnormal physiology. However, one of the very important uses of CPU is to allow the physician to decide when expensive and potentially harmful therapies may not be required. Case Presentation 1 illustrates a common scenario we observe where there is what appears to be clinical evidence of "PPHN" with high oxygen requirements and lability, but without ultrasound evidence of raised pulmonary pressures or right-to-left ductal shunting (the duct may often be closed).[23] Inhaled NO in this setting has a high chance of being ineffective and may cause harm by changing the vascular resistance in a baby with balanced physiology. Other examples might include excessive use of volume in an infant who already has adequate cardiac filling/preload or use of vasopressor-inotropes in a baby with low blood pressure but normal cardiac output.[29] Similarly, deciding when to wean an infant with significant hemodynamic support can be assisted by CPU. Key information, such as identifying when the cardiac function has improved to start weaning inotropes or when the pulmonary pressures have dropped and the PDA shunt direction is becoming predominantly left to right to allow weaning of iNO or when the PDA has closed to limit exposure to NSAID,[30] is available in real time to the clinician. This new way of managing the individual infant now has a name – precision or personalized medicine.[31]

Neonatal ultrasound tends to be focused on the heart and brain, but the point of care possibilities extend to many other organ systems including lung ultrasound, abdominal ultrasound, and assessment of line positions.

## Does CPU Make a Difference?

Introduction of a new diagnostic imaging technology is often accompanied by calls for validation and justification of the cost.[4] Ultrasound machines are large and costly, though in the last few years there has been reduction both in size and in cost, such that portable tablet-sized machines are now affordable to most neonatal intensive care units. Training in ultrasound also entails a significant time commitment. The introduction of CPU is different than introducing a new, high-level diagnostic imaging modality. It is the additive improvement in care that comes from having ultrasound easily available to help with treatment choices. There are several randomized trials that have utilized CPU in decision-making within the protocol and demonstrated improved outcomes. These include indomethacin dose minimization during PDA treatment,[30] identification of infants at high risk of pulmonary hemorrhage and reducing risk by early PDA treatment,[32] and prevention of postoperative cardiorespiratory lability following PDA ligation.[33,34] In addition, there are a number of services that have published the results of auditing the introduction of this practice – generally, these audits have shown benefits ranging from discovery of unexpected findings through to avoidance of planned interventions.[35,36] In 2020 the European Society of Paediatric and Neonatal Intensive Care released evidence-based guidelines on CPU for critically ill neonates and children, highlighting the roles of CPU in this setting and the supporting evidence.[37]

Other medical craft groups (anesthetists, intensivists, emergency physicians) have adopted CPU as part of clinical practice and there is a significant body of literature supporting use in children and adults in the intensive care setting. The approach in this setting has been toward a focused assessment with specific aims or goals specified.[38] This is similar to the way that CPU is taught in Australia/New Zealand.

## Conclusions

The use of CPU in the care of sick and preterm neonates is rapidly expanding. The benefits of a portable, bedside technique that provides real-time, longitudinal data regarding the physiology of individual patients are being progressively recognized. The role of CPU in managing the transitioning term or preterm infant, the septic/asphyxiated infant, the shocked or hypotensive infant, and the infant with suspected PPHN or congenital heart disease is increasingly recognized. With the acceptance of the usefulness of ultrasound in the clinical setting, the need for appropriate training programs and accreditation increases. Internationally, countries have adopted different approaches to these needs. In Australia/New Zealand a training program based on modular education with periods of self-directed learning under the supervision of an accredited and experienced neonatologist has been adopted. This has led to an increase in ultrasound education in trainees with a subsequent wide distribution of ultrasound skills in most NICUs in Australia/New Zealand. A similar program has been successfully running in North America and Europe with an increasing group of neonatologists with ultrasound skills.

## REFERENCES

1. Plomgaard AM, van Oeveren W, Petersen TH, et al. The SafeBoosC II randomized trial: treatment guided by near-infrared spectroscopy reduces cerebral hypoxia without changing early biomarkers of brain injury. *Pediatr Res.* 2016;79(4):528-535.
2. Kluckow M, Seri I, Evans N, Kluckow M, Seri I, Evans N. Echocardiography and the neonatologist. *Pediatr Cardiol.* 2008;29(6):1043-1047.
3. Kluckow M, Evans N. Point of care ultrasound in the NICU-training, accreditation and ownership. *Eur J Pediatr.* 2016;175(2):289-290.
4. Mertens L. Neonatologist performed echocardiography-hype, hope or nope. *Eur J Pediatr.* 2016;175(2):291-293.
5. Nguyen J, Cascione M, Noori S. Analysis of lawsuits related to point-of-care ultrasonography in neonatology and pediatric subspecialties. *J Perinatol.* 2016;36(9):784-786.
6. Marin JR, Lewiss RE, American Academy of Pediatrics, Committee on Pediatric Emergency Medicine, et al. Point-of-care ultrasonography by pediatric emergency medicine physicians. *Pediatrics.* 2015;135(4):e1113-e1122.
7. Marin JR, Lewiss RE, American Academy of Pediatrics, Committee on Pediatric Emergency Medicine, et al. Point-of-care ultrasonography by pediatric emergency physicians. Policy statement. *Ann Emerg Med.* 2015;65(4):472-478.

8. Australasian Society for Ultrasound in Medicine. *Certificate in Clinician Performed Ultrasound.* 2018. Available at: https://www.asum.com.au/education/ccpu-course/. Accessed October 1, 2018.

9. Mertens L, Seri I, Marek J, et al. Targeted neonatal echocardiography in the neonatal intensive care unit: practice guidelines and recommendations for training. *Eur J Echocardiogr.* 2011; 12(10):715-736.

10. Singh Y, Gupta S, Groves AM, et al. Expert consensus statement 'Neonatologist-performed Echocardiography (NoPE)'-training and accreditation in UK. *Eur J Pediatr.* 2016;175(2):281-287.

11. McNamara P, Lai W. Growth of neonatal hemodynamics programs and targeted neonatal echocardiography performed by neonatologists. *J Am Soc Echocardiogr.* 2020;33(10):A15-A16.

12. Mertens L, Seri I, Marek J, et al. Targeted neonatal echocardiography in the neonatal intensive care unit: practice guidelines and recommendations for training. writing group of the American Society of Echocardiography (ASE) in collaboration with the European Association of Echocardiography (EAE) and the Association for European Pediatric Cardiologists (AEPC). *J Am Soc Echocardiogr.* 2011;24(10):1057-1078.

13. Hebert A, Lavoie PM, Giesinger RE, et al. Evolution of training guidelines for echocardiography performed by the neonatologist: toward hemodynamic consultation. *J Am Soc Echocardiogr.* 2019;32(6):785-790.

14. Osborn DA, Evans N, Kluckow M. Clinical detection of low upper body blood flow in very premature infants using blood pressure, capillary refill time, and central-peripheral temperature difference. *Arch Dis Child Fetal Neonatal Ed.* 2004;89(2):F168-F173.

15. Cetin I, Kantar A, Unal S, Cakar N. The assessment of time-dependent myocardial changes in infants with perinatal hypoxia. *J Matern Fetal Neonatal Med.* 2012;25(9):1564-1568.

16. Kluckow M, Evans N. Low systemic blood flow in the preterm infant. *Semin Neonatol.* 2001;6(1):75-84.

17. Osborn DA, Evans N, Kluckow M. Hemodynamic and antecedent risk factors of early and late periventricular/intraventricular hemorrhage in premature infants. *Pediatrics.* 2003;112(1 Pt 1):33-39.

18. Semberova J, O'Donnell SM, Franta J, Miletin J. Inhaled nitric oxide in preterm infants with prolonged preterm rupture of the membranes: a case series. *J Perinatol.* 2015;35(4):304-306.

19. Shah DM, Kluckow M. Early functional echocardiogram and inhaled nitric oxide: usefulness in managing neonates born following extreme preterm premature rupture of membranes (PPROM). *J Paediatr Child Health.* 2011;47(6):340-345.

20. Kluckow M, Evans N. Early echocardiographic prediction of symptomatic patent ductus arteriosus in preterm infants undergoing mechanical ventilation. *J Pediatr.* 1995;127(5):774-779.

21. de Waal K, Evans N. Hemodynamics in preterm infants with late-onset sepsis. *J Pediatr.* 2010;156(6):918-922.e1.

22. Saini SS, Kumar P, Kumar RM. Hemodynamic changes in preterm neonates with septic shock: a prospective observational study*. *Pediatr Crit Care Med.* 2014;15(5):443-450.

23. Evans N, Kluckow M, Currie A. Range of echocardiographic findings in term neonates with high oxygen requirements. *Arch Dis Child Fetal Neonatal Ed.* 1998;78(2):F105-F111.

24. Roze JC, Storme L, Zupan V, Morville P, Dinh-Xuan AT, Mercier JC. Echocardiographic investigation of inhaled nitric oxide in newborn babies with severe hypoxaemia. *Lancet.* 1994; 344(8918):303-305.

25. Desandes R, Desandes E, Droulle P, Didier F, Longrois D, Hascoet JM. Inhaled nitric oxide improves oxygenation in very premature infants with low pulmonary blood flow. *Acta Paediatr.* 2004; 93(1):66-69.

26. Kabra NS, Kluckow MR. Survival after an acute pericardial tamponade as a result of percutaneously inserted central venous catheter in a preterm neonate. *Indian J Pediatr.* 2001; 68(7):677-680.

27. Browning Carmo K, Lutz T, Berry A, Kluckow M, Evans N. Feasibility and utility of portable ultrasound during retrieval of sick term and late preterm infants. *Acta Paediatr.* 2016; 105(12):e549-e554.

28. Browning Carmo K, Lutz T, Greenhalgh M, Berry A, Kluckow M, Evans N. Feasibility and utility of portable ultrasound during retrieval of sick preterm infants. *Acta Paediatr.* 2017; 106(8):1296-1301.

29. Kluckow M, Evans N. Relationship between blood pressure and cardiac output in preterm infants requiring mechanical ventilation. *J Pediatr.* 1996;129(4):506-512.

30. Carmo KB, Evans N, Paradisis M. Duration of indomethacin treatment of the preterm patent ductus arteriosus as directed by echocardiography. *J Pediatr.* 2009;155(6):819-822.

31. Cahan A, Cimino JJ. Improving precision medicine using individual patient data from trials. *CMAJ.* 2016;189(5):e204–e207.

32. Kluckow M, Jeffery M, Gill A, Evans N. A randomised placebo-controlled trial of early treatment of the patent ductus arteriosus. *Arch Dis Child Fetal Neonatal Ed.* 2014;99(2):F99-F104.

33. Jain A, Sahni M, El-Khuffash A, Khadawardi E, Sehgal A, McNamara PJ. Use of targeted neonatal echocardiography to prevent postoperative cardiorespiratory instability after patent ductus arteriosus ligation. *J Pediatr.* 2012;160(4): 584-589.

34. O'Rourke DJ, El-Khuffash A, Moody C, Walsh K, Molloy EJ. Patent ductus arteriosus evaluation by serial echocardiography in preterm infants. *Acta Paediatr.* 2008;97(5):574-578.

35. El-Khuffash A, Herbozo C, Jain A, Lapointe A, McNamara PJ. Targeted neonatal echocardiography (TnECHO) service in a Canadian neonatal intensive care unit: a 4-year experience. *J Perinatol.* 2013;33(9):687-690.

36. Harabor A, Soraisham AS. Utility of targeted neonatal echocardiography in the management of neonatal illness. *J Ultrasound Med.* 2015;34(7):1259-1263.

37. Singh Y, Tissot C, Fraga MV, et al. International evidence-based guidelines on Point of Care Ultrasound (POCUS) for critically ill neonates and children issued by the POCUS Working Group of the European Society of Paediatric and Neonatal Intensive Care (ESPNIC). *Crit Care.* 2020;24(1):65.

38. Via G, Hussain A, Wells M, et al. International evidence-based recommendations for focused cardiac ultrasound. *J Am Soc Echocardiogr.* 2014;27(7):683.e1-683.e33.

# Chapter 10

# Assessment of Systemic Blood Flow and Myocardial Function in the Neonatal Period Using Ultrasound

Eirik Nestaas, Drude Fugelseth, and Beate Horsberg Eriksen

## Key Points

- Echocardiography is useful for the assessment of systemic blood flow and myocardial function.
- Systemic blood flow is a dynamic and complex variable.
- Blood flow through persistent fetal shunts influences cardiac output measurements from both ventricles.
- Superior vena cava flow as a measure of cardiac input is a surrogate measure for global cerebral blood flow and systemic blood flow in the transitional period.
- Fractional shortening and ejection fraction are the most common cavity indices of the left ventricle.
- The echocardiographic assessment of the right ventricular size, volume, and function is controversial because of its complex geometric structure.
- Mitral and tricuspid annular plane systolic excursions assess the motion of the atrioventricular plane relative to the apex and are indices of left and right ventricular systolic function.
- All indices of heart function are dependent on loading conditions.
- It is important to interpret any echocardiographic index of heart function in the context of the clinical situation, loading conditions, and other echocardiographic indices.

## Introduction

Echocardiography is widely used to assess systemic blood flow and heart function in the newborn infant. This chapter gives an overview of conventional echocardiographic methods for the assessment of systemic blood flow, ventricular size, and myocardial function in newborns in the absence of congenital heart defects.

Reliable methods to monitor cardiovascular and hemodynamic function are important for assessment of circulatory disturbances and guide optimal therapy in the newborn infant.[1,2] Evidence of functional echocardiography improving neonatal outcome is emerging in the form of observational studies showing changes in care and reduced use of medications for patent ductus arteriosus (PDA) treatment and inotropes for borderline hypotension with normal systemic blood flow.[3,4] Two-dimensional (2D) and Doppler echocardiography is useful to assess hemodynamic status in routine clinical practice, as well as in clinical research. A complex integration of different echocardiographic modalities is necessary for the assessment of structure and dimension, blood flow, myocardial function, and loading conditions. Basic knowledge of physical and technical principles of the different modalities, sufficient operator skills, and experience in measuring relevant echocardiographic indices, as well as a comprehensive understanding of normal physiological and pathological processes, are essential for the optimal use of echocardiography.[5]

Echocardiography has a central role in diagnosing and monitoring congenital heart disease, screening for PDA in preterm neonates, assessing heart function and pulmonary hemodynamics, detecting pericardial or pleural effusion and thrombosis, and verifying central line placement.[6] The most common scenarios for functional echocardiography in neonates are circulatory assessment during the transitional circulation period in very premature infants, assessment of PDA beyond the early transitional period, exploration of the reasons for circulatory compromise and hypotension, and diagnosis and following of treatment for persistent pulmonary hypertension of the newborn.

Understanding the physiology of cardiovascular adaptation after birth and the effect of diseases and prematurity are key factors in interpretation. The complex and dramatic cardiorespiratory changes that take place during the transitional phase from fetal to neonatal circulation may be critical in both preterm and sick term infants. The onset of breathing promotes a rapid decrease in pulmonary vascular resistance, with a subsequent increase in pulmonary blood flow.[7] The augmentation in pulmonary venous return increases the left heart preload and enables the left heart to handle the raised afterload following cord clamping and disconnection of the low-resistance placenta circuit.[8-10] Chapter 6 discusses the effects of the timing of cord clamping on cardiovascular transition. While the right ventricle (RV) plays the dominant role in fetal life, the left ventricle (LV) gradually dominates after birth.

Closure of the fetal shunts normally starts with functional closure of the foramen ovale due to the altered pressure difference between the left and right atria, even though a small left-to-right shunt across the foramen ovale may be persistent over time. The changes in pulmonary and systemic vascular resistance after onset of breathing and cord clamping reverse the shunting of blood through the ductus arteriosus from right-to-left shunting to left-to-right.[11] In term neonates the functional closure of the ductus arteriosus normally takes place within the first 2–3 days of postnatal life, while the ductus venosus may be persistent for several days after birth.[12-14]

A variety of conditions in the perinatal period, such as asphyxia, respiratory distress, sepsis, and metabolic and hematological diseases, as well as positive pressure ventilation, may affect the cardiovascular system and hence disturb the transitional phase. Persistent high pulmonary vascular resistance might be due to fetal and/or perinatal hypoxia, resulting in abnormal pulmonary vascular development and/or responsiveness to local vascular mediators or to hypoxia caused by lung disease or apnea.[15] Typical findings in pulmonary hypertension are bidirectional flow across the foramen ovale, bidirectional or right-to-left flow across

the ductus arteriosus, and increased RV afterload, especially in the case of restrictive ductal flow. The latter may affect coronary blood flow and subsequently myocardial perfusion and function. The resultant decrease in left ventricular filling further affects myocardial function. Systemic circulatory failure (shock) may develop due to low systemic blood flow.[16]

Preterm infants are especially vulnerable in the transitional circulatory phase (see Chapter 7). The fetal myocardium has a higher water content and a less organized structure compared to later in life. Mononucleated cardiomyocytes, fewer sarcomeres, and different isoforms of contractile proteins make the heart less compliant, with reduced cardiac functional reserves and less contractile ability.[17-19] The immature heart is less tolerant to the abrupt changes in preload and afterload at birth.[20,21] In preterm neonates with a PDA the effect of the gradually increasing left-to-right ductal shunting on cardiac performance has opposite effects on the pulmonary and the systemic circulation. It contributes to the increased pulmonary blood flow immediately after birth,[22] but a significant left-to-right shunt may impair systemic blood flow and cause a deterioration in cardiac performance and organ perfusion.[23]

When the blood flow decreases, compensatory mechanisms redistribute the blood supply to vital organs by selective vasodilatation and vasoconstriction. In this compensatory phase of shock the blood pressure can remain normal, although the blood supply to the body is low.[24] As long as the net systemic vascular resistance is higher than normal, the blood pressure can remain normal despite reduced systemic blood flow. Applying the indices discussed in this chapter can help the intensivist to identify shock in this compensatory phase, enabling intervention at an early stage.

## Assessment of Systemic Blood Flow by Ultrasound

Systemic blood flow is a complex and dynamic variable with rapid fluctuations caused by the changes in activity and metabolic demand of the different organs. Doppler echocardiography offers direct and indirect measures of systemic and organ blood flow.[25]

Blood flow by Doppler echocardiography is calculated as the product of the displacement of the velocity profile, called the velocity-time integral (VTI) of blood flow velocity, the cross-sectional area of the vessel at the site of the measurement, and the heart rate. VTI is measured by tracing the pulsed Doppler velocity signal. The cross-sectional area is found by measuring the diameter (D) and calculating the area as $(\pi \times (D/2)^2)$.[26] Assuming a circular vessel with constant cross-sectional area, blood flow (volume per time, usually mL/min) is calculated as (VTI [for one heartbeat] × cross-sectional area × heart rate).[27,28] A prerequisite for this calculation is a laminar parabolic flow profile representative of long, straight blood vessels under steady flow conditions, meaning that blood in the entire cross-sectional area moves at the speed drawn as the outer edge of the VTI. This prerequisite is probably met to a less extent in venous than arterial vessels, as is the assumption of a circular cross-sectional shape of the vessel. Blood flow in neonates is usually indexed by weight (mL/kg/min) and not body surface area because neonates and children have a relatively larger body surface area compared with body weight than adults. This results in non-linear-indexed hemodynamic variables.[29] It is important to minimize the angle of insonation when obtaining the VTI and to assess the diameter with the ultrasound beam perpendicular to the vessel at the true (maximal) diameter. An inappropriate angle will underestimate the VTI and overestimate the diameter. Due to

the squaring of the radius in the formula, inaccurate measures of the diameter may have considerable influence. We recommend averaging the measurements from a minimum of three cardiac cycles to minimize measurement error.[30] Intra- and inter-observer variability significantly affects the Doppler flow measurements.[31] Variation between measurements may be within the range of 30% in arteries and 50% in veins.[32]

## LEFT VENTRICULAR OUTPUT

Left ventricular output (LVO) reflects the systemic blood flow in the absence of ductus arteriosus shunt. We measure the Doppler flow velocity from the left ventricle at the aortic valve or in the ascending aorta from an apical window (Figure 10.1). Measuring LVO in neonates may be challenging due to the curving of the ascending aorta, which leaves the heart ascending to the left- and backward, making the angle of insonation more inaccurate compared to adults. A reproducible left outflow diameter is easier to achieve. There are different opinions about where to measure the diameter; from the low parasternal window at the hinge of the aortic valve cusps or just beyond the sinus of Valsalva in the ascending aorta.[33] It is important to perform serial measures in a consistent way. Accurate measures require assessment of the VTI and cross-sectional area at the same locality.

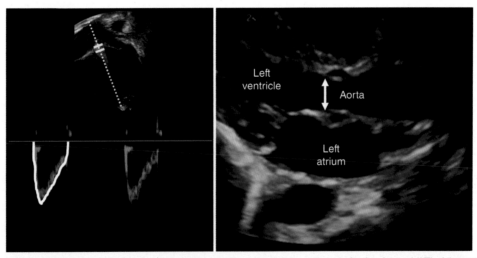

**Fig. 10.1  Assessment of left ventricular output from a term neonate.** The *left panel* shows the velocity time integral (*VTI*) of the aortic flow velocity for two heartbeats at the aortic valve hinges from the apical four-chamber view. The *white envelope* denotes tracing the VTI of the first heartbeat. The *right panel* shows a magnified parasternal long-axis view of the left ventricle. The *white arrow* denotes the diameter of the aortic valve "ring".

Several studies have validated flow measurements by VTI and cross-sectional area against other techniques.[27,30,34,35] Importantly, LVO will overestimate systemic blood flow if there is a large left-to-right shunting across the ductus arteriosus, which is especially relevant in preterm infants.[28] In the extreme situation of persistent pulmonary hypertension of the newborn with right-to-left shunting, LVO may underestimate true systemic blood flow.

## RIGHT VENTRICULAR OUTPUT

Right ventricular output (RVO) may be a more feasible index for systemic blood flow in neonates and especially in preterm babies.[36] Changes in RVO are associated with multiple factors, such as placental transfusion, gender, condition at birth, and early respiratory adaptation.[37]

Even though shunting of blood across the foramen ovale may contribute to RVO measurement, the magnitude of atrial shunting is usually less than the ductal shunting[28] and impaired systemic blood flow is therefore extremely rare when the RVO is normal. In the first 48 hours after birth, if the peak pulmonary valve velocity is more than 0.45 m/s, low systemic blood flow is unlikely.[36] Since the main pulmonary artery directs posteriorly, it is usually possible to obtain an optimal insonation angle for velocity measurements from the parasternal view (Figure 10.2). Measurement of pulmonary artery diameter may be challenging and is best obtained at the valve leaflet insertion from a slightly higher or tilted parasternal long-axis view.[38] The normal cardiac output from both left and right ventricle in neonates gradually increases after birth and is in the range of 150–300 mL/kg/min.[28]

## SUPERIOR VENA CAVA FLOW

Due to the influence of fetal shunts on cardiac output from both ventricles, assessment of cardiac input from the upper body by SVC is recommended as an additional measure for global cerebral and systemic blood flow in the transitional period.[39] As the brain is one of the main target organs for adequate perfusion, the focus on the return of blood from the upper body and brain may be justified, even though only 30% of the blood in the SVC may represent blood returning from the brain in preterm neonates.[39] Prolonged periods of low SVC flow indicate poor cerebral perfusion and are associated with increased risk of morbidity and mortality.[39-42]

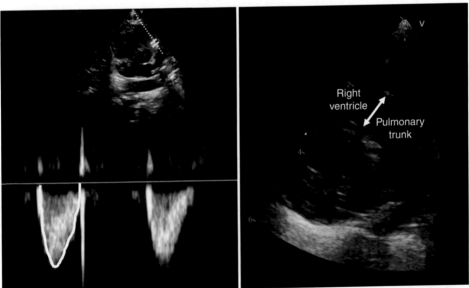

**Fig. 10.2 Assessment of right ventricular output from a term neonate.** The *left panel* shows the velocity time integral of the pulmonic flow velocity for two heartbeats at the pulmonary valve from the parasternal short-axis view. The *white envelope* denotes tracing the velocity time integral of the first heartbeat. The *right panel* shows a parasternal short-axis view of the outflow tract of the right ventricle. The *white arrow* denotes the diameter at the pulmonary valve.

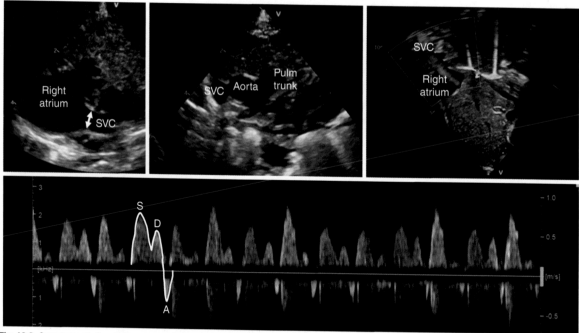

**Fig. 10.3 Assessment of superior vena cava flow.** The *left upper panel* shows a modified parasternal view, with a lengthwise view of the superior vena cava entering the right atrium. The *mid-panel* shows a modified parasternal view, with cross-sections of the superior vena cava and aorta. Note the ellipsoid cross-sectional shape of the superior vena cava. The *right upper panel* from a subcostal short-axis view with the *superimposed color flow image* shows blood entering the right atrium from the superior vena cava. The *lower panel* shows the superior vena cava velocity time integral over several heart cycles. The S and D peaks denote velocity peaks of flow into the right atrium during systole (*S*) and early diastole (*D*). The *negative A wave* denotes reversal of flow in the superior vena cava during atrial systole. The *white envelope* denotes tracing the velocity time integral of one heartbeat. *SVC,* Superior vena cava.

From the low subcostal window, a desirable angle of insonation for Doppler velocity measurement is obtained (Figure 10.3). Usually, the SVC VTI is biphasic with one positive peak in systole (S wave) and a smaller positive peak in early diastole (D wave), and a minimal positive or negative peak during atrial contraction (A wave). The negative A wave may increase in pathological situations, with increased pressure on the right side or high positive pressure ventilation. The original description of the technique recommends subtracting any significant negative peaks when assessing the VTI and averaging the VTI from 10 cardiac cycles due to the impact of respiration and the variations in the velocity profile (Figure 10.3).[39] As for the other estimates of blood flow, it is important to assess the VTI and the cross-sectional area of the vessel from the same place.

The preferred measurement of the SVC diameter is at the entrance to the right atrium just prior to the "funneling" or opening up of the vessel into the right atrium from the long-axis low to mid-parasternal view (Figure 10.3). Because SVC diameter varies more in size than the great arteries, it is recommended to measure the average of the maximum and minimum diameter over several heart cycles (minimum five) either on a 2D image or by use of M-mode.[39] Mean SVC flow is associated with gestation and increases from about 70 mL/kg/min to 90 mL/kg/min from 5 to 48 hours postnatally. The normal range is 40–120 mL/kg/min.[37,39]

The technique for measuring SVC flow by ultrasound has limitations. Although Doppler measures of arterial blood flow in the central circulation have good reproducibility and correlate well with invasive measures of blood flow, as discussed above, it is debated if the calculation developed for arterial flow is valid for venous flow. The most important methodological

**TABLE 10.1    Echocardiographic Assessment of Left Ventricular Internal Diameter (cm) in Diastole (LVIDd) and Systole (LVIDs) and Fractional Shortening (FS) in Newborn Infants by Weight.[52] Indices Are Given as Mean (Standard Deviation)**

| Echo Index | Birth Weight Cohort (g) | | | | | |
|---|---|---|---|---|---|---|
|  | 750–1249 | 1250–1749 | 1750–2249 | 2250–2749 | 2750–3249 | 3250–3749 |
| LVIDd | 1.26 (0.15) | 1.33 (0.12) | 1.52 (0.15) | 1.73 (0.22) | 1.79 (0.21) | 1.83 (0.20) |
| LVIDs | 0.85 (0.12) | 0.91 (0.10) | 0.98 (0.15) | 1.15 (0.14) | 1.17 (0.15) | 1.21 (0.17) |
| FS (%) | 33 (5) | 31 (4) | 36 (6) | 34 (4) | 34 (5) | 34 (4) |

problems with the assessment of SVC flow relate to the uncertainty of calculating the cross-section area of the vein. The formula pre-supposes a perfect round vessel and uses the square of the vessel radius to calculate a static cross-sectional area. These geometrical pre-suppositions, and the squaring of linear data, amplify measurement errors. A modification of the technique for measuring SVC flow has been published.[30] By interrogating the SVC Doppler flow from a suprasternal window, and measuring the cross-sectional area from a short axis view where the maximum and minimum cross-sectional area were directly traced, the agreement with magnetic resonance imaging–derived SVC flow was better. Additionally, the measure had less intra-user variation. The mid-panel of Figure 10.3 shows the SVC in cross-sectional view where a direct area tracing may be measured.

One magnetic resonance imaging study found the SVC method to be inaccurate[32] but others have criticized the study for not fulfilling standard criteria for repeated measurement validations.[43] Several guidelines for functional echocardiography in neonates do recommend the use of SVC flow, and low SVC flow is associated with adverse long-term outcome.[5,24,44,45]

## Cavity Measures

Calculation of cavity function indices involves assessment of changes between the largest and smallest cavity measurements in the cardiac cycle (usually end-diastole and end-systole). Indices based on percentage change between measurements or sizes describe heart function relatively independently of heart size. More geometrical assumptions are a prerequisite for the estimate of cavity sizes from unidimensional measurements compared to 2D measurements.

## CAVITY MEASURES OF THE LEFT VENTRICLE

LV function indices are the most frequently used indices of heart function in neonates. Despite growing evidence of its shortcomings and low ability to detect pathology and maturational changes,[46-51] the most frequently used cavity index in neonates is fractional shortening (FS). FS is assessed as the relative change during the cardiac cycle in the internal diameter of the LV. Diameters relate closely to bodyweight (Table 10.1) and normal FS values reported are often 30–45% in neonates[46-49,52] with little variation by weight. FS can be obtained from the parasternal or subcostal views[38,53] using M-mode or 2D images (Figure 10.4). The diameter is assessed perpendicular to the cavity at the tip of the mitral valve

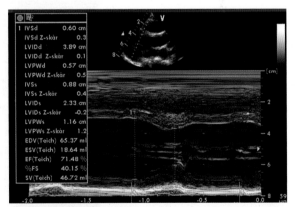

**Fig. 10.4. Fractional shortening of the left ventricle assessed by M-mode from a parasternal long-axis view.** The image shows assessment of the septum, internal diameter of the left ventricle, and the posterior wall. The fractional shortening is the change in diameter of the left ventricle cavity, relative to the diameter at end-diastole. (LVIDd – LVIDs)/LVIDd × 100. *LVIDd*, End-diastolic diameter of left ventricle; *LVIDs*, end-systolic diameter of left ventricle.

leaflets.[38] Its use as a cavity measure has, as a prerequisite, normal LV geometry and symmetric contraction, including normal septal motion.[38,53]

Ejection fraction (EF) is the fraction of end-diastolic volume ejected during systole. Published guidelines acknowledge estimation of EF by LV cavity areas from apical four-chamber and two-chamber views at end-systole and end-diastole by the Simpson biplane method (Figure 10.5).[38,54] Biplane EF has shown better discriminating capabilities than FS in neonates.[49,50] The Teich formula estimates the EF from FS.[55] The geometric assumptions for this formula are seldom met in pathological states and guidelines today do not recommend reporting EF estimates from FS.[54]

## CAVITY MEASURES OF THE RIGHT VENTRICLE

There are still controversies on how to assess RV size, volume, and function because of its complex geometric structure, and there is no accepted echocardiographic gold standard available.[38] Cavity measurements of the RV using ultrasound underestimate measurements by magnetic resonance imaging and the two modalities correlate poorly, especially in situations with volume overload.[56,57] The fractional area change (FAC) assesses the relative change in RV area during contraction, usually obtained from an RV-focused apical four-chamber recording by counter-clockwise rotation from the standard four-chamber view to expand the RV cavity to its maximum area.[54] RV FAC assessed from the RV-focused apical four-chamber view is hampered by low reproducibility, and better reproducibility has been obtained by assessing the RV FAC from the apical three-chamber view.[58] Some use the global RV FAC as the average of RV FAC from the apical three-chamber view and the RV-focused apical four-chamber view.[58]

Cavity measures assess myocardial function relative to the loading conditions and are not per se indices of the contractile properties of the myocardium. Preload has a direct impact on most diastolic cavity sizes. A high preload tends to increase diastolic chamber size. The diastolic cavity sizes are the denominator in the formulas and, if isolated, this would decrease the cavity functional indices. However, high preload also increases contraction due to the Frank-Starling effect,[59] and the net effect of the increased preload is increased cavity functional indices in most clinical situations.

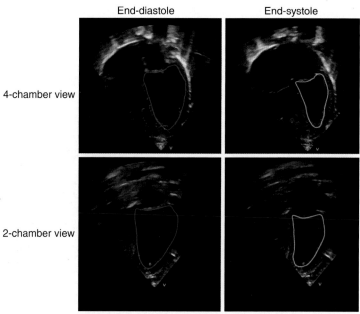

**Fig. 10.5 Assessment of left ventricle ejection fraction by Simpson biplane method.** Apical four-chamber (*upper panels*) and two-chamber (*lower panels*) at end-diastole (*left*) and end-systole (*right*). *Drawings* denote the cavity at end-diastole and end-systole. Biplane calculation involves calculating the ventricle volumes from areas at end of diastole and end of systole.

Increased afterload tends to increase end-systolic size and hence reduce the cavity functional indices. Factors within the myocardial wall can affect cavity measurements. Hypertrophic walls lead to smaller cavity measurements. The relative impact on the measurements is usually higher in systole, leading to higher cavity functional indices.

Severe preload and afterload alterations will influence the measurements in various hemodynamic scenarios. A premature neonate with normal LV contractility for gestational age and a large persistent ductus arteriosus might have LV function indices indicating normal or supernormal function because of the high preload and low afterload. A neonate with normal RV contractility and pulmonary hypertension might have reduced RV indices due to high afterload and possibly reduced LV indices due to low preload. In situations with reduced intrinsic myocardial contractility, cavity measures can be low in severe cases,[47] but several studies have shown that cavity measures (unidimensional measurements in particular) are relatively insensitive as heart function indices in clinical situations with reduced contractility.[46,47,51,60-63]

## Mitral and Tricuspid Annular Plane Systolic Excursion

The LV has a complex myocardial architecture. Fibers are principally longitudinally oriented in the sub-endocardial and sub-epicardial layer, and mostly circumferentially oriented in the mid-myocardial layer.[64] The intraventricular septum has a mixture of both longitudinal and circulatory fibers.[65] The longitudinal shortening of the LV relates closely to the LV stroke volume and EF.[66-68] In the RV longitudinal muscle fibers predominate in the free wall,[65] and longitudinal shortening contributes more than circumferential shortening to overall RV function.[69,70] Thus long-axis functions of both ventricles are important measures of global ventricular function.

The base of the heart descends toward the apex in systole due to the longitudinal shortening and ascends to its former position in diastole, while the apex is stationary due to tethering. Mitral annular plane systolic excursion (MAPSE) is now an accepted method for assessing LV long-axis systolic function.[64,71] Reference values for MAPSE have been published for term infants.[72]

Similarly, tricuspid annular plane systolic excursion (TAPSE) reflects the longitudinal systolic function of the RV.[73] TAPSE correlates well with EF, as measured by 2D echocardiography and radionuclide angiography in adults.[74] Cross-sectional studies providing reference values for term infants have also been published.[4,75,76]

The sonographer can assess atrioventricular annular excursions using the standard M-mode technique, with the interrogation line crossing the attachments of the MV (left lateral and septal MAPSE) and at the lateral attachment of the TV (TAPSE) from the four-chamber view. In adults it is generally advocated to average measurements of MAPSE at four standard points, namely septal and lateral in the four-chamber view and anterior and posterior in the two-chamber view.[77] However, a large study showed that the mean value of the two points of the four-chamber view resulted in the same mean as the four points of the two- and four-chamber views.[78] There is no clear recommendation to average MAPSE measurements in children and neonates. The septum is more dedicated to the dominant right ventricle in early postnatal age, and thereafter the dominance gradually shifts toward left ventricle, rendering the septal MAPSE more ambiguous to ventricular function. It is also possible to obtain the M-mode images by post-processing 2D B-mode recordings. The measurement at each hinge is the distance between the maximal backward excursion from the apex in diastole and the maximal systolic excursion in systole (Figure 10.6). Tables 10.2 and 10.3 show reference values for MAPSE and TAPSE, respectively, in neonates. It is important to emphasize that atrioventricular annulus excursions are, as cavity measures, dependent on loading conditions due to the Starling mechanism. Also, basal excursions will vary with heart size. Thus normalizing TAPSE and MAPSE by left ventricular end-diastolic length will appreciate this dependency and will also be a surrogate measurement for ventricular strain.[79,80]

Guidelines advise aligning the M-mode cursor parallel to the motion of the annulus.[54] Contrary to the effect on velocity using Doppler measurements, angle deviation will tend to overestimate M-mode measurements (Figure 10.7). Because M-mode images assess excursion along the hypotenuse, the excursion will be overestimated dependent on the cosine of the angle

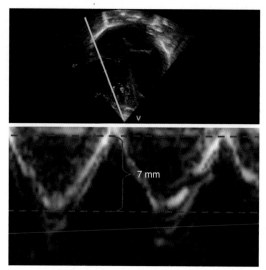

**Fig. 10.6 Post-processed M-mode tracing of tricuspid annular plane systolic excursion (TAPSE) in a term neonate.** The *upper panel* shows the grayscale image with the *solid line* denoting the direction of the M-mode line. The *white fluctuating line* in the *lower panel* is the signal from the right lateral hinge of the atrioventricular plane in two heart cycles. The *dotted horizontal lines* denote the positions at end-diastole and at end-systole. The distance between systolic and diastolic positions is the excursion, 7 mm in this example.

### TABLE 10.3 Measurements of Tricuspid Annular Plane Systolic Excursion (cm) by Gestational Age[81]

| GA | Mean − 2SD | Mean | Mean + 2SD |
|----|-----------|------|-----------|
| 26 | 0.30 | 0.44 | 0.59 |
| 27 | 0.36 | 0.48 | 0.61 |
| 28 | 0.37 | 0.52 | 0.68 |
| 29 | 0.41 | 0.57 | 0.73 |
| 30 | 0.48 | 0.60 | 0.71 |
| 31 | 0.53 | 0.63 | 0.74 |
| 32 | 0.51 | 0.68 | 0.85 |
| 33 | 0.58 | 0.70 | 0.83 |
| 34 | 0.60 | 0.73 | 0.87 |
| 35 | 0.61 | 0.74 | 0.88 |
| 36 | 0.65 | 0.78 | 0.92 |
| 37 | 0.68 | 0.82 | 0.96 |
| 38 | 0.75 | 0.86 | 0.97 |
| 39 | 0.77 | 0.90 | 1.02 |
| 40 | 0.81 | 0.95 | 1.10 |

*GA*, Gestational age; *Mean*, mean value; *Mean −2SD*, mean value minus 2 standard deviations; *Mean + 2SD*, mean value plus 2 standard deviations.

### TABLE 10.2 Measurements of Mitral Annular Plane Systolic Excursion (cm) From the Lateral Hinge of the Atrioventricular Plane by Gestational Age[88]

| GA | Mean − 2SD | Mean | Mean + 2SD |
|----|-----------|------|-----------|
| 26 | 0.26 | 0.36 | 0.46 |
| 27 | 0.28 | 0.38 | 0.48 |
| 23 | 0.25 | 0.4 | 0.55 |
| 29 | 0.29 | 0.42 | 0.54 |
| 30 | 0.26 | 0.42 | 0.58 |
| 31 | 0.32 | 0.45 | 0.58 |
| 32 | 0.27 | 0.43 | 0.59 |
| 33 | 0.24 | 0.44 | 0.64 |
| 34 | 0.36 | 0.48 | 0.6 |
| 35 | 0.34 | 0.49 | 0.64 |
| 36 | 0.33 | 0.48 | 0.63 |
| 37 | 0.31 | 0.5 | 0.68 |
| 38 | 0.41 | 0.53 | 0.65 |
| 39 | 0.32 | 0.52 | 0.71 |
| 40 | 0.40 | 0.56 | 0.73 |

*GA*, Gestational age; *Mean*, mean value; *Mean − 2SD*, mean value minus 2 standard deviations; *Mean + 2SD*, mean value plus 2 standard deviations.

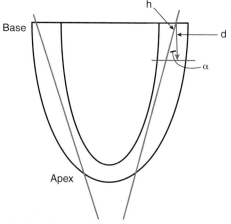

**Fig. 10.7 The effect of angle error on the measured atrioventricular plane excursion.** *Gray line*, direction of the ultrasound beam; *d*, true excursion; *h*, measured excursion (hypotenuse of the triangle, falsely high excursion); $\alpha$, the angle error. In measurements from an M-mode image the excursion is the hypotenuse of the triangle (h) measured along the direction of the ultrasound beam. The true excursion is the distance (d) that the atrioventricular plane moves during systole. $\alpha$ is the angle between the direction of the atrioventricular plane excursion and ultrasound beam, i.e., between the vector for the true excursion (d) and the vector for the ultrasound beam (h). The excursion assessed by M-mode (h in the figure) will overestimate the true excursion (d in the figure), with a factor of $1/\cos(\alpha)$ ($\alpha$ = angle error); the measured excursion (h) = true excursion $(d)/\cos(\alpha)$.

between the direction of the motion and the ultrasound beam. In general, angle deviation will be less in septal than in lateral recordings in apical four-chamber views due to better septal alignment with the ultrasound beam. TAPSE increases linearly with gestational age and body weight.[81]

Apart from reference values, there are also some data on TAPSE and MAPSE in clinical conditions in neonates. TAPSE improved and MAPSE was unchanged in premature neonates with RV afterload reduction after administration of surfactant.[82] It has also been shown that TAPSE may serve as a useful echocardiographic adjunct in assessing right ventricular myocardial function in infants with persistent pulmonary hypertension of the newborn[83] and give physiological real-time information to guide treatment in bronchopulmonary dysplasia.[84] TAPSE improved with reduction in pulmonary vascular resistance following transition after birth,[49,85] and TAPSE was lower in term neonates with persistent pulmonary hypertension of the newborn than in controls.[85] Impaired right ventricular outcome by TAPSE was associated with impaired outcome in infants with hypoxic-ischemic encephalopathy undergoing therapeutic hypothermia and infants with persistent pulmonary hypertension of the newborn.[4,87] MAPSE has also been shown to be suitable for assessing LV systolic function postoperatively after surgery for congenital heart defects in infants.[86]

## Conclusion

The most common scenarios for use of functional echocardiography in neonates are to assess the hemodynamic status during the transitional circulation period in very premature infants; assess the myocardial function, cardiac output, and significance of persistent fetal shunts in infants with circulatory compromise; and assess pulmonary circulation and hypertension throughout the neonatal course.

In line with most diagnostic tools there is no specific, single gold-standard echocardiographic measurement or index for assessing myocardial function and systemic blood flow in newborn infants. Evidence for echocardiography-guided improvements in neonatal outcomes is emerging. The neonatologist must always interpret an echocardiographic index in context with other indices and the clinical situation. Combining different methods

provides useful information about the hemodynamic situation in sick newborn infants to guide management. Systemic blood flow is most reliably assessed from the aortic or pulmonary blood flow when the fetal shunts are closed. If there is significant left-to-right shunt over either of the fetal shunts, the systemic blood flow is usually sufficient if the right heart output and Doppler flow velocity are within the normal range. Cavity measures of the left heart function are highly dependent on load. Longitudinal indices (MAPSE and TAPSE) are indices of left and right myocardial heart function.

## REFERENCES

1. Vincent JL, Rhodes A, Perel A, et al. Clinical review: update on hemodynamic monitoring – a consensus of 16. *Crit Care.* 2011;15(4):229.
2. Tissot C, Singh Y. Neonatal functional echocardiography. *Curr Opin Pediatr.* 2020;32(2):235-244.
3. Prasad R, Saha B, Kumar A. Ventricular function in congenital diaphragmatic hernia: a systematic review and meta-analysis. *Eur J Pediatr.* 2022;181(3):1071-1083.
4. Giesinger RE, El Shahed AI, Castaldo MP, et al. Neurodevelopmental outcome following hypoxic ischaemic encephalopathy and therapeutic hypothermia is related to right ventricular performance at 24-hour postnatal age. *Arch Dis Child Fetal Neonatal Ed.* 2022;107(1):70-75.
5. Mertens L, Seri I, Marek J, et al. Targeted neonatal echocardiography in the neonatal intensive care unit: practice guidelines and recommendations for training. *Eur J Echocardiogr.* 2011;12(10):715-736.
6. Kluckow M. Use of ultrasound in the haemodynamic assessment of the sick neonate. *Arch Dis Child Fetal Neonatal Ed.* 2014;99(4):F332-F337.
7. Teitel DF, Iwamoto HS, Rudolph AM. Changes in the pulmonary circulation during birth-related events. *Pediatr Res.* 1990;27(4 Pt 1):372-378.
8. Agata Y, Hiraishi S, Oguchi K, et al. Changes in left ventricular output from fetal to early neonatal life. *J Pediatr.* 1991;119(3):441-445.
9. Bhatt S, Alison BJ, Wallace EM, et al. Delaying cord clamping until ventilation onset improves cardiovascular function at birth in preterm lambs. *J Physiol.* 2013;591(8):2113-2126.
10. Hooper SB, Te Pas AB, Lang J, et al. Cardiovascular transition at birth: a physiological sequence. *Pediatr Res.* 2015;77(5):608-614.
11. Mott JC. Control of the foetal circulation. *J Exp Biol.* 1982;100:129-146.
12. Fugelseth D, Lindemann R, Liestol K, Kiserud T, Langslet A. Ultrasonographic study of ductus venosus in healthy neonates. *Arch Dis Child Fetal Neonatal Ed.* 1997;77(2):F131-F134.
13. Fugelseth D, Lindemann R, Liestol K, Kiserud T, Langslet A. Postnatal closure of ductus venosus in preterm infants < or = 32 weeks. An ultrasonographic study. *Early Hum Dev.* 1998;53(2):163-169.
14. Kondo M, Itoh S, Kunikata T, et al. Time of closure of ductus venosus in term and preterm neonates. *Arch Dis Child Fetal Neonatal Ed.* 2001;85(1):F57-F59.

15. Steinhorn RH. Neonatal pulmonary hypertension. *Pediatr Crit Care Med.* 2010;11(suppl 2):S79-S84.
16. Jain A, McNamara PJ. Persistent pulmonary hypertension of the newborn: advances in diagnosis and treatment. *Semin Fetal Neonatal Med.* 2015;20(4):262-271.
17. Paradis AN, Gay MS, Zhang L. Binucleation of cardiomyocytes: the transition from a proliferative to a terminally differentiated state. *Drug Discov Today.* 2014;19(5):602-609.
18. Iruretagoyena JI, Gonzalez-Tendero A, Garcia-Canadilla P, et al. Cardiac dysfunction is associated with altered sarcomere ultrastructure in intrauterine growth restriction. *Am J Obstet Gynecol.* 2014;210(6):550.e1-550.e7.
19. Bensley JG, Moore L, De Matteo R, Harding R, Black MJ. Impact of preterm birth on the developing myocardium of the neonate. *Pediatr Res.* 2018;83(4):880-888.
20. Eiby YA, Lumbers ER, Headrick JP, Lingwood BE. Left ventricular output and aortic blood flow in response to changes in preload and afterload in the preterm piglet heart. *Am J Physiol Regul Integr Comp Physiol.* 2012;303(7):R769-R777.
21. Lee A, Nestaas E, Liestol K, Brunvand L, Lindemann R, Fugelseth D. Tissue Doppler imaging in very preterm infants during the first 24 h of life: an observational study. *Arch Dis Child Fetal Neonatal Ed.* 2014;99(1):F64-F69.
22. Noori S, Wlodaver A, Gottipati V, McCoy M, Schultz D, Escobedo M. Transitional changes in cardiac and cerebral hemodynamics in term neonates at birth. *J Pediatr.* 2012;160(6):943-948.
23. Evans N, Moorcraft J. Effect of patency of the ductus arteriosus on blood pressure in very preterm infants. *Arch Dis Child.* 1992;67(10 Spec No):1169-1173.
24. de Boode WP, van der Lee R, Eriksen BH, et al. The role of neonatologist performed echocardiography in the assessment and management of neonatal shock. *Pediatr Res.* 2018;84(suppl 1):57-67.
25. Anavekar NS, Oh JK. Doppler echocardiography: a contemporary review. *J Cardiol.* 2009;54(3):347-358.
26. Ihlen H, Amlie JP, Dale J, et al. Determination of cardiac output by Doppler echocardiography. *Br Heart J.* 1984;51(1):54-60.
27. Alverson DC, Eldridge M, Dillon T, Yabek SM, Berman Jr W. Noninvasive pulsed Doppler determination of cardiac output in neonates and children. *J Pediatr.* 1982;101(1):46-50.
28. Evans N, Kluckow M. Early determinants of right and left ventricular output in ventilated preterm infants. *Arch Dis Child Fetal Neonatal Ed.* 1996;74(2):F88-F94.
29. Sigurdsson TS, Lindberg L. Indexing haemodynamic variables in young children. *Acta Anaesthesiol Scand.* 2021;65(2):195-202.
30. Ficial B, Bonafiglia E, Padovani EM, et al. A modified echocardiographic approach improves reliability of superior vena caval flow quantification. *Arch Dis Child Fetal Neonatal Ed.* 2017;102(1):F7-F11.
31. Lee A, Liestol K, Nestaas E, Brunvand L, Lindemann R, Fugelseth D. Superior vena cava flow: feasibility and reliability of the off-line analyses. *Arch Dis Child Fetal Neonatal Ed.* 2010;95(2):F121-F125.
32. Ficial B, Finnemore AE, Cox DJ, et al. Validation study of the accuracy of echocardiographic measurements of systemic blood flow volume in newborn infants. *J Am Soc Echocardiogr.* 2013;26(12):1365-1371.
33. Roman MJ, Devereux RB, Kramer-Fox R, O'Loughlin J. Two-dimensional echocardiographic aortic root dimensions in normal children and adults. *Am J Cardiol.* 1989;64(8):507-512.
34. Pugsley J, Lerner AB. Cardiac output monitoring: is there a gold standard and how do the newer technologies compare? *Semin Cardiothorac Vasc Anesth.* 2010;14(4):274-282.
35. Mellander M, Sabel KG, Caidahl K, Solymar L, Eriksson B. Doppler determination of cardiac output in infants and children: comparison with simultaneous thermodilution. *Pediatr Cardiol.* 1987;8(4):241-246.
36. Evans N. Which inotrope for which baby? *Arch Dis Child Fetal Neonatal Ed.* 2006;91(3):F213-F220.
37. Popat H, Robledo KP, Kirby A, et al. Associations of measures of systemic blood flow used in a randomized trial of delayed cord clamping in preterm infants. *Pediatr Res.* 2019;86(1):71-76.
38. Lopez L, Colan SD, Frommelt PC, et al. Recommendations for quantification methods during the performance of a pediatric echocardiogram: a report from the Pediatric Measurements Writing Group of the American Society of Echocardiography Pediatric and Congenital Heart Disease Council. *J Am Soc Echocardiogr.* 2010;23(5):465-577.
39. Kluckow M, Evans N. Superior vena cava flow in newborn infants: a novel marker of systemic blood flow. *Arch Dis Child Fetal Neonatal Ed.* 2000;82(3):F182-F187.
40. Azhibekov T, Soleymani S, Lee BH, Noori S, Seri I. Hemodynamic monitoring of the critically ill neonate: an eye on the future. *Semin Fetal Neonatal Med.* 2015;20(4):246-254.
41. de Waal K, Kluckow M. Superior vena cava flow: role, assessment and controversies in the management of perinatal perfusion. *Semin Fetal Neonatal Med.* 2020;25(5):101122.
42. Bischoff AR, Giesinger RE, Stanford AH, Ashwath R, McNamara PJ. Assessment of superior vena cava flow and cardiac output in different patterns of patent ductus arteriosus shunt. *Echocardiography.* 2021;38(9):1524-1533.
43. Kluckow MR, Evans NJ. Superior vena cava flow is a clinically valid measurement in the preterm newborn. *J Am Soc Echocardiogr.* 2014;27(7):794.
44. Singh Y, Gupta S, Groves AM, et al. Expert consensus statement "Neonatologist-performed Echocardiography (NoPE)"-training and accreditation in UK. *Eur J Pediatr.* 2016;175(2):281-287.
45. de Boode WP, Singh Y, Gupta S, et al. Recommendations for neonatologist performed echocardiography in Europe: consensus statement endorsed by European Society for Paediatric Research (ESPR) and European Society for Neonatology (ESN). *Pediatr Res.* 2016;80(4):465-471.
46. Nestaas E, Stoylen A, Brunvand L, Fugelseth D. Longitudinal strain and strain rate by tissue Doppler are more sensitive indices than fractional shortening for assessing the reduced myocardial function in asphyxiated neonates. *Cardiol Young.* 2011;21(1):1-7.
47. Wei Y, Xu J, Xu T, Fan J, Tao S. Left ventricular systolic function of newborns with asphyxia evaluated by tissue Doppler imaging. *Pediatr Cardiol.* 2009;30(6):741-746.
48. Abdel-Hady HE, Matter MK, El-Arman MM. Myocardial dysfunction in neonatal sepsis: a tissue Doppler imaging study. *Pediatr Crit Care Med.* 2012;13(3):318-323.
49. James AT, Corcoran JD, Jain A, et al. Assessment of myocardial performance in preterm infants less than 29 weeks gestation during the transitional period. *Early Hum Dev.* 2014;90(12):829-835.
50. Hirose A, Khoo NS, Aziz K, et al. Evolution of left ventricular function in the preterm infant. *J Am Soc Echocardiogr.* 2015;28(3):302-308.
51. Malowitz JR, Forsha DE, Smith PB, Cotten CM, Barker PC, Tatum GH. Right ventricular echocardiographic indices predict poor

outcomes in infants with persistent pulmonary hypertension of the newborn. *Eur Heart J Cardiovasc Imaging.* 2015;16(11): 1224-1231.

52. Walther FJ, Siassi B, King J, Wu PY. Echocardiographic measurements in normal preterm and term neonates. *Acta Paediatr Scand.* 1986;75(4):563-568.

53. Lai WW, Geva T, Shirali GS, et al. Guidelines and standards for performance of a pediatric echocardiogram: a report from the Task Force of the Pediatric Council of the American Society of Echocardiography. *J Am Soc Echocardiogr.* 2006;19(12):1413-1430.

54. Lang RM, Badano LP, Mor-Avi V, et al. Recommendations for cardiac chamber quantification by echocardiography in adults: an update from the American Society of Echocardiography and the European Association of Cardiovascular Imaging. *Eur Heart J Cardiovasc Imaging.* 2015;16(3):233-270.

55. Teichholz LE, Kreulen T, Herman MV, Gorlin R. Problems in echocardiographic volume determinations: echocardiographic-angiographic correlations in the presence of absence of asynergy. *Am J Cardiol.* 1976;37(1):7-11.

56. Helbing WA, Bosch HG, Maliepaard C, et al. Comparison of echocardiographic methods with magnetic resonance imaging for assessment of right ventricular function in children. *Am J Cardiol.* 1995;76(8):589-594.

57. Lai WW, Gauvreau K, Rivera ES, Saleeb S, Powell AJ, Geva T. Accuracy of guideline recommendations for two-dimensional quantification of the right ventricle by echocardiography. *Int J Cardiovasc Imaging.* 2008;24(7):691-698.

58. Jain A, Mohamed A, El-Khuffash A, et al. A comprehensive echocardiographic protocol for assessing neonatal right ventricular dimensions and function in the transitional period: normative data and z scores. *J Am Soc Echocardiogr.* 2014; 27(12):1293-1304.

59. Patterson SW, Starling EH. On the mechanical factors which determine the output of the ventricles. *J Physiol.* 1914;48(5): 357-379.

60. Nestaas E, Skranes JH, Stoylen A, Brunvand L, Fugelseth D. The myocardial function during and after whole-body therapeutic hypothermia for hypoxic-ischemic encephalopathy, a cohort study. *Early Hum Dev.* 2014;90(5):247-252.

61. Nestaas E, Stoylen A, Fugelseth D. Myocardial performance assessment in neonates by one-segment strain and strain rate analysis by tissue Doppler – a quality improvement cohort study. *BMJ Open.* 2012;2(4):e001636.

62. Czernik C, Rhode S, Helfer S, Schmalisch G, Buhrer C. Left ventricular longitudinal strain and strain rate measured by 2-D speckle tracking echocardiography in neonates during whole-body hypothermia. *Ultrasound Med Biol.* 2013;39(8):1343-1349.

63. Molicki J, Dekker I, de GY, van BF. Cerebral blood flow velocity wave form as an indicator of neonatal left ventricular heart function. *Eur J Ultrasound.* 2000;12(1):31-41.

64. Henein MY, Gibson DG. Normal long axis function. *Heart.* 1999;81(2):111-113.

65. Naito H, Arisawa J, Harada K, Yamagami H, Kozuka T, Tamura S. Assessment of right ventricular regional contraction and comparison with the left ventricle in normal humans: a cine magnetic resonance study with presaturation myocardial tagging. *Br Heart J.* 1995;74(2):186-191.

66. Simonson JS, Schiller NB. Descent of the base of the left ventricle: an echocardiographic index of left ventricular function. *J Am Soc Echocardiogr.* 1989;2(1):25-35.

67. Jones CJ, Raposo L, Gibson DG. Functional importance of the long axis dynamics of the human left ventricle. *Br Heart J.* 1990;63(4):215-220.

68. Pai RG, Bodenheimer MM, Pai SM, Koss JH, Adamick RD. Usefulness of systolic excursion of the mitral anulus as an index of left-ventricular systolic function. *Am J Cardiol.* 1991;67(2): 222-224.

69. Brown SB, Raina A, Katz D, Szerlip M, Wiegers SE, Forfia PR. Longitudinal shortening accounts for the majority of right ventricular contraction and improves after pulmonary vasodilator therapy in normal subjects and patients with pulmonary arterial hypertension. *Chest.* 2011;140(1):27-33.

70. Kukulski T, Hubbert L, Arnold M, Wranne B, Hatle L, Sutherland GR. Normal regional right ventricular function and its change with age: a Doppler myocardial imaging study. *J Am Soc Echocardiogr.* 2000;13(3):194-204.

71. Lundback S. Cardiac pumping and function of the ventricular septum. *Acta Physiol Scand Suppl.* 1986;550:1-101.

72. Koestenberger M, Nagel B, Ravekes W, et al. Left ventricular long-axis function: reference values of the mitral annular plane systolic excursion in 558 healthy children and calculation of z-score values. *Am Heart J.* 2012;164(1):125-131.

73. Rudski LG, Lai WW, Afilalo J, et al. Guidelines for the echocardiographic assessment of the right heart in adults: a report from the American Society of Echocardiography endorsed by the European Association of Echocardiography, a registered branch of the European Society of Cardiology, and the Canadian Society of Echocardiography. *J Am Soc Echocardiogr.* 2010;23(7): 685-788.

74. Kaul S, Tei C, Hopkins JM, Shah PM. Assessment of right ventricular-function using two-dimensional echocardiography. *Am Heart J.* 1984;107(3):526-531.

75. Koestenberger M, Ravekes W, Everett AD, et al. Right ventricular function in infants, children and adolescents: reference values of the tricuspid annular plane systolic excursion (TAPSE) in 640 healthy patients and calculation of z score values. *J Am Soc Echocardiogr.* 2009;22(6):715-719.

76. Jain A, El-Khuffash AF, van Herpen CH, et al. Cardiac function and ventricular interactions in persistent pulmonary hypertension of the newborn. *Pediatr Crit Care Med.* 2021;22(2):e145-e157.

77. Mondillo S, Galderisi M, Ballo P, Marino PN, Study Group of Echocardiography of the Italian Society of C. Left ventricular systolic longitudinal function: comparison among simple M-mode, pulsed, and M-mode color tissue Doppler of mitral annulus in healthy individuals. *J Am Soc Echocardiogr.* 2006; 19(9):1085-1091.

78. Dalen H, Thorstensen A, Vatten LJ, Aase SA, Stoylen A. Reference values and distribution of conventional echocardiographic Doppler measures and longitudinal tissue Doppler velocities in a population free from cardiovascular disease. *Circ Cardiovasc Imaging.* 2010;3(5):614-622.

79. Urheim S, Edvardsen T, Torp H, Angelsen B, Smiseth OA. Myocardial strain by Doppler echocardiography. Validation of a new method to quantify regional myocardial function. *Circulation.* 2000;102(10):1158-1164.

80. Eriksen BH, Nestaas E, Hole T, Liestol K, Stoylen A, Fugelseth D. Myocardial function in term and preterm infants. Influence of heart size, gestational age and postnatal maturation. *Early Hum Dev.* 2014;90(7):359-364.

81. Koestenberger M, Nagel B, Ravekes W, et al. Systolic right ventricular function in preterm and term neonates: reference values of the tricuspid annular plane systolic excursion (TAPSE) in 258 patients and calculation of Z-score values. *Neonatology.* 2011;100(1):85-92.

82. Vitali F, Galletti S, Aceti A, et al. Pilot observational study on haemodynamic changes after surfactant administration in

preterm newborns with respiratory distress syndrome. *Ital J Pediatr.* 2014;40(1):26.

83. Richardson C, Amirtharaj C, Gruber D, Hayes DA. Assessing myocardial function in infants with pulmonary hypertension: the role of tissue doppler imaging and tricuspid annular plane systolic excursion. *Pediatr Cardiol.* 2017;38(3):558-565.

84. Sehgal A, Blank D, Roberts CT, Menahem S, Hooper SB. Assessing pulmonary circulation in severe bronchopulmonary dysplasia using functional echocardiography. *Physiol Rep.* 2021;9(1):e14690.

85. Zakaria D, Sachdeva R, Gossett JM, Tang X, O'Connor MJ. Tricuspid annular plane systolic excursion is reduced in infants with pulmonary hypertension. *Echocardiography.* 2015;32(5):834-838.

86. Mądry W, Karolczak MA, Myszkowski M. Critical appraisal of MAPSE and TAPSE usefulness in the postoperative assessment of ventricular contractile function after congenital heart defect surgery in infants. *J Ultrason.* 2019;19(76):9-16.

87. Giesinger RE, El Shahed AI, Castaldo MP, et al. Impaired right ventricular performance is associated with adverse outcome after hypoxic ischemic encephalopathy. *Am J Respir Crit Care Med.* 2019;200(10):1294-1305.

88. Koestenberger M, Nagel B, Ravekes W, et al. Longitudinal systolic left ventricular function in preterm and term neonates: reference values of the mitral annular plane systolic excursion (MAPSE) and calculation of z-scores. *Pediatr Cardiol.* 2015;36(1):20-26.

# Chapter 11

# Advanced Cardiac Imaging in the Newborn: Tissue Doppler Imaging and Speckle Tracking Echocardiography

Philip T. Levy and Koert de Waal

## Key Points

- Tissue Doppler imaging (TDI) is a modality that employs the Doppler effect to assess muscle wall characteristics throughout the cardiac cycles including velocity, displacement, deformation, and event timings.

- Two-dimensional speckle tracking echocardiography (2DSTE) is a non-Doppler technique that applies computer software analysis of images generated by conventional ultrasound techniques to assess parameters of myocardial motion (displacement, velocity) and deformation (strain, strain rate) in all three axes.

- TDI and 2DSTE are feasible and reliable in the neonatal population, with recent literature describing normative and maturation values of the various measurements across a wide range of gestational ages that have significantly increased our knowledge of systolic and diastolic function and its development.

- Deformation parameters are more sensitive in detecting abnormalities in specific neonatal populations, such as severe growth restriction, maternal diabetes, hypoxic-ischemic encephalopathy, and congenital heart disease.

- Left atrial reservoir strain is a promising new feasible and reliable parameter to assess left atrial function.

- Blood speckle imaging is a new application of speckle tracking analysis that allows for imaging of intracardiac blood flow patterns.

## Introduction

Myocardial performance plays an important role in determining short- and long-term outcomes in term and preterm infants. Echocardiography is the most commonly used diagnostic modality for cardiovascular assessment in neonates; however, measuring the nature of cardiac mechanics is difficult due to the complex myocardial geometry and the interplay of cardiac loading conditions. In neonates myocardial performance can be characterized by three separate echocardiography techniques: (1) changes in cavity dimensions, (2) displacement and velocity of a single point along the myocardial wall, and (3) deformation of a segment of the wall. Until recently, the use of echocardiography in neonates to assess the adequacy of the cardiovascular system was largely dependent on either a subjective assessment of myocardial function, the use of measurements of cavity change during the cardiac cycle (e.g., shortening fraction, SF, and ejection fraction, EF), or blood flow velocity. However, not all aspects of cardiac mechanics can be identified using conventional echocardiography techniques; specifically, it is difficult to capture either the twisting motion or wall thickening for the whole ventricle. Furthermore, wall motion measurements cannot differentiate between active and passive movement of a myocardial segment. For example, on conventional echocardiography, a myocardial segment that has lost its function may still show movement due to the tethering effect of adjacent segments leading to misdiagnosis. Two emerging and validated modalities that

**189**

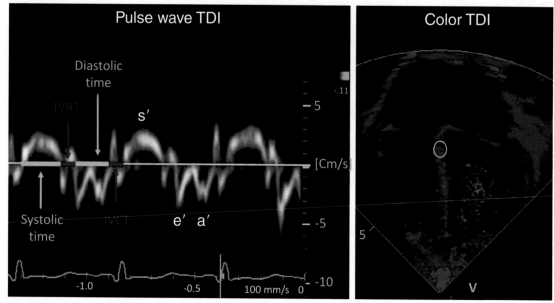

**Fig. 11.1 Pulsed wave tissue doppler imaging (TDI) and color TDI.** Pulsed wave TDI can be used to derive myocardial velocity during systole (s′) and diastole (e′ and a′), in addition to event timings (see text for further details) including isovolumic relaxation time (IVRT) and isovolumic contraction time (IVCT). Movement toward the probe is depicted as positive, and movement away from the probe is depicted as negative. Color TDI can be used to derive velocity and deformation values. Conventionally in color TDI, the muscle is colored *red* when traveling toward the probe and *blue* when traveling away from the probe.

directly assess muscle wall characteristics in neonates, tissue Doppler imaging (TDI) and two-dimensional (2D) speckle tracking echocardiography (2DSTE), enable acquisition of quantitative information that supersedes the qualitative impression provided by conventional methods.[1]

TDI is a modality that captures information on muscle movement velocity and cardiac cycle event timings using a high temporal resolution.[2] The Doppler effect is the term given to the change in frequency of a wave reflected by an acoustic source when there is relative movement between the source and the wave transmitter and can be applied in the assessment of heart muscle (tissue) characteristics. This was first demonstrated by Isaaz et al. in their assessment of the left ventricular (LV) wall using a pulse wave (pw) frequency signal.[3] TDI captures information using high frame rates (typically greater than 200 frames per second). The high temporal resolution achieved using this technique facilitates the measurement of a wide array of myocardial muscle characteristics including the velocity of muscle movement during systole and

diastole, deformation measurements (also known as strain and strain rate (SR) measurements), in addition to the measurements of the timing of events within the cardiac cycle (systolic and diastolic times/isovolumic contraction and relaxation times). Those measurements can now be derived by pw tissue Doppler imaging (pwTDI) and color TDI (cTDI) (Figure 11.1).

Myocardial deformation analysis is an emerging quantitative echocardiographic technique to characterize global and regional ventricular and atrial function in neonates. Cardiac strain is a measure of tissue deformation, and SR is the rate at which this deformation occurs. Myocardial strain can be measured in terms of three normal strains (longitudinal, radial strain, and circumferential) and six shear strains[4] (Figure 11.2). Currently, only normal strain and shear strain in the circumferential-longitudinal plane (rotational mechanics) have been investigated for clinical use in neonates.[1] These measurements can be obtained in neonates using TDI or 2DSTE.[1,5,6] Characterization of cardiac performance with myocardial deformation by 2DSTE is a validated method to assess

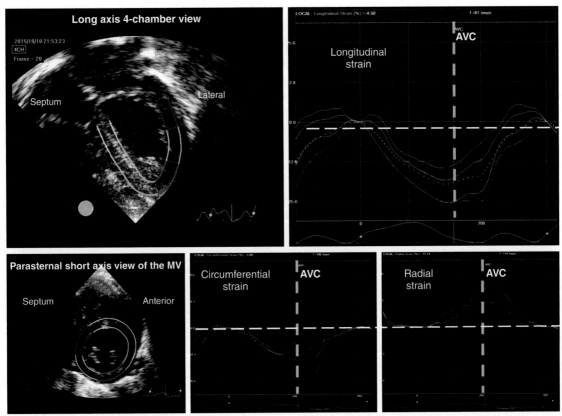

**Fig. 11.2 Two-dimensional speckle tracking echocardiography.** The *top panel* shows the assessment of the left ventricle (LV) by the offline analysis software in six segments (four-chamber view). The speckle-tracking algorithm divides the LV myocardium into six segments (basal septum, mid-septum, apical septum, basal lateral, mid-lateral, and apical lateral) and generates seven curves, six specific myocardial segments and one global value representing the combined strain from all segments. LV global longitudinal strain from a 17- or 18-segment model is calculated from segmental averaging of the three apical views, apical four-, three-, and two-chambers. The *bottom panel* demonstrated circumferential and radial strains obtained from the parasternal short-axis view at the level of the mitral valve. *AVC,* aortic valve closure.

both ventricular contractility and loading conditions in term and preterm infants and provides fundamental information on myocardial properties and mechanics that would otherwise be unavailable with conventional imaging.[1,5-8] 2DSTE is a non-Doppler technique that applies computer software analysis of images generated by conventional ultrasound techniques. The Doppler ultrasound signal generates artifacts due to random reflections, called speckles. These speckles stay stable during the cardiac cycle and can act as natural acoustic markers. Speckle tracking software defines and follows clusters of speckles from frame to frame to calculate parameters of motion (displacement and velocity) and parameters of deformation (strain and SR).[9,10]

There is an expanding body of literature describing longitudinal reference ranges and maturational patterns of TDI velocity– and 2DSTE-derived strain values in term and preterm infants.[1,2,10] Comprehension of principles, technical aspects, and clinical applicability of each modality is a prerequisite for its routine clinical use in neonates. This chapter will introduce the reader to TDI and 2DSTE of the LV and right ventricle (RV), as well as explore novel application of left atrial 2DSTE-derived strain, rotational mechanics, and blood speckle imaging (BSI). We discuss the expanding body of literature that details methodology (feasibility and reproducibility), terminology, and reference ranges and provides a practical guide to the acquisition and interpretation of data, and explore the diagnostic/predictive ability of all these parameters with respect to neonatal cardiopulmonary health and disease.

## Principles of Cardiac Function

In order to understand the relative strengths and weaknesses of all the measurements obtained using TDI and 2DSTE, a thorough understanding of the mechanics of cardiac performance is required. It is important to distinguish between intrinsic myocardial function (termed contractility) and pump function (termed myocardial performance). Contractility refers to the crosslinking of the actin and myosin filaments resulting in active myofiber force development and the shortening of sarcomeres. Myocardial performance or pump function describes the overall pressure development and deformation resulting in the ejection of blood from the ventricular cavity. Myocardial performance is therefore dependent on important physiological factors.

- *Preload:* defined as the amount of blood present in the ventricle at end-diastole before contraction begins. Up to a certain point, higher preload results in greater force generation and improved function (Frank-Starling relationship). Left and right ventricular preload are dependent primarily on pulmonary blood flow/pulmonary venous return and systemic venous return, respectively. Hydration and diastolic function are the two other important determinants.
- *Afterload:* also known as wall stress, is defined as the resistance against which the ventricle muscle must contract. This is primarily dependent on vascular resistance, blood viscosity, ventricular muscle wall thickness, and ventricular outflow tract obstruction. Higher afterload results in a reduction in deformation and myocardial performance, particularly in the preterm infant.
- *Contractility:* the intrinsic ability of the myocardial fibers to shorten as described above. This is determined by the efficiency of calcium-dependent crosslinking on the thick and thin filaments within the muscle fiber.[9]

## Tissue Doppler Velocity Imaging

The functional measurements obtained using TDI predominantly assess myocardial performance rather

than intrinsic function and as such, interpretation of values should be done in the context of the clinical situation and loading conditions. TDI filters out high-velocity signals obtained from movement of blood to focus on the lower-velocity Doppler signals of the muscle walls. TDI can be performed in pwTDI and cTDI modes (Figure 11.1).

## Pulsed Wave Tissue Doppler Velocity Measurements

Tissue Doppler velocities can be acquired by spectral analysis using a pw Doppler technique. Muscle tissue wall moves at a much slower velocity and a higher decibel amplitude range than blood, thus facilitating a high temporal resolution, with minimal artifact from blood.[1] Recent advances have enabled the distinction between the faster-moving blood (>50 cm/s) and slower-moving muscle tissue (<25 cm/s). pwTDI assesses longitudinal velocity of a ventricular wall segment from base to apex, providing a measure of systolic function that is recorded as the peak systolic velocity of the myocardial muscle (s′ wave).[11] The systolic wave is usually preceded by a short upstroke during isovolumic contraction. In addition, a measure of diastolic performance can be obtained as the ventricular wall moves away from the apex in the opposite direction. The diastolic wave is biphasic and is recorded as the peak early diastolic velocity (e′ wave) and the late diastolic peak velocity (a′ wave), which reflects the active ventricular relaxation and atrial contraction phases of diastole, respectively. The diastolic waves are usually preceded by another short upstroke during isovolumic relaxation time. The duration of the isovolumic relation and contraction phases, in addition to the systolic and diastolic times, can also be accurately obtained using this modality (Figure 11.1). pwTDI has high temporal resolution, but does not permit simultaneous analysis of multiple myocardial segments.

## Color Tissue Doppler Velocity

cTDI uses phase shift analysis to capture atrioventricular annular excursions. Compared with pwTDI, cTDI increases spatial resolution and provides visualization of multiple segments of the heart from one single view. It measures mean rather than peak systolic and diastolic velocities. As a result, velocities obtained using this technique are generally 20% lower in systole and diastole compared to pwTDI imaging. The two methods are therefore not interchangeable.[12] cTDI does have the advantage of combining the high temporal resolution seen with pwTDI, with a high spatial resolution. In addition to this, myocardial velocities recorded at the left and right ventricular base, and septal wall, can be obtained from a single image for later offline analysis. A comparison between left and right ventricular function can therefore be performed. Muscle tissue at the base moves at a higher velocity than that closer to the apex. cTDI can be used to assess this velocity gradient across the wall of interest (Figure 11.3). Data on cTDI values and clinical applicability in the neonatal setting are limited. This is likely due to the need for offline analysis to obtain those values and lower reproducibility when compared with pwTDI. The data presented below relate only to pwTDI.

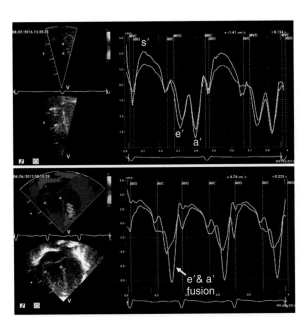

**Fig. 11.3 Color tissue Doppler imaging.** The *top panel* demonstrates an assessment of the velocity gradients of the septal wall in a term infant. Note that the velocities measured at the base (*yellow*) are higher in systole and diastole than those measured in the mid-segment of the wall (*green*). The *bottom panel* demonstrated the assessment of the septal wall and the right ventricular free wall in a preterm infant. Right ventricular velocities (*green*) are higher than septal velocities (*yellow*). Note the fusion of the e′ and a′ occurring due to the higher heart rate seen in preterm infants.

## Measurement of TDI Velocities

Accurate TDI velocity measurements are highly dependent on obtaining good-quality images. This may be challenging in the neonatal setting, particularly in premature infants, where lung artifact can interfere with obtaining clear images of the walls of interest. Images are most often obtained from an apical four-chamber view but can also be acquired from the apical three- and two-chamber views. The sector width of the field of view is usually narrowed to only include the wall of interest. This ensures that the temporal resolution is enhanced and a frame rate of over 200 frames per second is obtained. A pulsed wave Doppler sample is placed at the base of the LV free wall, the base of the septum, and the base of the RV free wall. The sample gate is narrowed to only capture the velocity of the area of interest (usually 1–2 mm). It is crucial to maintain an angle of insonation of <20° to prevent underestimation of velocities. This can be most challenging for the LV free wall in infants with marked ventricular enlargement due to volume overload (e.g., hsPDA). TDI velocity measurement modality will only assess muscle movement parallel to the probe beam. This is a limitation of this modality as muscle movement perpendicular to the line of interrogation will not be assessed, and as a result, TDI velocity measurements are reserved for longitudinal (base to apex) muscle tissue movement.

As outlined above, TDI velocity assessment measures myocardial performance rather than intrinsic contractility thus, the values are highly influenced by loading conditions (in addition to intrinsic contractility). Increased preload increases systolic tissue Doppler velocities, while increased afterload reduces those velocities.[13] Therefore clinical interpretation of those measurements must take into account the loading conditions likely to be present in the clinical situation. This has important implications for therapeutic interventions, where in some instances it may be more beneficial to improve preload (using volume support) or reduce afterload (using lusitropic medication) rather than targeting an improvement in intrinsic contractility. In addition, it is important to recognize that tissue Doppler velocity imaging cannot distinguish between active muscle movement and translational wall motion (a non-deforming segment tethered to a functioning segment). Tissue Doppler velocities may be falsely elevated, as they interrogate motion at a single point in the muscle wall with reference to the ultrasound transducer,[2] whereas deformation imaging (see later) easily differentiates the two.

## Clinical Application of TDI Velocity Measurements

The use of TDI has expanded in recent years as assessment is highly feasible in small infants and has been validated in term and premature neonatal populations[14,15] as well as in fetuses.[13] Reference values for term infants are shown in Table 11.1.[16-18]

Several studies have documented serial changes in those functional measurements over the first postnatal day and up to 1 year of age.[16-20] In term infants TDI can be used to assess RV function to provide important clinical prognostic information in infants with congenital diaphragmatic hernia[21] and may be used to

monitor treatment response in infants with acute pulmonary hypertension (aPH) of the newborn.[22] The superior sensitivity of TDI to subtle myocardial dysfunction when compared with shortening or ejection fraction in term infants was recently demonstrated. In infants born to mothers with diabetes mellitus (of any cause), left and right ventricular systolic function measured using TDI velocity is lower than control term infants. This occurs without differences in shortening fraction between the two groups.[23]

Providing reference ranges for preterm infants is more complex.[2] Tissue Doppler velocity imaging is dependent on the gestational age with lower myocardial velocities in both systole and diastole at lower gestations.[17,19,24] Furthermore, many preterm infants in the studies had conditions and treatments that influence preload and/or afterload, such as mechanical ventilation, PPHN, or a PDA. In premature infants pwTDI velocities have been used to predict clinical deterioration following patent ductus arteriosus (PDA)

**TABLE 11.1** "Reference ranges for pulse wave Tissue Doppler Imaging (pwTDI) in healthy term newborns. Peak Systolic (s′), Early Diastolic (e′), and Late Diastolic (a′) velocities and isovolumetric relaxation time" Velocities and Displacement of the AV-Valve Plane in Premature and Mature Neonates. Pulsed-Wave (pwTDI) and Color-Coded Tissue Doppler (cTDI) Indices – Mean (Standard Deviation). Reference Ranges for pwTDI in Healthy Term Newborns

|  | Day 1 | Days 2–3 | Day 28 |
|---|---|---|---|
| **s′ (cm/s)** | | | |
| LV free wall | 5.0 (3.5–7.0) | 5.0 (3.5–7.0) | 6.0 (5.0–8.0) |
| Septum | 4.5 (3.0–8.0) | 4.5 (3.0–8.0) | |
| RV free wall | 7.0 (5.5–9.0) | 7.0 (5.5–9.0) | 9.7 (6.0–12.0) |
| **e′ (cm/s)** | | | |
| LV free wall | 6.5 (5.0–8.5) | 6.8 (5.0–9.0) | 8.6 (6.0–11.0) |
| Septum | 5.0 (3.8–6.0) | 5.0 (4.0–7.0) | |
| RV free wall | 8.5 (6.0–11.0) | 8.0 (6.0–11.0) | 10.5 (6.0–14.0) |
| **a′ (cm/s)** | | | |
| LV free wall | 6.5 (4.5–10.0) | 5.5 (4.5–9.0) | 8.2 (6.0–11.0) |
| Septum | 4.5 (3.5–6.0) | 5.0 (4.0–8.0) | |
| RV free wall | 9.0 (7.0–12.0) | 8.5 (6.5–11.0) | 14.5 (6.0–18.0) |
| **Ee′ ratio** | | | |
| LV free wall | 8.5 (6.0–10.0) | 8.1 (6.0–9.8) | 7.5 (6.0–10.0) |
| Septum | 9.2 (7.0–11.0) | 9.5 (7.0–11.0) | |
| RV free wall | 5.8 (5.0–8.0) | 6.0 (5.0–8.0) | 6.0 (5.0–11.0) |
| IVRT (ms) | 54 (40–70) | 53 (40–70) | 42 (35–50) |

ligation and as a guide to institute targeted therapy. In addition, they can be used to assess treatment response in this scenario when conventional measures of function, including shortening and ejection fraction, are not sensitive enough.[25] Incorporating TDI for the assessment of myocardial performance in the setting of a PDA during the first few days of age may facilitate a more targeted approach to PDA treatment[25] and facilitate the development of prediction markers for adverse outcomes. Of note is that there is also an emerging association between lower diastolic function measured using TDI and chronic lung disease in premature infants.[25]

## Derived Deformation Measurements

### PRINCIPLES OF DEFORMATION IMAGING

Myocardial deformation refers to the change in shape of the myocardium in several planes, from its baseline shape in diastole to its deformed shape in systole. This occurs as a consequence of myofibril shortening. As the myocyte unit is not compressible, deformation of the ventricles occurs while maintaining the overall muscle volume resulting in a reduction of the ventricular cavity volume. Any shortening in one direction leads to expansion in other directions. The developing heart starts out as an isotropic tissue built of cardiomyocytes and supportive tissues and gradually develops into an anisotropic tissue where groups of cardiomyocytes are structured as laminar sheets of fibers.[26] In the subendocardial region the fibers are longitudinally oriented along the axis of the heart with an angle to the right (*right-handed helix*); in the midwall the fibers are circumferentially orientated; and in the subepicardial region they are longitudinal again but with an angle to the left (*left-handed helix*)[3] (Figure 11.4). This double helical structure of the heart is important for its function. Being able to

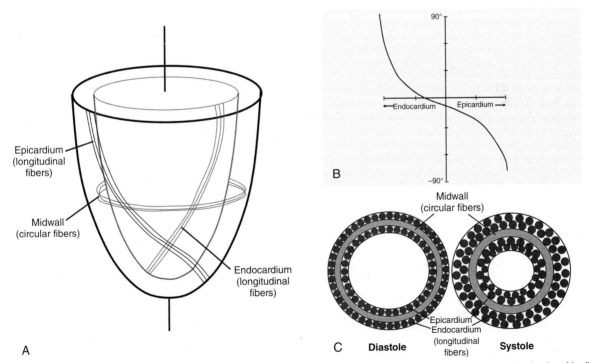

**Fig. 11.4** *Panel A:* Schematic representation of the left ventricle showing the longitudinal endocardial and epicardial fibers, and the circular midwall fibers. *Panel B:* The angle of the cardiac fibers according to the cardiac short axis changes from the endocardium to the epicardium. *Panel C:* Variable fiber angles help produce a shortening and twisting motion during systole, and a lengthening and untwisting motion during diastole. Wall thickening consists of thickening and inward shift of cardiac fibers.

shorten in longitudinal and circumferential directions simultaneously, thus creating a twisting motion greatly improves energy efficiency and the ability to empty and fill the heart with blood. Myocardial motion thus consists of narrowing, shortening, lengthening, widening, and twisting.

As mentioned, myocardial strain can be measured in terms of "normal" strain and "shear" strain.[4] Normal strain is caused by forces that act perpendicular to the surface of the myocardial wall, resulting in stretching or contraction without skewing of the volume.[27] There are three types of normal strain: longitudinal, radial, and circumferential. Conversely, forces causing shear strain act parallel to the surface of the wall and lead to a shift of volume borders relative to one another as delineated by a "shear" angle.[27] There are six forms of shear strain grouped into three categories: circumferential-longitudinal, circumferential-radial, and longitudinal-radial. Myocardial shear in the circumferential-longitudinal plane results in twist or torsional deformation of the LV during ejection. Only the three normal forms of strain and circumferential-longitudinal shear strain (rotational mechanics) have been investigated for clinical use in neonates.[1]

LV and RV deformation patterns differ based on their own unique myoarchitectural fiber orientation. The LV myocardium consists of circumferential fibers in the midwall layer and longitudinal fibers in the endocardial and epicardial layers.[28] The left ventricle (LV) deforms in three planes, including longitudinal (base to apex), radial, and circumferential. The LV shortens longitudinally and circumferentially but thickens in the radial plane. This facilitates the maintenance of muscle volume while reducing the volume of the ventricular cavity to facilitate the election of blood during systole. During diastole, the ventricle returns to its baseline un-deformed shape (Figure 11.5). In the circumferential-longitudinal plane the net difference in the systolic rotation of the myocardium between the apical and basal short-axis plane is referred to as twist (degrees) and represents the wringing motion of the LV during systole. If normalized to the distance between the respective image planes, it is referred to as torsion (degrees/cm). LV rotational mechanics (twist and torsion) are assessed by STE.

Compared with the LV, the RV myofiber architecture is composed of superficial oblique and dominant deep

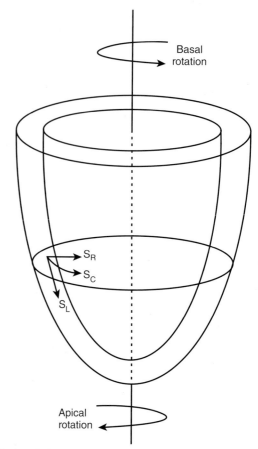

**Fig. 11.5 Deformation of the left ventricle.** Schematic representation of the left ventricle, showing the longitudinal (SL), circumferential (SC), and radial (SR) axis, and basal and apical rotation.

longitudinal layers. The myofibers in the RV are aligned in a more longitudinal direction than in the LV, and as the dominant pattern of RV deformation, longitudinal shortening provides the major contribution to stroke volume during systole and is a more sensitive indicator of RV dysfunction.[4,8,29] Deformation in the circumferential and radial directions in the RV may prove to be a valuable measure of function in certain neonatal conditions (i.e., congenital heart disease), but there is a paucity of studies that use these measures in clinical practice and those studies have not been able to demonstrate significant reliability in neonates.[30,31]

Deformation imaging has the advantage over velocity imaging in distinguishing between movement due to tethering and true deformation. Velocity imaging will register a displacement velocity of this non-deforming segment as it may be tethered by an adjacent functioning segment. However, an infarcted segment of the myocardium will not deform and its strain values will be close to zero. Strain can be used to assess regional and global myocardial performance. Strain is analogous to ejection fraction and as a result, it will be dependent on loading conditions as well as intrinsic contractility. SR on the other hand is thought to be less dependent on preload and afterload, and as a result, it may represent a more accurate reflection of intrinsic contractile function. Deformation imaging may therefore be used to distinguish between reduced performance resulting from loading conditions (which will affect strain but not SR) and reduced performance resulting from intrinsic contractile dysfunction (which will affect both strain and SR).[32]

There are two established methods for assessing and calculating deformation entitled Lagrangian strain and Eulerian (natural) strain.[33] Lagrangian strain refers to the change in length relative to an unstressed baseline length, against which all subsequent deformation will be measured.[34] Since Lagrangian strain is measured as the separation distance between two regions of myocardium relative to the original separation distance in end-diastole, it is not affected by the heart rate.[35] STE lends itself more readily to the calculation of Lagrangian strain, since the baseline length is always known and can easily be used as a reference. Eulerian strain calculation is based on a reference length that is different at each interrogation time point, for example, each color tissue Doppler frame, and is better suited for use with TDI. Natural and Lagrangian strains are related so that one can be converted into the other. STE software packages will report Lagrangian strain, but natural strain (i.e., tissue Doppler) can be derived from STE by conversion from the Lagrangian strain. Studies that utilized strain and SR measures to characterize function in neonates must therefore indicate the software package and the type of strain or SR. TDI-derived strain is not discussed in this chapter and is referenced elsewhere.[1,2]

## BASIC CONCEPTS AND TERMINOLOGY OF DEFORMATION

Strain (S) is the percent change from its original length, with negative values describing narrowing or shortening and positive values lengthening or thickening. SR is the average change in strain per unit time and is expressed as 1/s. Peak systolic strain occurs at the end of systole at aortic valve closure. Negative strain is used to express shortening (in the longitudinal and circumferential planes) and positive strain is used to express radial thickening. The nomenclature is longitudinal for base-to-apex, circumferential for rotational, and radial or transverse for inward motion and deformation. The difference in the rotation of the myocardium between the apical and basal short-axis plane is commonly referred to as twist and reported in degrees. If rotation is normalized to the distance between the respective image planes, it is referred to as torsion and reported in degrees/cm. Normalizing twist to LV length facilitates comparison of LV rotational mechanics across differing age groups, but this can only be done accurately with 3D imaging.

Recommended nomenclature, units, and abbreviations for 2DSTE-derived parameters are provided in an important recent consensus report.[8] The report also provides consensus on timing of mechanical events, essential for standardization of almost all derived parameters of motion and deformation. To be able to report on Lagrangian strain (where the original length is known), the software would need a reference point in time (the beginning of the cardiac cycle) and an endpoint where deformation is determined according to its reference point. End-diastole is commonly taken as beginning of the cardiac cycle, either determined from the four-chamber images as the frame before the mitral valve completely closes or using surrogates such as the R peak of the ECG or the largest volume of the LV. End-systole is the usual endpoint and coincides with aortic valve closure, determined from apical long-axis views or using surrogates such as the end of the T wave of the ECG, the end of the negative spike after ejection on the 2DSTE-derived velocity trace, or the minimum volume of the LV.[9,10] The current consensus in adult cardiology is to report on end-systolic strain, with other parameters reported in addition (Figure 11.6).

Most papers on neonates report on peak systolic strain (the first peak S value found) or maximum systolic strain (the highest S value found). Post-systolic strain has not been systematically reported in neonates but could prove to be an important parameter in

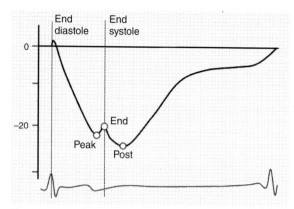

**Fig. 11.6 Representative curve showing cardiac time and the ECG trace on the x-axis and strain on the y-axis. End-diastole is determined from the R wave of the ECG. End-systole is marked in this example to show the difference between peak systolic strain, end-systolic strain, and post-systolic strain.**

fetal growth restriction.[36] As the heart contains layers of fibers in different directions, motion and deformation can vary depending on where in the myocardial wall it is measured. (i.e., at the endocardium, midwall, or averaged over the entire cardiac wall).[37] Whether this also plays a role in the analysis of the thin-walled and immature neonatal myocardium is unclear. Older software versions generally report on endocardial deformation, while the newer versions report on (the lower) global or midwall deformation, with separate reporting for each wall area.

To help interpret the data, it is important to understand the difference between global and segmental motion and deformation. The term global deformation should be reserved for the combined findings from the four-chamber, two-chamber, and long-axis apical views, or from the basal level of the papillary muscle and apical short-axis views. Segmental deformation can be vendor specific, as the segmental model used could describe 16, 17, or 18 segments.[38] Most software packages would divide the ventricular wall into six equidistant segments termed basal, mid, and apical segments for the apical views and anatomically for the short axis views (e.g., anteroseptal, anterior, lateral, posterior, inferior, and septal wall segment). Data can be reported as global (all segments of all views), four-chamber view alone (six segments), per ventricular wall (three segments of the LV free wall, RV free wall, and the septum, respectively), or

per individual segments (i.e., basal segments only for 2DSTE-derived myocardial velocities). Most 2DSTE data in neonates have been determined from the apical four-chamber view alone, as not all software can calculate global parameters when the heart rate varied too much between views.

## Image Acquisition

Speckle tracking analysis can be performed on normal 2D grayscale images but does require some adjustments to optimize feasibility of successful analysis. As mentioned earlier, 2DSTE tracks artifacts that are there because of random reflections of the Doppler signal; hence the optimal image should contain a combination of a perfect 2D grayscale image with enough artifacts (speckles) within the myocardial wall. This is not always easy to achieve. The feasibility of 2DSTE analysis in neonates has been reported to be between 70 and 95% of the images acquired, with the highest feasibility in the more recent studies.[1] As with any ultrasound imaging, the poorer the image quality, the less useful the analysis. Images selected for analysis should be reviewed for image quality before analysis is attempted. Using a subjective or objective image quality scoring sheet can assist in increasing the feasibility of 2DSTE analysis.[39] Quality items include completeness of the ventricle, how the endo- and epicardial borders appear, the presence of artifacts, the ECG trace, and frame rate used (Table 11.2). For optimal clarity of the endocardial borders, the overall gain setting and time-gain compensation should be adjusted to produce images that appear brighter than that typically used in conventional echocardiography. Neonates are often not sedated for image acquisition, so motion along with breathing can cause some segments to move in and out of the plane of view.

Reproducibility of neonatal deformation parameters was most robust when images were obtained with a frame rate to heart rate ratio between 0.7 and 0.9.[40] Low frame rate can cause under-sampling and thus underestimate peak systolic SR values. Strain is less frame rate sensitive, as the rate of change is lowest at end-systole. The operator can adjust depth and sector width to optimize frame rate, but reaching optimal frame rates might still be a challenge in neonates with very high heart rate and will require high-end

| TABLE 11.2 Image Quality Scoring Sheet for 2-Dimensional Speckle Tracking Echocardiography Image Analysis | |
|---|---|
| **Quality Item** | **Description** |
| Ventricle shape | No chamber foreshortening (apical views) |
| | Symmetry of the basal segments and valve (apical views) |
| | Contains circular images, not oblique cuts with ellipsoid shape (short axis views) |
| Endo- and epicardial borders | Enough speckles within each segment of interest |
| | Clear view of the endo- and epicardial borders of all segments throughout the cardiac cycle |
| Gain settings | Overall gain and image settings |
| | Distribution of gain over the myocardial segments |
| Artifacts | Reverberation, dropouts, breathing motion |
| Frame rate | Optimized to 0.7–0.9 frames/s per bpm |
| ECG signal | Clear R wave |

dedicated workstation. It is crucial to check the "send and storage" settings on the ultrasound machine before deformation imaging is started. The default setting for most older commercial ultrasound machines is to send all images in compressed format (DICOM) at a frame rate of 30 Hz. Some ultrasound machines now include a separate acquire button to send selected images in RAW format, but these images can only be analyzed using vendor-specific software. For vendor-independent software that uses DICOM images, the send and storage setting of the machine should be changed to "acquired frame rate". This setting will increase the need for server storage space and might cause network congestion depending on your local situation.

## Image Processing

Post-processing or the actual speckle tracking analysis is a semi-automated process of selecting a clip with optimal image quality and tracing the myocardial wall slightly within the endocardial border (or other areas of interest) as a sequence of points on a single frame. The software then generates a region of interest (ROI) to include the entire myocardial thickness. It is important to standardize settings for the width of the ROI if available. There is a learning curve for operators new to the technique to optimize imaging of the entire endocardial wall throughout the cardiac cycle and provide reproducible point selection for tracing. The software will track and trace the sequence of points from frame to frame throughout the cardiac cycle and renders a volume curve, and segmental, average, and global curves for velocity, displacement, S, and SR (Figure 11.7). After the first analysis, the operator should perform a visual frame-by-frame analysis of tracking accuracy by reviewing the underlying image loop with the superimposed tracking results. Some analysis software offers an automated measure of tracking accuracy, but it is recommended to always perform an operator check and, if needed, adjust the ROI.

## Interpretation of the Results

Three factors modulate variability in deformation imaging; these include variability in image acquisition, intra- and inter-observer variability in post-acquisition

ultrasound machines. A clear ECG signal is important for the speckle tracking software to allow proper gating of the images (i.e., capture 2–4 cardiac beats triggered by the R wave). On most modern equipment, the ECG trace can easily be obtained by connecting the ultrasound machine to the neonatal monitor without the need for machine-specific ECG leads. Although 2DSTE is angle independent, the angle of insonation can still make a small difference in S and SR.[41] This could be explained by differences in image quality and the appearance of the speckles under different angles. Parallel insonification of some segments of the apical views or the anterior and inferior-septal segments of the short axes images can lead to a reduction of speckles due to the fiber orientation.

## Sending and Storage of Acquired Images

After image acquisition, most operators would send and store selected images for offline analysis on a

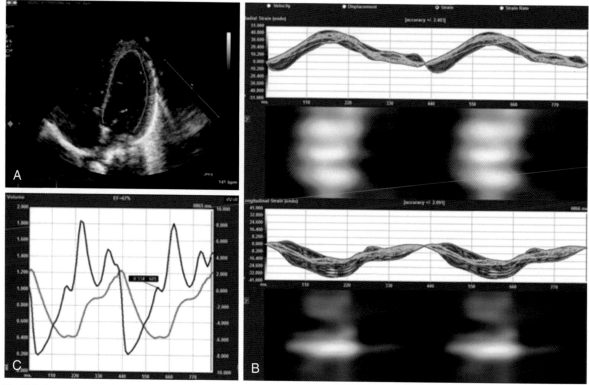

**Fig. 11.7  Screen capture of speckle tracking analysis (Tomtec Cardiac Performance Analysis software version 1.1) of a four-chamber clip with two cardiac beats.** *Panel A* shows the four-chamber clip with added tracking line placed along the endocardial border. *Panel B* shows radial (*top*) and longitudinal (*bottom*) motion and deformation data for each segment and as global average. Strain data are shown in this example. *Panel C* shows the data for volume (*orange line*) and rate of volume changes dVdt (*blue line*).

processing, and differences between echocardiographic equipment and proprietary software for image analysis.[8] This chapter discussed the first two factors (proper image acquisition and validation of deformation measurements), but in light of the push to standardize the acquisition of these measures and reduce inter-vendor differences and ambiguities,[34] it is important for the reader to review any details of hardware settings, manual settings, and local imaging protocols to get a better understanding of the values presented.

Strain is measured at end-systole, and thus at the end of ventricular contractile performance, and is closely related to stroke volume in healthy hearts.[42] SR is recorded earlier in the cardiac cycle and thus will not be subject to load during the entirety of systole. SR is measured at peak ventricular performance and is less load dependent, and thus SR is

considered to be closely related to myocardial contractility.[43]

The vendor's software package will determine how the results are presented, but most packages would show the data as color-coded parametric images, systolic numerical values, and time curves (Figure 11.7, Panel B). The patterns of S should be reviewed by exploring base-to-apex and left-to-right gradients. In neonates LV apical S and SR are usually higher compared to the mid and the basal segments, and the reverse is true for displacement and velocity. Deformation in the septum is usually lower compared to both the RV and LV free wall. Segmental abnormalities, as seen after myocardial infarcts, are rare in neonates. The curves should also be reviewed for diastolic events, best appreciated in the basal segments for 2DSTE-derived myocardial velocities and in the apex for S and SR. The reliability of diastolic 2DSTE parameters is not optimal, possibly due to the relative low frame rate per heartbeat as compared to TDI. Another issue with diastolic events in neonates is that fusion of the early and late diastolic events (EA fusion) commonly occurs at higher heart rates (>170/min). Such images would have to be omitted from analysis, prompting much data to be lost. It is not always clear how neonatal investigators handled this issue. One study in preterm infants reported all fusion events as late diastolic events instead of omitting the data.[25]

Circumferential motion and deformation and rotational mechanics are derived from the short-axis images (see below). Cardiac mechanical dysfunction is usually present in all directions in neonates, but under certain circumstances, rotational deformation can be a compensatory mechanism and provide clues for early detection of disease. All software also reports on radial and transverse deformation. The reliability for these parameters in neonates has been poor,[44] but improving,[45] possibly due to the small area changes, and is not routinely reported in neonatal studies.

Deformation is affected by a number of additional factors that should be considered when using strain imaging in clinical practice. Specifically, global and regional strain (%) are influenced by preload (which increases wall strain) and afterload (which reduces wall strain). Compared to strain, SR is thought to be less dependent on loading conditions and is a more accurate reflection of intrinsic myocardial contractile function.[46] Preclinical studies in animal models have demonstrated that preload has a positive impact on strain, whereas increasing afterload is associated with its reduction.[46,47] In preterm clinical studies surgical ligation of the PDA resulted in a sudden elevation in LV afterload and a reduction in LV preload that decreased LV strain in the immediate postoperative period.[48] In the early transitional period in preterm infants, there is negative correlation between strain and measures of afterload and positive correlation between strain and measures of preload.[30,32] Antenatal magnesium sulfate administration is associated with lower SVR and higher myocardial function as measured by strain imaging, but SR appeared to be less influenced by loading conditions, further validating the lower SR dependency on loading conditions.[49]

Cantinotti et al. suggested that deformation parameters should be normalized to age and body size.[50] We, and others, do not think that this is necessary for S and SR measurements.[51] Deformation parameters are fractional changes in length of a cardiac segment relative to its original length, and thus values are already normalized for cardiac size. In adult hearts there is a clear relationship between cardiac size, stroke volume, and deformation parameters, with a dilated heart able to generate a larger stroke volume with the same contractile force. Only when the observed changes deviate from the predicted changes is myocardial contractility reduced.[52] We could replicate some of these findings in a cohort of preterm infants with volume load due to a PDA, suggesting that cardiac remodeling and subsequent mechanical changes are already present from very early cardiac developmental stages.[53]

Deformation parameters are load dependent and should be interpreted in the context of existing or changing loading conditions. Strain and SR are positively influenced by preload and negatively by afterload.[54] In a meta-analysis of normal ranges of longitudinal strain ($S_L$) in adult studies, systolic blood pressure (an important determinant of LV afterload) at the time of the study was associated with normal variation and should be considered in the interpretation of S.[55]

## Clinical Application of 2DSTE-Derived Deformation Measurements

### REFERENCE RANGES AND CLINICAL UTILITY IN THE NEONATAL POPULATION

Normative data and reference ranges are still emerging for deformation parameters obtained using 2DSTE in the preterm and term infants (Table 11.3). Reference ranges have been published in healthy uncomplicated term[5,56-64] and preterm populations,[6,30,32,59,65-68] or reported results from control groups of neonates (who were recruited for specific studies).[23,69-75] The process of standardization and reference values in neonates stems from a relatively small number of infants included in each study, the varying time points at which echocardiograms were acquired in the first year of age, and the multitude of vendors and software versions utilized for acquisition and post-processing. In addition, only

**TABLE 11.3    Reference Ranges for Speckle Tracking Echocardiography Deformation Parameters in the Neonatal Population**

| Study and Equipment | Population | Values |
|---|---|---|
| Klitsie et al.[63] General electric | Gest: 40 weeks ± 1.2 Wt = 3.5 kg ± 0.5 N = 28 2 days 23 days 48 days | LV four-chamber view only for longitudinal strain LV parasternal short axis view (papillary muscles) for circ strain |

| | 1–3 Days | 3 Weeks | 6–7 Weeks |
|---|---|---|---|
| Longitudinal Strain | −18.8 ± 3.5 | −18.6 ± 2.5 | −19.4 ± 2.3 |
| Circ Strain | −19.7 ± 4.3 | −20.5 ± 4.5 | −19.6 ± 4.9 |

| Study and Equipment | Population | Values |
|---|---|---|
| Schubert et al.[64] General electric | Gest: Term Wt = No SGA N = 30 170 h (135–207) | Four-chamber view only was used |

| | LV | Septum | RV |
|---|---|---|---|
| Longitudinal Strain | −19.5 ± 2.1 | −19.5 ± 2.1 | −23.0 ± 4.3 |
| Systolic Strain Rate* | −2.94 ± 1.05 | −2.23 ± 0.77 | −3.61 ± 1.59 |

*Basal values presented. Refer to manuscript for further details.

| Study and Equipment | Population | Values |
|---|---|---|
| Jain et al.[5] General electric | Gest: 40 weeks ± 1.2 Wt: 3.49 kg ± 0.44 N = 50 Day 1: 15 h Day 2: 35 h | RV parameters[5] LV parameters[62]* |

| | Day 1 | Day 2 |
|---|---|---|
| RV Four-Chamber Strain | −21.2 ± 5.3 | −21.3 ± 5.4 |
| RV Three-Chamber Strain | −21.4 ± 4.4 | −20.6 ± 4.2 |
| RV Global Strain | −21.2 ± 3.9 | −21.2 ± 4.2 |
| LV Global Strain | −21.7 ± 1.9 | −21.2 ± 1.8 |
| LV Global SRs | 2.05 ± 2.0 | 2.17 ± 2.3 |

*Early and late LV SR in Ref. 62.

| Study and Equipment | Population | Values |
|---|---|---|
| Nasu et al.[66] QLAB, Philips | Gest: 33 weeks ± 2 Wt = 1.9 kg ± 0.21 N = 21 Serial data | Four-chamber view used. Septum was divided into LV and RV sides. |

| | 1 h | 24 h | 48 h | 72 h |
|---|---|---|---|---|
| LV | −23.8 ± 4.0 | −23.4 ± 3.2 | −23.8 ± 5.1 | −24.9 ± 3.2 |
| Sep-LV | −22.7 ± 5.7 | −21.0 ± 5.1 | −19.8 ± 3.1 | −20.9 ± 3.0 |
| RV | −22.0 ± 4.7 | −24.7 ± 4.7 | −20.8 ± 2.6 | −22.9 ± 5.1 |
| Sep-RV | −17.9 ± 4.5 | −17.7 ± 4.6 | −17.3 ± 4.5 | −14.7 ± 4.6 |

More time points available in the manuscript.

| Study and Equipment | Population | Values |
|---|---|---|
| Hirose et al.[73] General electric | Preterm group Gest: 27 weeks ± 1.2 Wt = 1.1 kg ± 0.2 N = 30 Age: 28 days Control group Gest > 37 weeks Wt = 3.3 kg ± 0.6 N = 30 Age: 28 days | Four-chamber view only used for LS LV base and apex planes were used for CS |

| | Preterm | Term |
|---|---|---|
| Longitudinal Strain | −16.0 ± 3.3 | −17.6 ± 3.7 |
| Longitudinal SRs | −1.63 ± 0.26 | −1.59 ± 0.26 |
| Circ Strain (Basal) | −15.5 ± 3.2 | −15.3 ± 4.7 |
| Circ SRs (Basal) | −1.75 ± 0.39 | −1.79 ± 0.41 |
| Circ Strain (Apical) | −24.0 ± 3.9 | −23.7 ± 5.9 |
| Circ SRs (Apical) | −2.58 ± 0.68 | −2.35 ± 0.69 |

16 preterm infants had repeat scans near term. There was no difference in the values when compared with 28 days.

**TABLE 11.3 Reference Ranges for Speckle Tracking Echocardiography Deformation Parameters in the Neonatal Population (Continued)**

| Study and Equipment | Population | Values |
|---|---|---|
| de Waal et al.[30] TomTec imaging system | Gest: 27 weeks (23–29)* Wt = 965 g (550–1530)* N = 54 Serial data *Ranges | Four-chamber view only used for LS LV mid-ventricular level (papillary muscle) used for CS |

| | Day 3 | Day 7 | Day 14 | Day 21 | Day 28 |
|---|---|---|---|---|---|
| LV LS | −22.9 ± 2.5 | −23.2 ± 2.6 | −23.4 ± 2.5 | −23.2 ± 2.7 | −23.3 ± 2.4 |
| LV SRs | −2.64 ± 0.41 | −2.70 ± 0.55 | −2.65 ± 0.4 | −2.60 ± 0.4 | −2.60 ± 0.6 |

| Study and Equipment | Population | Values |
|---|---|---|
| de Waal et al.[68] TomTec imaging system | Gest: 28 weeks (25–29)* Wt = 1062 g (630–1530)* N = 25 (uncomplicated) Serial data *Ranges | Four-chamber view only used for LS LV mid-ventricular level (papillary muscle) used for CS |

| | Day 3 | Day 7 | Day 14 | Day 21 | Day 28 |
|---|---|---|---|---|---|
| LV LS | −21.1 ± 2.3 | −21.5 ± 2.1 | −21.4 ± 2.2 | −23.0 ± 2.0 | −22.3 ± 2.3 |
| LV SRs | −2.37 ± 0.38 | −2.58 ± 0.52 | −2.36 ± 0.36 | −2.70 ± 0.55 | −2.52 ± 0.49 |
| Circ S | −28.5 ± 5.0 | −28.2 ± 4.6 | −28.0± 4.9 | −30.5 ± 5.9 | −28.9 ± 2.9 |
| Circ SRs | −3.72 ± 0.97 | −3.75 ± 0.74 | −3.27 ± 0.76 | −4.18 ± 0.96 | −4.71 ± 0.96 |

| Study and Equipment | Population | Values |
|---|---|---|
| Czernik et al.[74] General electric | Gest: 27 weeks (26–29)* Wt = 996 g (745–1200)* N = 119 Serial data *IQR | Four-chamber view only used (median values) |

| | Day 1 | Day 7 | Day 14 | Day 28 |
|---|---|---|---|---|
| LV LS | −15.5 | −15.1 | −15.5 | −15.1 |
| LV SRs | −1.4 | −1.5 | −1.6 | −1.6 |

| Study and Equipment | Population | Values |
|---|---|---|
| Schubert et al.[67] General electric | Preterm group Gest: 27 weeks ± 1.2 Wt = 1153 g ± 258 N = 25 Age 28 weeks corrected Control group Gest: 39.0 weeks ± 1.2 Wt = 3456 g ± 437 | Four-chamber view only was used |

| | 28 Weeks | 40 Weeks PMA | | 53 Weeks PMA | | |
|---|---|---|---|---|---|---|
| | Preterm | Preterm | Term | Preterm | Term | p* |
| LV LS | −17.9 | −18.7 | −19.5 | −20.0 | −22.0† | 0.03 |
| LV SRs | −2.33 | −2.60 | −2.40 | −3.37† | −3.06† | 0.53 |
| LV SRe | 2.78 | 3.51 | 3.05 | 3.33 | 4.33† | 0.28 |
| LV SRa | 2.28 | 2.76 | 2.10 | 2.52 | 3.22† | 0.28 |
| Sep LS | −19.0 | −20.3 | −20.1 | −21.9 | −22.5† | 0.44 |
| Sep SRs | −2.12 | −2.32 | −2.08 | −2.62 | −2.60† | 0.75 |
| Sep SRe | 2.72 | 2.62 | 2.32 | 3.22† | 3.44† | 0.93 |
| Sep SRa | 2.45 | 2.47 | 1.88 | 2.56 | 2.57† | 0.23 |
| RV LV | −20.5 | −23.3 | −23.0 | −23.9 | −24.4 | 0.69 |
| RV SRs | −2.79 | −3.81 | −2.70 | −4.17 | −3.79† | 0.38 |
| RV SRe | 3.20 | 3.59 | 3.00 | 4.54† | 4.16† | 0.82 |
| RV SRa | 2.64 | 3.33 | 2.30 | 2.90 | 3.53† | 0.38 |

*For the difference between groups at 53 weeks PMA.
†Within group P < 0.05 from 40 to 53 weeks PMA.

*Continued on following page*

**TABLE 11.3** **Reference Ranges for Speckle Tracking Echocardiography Deformation Parameters in the Neonatal Population (Continued)**

| Study and Equipment | Population | Values |
|---|---|---|
| Levy et al.[6] General electric | Preterm group Gest: 27 weeks (26–28)* Wt = 960 g (800–138)* N = 239 N = 103 (uncomplicated) * IQR | Four-, three-, and two-chamber views for LV RV focus 4-chamber view for RV |

| | Day 1 | Day 2 | Days 5–7 | 32 Weeks PMA | 36 Weeks PMA | 1 Year |
|---|---|---|---|---|---|---|
| LV GLS | −18.4 ± 3.5 | −20.3 ± 3.2 | −20.7 ± 3.0 | −19.8 ± 3.1 | −20.5 ± 2.2 | −20.2 ± 2.0 |
| LV GLSRs | −1.8 ± 0.3 | −2.1 ± 0.3 | −2.3 ± 0.4 | −1.8 ± 0.3 | −2.1 ± 0.3 | −2.3 ± 0.4 |
| IVS GLS | −17.7 ± 2.1 | −18.0 ± 2.1 | −18.4 ± 2.1 | −19.1 ± 2.3 | −20.7 ± 1.9 | −22.47 ± 2.0 |
| IVS GLSR | −1.7 ± 0.2 | −1.8 ± 0.2 | −1.9 ± 0.2 | −2.1 ± 0.2 | −2.3 ± 0.2 | −2.5 ± 0.2 |
| RV FWLS | −18.1 ± 4.0 | −20.3 ± 3.2 | −20.5 ± 3.2 | −22.0 ± 3.0 | −23.0 ± 3.1 | −26.5 ± 3.4 |
| RV FWLSRs | −1.9 ± 0.5 | −2.2 ± 0.6 | −2.7 ± 0.7 | −2.9 ± 0.5 | −3.1 ± 0.4 | −3.2 ± 0.3 |

*FW*, free wall; *GLS*, global longitudinal strain; *IVS*, interventricular septum.

two studies have assessed true "global" LV longitudinal (from the three apical chamber views) strain,[6,62] while most have reported LV longitudinal strain values from a single LV four-chamber view.[5,30,63,64,66,73,74] Very few studies have reported circumferential strain in neonates.[45,68,73] Radial deformation values and diastolic SR parameters (early and atrial) measured using 2DSTE remain unreliable in the neonatal population.[76] In general, LV deformation parameters measured using 2DSTE appear to remain stable during the transitional period and up to 28 days.[6,30,74,76] RV strain parameters gradually increase beyond the transitional period and through the first year of age.[6,67,76] Strain and SRs values are higher in the RV than the LV, reflective of the changing loading conditions specific to each ventricle.[6,76] In the LV circumferential deformation parameters appear to be slightly higher than longitudinal deformation.[68,73]

2DSTE has also been examined in various disease states in neonates.[23,48,49,69,71,72,75,77] One of the first studies of 2D STE in preterm infants illustrated the negative impact of PDA ligation on LV GLS in the immediate postoperative period, followed by recovery 24 hours later.[48] The reduction in LV GLS postoperatively was mostly attributed to the increase in afterload upon PDA closure. In the early transitional period another study demonstrated that the administration of antenatal magnesium sulfate is associated with lower SVR and higher LV GLS on postnatal day 1.[49] Those studies further highlight the load dependency of strain.

The influence of common cardiopulmonary abnormalities in preterm infants (such as CLD and pulmonary hypertension) appears to leave a negative effect on RV and septal strain, with preservation of LV strain patterns.[6,69,74] LV and RV function have also been evaluated in term infants of diabetic mothers (gestational and pre-gestational diabetes).[23,72,77] LV GLS is lower in pre-gestational (−10.4 ± 3.2, n = 20) and gestational (−13.1 ± 4.7, n = 25) groups when compared with the control group (−19 ± 2, n = 45) ($P < 0.01$).[23] Similarly, LV GLS can identify dysfunction in severely asphyxiated term infants who are undergoing therapeutic hypothermia when compared with healthy controls (−11.01% ± 2.48 vs. −21.45% ± 2.74, $P < 0.001$).[75]

LV GLS has a significant correlation with troponin levels ($R^2 = 0.64$, $P < 0.001$), suggesting that LV GLS is also capable of grading disease severity.[75] 2DSTE strain was found to be significantly lower in term infants with proven sepsis in the first month of age when compared to age- and weight-matched controls.[71] Finally, 2DSTE has been deployed in neonates with encephalopathy undergoing therapeutic hypothermia where abnormal RV strain at 24 hours of age has been associated with death, abnormal MRI, and abnormal neurodevelopment at 2 years of age.

## Left Atrium Strain

The left atrium (LA) is an anatomically complex, highly dynamic structure that allows for venous blood flow into the LV. Its function has been conventionally divided into three phases timed to the ventricular QRS complex. During ventricular contraction, the LA functions as reservoir by storing incoming pulmonary venous blood. During early ventricular relaxation, blood flows passively into the ventricle with the help of the suction forces of the ventricle, and the LA acts as conduit by transferring blood directly from the pulmonary veins into the LV. In the last phase the atrium contracts and provides additional transfer of blood into the LV.[78,79]

LA function can be assessed by measurement of changes in cavity size (volumetric measurements), conventional Doppler, tissue Doppler (TDI), and, more recently, deformation imaging using 2DSTE.[80,81] 2DSTE allows for measurement of important aspects of LA function (volume and deformation) and is able to quantify the contribution of reservoir, conduit, and active pump function. In adults STE is quick and reliable and can greatly facilitate ease of functional LA assessments. LA deformation parameters are more sensitive compared to conventional measurements to predict cardiovascular events in a wide range of adult patient populations and diseases and have incremental value in detecting increased LV filling pressure in patients with heart failure.

Images should be acquired from the apical four and either three- or two-chamber views, with special emphasis on avoiding LA foreshortening. Using the apical four-chamber, tracing starts at the endocardial border of the mitral annulus and traverses the LA endocardial border while excluding the pulmonary veins and vein confluence and the LA appendage orifices, up to the opposite mitral annulus side.

Longitudinal LA strain can be analyzed using the P wave or QRS as trigger onset, and values will vary accordingly (Figure 11.8). Although using the P wave would be more physiological, the current consensus is to trigger using the QRS, as the change from conduit to contraction phase can be difficult to appreciate in patients with high heart rate and short conduit time. The available literature has reported LA strain and SR using numerous (and sometimes confusing) nomenclature. The latest consensus document suggests using LA peak strain during the reservoir phase (LAS$_R$), LA peak strain during the conduit phase (LAS$_{CD}$), and LA peak strain during the contraction phase (LAS$_{CT}$).[81]

Few studies have collected reference values of LA strain in neonates, summarized in Table 11.4.[82,83] Feasibility in obtaining images and completing analysis was >95% in both neonatal studies. Reliability was good to excellent and better for images timed to QRS compared to images timed to the P wave. A moderate increase in LA strain can be seen during the early transitional phase, where the LA increases in size and manages an increasing volume throughput with stable

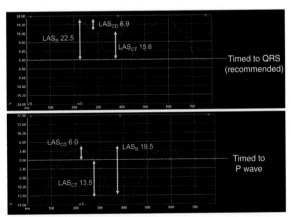

**Fig. 11.8 Measurement of left atrial strain components.** *Top panel:* with the zero strain reference at end-diastole (recommended). *Bottom panel:* with zero strain reference at the onset of atrial contraction. Note that the entire strain curve changes its amplitude depending on the definition of the zero reference. In both cases three measurement points are needed to calculate the deformation during the three phases of the LA cycle: *LAS$_{CD}$*, conduit phase; *LAS$_{CT}$*, contraction phase; *LAS$_R$*, reservoir phase.

**TABLE 11.4   Reference Values for Atrial Strain in Stable Preterm Infants and Healthy Term Infants**

|  | Preterm Day 1 | Preterm Day 2 | Preterm Day 3 | Preterm Day 28 | Term Day 1 | Term Day 2 |
|---|---|---|---|---|---|---|
| LAS$_R$ | 32(5) | 37(6) | 41(3) | 44(5) | 33(4) | 37(5) |
| LAS$_{CD}$ | 19(21) | 20(19) | 13(3) | 14(4) | 20(11) | 22(12) |
| LAS$_{CT}$ | 11(10) | 14(17) | 28(2) | 29(3) | 13(9) | 13(10) |

*LAS$_{CD}$*, conduit phase; *LAS$_{CT}$*, contraction phase; *LAS$_R$*, reservoir phase.
Adapted from de Waal et al.[82] (P wave timed values converted into QRS timed values) and Ficial et al.

reservoir LA strain values thereafter. Findings were comparable to those seen in children and adults, but values can vary significantly depending on acquisition method, equipment, and analysis software version used.[84,85]

Several neonatal diseases are associated with atrial dysfunction and where LA strain can assist in diagnosis and help guide treatments. Prolonged volume overload due to a PDA is a common cause for reduced atrium strain.[82] Figure 11.9 shows LAS$_R$ in infants with no PDA compared to infants with a PDA >1.5 mm diameter. Some infants with a PDA have normal LA function, but many infants with a PDA showed significant atrial dysfunction and might benefit from timely treatments.

LA strain can help differentiate between preterm infants with indeterminate diastolic function and abnormal diastolic function as determined by an adapted multi-parameter approach for the classification of diastolic dysfunction and the diagnosis of Heart Failure with Preserved Ejection Fraction (HFpEF).[86] The left atrium is the last bulwark before overt clinical heart failure occurs, and LA strain is a promising new parameter to select patients for trials and treatments in clinical conditions where increased LA pressure or LA dysfunction is expected.

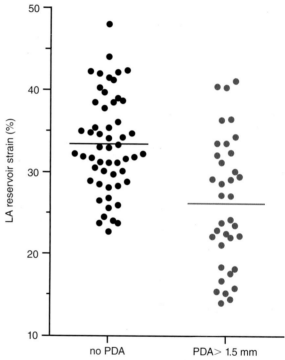

**Fig. 11.9 LA reservoir strain in preterm infants with no PDA (*black*) compared to infants with a PDA >1.5 mm. A significant reduction in LA reservoir strain can be appreciated in some of the infants with a PDA.** (Adapted from de Waal K, Phad N, Boyle A. Left atrium function and deformation in very preterm infants with and without volume load. *Echocardiography.* 2018;35:1818–1826. doi:10.1111/echo.14140.)

## Left Ventricular Rotational Mechanics

LV twist describes the wringing motion of the LV during systole and is the net result of the contrasting rotation of the apex (in an anti-clockwise direction, depicted as a positive rotation) and the base (in a clockwise direction, depicted as a negative rotation) along the long axis of the left ventricle; both are expressed in degrees. LV torsion is the term given to LV

twist indexed to its length. This wringing motion, which is also expressed in degrees, improves the ejection of blood from the LV cavity during systole. LV untwist contributes directly to early diastolic filling and is influenced by muscle fiber compliance and elastic recoil properties. The speed at which LV twist occurs (LV twist rate) and LV untwist occurs (LV untwist rate) can also be measured and expressed as degrees per second (Figure 11.10). These rotational parameters can add important information on myocardial performance.[87] The twisting motion of the LV is aided by the helical arrangement of the subepicardial (left-handed) and subendocardial (right-handed) fibers.[88] Untwist is facilitated by the kinetic energy stored in those twisted fibers, which is released during diastole due to elastic recoil. Therefore LV untwist rate in early diastole is highly influenced by LV twist in systole. Reduced LV twist will therefore translate to reduced LV untwist rate.[89] Increased afterload appears to decrease LV twist and untwist rate in experimental animal models (mongrel dogs) and human adults.[54] Similarly, in the preterm neonatal population increased afterload appears to negatively impact those measurements.[49]

Rotational mechanics can be assessed by STE in a similar fashion to the method described above. STE measures apical and basal rotation from the parasternal short axis views and demonstrates acceptable agreements with twist measured by magnetic resonance imaging (MRI).[87,90] Twist as a marker of cardiac function has been validated in adults and children.[91,92] Rotational mechanics data in term neonates during the early transitional period is lacking. There are limited studies of those parameters in preterm infants. Our group have recently demonstrated the feasibility and acceptable reproducibility of measuring LV twist in the premature population, in addition to the changes occurring over the first week of age.[89] We also demonstrated that increased systemic vascular resistance over the first day of age has a negative impact on LV twist and untwist.[49]

## Intracardiac Blood Flow Imaging and Analysis

Intracardiac blood flow patterns play a key role in cardiac development, starting in fetal morphogenesis and continuing throughout life.[93] Fluctuations in shear stress on the cardiac wall can stimulate cardiac growth by different expression patterns of shear responsive genes. Hence intracardiac blood flow helps modulate and shape the fetal heart into the normal four-chamber structure during early cardiac development and into normal neonatal proportions during later intra-uterine life.[94] The laws of fluid dynamics dictate that blood passing along a vessel wall will move slower when closest to the wall and faster when in the middle of a vessel where resistance is lower. This phenomenon can be captured in any large artery or vein with pulse wave Doppler as the typical Doppler velocity time integral envelope. When blood enters a larger cavity such as the heart, the blood furthest from the wall will continue to increase its velocity relative to the blood closest to the wall and create a rotational body of fluid known as a vortex. Once generated, vortices are relatively longstanding inertial flow structures capable of drawing in surrounding fluid by decreasing pressure in their vicinity without an energetic cost of the driving system. Thus a vortex can transport more mass than an equivalent straight jet of fluid; promote greater cardiac efficiency; and optimize atrial, ventricular, and vascular interactions.[95] The evolutionary purpose of vortices in nature is to conserve kinetic energy, to minimize shear stress, and to maximize flow efficiency. Specifically for the heart, this includes storing of energy in a rotary motion, facilitation of valve closure, and propagation of blood flow toward the outflow tract (Figure 11.11). Altered intracardiac blood flow patterns are expected in pathological situations, and this is where vortices have proven their diagnostic potential as early predictors of cardiovascular outcomes in adults.[96]

Intracardiac blood flow patterns can be visualized by using cardiac MRI, echo particle imaging velocimetry, vector flow mapping, and BSI.[97] In neonates BSI has the most advantages and uses high-frame-rate ultrasound techniques with unfocused pulses emitted to each region to track the blood speckles. This allows for a high temporal resolution, fewer mathematical assumptions, and angle-independent imaging compared to other color Doppler techniques. Its disadvantage is a higher loss of signal-to-noise ratio and less penetrating depth, currently up to 10 cm. The speckle-tracking features are analogous to those used in tissue speckle tracking used to study myocardial deformation. Because red blood cells tend to move faster than the surrounding tissue, their Doppler frequency is generally higher, and the two signals can be separated by applying a temporal filter. BSI uses a best-match algorithm to quantify the movement of blood speckles directly without the use of contrast agents.[98] The

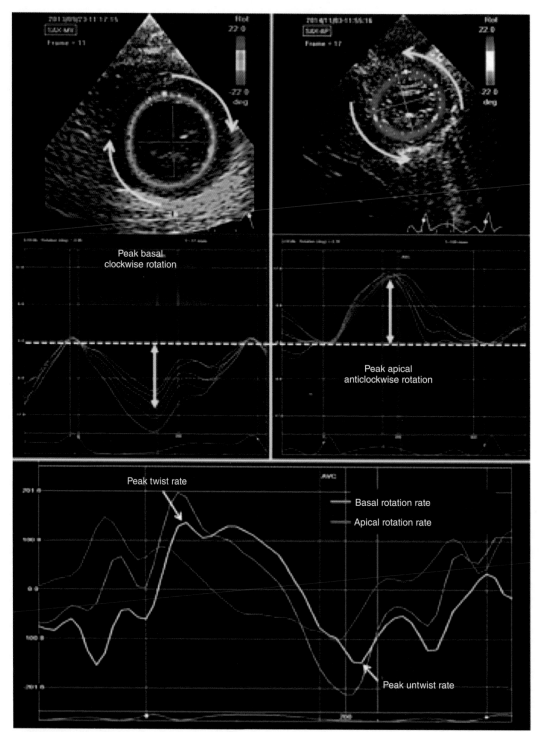

**Fig. 11.10 Left ventricle rotational mechanics.** The base of the LV rotates in a clockwise fashion (depicted as a negative rotation) and the apex of the LV rotates in an anti-clockwise fashion (depicted as a positive rotation). The net difference between those opposing rotational movements if LV twist. The rate of twist (o/s) in systole and early untwist in diastole are illustrated as well.

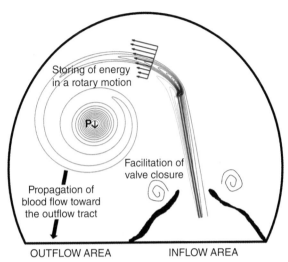

**Fig. 11.11** Schematic representation of intracardiac blood flow patterns and vortex formation.

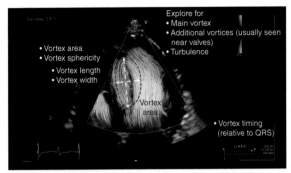

**Fig. 11.12 Blood speckle tracking image of the left ventricle in a 1080 g preterm infant.** The main vortex can be seen in the *upper left quadrant* of the left ventricle near the septum as an elongated *oval-shaped* anti-clockwise rotating structure. A residual small clockwise rotating vortex can be appreciated lateral from the mitral valve leaflet. This example image does not show any turbulence, and the vortex sphericity can be measured from vortex length and width.

blood velocity measurements can be visualized as arrows, streamlines, or path lines, with or without underlying color Doppler images and highlight areas of complex flow. BSI also allows for the measurement of quantitative flow measures such as velocity magnitude, vorticity, energy loss, and kinetic energy. Imaging techniques, vortex properties, and terminology are summarized in an excellent review by Mele et al.[97]

Image acquisition is comparable to color Doppler imaging. Acquisition frame rate is between 400 and 600 Hz and the color box should narrowly cover the area of interest to optimize tracking quality. Most intracardiac complex flow occurs in diastole, thus scale should be adjusted to the lowest velocities and loops saved from at least two cardiac cycles to capture the blood flow changes from diastole into systole. Image analysis of the LV includes vortex number and location, morphology, and timing (Figure 11.12). In stable preterm infants the main vortex is an elongated oval-shaped anti-clockwise rotating structure located in the upper left quadrant of the LV near the septum, with the maximum vortex area found in late diastole.[99] In older children the maximum LV vortex area is more likely seen in early diastole, as would be expected from the changes in early and late diastolic function with increasing age.[84] Each cardiac chamber has its typical blood flow pattern, vortex morphology, and vortex location.

The clinical applications of BSI include analysis of complex flow in infants with congenital heart disease.[84] Adding kinetic energy and energy loss might be promising to help determine optimal timing of surgery in selected abnormalities.[100] BSI parameters are used in a research setting as a supplementary tool to assess cardiac function and cardiac remodeling after preterm birth. At least one in four very preterm infants show signs of cardiac remodeling at the time of discharge, but there is limited information available on the underlying mechanisms.[101] We found that vortices were less elongated at day 7 after preterm birth in infants who later developed cardiac remodeling.[102] This finding supports the hypothesis that intracardiac blood flow patterns that could reflect abnormal hemodynamics disease states may play an important role in cardiac development after preterm birth, and further studies are needed to test where an early and short-term intervention has the potential to prevent the pathway of abnormal cardiac development.

## Conclusion

The assessment of tissue Doppler–derived velocity and deformation measurements in neonates continues to gain considerable interest. The emerging literature has clearly demonstrated their feasibility and reproducibility in the neonatal population and the relative advantages of those techniques when compared or added to conventional measures. In addition, with reference ranges and normative data continuing to emerge and studies assessing their diagnostic and prognostic values and their ability to monitor treatment response, their routine clinical use is likely to become more common. In summary, muscle tissue velocities obtained using pwTDI and deformation using 2DSTE are feasible and reliable and valid modalities for the assessment of myocardial performance in the premature and term neonatal population. Those measurements are highly influenced by loading conditions and therefore do not represent intrinsic function (contractility). Reference ranges across a wide variety of gestations have emerged, and their use in detecting myocardial dysfunction, guiding therapeutic interventions, predicting important clinical outcomes, and monitoring response to treatment is expanding in the neonatal population.

## REFERENCES

1. Breatnach CR, Levy PT, James AT, Franklin O, El-Khuffash A. Novel echocardiography methods in the functional assessment of the newborn heart. *Neonatology*. 2016;110(4):248-260.
2. Nestaas E, Schubert U, de Boode WP, El-Khuffash A. Tissue Doppler velocity imaging and event timings in neonates: a guide to image acquisition, measurement, interpretation, and reference values. *Pediatr Res*. 2018;84(suppl 1):18-29.
3. Isaaz K, Thompson A, Ethevenot G, Cloez JL, Brembilla B, Pernot C. Doppler echocardiographic measurement of low velocity motion of the left ventricular posterior wall. *Am J Cardiol*. 1989;64(1):66-75.
4. Tee M, Noble JA, Bluemke DA. Imaging techniques for cardiac strain and deformation: comparison of echocardiography, cardiac magnetic resonance and cardiac computed tomography. *Expert Rev Cardiovasc Ther*. 2013;11:221-231.
5. Jain A, Mohamed A, El-Khuffash A, et al. A comprehensive echocardiographic protocol for assessing neonatal right ventricular dimensions and function in the transitional period: normative data and z scores. *J Am Soc Echocardiogr*. 2014; 27:1293-1304.
6. Levy PT, El-Khuffash A, Patel MD, et al. Maturational patterns of systolic ventricular deformation mechanics by two-dimensional speckle tracking echocardiography in preterm infants over the first year of age. *J Am Soc Echocardiogr*. 2017;30(7):685-698.e1.
7. James A, Corcoran JD, Mertens L, Franklin O, El-Khuffash A. Left ventricular rotational mechanics in preterm infants less than 29 weeks' gestation over the first week after birth. *J Am Soc Echocardiogr*. 2015;28(7):808–817.e1.
8. Levy PT, Holland MR, Sekarski TJ, Hamvas A, Singh GK. Feasibility and reproducibility of systolic right ventricular strain measurement by speckle-tracking echocardiography in premature infants. *J Am Soc Echocardiogr*. 2013;26(10):1201-1213.
9. Bussmann N, El-Khuffash A. Future perspectives on the use of deformation analysis to identify the underlying pathophysiological basis for cardiovascular compromise in neonates. *Pediatr Res*. 2019;85(5):591-595.
10. El-Khuffash A, Schubert U, Levy PT, Nestaas E, de Boode WP. Deformation imaging and rotational mechanics in neonates: a guide to image acquisition, measurement, interpretation, and reference values. *Pediatr Res*. 2018;84(suppl 1):30-45.
11. Hiarada K, Orino T, Yasuoka K, Tamura M, Takada G. Tissue doppler imaging of left and right ventricles in normal children. *Tohoku J Exp Med*. 2000;191(1):21-29.
12. Nagueh SF, Middleton KJ, Kopelen HA, Zoghbi WA, Quinones MA. Doppler tissue imaging: a noninvasive technique for evaluation of left ventricular relaxation and estimation of filling pressures. *J Am Coll Cardiol*. 1997;30(6):1527-1533.
13. Iwashima S, Sekii K, Ishikawa T, Itou H. Serial change in myocardial tissue Doppler imaging from fetus to neonate. *Early Hum Dev*. 2013;89(9):687-692.
14. Negrine RJ, Chikermane A, Wright JG, Ewer AK. Assessment of myocardial function in neonates using tissue Doppler imaging. *Arch Dis Child Fetal Neonatal Ed*. 2012;97(4):F304-F306.
15. Alp H, Karaarslan S, Baysal T, Cimen D, Ors R, Oran B. Normal values of left and right ventricular function measured by M-mode, pulsed doppler and Doppler tissue imaging in healthy term neonates during a 1-year period. *Early Hum Dev*. 2012;88(11):853-859.
16. Murase M, Morisawa T, Ishida A. Serial assessment of right ventricular function using tissue Doppler imaging in preterm infants within 7 days of life. *Early Hum Dev*. 2015;91(2):125-130.
17. Murase M, Morisawa T, Ishida A. Serial assessment of left-ventricular function using tissue Doppler imaging in premature infants within 7 days of life. *Pediatr Cardiol*. 2013;34(6):1491-1498.
18. Di Maria MV, Younoszai AK, Sontag MK, et al. Maturational changes in diastolic longitudinal myocardial velocity in preterm infants. *J Am Soc Echocardiogr*. 2015;28(9):1045-1052.
19. Eriksen BH, Nestaas E, Hole T, Liestøl K, Støylen A, Fugelseth D. Myocardial function in term and preterm infants. Influence of heart size, gestational age and postnatal maturation. *Early Hum Dev*. 2014;90(7):359-364.
20. Torres E, Levy PT, El-Khuffash A, Gu H, Hamvas A, Singh GK. Left ventricle phenotyping utilizing tissue Doppler imaging in premature infants with varying severity of Bronchopulmonary Dysplasia. *J Clin Med*. 2021;10(10):2211.
21. Patel N, Mills JF, Cheung MM. Assessment of right ventricular function using tissue Doppler imaging in infants with pulmonary hypertension. *Neonatology*. 2009;96(3):193-199; discussion 200-202.
22. James AT, Corcoran JD, McNamara PJ, Franklin O, El-Khuffash AF. The effect of milrinone on right and left ventricular function when used as a rescue therapy for term infants with pulmonary hypertension. *Cardiol Young*. 2016;26(1):90-99.
23. Al-Biltagi M, Tolba OA, Rowisha MA, Mahfouz Ael S, Elewa MA. Speckle tracking and myocardial tissue imaging in infant of diabetic mother with gestational and pregestational diabetes. *Pediatr Cardiol*. 2015;36(2):445-453.
24. Lee A, Nestaas E, Liestøl K, Brunvand L, Lindemann R, Fugelseth D. Tissue Doppler imaging in very preterm infants during the first 24 h of life: an observational study. *Arch Dis Child Fetal Neonatal Ed*. 2014;99(1):F64-F69.
25. El-Khuffash A, James AT, Corcoran JD, et al. A patent ductus arteriosus severity score predicts chronic lung disease or death before discharge. *J Pediatr*. 2015;167(6):1354-1361.e2.
26. Omoto R, Yokote Y, Takamoto S, et al. The development of real-time two-dimensional Doppler echocardiography and its clinical significance in acquired valvular diseases. With special reference to the evaluation of valvular regurgitation. *Jpn Heart J*. 1984;25(3):325-340.

27. Blessberger H, Binder T. Two dimensional speckle tracking echocardiography: clinical applications. *Heart.* 2010;96(24): 2032-2040.

28. Greenbaum RA, Ho SY, Gibson DG, Becker AE, Anderson RH. Left ventricular fibre architecture in man. *Br Heart J.* 1981; 45(3):248-263.

29. Petitjean C, Rougon N, Cluzel P. Assessment of myocardial function: a review of quantification methods and results using tagged MRI. *J Cardiovasc Magn Reson.* 2005;7:501-516.

30. de Waal K, Phad N, Lakkundi A, Tan P. Cardiac function after the immediate transitional period in very preterm infants using speckle tracking analysis. *Pediatr Cardiol.* 2016;37(2):295-303.

31. Levy PT, Sanchez Mejia AA, Machefsky A, Fowler S, Holland MR, Singh GK. Normal ranges of right ventricular systolic and diastolic strain measures in children: a systematic review and meta-analysis. *J Am Soc Echocardiogr.* 2014;27(5):549-560.e3.

32. James AT, Corcoran JD, Breatnach CR, Franklin O, Mertens L, El-Khuffash A. Longitudinal assessment of left and right myo- cardial function in preterm infants using strain and strain rate imaging. *Neonatology.* 2016;109(1):69-75.

33. Lorch SM, Ludomirsky A, Singh GK. Maturational and growth- related changes in left ventricular longitudinal strain and strain rate measured by two-dimensional speckle tracking echocar- diography in healthy pediatric population. *J Am Soc Echocar- diogr.* 2008;21(11):1207-1215.

34. Voigt JU, Pedrizzetti G, Lysyansky P, et al. Definitions for a com- mon standard for 2D Speckle tracking echocardiography: consen- sus document of the EACVI/ASE/industry task force to standardize deformation imaging. *J Am Soc Echocardiogr.* 2015;28:183-193.

35. Boettler P, Hartmann M, Watzl K, et al. Heart rate effects on strain and strain rate in healthy children. *J Am Soc Echocardiogr.* 2005;18:1121-1130.

36. Crispi F, Bijnens B, Sepulveda-Swatson E, et al. Postsystolic shortening by myocardial deformation imaging as a sign of cardiac adaptation to pressure overload in fetal growth restric- tion. *Circ Cardiovasc Imaging.* 2014;7(5):781-787.

37. Shi J, Pan C, Kong D, Cheng L, Shu X. Left ventricular longitu- dinal and circumferential layer-specific myocardial strains and their determinants in healthy subjects. *Echocardiography.* 2016; 33(4):510-518.

38. Levy PT, Machefsky A, Sanchez AA, et al. Reference ranges of left ventricular strain measures by two-dimensional speckle- tracking echocardiography in children: a systematic review and meta-analysis. *J Am Soc Echocardiogr.* 2016;29(3):209-225.e6.

39. Colan SD, Shirali G, Margossian R, et al. The ventricular vol- ume variability study of the Pediatric Heart Network: study design and impact of beat averaging and variable type on the reproducibility of echocardiographic measurements in children with chronic dilated cardiomyopathy. *J Am Soc Echocardiogr.* 2012;25(8):842-854.e6.

40. Sanchez AA, Levy PT, Sekarski TJ, Hamvas A, Holland MR, Singh GK. Effects of frame rate on two-dimensional speckle tracking-derived measurements of myocardial deformation in premature infants. *Echocardiography.* 2015;32(5):839-847.

41. Forsha D, Risum N, Rajagopal S, et al. The influence of angle of insonation and target depth on speckle-tracking strain. *J Am Soc Echocardiogr.* 2015;28(5):580-586.

42. Thorstensen A, Dalen H, Amundsen BH, Støylen A. Peak sys- tolic velocity indices are more sensitive than end-systolic indi- ces in detecting contraction changes assessed by echocardiog- raphy in young healthy humans. *Eur J Echocardiogr.* 2011; 12(12):924-930.

43. Breatnach CR, Levy PT, Franklin O, El-Khuffash A. Strain rate and its positive force-frequency relationship: further evidence from a premature infant cohort. *J Am Soc Echocardiogr.* 2017;30(10):1045-1046.

44. Laser KT, Haas NA, Fischer M, et al. Left ventricular rotation and right-left ventricular interaction in congenital heart disease: the acute effects of interventional closure of patent arterial ducts and atrial septal defects. *Cardiol Young.* 2014;24(4):661-674.

45. Smith A, Bussmann N, Levy P, Franklin O, McCallion N, El-Khuffash A. Comparison of left ventricular rotational me- chanics between term and extremely premature infants over the first week of age. *Open Heart.* 2021;8(1):e001458).

46. Greenberg NL, Firstenberg MS, Castro PL, et al. Doppler- derived myocardial systolic strain rate is a strong index of left ventricular contractility. *Circulation.* 2002;105(1):99-105.

47. Ferferieva V, Van den Bergh A, Claus P, et al. The relative value of strain and strain rate for defining intrinsic myocardial function. *Am J Physiol Heart Circ Physiol.* 2012;302(1):H188-H195.

48. El-Khuffash AF, Jain A, Dragulescu A, McNamara PJ, Mertens L. Acute changes in myocardial systolic function in preterm in- fants undergoing patent ductus arteriosus ligation: a tissue Doppler and myocardial deformation study. *J Am Soc Echocar- diogr.* 2012;25(10):1058-1067.

49. James AT, Corcoran JD, Hayes B, Franklin O, El-Khuffash A. The effect of antenatal magnesium sulfate on left ventricular afterload and myocardial function measured using deformation and rotational mechanics imaging. *J Perinatol.* 2015;35(11): 913-918.

50. Cantinotti M, Kutty S, Giordano R, et al. Review and status report of pediatric left ventricular systolic strain and strain rate nomograms. *Heart Fail Rev.* 2015;20(5):601-612.

51. Oxborough D, Batterham AM, Shave R, et al. Interpretation of two-dimensional and tissue Doppler-derived strain (epsilon) and strain rate data: is there a need to normalize for individual variability in left ventricular morphology? *Eur J Echocardiogr.* 2009;10(5):677-682.

52. Marciniak A, Claus P, Sutherland GR, et al. Changes in systolic left ventricular function in isolated mitral regurgitation. A strain rate imaging study. *Eur Heart J.* 2007;28(21):2627-2636.

53. de Waal K, Phad N, Collins N, Boyle A. Cardiac remodeling in preterm infants with prolonged exposure to a patent ductus arteriosus. *Congenit Heart Dis.* 2017;12(3):364-372.

54. Burns AT, La GA, Prior DL, Macisaac AI. Left ventricular torsion parameters are affected by acute changes in load. *Echocardiog- raphy.* 2010;27(4):407-414.

55. Yingchoncharoen T, Agarwal S, Popović ZB, Marwick TH. Nor- mal ranges of left ventricular strain: a meta-analysis. *J Am Soc Echocardiogr.* 2013;26(2):185-191.

56. Pena JL, da Silva MG, Faria SC, et al. Quantification of regional left and right ventricular deformation indices in healthy neo- nates by using strain rate and strain imaging. *J Am Soc Echocar- diogr.* 2009;22(4):369-375.

57. Nestaas E, Støylen A, Fugelseth D. Myocardial performance assessment in neonates by one-segment strain and strain rate analysis by tissue Doppler – a quality improvement cohort study. *BMJ Open.* 2012;2(4):e001636).

58. Maskatia SA, Pignatelli RH, Ayres NA, Altman CA, Sangi- Haghpeykar H, Lee W. Longitudinal changes and interobserver variability of systolic myocardial deformation values in a pro- spective cohort of healthy fetuses across gestation and after delivery. *J Am Soc Echocardiogr.* 2016;29(4):341–349.

59. Elkiran O, Karakurt C, Kocak G, Karadag A. Tissue Doppler, strain, and strain rate measurements assessed by two-dimensional speckle-tracking echocardiography in healthy newborns and infants. *Cardiol Young.* 2013;24(2):201–211.

60. Marcus K, Mavinkurve-Groothuis AMC, Barends M, et al. Reference values for myocardial two-dimensional strain echocardiography in a healthy pediatric and young adult cohort. *J Am Soc Echocardiogr.* 2011;24:625-636.

61. Nestaas E, Støylen A, Brunvand L, Fugelseth D. Tissue Doppler derived longitudinal strain and strain rate during the first 3 days of life in healthy term neonates. *Pediatr Res.* 2009;65: 357-362.

62. Jain A, EL-Khuffash AF, Kuipers BCW, et al. Left ventricular function in healthy term neonates during the transitional period. *J Pediatr.* 2016;182:197-203.e2.

63. Klitsie LM, Roest AA, Haak MC, Blom NA, Ten Harkel AD. Longitudinal follow-up of ventricular performance in healthy neonates. *Early Hum Dev.* 2013;89(12):993-997.

64. Schubert U, Muller M, Norman M, Abdul-Khaliq H. Transition from fetal to neonatal life: changes in cardiac function assessed by speckle-tracking echocardiography. *Early Hum Dev.* 2013;89(10):803-808.

65. de Waal K, Lakkundi A, Othman F. Speckle tracking echocardiography in very preterm infants: feasibility and reference values. *Early Hum Dev.* 2014;90(6):275-279.

66. Nasu Y, Oyama K, Nakano S, et al. Longitudinal systolic strain of the bilayered ventricular septum during the first 72 hours of life in preterm infants. *J Echocardiogr.* 2015;13(3):90-99.

67. Schubert U, Muller M, Abdul-Khaliq H, Norman M. Preterm birth is associated with altered myocardial function in infancy. *J Am Soc Echocardiogr.* 2016;29(7):670–678.

68. de Waal K, Phad N, Lakkundi A, Tan P. Post-transitional adaptation of the left heart in uncomplicated, very preterm infants. *Cardiol Young.* 2017;27(6):1167–1173.

69. Haque U, Stiver C, Rivera BK, et al. Right ventricular performance using myocardial deformation imaging in infants with bronchopulmonary dysplasia. *J Perinatol.* 2017;37(1):81–87.

70. Sehgal A, Doctor T, Menahem S. Cyclooxygenase inhibitors in preterm infants with patent ductus arteriosus: effects on cardiac and vascular indices. *Pediatr Cardiol.* 2014;35:1429-1436.

71. Awny MA, Tolba OA, Al-Biltagi MA, Al-Asy HM, El-Mahdy HS. Cardiac functions by tissue Doppler and speckle tracking echocardiography in neonatal sepsis and its correlation with sepsis markers and cardiac Troponin-T. *J Pediatr Neonatal Care.* 2016; 5(3):00184. doi:10.15406/jpnc.2016.05.00184.

72. Cade WT, Tinius RA, Reeds DN, Patterson BW, Cahill AG. Maternal glucose and fatty acid kinetics and infant birth weight in obese women with type 2 diabetes. *Diabetes.* 2016:65(4): 893-901.

73. Hirose A, Khoo NS, Aziz K, et al. Evolution of left ventricular function in the preterm infant. *J Am Soc Echocardiogr.* 2015; 28(3):302-308.

74. Czernik C, Rhode S, Helfer S, Schmalisch G, Buhrer C, Schmitz L. Development of left ventricular longitudinal speckle tracking echocardiography in very low birth weight infants with and without bronchopulmonary dysplasia during the neonatal period. *PLoS One.* 2014;9(9):e106504.

75. Sehgal A, Wong F, Menahem S. Speckle tracking derived strain in infants with severe perinatal asphyxia: a comparative case control study. *Cardiovasc Ultrasound.* 2013;11:34.

76. James AT, Corcoran JD, Breatnach CR, Franklin O, Mertens L, El-Khuffash A. Longitudinal assessment of left and right myocardial function in preterm infants using strain and strain rate imaging. *Neonatology.* 2015;109:69-75.

77. Liao WQ, Zhou HY, Chen GC, Zou M, Lv X. Left ventricular function in newborn infants of mothers with gestational diabetes mellitus. *Zhongguo Dang Dai Er Ke Za Zhi.* 2012;14:575-577.

78. Blume GG, McLeod CJ, Barnes ME, et al. Left atrial function: physiology, assessment, and clinical implications. *Eur J Echocardiogr.* 2011;12(6):421-430.

79. Vieira MJ, Teixeira R, Gonçalves L, Gersh BJ. Left atrial mechanics: echocardiographic assessment and clinical implications. *J Am Soc Echocardiogr.* 2014;27(5):463-478.

80. Cameli M, Mandoli GE, Mondillo S. Left atrium: the last bulwark before overt heart failure. *Heart Fail Rev.* 2017;22(1):123-131.

81. Badano LP, Kolias TJ, Muraru D, et al. Standardization of left atrial, right ventricular, and right atrial deformation imaging using two-dimensional speckle tracking echocardiography: a consensus document of the EACVI/ASE/Industry Task Force to standardize deformation imaging. *Eur Heart J Cardiovasc Imaging.* 2018;19(6):591-600.

82. de Waal K, Phad N, Boyle A. Left atrium function and deformation in very preterm infants with and without volume load. *Echocardiography.* 2018;35(11):1818-1826.

83. Ficial B, Corsini I, Clemente M, et al. Feasibility, reproducibility and reference ranges of left atrial strain in preterm and term neonates in the first 48 h of life. *Diagnostics (Basel).* 2022; 12(2):350.

84. Marchese P, Cantinotti M, Van den Eynde J, et al. Left ventricular vortex analysis by high-frame rate blood speckle tracking echocardiography in healthy children and in congenital heart disease. *Int J Cardiol Heart Vasc.* 2021;37:100897.

85. Pathan F, D'Elia N, Nolan MT, Marwick TH, Negishi K. Normal ranges of left atrial strain by speckle-tracking echocardiography: a systematic review and meta-analysis. *J Am Soc Echocardiogr.* 2017;30(1):59-70.e8.

86. de Waal K, Costley N, Phad N, Crendal E. Left ventricular diastolic dysfunction and diastolic heart failure in preterm infants. *Pediatr Cardiol.* 2019;40(8):1709-1715.

87. Buckberg G, Hoffman JI, Nanda NC, Coghlan C, Saleh S, Athanasuleas C. Ventricular torsion and untwisting: further insights into mechanics and timing interdependence: a viewpoint. *Echocardiography.* 2011;28(7):782-804.

88. Alagarsamy S, Chhabra M, Gudavalli M, Nadroo AM, Sutija VG, Yugrakh D. Comparison of clinical criteria with echocardiographic findings in diagnosing PDA in preterm infants. *J Perinat Med.* 2005;33(2):161-164.

89. James A, Corcoran JD, Mertens L, Franklin O, El-Khuffash A. Left ventricular rotational mechanics in preterm infants less than 29 weeks' gestation over the first week after birth. *J Am Soc Echocardiogr.* 2015;28(7):808-817.

90. Huang SJ, Orde S. From speckle tracking echocardiography to torsion: research tool today, clinical practice tomorrow. *Curr Opin Crit Care.* 2013;19(3):250-257.

91. Kaku K, Takeuchi M, Tsang W, et al. Age-related normal range of left ventricular strain and torsion using three-dimensional speckle-tracking echocardiography. *J Am Soc Echocardiogr.* 2014;27(1):55-64.

92. Zhang Y, Zhou QC, Pu DR, Zou L, Tan Y. Differences in left ventricular twist related to age: speckle tracking echocardiographic data for healthy volunteers from neonate to age 70 years. *Echocardiography.* 2010;27(10):1205-1210.

93. Poelmann RE, Gittenberger-de Groot AC. Hemodynamics in cardiac development. *J Cardiovasc Dev Dis.* 2018;5(4):54.

94. Lindsey SE, Butcher JT, Yalcin HC. Mechanical regulation of cardiac development. *Front Physiol.* 2014;5:318.

95. Pedrizzetti G, La Canna G, Alfieri O, Tonti G. The vortex – an early predictor of cardiovascular outcome? *Nat Rev Cardiol.* 2014;11:545-553.

96. Kheradvar A, Houle H, Pedrizzetti G, et al. Echocardiographic particle image velocimetry: a novel technique for quantification of left ventricular blood vorticity pattern. *J Am Soc Echocardiogr.* 2010;23(1):86-94.

97. Mele D, Smarrazzo V, Pedrizzetti G, et al. Intracardiac flow analysis: techniques and potential clinical applications. *J Am Soc Echocardiogr.* 2019;32(3):319-332.

98. Nyrnes SA, Fadnes S, Wigen MS, Mertens L, Lovstakken L. Blood speckle-tracking based on high-frame rate ultrasound imaging in pediatric cardiology. *J Am Soc Echocardiogr.* 2020;33(4):493-503.e5.

99. de Waal K, Crendal E, Boyle A. Left ventricular vortex formation in preterm infants assessed by blood speckle imaging. *Echocardiography.* 2019;36(7):1364-1371.

100. Mawad W, Løvstakken L, Fadnes S, et al. Right ventricular flow dynamics in dilated right ventricles: energy loss estimation based on blood speckle tracking echocardiography – a pilot study in children. *Ultrasound Med Biol.* 2021;47(6):1514-1527.

101. Phad NS, de Waal K, Holder C, Oldmeadow C. Dilated hypertrophy: a distinct pattern of cardiac remodeling in preterm infants. *Pediatr Res.* 2020;87(1):146-152.

102. de Waal K, Phad N, Crendal E. Intracardiac Blood Flow Patterns Detemine the Development of the Preterm Heart [abstract only]. Sydney: ASUM; 2021.

# ASSESSMENT OF HEMODYNAMICS AND CARDIAC FUNCTION: OTHER METHODS

# Chapter 12

# Assessment of Cardiac Output in Neonates: Techniques Using the Fick Principle, Indicator Dilution Technology, Doppler Ultrasound, Electrical Biosensing Technology, and Arterial Pulse Contour Analysis

Willem-Pieter de Boode and Shahab Noori

## Key Points

- Cardiac output monitoring in preterm and term neonates is feasible but remains challenging despite the availability of different technologies.
- The best systems to monitor cardiac output in the clinical setting in neonatal intensive care at present are transthoracic echocardiography, transpulmonary indicator dilution, electrical biosensing technology, and arterial pulse contour analysis.
- Noninvasive cardiac output monitoring is inversely related to accuracy; hence there will always be a compromise between these two characteristics.
- A normal cardiac output does not imply adequate perfusion of all tissues; cardiac output assessment will only provide information about global blood flow.
- Advanced hemodynamic monitoring in itself will not improve outcome; it is the correct interpretation of the acquired variables and the resultant, appropriately tested hemodynamic management approaches that may result in better outcomes.

## Introduction

Appropriate monitoring of the cardiovascular system and thus treatment of critically ill neonates with cardiovascular compromise hinge on the ability to monitor at least two of the three interdependent cardiovascular parameters (blood pressure, cardiac output, and systemic vascular resistance), determining systemic blood flow and thus systemic oxygen delivery. In the following equation the Hagen-Poiseuille law is applied to systemic blood flow (similar to Ohm law in electrical circuits):

$$SVR = \frac{SABP - RAP}{CO} \tag{12.1}$$

where CO is the cardiac output (i.e., systemic blood flow); (SABP − RAP) is the pressure difference between systolic arterial blood pressure (SABP) and right atrial pressure (RAP); and SVR is systemic vascular resistance.

Oxygen delivery can be calculated when cardiac output and arterial oxygen content are known:

$$DO_2 = CO \times CaO_2 \tag{12.2}$$

where $DO_2$ denotes oxygen delivery to the tissues, CO is the cardiac output, and $CaO_2$ is the arterial oxygen content.

At present, only blood pressure can be monitored continuously in absolute numbers in real time, albeit only invasively (see Chapter 3). Since reliable monitoring of SVR is not possible at present, continuous, noninvasive real-time assessment of beat-to-beat cardiac output has become the "holy grail" of modern-day neonatal intensive care. This is even more relevant considering the limited ability to clinically assess cardiac output using indirect parameters of systemic blood flow irrespective of the experience level of the clinician.[1-3] With the ability to continuously monitor both blood pressure and cardiac output in real time, the neonatologist is able to more accurately diagnose and perhaps treat neonatal shock (see Chapters 1, 21-24).

Several methods of cardiac output measurement are available. However, not all technologies are feasible in neonates due to size restraints, potential indicator toxicity, risk of fluid overload, difficulties in vascular access, and the presence of shunts during the transitional phase and in patients with congenital heart defects. A classification of the different methods used for cardiac output measurement is depicted in Box 12.1.

## BOX 12.1  CLASSIFICATION OF METHODS FOR CARDIAC OUTPUT ASSESSMENT

### FICK PRINCIPLE–BASED METHODS
Oxygen Fick ($O_2$-Fick)
Carbon dioxide Fick ($CO_2$-Fick)
- Modified carbon dioxide Fick method (m$CO_2$F)
- Carbon dioxide rebreathing technology ($CO_2$-R)

### INDICATOR DILUTION TECHNIQUES
Pulmonary artery thermodilution (PATD)
Transpulmonary thermodilution (TPTD)
Transpulmonary lithium dilution (TPLiD)
Transpulmonary ultrasound dilution (TPUD)
Pulse dye densitometry (PDD)

### DOPPLER ULTRASOUND
Transesophageal echocardiography/Doppler (TEE/TED)
Transcutaneous Doppler (TCD)
Transthoracic echocardiography (TTE)

### ELECTRICAL BIOSENSING TECHNIQUES (EBTS)
Thoracic bioimpedance (TBI)
Thoracic bioreactance (TBR)
Whole-body bioimpedance (WBBI)

### ARTERIAL PULSE CONTOUR ANALYSIS (APCA)
As an adjunct to and calibrated by indicator dilution methods
Modelflow method
Pressure recording analytical method (PRAM)

### CARDIAC MAGNETIC RESONANCE IMAGING (MRI)

*In this box different methods used for cardiac output measurement are summarized, divided into six categories.*

An ideal method for the assessment of cardiac output is expected to include appropriate validation for accuracy and precision in real-time and absolute numbers, as well as trending ability. In addition, the ideal method should be continuous, reliable, practical, affordable, and easy to use and document. Finally, its ability to assess systemic blood flow in neonates with extra- and intracardiac shunting is an important requirement. Currently, none of the available methods are even close to fulfilling all these requirements.

## The Importance of Validation

It is of the utmost importance to pay attention to the validation of cardiac output monitoring systems prior to their introduction into clinical practice. Validation studies, especially in preterm neonates, are scarce and generally include only small numbers of patients. A new technology for cardiac output measurement must be validated against a gold standard reference method that is known to be accurate and precise and does not affect the technology being tested. Ideally, this means validation against transit time flow probes, since this is considered the optimal in vivo reference method with a variability of less than 10%.[4-6] The flow probe should be positioned around the pulmonary artery, since this will represent true systemic blood flow in the absence of shunts. Placing the flow probe around the ascending aorta will underestimate systemic blood flow, because coronary blood flow is not taken into account.[7] Given the invasiveness of this reference method, its use is generally limited to animal studies. The Fick technology and the transpulmonary thermodilution (TPTD) cardiac output measurement are considered the clinical gold-standard methods in pediatric critical care.[8-10] However, these technologies are not feasible in newborn infants.

Bland-Altman analysis is the most appropriate statistical method for comparing cardiac output measurements using two different technologies.[11] Correlation and regression analysis are not sufficient for this purpose. With Bland-Altman analysis, the difference between the two methods (bias) is plotted against their mean. The accuracy is expressed as the mean bias, while precision is defined as the limits of agreement (LOA). The LOA can be calculated from the standard deviation (SD) of the mean bias (LOA = ±1.96 × SD). The LOA provides us with a range of the difference in cardiac output between two methods for 95% of the study population. It is recommended to express both accuracy and precision as a percentage of mean cardiac output instead of an absolute value.[12] Bias percentage (bias%) is defined as the mean bias divided by mean cardiac output multiplied by 100 (%), while the error percentage (error%) is calculated as 100% × LOA/mean cardiac output. The difference between accuracy and precision is further explained in Figure 12.1.[13]

For acceptance of a new technology, the accuracy (bias%) and precision (error%) should at least be comparable with the reference method. This stresses the importance of the use of a valid, and preferably gold-standard, technique for reference. A new technology is generally accepted when the error% is ±30% or less.[12] However, this cutoff value is based on the assumption that the precision of the reference method is ±10% to 20% with the acceptance of a new technology when the error% is no more than ±20%. When using a reference method with an error% of more than 20%, the cutoff value for acceptance of the tested technique should be adjusted.[12,13]

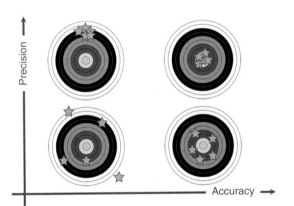

**Fig. 12.1 Validation of the new method of cardiac output measurement expressed as accuracy and precision.** The closer every measurement with the new technique (comparator) is to the bull's eye (gold-standard reference technology), the more accurate the comparator is; the more the spread between multiple measurements, the more imprecise the comparator is. (From Cecconi M, Rhodes A, Poloniecki J, et al. Bench-to-bedside review: the importance of the precision of the reference technique in method comparison studies – with specific reference to the measurement of cardiac output. *Crit Care*. 2009;13(1):201. doi:10.1186/cc7129.)

The combined error% can be calculated using the following formula:

$$error_{COMP+REF} = \sqrt{(error_{COMP})^2 + (error_{REF})^2} \quad (12.3)$$

where error%$_{COMP+REF}$ is the combined error%, error%$_{COMP}$ is the error% of the comparator (new method), and error%$_{REF}$ is the error% of the reference method.

The resultant error percentage as a function of the error percentage of the tested method (comparator) and the reference method, respectively, is displayed as an error-gram, as shown in Figure 12.2.[12]

In addition, the agreement in monitoring temporal changes in cardiac output (trending ability) should be studied by analysis of four-quadrant plots and polar plot methodology.[14-16] In a concordance plot the changes in cardiac output, assessed with the comparator ($\Delta CO_{COMP}$), are plotted against the changes in cardiac output, assessed with the reference method ($\Delta CO_{REF}$). When the changes in cardiac output are in the same direction within the two methods, these changes are concordant. Discordant measurements occur when the changes in one method are in the opposite direction of the other technology. The concordance rate is calculated as the number of concordant measurements divided by the total number of measurements (concordant plus discordant). A concordance rate of >95% is considered good, 90–95% marginal, and <90% poor trending ability.[14] Polar plot analysis considers not only the direction but also the magnitude of temporal changes in cardiac output. In a polar plot each data point ($\Delta CO_{REF}$ vs $\Delta CO_{COMP}$) is determined by an angle (the direction of change) and a radius (the magnitude of change). This enables the calculation of:

- the *angular bias*, that is, the average angle between all polar plot data and the polar axis (0°). An angular bias ≤±5° is considered a good trending ability.[16]
- the *radial limits of agreement* (LOA), the radial sector that encompasses 95% of all data points, defined as mean angular bias ± 1.96 SD. Radial LOA ±27 to 37° is classified as good, ±37 to 45° as moderate, and ≥±45° as poor trending.[16] In general, radial LOA of <±30° is acceptable.

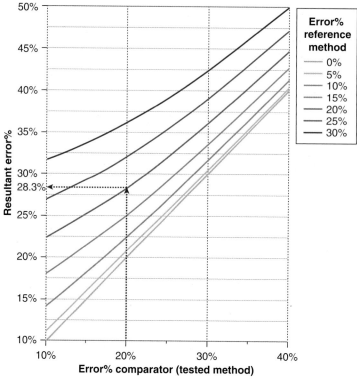

**Fig. 12.2** Resultant error% as a function of the error percentages of the used reference method and tested comparator (error-gram). *X*-axis: error% of the tested method (comparator). *Y*-axis: resultant error% dependent on the precision of the used reference method (isolines).[12] For example, when the limits of agreement of the comparator are ±20%, and the used reference method has an error% of 20% (*red line*), and the resultant error% is 28.3% (*red arrows*).

- the *angular concordance rate*, that is, the percentage of data points within the ±30° radial zone. An angular concordance rate of >92% represents a good trending ability.[16]

This chapter will provide an overview of all available technologies for the assessment of cardiac output, with emphasis on their applicability in (preterm) newborn infants. A summary of the characteristics, advantages, and limitations of each method is presented in Table 12.1. When available, the results of neonatal validation studies are shown in tables within the appropriate paragraphs.

## Fick Principle

Methods using the Fick principle might utilize the direct Fick method or one of its modifications to render the technique more clinically applicable. However, the modifications often come at the expense of accuracy. In 1870 German physiologist Adolf Eugen Fick stated that the volume of blood flow in a given period (cardiac output) equals the amount of a substance entering the bloodstream in the same period divided by the difference in concentrations of the substance upstream and downstream, respectively.[17]

### OXYGEN FICK

Determination of cardiac output according to the original or direct Fick method requires the application of a face mask (or some means of assessing oxygen consumption) and consideration of arterial and venous oxygen concentration, which is usually obtained by taking blood samples for laboratory analysis. The direct Fick method employing a measurement of pulmonary

**TABLE 12.1 Overview of Different Methods of Cardiac Output Monitoring**

| Method | Invasive? | Continuous (C) or Intermittent (I) | Equipment | Feasible in Neonates? | Validation Studies in Neonates? | Advantages | Limitations |
|---|---|---|---|---|---|---|---|
| **Fick Principle** | | | | | | | |
| $O_2$-Fick | + | I | AC, CVC | + | – | Accurate, especially in low flow state | Need for multiple, multisite blood sampling; accuracy limited in the presence of cardiopulmonary disease, air leakage, and enhanced pulmonary oxygen consumption (as in preterms with bronchopulmonary dysplasia); affected by shunts; less reliable in high flow state |
| $mCO_2F$ | + | I | AC, CVC | + | – | No specific additional equipment required; reliable in the presence of significant left-to-right shunt; use of regular arterial and central venous catheters | Need for multiple, multisite blood sampling; inaccuracy related to calculation error of carbon dioxide concentration in blood |
| $CO_2$-R | – | I | ET | – | – | Easy to use; noninvasive | Not feasible/accurate in children with BSA <0.6 m$^2$ and tidal volume <300 mL; only applicable in intubated patients; contraindicated in patients susceptible to fluctuating arterial carbon dioxide levels |
| **Indicator Dilution** | | | | | | | |
| PATD | +++ | I (& C) | PAC | – | – | Clinical gold standard of cardiac output monitoring in adults; ancillary hemodynamic variables provided | Very invasive; not feasible in small children; relatively high complication rate; transient bradycardia in response to fast injection of cold saline; results affected by shunt |
| TPTD | ++ | I (& C) | Dedicated AC, CVC | – | – | Clinical gold standard in pediatric patients; continuous monitoring when used to calibrate APCA; ancillary hemodynamic variables provided; reliable in presence of significant LtR-shunt | Dedicated thermistor-tipped arterial catheter required; catheterization of femoral, brachial, or axillary artery needed; repetitive measurements affect fluid balance |

*Continued on following page*

**TABLE 12.1** Overview of Different Methods of Cardiac Output Monitoring (Continued)

| Method | Invasive? | Continuous (C) or Intermittent (I) | Equipment | Feasible in Neonates? | Validation Studies in Neonates? | Advantages | Limitations |
|---|---|---|---|---|---|---|---|
| TPLiD | ++ | I (& C) | AC, CVC | − | − | Regular catheters used; continuous monitoring when used to calibrate APCA; ancillary hemodynamic variables provided | Lithium toxicity; need to withdraw blood; limited repeated measurements possible; not compatible with non-depolarizing muscle relaxants; influenced by hyponatremia; results affected by shunts |
| TPUD | ++ | I (& C) | AC, CVC | + | − | Nontoxic indicator; small indicator volume; ancillary hemodynamic variables provided; safe with regard to cerebral and systemic oxygenation and circulation; reliable in presence of significant LtR-shunt or heterogeneous lung injury | Repetitive measurements affect fluid balance; necessity to use extracorporeal loop |
| PDD | + | I | CVC | + | − | Noninvasive detection of indocyanine green; intravascular volume measurement possible | Limited repeated measurements possible; inaccuracy due to poor peripheral perfusion, motion artifact, or excess light; rarely side effects; difficulty in the acquisition of reliable pulse waveforms in small children and newborns |
| **Doppler Ultrasound** | | | | | | | |
| TEE | + | I | Esophageal probe | ± | − | Less invasive; evaluation of cardiac function and structure | Significant training required; highly operator dependent; inaccuracy due to errors in the calculation of velocity time integral, cross-sectional area and angle of insonation; not feasible in infants <3 kg; small risk of complications; not tolerated by conscious patients |
| TED | + | I | Esophageal probe | ± | − | Less invasive; continuous monitoring | Inaccuracy due to errors in the calculation of velocity time integral, cross-sectional area, and angle of insonation; not feasible in infants <3 kg; small risk of complications; not tolerated by conscious patients |

| Method | | | | | Device | Advantages | Limitations |
|---|---|---|---|---|---|---|---|
| TCD | – | | + | + | External probe | Noninvasive; easy to use | Blind aiming of transducer for signal acquisition; error due to insonation angle deviation; no real measurement of cross-sectional area of outflow tract; large interobserver variability; questionable accuracy and precision |
| TTE | – | | + | + | Echocardiograph | Noninvasive; evaluation in detail of cardiac function and structure; additional information about potential intra- and extracardiac shunting; most used method of cardiac output monitoring in neonatal clinical care | Significant training required; highly operator dependent; not an easy, bedside method; high intra- and interobserver variability; inaccuracy due to errors in the calculation of velocity time integral, cross-sectional area, and angle of insonation |
| **Electrical Biosensing Technology** | | | | | | | |
| EC | – | C | + | + | Surface electrodes on thorax | Only real noninvasive technology; continuous monitoring; user-independent; ancillary hemodynamic variables provided; easy to apply | Sensitive to motion artifact; inaccuracy due to alteration in position or contact of the electrodes, irregular heart rates, and acute changes in tissue water content; compromised reliability on high-frequency ventilation; questionable accuracy and precision |
| BR | – | C | + | + | Surface electrodes on thorax | | Sensitive to motion artifact; inaccuracy due to alteration in position or contact of the electrodes, irregular heart rates, and acute changes in tissue water content |
| WBEBT | – | C | + | – | Surface electrodes on wrist and contralateral ankle | | |
| **Arterial Pulse Contour Analysis** | | | | | | | |
| PulseCO | ++ | C | – | – | AC, CVC | Less invasive; continuous monitoring | Repeated calibration required; use of small arterial catheters can cause distortion of the shape of the pressure wave and overdamped curves; accuracy influenced by changes in arterial compliance, changes in vasomotor tone, and irregular heart rate |

*Continued on following page*

| TABLE 12.1 | Overview of Different Methods of Cardiac Output Monitoring (Continued) | | | | | |
|---|---|---|---|---|---|---|
| Method | Invasive? | Continuous (C) or Intermittent (I) | Equipment | Feasible in Neonates? | Validation Studies in Neonates? | Advantages | Limitations |
| PICCO | ++ | C | Dedicated AC, CVC | – | – | Less invasive; continuous monitoring | Repeated calibration required; accuracy influenced by changes in arterial compliance, changes in vasomotor tone, and irregular heart rate |
| PRAM | + | C | AC | + | + | Less invasive; continuous monitoring; no calibration required | Use of small arterial catheters can cause distortion of the shape of the pressure wave and overdamped curves; accuracy influenced by changes in arterial compliance, changes in vasomotor tone, and irregular heart rate; questionable accuracy and precision |

*AC*, Arterial catheter; *APCA*, arterial pulse contour analysis; *BR*, bioreactance; *BSA*, body surface area; *CO₂-R*, $CO_2$ rebreathing; *CVC*, central venous catheter; *EC*, electrical cardiometry; *ET*, endotracheal tube; *LtR*, left-to-right; *mCO₂F*, modified $CO_2$-Fick method; *O₂-Fick*, oxygen Fick; *PAC*, pulmonary artery catheter; *PATD*, pulmonary artery thermodilution; *PDD*, pulse dye densitometry; *PICCO*, APCA calibrated by TPTD; *PRAM*, pressure recording analytical method; *PulseCO*, APCA calibrated by TPLID; *TCD*, transcutaneous Doppler; *TED*, transesophageal Doppler; *TEE*, transesophageal echocardiography; *TPLiD*, transpulmonary lithium dilution; *TPTD*, transpulmonary thermodilution; *TPUD*, transpulmonary ultrasound dilution; *TTE*, transthoracic echocardiography; *WBEBT*, whole-body electrical biosensing technology.

oxygen uptake (discussed later) is considered the gold standard for assessing cardiac output, despite several disadvantages. It is of note though that recent advances in magnetic resonance imaging (MRI) technology have initiated a shift in our thinking; specifically, MRI-derived estimates of cardiac output measurement are now considered by many experts as the gold standard for the measurement of cardiac output. However, MRI-based cardiac output measurement is only feasible in stable patients who are fit enough to undergo MRI scanning (see Chapter 13). According to the direct Fick principle, cardiac output is calculated by dividing oxygen consumption ($VO_2$) by the difference in the oxygen content of the aortic blood ($CaO_2$) and the mixed venous blood ($CmvO_2$).

The applicability in its original form, measuring $VO_2$ instead of assuming it, is limited by the fact that in non-intubated patients a face mask must be used. With respect to the application in neonates, a further limitation is that multiple and multisite blood sampling is required. With oxygen being the substance for this method, the Fick principle states that during steady state, oxygen uptake in the pulmonary system equals the oxygen consumption in the tissues (Figure 12.3). Cardiac output (pulmonary blood flow) can be calculated by dividing the pulmonary oxygen uptake by the oxygen concentration gradient (difference) between arterial blood ($CaO_2$) and $CmvO_2$. Under steady-state condition, tissue oxygen consumption is equal to pulmonary oxygen uptake ($VO_2$). Hence

$$CO = \frac{VO_2}{CaO_2 - CmvO_2} \qquad (12.4)$$

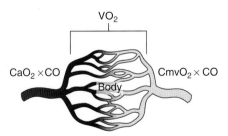

**Fig. 12.3 Fick principle.** See text for details. $CaO_2$, arterial oxygen concentration; $CmvO_2$, mixed venous oxygen concentration; $CO$, cardiac output; $VO_2$, pulmonary oxygen uptake ($O_2$ consumption).

where CO is the cardiac output in L/min, $VO_2$ is pulmonary oxygen uptake in mL $O_2$/min, $CaO_2$ is oxygen concentration of arterial blood in mL $O_2$/L, and $CmvO_2$ is oxygen concentration of mixed venous blood (preferably determined in the pulmonary artery) in mL $O_2$/L.

Pediatric and adult patients differ in oxygen consumption. Cardiac index is 30–60% higher in neonates and infants to help meet their increased oxygen consumption. Fetal hemoglobin is present in decreasing concentration up to 3–6 months following birth, has higher oxygen affinity, and thus does not deliver oxygen to the tissues as effectively as does adult hemoglobin, when arterial oxygen saturation increases from the fetal levels of 75% in the ascending aorta to 98–100% after birth. In neonates the combination of a higher hemoglobin concentration (16–19 g/dL compared with 13.5–17.5 g/dL in men and 12–16 g/dL in women), higher blood volume per kilogram of body weight, and increased cardiac output compensate for the decreased release of oxygen from hemoglobin to the tissues.

### Pulmonary Oxygen Uptake

Pulmonary oxygen uptake ($VO_2$), or oxygen consumption, can be measured via a Douglas bag, by mass spectrometry, spirometry, or metabolic monitors (indirect calorimetry).[18] Table 12.2 depicts $VO_2$ measurements obtained in different patient populations and under different clinical conditions.[19-22] Instead of actually measuring $VO_2$, this can also be estimated with the use of different regression equations.[23,24] However, the estimation of $VO_2$, which is also referred to as the indirect Fick method, is subject to errors in the determination of cardiac output potentially exceeding 50%. Because of the potential errors and its questionable adaptability to neonates, the cardiac output obtained by the indirect Fick method may be used in neonates for orientation purposes only.

### Oxygen Concentration Gradient

Oxygen concentration ($cO_2$) is calculated by determining hemoglobin concentration (Hb) and oxygen saturation ($sO_2$), which traditionally is obtained by blood gas analysis:

$$cO_2 = (Hb \times sO_2 \times 1.36) + (pO_2 \times 0.0032) \quad (12.5)$$

**TABLE 12.2 Pulmonary Oxygen Uptake or Oxygen Consumption ($VO_2$) in Different Patient Populations**

| Group | $VO_2$ (Mean $\pm$ SD) | Notes |
|---|---|---|
| Adults | 125 mL $O_2$/min/m² | Indexed for body surface area |
| Healthy newborns (Bauer, 2002)[20] | 6.7 $\pm$ 0.6 to 7.1 $\pm$ 0.4 mL $O_2$/min/kg | Indexed for body weight ($n = 7$) |
| Neonates with sepsis (Bauer, 2002)[20] | 7.0 $\pm$ 0.3 to 8.2 $\pm$ 0.4 mL $O_2$/min/kg | $n = 10$ |
| Mechanically ventilated preterm infants (Shiao, 2006)[21] | 8.0 $\pm$ 3.73 mL $O_2$/min/kg | <8 h after blood drawn ($n = 202$) |
| | 11.3 $\pm$ 5.65 mL $O_2$/min/kg | $\geq$8 h after blood drawn ($n = 65$) |
| Preterm and term infants before and 1 h after feeding (Stothers and Warner, 1979)[19] | 4.8 mL $O_2$/min/kg (estimated from Figure 6.1) | $n = 9$ preterm infants<br>$n = 9$ term infants |
| Term infants during sleep[22] | 5.97 mL $O_2$/min/kg during REM sleep<br>5.72 mL $O_2$/min/kg during non-REM sleep | $n = 30$ |

Pulmonary oxygen uptake in adults, healthy term newborns, neonates with sepsis, mechanically ventilated preterm neonates, and preterm and term neonates before and after feeding.[19-21] See text for details.

where Hb is hemoglobin in g/dL, $sO_2$ is oxygen saturation as gradient, 1.36 is the oxygen binding capacity of hemoglobin in mL $O_2$/g, 0.0032 is the solubility coefficient of oxygen in mL $O_2$/mmHg, and $pO_2$ is the partial pressure of oxygen in mmHg.

Note that the aforementioned equation obtains oxygen content ($cO_2$) in mL $O_2$/dL. To obtain oxygen concentration ($cO_2$) in mL $O_2$/L, one needs to multiply the result by 10 (1 L = 10 dL). Because dissolved oxygen contributes very little to the total oxygen-carrying capacity in the normal range of $pO_2$, oxygen content can be approximated by

$$cO_2 = Hb \times sO_2 \times 1.36 \qquad (12.6)$$

and the gradient by

$$c_{(a - mv)}O_2 = Hb \times sO_2 \times (SaO_2 - SmvO_2) \qquad (12.7)$$

where Hb is hemoglobin in g/dL, $SaO_2$ is arterial (pulmonary vein) oxygen saturation as gradient, and $SmvO_2$ is mixed venous (pulmonary artery) oxygen saturation as gradient.

Alternative to blood gas analysis, $SaO_2$ and $SvO_2$ may be obtained via catheters (e.g., Opticath catheter in combination with Oximetric-3 monitors, Abbott Critical Care Systems, Abbott Laboratories, Abbott Park, Illinois). The limitation is, however, that not

mixed venous but central venous blood is sampled, and these are not interchangeable regarding oxygen saturation or oxygen content. Arterial oxygen saturation ($SaO_2$) may be approximated noninvasively by $SpO_2$ obtained via pulse oximetry.

### Cardiac Output (Calculation Examples)

Assuming a neonate with $VO_2$ of 7 mL $O_2$/min/kg, Hb of 17 g/dL, $SaO_2$ of 99%, and $SmvO_2$ of 75%,

$$c_{(a - mv)}O_2 = Hb \times 1.36 \times (SaO_2 - SmvO_2)$$

$$= 17\left(\frac{g}{dl}\right) \times 1.36\left(\frac{mLO_2}{g}\right) \times (0.99 - 0.75)$$

$$= 5.55\frac{mLO_2}{dL}$$

With $VO_2$ normalized for weight, the cardiac output is

$$CI = \frac{VO_2}{CaO_2 - CmvO_2} = \frac{7.0\left(\frac{mL\ O_2}{min.kg}\right)}{5.55\left(\frac{mL\ O_2}{dL}\right)}$$

$$= 1.26\left(\frac{dL}{min.kg}\right) = 0.126\frac{L}{min.kg}$$

According to this calculation, cardiac output is 126 mL/kg/min in a neonate under physiologic circumstances. In a study by Tibby and colleagues, in five neonates with birth weights of 3.2 kg or less, the median CO following surgical correction of their congenital heart disease was 138 mL/kg/min.[8] However, CO measured by echocardiography in neonates averages around 200 mL/kg/min. There are several reasons why our calculation suggests lower cardiac output compared with the CO assessed by echocardiography. While the Hb concentration assumed in the equation is normal for term neonates in the transitional period, it is likely too high for neonates who underwent cardiac catheterization for clinical reasons and had their CO determined using the Fick principle. In these patients oxygen consumption is also likely to be higher than that of a healthy term neonate. In addition, the methods using the direct Fick principle yield a lower CO compared with that assessed by echocardiography because of the physiologic shunting (approximately 20%) present in the lungs. Indeed, if we change the Hb concentration and the $VO_2$ to 15 g/dL and 8 mL $O_2$/min/kg, respectively, and add 20% to compensate for the physiologic shunting in the lungs, we get a CO of 196 mL/kg/min, which is the same as the estimated 200 mL/kg/min of average CO determined by echocardiography.

## CARBON DIOXIDE FICK

With the $CO_2$-Fick method, instead of using oxygen as a marker, the exchange of carbon dioxide may be used. This principle is used in the *modified carbon dioxide Fick method* (m$CO_2$F) and the *carbon dioxide rebreathing technology* (CO_2R).

### Modified Carbon Dioxide Fick Method

The m$CO_2$F is based on the principle that steady-state carbon dioxide production in the tissue is equal to pulmonary carbon dioxide exchange ($VCO_2$):

$$CO = \frac{VCO_2}{CvCO_2 - CaCO_2} \quad (12.8)$$

where CO is the cardiac output in L/min, $VCO_2$ is the pulmonary carbon dioxide exchange in mL $CO_2$/min, $CaCO_2$ is the carbon dioxide concentration in arterial blood in mL $CO_2$/min, and $CvCO_2$ is the carbon diox-

ide concentration of venous blood (preferably determined in the pulmonary artery), measured in mL $CO_2$/L.

Pulmonary carbon dioxide exchange ($VCO_2$) may be measured using volumetric capnography. In a ventilated patient $VCO_2$ can be determined by analysis of the expiratory airflow ($Q_{exp}$) and carbon dioxide fraction in the expiratory air ($FeCO_2$):

$$VCO_2 = \left\{ \int Q_{exp(t)} \cdot FeCO_2(t) \cdot dt \right\} \cdot T^{-1} \quad (12.9)$$

where $Q_{exp}$ is expiratory airflow in L/min, $FeCO_2$ is carbon dioxide fraction in expiratory air in mL $CO_2$/L, and T is time in minutes.

Carbon dioxide in an arterial or venous blood sample ($CbCO_2$) can be measured by the Douglas equation.[25] The amount of both pulmonary $CO_2$ exchange and systemic $CO_2$ production must be converted to *standard temperature pressure, dry conditions*. This method has been validated in an animal model, and the site of venous blood sampling has been shown to be of minor importance.[26] Interestingly, the presence of a significant left-to-right shunt through an artificial ductus arteriosus did not influence the accuracy of the m$CO_2$F method in another study using a juvenile animal model.[27] No studies in newborn infants have been published, probably related to the limitation of the need for frequent and multisite blood sampling.

### Carbon Dioxide Rebreathing Technology

In the rebreathing method mixed venous $CO_2$ concentration is estimated from exhaled gas and in this way obviates the need for direct measurement. The change in $CO_2$ exchange and resultant change in arterial $CO_2$ concentration secondary to an end-expiratory hold or addition of dead space is used in the $CO_2$-Fick equation:

$$Q_{PCBF} = \frac{VCO_2 n}{CmvCO_2 n - CaCO_2 n} = \frac{VCO_2 r}{CmvCO_2 r - CaCO_2 r} \quad (12.10)$$

where $Q_{PCBF}$ is the pulmonary capillary blood flow in L/min, $VCO_2$ is the pulmonary carbon dioxide exchange in mL $CO_2$/min, n denotes normal situation, r denotes rebreathing, $CaCO_2$ is the carbon dioxide concentration in arterial blood in mL $CO_2$/min, and $CmvCO_2$ is the carbon dioxide concentration of mixed venous blood in ml $CO_2$/L.

Pulmonary blood flow is considered constant during the measurements. Another assumption is that $CmvCO_2$ is not significantly changed throughout the period of rebreathing and nonrebreathing, implying that

$$CmvCO_2 n \cong CmvCO_2 r \qquad (12.11)$$

Therefore

$$Q_{PCBF} = \frac{VCO_2 n - VCO_2 r}{(CmvCO_2 n - CaCO_2 n) - (CmvCO_2 r - CaCO_2 r)} \qquad (12.12)$$
$$= \frac{\Delta VCO_2}{\Delta CaCO_2}$$

where $\Delta VCO_2$ denotes the change in pulmonary $CO_2$ exchange and $\Delta CaCO_2$ the change in arterial carbon dioxide concentration.

Pulmonary capillary blood flow only yields an estimate of the non-shunted blood flow participating in gas exchange. The blood bypassing the lung (shunted blood flow) may be estimated and added to $Q_{PCBF}$ to determine overall cardiac output as follows[28]:

$$CO = Q_{PCBF} + Q_{SHUNT}. \qquad (12.13)$$

Moreover, it is not the change in $CaCO_2$ that is measured in clinical practice, but the change in the partial pressure of carbon dioxide ($pCO_2$) at the endotracheal tube, assuming that endotracheal $\Delta pCO_2$, alveolar $\Delta pCO_2$, and arterial $\Delta CaCO_2$ are interchangeable. This may lead to errors in cardiac output calculation, especially in situations with large dead space ventilation.

The NICO system (Philips Respironics, Pittsburgh, Pennsylvania) is an example of a monitor incorporating the carbon dioxide rebreathing method. However, this device is not feasible in small children because of the large dead space of the rebreathing valve. In newborn infants, particularly in premature infants, partial rebreathing is contraindicated, since the technology is based on changes in arterial carbon dioxide concentrations causing significant changes in cerebral blood flow. Indeed, significant alterations in $PaCO_2$ have been shown to be associated with an increased risk of intraventricular hemorrhage, periventricular leukomalacia, and impaired neurodevelopmental outcome (see Chapters 1, 2, and 7).[29-31]

## Indicator Dilution Techniques

In 1761 Haller reported a new methodology to measure pulmonary circulation time with the use of a colored dye in an animal model.[32] This principle was adopted and modified initially by Stewart[33,34] and later by Hamilton,[35,36] and it's now known as the indicator dilution technique. An indicator dilution curve can be obtained by measuring the change in time of the concentration of a known quantity of indicator that is injected proximal to the point of measurement. With the use of the Stewart-Hamilton equation, blood flow (cardiac output) can be derived from the dilution curve:

$$CO = \frac{60 \cdot i}{\int C(t)dt}, \qquad (12.14)$$

where CO is the cardiac output in L/min, $i$ is the injected quantity of indicator in mg, $C$ is the concentration of indicator in mg/L (area under the indicator dilution curve), and $t$ indicates time in seconds.

Cardiac output is inversely proportional to the area under the dilution curve. The lower the blood flow, the higher the measured indicator concentration – hence the larger the area under the dilution curve (Figure 12.4A). Different indicators are used to obtain dilution curves, such as indocyanine green (ICG), Evans blue and brilliant red in dye dilution, cold solutions in thermodilution, lithium in lithium dilution, and isotonic saline in ultrasound dilution.

The following prerequisites need to be met for a reliable interpretation of the indicator dilution technique: fast, instantaneous injection of a small volume of indicator; fast and complete mixing of indicator and blood; no indicator loss between site of injection and detection; no changes in blood volume; uniform volume flow; no shunting; minimal valve regurgitation; flow of indicator identical to blood flow; blood flow not influenced by the volume of injected indicator; steady-state status; and stable hemodynamics during the measurement.[18] Potential limitations of this technology include the lack of indicator stability, inaccuracy in indicator measurement, and accumulation of indicator. The influence of a left-to-right shunt and right-to-left shunt on the indicator dilution curve is shown in Figures 12.4B and C, respectively.

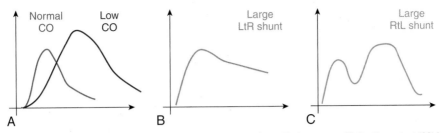

**Fig. 12.4 Indicator dilution curves.** Several configurations of transpulmonary indicator dilution curves. (A) Cardiac output (CO) is inversely proportional to the area under the dilution curve. (B) Large left-to-right (LtR) shunt will lead to early recirculation and therefore a prolonged detection of the indicator. (C) Large right-to-left (RtL) shunt will in fact lead to two dilution curves. The first curve is caused by the indicator that is bypassing the pulmonary circulation and is detected very soon; the non-shunted, transpulmonary passage of the indicator is detected as a second curve.

## PULMONARY ARTERY THERMODILUTION

A specific thermistor-tipped pulmonary artery catheter, also known as a Swan-Ganz catheter, is used to measure the change in blood temperature downstream after the injection of a cold solution in the right atrium. This change in blood temperature is used to obtain an indicator dilution curve from which the cardiac output is calculated. Despite many sources of potential errors, pulmonary artery thermodilution (PATD) is regarded as one of the clinical gold-standard technologies in adult critical care. For obvious reasons, the insertion of a flow-directed pulmonary catheter is not feasible in small infants.

## TRANSPULMONARY INDICATOR DILUTION AND THERMODILUTION

The technique of *transpulmonary indicator dilution* (TPID) has been developed in order to avoid the potential complications associated with the insertion and use of a pulmonary artery catheter. In this method the indicator is injected into a central vein and detected after passing the pulmonary circulation in a systemic artery. However, the increased path length between the sites of injection and detection implies a higher risk of indicator loss, as well as less variation in cardiac output measurements induced by cardiopulmonary interaction.

Cardiac output assessment with *transpulmonary thermodilution* (TPTD) is done by the injection of 3–5 mL of isotonic saline (cold or at body temperature) via a central venous catheter, which is subsequently detected by a dedicated, thermistor-tipped catheter positioned in the femoral, brachial, or axillary artery. Cardiac output is calculated by using blood temperature, temperature and volume of injected saline, area under the thermodilution curve, and a "correction factor" in the modified Stewart-Hamilton equation. TPTD has been validated in animal studies[9,37] and in children in the pediatric intensive care setting.[8,38,39] The central venous catheter should not be placed in close proximity to the arterial catheter – for example, in the femoral vein and artery on the same side. This is due to cross-talk phenomenon causing possible direct interference and erroneous cardiac output calculation.[40] TPTD is regarded as the clinical gold standard for pediatric cardiac output measurement.[10] TPTD can be used to calibrate software for continuous cardiac output monitoring using arterial pulse contour analysis (APCA; PiCCO, Pulsion Medical Systems, Feldkirchen, Germany). Validation studies in newborn infants are lacking, but the use of TPTD has been described in newborn infants (3.0–4.9 kg) undergoing arterial switch surgery.[41] Because of the preferred position of a dedicated arterial catheter, this technique is not safely applicable in smaller infants.

## TRANSPULMONARY LITHIUM DILUTION

The use of lithium as an indicator to obtain a dilution curve for cardiac output calculations was first described in 1993.[42] The choice of lithium was based on the minimal loss of this substance during the first passage and the rapid distribution, which enables multiple measurements.[43,44] Lithium is injected intravenously in a known quantity and detected by a lithium-ion sensitive electrode that is attached to a peripheral arterial catheter. Blood is drawn through this sensor at a specific rate by a roller pump. For an accurate calculation of cardiac output, a correction is needed for blood sodium concentration, since sodium

**TABLE 12.3   Validation Study of Transpulmonary Lithium Dilution in Neonates and Children**

| Subjects | Comparison | CO, Mean | Mean Bias (Absolute) | LOA (Absolute) | Bias% | Error% |
|---|---|---|---|---|---|---|
| 17 patients (3 weeks to 9 years; 2.6–28 kg); PICU; 48 paired measurements | TPLiD vs. TPTD | 1.9 L/min | −0.1 L/min | ±0.61 L/min | 5% | 32% |

From Linton RA, Jonas MM, Tibby SM, et al. Cardiac output measured by lithium dilution and transpulmonary thermodilution in patients in a pediatric intensive care unit. *Intensive Care Med*. 2000;26(10):1507–1511.

is the main determinant of the potential difference across the sensor in the absence of lithium, and therefore it determines the baseline voltage. Since lithium is only distributed in plasma, a correction is also needed for hematocrit.

The first feasibility study of transpulmonary lithium dilution (TPLiD) in 17 children receiving intensive care (2.6–28.2 kg) was performed by Linton et al. and validated against TPTD (Table 12.3).[45] TPLiD can be used to calibrate software for continuous cardiac output monitoring using APCA (LiDCOplus, LiDCO, London, United Kingdom). The potential toxicity of lithium in newborns is of major concern, especially after repeated measurements, and therefore this technology is not feasible in newborn infants.

## TRANSPULMONARY ULTRASOUND DILUTION

Since ultrasound travels slower through normal saline (1533 m/s) in comparison with blood (1560–1585 m/s), injection of isotonic saline via a central vein will lead to a decrease in ultrasound velocity in blood that can be detected in a systemic artery. Sensors must be placed on both the arterial and venous sides of the circulation for measurement of flow and ultrasound dilution by means of an extracorporeal circuit. This is constructed by connecting a disposable, arteriovenous (AV) loop in between regular arterial and central venous catheters. Isotonic saline at body temperature is rapidly injected in a volume of 0.5 to 1.0 mL/kg into the venous limb of the AV loop. The decrease in ultrasound velocity is detected after transpulmonary passage through the body in the arterial limb of the AV loop, from which an ultrasound dilution curve is obtained. With the use of the Stewart-Hamilton equation, the cardiac output is calculated. Transpulmonary ultrasound dilution (TPUD) has been validated in vitro[46] and in animal

models.[47-51] In an animal model the interventions needed to measure cardiac output using TPUD, such as starting and stopping blood flow through the AV loop and the fast injection of isotonic saline at body temperature, did not cause clinically relevant changes in cerebral and systemic circulation and oxygenation.[52] The accuracy of cardiac output calculation by TPUD is not influenced by the presence of a significant left-to-right shunt[49] or heterogeneous lung injury.[48] TPUD has also been shown to accurately detect a left-to-right shunt.[51,53] Hemodynamic volumetry by TPUD is a promising technique for monitoring changes in active circulating blood volume, central blood volume, and total end-diastolic volume.[50] Validation studies have been published in children (Table 12.4) but are lacking in newborns.[53-56] TPUD has been shown to accurately detect small anatomical shunts in a pediatric (cardiac) intensive care setting.[57,58]

## PULSE DYE DENSITOMETRY

The original dye dilution technology requires direct, continuous, and invasive blood sampling through a cuvette for measurement of the injected indicator (e.g., ICG) in arterial blood for the acquisition of a dye dilution curve. Consequently, this cannot be regarded as a clinical method of cardiac output estimation, especially in small children.

Interestingly, the problem of unacceptable blood withdrawal has been overcome with the use of a new technology, *pulse dye densitometry* (PDD). The injected ICG is noninvasively detected in this method via a fingertip sensor by analyzing the pulsatile changes in ICG concentration. However, PDD for cardiac output calculation has not been validated in newborn infants, most probably because of the difficulty in the acquisition of reliable pulse waveforms in small children and newborns.[59]

**TABLE 12.4  Validation Study of Transpulmonary Ultrasound Dilution in Neonates and Children**

| Reference | Subjects | Comparison | CO, Mean | Mean Bias (Absolute) | LOA (Absolute) | Bias% | Error% |
|---|---|---|---|---|---|---|---|
| Crittendon, 2012[54] | 28 patients (1–17 years; 9–74 kg) in cardiac catheterization laboratory; 28 paired measurements | TPUD vs. PATD | 3.18 L/min | −0.004 L/min | ±0.8 L/min | 0.1% | 25% |
| Floh, 2013[55] | 35 children after cardiac surgery (median age 147 days; median weight 4.98 kg); 66 paired measurements | TPUD vs. O$_2$-Fick | NA | 0.00 L/min | ±0.76 L/min | 0% | 97% |
| Lindberg, 2014[53] | 21 children (mean weight 6.1 kg; median age 8.1 months) undergoing cardiac surgery; 90 paired measurements | TPUD vs. TTFP | | | | | |
| | *All data* | | 1.02 L/min | −0.02 L/min | ±0.32 L/min | −1.9% | 31% |
| | *Before correction, large shunts* | | 0.94 L/min | −0.02 L/min | ±0.25 L/min | −2.1% | 27% |
| | *After correction, no shunts* | | 1.29 L/min | −0.04 L/min | ±0.24 L/min | −3.1% | 19% |
| | *After correction, residual shunts* | | 0.83 L/min | 0.03 L/min | ±0.56 L/min | 3.6% | 67% |
| Boehne, 2014[56] | 26 children (median age 6 years 2 months; median weight 19.2 kg) during diagnostic heart catheterization | TPUD vs. O$_2$-Fick | 3.76 L/min | 0.26 L/min | ±0.92 L/min | 6.9% | 24% |

## Doppler Ultrasound

The principle underlying ultrasonic measurement of stroke volume (SV) is quite simple: if the distance (d, measured in cm) traversed by a cylindrical column of blood is measured over its ejection interval (t, measured in seconds) and multiplied by the measured cross-sectional area conduit (CSA, measured in cm$^2$) through which it flows, then SV (measured in mL) can be calculated as

$$SV = CSA \cdot d \qquad (12.15)$$

where CSA of the right or left ventricular outflow tract (pulmonary or aortic valve) is calculated via diameter measurements employing ultrasonic echo imaging. The distance (d) is calculated using the Doppler envelope of blood velocity extracted from ultrasonic Doppler velocimetry (see Chapter 10).

According to the Doppler principle, when an emitted ultrasonic wave of constant magnitude is reflected (backscattered) from a moving object (red blood cell), the frequency of the reflected ultrasound is altered. The frequency difference between the ultrasound emitted ($f_0$) and that received ($f_R$) by the Doppler transducer is called frequency shift: $\Delta f = f_R - f_0$. This instantaneous frequency shift depends upon the magnitude of the instantaneous velocity of the reflecting targets, their direction with respect to the Doppler transducer, and the cosine of angle at which the emitted ultrasound intersects these targets[60]:

$$\Delta f = \frac{2f_0 \cdot v_i \cdot \cos\theta}{C} \qquad (12.16)$$

where $\Delta f$ is the instantaneous frequency shift; $f_0$ is the emitted constant magnitude ultrasonic frequency; $C$ is the speed (propagation velocity) of ultrasound in tissue (blood); $\theta$ is the incident angle formed by the axial flow of red blood cells and the emitted ultrasonic signal; and $v_i$ is the instantaneous velocity of red cells within the scope of the interrogating ultrasound perimeter or target volume.

By algebraic rearrangement,

$$v_i = \frac{C}{2f_0} \cdot \frac{\Delta f}{\cos\theta}. \qquad (12.17)$$

Since C and $f_0$ are constants,

$$v_i = K \cdot \frac{\Delta f}{\cos\theta}. \qquad (12.18)$$

If the angle of incidence between the axial flow of blood and the ultrasonic beam is 0° (i.e., $\theta = 0°$), then cosine $\theta$ equals 1, and thus

$$\begin{aligned} v_i &= K \cdot \Delta f. \\ v_i &\propto \Delta f \end{aligned} \qquad (12.19)$$

After the opening of the ventriculo-arterial (VA) valve, blood velocity rapidly accelerates from zero to reach a maximum (peak velocity) during the first one-third or one-half of the ejection phase of systole, followed by a more gradual deceleration phase back to zero; velocity that occurs with the closure of the VA valve, hence $v_i$ is not constant. Therefore, to obtain the distance $d$ traversed by the cylindrical column of blood according to the model described earlier, $vi$ has to be integrated over time – that is, from the point in time $t_0$ representing the opening of the valve to $t_1$ representing the closure of the valve:

$$d(t) = \int_{t_0}^{t_1} v_i(t)dt = VTI \qquad (12.20)$$

where this integral is called the velocity time integral (VTI) and defines the stroke distance in centimeters.

SV is then calculated as

$$SV = CSA \cdot VTI. \qquad (12.21)$$

Cardiac output is subsequently calculated by multiplying SV by heart rate (HR):

$$CO = SV \cdot HR. \qquad (12.22)$$

A number of assumptions are made when developing Eq. 12.21. A first assumption is that blood flows through the ventricular outflow tract in an undisturbed laminar flow. Because under certain conditions, the flow can be turbulent (valve stenosis, outflow tract obstruction), this assumption has questionable validity.

Another important consideration is the assumption that flow occurs in a circular vessel of constant internal diameter, only fulfilled superficially in a largely undetermined patient population. In fact, aortic shape in some patients can be, for example, oval or have the shape of an irregular circle. Furthermore, the ascending aorta is not rigid, as assumed, since it pulsates during systolic ejection, producing 5 to 17% changes in the CSA from its diastolic to systolic pressure extremes.[61]

Moreover, even if the aorta were circular, the accuracy of any echocardiographic method is limited by spatial resolution. Indeed, poor correlation has been found between aortic diameters measured intraoperatively and those measured by a commercially available A-mode echo device preoperatively.[62] In addition, errors in echocardiographic diameter (D) are magnified to the second power (CSA $= \pi \cdot D^2/4$). This becomes more of an issue with the smaller diameter of the aorta in the neonate. Table 12.5 presents a range of aortic radiuses and diameters and for each range the corresponding CSA. The last column refers to the relative change of CSA if the diameter of the aorta were assessed to be larger by 1 mm. (For example, the 5-mm aortic diameter of neonates, especially preterm neonates, the echocardiographically "measured" CSA would indeed be 44% larger than the actual value.) To avoid the use of major erroneous estimates of outflow tract diameters, one is advised to use a consistent landmark for diameter assessment, preferably the hinge point of the respective valves, with high-quality imaging, and check with published reference values.[63] For this reason, one should consider using the same estimated diameter for recurrent assessments within a short time frame.

Errors in the velocity measurement are increased by interrogating the axial blood flow at an angle greater than 0° by the emitted ultrasonic signal. However, because the cosine of $\theta <20°$ is close to 1 (Table 12.6), determining velocity with an acceptable accuracy is still possible. With the increase in angle of insonation ($\theta$) beyond 20°, the velocity is progressively underestimated and therefore angle correction is needed.

**TABLE 12.5** **Aortic Radius/Diameter and Corresponding Cross-Sectional Area, Assuming a Circular-Shaped Aorta**

| Radius (r) (mm) | Diameter (d) (mm) | CSA mm² | Relative Change of CSA |
|---|---|---|---|
| 2.5 | 5.0 | 19.6 | |
| 3.0 | 6.0 | 28.3 | 44% larger than when r = 2.5 mm |
| 3.5 | 7.0 | 38.5 | 36% larger than when r = 3.0 mm |
| 4.0 | 8.0 | 50.3 | 31% larger than when r = 3.5 mm |
| 4.5 | 9.0 | 63.6 | 27% larger than when r = 4.0 mm |

Relatively small errors in determining the true diameter of the aorta result in significant errors when calculating the CSA and in turn stroke volume and cardiac output. *CSA*, Cross-sectional area.

**TABLE 12.6** **Underestimation of Velocity per Angle of Insonation**

| Angle of Insonation (θ) | Cosθ | Underestimation of Velocity |
|---|---|---|
| 0 | 1 | 0 |
| 10 | 0.98 | 2% |
| 20 | 0.94 | 6% |
| 30 | 0.87 | 13% |
| 40 | 0.77 | 23% |

*Cos*, Cosine.

## TRANSTHORACIC ECHOCARDIOGRAPHY

Echocardiography has its first and foremost use as an imaging technique to evaluate the mechanical function of the neonate's heart. The use of echocardiography for Doppler velocimetry and determination of SV and cardiac output is a readily available and frequently utilized option at the bedside. The accuracy of SV and cardiac output measurements using echocardiography, however, depend on the skills of the operator, and the various sources of errors must be considered when utilizing this method. Transthoracic echocardiography (TTE) – derived cardiac output measurements have been validated against several reference techniques, such as dye dilution, direct Fick, and thermodilution, and yielded a bias of less than 10%, with a relatively wide range (−37% to +16%) and a precision (±1.96 SD) of ±30%.[64] The intra- and inter-observer variabilities have been reported in the range of 2.1–22% and 3.1–21.7%, respectively. The use of TTE for neonatal hemodynamic assessment is beyond the scope of this chapter and is extensively described in Chapters 9–11.

## TRANSESOPHAGEAL ECHOCARDIOGRAPHY

Real-time imaging of the heart can be acquired by transesophageal echocardiography (TEE), from which both the VTI in the left and/or right ventricular outflow tract and the CSA of the aortic and/or pulmonary valve can be measured. Besides cardiac output calculation, the cardiac anatomy, preload status, and myocardial performance can be assessed. TEE is mainly used perioperatively for functional and structural imaging in children with congenital heart defects. Although anecdotal cases have been described where intraoperative TEE has been successfully used in low-birth-weight infants less than 1.6 kg,[65,66] it is advised to only consider TEE in children weighing 3 kg or more, since the smallest patients have an increased risk of complications, such as esophageal perforation, tracheal and bronchial compression, inadvertent endotracheal tube dislodgment, and compression of the aorta or left atrium.

## TRANSESOPHAGEAL DOPPLER

With transesophageal Doppler (TED), the blood flow velocity in the descending aorta is measured with the use of an ultrasound probe that is positioned in the esophagus. An essential difference with TEE is that no direct imaging of cardiovascular structures is acquired, so the ultrasound beam has to be aimed toward the aorta without direct visualization of the vessel by checking the signal quality. This also implies that the CSA of the aorta has to be acquired separately by M-mode echocardiography, although it is usually estimated using a nomogram based on age, sex, height, weight, or body surface area. However, it is understood that the aortic diameter is not a static value, since it varies with changes in blood pressure.[67] TED is mainly used intraoperatively to assess fluid responsiveness in children.[68,69] As with TEE, this method is mainly applicable in infants greater than 3 kg.

## TRANSCUTANEOUS DOPPLER

Transcutaneous Doppler (TCD) technology (USCOM 1A, USCOM, Sydney, Australia) uses the conventional Doppler method of acquiring a Doppler velocity time flow profile across the semilunar valves. This signal can be acquired from the suprasternal window angling down into the mediastinum, perpendicular to the aortic valve and parallel to the transaortic blood flow. In addition, the Doppler beam can be angled perpendicular to the pulmonary valve and parallel to the transvalvular flow through the parasternal acoustic access in the third to fifth anterior intercostal spaces. This allows the acquisition of a simple Doppler velocity time flow profile for both the transaortic and transpulmonary blood flow, and from each flow profile, the VTI can be calculated.

Since there is no direct visualization of the semilunar valve, correct position of the ultrasound beam must be assumed based on the acquired signal quality, and the cross-sectional area of the aortic and pulmonary valve is derived from an anthropometric algorithm, based on weight, height, and age.

The intra-observer variability ranges from 4 to 11%.[70-72] A limited number of validation studies in newborn infants of TCD have been published, which show a high error percentage (Table 12.7).[71,73-75] This is in agreement with the conclusions from a systematic review of clinical studies comparing TCD with thermodilution as a reference method finding an error percentage of 43%.[76]

## Electrical Biosensing Technology

Electrical biosensing technology (EBT) is currently probably the only true noninvasive method of continuous

| TABLE 12.7 | Validation Studies of Transcutaneous Doppler in Children and Newborns | | | | | | |
|---|---|---|---|---|---|---|---|
| Reference | Subjects | Comparison | CO, Mean | Mean Bias (Absolute) | LOA (Absolute) | Bias% | Error% |
| Phillips, 2006 | 37 preterm infants (1.13 ± 0.47 kg); 66 paired measurements | TCD vs. TTE (LVO) | 0.37 L/min | 0.00 L/min | ±0.16 L/min | 0% | 43% |
| Knirsch, 2008 | 24 children with CHD without shunt undergoing heart catheterization (0.1–16.7 years; 3.4–51 kg); 72 paired measurements | TCD vs. PATD | 3.68 L/min | −0.13 L/min | ±1.34 L/min | −3.5% | 36% |
| Patel, 2011 | 56 (pre)term infants; median (range) 39 (31–41) weeks, 3.4 (1.4–4.9 kg); 56 paired measurements | TCD vs. TTE (LVO) | 251 mL/kg/min | 14 mL/kg/min | ±108 mL/kg/min | 6% | 43% |
| | | TCD vs. TTE (RVO) | 279 mL/kg/min | −59 mL/kg/min | ±160 mL/kg/min | 21% | 57% |
| Chaiyakulsil, 2018 | 121 children (mean age 4.9 years; mean weight 19.8 kg); 726 paired measurements | TCD vs. TTE (LVO) | 3.4 L/min | −0.5 L/min | ±2.16 L/min | −14.7% | 64% |

*CHD*, congenital heart disease; *CO*, cardiac output; *LOA*, limits of agreement; *LVO*, left ventricular output; *PATD*, pulmonary artery thermodilution; *RVO*, right ventricular output; *TCD*, transcutaneous Doppler; *TTE*, transthoracic echocardiography. See Refs. 70, 72–74.

cardiac output assessment. The first study of the application of impedance cardiography was published in 1949 by Kedrov and Liberman.[77] Further development of this technique, designed to analyze the effect of weightlessness on cardiac output, was published in 1966.[78]

The noninvasive and easy-to-apply impedance-based methods for determining cardiac output extract the changes in electrical impedance caused by the cardiac cycle when a high-frequency, low-amplitude current is applied across the thorax (thoracic electrical biosensing technology, TEBT) or the whole body (whole-body electrical biosensing technology, WBEBT). The methods differ in which component of bioimpedance is utilized to create the impedance cardiogram and in the interpretation of the waveform.

*Bioimpedance* has two orthogonal components, bioresistance and bioreactance, the value of which depends on the frequency of the current or voltage applied. Bioimpedance is a property of the particular tissue. Each tissue in the thoracic compartment, such as blood, tissue of the different organs, or bone, has specific bioimpedance – that is, specific bioresistance and specific *bioreactance*. Blood has very low bioresistance and thus bioimpedance in contrast with bone tissue or compartments filled with air, such as the lungs at peak inspiration. Accordingly, one possible embodiment of bioimpedance measurement is to obtain the respiration rate.

In order to obtain hemodynamic parameters (i.e., parameters related to blood flow), bioimpedance measurement must encompass a major artery such as the aorta or even the brachial artery. If the intention is to derive SV or cardiac output from the blood flow in the aorta, then sensors for applying an electrical field are generally placed between a patient's neck and lower thorax (thus encompassing the aorta).

Obtaining hemodynamic parameters from bioimpedance measurements is a two-step process. In the first step signal acquisition and processing have to acquire and record the portion of the change of bioimpedance specifically related to cardiac activity, referred to as the *impedance cardiogram*. The surface electrocardiogram (ECG), which is usually recorded in parallel, can serve as a reference for specific landmarks occurring in the course of the impedance cardiogram. The second step is to apply a model which converts the measured bioimpedance into a meaningful hemodynamic variable.

Therefore a model and related assumptions are applied to derive from the measured bioimpedance a hemodynamic parameter. The same applies to the impedance cardiogram, no matter how it was derived and which component of bioimpedance (bioresistance or bioreactance) was pursued.

The estimation of SV and cardiac output by means of EBT requires the application of a low-magnitude (~2 mA), high-frequency (30–100 KHz) alternating current (AC) to the thorax (TEBT) or the whole body (WBEBT). Bioimpedance is calculated as the ratio of the measured voltage U(t) and the applied current I(t):

$$Z(t) = \frac{U(t)}{I(t)} \ (Ohm \ Law). \qquad (12.23)$$

If the current I(t) is of constant amplitude, the bioimpedance Z(t) is proportional to the measured voltage U(t):

$$Z(t) \approx U(t). \qquad (12.24)$$

Upon application of an AC, in contrast to a direct current (DC), such as provided by a battery, the bioimpedance (Z) of tissue comprises not only a resistive component but also a reactive component. The reactive component causes a shift in phase between the AC applied and the alternating voltage measured. This occurs because biologic tissue can be modeled as a network of electrical resistances (e.g., blood plasma) and capacitors (e.g., cell membranes). As stated before, bioimpedance and its components are dependent on the frequency of the electric current applied. Imagine a cell membrane that cannot be "crossed" by an AC of low frequency but becomes more and more "permeable" to a current with increasing frequency. This applies to electrical impedance and is one of the reasons why bioimpedance-based methods use an electrical current, usually in the range of 30–100 KHz and not much higher or lower.

EBT is usually measured in the longitudinal direction of the human body, with surface electrodes (or sometimes electrodes on an esophageal catheter) placed in such a way that the electrical field established by the application of an AC encompasses the heart and, more preferably, the ascending aorta and a portion of the descending aorta. The reason for the focus on the aorta rather than the heart is that the most significant and rapid change in bioimpedance related to the blood circulation occurs shortly (50–70 ms) after aortic valve opening; thus this change is considered to be a phenomenon related to the aorta. This rapid change in bioimpedance with time can be observed in both of its components, bioresistance R(t) and bioreactance X(t), which can also be expressed in magnitude |Z(t)| and phase $\theta(t)$:

$$|Z(t)| = \sqrt{(R(t)^2) + (X(t)^2)} \qquad (12.25)$$

$$\theta(t) = \arctan\left(\frac{X(t)}{R(t)}\right) \qquad (12.26)$$

Electrical cardiometry (EC) measures bioresistance R(t) and bioreactance X(t) and employs the temporal course of magnitude of impedance |Z(t)| for determination of SV. In contrast, the BR focuses on the temporal course of the phase $\theta(t)$ of bioimpedance. Both methods reveal an impedance cardiogram that is to some extent similar to an arterial pressure waveform.

## ELECTRICAL CARDIOMETRY

An example of a bioimpedance method is electrical cardiometry (EC; ICON, AESCULON; Osypka Medical, Berlin, Germany). When measuring the temporal course of bioimpedance of the thorax, Z(t), the result is the sum of the arrangement of tissue impedances in series and in parallel to each other. Most prevalent are the static and quasistatic impedances, referred to as $Z_0$, followed by a fairly significant dynamic change in bioimpedance corresponding to the respiratory cycle, $\Delta Z_R(t)$, and, to a lesser degree, a change in bioimpedance corresponding to the cardiac cycle, $\Delta Z_C(t)$, all of which are superimposed:

$$Z(t) = Z_0 + \Delta Z_R(t) + \Delta Z_c(t). \qquad (12.27)$$

Because the determination of SV and cardiac output is of interest, the respiratory component of thoracic bioimpedance is omitted (practically by applying high-pass filters), thus reducing bioimpedance to

$$Z(t) = Z_0 + \Delta Z_c(t). \qquad (12.28)$$

Thoracic fluid content (TFC) is calculated from base impedance $Z_0$,

$$TFC = \frac{1000}{Z_0}, \qquad (12.29)$$

and is indicative of excess fluids in the thorax such as pulmonary edema, pleural effusion, and pericardial effusion.

EC is based on the phenomenon that the conductivity of the blood in the aorta changes during the cardiac cycle. Prior to opening of the aortic valve, the red blood cells (erythrocytes) assume a random orientation – there is no blood flow in the ascending aorta (Figure 12.5). The electrical current applied must circumvent the red blood cells for passing through the aorta, which results in a higher voltage measurement and thus lower conductivity. Very shortly after aortic valve opening, the pulsatile blood flow forces the red blood cells to align in parallel with the blood flow (mechanical properties of the disc-shaped red blood cells). The electrical current applied (f = 50 kHz) passes through the red blood cells more easily, which results in a lower voltage measurement and thus in a higher conductivity.

Figure 12.6 illustrates the course of the surface ECG (waveform on top); −dZ(t) (second waveform from top); the calculated, artificial −dZ(t)/dt signal (third waveform from top); and the pulse plethysmogram (obtained by pulse oximetry; bottom waveform). The change from random orientation to alignment of red blood cells upon opening of the aortic valves generates a characteristic steep, beat-to-beat increase of conductivity (corresponding to a steep decrease of impedance). The red arrows point to the two states shown in the change-of-conductivity signal. The steeper the slope of the −dZ(t) signal, or the higher the peak amplitude of −dZ(t)/dt, the quicker the alignment process and thus the higher the contractility of the heart.

The general formula to determine SV by means of bioimpedance ($SV_{TEB}$) is

$$SV_{TEB} = C_P \cdot \bar{v}_{FT} \cdot FT \qquad (12.30)$$

where $C_P$ is a patient constant, primarily derived from body mass and height; $\bar{v}_{FT}$ is the mean blood velocity during flow time; and FT is the flow time (left

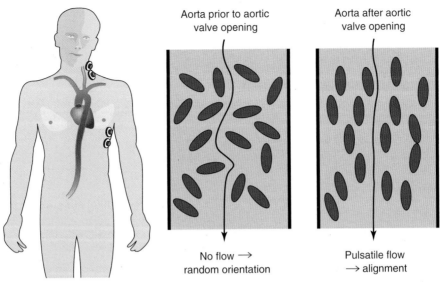

Aorta prior to aortic valve opening

Aorta after aortic valve opening

No flow →
random orientation

Pulsatile flow
→ alignment

**Fig. 12.5** Electrode arrangement and proposed orientation of red blood cells in the aorta prior to and shortly after aortic valve opening are shown.

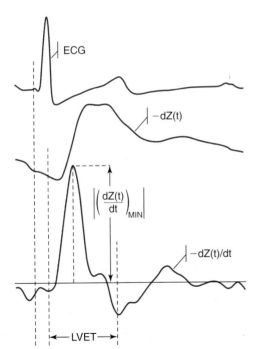

ECG

$-dZ(t)$

$\left|\left(\dfrac{dZ(t)}{dt}\right)_{MIN}\right|$

$-dZ(t)/dt$

←— LVET —→

**Fig. 12.6** Temporal course of surface electrocardiogram (*ECG*), the cardiac-related change of bioimpedance [−dZ(t)], and the rate of change of bioimpedance |−dZ(t)/dt|. The rate of change of bioimpedance is a calculated (i.e., artificial) signal waveform and is used for waveform analysis (such as determination of minima and maxima). *LVET*, Left ventricular ejection time.

ventricular ejection time). $\overline{v}_{FT}$ is derived from the ohmic equivalent to peak aortic acceleration, $[-dZ(t)/dt]/Z_0$.[79]

## BIOREACTANCE METHOD

Blood flow changes are probably related not only to temporal changes in bioimpedance but also to changes in capacitance (ability to store an electrical current) and inductance (ability to store energy in a non-electrical form).[80] The bioreactance (BR) method (Starling SV, NICOM; Baxter, Deerfield, Illinois, USA) obtains its impedance cardiogram by looking at the phase of impedance – that is, the continuously changing shift of the voltage compared to the applied current (f = 75 kHz). The understanding is that a higher SV corresponds to a higher change of phase shift.

The general formula to determine SV by means of bioreactance (SV$_X$) is

$$SV_x = C_{px} \times VET \times d\varphi/dt_{max} \qquad (12.31)$$

where SV$_x$ is stroke volume, C$_{PX}$ is a patient constant, VET is the ventricular ejection time, $d\varphi/dt_{max}$, and is the peak rate of change of phase shift ($\varphi$).[81]

Compared with methods relying on the magnitude of bioimpedance, it is claimed that the BR is less prone to artifacts caused by motion, sensor placement, and excess thoracic fluids. However, the measurement of bioreactance or phase of bioimpedance does not reveal any information about quasi-static fluids.

## WHOLE-BODY ELECTRICAL BIOSENSING TECHNOLOGY

In whole-body electrical biosensing technology (NICaS, NI Medical, Petah Tikva, Israel), an alternating electrical current (1.4 mA; 30 kHz) is applied through the body via two pairs of sensors (one on a wrist and one on the contralateral ankle). The acquired peripheral impedance signal is used to estimate stroke volume.

$$SV = \frac{dR}{r} \times \rho \times \frac{L^2}{Ri} \times \frac{(\alpha + \beta)}{\beta} \times K_w \times HF \quad (12.32)$$

where SV is stroke volume, dR is the change in impedance of the arterial system because of systolic expansion, R is basal resistance, $\rho$ is blood electrical resistance, L is the patient's height, Ri is the corrected basal resistance according to gender and age, $(\alpha + \beta)$ is the ECG R-R interval, $\beta$ is the diastolic time interval, $K_w$ is the correction of weight according to ideal values, and HF is the hydration factor which considers the body water composition.

Validation studies of EBT are listed in Table 12.8.[82-93] In newborns thoracic electrical bioimpedance and bioreactance technologies have only been validated against transthoracic echocardiography, and a recent systematic review demonstrated poor interchangeability.[80] Although EBT is regularly used in clinical observational studies as trend monitoring, validation studies for trending ability are scarce. Van Wyk et al. demonstrated poor trending ability for BR in preterm infants in comparison with transthoracic echocardiography.[94]

## Arterial Pulse Contour Analysis

Arterial pulse contour analysis (APCA) is based on the real-time estimation of SV derived from the arterial pressure wave form. This concept was first postulated by Frank in 1899, who suggested that the total peripheral resistance could be calculated from the time constant of diastolic aortic pressure decay and arterial compliance estimated by measuring aortic pulse wave

velocity.[95] Cardiac output could subsequently be calculated by dividing blood pressure by the total peripheral resistance. The calculation of SV by calculating the area under the systolic part of the arterial pressure wave was described by Kouchoukos et al.[96] Wesseling et al. introduced the technique to calculate SV from the change in arterial blood pressure during systole and the aortic impedance,[97,98]

$$SV = \frac{\int dP/dt}{Z} \quad (12.33)$$

where SV is the stroke volume, P is the arterial pressure, $t$ is the time from end-diastole to end-systole, and Z is the aortic impedance.

It should be noted that the configuration of the arterial pressure wave form can vary under different physiologic and pathologic circumstances. The arterial pressure wave form is the result of an initial pressure wave that is proportional to the SV and the pressure wave reflected back from the peripheral vasculature. The site of pressure registration will also influence the pressure wave configuration. Indeed, for the more distal vasculature, a higher systolic peak pressure, decreased diastolic pressure, higher pulse pressure, and nearly unchanged mean blood pressure are characteristic. However, this has been disputed by others, based on their work in mathematical modeling demonstrating that peripheral blood pressure resembles central blood pressure.[99] Unfortunately, there is no linear relationship between blood pressure and blood flow. This is primarily due to aortic impedance, which is influenced by aortic compliance, (vascular) resistance, and inductance (inertia of blood). The complexity of APCA is related to the dependency of the aortic impedance on both cardiac output and aortic compliance. However, APCA could be very useful in monitoring the trend in SV or cardiac output, especially when it is calibrated by another (invasive) technology, such as TPTD (PiCCO) and lithium dilution (PulseCO). The ability to track fast changes in cardiac output by pulse contour analysis is limited, so a rather high frequency of calibration procedure might be needed.[37] PiCCO and PulseCO have been validated in children, but not in neonates.[100-102]

There are also systems available (PRAM, Mostcare, Vygon, France; and Vigileo/FloTrac system, Edwards Life Sciences, Irvine [CA], USA) that claim not to need

**TABLE 12.8** Validation Studies of Electrical Biosensing Technologies in Newborns

| Reference | Subjects | Comparison | CO, Mean | Mean Bias (Absolute) | LOA (Absolute) | Bias% | Error% |
|---|---|---|---|---|---|---|---|
| Tibballs, 1989 | 26 newborns post cardiac surgery (BW 0.75–4.95 kg, mean 3.10 kg); 78 paired measurements | BI vs. TTE (LVO) | 239 mL/kg/min | 0.23 mL/kg/min | ±13.5 mL/kg/min | 1.0% | 6% |
| Noori, 2012 | 20 healthy newborns (39.2 ± 1.1 weeks; 3094 ± 338 g); PNA <48 h; PDA included 115 paired measurements | EC vs. TTE (LVO) | 538 mL/min | −4 mL/min | ±238 mL/min | 1% | 44% |
| Weisz, 2012 | 10 term neonates (median 37 weeks; 2.72 kg); 97 paired measurements | BR vs. TTE (LVO) | 559 mL/min | 153 mL/min | ±155 mL/min | 27% | 28% |
| Song, 2014 | 40 preterms (mean 27 weeks); 108 paired measurements | EC vs. TTE (LVO) | 218 mL/kg/min | | | | |
| | • *Overall* | | | −18.8 mL/kg/min | ±133 mL/kg/min | 9% | 61% |
| | • *Nonventilated* | | | −20.4 mL/kg/min | ±105 mL/kg/min | 9% | 48% |
| | • *Room air* | | | −25.0 mL/kg/min | ±44.6 mL/kg/min | 11% | 20% |
| | • *nCPAP* | | | −18.2 mL/kg/min | ±125 mL/kg/min | 8% | 57% |
| | • *Ventilated* | | | −17.5 mL/kg/min | ±156 mL/kg/min | 8% | 72% |
| | • *SIMV* | | | −30.2 mL/kg/min | ±145 mL/kg/min | 14% | 67% |
| | • *HFJV* | | | −10.9 mL/kg/min | ±160 mL/kg/min | 5% | 73% |
| | • *HFOV* | | | 38.2 mL/kg/min | ±179 mL/kg/min | 18% | 82% |
| Weisz, 2014 | 25 preterm infants (median 25 weeks) post-PDA ligation; 78 paired measurements | BR vs. TTE (LVO) | 227 mL/kg/min | NA | NA | 39% | 32% |
| Grollmuss, 2014 | 28 preterms (mean 31.7 weeks); 228 paired measurements | EC vs. TTE (LVO) | 256 mL/kg/min | | | | |
| | • *All* | | | 8.9 mL/kg/min | ±63 mL/kg/min | 3% | 24% |
| | • *LBW (<2500 g)* | | | 10.4 mL/kg/min | ±61 mL/kg/min | 4% | 24% |
| | • *VLBW (<1500 g)* | | | 5.3 mL/kg/min | ±59 mL/kg/min | 2% | 23% |
| Torigoe, 2015 | 28 preterms (median 32 weeks); 81 paired measurements | EC vs. TTE (LVO) | 317 mL/min | | | | |
| | • *Overall* | | | −6 mL/min | ±92 mL/min | 2% | 29% |
| | • *No hsPDA* | | | 6 mL/min | ±67 mL/min | 2% | 21% |
| | • *hsPDA* | | | −36 mL/min | ±120 mL/min | 11% | 38% |
| | • *Nonventilated* | | | −14 mL/min | ±103 mL/min | 4% | 32% |
| | • *nCPAP* | | | 6.3 mL/min | ±73 mL/min | 2% | 23% |
| | • *SIMV* | | | −29.6 mL/min | ±98 mL/min | 9% | 31% |
| | • *HFOV* | | | −12.0 mL/min | ±106 mL/min | 4% | 33% |

*Continued on following page*

| TABLE 12.8 | Validation Studies of Electrical Biosensing Technologies in Newborns (Continued) | | | | | | |
|---|---|---|---|---|---|---|---|
| Reference | Subjects | Comparison | CO, Mean | Mean Bias (Absolute) | LOA (Absolute) | Bias% | Error% |
| Boet, 2016 | 79 preterms (31 ± 3.2 weeks); 451 paired measurements | EC vs. TTE (LVO) | NA | −0.21 L/min | ±0.35 L/min (?) estimated (graph) | NA | NA |
| Hsu, 2017 | 36 preterm infants (GA 27.2 ± 6.6 weeks; BW 1.01 ± 1.00 kg); 105 paired measurements | EC vs. TTE | 258 mL/kg/min | −5.3 mL/kg/min | ±72.9 mL/kg/min | −2.1% | 28% |
| van Wyk, 2020 | 63 neonates (GA 31.3 ± 2.7 weeks; BW 1.56 ± 0.41 kg); 754 paired measurements | BR vs. TTE | 124 mL/kg/min | −18.5 mL/kg/min | ±87.6 mL/kg/min | −15% | 71% |
| Hassan, 2021 | 38 preterm infants (22.3–31.6 weeks; BW 668 ± 157 g); 85 paired measurements | EC vs. TTE | 271 mL/min | −126 mL/min | ±178.5 mL/min | −46% | 66% |
| Wu, 2021 | 30 neonates (GA 37.5 ± 1.9 weeks; BW 2913 ± 423 g) | NICaS vs. TTE | 615 mL/min | 10 mL/min | ±320 mL/min | 1.6% | 53% |

*BR*, Bioreactance method; *BW*, birth weight; *CO*, cardiac output; *EC*, electrical cardiometry; *GA*, gestational age; *HFJV*, high-frequency jet ventilation; *HFOV*, high-frequency oscillatory ventilation; *hsPDA*, hemodynamically significant PDA; *LBW*, low birth weight; *LOA*, limits of agreement; *LVO*, left ventricular output; *NA*, not available; *nCPAP*, nasal continuous positive airway pressure; *PDA*, patent ductus arteriosus; *PNA*, postnatal age; *SIMV*, synchronized intermittent mandatory ventilation; *TTE*, transthoracic echocardiography; *VLBW*, very low birth weight. See Refs. 81–92.

| TABLE 12.9 | Validation Studies of Arterial Pulse Contour Analysis in Newborns and Infants | | | | | | |
|---|---|---|---|---|---|---|---|
| Reference | Subjects | Comparison | CO, Mean | Mean Bias (Absolute) | LOA (Absolute) | Bias% | Error% |
| Calamandrei, 2008 | 48 patients (2–45 kg); PICU; 48 paired measurements | PRAM vs. TTE | 2.7 L/min | 0.12 L/min | ±0.66 L/min | 4% | 24% |
| Saxena, 2013 | 48 patients (median weight 10.7 kg); 210 paired measurements | PRAM vs. TPUD | 1.9 L/min | 0.02 L/min | ±2.21 L/min | 1% | 116% |
| Garisto, 2015 | 20 patients (4.1–7.8 kg): cardiac surgery; 80 paired measurements | PRAM vs. BR | NA | 5.7 mL/m² | ±18.5 mL/m² | NA | 92% |

*BR*, Bioreactance; *CO*, cardiac output; *LOA*, limits of agreement; *NA*, not available; *PICU*, pediatric intensive care unit; *PRAM*, pressure recording analytical method; *TPUD*, transpulmonary ultrasound dilution; *TTE*, transthoracic echocardiography. See Refs. 102–104.

prior calibration because of advanced algorithms used to translate the arterial pressure waveform to SV. The pressure recording analytical method (PRAM) has been validated in three studies in children, but the number of small infants was rather limited in these studies (Table 12.9).[103-105]

## Conclusion

Despite the availability of several technologies, cardiac output monitoring remains challenging in newborn infants. Unfortunately, none of the monitoring devices fulfill the characteristics of an ideal system (i.e., being accurate, precise, noninvasive, continuous, operator-independent, and inexpensive). Clinicians who use any method of cardiac output monitoring are obliged to thoroughly understand the basic principles of the applied technology and its respective advantages and limitations to prevent erroneous hemodynamic management. Newly designed systems of cardiac output monitoring must be carefully validated and evaluated for safety. The best candidates for cardiac output monitoring systems for clinical use in neonatal intensive care are TPID, TTE, TCD, TEB, and APCA.

In the selection of an appropriate cardiac output monitoring device, one should pay close attention to the accuracy and precision of the device, as well as to its feasibility and the safety risk it might pose to newborn infants. One needs to also consider whether measurement of precise intermittent absolute values or a reliable trend monitoring system would be the most appropriate in the given situation. In most cur-

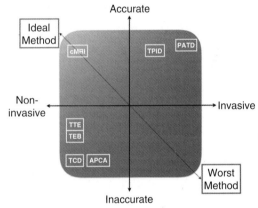

**Fig. 12.7 Relation between invasiveness and accuracy.** The level of invasiveness is shown on the *X*-axis, with the degree of accuracy on the *Y*-axis. Different methods of cardiac output monitoring are placed in this diagram. Of note, this classification is based on the subjective estimation of the authors and not on solid evidence. cMRI is almost an ideal method, but only in terms of accuracy and noninvasiveness. On the contrary, its feasibility in daily clinical practice is extremely limited. *APCA*, arterial pulse contour analysis; *cMRI*, cardiac magnetic resonance imaging; *PATD*, pulmonary artery thermodilution; *TCD*, transcutaneous Doppler; *TEB*, thoracic electrical bioimpedance; *TPID*, transpulmonary indicator dilution; *TTE*, transthoracic echocardiography. (Modified from Vincent JL, Pelosi P, Pearse R, et al. Perioperative cardiovascular monitoring of high-risk patients: a consensus of 12. *Crit Care.* 2015;19(1):224.)

rently available monitoring systems, noninvasiveness is unfortunately inversely related to accuracy; hence there will always be a compromise between these characteristics, as shown in Figure 12.7.[106] Unfortunately, at present, there is still no clinical gold standard for neonatal cardiac output monitoring that can be used to guide hemodynamic management.

It is also important to understand that an accurately measured cardiac output in the normal or even high reference range does not automatically imply adequate perfusion in all tissues. Cardiac output assessment will only provide information about global blood flow and oxygen delivery (see Chapters 1 and 2). The hemodynamic status of a newborn can only be adequately assessed with comprehensive hemodynamic monitoring, including cardiac output measurement (see Chapter 14).

Finally, it needs to be emphasized that without developing an accurate, noninvasive, continuous, easy-to-use, and appropriately validated technique to monitor cardiac output in the neonate, further advances in our understanding of transitional cardiovascular physiology and neonatal cardiovascular compromise and its treatment are unlikely to be achieved.

## REFERENCES

1. Tibby SM, Hatherill M, Marsh MJ, Murdoch IA. Clinicians' abilities to estimate cardiac index in ventilated children and infants. *Arch Dis Child.* 1997;77(6):516-518.
2. Egan JR, Festa M, Cole AD, Nunn GR, Gillis J, Winlaw DS. Clinical assessment of cardiac performance in infants and children following cardiac surgery. *Intensive Care Med.* 2005;31(4):568-573. doi:10.1007/s00134-005-2569-5.
3. de Boode WP. Clinical monitoring of systemic hemodynamics in critically ill newborns. *Early Hum Dev.* 2010;86(3):137-141. doi:10.1016/j.earlhumdev.2010.01.031.
4. Lundell A, Bergqvist D, Mattsson E, Nilsson B. Volume blood flow measurements with a transit time flowmeter: an in vivo and in vitro variability and validation study. *Clin Physiol.* 1993;13(5):547-557.
5. Hartman JC, Olszanski DA, Hullinger TG, Brunden MN. In vivo validation of a transit-time ultrasonic volume flow meter. *J Pharmacol Toxicol Methods.* 1994;31(3):153-160.
6. Dean DA, Jia CX, Cabreriza SE, et al. Validation study of a new transit time ultrasonic flow probe for continuous great vessel measurements. *ASAIO J.* 1996;42(5):M671-M676.
7. Gratama JW, Meuzelaar JJ, Dalinghaus M, et al. Myocardial blood flow and $VO_2$ in lambs with an aortopulmonary shunt during strenuous exercise. *Am J Physiol.* 1993;264(3 Pt 2): H938-H945.
8. Tibby SM, Hatherill M, Marsh MJ, Morrison G, Anderson D, Murdoch IA. Clinical validation of cardiac output measurements using femoral artery thermodilution with direct Fick in ventilated children and infants. *Intensive Care Med.* 1997; 23(9):987-991.
9. Lemson J, de Boode WP, Hopman JCW, Singh SK, van der Hoeven JG. Validation of transpulmonary thermodilution cardiac output measurement in a pediatric animal model. *Pediatr Crit Care Med.* 2008;9(3):313-319. doi:10.1097/PCC.0b013e31816c6fa1.
10. Tibby S. Transpulmonary thermodilution: finally, a gold standard for pediatric cardiac output measurement. *Pediatr Crit Care Med.* 2008;9(3):341-342. doi:10.1097/PCC.0b013e318172ea56.
11. Bland JM, Altman DG. Statistical methods for assessing agreement between two methods of clinical measurement. *Lancet.* 1986;1(8476):307-310.
12. Critchley LA, Critchley JA. A meta-analysis of studies using bias and precision statistics to compare cardiac output measurement techniques. *J Clin Monit Comput.* 1999;15(2):85-91.
13. Cecconi M, Rhodes A, Poloniecki J, Della Rocca G, Grounds RM. Bench-to-bedside review: the importance of the precision of the reference technique in method comparison studies – with specific reference to the measurement of cardiac output. *Crit Care.* 2009;13(1):201. doi:10.1186/cc7129.
14. Critchley LA, Lee A, Ho AM. A critical review of the ability of continuous cardiac output monitors to measure trends in cardiac output. *Anesth Analg.* 2010;111(5):1180-1192. doi:10.1213/ANE.0b013e3181f08a5b.
15. Saugel B, Grothe O, Wagner JY. Tracking changes in cardiac output: statistical considerations on the 4-quadrant plot and the polar plot methodology. *Anesth Analg.* 2015;121(2): 514-524. doi:10.1213/ANE.0000000000000725.
16. Critchley LA, Yang XX, Lee A. Assessment of trending ability of cardiac output monitors by polar plot methodology. *J Cardiothorac Vasc Anesth.* 2011;25(3):536-546. doi:10.1053/j.jvca.2011.01.003.
17. Fick A. On the measurement of the blood quantity in the ventricles of the heart [Uber die Messung des Blutquantums in den Herzventrikeln]. *Wurzburg Physikalische Medizinische Gesellschaft.* 1870;36:290-291.
18. de Boode WP. *Neonatal Hemodynamic Monitoring. Validation in an Experimental Animal Model.* Thesis. Radboud University; 2010.
19. Stothers JK, Warner RM. Effect of feeding on neonatal oxygen consumption. *Arch Dis Child.* 1979;54(6):415-420.
20. Bauer J, Hentschel R, Linderkamp O. Effect of sepsis syndrome on neonatal oxygen consumption and energy expenditure. *Pediatrics.* 2002;110(6):e69.
21. Shiao SY. Oxygen consumption monitoring by oxygen saturation measurements in mechanically ventilated premature neonates. *J Perinat Neonatal Nurs.* 2006;20(2):178-189.
22. Stothers JK, Warner RM Oxygen consumption and neonatal sleep states. J Physiol. 1978;278:435–440.
23. LaFarge CG, Miettinen OS. The estimation of oxygen consumption. *Cardiovasc Res.* 1970;4(1):23-30.
24. Krovetz LJ, Goldbloom S. Normal standards for cardiovascular data. I. Examination of the validity of cardiac index. *Johns Hopkins Med J.* 1972;130(3):174-186.
25. Douglas AR, Jones NL, Reed JW. Calculation of whole blood $CO_2$ content. *J Appl Physiol (1985).* 1988;65(1):473-477.
26. De Boode WP, Hopman JCW, Daniels O, Van der Hoeven HG, Liem KW. Cardiac output measurement using a modified carbon dioxide Fick method: A validation study in ventilated lambs. *Pediatric research.* 2007;61(3):279-283. doi:10.1203/pdr.0b013e318030d0c6.
27. de Boode WP, Hopman JCW, Wijnen M, Tanke RB, van der Hoeven HG, Liem KD. Cardiac output measurement in ventilated lambs with a significant left-to-right shunt using the modified carbon dioxide Fick method. *Neonatology.* 2010; 97(2):124-131. doi:10.1159/000237223.
28. Jaffe MB. Partial $CO_2$ rebreathing cardiac output – operating principles of the NICO system. *J Clin Monit Comput.* 1999; 15(6):387-401.
29. Thome UH, Carroll W, Wu TJ, et al. Outcome of extremely preterm infants randomized at birth to different $PaCO_2$ targets

during the first seven days of life. *Biol Neonate*. 2006;90(4): 218-225. doi:10.1159/000092723.

30. Fabres J, Carlo WA, Phillips V, Howard G, Ambalavanan N. Both extremes of arterial carbon dioxide pressure and the magnitude of fluctuations in arterial carbon dioxide pressure are associated with severe intraventricular hemorrhage in preterm infants. *Pediatrics*. 2007;119(2):299-305. doi:10.1542/peds.2006-2434.

31. McKee LA, Fabres J, Howard G, Peralta-Carcelen M, Carlo WA, Ambalavanan N. PaCO$_2$ and neurodevelopment in extremely low birth weight infants. *J Pediatr*. 2009;155(2):217-221.e1. doi:10.1016/j.jpeds.2009.02.024.

32. Jhanji S, Dawson J, Pearse RM. Cardiac output monitoring: basic science and clinical application. *Anaesthesia*. 2008;63(2): 172-181. doi:10.1111/j.1365-2044.2007.05318.x.

33. Stewart GN. Researches on the circulation time and on the influences which affect it. *J Physiol*. 1897;22(3):159-183.

34. Stewart GN. The measurement of output of the heart. *Science*. 1897;5:137.

35. Hamilton WF. Simultaneous determination of the greater and lesser circulation time, of the mean velocity of blood flow through the heart and lungs and an approximation of the amount of blood actively circulating in the heart and lungs. *Am J Physiol*. 1928;85:337-378.

36. Hamilton WF, Moore JW, Kinsman JM, et al. Studies on the circulation IV. Further analysis of the injection method, and changes in hemodynamics under physiological and pathological conditions. *Am J Physiol*. 1932;99:534-542.

37. Proulx F, Lemson J, Choker G, Tibby SM. Hemodynamic monitoring by transpulmonary thermodilution and pulse contour analysis in critically ill children. *Pediatr Crit Care Med*. 2011;12(4):459-466. doi:10.1097/PCC.0b013e3182070959.

38. McLuckie A, Murdoch IA, Marsh MJ, Anderson D. A comparison of pulmonary and femoral artery thermodilution cardiac indices in paediatric intensive care patients. *Acta Paediatr*. 1996;85(3):336-338.

39. Pauli C, Fakler U, Genz T, Hennig M, Lorenz HP, Hess J. Cardiac output determination in children: equivalence of the transpulmonary thermodilution method to the direct Fick principle. *Intensive Care Med*. 2002;28(7):947-952. doi:10.1007/s00134-002-1334-2.

40. Lemson J, Eijk RJ, van der Hoeven JG. The "cross-talk phenomenon" in transpulmonary thermodilution is flow dependent. *Intensive Care Med*. 2006;32(7):1092. doi:10.1007/s00134-006-0162-1.

41. Szekely A, Breuer T, Sapi E, et al. Transpulmonary thermodilution in neonates undergoing arterial switch surgery. *Pediatr Cardiol*. 2011;32(2):125-130. doi:10.1007/s00246-010-9828-0.

42. Linton RA, Band DM, Haire KM. A new method of measuring cardiac output in man using lithium dilution. *Br J Anaesth*. 1993;71(2):262-266.

43. Band DM, Linton RA, O'Brien TK, Jonas MM, Linton NW. The shape of indicator dilution curves used for cardiac output measurement in man. *J Physiol*. 1997;498(Pt 1):225-229.

44. Kurita T, Morita K, Kawasaki H, Fujii K, Kazama T, Sato S. Lithium dilution cardiac output measurement in oleic acid-induced pulmonary edema. *J Cardiothorac Vasc Anesth*. 2002; 16(3):334-337.

45. Linton RA, Jonas MM, Tibby SM, et al. Cardiac output measured by lithium dilution and transpulmonary thermodilution in patients in a paediatric intensive care unit. *Intensive Care Med*. 2000;26(10):1507-1511.

46. Krivitski NM, Kislukhin VV, Thuramalla NV. Theory and in vitro validation of a new extracorporeal arteriovenous loop approach for hemodynamic assessment in pediatric and neonatal intensive care unit patients. *Pediatr Crit Care Med*. 2008;9(4):423-428. doi:10.1097/01.PCC.0b013e31816c71bc.

47. de Boode WP, van Heijst AFJ, Hopman JCW, Tanke RB, van der Hoeven HG, Liem KD. Cardiac output measurement using an ultrasound dilution method: A validation study in ventilated piglets. *Pediatr Crit Care Med*. 2010;11(1):103-108. doi:10.1097/PCC.0b013e3181b064ea.

48. Vrancken SL, de Boode WP, Hopman JC, Looijen-Salamon MG, Liem KD, van Heijst AF. Influence of lung injury on cardiac output measurement using transpulmonary ultrasound dilution: a validation study in neonatal lambs. *Br J Anaesth*. 2012;109(6):870-878. doi:10.1093/bja/aes297.

49. Vrancken SL, de Boode WP, Hopman JC, Singh SK, Liem KD, van Heijst AF. Cardiac output measurement with transpulmonary ultrasound dilution is feasible in the presence of a left-to-right shunt: a validation study in lambs. *Br J Anaesth*. 2012; 108(3):409-416. doi:10.1093/bja/aer401.

50. Vrancken SL, van Heijst AF, Hopman JC, Liem KD, van der Hoeven JG, de Boode WP. Hemodynamic volumetry using transpulmonary ultrasound dilution (TPUD) technology in a neonatal animal model. *J Clin Monit Comput*. 2015;29(5): 643-652. doi:10.1007/s10877-014-9647-6.

51. Vrancken SL, van Heijst AF, Hopman JC, Liem KD, van der Hoeven JG, de Boode WP. Detection and quantification of left-to-right shunting using transpulmonary ultrasound dilution (TPUD): a validation study in neonatal lambs. *J Perinat Med*. 2016;44(8):925-932. doi:10.1515/jpm-2015-0310.

52. de Boode WP, van Heijst AFJ, Hopman JCW, Tanke RB, van der Hoeven HG, Liem KD. Application of ultrasound dilution technology for cardiac output measurement: Cerebral and systemic hemodynamic consequences in a juvenile animal model. *Pediatr Crit Care Med*. 2010;11(5):616-623. doi:10.1097/PCC.0b013e3181c517b3.

53. Lindberg L, Johansson S, Perez-de-Sa V. Validation of an ultrasound dilution technology for cardiac output measurement and shunt detection in infants and children. *Pediatr Crit Care Med*. 2014;15(2):139-147. doi:10.1097/PCC.0000000000000053.

54. Crittendon I, 3rd, Dreyer WJ, Decker JA, Kim JJ. Ultrasound dilution: an accurate means of determining cardiac output in children. *Pediatr Crit Care Med*. 2012;13(1):42-46. doi:10.1097/PCC.0b013e3182196804.

55. Floh AA, La Rotta G, Wermelt JZ, Bastero-Minon P, Sivarajan VB, Humpl T. Validation of a new method based on ultrasound velocity dilution to measure cardiac output in paediatric patients. *Intensive Care Med*. 2013;39(5):926-933. doi:10.1007/s00134-013-2848-5.

56. Boehne M, Baustert M, Paetzel V, et al. Determination of cardiac output by ultrasound dilution technique in infants and children: a validation study against direct Fick principle. *Br J Anaesth*. 2014;112(3):469-476. doi:10.1093/bja/aet382.

57. Saxena R, Krivitski N, Peacock K, Durward A, Simpson JM, Tibby SM. Accuracy of the transpulmonary ultrasound dilution method for detection of small anatomic shunts. *J Clin Monit Comput*. 2015;29(3):407-414. doi:10.1007/s10877-014-9618-y.

58. Boehne M, Baustert M, Paetzel V, et al. Feasibility and accuracy of cardiac right-to-left-shunt detection in children by new transpulmonary ultrasound dilution method. *Pediatr Cardiol*. 2017;38(1):135-148. doi:10.1007/s00246-016-1494-4.

59. Taguchi N, Nakagawa S, Miyasaka K, Fuse M, Aoyagi T. Cardiac output measurement by pulse dye densitometry using three wavelengths. *Pediatr Crit Care Med*. 2004;5(4):343-350.

60. Milnor W. *Methods of Measurement. Hemodynamics*. Philadelphia: Williams & Wilkins; 1982.

61. Greenfield Jr JC, Patel DJ. Relation between pressure and diameter in the ascending aorta of man. *Circ Res*. 1962;10:778-781.

62. Mark JB, Steinbrook RA, Gugino LD, et al. Continuous noninvasive monitoring of cardiac output with esophageal Doppler ultrasound during cardiac surgery. *Anesth Analg*. 1986;65(10):1013-1020.

63. de Waal K, Kluckow M, Evans N. Weight corrected percentiles for blood vessel diameters used in flow measurements in preterm infants. *Early Hum Dev*. 2013;89(12):939-942. doi:10.1016/j.earlhumdev.2013.09.017.

64. Chew MS, Poelaert J. Accuracy and repeatability of pediatric cardiac output measurement using Doppler: 20-year review of the literature. *Intensive Care Med*. 2003;29(11):1889-1894. doi:10.1007/s00134-003-1967-9.

65. Kawahito S, Kitahata H, Tanaka K, Nozaki J, Oshita S. Intraoperative transoesophageal echocardiography in a low birth weight neonate with atrioventricular septal defect. *Paediatr Anaesth*. 2003;13(8):735-738.

66. Mart CR, Fehr DM, Myers JL, Rosen KL. Intraoperative transesophageal echocardiography in a 1.4-kg infant with complex congenital heart disease. *Pediatr Cardiol*. 2003;24(1):84-85. doi:10.1007/s00246-002-0239-8.

67. Tibby SM, Hatherill M, Murdoch IA. Use of transesophageal Doppler ultrasonography in ventilated pediatric patients: derivation of cardiac output. *Crit Care Med*. 2000;28(6):2045-2050.

68. Tibby SM, Hatherill M, Durward A, Murdoch IA. Are transesophageal Doppler parameters a reliable guide to paediatric haemodynamic status and fluid management? *Intensive Care Med*. 2001;27(1):201-205.

69. Raux O, Spencer A, Fesseau R, et al. Intraoperative use of transoesophageal Doppler to predict response to volume expansion in infants and neonates. *Br J Anaesth*. 2012;108(1):100-107. doi:10.1093/bja/aer336.

70. Cattermole GN, Leung PY, Mak PS, Chan SS, Graham CA, Rainer TH. The normal ranges of cardiovascular parameters in children measured using the Ultrasonic Cardiac Output Monitor. *Crit Care Med*. 2010;38(9):1875-1881. doi:10.1097/CCM.0b013e3181e8adee.

71. Patel N, Dodsworth M, Mills JF. Cardiac output measurement in newborn infants using the ultrasonic cardiac output monitor: an assessment of agreement with conventional echocardiography, repeatability and new user experience. *Arch Dis Child Fetal Neonatal Ed*. 2011;96(3):F206-F211. doi:10.1136/adc.2009.170704.

72. Kanmaz HG, Sarikabadayi YU, Canpolat E, Altug N, Oguz SS, Dilmen U. Effects of red cell transfusion on cardiac output and perfusion index in preterm infants. *Early Hum Dev*. 2013;89(9):683-686. doi:10.1016/j.earlhumdev.2013.04.018.

73. Phillips RA, Paradisis M, Evans NJ, Southwell DL, Burstow DJ, West MJ. Cardiac output measurement in preterm neonates: validation of USCOM against echocardiography [abstract]. *Crit Care*. 2006;10(suppl 1):144. doi:10.1186/cc4690.

74. Knirsch W, Kretschmar O, Tomaske M, et al. Cardiac output measurement in children: comparison of the Ultrasound Cardiac Output Monitor with thermodilution cardiac output measurement. *Intensive Care Med*. 2008;34(6):1060-1064. doi:10.1186/cc4690.

75. Chaiyakulsil C, Chantra M, Katanyuwong P, Khositseth A, Anantasit N. Comparison of three non-invasive hemodynamic monitoring methods in critically ill children. *PLoS One*. 2018;13(6):e0199203. doi:10.1371/journal.pone.0199203.

76. Chong SW, Peyton PJ. A meta-analysis of the accuracy and precision of the ultrasonic cardiac output monitor (USCOM). *Anaesthesia*. 2012;67(11):1266-1271. doi:10.1111/j.1365-2044.2012.07311.x.

77. Kedrov AA, Liberman TU. O tak nazyvaemoi reokardiografii [Rheocardiography]. *Klin Med (Mosk)*. 1949;27(3):40-46.

78. Kubicek WG, Karnegis JN, Patterson RP, Witsoe DA, Mattson RH. Development and evaluation of an impedance cardiac output system. *Aerosp Med*. 1966;37(12):1208-1212.

79. Bernstein DP, Osypka MJ. Apparatus and method for determining an approximation of the stroke volume and the cardiac output of the heart. U.S. Patent No. 6,511,438. 2003.

80. Van Wyk L, Gupta S, Lawrenson J, de Boode WP. Accuracy and trending ability of electrical biosensing technology for non-invasive cardiac output monitoring in neonates: a systematic qualitative review. *Front Pediatr*. 2022;10:851850. doi:10.3389/fped.2022.851850.

81. Keren H, Simon AB. System, method and apparatus for measuring blood flow and blood volume. U.S. Patent No. 8,388,545. 2013.

82. Tibballs J. A comparative study of cardiac output in neonates supported by mechanical ventilation: measurement with thoracic electrical bioimpedance and pulsed Doppler ultrasound. *J Pediatr*. 1989;114(4):632-635. doi:10.1016/s0022-3476(89)80710-3.

83. Noori S, Drabu B, Soleymani S, Seri I. Continuous non-invasive cardiac output measurements in the neonate by electrical velocimetry: a comparison with echocardiography. *Arch Dis Child Fetal Neonatal Ed*. 2012;97(5):F340-F343. doi:10.1136/fetalneonatal-2011-301090.

84. Weisz DE, Jain A, McNamara PJ, EL-Khuffash A. Non-invasive cardiac output monitoring in neonates using bioreactance: a comparison with echocardiography. *Neonatology*. 2012;102(1):61-67. doi:10.1159/000337295.

85. Song R, Rich W, Kim JH, Finer NN, Katheria AC. The use of electrical cardiometry for continuous cardiac output monitoring in preterm neonates: a validation study. *Am J Perinatol*. 2014;31(12):1105-1110. doi:10.1055/s-0034-1371707.

86. Weisz DE, Jain A, Ting J, McNamara PJ, El-Khuffash A. Non-invasive cardiac output monitoring in preterm infants undergoing patent ductus arteriosus ligation: a comparison with echocardiography. *Neonatology*. 2014;106(4):330-336. doi:10.1159/000365278.

87. Grollmuss O, Gonzalez P. Non-invasive cardiac output measurement in low and very low birth weight infants: a method comparison. *Front Pediatr*. 2014;2:16. doi:10.3389/fped.2014.00016.

88. Torigoe T, Sato S, Nagayama Y, Sato T, Yamazaki H. Influence of patent ductus arteriosus and ventilators on electrical velocimetry for measuring cardiac output in very-low/low birth weight infants. *J Perinatol*. 2015;35(7):485-489. doi:10.1038/jp.2014.245.

89. Boet A, Jourdain G, Demontoux S, De Luca D. Stroke volume and cardiac output evaluation by electrical cardiometry: accuracy and reference nomograms in hemodynamically stable preterm neonates. *J Perinatol*. 2016;36(9):748-752. doi:10.1038/jp.2016.65.

90. Hsu KH, Wu TW, Wu IH, et al. Electrical cardiometry to monitor cardiac output in preterm infants with patent ductus

arteriosus: a comparison with echocardiography. *Neonatology.* 2017;112(3):231-237. doi:10.1159/000475774.

91. Van Wyk L, Smith J, Lawrenson J, de Boode WP. Agreement of cardiac output measurements between bioreactance and transthoracic echocardiography in preterm infants during the transitional phase: a single-centre, prospective study. *Neonatology.* 2020:117:271-278. doi:10.1159/000506203.

92. Hassan MA, Bryant MB, Hummler HD. Comparison of cardiac output measurement by electrical velocimetry with echocardiography in extremely low birth weight neonates. *Neonatology.* 2022;119(1):18-25. doi:10.1159/000519713.

93. Wu W, Lin S, Xie C, Li J, Lie J, Qiu S. Consistency between impedance technique and echocardiogram hemodynamic measurements in neonates. *Am J Perinatol.* 2021;38(12):1259-1262. doi:10.1055/s-0040-1710030.

94. Van Wyk L, Smith J, Lawrenson J, Lombard CJ, de Boode WP. Bioreactance cardiac output trending ability in preterm infants: a single centre, longitudinal study. *Neonatology.* 2021;118:600-608. doi:10.1159/000518656.

95. Frank O. Die Grundform des arteriellen Pulses. Erste Abhandlung. Mathematische Analyze. *Zeitschrift fur Biologie.* 1899;37:483-526.

96. Kouchoukos NT, Sheppard LC, McDonald DA. Estimation of stroke volume in the dog by a pulse contour method. *Circ Res.* 1970;26(5):611-623.

97. Wesseling KH, de Witt B, Weber AP, Smith NT. A simple device for the continuous measurement of cardiac output. Its model basis and experimental verification. Advanced Cardiovascular Physiology. 1983;5:1-52.

98. Jansen JR, Wesseling KH, Settels JJ, Schreuder JJ. Continuous cardiac output monitoring by pulse contour during cardiac surgery. *Eur Heart J.* 1990;11(suppl I):26-32.

99. Westerhof BE, van Gemert MJC, van den Wijngaard JP. Pressure and flow relations in the systemic arterial tree throughout development from newborn to adult. *Front Pediatr.* 2020;8:251. doi:10.3389/fped.2020.00251.

100. Mahajan A, Shabanie A, Turner J, Sopher MJ, Marijic J. Pulse contour analysis for cardiac output monitoring in cardiac surgery for congenital heart disease. *Anesthesia & Analgesia.* 2003;97:1283-1288. doi:10.1213/01.ane.0000081797.61469.12.

101. Kim JJ, Dreyer WJ, Chang AC, Breinholt JP III, Grifka RG. Arterial pulse wave analysis: An accurate means of determining cardiac output in children. *Pediatr Crit Care Med.* 2006;7(6):532-535. doi:10.1097/01.PCC.0000243723.47105.A2.

102. Fakler U, Pauli C, Balling G, et al. Cardiac index monitoring by pulse contour analysis and thermodilution after pediatric cardiac surgery. *J Thorac Cardiovasc Surg.* 2007;133(1):224-228. doi:10.1016/j.jtcvs.2006.07.038.

103. Calamandrei M, Mirabile L, Muschetta S, Gensini GF, De Simone L, Romano SM. Assessment of cardiac output in children: a comparison between the pressure recording analytical method and Doppler echocardiography. *Pediatr Crit Care Med.* 2008;9(3):310-312. doi:10.1097/PCC.0b013e31816c7151.

104. Saxena R, Durward A, Puppala NK, Murdoch IA, Tibby SM. Pressure recording analytical method for measuring cardiac output in critically ill children: a validation study. *Br J Anaesth.* 2013;110(3):425-431. doi:10.1093/bja/aes420.

105. Garisto C, Favia I, Ricci Z, et al. Pressure recording analytical method and bioreactance for stroke volume index monitoring during pediatric cardiac surgery. *Paediatr Anaesth.* 2015;25(2):143-149. doi:10.1111/pan.12360.

106. Vincent JL, Pelosi P, Pearse R, et al. Perioperative cardiovascular monitoring of high-risk patients: a consensus of 12. *Crit Care.* 2015;19(1):224. doi:10.1186/s13054-015-0932-7.

# Chapter 13

# Cardiac Magnetic Resonance Imaging in the Assessment of Systemic and Organ Blood Flow and the Function of the Developing Heart

Anthony N. Price, David J. Cox, and Alan M. Groves

## Key Points

- Cardiac magnetic resonance (CMR) Imaging techniques provide noninvasive assessments of the newborn circulation with high accuracy and repeatability.
- Cine CMR produces three-dimensional assessments of chamber volumes and myocardial mass.
- Phase contrast CMR can quantify blood flow in any major vessel.
- CMR techniques have provided normative ranges for neonatal left and right ventricular development and quantification of PDA shunt volume and have guided optimization of echo techniques.

## Introduction

This chapter describes the evolving role of cardiovascular magnetic resonance (CMR) in the assessment of neonatal hemodynamics. Although CMR currently occupies only a niche role in circulatory assessments in the neonatal intensive care unit (NICU), the technique has begun to demonstrate its value in providing highly detailed insights into the pathophysiology of the fetal and neonatal circulations.

CMR has become a standard imaging modality in assessments of structural congenital heart disease. A 2022 consensus statement, endorsed among others by the Society of Cardiovascular Magnetic Resonance, American Society of Echocardiography, and the American Heart Association, describes recent advances in CMR capabilities as "spectacular" and highlights the value of a single imaging modality in providing noninvasive assessments of cardiac structure, function, and blood flow.[1]

The evolution of brain magnetic resonance imaging (MRI) from a research tool into a core clinical imaging modality shows the potential path forward for CMR in the newborn. The widespread use of brain MRI can also facilitate the growth of CMR, as NICU team members have become comfortable with MR technology, clinical monitoring in the scanner environment, and the widespread use of non-pharmacologic approaches to obtain usable images.[2]

CMR assessments of neonatal hemodynamic function are neither simple nor inexpensive but are highly detailed, highly accurate, and entirely noninvasive. This chapter summarizes areas of neonatal hemodynamics where there is residual uncertainty over pathophysiology and management, provides a background to application of CMR in adults and newborns, discusses the current and emerging CMR techniques, and describes areas where CMR has already advanced understanding of developmental cardiovascular physiology and where in the future it may contribute to changes in the care of critically ill preterm and term neonates with cardiovascular compromise.

Our hope is that as co-location of MRI technology within NICUs becomes more common,[3-5] CMR will fulfill its significant promise to advance clinical research and support improvements in mortality and morbidity in the vulnerable newborn through enhanced hemodynamic monitoring and support.

# Current Understanding of Neonatal Hemodynamics

As discussed in a number of chapters in this book, the most prematurely born infants remain at high risk of death and disability.[6] While in the past respiratory disease was the primary cause of death, high-quality research has improved preterm respiratory care, such that an increasing proportion of deaths occur due to episodes of sepsis or necrotizing enterocolitis,[7] where impaired myocardial function[8] and failing peripheral vascular control often make circulatory failure the final mechanism of death.

Circulatory failure is also central to the pathophysiology of the key morbidities of premature birth. The long-term sequelae of preterm birth carry an estimated annual socioeconomic burden of >£3 billion in the UK[9] and >$26 billion in the United States.[10] Failing cardiac function causes cerebral hypoperfusion,[11] and episodes of low cerebral blood flow are central to the pathophysiology of preterm brain injury, which causes long-term disability (Chapters 7 and 8).[12] Limitations in clinicians' ability to adequately assess circulatory function[13] impair both the ability to tailor care in individual infants and the conduct of adequate trials of the impact of potential therapies. Improving circulatory management is therefore a research priority in preterm infants.[14]

## CIRCULATORY PHYSIOLOGY AND ASSESSMENT

All circulatory function relies on the interplay of preload, contractility, and afterload (Chapter 1). The preterm transitional circulation is further complicated by the persistence of fetal shunt pathways (foramen ovale and ductus arteriosus), which may alter circulatory dynamics. A robust assessment of the newborn circulation therefore needs to quantify preload, contractility, afterload, and systemic and organ perfusion.

Unfortunately, the current methods fall short of this ideal; in particular, routine clinical monitoring of circulatory status in the neonatal unit still relies heavily on arterial blood pressure.[15,16] However, systemic arterial blood pressure is the product of systemic blood flow and systemic vascular resistance, but it cannot itself distinguish between the two. While clinicians presumably feel that monitoring systemic blood pressure is a screening tool for low systemic perfusion,

in fact, blood pressure in itself is at best weakly predictive of volume of blood flow,[17] and some studies have suggested no,[18] or even an inverse,[19] relationship between blood pressure and flow in newborn preterm infants. Other clinical assessments, such as capillary refill time or volume of urine output, also have limited value in indicating circulatory health.[17]

A range of technologies are now entering "prime time" for hemodynamic assessment in the neonatal unit. Point of care cardiac ultrasound/echocardiography (Chapters 9–11) leads the way, has produced important advances in the understanding of circulatory physiology, and has an increasing role in the assessment of circulatory status at the bedside. Established techniques are being improved upon[20,21] and newer modalities are emerging and undergoing optimization.[22,23] Bedside cardiac imaging currently provides only snapshots of hemodynamic status, so continuous monitoring techniques such as impedance monitoring[24] (Chapter 12) and near-infrared spectroscopy[25] are also reaching the point of clinical utility. Finally, the evolving systems capable of real-time, comprehensive, and mostly noninvasive, continuous cardiorespiratory and neurocritical care monitoring and data acquisition at the bedside provide an approach with the potential of addressing many of the presently unanswered questions and unresolved controversies (Chapter 14). CMR will again play a key role in helping to improve our understanding of the interplay among important hemodynamic factors during transition and in pathological conditions, as well as assessing the response to various treatment approaches in neonates with hemodynamic compromise.

A key step for all new modalities is robust validation in the population of interest. In the current absence of a gold-standard assessment of cardiac function in the premature infant, CMR has a role as a validation tool – its accuracy and repeatability in newborns[26-29] are consistently outperforming that of cardiac ultrasound,[30] near-infrared spectroscopy,[31] and impedance monitoring.[32] Outside the early newborn period (where transfer of a sick newborn to an MRI scanner, even one located on the NICU, is challenging), the accuracy of CMR in quantifying volume of blood flow and myocardial mass provides valuable insights into circulatory physiology and cardiac development.

# Cardiac Magnetic Resonance in Adults and Newborns

A comprehensive discussion of magnetic resonance (MR) physics is beyond the scope of this textbook, but a few basic principles may be pertinent. The underlying principle of MR relies upon the fact that certain atomic nuclei possess an intrinsic magnetic moment, if they contain an odd number of protons or neutrons. This is also identified as nuclei having the property of non-zero spin. When placed in a strong magnetic field, these nuclei align either with, or against, the field; a slightly higher proportion align with rather than against the field, leading to a net magnetization. The effect is proportional to the field strengh and ultimately leads to the level of signal available in MRI, hence the drive to increase field strength magnets in clinical imaging. The resulting net magnetization rotates or "precesses around the axis of the feld at a set rate, depending on the field strength and the gyromagnetic ratio of the nuclei. This rate of precession (or resonance) is known as the *Larmor* frequency.

The aligned equilibrium magnetization can be manipulated by radiofrequency (RF) pulses applied at the resonant frequency; subsequently, the perturbed magnetization will then emit its own RF signal as it rotates in the magnetic field; this is measured using closely coupled receiver coils. Images are produced by localizing the abundance of spins by use of magnetic field gradients. Hydrogen atoms, consisting of a single proton, provide the strongest signal of all relevant atoms and are also the most abundant in the body. Image contrast may be based on the concentrations of protons or how they interact with their magnetic environment, which is detected by changes in their relaxation rate. In-flow effects can provide additional contrast; this is particularly useful to CMR, where blood flow provides "fresh" magnetization compared to saturated signal of more static tissue. Alternatively, in phase contrast (PC) MR spins are "labeled" according to their velocity by applying additional encoding magnetic field gradients, producing a signal dependent on their velocity through the direction of the applied field, analogous to that achieved with Doppler ultrasound.

## CMR IN ADULTS

Cardiac magnetic resonance techniques have significantly advanced understanding of cardiovascular physiology and pathophysiology in adults and are now considered the gold-standard functional assessment tool.[33] These noninvasive assessments of cardiac health are now being gained faster, in more detail, and with greater sophistication than ever before. The range of techniques available have been summarized in recent reviews.[1,34] The key benefits of CMR in the adult population are the ability to quantify the component factors of circulatory function and the improved repeatability over echocardiography for assessment of quantitative measures. Critically, improved repeatability also translates into a reduction in the patient numbers required to prove a hypothesis in research studies.[35]

## CMR IN NEWBORNS

It is clear that functional CMR will not become a routine clinical assessment tool for the sick newborn infant in the foreseeable future – imaging acutely ill children and infants remains challenging. It is more feasible, especially for more stable newborns, when an MR scanner is located within the neonatal unit – a growing number of centers are installing either dedicated neonatal[3,4] or full-size adult scanners,[36] bringing "point-of-care MRI" closer to reality. It is now well established[36] that MR scans can safely be performed in the newborn population while maintaining respiratory, circulatory, and thermal stability. We have now performed cardiac MR examinations in over 350 newborn preterm and term infants without any adverse events. Functional CMR images have been successfully obtained in infants weighing under 600 g and at 25 weeks' corrected gestation.

Our belief is that virtually all infants undergoing CMR imaging can lay still after they have been fed and allowed to fall into a natural sleep after a feed. A recent systematic review of this "feed and wrap" approach reports very high success rates.[2] Infants should be scanned with oxygen saturation, heart rate, and continuous temperature monitoring; a pediatrician/neonatologist or trained neonatal nurse should be in attendance throughout each scan. Protection from acoustic noise is achieved by applying moldable dental putty or ear plugs and then covering with neonatal ear muffs.[36] Application of an acoustic hood can further reduce disturbance from scanner noise.[37] Scans can be performed free-breathing or, with the provision of mechanical ventilation, with nasal continuous positive airway pressure and high-flow or low-flow oxygen therapy as clinically indicated. In older subjects respiratory motion causes significant image degradation requiring breath-holds, use of image navigators to coordinate acquisition with diaphragmatic movement, or advanced post-processing to account for respiratory motion.[38] In neonates relatively high-quality cardiac images are obtainable without the use of respiratory navigation, presumably due to the relatively small degrees of diaphragmatic excursion. However, the widespread implementation of free-breathing techniques in older subjects[38] is making their application in newborns feasible (see below).

Gating of scan acquisitions to the infant's cardiac cycle remains vital for adequate imaging. This is relatively easily achieved using a four-lead vector cardiogram (VCG) (standard three-lead ECGs tend to be significantly degraded by the magnetic fields in the MRI environment). VCG gating can be carried out prospectively or retrospectively. In general, retrospective gating is preferred as this technique allows imaging throughout the entire cardiac cycle and gives additional flexibility to adapt to the variable heart rate seen in the newborn. Novel approaches to cardiac self-gating[39] and real-time sequences[40] are emerging, which may have particular benefits in newborns with unpredictable heart rates and whole-body motion patterns.

Adult CMR studies are increasingly performed at higher (3.0 Tesla) field strengths. Discussion on the specific challenges faced when imaging at higher field strengths is outside the scope of this review.[41] However, in brief, the main drive to higher field systems comes from the increased signal offered as field strength increases, which may confer a substantial benefit for imaging small neonates. The major challenges faced in performing CMR in neonates arise from the need to significantly increase image resolution, both spatially – due to the size of the heart – and temporally – due to the rapid heart rates. These requirements place significant increased demands on the scanner hardware. In addition, the standard imaging protocols applied to adults may not be directly transferable and thus require modification to be used for scanning small neonates. The initial process of image optimization which we have undergone to improve image quality has previously been described.[26,29]

## Current and Emerging CMR Techniques

### CINE CMR

Cine CMR plays a central role in any CMR assessment by producing time-resolved images of the heart that can be used to analyze cardiac function. Typically, in adults an MR acquisition method known as steady-state free procession (SSFP) is used because it provides images with excellent contrast between blood and muscle while also having very high signal-to-noise efficiency. The technique applies rapid repetitive RF pulses and subsequently acquires data, referenced relative to the VCG trace to allow retrospective reordering, that can produce dynamic images of the beating heart. Applying this technique at higher fields (3.0 Tesla and above) is, however, challenging and requires maintenance of a very uniform background magnetic field through careful shimming of field inhomogeneities. Cine images acquired in the newborn infant typically have a temporal resolution of around 10–20 milliseconds, a spatial (in-plane) resolution of 1 mm, and a slice thickness of 4–5 mm and can be acquired in around 30 seconds per slice, with multiple averages. Scans can be acquired in any imaging plane, such as the four-chamber and short-axis views shown in Figure 13.1.[29,42]

However, the key utility of cine CMR comes from acquiring a stack of contiguous short-axis images to encompass the entire volume of the left and right ventricles. Endocardial and epicardial borders can be traced at end-diastole and end-systole at each level of the stack of images to reconstruct three-dimensional (3D) models of ventricular function using freely available software packages (e.g., Segment [http://medviso.com/products/segment/]) (Figure 13.2). These models are constructed directly from imaging of the whole heart, and without the assumptions on ventricular geometry, which weaken the equivalent two-dimensional (2D) echocardiographic estimations.

Cine CMR techniques can therefore provide data on cardiac preload (end-diastolic volume), cardiac contractility (ejection fraction), cardiac output (stroke volume), and myocardial volume from these 3D models. In addition to enabling assessments of cardiac preload and ejection fraction, which have not previously been readily assessed by echocardiography, our data demonstrates that these quantitative CMR measures have improved

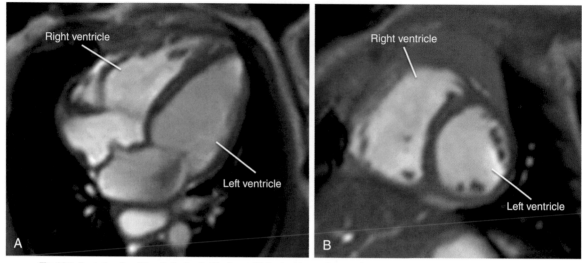

Fig. 13.1 Four-chamber (A) and short-axis (B) views obtained with steady-state free procession sequences in a preterm infant.

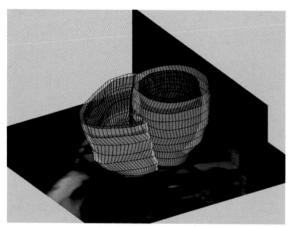

Fig. 13.2 Quantification of left and right ventricular chamber and myocardial volumes from a stack of cine images using "Segment" software.

repeatability compared to traditional echocardiographic methods[26] (see below).

## PHASE CONTRAST CMR

PC CMR techniques require additional flow encoding gradients alongside a reference acquisition collected in quick succession. Any static tissue will have the same phase between acquisitions. Moving objects experience a different magnetic field between the flow encoded and reference acquisition and therefore accumulate a phase directly (and quantifiably) proportional to the velocity of tissue or (more often) blood. Utilizing this technique with a VCG-synchronized cine (time-resolved) acquisition means that the flow of blood can be directly measured throughout the cardiac cycle. PC slices can be again placed in any orientation, allowing quantification of volume of flow in any large blood vessel. PC images acquired in the newborn infant have a temporal resolution of 10–20 milliseconds and, with sequence optimization and dedicated receiver coil technology images, can now be acquired with a spatial (in-plane) resolution of 0.4–0.6 mm and a slice thickness of 4 mm in around 90 seconds.[27]

The value of PC imaging in the neonate lies in quantification of flow at multiple points in the circulation. The persistence of fetal shunt pathways in the preterm neonate means that neither left nor right ventricular output represents "true" systemic or pulmonary perfusion. Cardiac MR allows quantification of flow in the superior vena cava (SVC) and descending aorta (DAo), both of which are considered markers of true systemic perfusion in the preterm neonate.[43,44] In addition, flow can be assessed in the internal carotid and basilar arteries,[28,45] the sum of which equates to total brain blood flow.

PC MRI is a highly validated technique in the adult. Our data also demonstrate that quantification of SVC and DAo flow with PC CMR has improved repeatability[26,27] compared to prior echocardiography cohorts[43,44] (see below). This may be because echocardiographic techniques measure diameter, which then must be squared to estimate area and then multiplied by the measured velocity time integral of blood flow, producing a potential multiplication of errors.[21,46] In contrast, PC MRI techniques measure velocity in each voxel across the vessel area, and total flow is estimated by summation of signal over each of these voxels, so potentially smoothing out errors. The sum of SVC and DAo flow volumes correlates closely with left ventricular (LV) output when the ductus is closed,[27] providing further validation of the techniques and supporting the notion that both SVC flow and DAo flow are reasonable surrogates for systemic perfusion.

### 3D PHASE CONTRAST CMR

While 2D PC techniques allow quantification of flow within a single blood vessel, 3D techniques allow visualization of flow in entire regions of the body. Specialist post-processing software is commercially available, which allows the user to trace the path of a notional bolus of blood from within any vessel, throughout the cardiac cycle. We have applied these techniques in newborn infants and utilized MRI flow software (GTFlow, GyroTools, Zurich, Switzerland) to visualize flow in the aortic arch and pulmonary arteries (Figure 13.3). The technique has also allowed visualization of flow through a patent ductus arteriosus in neonates[47] and demonstrated neonatal disruption of the adult physiologic intra-cardiac flow patterns, which theoretically maintain the kinetic energy of blood flow within the cardiac chambers.[48] 3D PC techniques may have the greatest value in visualization of flow in infants with structural congenital heart disease (see below).

### ASSESSMENT OF MYOCARDIAL MOTION

Several MR techniques give the potential for noninvasive quantification of myocardial motion. Myocardial tagging techniques use "magnetization preparation" pulses to transiently saturate myocardial tissue along set lines or grids, producing low signal areas. These "tags" are then distorted by the motion of the cardiac musculature. Several techniques are in use in adults, though these require adaptation for use in the neonate. Further candidates for development in the newborn are complementary spatial modulation of magnetization (CSPAMM),[49] which has been shown to have improved tag persistence and temporal resolution in adults, automated analysis packages such as harmonic phase (HARP),[50] and automated feature tracking applications.[51] Once adapted for use in the newborn infant, motion assessment techniques may be able to provide quantitative measures of radial, longitudinal, and rotational motion of the heart, enhancing understanding of development of intrinsic myocardial contractility.

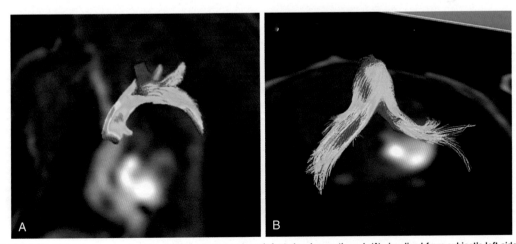

**Fig. 13.3** Three-dimensional phase contrast imaging in a term newborn infant showing aortic arch (A) visualized from subject's left side and pulmonary bifurcation (B) visualized from subject's back.

## "ATLASING" OF CINE CMR IMAGES

The definition of an imaging atlas is an alignment of data from different domains, which enables the querying of relations from multiple domains to create "the big picture". Atlases help overcome the significant inter-subject variability in anatomy and function, which makes medical image interpretation challenging through the creation and use of common reference spaces, which provide frameworks facilitating inter-and intra-subject comparison. The concept of an atlas can be applied to examine anatomical or functional differences within individuals in a population or provide robust longitudinal assessment of a subject or cohort over time. Though image post-processing is required, atlases provide statistically powerful representations of normal and abnormal cardiac anatomy, geometry, function, and development.[52] Application of atlasing technology in the adult has already provided unique insights into cardiac remodeling occurring as a response to hypertension,[53] obesity,[54] and preterm birth[55] (see below).

## VALIDATION OF CMR IN THE NEWBORN

As previously mentioned, robust validation is a key step in the development of all new imaging modalities. We have previously shown robust validation of neonatal PC MRI sequences against a gold-standard ex vivo flow phantom ($R^2 = 0.995$).[26] We have validated

PC MRI against volumes of cardiac output generated from stacks of cine MR images (95% limits of agreement ± 16.6%)[29] and have internally validated PC sequences of systemic perfusion by comparing LVO with the sum of SVC and descending aortic flow in neonates without a ductus arteriosus (95% limits of agreement ± 13.2%).[27] Lastly, we have demonstrated that the scan-rescan repeatability of flow estimates from PC CMR is significantly better than flow estimates from echocardiography (95% limits of agreement for MRI ± 12%,[27] limits of agreement for echocardiography 30–50%[21,30,44,46]).

## Role of CMR in Diagnosis of Structural Congenital Heart Disease

The advances in neonatal CMR acquisition and post-processing in the last decade have been truly remarkable and have resulted in vast improvements in image quality and diagnostic utility. CMR is now the modality of choice for assessments of biventricular size and function and is frequently utilized for defining optimal surgical approach in single ventricle circulations, estimation of pulmonary and systemic flow (Figure 13.4), and diagnosis of pulmonary venous, aortic arch, and other structural anomalies.[1] 3D models printed from CMR datasets have been shown to enhance surgical training and to assist in the design of surgical shunts.[56]

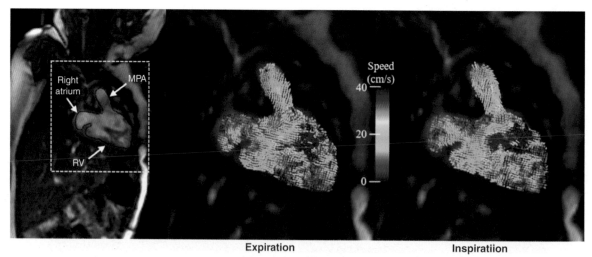

Expiration                    Inspiratiion

**Fig. 13.4** 3D phase contrast MRI image in an infant post Norwood repair, in which the right ventricle (RV) is used as a systemic ventricle and the main pulmonary artery (MPA) is used to augment the aorta. (Reproduced with permission.[82])

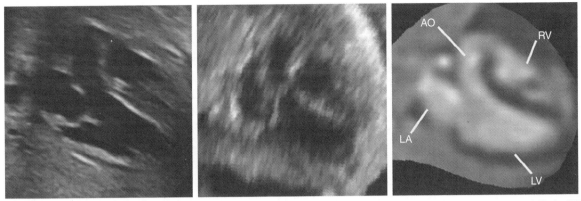

**Fig. 13.5** 2D echocardiogram (left column), 4D spatio-temporal image correlation (STIC) ultrasound (center column), and reconstructed 4D cine MRI (right column) of the left ventricle in a 32-week gestation fetus. (Reproduced under a Creative Commons Licence.[83])

Cardiac imaging is now increasingly being applied in the fetus with structural congenital heart disease, with advanced motion correction algorithms allowing generation of high-quality cine (Figure 13.5) and flow (Figure 13.6) images. Fetal assessments of cardiac anatomy have been shown to reliably predict postnatal surgical intervention.[57] 3D PC acquisitions also allow mapping and quantification of the distribution of flow within the fetal circulation.[58,59] Estimation of MRI relaxation times also allows quantification of oxygen saturations in the fetal great vessels.[60]

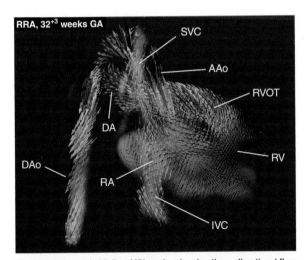

**Fig. 13.6** Volumetric 3D flow MRI render showing three-directional flow velocity vectors in a fetus with right-sided aortic arch at 32 weeks' gestational age. (Reproduced under a Creative Commons Licence.[84])

## Role of CMR in the Study of Neonatal Hemodynamics

As acknowledged previously, functional CMR will not become a routine clinical assessment tool for the sick newborn infant in the foreseeable future. However, as a research tool, the technique can add significantly to the study of neonatal hemodynamics. The feasibility of CMR in the newborn and even the fetus with structural congenital heart disease illustrates that these techniques should also be implementable in the NICU patient.

### PROVISION OF NORMATIVE DATA

Our group has constructed normal ranges for LV output, end-diastolic volume, end-systolic volume, and ejection fraction from cine MR images (Figure 13.7).

These data were produced from a cohort of 75 infants with median (range) birth weight of 1886 (790–4140) g, birth gestation of 33 (25–42) weeks, postnatal age at scan of 9 (1–73) days, weight at scan of 2192 (790–4140) g, and gestation at scan of 35 (28–42) weeks. In total, 46 infants had been admitted to the neonatal unit, of whom 29 were term or near-term infants from the postnatal ward. The normal range for LV output decreased with increasing gestation, while chamber volumes and ejection fraction were stable across gestations. The lower limits of the population normal (2.5th centile) were 1.8 mL/kg, 0.4 mL/kg, and 58% for end-diastolic volume, end-systolic volume, and ejection fraction, respectively. We have

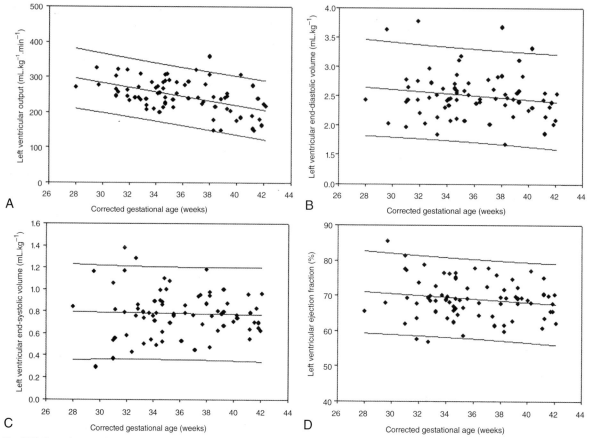

**Fig. 13.7** Normal ranges by corrected gestational age at scan for steady-state free precession assessment of LV output (A), end-diastolic volume (B), end-systolic volume (C), and ejection fraction (D). (Reproduced with permission.[26])

similarly constructed a nomogram for left and right ventricular outputs and SVC and DAo flow volumes from a cohort of 28 newborns with confirmed ductal closure (Figure 13.8). Once again, normal ranges for cardiac output and systemic blood flow volume decreased with increasing gestation at scan.

## QUANTIFICATION OF PDA SHUNT VOLUME

We have previously demonstrated that the sum of SVC and DAo flow volumes correlates closely with LV output when the ductus arteriosus is closed.[27] By extrapolation, when the ductus arteriosus is patent, the volume of shunt can be estimated as the difference between LV output and the sum of SVC and DAo flow (Figure 13.9).[27] Using this approach, we have been able to demonstrate that shunt through the PDA can

account for up to 74% of the LV output in preterm infants. Despite this high shunt volume, at least outside the transitional period, LV output increases significantly such that the volume of systemic blood flow approximates the normal range.[27] By examining the relationship between ductal shunt volume quantified by MRI and commonly used echocardiographic markers of PDA shunt volume, we have also demonstrated that presence of diastolic flow reversal in the descending aorta is the most predictive marker of high-volume ductal steal (Table 13.1).[27]

## ASSESSMENT OF PULMONARY HYPERTENSION

In adults CMR has been demonstrated to produce reliable estimates of right ventricular chamber size and strain, as well as pulmonary perfusion and pulmonary

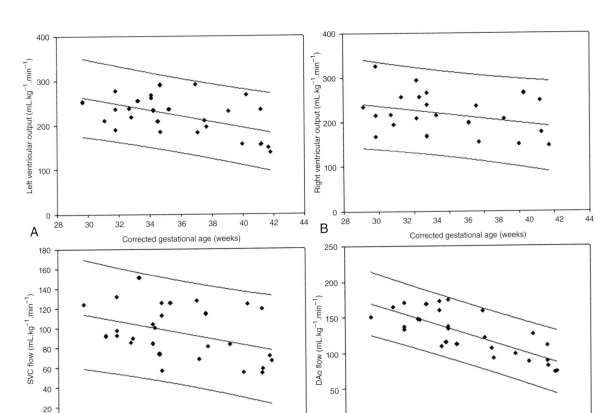

**Fig. 13.8** Normal ranges by corrected gestational age at scan for phase contrast MRI assessment of LV output (A), right ventricular output (B), superior vena caval flow (C), and descending aortic flow (D). (Reproduced with permission.[26])

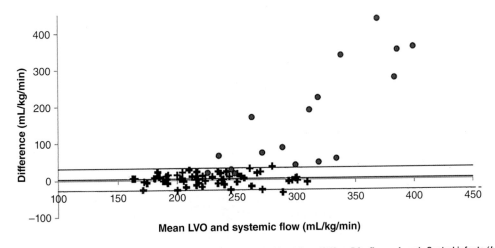

**Fig. 13.9** Ductal shunt volume: Bland-Altman plot of LVO and total systemic blood flow (SVC + DAo flow volume). Control infants (*blue crosses*) and PDA infants (*red circles*). Ductal shunt ranged between 6.4 and 74.2% of LVO. (Reproduced with minor alterations.[27])

**TABLE 13.1** $R^2$ **and** $P$ **Values for the Linear Regression Between Ductal Shunt Volume as a Percentage of LVO and the Four Echo Measures: DAo Regurgitant Fraction, Duct Diameter, LA:Ao Ratio, and ED/Max. Ductal Flow**

| Echocardiography Measures | $R^2$ | $P$ Value |
|---|---|---|
| DAo regurgitant fraction | 0.84 | <0.001 |
| PDA diameter | 0.63 | <0.001 |
| LA:Ao ratio | 0.59 | 0.001 |
| End-diastolic/max. ductal flow velocity | 0.55 | 0.004 |

arterial pressure.[61] 3D PC imaging methods allow not only quantification of flow within the main and branch pulmonary arteries but also estimation of pulmonary arterial pressure from presence and duration of vortical flow patterns in the pulmonary trunk.[61] With increasing survival of infants born at earlier gestations[62] and the high rates of pulmonary hypertension in these infants,[63] noninvasive assessments of pulmonary hypertension in survivors of preterm birth will be of great utility. A number of studies have already demonstrated the feasibility of quantification of right ventricular function and pulmonary blood flow in infants with bronchopulmonary dysplasia (BPD) and pulmonary hypertension.[64] Combined MRI assessments of lung ventilation and perfusion are also now available on commercial imaging platforms (Figure 13.10)[65] and have also been applied to infants with congenital diaphragmatic hernia.[66]

## GUIDING THE DEVELOPMENT OF EMERGING CARDIAC ULTRASOUND TECHNIQUES

As discussed above and in Chapters 9–11, point-of-care cardiac ultrasound has produced important advances in the understanding of circulatory physiology and plays a leading role in the assessment of circulatory status at the bedside. Traditional techniques are evolving, and newer modalities are emerging. A central aim of our drive to develop cardiac MRI in the newborn was to use it to power improvements in cardiac ultrasound measurements, an approach also applied in older subjects.[67-72] As proof of concept, we performed paired MRI and ultrasound assessments of LV output and SVC flow volume in a cohort of newborns. While echocardiography and MRI showed good agreement for LVO ($R^2 = 0.83$), the agreement between measures of SVC flow was much weaker ($R^2 = 0.22$).[73] MRI also suggested that the cause for some of this variability may be the non-circular outline of the SVC (Figure 13.11A).

We therefore proposed that quantification of SVC area directly from an axial rather than the traditional sagittal view might reduce measurement variability.[73] In a subsequent cohort of infants we demonstrated that combining ultrasound quantification of SVC area from axially oriented imaging (Figure 13.11B) with quantification of SVC flow velocity from images acquired in a plane superior to the vessel (as previously suggested by Harabor et al.[74]) produces improvements in correlation with MRI ($R^2 = 0.77$ vs. 0.26).[21] This modified ultrasound approach also shows improved scan-rescan repeatability and improved repeatability of offline analysis.[21] While normative data using this

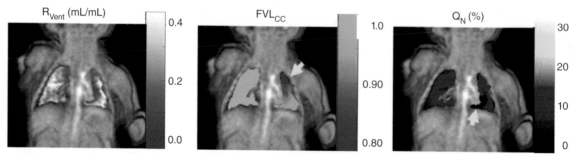

**Fig. 13.10** Regional Ventilation (R$_{Vent}$), Flow-Volume Loop (FVL$_{cc}$), and normalized perfusion (Q$_N$) maps overlaid on registered grayscale MR images in a 4-day-old infant. *Yellow arrows* highlight regions of low FVL$_{cc}$ and Q$_N$ in the left lung. (Reproduced with minor alterations.[65])

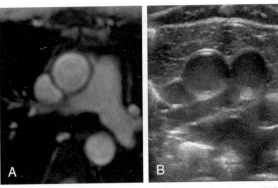

**Fig. 13.11** Axial (cross-sectional) view of the superior vena cava (SVC) adjacent to the ascending aorta (Ao) at the level of the right pulmonary artery (RPA) visualized by magnetic resonance imaging (A) and echocardiography (B).

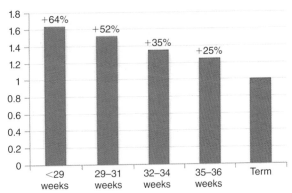

**Fig. 13.12** LV mass at term corrected age by gestational age at birth.

modified approach are currently limited, and validation in the hands of other operators has not yet been demonstrated, at least one expert in the field is suggesting that the modified approach, standardized against MRI measures, could be adopted as the new standard approach.[20]

In future, we hope that highly detailed CMR assessments of cardiac volumes and blood flows will be applied to power improvements in other cardiac ultrasound measures such as 3D ultrasound, tissue Doppler imaging, and speckle tracking modalities.

## CARDIAC GROWTH AND REMODELING

There is currently data emerging that suggests that the long-term pattern of heart growth and function may be altered by premature birth. Lewandowski et al have assessed young adults with cardiac MRI and demonstrated significant increases in biventricular mass and decreases in biventricular contractility and response to exercise in those born prematurely.[55,75,76]

Our group has begun to study the phenomenon of early preterm ventricular remodeling through the creation of computational atlases of the preterm ventricles in the neonatal period. Our initial data suggests that altered ventricular postnatal development, associated with prematurity, can be observed in the newborn period. By term corrected age, infants born prematurely have an increase in their LV mass that is proportional to their degree of prematurity (Figure 13.12) and specific alterations in LV geometry identified by principal component analysis. The predominant alteration in

geometry is increased sphericity of the left ventricle, a finding which has now been replicated by echocardiography in preterm infants with patent ductus arteriosus.[77] Prolonged patency of the ductus arteriosus also appears to be associated with increased LV mass as assessed by both MRI[42] and echocardiography.[77] However, LV mass may return to normal following spontaneous or forced closure of the PDA.[42,77]

Computational atlasing of preterm neonatal MR images also allows for multiple regression analysis of associations of altered ventricular wall thickness, with degree of prematurity, duration of respiratory support, and antenatal steroid administration showing the strongest independent associations with increased LV wall thickness (Figure 13.13).

Quantitative CMR assessments have now also been performed in term infants showing a potential impact of maternal obesity on cardiac growth.[78]

## ADVANTAGES AND DISADVANTAGES OF FUNCTIONAL CMR IMAGING

The multiple advantages of CMR imaging in terms of the complexity and repeatability of circulatory assessment have been described above. It is important to also acknowledge the disadvantages of the technique, the most significant being access to the MR scanner. In addition, specialist cardiac radiographers are required for optimal image acquisition, and MR physicists have an important role to play in optimizing methodology. The process of CMR requires physical movement of the neonate from the NICU to the MR scanning suite. While this is an additional handling episode, we have

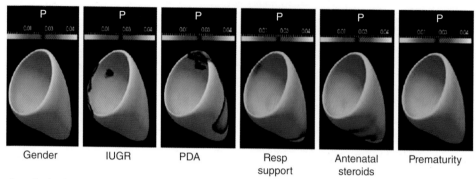

**Fig. 13.13** **Cardiac atlasing facilitates generalized linear modeling of associations with LV remodeling in the newborn.** Prematurity, antenatal steroid use, and duration of respiratory support are independently associated with statistically significant (*blue*) increases in LV wall thickness. Gender, growth restriction, and patency of the ductus arteriosus have less significant impact.

been able to demonstrate that the process can occur without apparent adverse effect.[36] The potential for adverse effects from the imaging modality itself must be considered. MR imaging is safe, provided it is performed within internationally agreed limits, but this may require a more detailed understanding of the MR safety systems when scanning infants; for example, the use of non-specific RF coils should be used with caution to ensure SAR predictions are not violated for such small patients.[79] The risk of metallic objects either causing skin burns during the scan or becoming a projectile as they approach the main magnetic field is significant. A thorough metal checking process, including for implanted objects such as PDA clips and ventriculo-peritoneal drains, to prevent these complications is mandatory.[79]

## Conclusion

Functional CMR imaging is feasible in the newborn infant and may contribute significantly to understanding of circulatory function and development in this population. The detailed assessments provided and the robust repeatability of the techniques may allow conclusions to be drawn from interventional studies in relatively small numbers of infants. Future advances in imaging hardware[80] and sequence design[81] will likely continue to drive improvements in fetal and neonatal CMR, leading to further clinical and research applications.

## Acknowledgments

We are grateful to Prof David Edwards, Prof Reza Razavi, Prof Jo Hajnal, Miss Giuliana Durighel, Dr Kathryn Broadhouse, Dr Anna Finnemore, and the staff of Queen Charlotte's and Chelsea Hospital and St Thomas' Hospital Neonatal Units for their assistance with the project.

## REFERENCES

1. Fogel MA, Anwar S, Broberg C, et al. Society for Cardiovascular Magnetic Resonance/European Society of Cardiovascular Imaging/American Society of Echocardiography/Society for Pediatric Radiology/North American Society for Cardiovascular Imaging Guidelines for the use of cardiac magnetic resonance in pediatric congenital and acquired heart disease: endorsed by the American Heart Association. *Circ Cardiovasc Imaging.* 2022;15(6):e014415. doi:10.1161/CIRCIMAGING.122.014415.
2. Torres ER, Tumey TA, Dean DC III, Kassahun-Yimer W, Lopez-Lambert ED, Hitchcock ME. Non-pharmacological strategies to obtain usable magnetic resonance images in non-sedated infants: systematic review and meta-analysis. *Int J Nurs Stud.* 2020; 106:103551. doi:10.1016/j.ijnurstu.2020.103551.
3. Tkach JA, Merhar SL, Kline-Fath BM, et al. MRI in the neonatal ICU: initial experience using a small-footprint 1.5-T system. *AJR Am J Roentgenol.* 2014;202(1):W95-W105. doi:10.2214/AJR.13.10613.
4. Thiim KR, Singh E, Mukundan S, et al. Clinical experience with an in-NICU magnetic resonance imaging system. *J Perinatol.* 2022;42(7):873-879. doi:10.1038/s41372-022-01387-5.
5. Hughes EJ, Winchman T, Padormo F, et al. A dedicated neonatal brain imaging system. *Magn Reson Med.* 2017;78(2):794-804. doi:10.1002/mrm.26462.
6. Marlow N, Wolke D, Bracewell MA, Samara M. Neurologic and developmental disability at six years of age after extremely preterm birth. *N Engl J Med.* 2005;352(1):9-19.

7. Doyle LW, Gultom E, Chuang SL, James M, Davis P, Bowman E. Changing mortality and causes of death in infants 23–27 weeks' gestational age. *J Paediatr Child Health*. 1999;35(3):255-259.

8. Ng PC, Li K, Wong RP, et al. Proinflammatory and anti-inflammatory cytokine responses in preterm infants with systemic infections. *Arch Dis Child Fetal Neonatal Ed*. 2003;88(3):F209-F213.

9. Mangham LJ, Petrou S, Doyle LW, Draper ES, Marlow N. The cost of preterm birth throughout childhood in England and Wales. *Pediatrics*. 2009;123(2):e312-e327. doi:10.1542/peds. 2008-1827.

10. Behrman R, Stith Butler A. *Preterm Birth: Causes, Consequences, and Prevention/Committee on Understanding Premature Birth and Assuring Healthy Outcomes, Board on Health Sciences Policy*. Washington, DC: The National Academies Press; 2007.

11. Kusaka T, Okubo K, Nagano K, Isobe K, Itoh S. Cerebral distribution of cardiac output in newborn infants. *Arch Dis Child Fetal Neonatal Ed*. 2005;90(1):F77-F78.

12. Volpe JJ. Neurobiology of periventricular leukomalacia in the premature infant. *Pediatr Res*. 2001;50(5):553-562.

13. Kluckow M. Low systemic blood flow and pathophysiology of the preterm transitional circulation. *Early Hum Dev*. 2005; 81(5):429-437.

14. Jobe AH. The cardiopulmonary system: research and training opportunities. *J Perinatol*. 2006;(26 Suppl 2):S5-S7.

15. Sehgal A, Osborn D, McNamara PJ. Cardiovascular support in preterm infants: a survey of practices in Australia and New Zealand. *J Paediatr Child Health*. 2012;48(4):317-323. doi:10.1111/ j.1440-1754.2011.02246.x.

16. Stranak Z, Semberova J, Barrington K, et al. International survey on diagnosis and management of hypotension in extremely preterm babies. *Eur J Pediatr*. 2014;173(6):793-798. doi:10. 1007/s00431-013-2251-9.

17. Osborn DA, Evans N, Kluckow M. Clinical detection of low upper body blood flow in very premature infants using blood pressure, capillary refill time, and central-peripheral temperature difference. *Archives of DIsease in Childhood Fetal and Neonatal Edition*. 2004;89(2):F168-F173.

18. Tyszczuk L, Meek J, Elwell C, Wyatt JS. Cerebral blood flow is independent of mean arterial blood pressure in preterm infants undergoing intensive care. *Pediatrics*. 1998;102(2 Pt 1):337-341.

19. Groves AM, Kuschel CA, Knight DB, Skinner J. The relationship between blood pressure and blood flow in newborn preterm infants. *Arch Dis Child Fetal Neonatal Ed*. 2008;93(1):F29-F32.

20. Evans N. Towards more accurate assessment of preterm systemic blood flow. *Arch Dis Child Fetal Neonatal Ed*. 2017; 102(1):F2-F3. doi:10.1136/archdischild-2016-311129.

21. Ficial B, Bonafiglia E, Padovani EM, et al. A modified echocardiographic approach improves reliability of superior vena caval flow quantification. *Arch Dis Child Fetal Neonatal Ed*. 2017; 102(1):F7-F11. doi:10.1136/archdischild-2015-309523.

22. Levy PT, Dioneda B, Holland MR, et al. Right ventricular function in preterm and term neonates: reference values for right ventricle areas and fractional area of change. *J Am Soc Echocardiogr*. 2015;28(5):559-569. doi:10.1016/j.echo.2015.01.024.

23. Levy PT, Machefsky A, Sanchez AA, et al. Reference ranges of left ventricular strain measures by two-dimensional speckle-tracking echocardiography in children: a systematic review and meta-analysis. *J Am Soc Echocardiogr*. 2016;29(3):209-225.e6. doi:10.1016/j.echo.2015.11.016.

24. Noori S, Drabu B, Soleymani S, Seri I. Continuous non-invasive cardiac output measurements in the neonate by electrical velocimetry: a comparison with echocardiography. *Arch Dis Child*

*Fetal Neonatal Ed*. 2012;97(5):F340-F343. doi:10.1136/fetal-neonatal-2011-301090.

25. Hyttel-Sorensen S, Pellicer A, Alderliesten T, et al. Cerebral near infrared spectroscopy oximetry in extremely preterm infants: phase II randomised clinical trial. *BMJ*. 2015;350:g7635. doi:10.1136/bmj.g7635.

26. Groves AM, Chiesa G, Durighel G, et al. Functional cardiac MRI in preterm and term newborns. *Arch Dis Child Fetal Neonatal Ed*. 2011;96(2):F86-F91. doi:10.1136/adc.2010.189142.

27. Broadhouse KM, Price AN, Durighel G, et al. Assessment of PDA shunt and systemic blood flow in newborns using cardiac MRI. *NMR Biomed*. 2013;26:1135-1141. doi:10.1002/nbm.2927.

28. Varela M, Groves AM, Arichi T, Hajnal JV. Mean cerebral blood flow measurements using phase contrast MRI in the first year of life. *NMR Biomed*. 2012;25(9):1063-1072. doi:10.1002/ nbm.2771.

29. Price AN, Malik SJ, Broadhouse KM, et al. Neonatal cardiac MRI using prolonged balanced SSFP imaging at 3T with active frequency stabilization. *Magn Reson Med*. 2013;70(3):776-784. doi:10.1002/mrm.24518.

30. Chew MS, Poelaert J. Accuracy and repeatability of pediatric cardiac output measurement using Doppler: 20-year review of the literature. *Intensive Care Med*. 2003;29(11):1889-1894.

31. Hessel TW, Hyttel-Sorensen S, Greisen G. Cerebral oxygenation after birth – a comparison of INVOS® and FORE-SIGHT™ near-infrared spectroscopy oximeters. *Acta Paediatr*. 2014; 103(5):488-493. doi:10.1111/apa.12567.

32. Taylor K, Manlhiot C, McCrindle B, Grosse-Wortmann L, Holtby H. Poor accuracy of noninvasive cardiac output monitoring using bioimpedance cardiography [PhysioFlow(R)] compared to magnetic resonance imaging in pediatric patients. *Anesth Analg*. 2012;114(4):771-775. doi:10.1213/ANE.0b013e318246c32c.

33. Finn JP, Nael K, Deshpande V, Ratib O, Laub G. Cardiac MR imaging: state of the technology. *Radiology*. 2006;241(2):338-354.

34. Guo R, Weingartner S, Siuryte P, et al. Emerging techniques in cardiac magnetic resonance imaging. *J Magn Reson Imaging*. 2022;55(4):1043-1059. doi:10.1002/jmri.27848.

35. Grothues F, Smith GC, Moon JC, et al. Comparison of inter-study reproducibility of cardiovascular magnetic resonance with two-dimensional echocardiography in normal subjects and in patients with heart failure or left ventricular hypertrophy. *Am J Cardiol*. 2002;90(1):29-34.

36. Merchant N, Groves A, Larkman DJ, et al. A patient care system for early 3.0 Tesla magnetic resonance imaging of very low birth weight infants. *Early Hum Dev*. 2009;85(12):779-783. doi:10.1016/j.earlhumdev.2009.10.007.

37. Hughes EJ, Winchman T, Padormo F, et al. A dedicated neonatal brain imaging system. *Magn Reson Med*. 2017;78(2): 794-802. doi:10.1002/mrm.26462.

38. Zucker EJ, Sandino CM, Kino A, Lai P, Vasanawala SS. Free-breathing accelerated cardiac MRI using deep learning: validation in children and young adults. *Radiology*. 2021;300(3): 539-548. doi:10.1148/radiol.2021202624.

39. von Kleist H, Buehrer M, Kozerke S, et al. Cardiac self-gating using blind source separation for 2D cine cardiovascular magnetic resonance imaging. *Magn Reson Imaging*. 2021;81:42-52. doi:10.1016/j.mri.2021.04.008.

40. Nayak KS, Lim Y, Campbell-Washburn AE, Steeden J. Real-time magnetic resonance imaging. *J Magn Reson Imaging*. 2022; 55(1):81-99. doi:10.1002/jmri.27411.

41. Gutberlet M, Noeske R, Schwinge K, Freyhardt P, Felix R, Niendorf T. Comprehensive cardiac magnetic resonance imaging

at 3.0 Tesla: feasibility and implications for clinical applications. *Invest Radiol.* 2006;41(2):154-167.

42. Broadhouse KM, Finnemore AE, Price AN, et al. Cardiovascular magnetic resonance of cardiac function and myocardial mass in preterm infants: a preliminary study of the impact of patent ductus arteriosus. *J Cardiovasc Magn Reson.* 2014;16:54. doi:10.1186/s12968-014-0054-4.

43. Groves AM, Kuschel CA, Knight DB, Skinner JR. Echocardiographic assessment of blood flow volume in the SVC and descending aorta in the newborn infant. *Arch Dis Child Fetal Neonatal Ed.* 2008;93(1):F24-F28.

44. Kluckow M, Evans N. Superior vena cava flow in newborn infants: a novel marker of systemic blood flow. *Arch Dis Child Fetal Neonatal Ed.* 2000;82(3):F182-F187.

45. Benders MJ, Hendrikse J, De Vries LS, Van Bel F, Groenendaal F. Phase-contrast magnetic resonance angiography measurements of global cerebral blood flow in the neonate. *Pediatr Res.* 2011;69(6):544-547. doi:10.1203/PDR.0b013e3182176aab.

46. Lee A, Liestol K, Nestaas E, Brunvand L, Lindemann R, Fugelseth D. Superior vena cava flow: feasibility and reliability of the off-line analyses. *Arch Dis Child Fetal Neonatal Ed.* 2010;95(2):F121-F125. doi:10.1136/adc.2009.176883.

47. Broadhouse KM, Price AN, Finnemore AE, et al. 4D phase contrast MRI in the preterm infant: visualisation of patent ductus arteriosus. *Arch Dis Child Fetal Neonatal Ed.* 2015;100(2):F164. doi:10.1136/archdischild-2013-305281.

48. Groves AM, Durighel G, Finnemore A, et al. Disruption of intracardiac flow patterns in the newborn infant. *Pediatr Res.* 2012;71(4 Pt 1):380-385. doi:10.1038/pr.2011.77.

49. Ibrahim el-SH, Stuber M, Schar M, Osman NF. Improved myocardial tagging contrast in cine balanced SSFP images. *J Magn Reson Imaging.* 2006;24(5):1159-1167. doi:10.1002/jmri.20730.

50. Pan L, Prince JL, Lima JA, Osman NF. Fast tracking of cardiac motion using 3D-HARP. *IEEE Trans Biomed Eng.* 2005;52(8):1425-1435.

51. Claus P, Omar AM, Pedrizzetti G, Sengupta PP, Nagel E. Tissue tracking technology for assessing cardiac mechanics: principles, normal values, and clinical applications. *JACC Cardiovasc Imaging.* 2015;8(12):1444-1460. doi:10.1016/j.jcmg.2015.11.001.

52. Young AA, Frangi AF. Computational cardiac atlases: from patient to population and back. *Exp Physiol.* 2009;94(5):578-596. doi:10.1113/expphysiol.2008.044081.

53. de Marvao A, Dawes TJ, Shi W, et al. Precursors of hypertensive heart phenotype develop in healthy adults: a high-resolution 3D MRI study. *JACC Cardiovasc Imaging.* 2015;8(11):1260-1269. doi:10.1016/j.jcmg.2015.08.007.

54. Corden B, de Marvao A, Dawes TJ, et al. Relationship between body composition and left ventricular geometry using three dimensional cardiovascular magnetic resonance. *J Cardiovasc Magn Reson.* 2016;18(1):32. doi:10.1186/s12968-016-0251-4.

55. Lewandowski AJ, Augustine D, Lamata P, et al. Preterm heart in adult life: cardiovascular magnetic resonance reveals distinct differences in left ventricular mass, geometry, and function. *Circulation.* 2013;127(2):197-206. doi:10.1161/CIRCULATIONAHA.112.126920.

56. Yoo SJ, Hussein N, Peel B, et al. 3D modeling and printing in congenital heart surgery: entering the stage of maturation. *Front Pediatr.* 2021;9:621672. doi:10.3389/fped.2021.621672.

57. Lloyd DFA, van Poppel MPM, Pushparajah K, et al. Analysis of 3-dimensional arch anatomy, vascular flow, and postnatal outcome in cases of suspected coarctation of the aorta using fetal

cardiac magnetic resonance imaging. *Circ Cardiovasc Imaging.* 2021;14(7):e012411. doi:10.1161/CIRCIMAGING.121.012411.

58. Seed M, van Amerom JF, Yoo SJ, et al. Feasibility of quantification of the distribution of blood flow in the normal human fetal circulation using CMR: a cross-sectional study. *J Cardiovasc Magn Reson.* 2012;14:79. doi:10.1186/1532-429X-14-79.

59. Prsa M, Sun L, van Amerom J, et al. Reference ranges of blood flow in the major vessels of the normal human fetal circulation at term by phase-contrast magnetic resonance imaging. *Circ Cardiovasc Imaging.* 2014;7(4):663-670. doi:10.1161/CIRCIMAGING.113.001859.

60. Saini BS, Darby JRT, Portnoy S, et al. Normal human and sheep fetal vessel oxygen saturations by T2 magnetic resonance imaging. *J Physiol.* 2020;598(15):3259-3281. doi:10.1113/JP279725.

61. Alabed S, Garg P, Johns CS, et al. Cardiac magnetic resonance in pulmonary hypertension-an update. *Curr Cardiovasc Imaging Rep.* 2020;13(12):30. doi:10.1007/s12410-020-09550-2.

62. Rysavy MA, Mehler K, Oberthur A, et al. An immature science: intensive care for infants born at ≤23 weeks of gestation. *J Pediatr.* 2021;233:16-25.e1. doi:10.1016/j.jpeds.2021.03.006.

63. Sallmon H, Koestenberger M, Avian A, et al. Extremely premature infants born at 23-25 weeks gestation are at substantial risk for pulmonary hypertension. *J Perinatol.* 2022;42(6):781-787. doi:10.1038/s41372-022-01374-w.

64. Critser PJ, Higano NS, Tkach JA, et al. Cardiac magnetic resonance imaging evaluation of neonatal bronchopulmonary dysplasia-associated pulmonary hypertension. *Am J Respir Crit Care Med.* 2020;201(1):73-82. doi:10.1164/rccm.201904-0826OC.

65. Zanette B, Schrauben EM, Munidasa S, et al. Clinical feasibility of structural and functional MRI in free-breathing neonates and infants. *J Magn Reson Imaging.* 2022;55(6):1696-1707. doi:10.1002/jmri.28165.

66. Tkach JA, Higano NS, Taylor MD, et al. Quantitative cardiopulmonary magnetic resonance imaging in neonatal congenital diaphragmatic hernia. *Pediatr Radiol.* 2022;52(12):2306-2318. doi:10.1007/s00247-022-05384-w.

67. Muraru D, Spadotto V, Cecchetto A, et al. New speckle-tracking algorithm for right ventricular volume analysis from three-dimensional echocardiographic data sets: validation with cardiac magnetic resonance and comparison with the previous analysis tool. *Eur Heart J Cardiovasc Imaging.* 2016;17(11):1279-1289. doi:10.1093/ehjci/jev309.

68. Choi J, Hong GR, Kim M, et al. Automatic quantification of aortic regurgitation using 3D full volume color doppler echocardiography: a validation study with cardiac magnetic resonance imaging. *Int J Cardiovasc Imaging.* 2015;31(7):1379-1389. doi:10.1007/s10554-015-0707-x.

69. Laser KT, Houben BA, Korperich H, et al. Calculation of pediatric left ventricular mass: validation and reference values using real-time three-dimensional echocardiography. *J Am Soc Echocardiogr.* 2015;28(3):275-283. doi:10.1016/j.echo.2014.11.008.

70. Ebtia M, Murphy D, Gin K, et al. Best method for right atrial volume assessment by two-dimensional echocardiography: validation with magnetic resonance imaging. *Echocardiography.* 2015;32(5):734-739. doi:10.1111/echo.12735.

71. Zhang QB, Sun JP, Gao RF, et al. Feasibility of single-beat full-volume capture real-time three-dimensional echocardiography for quantification of right ventricular volume: validation by cardiac magnetic resonance imaging. *Int J Cardiol.* 2013;168(4):3991-3995. doi:10.1016/j.ijcard.2013.06.088.

72. Borzage M, Heidari K, Chavez T, Seri I, Wood J, Blüml S. Phase-contrast MR imaging contradicts impedance cardiography stroke volume determination. *Am J Crit Care.* 2017;26(5):408-415.

73. Ficial B, Finnemore AE, Cox DJ, et al. Validation study of the accuracy of echocardiographic measurements of systemic blood flow volume in newborn infants. *J Am Soc Echocardiogr.* 2013;26(12):1365-1371. doi:10.1016/j.echo.2013.08.019.

74. Harabor A, Fruitman D. Comparison between a suprasternal or high parasternal approach and an abdominal approach for measuring superior vena cava Doppler velocity in neonates. *J Ultrasound Med.* 2012;31(12):1901-1907.

75. Lewandowski AJ, Bradlow WM, Augustine D, et al. Right ventricular systolic dysfunction in young adults born preterm. *Circulation.* 2013;128(7):713-720. doi:10.1161/CIRCULATIONAHA.113.002583.

76. Huckstep OJ, Williamson W, Telles F, et al. Physiological stress elicits impaired left ventricular function in preterm-born adults. *J. Am Coll Cardiol.* 2018;71(12):1347-1356. doi:10.1016/j.jacc.2018.01.046.

77. de Waal K, Phad N, Collins N, Boyle A. Cardiac remodeling in preterm infants with prolonged exposure to a patent ductus arteriosus. *Congenit Heart Dis.* 2017;12(3):364-372. doi:10.1111/chd.12454.

78. Groves AM, Price AN, Russell-Webster T, et al. Impact of maternal obesity on neonatal heart rate and cardiac size. *Arch Dis Child Fetal Neonatal Ed.* 2022;107(5):481-487. doi:10.1136/archdischild-2021-322860.

79. Shellock FG, Crues JV. MR procedures: biologic effects, safety, and patient care. *Radiology.* 2004;232(3):635-652. doi:10.1148/radiol.2323030830.

80. Clement J, Tomi-Tricot R, Malik SJ, Webb A, Hajnal JV, Ipek O. Towards an integrated neonatal brain and cardiac examination capability at 7 T: electromagnetic field simulations and early phantom experiments using an 8-channel dipole array. *MAGMA.* 2022;35(5):765-778. doi:10.1007/s10334-021-00988-z.

81. van Amerom JF, Lloyd DF, Price AN, et al. Fetal cardiac cine imaging using highly accelerated dynamic MRI with retrospective motion correction and outlier rejection. *Magn Reson Med.* 2018;79(1):327-338. doi:10.1002/mrm.26686.

82. Schrauben EM, Lim JM, Goolaub DS, Marini D, Seed M, Macgowan CK. Motion robust respiratory-resolved 3D radial flow MRI and its application in neonatal congenital heart disease. *Magn Reson Med.* 2020;83(2):535-548. doi:10.1002/mrm.27945.

83. van Amerom JFP, Lloyd DFA, Deprez M, et al. Fetal whole-heart 4D imaging using motion-corrected multi-planar real-time MRI. *Magn Reson Med.* 2019;82(3):1055-1072. doi:10.1002/mrm.27798.

84. Roberts TA, van Amerom JFP, Uus A, et al. Fetal whole heart blood flow imaging using 4D cine MRI. *Nat Commun.* 2020;11(1):4992. doi:10.1038/s41467-020-18790-1.

# Comprehensive, Real-Time Hemodynamic Monitoring and Data Acquisition: An Essential Component of the Development of Individualized Neonatal Intensive Care

Willem-Pieter de Boode, Shahab Noori, David van Laere, Eugene Dempsey, and Istvan Seri

## Key Points

- Accurate assessment of the hemodynamic status in critically ill neonates requires blood pressure measurements to be interpreted in the context of indirect (clinical signs) and direct (measurements and assessments) indicators of systemic circulation (cardiac output) and regional organ blood flow.
- Further judiciary validation of emerging technological approaches to evaluate systemic circulation and regional blood flow in a continuous and noninvasive manner is necessary.
- Comprehensive monitoring systems allow continuous and simultaneous collection of physiologic data on multiple hemodynamic parameters in real time. Inclusion of motion-activated video-recording device enables analyzing objectively collected information in the context of the various clinical events taking place at the bedside.
- Addition of the modules to assess functional status of a given organ allows correlation of the hemodynamic changes with functional activity of the interrogated organ (with a primary focus on the brain).
- In a neonate complex physiologic interactions such as baroreceptor reflex sensitivity, an indicator of the autonomic control of the circulation (heart and peripheral vascular resistance), and cerebral autoregulation can only be reliably evaluated using comprehensive monitoring systems.
- Computational modeling utilizing large amounts of the physiometric data obtained is the next step in identifying physiologic trends that predict the development

of cardiovascular compromise. The development of algorithms then enables timely application of pathophysiology- and evidence-based interventions.

- Relevant genetic information obtained via genome sequencing coupled with physiometric data may allow further stratification of patient subpopulations based on their individual risk of developing cardiovascular compromise and subsequent complications such as peri-/intraventricular hemorrhage and allows prediction of the potential response to particular interventions. This approach will serve as the foundation of the development of individualized medicine in neonatology.

## Introduction

Recent advances in biomedical research and technology have allowed clinicians to obtain more clinically relevant physiologic, biochemical, and genetic information that could be useful in the diagnosis and management of various conditions. Neonatology has become one of the rapidly evolving subspecialties at the frontier of this progress. However, the field of neonatal hemodynamics, while being extensively investigated in basic/animal laboratory and clinical research settings, remains inadequately understood. Accordingly, we continue to have difficulties in establishing reliable criteria for the diagnosis of the most common deviations from physiology, such as neonatal hypotension, especially during the period of immediate postnatal transition. This, in turn, leads to a paucity of established, evidence-based guidelines on when and how to intervene in a neonate presenting with these conditions.[1] Thus we must recognize the significant limitations of our current understanding of a number of clinically relevant aspects of neonatal cardiovascular physiology and pathophysiology and acknowledge the existing vast differences in opinions on diagnostic criteria and treatment approaches in neonatal intensive care and neonatal cardiovascular pathophysiology in particular.

The next logical step in identifying individual patients with early signs of hemodynamic compromise is to develop and implement comprehensive objective hemodynamic monitoring systems that enable continuous and real-time monitoring and acquisition of multiple hemodynamic parameters of systemic and regional blood flow and oxygen demand-delivery coupling. The information obtained can then be used to design and execute clinical trials in subpopulations of neonates exhibiting common hemodynamic features and targeted by a given intervention. This approach will enable timely identification of the individual patient in the future in whom a trial-tested, individualized management plan can be utilized and the response to the pathophysiology- and evidence-based interventions monitored.

## Limitations of Conventional Monitoring

Multiple studies have shown an association between severe cardiovascular compromise and increased morbidity and mortality in affected patients.[2-6] Although there is some evidence for improved outcome in hypotensive preterm infants responding to vasopressor-inotropes with increases in blood pressure and cerebral blood flow,[7,8] essentially none of the suggested interventions or medications used (dopamine, epinephrine, dobutamine, milrinone or vasopressin) has been properly studied to determine the actual impact of the treatment on clinically relevant medium- and long-term outcomes.[9-13]

The failure to identify effective interventions for the treatment of neonatal hemodynamic compromise stems from several unresolved challenges. The cardiovascular system of the newborn undergoes rapid changes during transition to extrauterine life, and these changes are greatly affected by multiple intrinsic and extrinsic factors. Such factors include, but are not limited to, individual variations in the degree of immaturity based on gestational and postnatal age, coexisting comorbidities including the need for positive pressure ventilation, the complex interactions between systemic and regional blood flow, and underlying genetic heterogeneity.

Another fundamental challenge is the lack of pathophysiology- and evidence-based definition of neonatal hypotension (see Chapters 1 and 3). Measurements of blood pressure with or without the use of indirect clinical indicators of perfusion remain the major criterion in the assessment of the hemodynamic status and the need for interventions.[13-15] Normative blood pressure values in preterm and term infants have been reported in population-based studies, and mean arterial blood pressure increases with increasing gestational and postnatal age (Chapter 3).[16,17] However, blood pressure within the normal range for a given gestational and postnatal age does not necessarily reflect normal organ blood flow. And, similarly, abnormally low blood pressure values do not automatically translate into compromised organ blood flow (see Chapters 1 and 3). So, for patients of the same gestational age and degree of maturity, the same blood pressure values can be associated with either adequate or compromised systemic and organ perfusion. More so, even for the same patient under different conditions and points in time, the same blood pressure values may represent adequate or compromised systemic and/or organ perfusion. The reason for such limitations of using the blood pressure alone as an indicator of hemodynamic compromise lies in the fact that blood pressure is determined by the interaction between systemic blood flow (represented by effective cardiac output) and systemic vascular resistance. Thus the same values of blood pressure, the dependent variable, can result from different combinations of the other two, independent, variables. In the early, compensated phase of shock, blood pressure remains within the normal range while non-vital organ perfusion has, by definition, decreased. As many pathophysiologic mechanisms may lead to inadequate organ blood flow, whether they affect effective cardiac output, systemic vascular resistance, or both, failure to recognize these changes potentially leads to delay in initiation of treatment, exhaustion of limited compensatory mechanisms, and a resultant progression to the uncompensated phase of shock, with obvious signs of decreased organ perfusion and oxygen delivery. On the other hand, unnecessary treatment might also be started if the condition is thought to have reached the treatment threshold when, in reality, systemic and/or regional blood flow is maintained. In addition, identification of the primary pathophysiologic mechanism that could prompt appropriately targeted intervention becomes more challenging when reliable information on the status of the macro-circulation and/or tissue oxygen delivery is not readily available.

Other conventional hemodynamic parameters (heart rate and arterial oxygen saturation), even if continuously monitored along with blood pressure, as well as capillary refill time, urine output, and serum lactate levels, have significant limitations for timely and accurate assessment of both the cardiovascular status and the response to interventions aimed to treat the hemodynamic compromise. Therefore inclusion of targeted assessment of systemic blood flow and regional organ perfusion becomes paramount to overcome these limitations and identify at-risk patients in a timely manner and intervene appropriately.

## Assessment Of Systemic And Regional Blood Flow

### SYSTEMIC BLOOD FLOW

The essential component in bedside assessment of systemic perfusion is measurement of cardiac output (CO). Several diagnostic modalities are available for such measurements, with functional cardiac MRI (fcMRI) being now considered a "gold standard". However, several factors, such as the need for expensive equipment and highly trained personnel and sedation and transportation of the patient to the MRI suite, as well as its non-continuous nature limit the use of fcMRI for routine bedside assessment.[18] Accordingly, fcMRI remains mostly utilized in research settings (see Chapter 13).

Bedside echocardiography (ECHO) offers noninvasive, real-time, yet non-continuous assessment of CO in addition to other important parameters such as myocardial contractility, estimates of preload and afterload, etc. (see Chapters 9, 10, 11, and 12) The precision of echocardiographically estimated cardiac output is within the acceptable range for technology utilized for clinical applications, albeit approximately ±30%.[19] It has become an integral part of routine bedside neonatal assessment[20-22]; however, to ensure accurate and reliable measurements, it requires appropriate training and sufficient practice.[23,24] More so, a number of important limitations of ECHO need to be accounted for when assessment of systemic circulation is performed at the bedside. Unlike in older children and adults when left ventricular output (LVO) can be used as a surrogate of systemic blood flow with confidence, transitional changes of the cardiovascular system in a neonate may significantly affect LVO as it will no longer only represent systemic blood flow. For example, in the presence of a hemodynamically significant PDA (hsPDA) when substantial left-to-right shunting takes place, the resultant increase in LVO represents both systemic and ductal (pulmonary) blood flow. Relying on LVO in such cases will lead to overestimation of true systemic blood flow that can, in reality, be either within the normal range or decreased. Right ventricular output (RVO) has also been utilized as an assessment of systemic perfusion. However, with significant left atrial overload from pulmonary over-circulation in the presence of a hsPDA, left-to-right atrial shunting via the patent foramen ovale (PFO) will result in an increased RVO.[25,26] Thus RVO in such cases reflects both systemic venous return and trans-atrial left-to-right flow through the PFO. Therefore a normal or increased LVO or RVO in the presence of hsPDA does not ensure adequate systemic blood flow. However, it is important to point out that a low LVO or RVO in the presence of a hsPDA indicates low systemic blood flow. Alternatively, superior vena cava (SVC) flow, which is not affected by the presence of either interatrial or transductal shunts, has been studied and proposed as a surrogate of systemic perfusion.[27] While not without its own limitations, decreased SVC flow has been associated with adverse short- and long-term outcomes.[2,4] Finally, and of utmost importance, in any situation when congenital heart disease is suspected clinically or has been prenatally diagnosed, a comprehensive anatomic echocardiography evaluation must be performed and then interpreted by a pediatric cardiologist.

Electrical biosensing technologies (EBT) enable continuous and noninvasive assessment of CO, utilizing the changes in bioimpedance or bioreactance during the cardiac cycle (Chapter 12). It should, however, be noted that the interchangeability of EBT with transthoracic echocardiography is poor and evidence of accurate trending ability is lacking.[28,29] Many other modalities of cardiac output monitoring are described in Chapter 12.

## ORGAN BLOOD FLOW

Near-infrared spectroscopy (NIRS) utilizes the principle of the different absorbency patterns of near-infrared light by oxyhemoglobin and deoxyhemoglobin to measure tissue oxygenation index (TOI) or regional tissue oxygen saturation ($rSO_2$). Thus NIRS also provides information on tissue oxygen extraction in vital and non-vital organs. Therefore it allows the indirect assessment of organ blood flow noninvasively, and in a continuous manner. Indeed, with caution, it can be used as a surrogate of organ blood flow[30,31] provided that arterial oxygen saturation ($SpO_2$), the metabolic rate for oxygen, the ratio of arterial-to-venous blood flow in the target organ, and hemoglobin concentration during the assessment remain stable.

A growing body of evidence supports the clinical use of NIRS in neonates, particularly for assessment of cerebral tissue oxygen saturation ($CrSO_2$). A number of studies have reported on the changes in $CrSO_2$ in preterm and term neonates during transition[32-34] and investigated the association between changes in $CrSO_2$ and adverse short- and long-term outcomes.[35-38] Of note is the fact that earlier studies have important limitations due to the non-continuous assessment of $CrSO_2$. This methodological problem has, for instance, resulted in contradicting reports on the association between changes in $CrSO_2$ and the development of peri-/intraventricular hemorrhage (P/IVH) in preterm neonates (see Chapters 7 and 8). Both increased mean $CrSO_2$ along with decreased mean fractional tissue oxygen extraction (FTOE)[35] and, conversely, decreased $CrSO_2$ along with increased FTOE values[37] have been reported in preterm neonates that developed P/IVH during the first few postnatal days compared to controls. When the systemic and cerebral hemodynamic changes were investigated in extremely preterm neonates using intermittent assessment of cardiac function by ECHO and mean velocity in the middle cerebral artery (MCA) by Doppler ultrasound

along with continuous $CrSO_2$ monitoring, the identified early pattern of hemodynamic changes in preterm neonates later affected by P/IVH suggested a plausible pathophysiologic explanation for such discrepancies in the reported findings (Chapter 7).[36] Affected neonates demonstrated initial systemic and cerebral hypoperfusion, followed by improvement in both systemic and cerebral blood flow as indicated by the increase in CO, MCA mean velocity, and $CrSO_2$ during the subsequent 20–44 hours and preceding detection of P/IVH. Of note, partial pressure of arterial carbon dioxide ($PaCO_2$) also increased prior to detection of P/IVH. These observations support the hypoperfusion-reperfusion hypothesis as the major hemodynamic pathophysiological factor in the development of P/IVH and underscore the advantages of continuous $rSO_2$ monitoring in neonates using NIRS technology. Furthermore, findings of several recent studies investigating the changes in $CrSO_2$ in conjunction with other hemodynamic parameters and brain functional activity have enabled the assessment of cerebral autoregulation dynamics and its potential clinical implications in preterm and term neonates under different conditions (see below). The role of cerebral NIRS as a routine monitoring tool in extremely preterm infants is currently being evaluated in the SafeBoosC-III trial.

## PERIPHERAL PERFUSION AND MICROCIRCULATION

The observations on the gender-specific differences in vascular tone regulation and peripheral perfusion in preterm and term neonates and the findings that, in patients with sepsis or anemia, changes in microcirculation precede the changes in other hemodynamic parameters or laboratory values indicate the importance of the assessment of microcirculation in the overall evaluation of the neonate.

Perfusion index (PI), defined as the ratio of the pulsatile and non-pulsatile components of the photoelectric plethysmographic signal of pulse oximetry, has been used as a marker of peripheral perfusion.[39-43] It is an appealing measurement as it is noninvasive and continuous and theoretically should provide insight into the circulatory status as it is expected to be affected by a reduction in stroke volume. The signal is readily available at a low cost in many NICUs, with good signal quality in the first 24 hours and without the need for additional monitoring equipment.[44] Interpretation of crude PI values at the bedside is complex due to its dependency on different clinical variables such as positioning of the sensor, the presence of a hsPDA, influence of ventilation strategy, and both gestational and postnatal age.[45] Although the raw PI signal might not be considered informative during early transition in both preterm and term neonates,[46-48] multiple features of a processed PI sub-signal in the first 72 hours of life are associated with adverse outcome in extremely preterm infants.[49,50] There is also strong evidence that preductal values of PI are strongly correlated with low cardiac output states in preterm infants, which advocates the use of the PI signal in trend monitoring.[51] In addition, there is emerging evidence that PI can detect early microcirculatory changes associated with late onset in preterm infants.[52] Whether the PI can be used reliably in the clinical setting for monitoring of perfusion in patients with hsPDA remains uncertain. While, compared to neonates with a non-hsPDA or no PDA, some studies reported a difference in pre- and post-ductal PI values in patients with a hsPDA during the early transitional period,[53] others reported no effect of ductal flow and/or its persistence on PI.[54] Moreover, the presence of the reported pre- and post-ductal gradient in both preterm[55] and term neonates resolved by postnatal day 5.[56] More recently, Gomez-Pomar identified that the mean ΔPI, mean pre-PI, and the ΔPI variability were lower in infants with a PDA, many of whom had echocardiography studies performed after 5 days of postnatal life.[57] PI has also been evaluated as a tool to help identify critical congenital heart disease, in particular for infants with left heart obstruction.[58]

Several other methods are currently available to assess peripheral perfusion and the microcirculation. They include but are not limited to orthogonal polarization (OPS) and side-stream dark-field (SDF) imaging,[59-64] laser Doppler flowmetry,[65-68] and visible light technology.[69,70] Videomicroscopy techniques (OPS and SDF) allow direct visualization of the microcirculation. However, their bedside use in neonates has been limited to intermittent assessments of peripheral perfusion rather than continuous monitoring. While continuous recording of the images can be done, real-time assessment and interpretation remain challenging at this point, with motion and pressure artifacts

posing a significant problem. A newer technique, incident dark field imaging (IDF), appears to be superior to SDF in image quality and accuracy of assessment of the microcirculation in preterm neonates but also bears the limitation of non-continuous evaluation.[71] Laser Doppler flowmetry, on the other hand, offers the capability of continuous monitoring and has been also used in the neonatal population. The main limitations of the technology include inability to evaluate absolute flow properties and thus only allowing assessment of the relative changes in flow over time, low temporal resolution requiring measurement times of ~1 minute, and technical challenges (motion artifacts) to maintain proper probe position on the patient for an extended period of time. A newer laser-based technology, laser speckle contrast imaging (LSCI),[72-75] addresses the issue of temporal resolution with significantly faster measurement times. However, similar to laser Doppler flowmetry, it provides only relative measurements of flux. In addition, LSCI has not been studied in the neonate yet. Assessment of the microcirculation utilizing visible light technology has been reported.[76] However, little is known about its utility in the neonatal population.[77]

Table 14.1 summarizes the tools available for bedside monitoring of the various physiologic parameters discussed in this section.

## COMPREHENSIVE MONITORING SYSTEMS

A growing body of evidence underscores the importance of, and the need for, incorporating multiple physiologic parameters when evaluating the hemodynamic status of neonates. Increasingly, investigators have combined data from different monitoring tools to improve their diagnostic and prognostic value. Such an approach frequently provides valuable insights into the underlying physiological processes as well as the pathophysiology of the cardiovascular compromise that would not be possible with monitoring tools employed in isolation.[78-81] As an example, cerebral autoregulation, that is, the ability of the brain to maintain cerebral blood flow during fluctuations of blood pressure within a certain blood pressure range (Chapters 2, 3, and 8),[82] has been studied using the interaction between the two aforementioned parameters (blood pressure and cerebral blood flow). Significant advances have been made in both studying cerebral autoregulation[83] and improving our

**TABLE 14.1   Systemic and Regional Hemodynamic Parameters Frequently Monitored in Neonates**

| | Parameter | Technology/Method | Purpose and Acquisition [C, I, or C/I] |
|---|---|---|---|
| Systemic perfusion (BP and CO) | Heart rate | ECG (electrodes) | In conjunction with stroke volume gives flow status [C] |
| | BP | Arterial line/cuff (oscillometry; Doppler-US) | Perfusion pressure [C/I] |
| | Stroke volume/CO[138-140] | Echocardiography | Systemic, pulmonary (CO) and organ blood flow, cardiac function [I] |
| | | EBT | Systemic blood flow (CO) and stroke volume (SV) [I] |
| Systemic oxygenation CO$_2$ status | SpO$_2$ | Pulse oximetry | Oxygenation on the arterial side [C] |
| | TCOM | CO$_2$ diffusion through skin | Potential effect on cerebral vasculature (changes in CBF) [C] |
| Regional perfusion | Regional O$_2$ saturation | NIRS | Tissue oxygenation and (indirectly) organ perfusion [C] |
| Peripheral perfusion | Microcirculation (oxygenation; blood flow velocity; capillary recruitment) | Visible light technology | Peripheral perfusion [C] |
| | | Laser Doppler flowmetry | Peripheral perfusion [C] |
| | | OPS, SDF, and IDF | Peripheral perfusion [I] |
| Indirect assessment of perfusion | Capillary refill time | Visual[141] | Systemic perfusion (indirectly) [I] |
| | Delta T (C-P) | Temperature | Systemic perfusion (indirectly) [I] |
| | Color | Visual | Peripheral perfusion [I] |
| Organ function | Brain electrical activity | aEEG[142,143,] | Assessment of brain activity [C] |
| | Urine Output | Urinary catheter | Assessment of renal function [I] |

Legend to Table 14.1.
Physiologic parameters of systemic blood flow (BP and CO) and oxygenation, carbon dioxide production and elimination, regional (organ) and peripheral (microcirculation) blood flow, and organ (brain) function (aEEG) with corresponding assessment tools are listed that can be monitored at the bedside along with the indirect methods used in clinical practice to evaluate perfusion and organ function. Data acquisition can be continuous [C], intermittent [I], or both [C/I]. Adapted from Azhibekov et al., 2014.[31]
*aEEG*, Amplitude-integrated electroencephalography; *CBF*, cerebral blood flow; *Delta T (C – P)*, difference between core and peripheral temperature; *EBT*, electrical biosensing technology; *IDF*, incident dark field (imaging); *IEC*, impedance electrical cardiometry; *OPS*, orthogonal polarization spectral (imaging); *SDF*, Side-stream dark-field (imaging); *TCOM*, transcutaneous CO$_2$ monitoring; *US*, Ultrasonography.

prognostic capability in preterm neonates,[84] especially in those at risk for the development of P/IVH and in term neonates with hypoxic-ischemic encephalopathy undergoing therapeutic hypothermia.[85,86] Inclusion of continuous monitoring of PaCO$_2$, the most important and powerful regulator of cerebral blood flow,[87-89] has the potential to provide additional information about the complex interactions between PaCO$_2$, cerebral blood flow, and other hemodynamic parameters. This is of importance as significant alterations in PaCO$_2$ (both

hypo- and hypercapnia) have been associated with adverse short- and long-term outcomes.[36,90,91]

Currently, clinical and conventional physiologic data are collected and documented manually in the patient's chart or recorded automatically from the bedside monitors to the patient's electronic medical records (EMR). This information, however, is typically documented on an hourly or bi-hourly basis only and may be subject to human error. These intervals are probably inadequate for appropriate monitoring of the rapid and dynamic changes characteristic of the cardiovascular system. To be able to accurately assess the overall hemodynamic status, identify relevant changes in a timely manner, and understand the intricate interplay among the different hemodynamic parameters, these data need to be collected at much higher frequencies (sampling rates) and be time-stamped to other relevant clinical events. The development of comprehensive hemodynamic monitoring systems enables real-time, simultaneous, and continuous collection of physiologic data in a reliable and comprehensive manner for subsequent analysis and assessment of the complex interactions among multiple hemodynamic parameters that may change significantly in a matter of seconds or minutes. Such systems include various monitoring tools, enabling concomitant evaluation of both systemic and regional perfusion and oxygen delivery and other physiologic parameters that play a role in cardiovascular regulation and adaptation, along with monitoring the functional status of specific organs (Figure 14.1). Advances in biomedical technology and computer science have improved the capabilities of comprehensive monitoring systems to collect and store increasing sets of complex physiometric data. Training computer algorithms using hemodynamic high-frequency monitoring data, in combination with nursing observation parameters and patient history details, has the potential to uncover disease-associated patterns in clinical data that are not (always) visible to the human eye. Machine learning techniques could aid clinicians in targeting treatment in an individualized manner, and artificial intelligence software solutions will become available over time.

For these models to be developed correctly and to be deemed clinically relevant, the medical and neonatal community urgently needs to develop a strategy for the critical appraisal and assessment of the technology aids that use modeling on time series data. However, the caveats regarding their accuracy, feasibility, reliability, and need for validation across various subpopulations must be emphasized.[92,93] Finally, and as previously discussed, the utility of the monitoring systems is determined by the comprehensiveness of the monitored hemodynamic parameters.

A previously described hemodynamic monitoring "tower" developed by some of the authors[91,92] was the first step in the process to enable practical, continuous,

and simultaneous monitoring and acquisition of neonatal hemodynamic data at high sampling rates in real time, initially designed for research applications. It integrates conventionally used technologies to continuously monitor heart rate, blood pressure, $SpO_2$, transcutaneous $CO_2$ tension (TCOM), and respiratory rate with other technologies such as EBT for beat-to-beat measurements of SV and CO and NIRS for continuous monitoring of $rSO_2$ changes in vital (brain) and nonvital (kidney, intestine, and/or muscle) organs. The "tower" incorporates these various parameters onto a comprehensive patient monitor using conventional or VueLink modules (Phillips, Palo Alto, CA). The continuous stream of measurements is then acquired through the analog output of the monitor via the use of an analog-to-digital converter and data-acquisition system onto a laptop computer. A motion-activated camera with the same time stamp is used to capture the bedside events that could affect the accuracy and interpretation of the collected data. This functionality aids in differentiating between true fluctuations of physiologic data versus equipment malfunction (lead disconnection, electrode/optode displacement) or other potential artifacts related to provision of routine clinical care and procedures. Another unique advantage of the "tower" is its ability to operate as a mobile, stand-alone unit that could be utilized at any bedside, space permitting. With the increasing recognition of the importance of comprehensive monitoring in intensive care settings in the last decade, several central data collecting systems have become available (for example, Sickbay and Etiometry). These platforms allow for display of interaction of various physiological (including hemodynamic) parameters in graphic formats at bedside.

Collection of all the data with a single monitoring device enables automatic data synchronization and avoids the need to match different time stamps so that simultaneous minute-to-minute changes and interactions between various parameters can be reliably analyzed. Relevant clinical events such as fluid bolus administration, titration of vasoactive medications or treatment of a PDA, transfusion of blood products, intubation/extubation, and change in respiratory support are manually documented by the bedside nurse on a dedicated flowsheet. Figure 14.2 demonstrates an example of a 1-hour period of processed patient

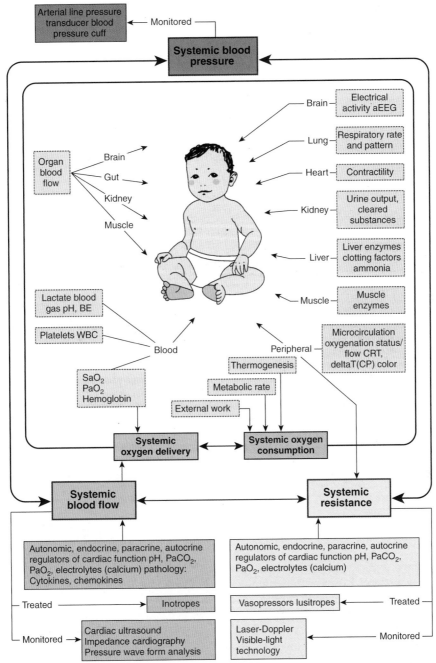

**Fig. 14.1 Comprehensive Neonatal Hemodynamic Monitoring.** Physiologic parameters and tools available to provide a global (outside the circle) and regional (inside the circle) assessment of developmental hemodynamics. Global monitoring of the relationship among systemic flow, blood pressure and resistance, and arterial/venous oxygen content provides information on systemic oxygen delivery and consumption. Regionally monitored parameters provide direct or indirect information on specific organ blood flow and function and vital versus non-vital blood flow regulatory assignment. *aEEG*, amplitude-integrated electroencephalography; *BE*, base excess; *CRT*, capillary refill time; *PaCO₂*, arterial partial pressure of carbon dioxide; *PaO₂*, arterial partial pressure of oxygen; *SaO₂*, arterial oxygen saturation; *WBC*, white blood cells. (Adapted from Azhibekov et al., 2014[31])

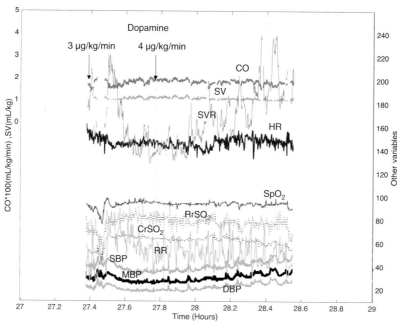

**Fig. 14.2 An approximately 1-hour and 10-minute tracing selected from the comprehensive monitor recording of a 1-day-old 27 weeks' gestation (BW 1020 g) preterm infant with respiratory failure on volume-guarantee ventilation.** Patient received low doses of dopamine as she was considered to be hypotensive. Yet, renal rSO2 was consistently higher than cerebral rSO2, a pattern frequently seen in normotensive neonates, suggesting that the patient's mean blood pressure in the high 20 mmHg range with a cardiac output of ±200 mL/kg/min was most likely appropriate to ensure normal oxygen delivery to the organs. Accordingly, based on the data obtained by the comprehensive monitoring system, this patient did not meet the criteria of systemic hypotension. During the recording shown, cardiac output remained unchanged while the blood pressure and thus calculated systemic vascular resistance (SVR) increased. The increase in blood pressure from ±25 mmHg to ±40 mmHg was associated with a small but apparent decrease in cerebral and renal rSO2 from ±65% and 82% to ±60% and ±77%, respectively, while SpO2 remained unchanged. At the time of these changes, dopamine was being delivered at 3 and 4 μg/kg/min at 27.4 and 27.8 hours, respectively. The findings might be explained by the development of slight vasoconstriction in response to low-dose dopamine or it might be due to spontaneous changes in SVR due to autonomic nervous system immaturity/dysregulation and/or physiologic fluctuations in vascular resistance. *CO*, cardiac output (×100 mL/kg/min); *CrSO2*, cerebral regional tissue oxygen saturation (%); *DBP*, diastolic blood pressure (mmHg); *HR*, heart rate (beats/min); *MBP*, mean blood pressure (mmHg); *RR*, respiratory rate (breaths/min); *RrSO2*, renal regional tissue oxygen saturation (%); *SBP*, systolic blood pressure (mmHg); *SpO2*, peripheral oxygen saturation (%); *SV*, stroke volume (mL/kg); *SVR*, calculated systemic vascular resistance (mmHg × min × mL⁻¹).

data that was acquired using the hemodynamic monitoring "tower" of a preterm infant with respiratory failure on volume-guarantee ventilation. Figure 14.3 demonstrates the hemodynamic changes that were observed during various events related to routine patient care and extubation. Retrospective review of the video data captured by the motion-activated camera during the study period enabled identification and accurate time-stamping of these events. Without the concomitant video component, proper interpretation of the physiologic data would have been challenging, if not impossible.

On a larger scale, hospital-wide systems are now also available from third-party vendors (e.g., Bernoulli Enterprise [Cardiopulmonary Corporation, Milford, CT, USA] or BedMaster [Excel Medical Electronics, Jupiter, FL, USA]). Using hospital data networks, these systems acquire output data from bedside monitors and other devices (e.g., ventilators, infusion pumps, etc.) from multiple patients and route it to central servers for storage and subsequent data processing and analysis. The collected physiologic data can then be retrieved in real time or retrospectively as a data spreadsheet or as waveforms when applicable. Various software packages are

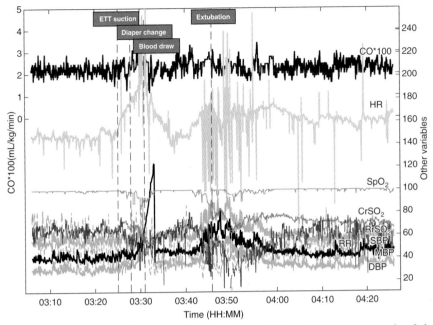

**Fig. 14.3 A 90-minute segment of prospectively collected continuous recording of 9 hemodynamic parameters in a 3-day-old preterm neonate born at 28 weeks' gestation (birth weight [BW] 920 g).** Retrospective review of the data from the motion-activated camera allowed time stamping of the clinical events on the figure. The video recording revealed that the increase in heart rate along with changes in blood pressure at around the 03:25 mark corresponded to the time of endotracheal tube (ETT) suctioning, followed by a diaper change and then a blood draw. Increased heart rate and blood pressure variability 10 minutes later corresponds to the time of extubation. *CO*, cardiac output; *CrSO₂*, cerebral regional tissue oxygen saturation (%); *DBP*, diastolic blood pressure (mmHg); *HR*, heart rate (beats/min); *MBP*, mean blood pressure (mmHg); *RR*, respiratory rate (breaths/min); *RrSO₂*, renal regional tissue oxygen saturation (%); *SBP*, systolic blood pressure (mmHg); *SpO₂*, peripheral oxygen saturation (%).

available to process these data so that the parameters of interest can be viewed, scored, transformed, and/or analyzed. Flexibility of the output format allows analyzing various combinations of parameters, such as blood pressure and cerebral rSO₂ (CrSO₂) to evaluate cerebral autoregulation, or rSO₂ and SpO₂ to calculate fractional tissue oxygen extraction (FTOE).

Automated collection of physiologic datasets has a number of inherent challenges. These include but are not limited to intermittent data fall-out (patient movements or maneuvers by the care team, sensor dislodgement, or erroneous measurements during sensor calibration) and the presence of noise and artifacts. Thorough and systematic cleaning of the data is a time-consuming and challenging task but it is crucial to address these issues prior to data analysis. Furthermore, information about data variability such as the coefficient of variation should also be available for all

variables studied. Without this information, one would not be able to interpret changes in the trend of a given hemodynamic parameter, as we need to know what level of changes can be considered normal variability and which are pathological.

The next step in the process is performing the analysis of the processed data that can potentially advance our understanding of the physiologic characteristics of a parameter and/or a relationship between two or more parameters. As an example, heart rate and blood pressure characteristics can be used to assess autonomic nervous system function; indeed, heart rate variability (HRV) and baroreflex sensitivity can indirectly quantify autonomic activity.

Heart rate variability is a well-established noninvasive measure of autonomic control of the heart. It provides a powerful means of monitoring the interplay between the sympathetic and parasympathetic nervous systems.[94,95] Both parasympathetic and sympathetic activities modulate the R-R interval at low frequency (LF) range, while parasympathetic activity modulates it in the higher frequency (HF) range. Fast Fourier transformation (FFT) for power spectral density (PSD) analysis can be used to measure RR interval variability distribution as a function of the frequency.[94] LF and HF components are calculated based on the frequency bands identified for infants as 0.03–0.2 Hz and 0.3–2 Hz, respectively.[96,97]

The baroreceptor reflex buffers change in systemic blood pressure by adjusting HR and peripheral vascular resistance (Figure 14.4). Evaluation of baroreceptor sensitivity can provide insights into the ability of a neonate to redistribute blood flow via changes in peripheral vascular resistance. HR changes are mediated by both the parasympathetic and sympathetic nervous systems, whereas a change in vascular resistance is mediated through the sympathetic system.[98,99] Baroreceptor function is measured as the slope of the sigmoid-shaped blood pressure and R-R interval relationship at the operating physiological point, referred to as

baroreceptor reflex sensitivity (Figure 14.5).[100] It is typically measured during a change (increase or decrease) in the blood pressure that is pharmacologically induced. Since it is rarely practical or ethical to pharmacologically modify the blood pressure in neonates for diagnostic purposes, researchers have used spontaneous fluctuation in blood pressure and the R-R interval. Using transfer function analysis, baroreceptor reflex sensitivity is then calculated as a transfer gain using the ratio of the amplitude of the output signal (R-R interval) to that of the input signal (systolic blood pressure) at low frequency range.[100] Table 14.2 summarizes the available information on baroreceptor reflex sensitivity in neonates.[100,101]

Another example includes cerebral autoregulation. Newer analytic approaches have laid the ground for further improvements in our understanding of cerebral hemodynamics and its autoregulation (Chapter 2).[102,103] In addition, a number of other approaches to studying cerebral autoregulation have been reported in the literature, including correlation analysis using statistical principles,[104] spectral analysis techniques of coherence

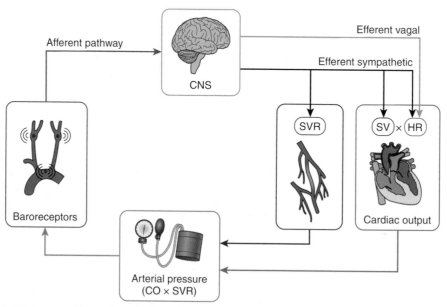

**Fig. 14.4 Interactions between cardiovascular and autonomic nervous systems.** Changes in blood pressure are sensed by baroreceptors in the aorta or carotid sinus. The information is sent, via afferent nerves, to the cardiac regulatory center in the brain, which in turn initiates changes in vagal and sympathetic tone. In response to a sudden increase in blood pressure, a decrease in sympathetic tone and an increase in parasympathetic tone ensues. Decrease in sympathetic signal causes vasodilation in the vessels (↓ SVR), decrease in contractility (↓ SV), and slower firing rate of the SA node (↓ HR), all of which result in lowering blood pressure. The elevated parasympathetic tone decreases the SA node firing rate and also contributes to lowering the blood pressure by decreasing the heart rate.

**Baroreceptor reflex**

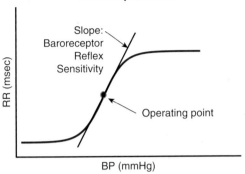

Fig. 14.5 Baroreceptor function is measured as the slope of the sigmoid-shaped blood pressure and R-R interval relationship at the operating physiological point, referred to as baroreceptor reflex sensitivity.[100]

function or the transfer function analysis,[80,105-108] and, more recently, wavelet coherence analysis.[109]

## From Research to Individualized Neonatal Intensive Care

Due to a number of limitations, comprehensive hemodynamic monitoring systems are still being utilized mostly for research purposes. Overall, the implementation and maintenance of such a system is a challenging and time-consuming process that, in addition to the financial cost, requires very close collaboration between the vendor, the institution's biomedical engineering and information technology departments, hospital administration, and

the members of the multidisciplinary team of healthcare providers (physicians, respiratory therapists, and nurses). The enormous amount of continuously growing data requires additional infrastructure to store and organize the data, as well as the involvement of computer scientists and experts in bioinformatics to assist with large data handling and analysis. In addition, since the collected data represent protected health information, protection of patients' rights and confidentiality is mandatory, and all related processes to access the data for research and quality improvement purposes must comply with federal, state, and hospital-wide regulations, policies, and procedures. Once established, however, accurately collected and appropriately stored data from such multi-modular monitoring systems will serve as an invaluable resource for multiple research ideas and quality improvement activities that extend far beyond cardiovascular physiology alone.

For clinical application, with close collaboration among researchers in basic science and translational and clinical research, biostatisticians, computer and bioinformatics scientists, biomedical engineers, and scientists in other specialties, analysis of the information obtained via comprehensive hemodynamic monitoring can potentially reveal pathognomonic trends and patterns that may precede changes in systemic and organ perfusion. Therefore such a system with the required infrastructural support enables the development of algorithms to predict impending hemodynamic compromise and the responsiveness of a given patient to a particular intervention. As an example of

| TABLE 14.2 | **Baroreceptor Reflex Sensitivity in Neonates** | | | | |
|---|---|---|---|---|---|
| Method | Sequence Method (Drouin et al., 1997[101]) | | Spectral Method (Andriessen et al., 2005[100]) | | |
| GA | GA: 26–39 N = 14 | GA: 40–41 N = 5 | PMA 28–32 (n = 16) | PMA 32–37 (n = 10) | PMA 37–42 (n = 6) |
| Baroreceptor reflex sensitivity value (ms/mmHg) Mean (SD) or median (range) | 4.07 (2.19) | 10.23 (2.92) | 4.6 (3.1–5.4) | 7.5 (5.2–10.1) | 15.0 (11.8–19.7) |

Legend to Table 14.2.
Comparison of baroreceptor reflex sensitivity (BRS) value using the sequence and spectral methods in neonates. In the sequence method BRS is calculated using the mean slope of the linear regression of the R-R intervals vs. systolic blood pressure (SBP). In the spectral method BRS is calculated using the low-frequency (0.04–0.15 Hz) transfer function gain between SBP and the R-R interval.

such an effort, analysis of heart rate variability allowed developing a heart rate characteristics monitoring system to identify neonates at risk for developing sepsis, and it has subsequently been shown to decrease mortality from late-onset neonatal sepsis.[110,111] In the pediatric and adult critical care literature, similar findings of continuous monitoring of dynamic changes in cardiovascular parameters in response to various factors have also been reported.[112] Clinical applications of hemodynamic monitoring data include the ability to detect shock in the compensated phase prior to decompensation[113,114] and the prediction of the patient's responsiveness to fluid administration.[115-119] The feasibility of the use of arterial blood pressure variation to predict fluid responsiveness in newborn infants has been questioned, because of a physiologic aliasing effect secondary to a reduced heart rate/respiratory rate ratio in these patients.[120]

Computational modeling is one of the approaches that enable such transition from research findings to advances in intensive care, where decision-making needs to take place quickly in the setting of large amounts of patient data that have to be included and analyzed. Computational models serve as a mathematical representation of human physiology and/or pathophysiology and assist in improving our understanding of the inter-relationship among various parameters or estimating the unknown ones, thus aiding in the diagnosis and management of certain conditions. They also allow experimentation with potential interventions and procedures in the model before trialing them in patient care.[121] Hemodynamic data obtained via comprehensive monitoring can be used to validate mathematical models aiming at predicting cardiovascular responses to distinct stimuli. As an example of such mathematical models, PNEUMA, a comprehensive and physiologically realistic computer model, has been developed and described in the adult literature.[122] It incorporates cardiovascular, respiratory, and autonomous nervous systems and was originally designed to study cardiorespiratory mechanisms of breathing in adults with sleep disorders. The model has been adapted by the authors to neonatal physiology to study the effects of PDA on systemic, pulmonary, and organ blood flow, as well as the ability to predict hemodynamic and autonomic nervous system changes in response to surgical closure of the PDA.

Hemodynamic and/or respiratory changes associated with PDA ligation have been studied in both animal models[123] and premature infants.[124,125] Despite differences in the study designs, measurement techniques, and time intervals, all studies reported similar changes, with decreases in SV and CO and increases in SVR immediately following ductal closure. These changes, when monitored for up to 24 hours, gradually improved over time. Figure 14.6 demonstrates the acute hemodynamic and autonomic changes following PDA ligation as predicted by a modified PNEUMA model[126] that align with the published literature (Figure 14.7). Data from the authors' institution provide an example of the hemodynamic changes observed in a preterm neonate when PDA ligation was captured using the Bernoulli system (Figure 14.8). Of note is that validation of the predictive capabilities of the model in neonates still requires further work.

Another important factor being increasingly recognized is genetic variability and its impact on individual susceptibility to certain external adverse factors, characteristics of the disease process, and response to particular interventions. Advances in molecular genetics and genetic epidemiology and the increasingly simplified access to data provided by whole genome sequencing will open another era of hemodynamic research and aid in the appreciation and better understanding of the multi-layered nature of cardiovascular physiology and pathophysiology. Theoretically, the advantages of studying the neonatal population[127] and exploring the associations between genetic variability and phenotypic presentations will likely lead to identification of genetic variants associated with particular cardiovascular disease processes in discrete subpopulations of neonates or to understanding of therapeutic efficacy or inefficacy of the pharmacologic agents used in the treatment of neonatal cardiovascular compromise.

To support this hypothesis, an increasing number of genome-wide association studies (GWASs) report identified genetic polymorphisms that are associated with certain hemodynamic parameters such as blood pressure,[128] resting heart rate,[129,130] heart rate variability,[131] and cardiac function.[132] These findings provide new insights into underlying biological mechanisms of the inter-individual variability of the hemodynamic parameters and their interaction with potentially important diagnostic and therapeutic applications. For

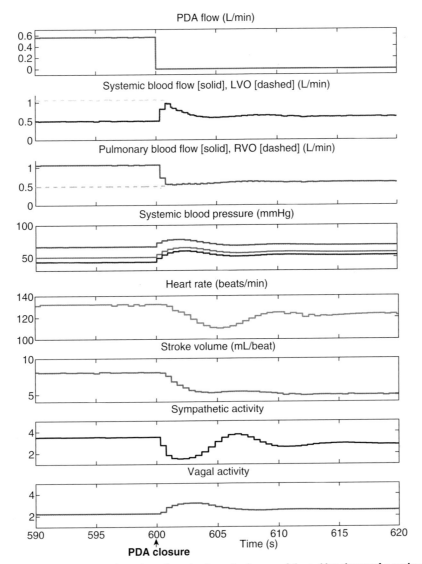

**Fig. 14.6  Computer simulation of the acute hemodynamic and autonomic changes of the sudden closure of a moderate PDA.** Systolic, mean, and diastolic blood pressure is represented in the systemic blood pressure panel. See text for details. *LVO*, left ventricular output; *PDA*, patent ductus arteriosus; *RVO*, right ventricular output. (Adapted from Soleymani et al., 2015[126] and Azhibekov et al., 2015.[127])

example, single nucleotide polymorphisms (SNPs) have recently been identified that are associated with the response pattern to different classes of antihypertensive medications such as diuretics and angiotensin II receptor blockers.[133,134] Moreover, SNPs associated with genetic predisposition to presenting with a patent ductus arteriosus in preterm neonates have been reported as well.[135,136]

Lastly, inclusion of the tools that assess functional status of target organs, such as amplitude-integrated electroencephalography (aEEG), into comprehensive hemodynamic monitoring systems will allow the development of predictive models for short-term neonatal outcomes such as P/IVH and long-term outcomes such as neurodevelopmental scores. With the incorporation of additional data such as neuroimages, biomarkers,

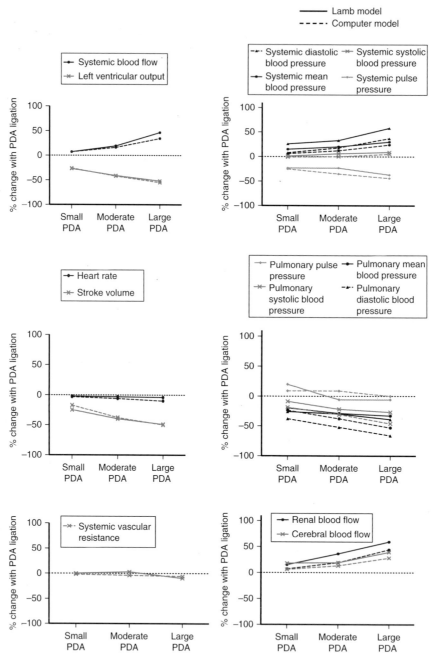

**Fig. 14.7 Changes in various cardiovascular and respiratory parameters in response to PDA ligation as determined in a lamb model[123]** (*solid lines*) **and predicted by PNEUMA computer model (d***ashed lines***).** The data are presented as percent change from baseline occurring once the PDA is closed. Stratification is based on the size of the duct: small, moderate, and large PDA.

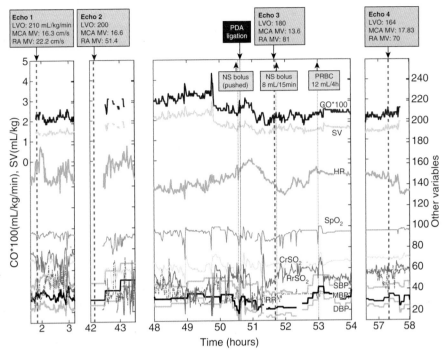

**Fig. 14.8 Real-time recording of 10 hemodynamic parameters prospectively collected in an 11-day-old preterm neonate born at 25 weeks' gestation (BW 810 g) undergoing PDA ligation.** This mechanically ventilated neonate had received two courses of indomethacin without success. PDA ligation is marked in red at approximately the 50.5-hour mark. The four functional echocardiographic/Doppler ultrasound assessments of left ventricular output (LVO), middle cerebral artery and renal artery mean velocity (MCA MV and RA MV, respectively) are displayed in light red boxes. Administration of normal saline (NS Bolus) and packed red blood cells (PRBC) are displayed in grey boxes. Immediately prior to ligation, the significant decrease in blood pressure was likely precipitated by the anesthesia and mediated via a decrease in the SVR. Administration of a normal saline bolus (possibly through an increase in preload) and ligation of PDA (by the sudden removal of the shunt) resulted in a blood pressure increase primarily via an increase in the effective CO (both SV and HR increased). The subsequent decrease in HR to the "pre-ligation range" accompanied by a more prominent decrease in SV (below the pre-ligation values) within 1 hour resulted in a significant decrease in the CO and thus in BP. $CrSO_2$ did not show significant changes in absolute values. However, the fluctuations in $CrSO_2$ following the ligation appear to be less related to changes in $SpO_2$ and BP, suggesting an improvement in cerebral autoregulation. $RrSO_2$, instead, increased significantly following PDA ligation and fluid administration, concomitantly with an increase in RA MV as estimated by Doppler ultrasound. These changes likely represent improved non-vital organ blood flow after removal of the left-to-right PDA shunt. Hemodynamic parameters: Left y-axis depicts SV (mL) and CO (100 mL/min) and the right y-axis shows the values for $SpO_2$, $CrSO_2$ and $RrSO_2$ (%), HR and RR (1/min), SPB, MBP, and DBP (mmHg). *CO,* Cardiac output; *$CrSO_2$,* cerebral regional tissue oxygen saturation; *DBP,* diastolic blood pressure; *HR,* heart rate; *MBP,* mean blood pressure; *RR,* respiratory rate; *$RrSO_2$,* renal regional tissue oxygen saturation; *SBP,* systolic blood pressure; *$SpO_2$,* arterial oxygen saturation; *SV,* stroke volume.

and single nucleotide polymorphisms, these multi-modular monitoring systems will contribute to the creation of a new generation of real-time clinical decision support tools to refine individualized medical care plans and improve survival and quality of life for critically ill neonates.

In order to change from population-focused medicine, using evidence from large clinical trials enrolling patients with little to no consideration for individual patient characteristics to individualized medicine, we need to make radical changes in our approach, and a starting point would be for patients requiring intensive or complex clinical care. Indeed, the recent recognition of the need to develop and utilize comprehensive monitoring and data acquisition systems, harness mathematical analysis to develop predictive algorithms, and incorporate machine learning and artificial intelligence allows us to advance our ability to predict the future and are the first steps in this direction.[31,137]

## Conclusion

In summary, despite multiple attempts to define cardiovascular failure, develop criteria for initiating interventions, and/or identify the most appropriate, pathophysiology-targeted treatment to normalize blood pressure and organ perfusion, these and other related questions remain mostly unanswered. The challenges to define hypotension include variations in blood pressure values based on gestational and postnatal age and existing comorbidities (lung disease, infection, etc.) and the fact that, in patients of the same gestational and postnatal age and degree of maturity, the same blood pressure value can be associated with either adequate or compromised systemic and organ perfusion. Even in the same patient under different conditions and at different points in time, the same blood pressure value can represent adequate or compromised systemic and/or organ perfusion. Without comprehensive evaluation using additional data that accurately represent both blood pressure and systemic and organ blood flow and oxygen delivery in neonates at risk, timely diagnosis of impending cardiovascular compromise and appropriate, pathophysiology-targeted decision to intervene with the most appropriate medication in the given individual remains challenging, if not impossible.

At present, comprehensive hemodynamic monitoring systems are being utilized primarily for research applications. The use of these novel systems capable of continuous data monitoring and acquisition, sophisticated data handling, and analysis of large physiologic data sets with validation of the findings followed by the development of management algorithms requires a truly multidisciplinary approach with close collaboration among clinicians and researchers of different specialties, biomedical engineers, statisticians, and computer scientists. The ultimate goal is to be able to predict potential adverse events with reasonable certainty. This goal can be accomplished by identifying discrete neonatal subpopulations that have a significantly higher risk for the development of severe hemodynamic instability or its complications based on genetic susceptibility, perinatal factors, and/or the presence of early signs of impending compromise and applying pathophysiology-targeted interventions that are the most beneficial and the least harmful in the given patient. As a result, the novel information obtained may contribute to clinically relevant improvements in neonatal care, including a decrease in morbidity and mortality associated with cardiovascular instability in the neonatal period and improvement in relevant long-term outcomes. Comprehensive hemodynamic monitoring will not improve outcome alone and requires early detection of circulatory failure followed by optimized and individualized hemodynamic management. Gaining insight into the underlying pathophysiology and monitoring the effects of therapeutic interventions will further contribute to the benefits gained from the use of comprehensive hemodynamic monitoring and data acquisition. Finally, these systems and the inherent need for the use of a multidisciplinary approach will serve as the foundation to utilize mathematical analysis to develop predictive algorithms and employ machine learning and artificial intelligence to predict the future instead of continuing to only react to advancing pathophysiological events.

## Acknowledgment

The authors acknowledge the contributions of Timur Azhibekov and Sadaf Soleymani to the chapter in the previous editions.

## REFERENCES

1. Seri I, Evans J. Controversies in the diagnosis and management of hypotension in the newborn infant. *Curr Opin Pediatr.* 2001;13(2):116-123.
2. Kluckow M, Evans N. Low superior vena cava flow and intraventricular haemorrhage in preterm infants. *Arch Dis Child Fetal Neonatal Ed.* 2000;82(3):F188-F194. doi:10.1136/fn.82.3.F188.
3. Osborn DA, Evans N, Kluckow M. Hemodynamic and antecedent risk factors of early and late periventricular/intraventricular hemorrhage in premature infants. *Pediatrics.* 2003;112(1 Pt 1):33-39.
4. Hunt RW, Evans N, Rieger I, Kluckow M. Low superior vena cava flow and neurodevelopment at 3 years in very preterm infants. *J Pediatr.* 2004;145(5):588-592. doi:10.1016/j.jpeds.2004.06.056.
5. Fanaroff JM, Wilson-Costello DE, Newman NS, Montpetite MM, Fanaroff AA. Treated hypotension is associated with neonatal morbidity and hearing loss in extremely low birth weight infants. *Pediatrics.* 2006;117(4):1131-1135. doi:10.1542/peds.2005-1230.
6. Pellicer A, Bravo MC, Madero R, Salas S, Quero J, Cabanas F. Early systemic hypotension and vasopressor support in low birth weight infants: impact on neurodevelopment. *Pediatrics.* 2009;123(5):1369-1376. doi:10.1542/peds.2008-0673.
7. Pellicer A, Valverde E, Elorza MD, et al. Cardiovascular support for low birth weight infants and cerebral hemodynamics: a

randomized, blinded, clinical trial. *Pediatrics.* 2005;115(6): 1501-1512. doi:10.1542/peds.2004-1396.

8. Vesoulis ZA, Ters NE, Foster A, Trivedi SB, Liao SM, Mathur AM. Response to dopamine in prematurity: a biomarker for brain injury? *J Perinatol.* 2016;36(6):453-458. doi:10.1038/jp.2016.5.

9. Roze JC, Tohier C, Maingueneau C, Lefevre M, Mouzard A. Response to dobutamine and dopamine in the hypotensive very preterm infant. *Arch Dis Child.* 1993;69(1 Spec No):59-63.

10. Tibballs J, Hochmann M, Osborne A, Carter B. Accuracy of the BoMED NCCOM3 bioimpedance cardiac output monitor during induced hypotension: an experimental study in dogs. *Anaesth Intensive Care.* 1992;20(3):326-331. doi:10.1177/0310057X9202000309.

11. Paradisis M, Evans N, Kluckow M, Osborn D. Randomized trial of milrinone versus placebo for prevention of low systemic blood flow in very preterm infants. *J Pediatr.* 2009;154(2): 189-195. doi:10.1016/j.jpeds.2008.07.059.

12. Bidegain M, Greenberg R, Simmons C, Dang C, Cotten CM, Smith PB. Vasopressin for refractory hypotension in extremely low birth weight infants. *J Pediatr.* 2010;157(3):502-524. doi:10.1016/j.jpeds.2010.04.038.

13. Batton B, Li L, Newman NS, et al. Use of antihypotensive therapies in extremely preterm infants. *Pediatrics.* 2013;131(6): e1865-e1873. doi:10.1542/peds.2012-2779.

14. Dempsey EM, Barrington KJ. Diagnostic criteria and therapeutic interventions for the hypotensive very low birth weight infant. *J Perinatol.* 2006;26(11):677-681. doi:10.1038/sj.jp.7211579.

15. Stranak Z, Semberova J, Barrington K, et al. International survey on diagnosis and management of hypotension in extremely preterm babies. *Eur J Pediatr.* 2014;173(6):793-798. doi:10.1007/s00431-013-2251-9.

16. Batton B, Batton D, Riggs T. Blood pressure during the first 7 days in premature infants born at postmenstrual age 23 to 25 weeks. *Am J Perinatol.* 2007;24(2):107-115. doi:10.1055/s-2007-970178.

17. Lee J, Rajadurai VS, Tan KW. Blood pressure standards for very low birthweight infants during the first day of life. *Arch Dis Child Fetal Neonatal Ed.* 1999;81(3):F168-F170. doi:10.1136/fn.81.3.f168.

18. Groves AM, Chiesa G, Durighel G, et al. Functional cardiac MRI in preterm and term newborns. *Arch Dis Child Fetal Neonatal Ed.* 2011;96(2):F86-F91. doi:10.1136/adc.2010.189142.

19. Chew MS, Poelaert J. Accuracy and repeatability of pediatric cardiac output measurement using Doppler: 20-year review of the literature. *Intensive Care Med.* 2003;29(11):1889-1894. doi:10.1007/s00134-003-1967-9.

20. Kluckow M, Seri I, Evans N. Functional echocardiography: an emerging clinical tool for the neonatologist. *J Pediatr.* 2007;150(2):125-130. doi:10.1016/j.jpeds.2006.10.056.

21. Kluckow M. Functional echocardiography in assessment of the cardiovascular system in asphyxiated neonates. *J Pediatr.* 2011;158(suppl 2):e13-e18. doi:10.1016/j.jpeds.2010.11.007.

22. de Waal K, Kluckow M. Functional echocardiography; from physiology to treatment. *Early Hum Dev.* 2010;86(3):149-154. doi:10.1016/j.earlhumdev.2010.01.030.

23. Mertens L, Seri I, Marek J, et al. Targeted neonatal echocardiography in the neonatal intensive care unit: practice guidelines and recommendations for training. Writing Group of the American Society of Echocardiography (ASE) in collaboration with the European Association of Echocardiography (EAE) and the Association for European Pediatric Cardiologists (AEPC).

*J Am Soc Echocardiogr.* 2011;24(10):1057-1078. doi:10.1016/j.echo.2011.07.014.

24. de Boode WP, Singh Y, Gupta S, et al. Recommendations for neonatologist performed echocardiography in Europe: consensus statement endorsed by European Society for Paediatric Research (ESPR) and European Society for Neonatology (ESN). *Pediatr Res.* 2016;80(4):465-471. doi:10.1038/pr.2016.126.

25. Evans N, Iyer P. Assessment of ductus arteriosus shunt in preterm infants supported by mechanical ventilation: effect of interatrial shunting. *J Pediatr.* 1994;125(5 Pt 1):778-785.

26. Evans N, Iyer P. Incompetence of the foramen ovale in preterm infants supported by mechanical ventilation. *J Pediatr.* 1994; 125(5 Pt 1):786-792.

27. Kluckow M, Evans N. Superior vena cava flow in newborn infants: a novel marker of systemic blood flow. *Arch Dis Child Fetal Neonatal Ed.* 2000;82(3):F182-F187.

28. Van Wyk L, Gupta S, Lawrenson J, de Boode WP. Accuracy and trending ability of electrical biosensing technology for non-invasive cardiac output monitoring in neonates: a systematic qualitative review. *Frontiers in Pediatrics.* 2022;10:851850. doi:10.3389/fped.2022.851850.

29. Van Wyk L, Smith J, Lawrenson J, Lombard CJ, de Boode WP. Bioreactance cardiac output trending ability in preterm infants: a single centre, longitudinal study. *Neonatology.* 2021:118: 600-608. doi:10.1159/000518656.

30. van Bel F, Lemmers P, Naulaers G. Monitoring neonatal regional cerebral oxygen saturation in clinical practice: value and pitfalls. *Neonatology.* 2008;94(4):237-244. doi:10.1159/000151642.

31. Azhibekov T, Noori S, Soleymani S, Seri I. Transitional cardiovascular physiology and comprehensive hemodynamic monitoring in the neonate: relevance to research and clinical care. *Semin Fetal Neonatal Med.* 2014;19(1):45-53. doi:10.1016/j.siny.2013.09.009.

32. Binder C, Urlesberger B, Avian A, Pocivalnik M, Müller W, Pichler G. Cerebral and peripheral regional oxygen saturation during postnatal transition in preterm neonates. *J Pediatr.* 2013;163(2):394-399. doi:10.1016/j.jpeds.2013.01.026.

33. Mukai M, Uchida T, Itoh H, Suzuki H, Niwayama M, Kanayama N. Tissue oxygen saturation levels from fetus to neonate. *J Obstet Gynaecol Res.* 2017;43(5):855-859. doi:10.1111/jog.13295.

34. Tamussino A, Urlesberger B, Baik N, et al. Low cerebral activity and cerebral oxygenation during immediate transition in term neonates-A prospective observational study. *Resuscitation.* 2016;103:49-53. doi:10.1016/j.resuscitation.2016.03.011.

35. Alderliesten T, Lemmers PMA, Smarius JJM, van de Vosse RE, Baerts W, van Bel F. Cerebral oxygenation, extraction, and autoregulation in very preterm infants who develop peri-intraventricular hemorrhage. *J Pediatr.* 2013;162(4):698-704. doi:10.1016/j.jpeds.2012.09.038.

36. Noori S, McCoy M, Anderson MP, Ramji F, Seri I. Changes in cardiac function and cerebral blood flow in relation to peri/intraventricular hemorrhage in extremely preterm infants. *J Pediatr.* 2014;164(2):264-270.e1-e3. doi:10.1016/j.jpeds.2013.09.045.

37. Verhagen EA, Ter Horst HJ, Keating P, Martijn A, Van Braeckel KN, Bos AF. Cerebral oxygenation in preterm infants with germinal matrix-intraventricular hemorrhages. *Stroke.* 2010;41(12): 2901-2907. doi:10.1161/STROKEAHA.110.597229.

38. Verhagen EA, Van Braeckel KN, van der Veere CN, et al. Cerebral oxygenation is associated with neurodevelopmental outcome of preterm children at age 2 to 3 years. *Dev Med Child Neurol.* 2015;57(5):449-455. doi:10.1111/dmcn.12622.

39. Lima AP, Beelen P, Bakker J. Use of a peripheral perfusion index derived from the pulse oximetry signal as a noninvasive indicator of perfusion. *Crit Care Med.* 2002;30(6):1210-1213. doi:10.1097/00003246-200206000-00006.

40. De Felice C, Latini G, Vacca P, Kopotic RJ. The pulse oximeter perfusion index as a predictor for high illness severity in neonates. *Eur J Pediatr.* 2002;161(10):561-562. doi:10.1007/s00431-002-1042-5.

41. De Felice C, Del Vecchio A, Criscuolo M, Lozupone A, Parrini S, Latini G. Early postnatal changes in the perfusion index in term newborns with subclinical chorioamnionitis. *Arch Dis Child Fetal Neonatal Ed.* 2005;90(5):F411-F414. doi:10.1136/adc.2004.068882.

42. Takahashi S, Kakiuchi S, Nanba Y, Tsukamoto K, Nakamura T, Ito Y. The perfusion index derived from a pulse oximeter for predicting low superior vena cava flow in very low birth weight infants. *J Perinatol.* 2010;30(4):265-269. doi:10.1038/jp.2009.159.

43. Bagci S, Muller N, Muller A, Heydweiller A, Bartmann P, Franz AR. A pilot study of the pleth variability index as an indicator of volume-responsive hypotension in newborn infants during surgery. *J Anesth.* 2013;27(2):192-198. doi:10.1007/s00540-012-1511-6.

44. Schwarz CE, O'Toole JM, Livingstone V, Pavel AM, Dempsey EM. Signal quality of electrical cardiometry and perfusion index in very preterm infants. *Neonatology.* 2021;118(6):672-677. doi:10.1159/000518061.

45. Alderliesten T, Lemmers PM, Baerts W, Groenendaal F, van Bel F. Perfusion index in preterm infants during the first 3 days of life: reference values and relation with clinical variables. *Neonatology.* 2015;107(4):258-265. doi:10.1159/000370192.

46. Unal S, Ergenekon E, Aktas S, et al. Perfusion index assessment during transition period of newborns: an observational study. *BMC Pediatr.* 2016;16(1):164. doi:10.1186/s12887-016-0701-z.

47. Kroese JK, van Vonderen JJ, Narayen IC, Walther FJ, Hooper S, te Pas AB. The perfusion index of healthy term infants during transition at birth. *Eur J Pediatr.* 2016;175(4):475-479. doi:10.1007/s00431-015-2650-1.

48. Hawkes GA, O'Toole JM, Kenosi M, Ryan CA, Dempsey EM. Perfusion index in the preterm infant immediately after birth. *Early Hum Dev.* 2015;91(8):463-465. doi:10.1016/j.earlhumdev.2015.05.003.

49. Van Laere D, O'Toole JM, Voeten M, McKiernan J, Boylan GB, Dempsey E. Decreased variability and low values of perfusion index on day one are associated with adverse outcome in extremely preterm infants. *J Pediatr.* 2016;178:119-124.e1. doi:10.1016/j.jpeds.2016.08.008.

50. O'Toole JM, Dempsey EM, Van Laere D. Nonstationary coupling between heart rate and perfusion index in extremely preterm infants in the first day of life. *Physiol Meas.* 2021;42(3). doi:10.1088/1361-6579/abe3de.

51. Janaillac M, Beausoleil TP, Barrington KJ, et al. Correlations between near-infrared spectroscopy, perfusion index, and cardiac outputs in extremely preterm infants in the first 72 h of life. *Eur J Pediatr.* 2018;177(4):541-550. doi:10.1007/s00431-018-3096-z.

52. Singh J, Jain S, Chawla D, Randev S, Khurana S. Peripheral perfusion index as a marker of sepsis in preterm neonates. *J Trop Pediatr.* 2022;68(2):fmac014. doi:10.1093/tropej/fmac014.

53. Khositseth A, Muangyod N, Nuntnarumit P. Perfusion index as a diagnostic tool for patent ductus arteriosus in preterm infants. *Neonatology.* 2013;104(3):250-254. doi:10.1159/000353862.

54. Vidal M, Ferragu F, Durand S, Baleine J, Batista-Novais AR, Cambonie G. Perfusion index and its dynamic changes in preterm neonates with patent ductus arteriosus. *Acta Paediatr.* 2013;102(4):373-378. doi:10.1111/apa.12130.

55. Kinoshita M, Hawkes CP, Ryan CA, Dempsey EM. Perfusion index in the very preterm infant. *Acta Paediatr.* 2013;102(9):e398-e401. doi:10.1111/apa.12322.

56. Hakan N, Dilli D, Zenciroglu A, Aydin M, Okumus N. Reference values of perfusion indices in hemodynamically stable newborns during the early neonatal period. *Eur J Pediatr.* 2014;173(5):597-602. doi:10.1007/s00431-013-2224-z.

57. Gomez-Pomar E, Makhoul M, Westgate PM, et al. Relationship between perfusion index and patent ductus arteriosus in preterm infants. *Pediatric Research.* 2017;81(5):775-779. doi:10.1038/pr.2017.10.

58. Uygur O, Koroglu OA, Levent E, et al. The value of peripheral perfusion index measurements for early detection of critical cardiac defects. *Pediatr Neonatol.* 2019;60(1):68-73. doi:10.1016/j.pedneo.2018.04.003.

59. Groner W, Winkelman JW, Harris AG, et al. Orthogonal polarization spectral imaging: a new method for study of the microcirculation. *Nat Med.* 1999;5(10):1209-1212. doi:10.1038/13529.

60. Genzel-Boroviczeny O, Strotgen J, Harris AG, Messmer K, Christ F. Orthogonal polarization spectral imaging (OPS): a novel method to measure the microcirculation in term and preterm infants transcutaneously. *Pediatr Res.* 2002;51(3):386-391. doi:10.1203/00006450-200203000-00019.

61. Genzel-Boroviczeny O, Seidl T, Rieger-Fackeldey E, Abicht J, Christ F. Impaired microvascular perfusion improves with increased incubator temperature in preterm infants. *Pediatr Res.* 2007;61(2):239-242. doi:10.1203/pdr.0b013e31802d77a2.

62. Genzel-Boroviczeny O, Christ F, Glas V. Blood transfusion increases functional capillary density in the skin of anemic preterm infants. *Pediatr Res.* 2004;56(5):751-755. doi:10.1203/01.PDR.0000141982.38959.10.

63. Weidlich K, Kroth J, Nussbaum C, et al. Changes in microcirculation as early markers for infection in preterm infants – an observational prospective study. *Pediatr Res.* 2009;66(4):461-465. doi:10.1203/PDR.0b013e3181b3b1f6.

64. van den Berg VJ, van Elteren HA, Buijs EA, et al. Reproducibility of microvascular vessel density analysis in Sidestream dark-field-derived images of healthy term newborns. *Microcirculation.* 2015;22(1):37-43. doi:10.1111/micc.12163.

65. Kubli S, Feihl F, Waeber B. Beta-blockade with nebivolol enhances the acetylcholine-induced cutaneous vasodilation. *Clin Pharmacol Ther.* 2001;69(4):238-244. doi:10.1067/mcp.2001.114670.

66. Yvonne-Tee GB, Rasool AH, Halim AS, Rahman AR. Reproducibility of different laser Doppler fluximetry parameters of postocclusive reactive hyperemia in human forearm skin. *J Pharmacol Toxicol Methods.* 2005;52(2):286-292. doi:10.1016/j.vascn.2004.11.003.

67. Stark MJ, Clifton VL, Wright IM. Neonates born to mothers with preeclampsia exhibit sex-specific alterations in microvascular function. *Pediatr Res.* 2009;65(3):292-295. doi:10.1203/pdr.0b013e318193edf1.

68. Stark MJ, Clifton VL, Wright IM. Sex-specific differences in peripheral microvascular blood flow in preterm infants. *Pediatr Res.* 2008;63(4):415-419. doi:10.1203/01.pdr.0000304937.38669.63.

69. Benaron DA, Parachikov IH, Friedland S, et al. Continuous, noninvasive, and localized microvascular tissue oximetry using

visible light spectroscopy. *Anesthesiology*. 2004;100(6): 1469-1475. doi:10.1097/00000542-200406000-00019.

70. Benaron DA, Parachikov IH, Cheong WF, et al. Design of a visible-light spectroscopy clinical tissue oximeter. *J Biomed Opt*. 2005;10(4):44005. doi:10.1117/1.1979504.

71. van Elteren HA, Ince C, Tibboel D, Reiss IK, de Jonge RC. Cutaneous microcirculation in preterm neonates: comparison between sidestream dark field (SDF) and incident dark field (IDF) imaging. *J Clin Monit Comput*. 2015;29(5):543-548. doi:10.1007/s10877-015-9708-5.

72. Briers D, Duncan DD, Hirst E, et al. Laser speckle contrast imaging: theoretical and practical limitations. *J Biomed Opt*. 2013;18(6):066018. doi:10.1117/1.JBO.18.6.066018.

73. Sun S, Hayes-Gill BR, He D, Zhu Y, Huynh NT, Morgan SP. Comparison of laser Doppler and laser speckle contrast imaging using a concurrent processing system. *Opt Lasers Eng*. 2016;83:1-9. doi:10.1016/j.optlaseng.2016.02.021.

74. Ansari MZ, Humeau-Heurtier A, Offenhauser N, Dreier JP, Nirala AK. Visualization of perfusion changes with laser speckle contrast imaging using the method of motion history image. *Microvasc Res*. 2016;107:106-109. doi:10.1016/j.mvr.2016.06.003.

75. Ansari MZ, Kang EJ, Manole MD, Dreier JP, Humeau-Heurtier A. Monitoring microvascular perfusion variations with laser speckle contrast imaging using a view-based temporal template method. *Microvasc Res*. 2017;111:49-59. doi:10.1016/j.mvr.2016.12.004.

76. Amir G, Ramamoorthy C, Riemer RK, Davis CR, Hanley FL, Reddy VM. Visual light spectroscopy reflects flow-related changes in brain oxygenation during regional low-flow perfusion and deep hypothermic circulatory arrest. *J Thorac Cardiovasc Surg*. 2006;132(6):1307-1313. doi:10.1016/j.jtcvs.2006.04.056.

77. Noori S, Drabu B, McCoy M, Sekar K. Non-invasive measurement of local tissue perfusion and its correlation with hemodynamic indices during the early postnatal period in term neonates. *J Perinatol*. 2011;31(12):785-788. doi:10.1038/jp.2011.34.

78. Verhagen EA, Hummel LA, Bos AF, Kooi EMW. Near-infrared spectroscopy to detect absence of cerebrovascular autoregulation in preterm infants. *Clin Neurophysiol*. 2014;125(1):47-52. doi:10.1016/j.clinph.2013.07.001.

79. Tsuji M, Saul JP, du Plessis A, et al. Cerebral intravascular oxygenation correlates with mean arterial pressure in critically ill premature infants. *Pediatrics*. 2000;106(4):625-632.

80. Soul JS, Hammer PE, Tsuji M, et al. Fluctuating pressure-passivity is common in the cerebral circulation of sick premature infants. *Pediatr Res*. 2007;61(4):467-473. doi:10.1203/pdr.0b013e31803237f6.

81. ter Horst HJ, Verhagen EA, Keating P, Bos AF. The relationship between electrocerebral activity and cerebral fractional tissue oxygen extraction in preterm infants. *Pediatr Res*. 2011; 70(4):384-388. doi:10.1203/PDR.0b013e3182294735.

82. Greisen G. Autoregulation of cerebral blood flow in newborn babies. *Early Hum Dev*. 2005;81(5):423-428. doi:10.1016/j.earlhumdev.2005.03.005.

83. Caicedo A, De Smet D, Naulaers G, et al. Cerebral tissue oxygenation and regional oxygen saturation can be used to study cerebral autoregulation in prematurely born infants. *Pediatr Res*. 2011;69(6):548-553. doi:10.1203/PDR.0b013e3182176d85.

84. Alderliesten T, Lemmers PMA, van Haastert IC, et al. Hypotension in preterm neonates: low blood pressure alone does not affect neurodevelopmental outcome. *J Pediatr*. 2014;164(5): 986-991. doi:10.1016/j.jpeds.2013.12.042.

85. Ancora G, Maranella E, Grandi S, et al. Early predictors of short term neurodevelopmental outcome in asphyxiated cooled infants.

A combined brain amplitude integrated electroencephalography and near infrared spectroscopy study. *Brain Dev*. 2013;35(1): 26-31. doi:10.1016/j.braindev.2011.09.008.

86. Gucuyener K, Beken S, Ergenekon E, et al. Use of amplitude-integrated electroencephalography (aEEG) and near infrared spectroscopy findings in neonates with asphyxia during selective head cooling. *Brain Dev*. 2012;34(4):280-286. doi:10.1016/j.braindev.2011.06.005.

87. Wolf ME. Functional TCD: regulation of cerebral hemodynamics – cerebral autoregulation, vasomotor reactivity, and neurovascular coupling. *Front Neurol Neurosci*. 2015;36:40-56. doi:10.1159/000366236.

88. Kaiser JR, Gauss CH, Williams DK. The effects of hypercapnia on cerebral autoregulation in ventilated very low birth weight infants. *Pediatr Res*. 2005;58(5):931-935. doi:10.1203/01.pdr.0000182180.80645.0c.

89. Noori S, Anderson M, Soleymani S, Seri I. Effect of carbon dioxide on cerebral blood flow velocity in preterm infants during postnatal transition. *Acta Paediatr*. 2014;103(8): e334-e339. doi:10.1111/apa.12646.

90. Kaiser JR, Gauss CH, Pont MM, Williams DK. Hypercapnia during the first 3 days of life is associated with severe intraventricular hemorrhage in very low birth weight infants. *J Perinatol*. 2006;26(5):279-285. doi:10.1038/sj.jp.7211492.

91. McKee LA, Fabres J, Howard G, Peralta-Carcelen M, Carlo WA, Ambalavanan N. PaCO$_2$ and neurodevelopment in extremely low birth weight infants. *J Pediatr*. 2009;155(2): 217-221.e1. doi:10.1016/j.jpeds.2009.02.024.

92. Soleymani S, Borzage M, Seri I. Hemodynamic monitoring in neonates: advances and challenges. *J Perinatol*. 2010;(suppl 30):S38-S45. doi:10.1038/jp.2010.101.

93. Soleymani S, Borzage M, Noori S, Seri I. Neonatal hemodynamics: monitoring, data acquisition and analysis. *Expert Rev Med Devices*. 2012;9(5):501-511. doi:10.1586/erd.12.32.

94. Malik M, Bigger JT, Camm AJ, et al. Heart rate variability: Standards of measurement, physiological interpretation, and clinical use. *European Heart Journal*. 1996;17(3):354-381. doi:10.1093/oxfordjournals.eurheartj.a014868.

95. Rajendra Acharya U, Paul Joseph K, Kannathal N, Lim CM, Suri JS. Heart rate variability: a review. *Med Biol Eng Comput*. 2006;44(12):1031-1051. doi:10.1007/s11517-006-0119-0.

96. Schechtman VL, Harper RM, Kluge KA, Wilson AJ, Southall DP. Correlations between cardiorespiratory measures in normal infants and victims of sudden infant death syndrome. *Sleep*. 1990;13(4):304-317. doi:10.1093/sleep/13.4.304.

97. Regalado MG, Schechtman VL, Khoo MC, Bean XD. Spectral analysis of heart rate variability and respiration during sleep in cocaine-exposed neonates. *Clin Physiol*. 2001;21(4): 428-436. doi:10.1046/j.1365-2281.2001.00353.x.

98. Ursino M. Interaction between carotid baroregulation and the pulsating heart: a mathematical model. *Am J Physiol*. 1998;275(5):H1733-H1747. doi:10.1152/ajpheart.1998.275.5.H1733.

99. Dat M, Jennekens W, Bovendeerd P, et al. *Modeling Cardiovascular Autoregulation of the Preterm Infant*. Eindhoven, the Netherlands: Eindhoven University of Technology; 2010.

100. Andriessen P, Oetomo SB, Peters C, Vermeulen B, Wijn PF, Blanco CE. Baroreceptor reflex sensitivity in human neonates: the effect of postmenstrual age. *J Physiol*. 2005;568(Pt 1): 333-341. doi:10.1113/jphysiol.2005.093641.

101. Drouin E, Gournay V, Calamel J, Mouzard A, Roze JC. Assessment of spontaneous baroreflex sensitivity in neonates. *Arch*

*Dis Child Fetal Neonatal Ed.* 1997;76(2):F108-F112. doi:10.1136/fn.76.2.f108.

102. Caicedo A, Alderliesten T, Naulaers G, Lemmers P, van Bel F, Van Huffel S. A new framework for the assessment of cerebral hemodynamics regulation in neonates using NIRS. *Adv Exp Med Biol.* 2016;876:501-509. doi:10.1007/978-1-4939-3023-4_63.

103. Kleiser S, Pastewski M, Hapuarachchi T, et al. Characterizing fluctuations of arterial and cerebral tissue oxygenation in preterm neonates by means of data analysis techniques for nonlinear dynamical systems. *Adv Exp Med Biol.* 2016;876:511-519. doi:10.1007/978-1-4939-3023-4_64.

104. Lemmers PMA, Toet M, van Schelven LJ, van Bel F. Cerebral oxygenation and cerebral oxygen extraction in the preterm infant: the impact of respiratory distress syndrome. *Exp Brain Res.* 2006;173(3):458-467. doi:10.1007/s00221-006-0388-8.

105. De Smet D, Jacobs J, Ameye L, et al. The partial coherence method for assessment of impaired cerebral autoregulation using near-infrared spectroscopy: potential and limitations. *Adv Exp Med Biol.* 2010;662:219-224. doi:10.1007/978-1-4419-1241-1_31.

106. Kuo TB, Chern CM, Sheng WY, Wong WJ, Hu HH. Frequency domain analysis of cerebral blood flow velocity and its correlation with arterial blood pressure. *J Cereb Blood Flow Metab.* 1998;18(3):311-318. doi:10.1097/00004647-199803000-00010.

107. Wong FY, Leung TS, Austin T, et al. Impaired autoregulation in preterm infants identified by using spatially resolved spectroscopy. *Pediatrics.* 2008;121(3):e604-e611. doi:10.1542/peds.2007-1487.

108. Zhang R, Zuckerman JH, Giller CA, Levine BD. Transfer function analysis of dynamic cerebral autoregulation in humans. *Am J Physiol.* 1998;274(1 Pt 2):H233-H241. doi:10.1152/ajpheart.1998.274.1.h233.

109. Tian F, Tarumi T, Liu H, Zhang R, Chalak L. Wavelet coherence analysis of dynamic cerebral autoregulation in neonatal hypoxic-ischemic encephalopathy. *Neuroimage Clin.* 2016;11:124-132. doi:10.1016/j.nicl.2016.01.020.

110. Fairchild KD, O'Shea TM. Heart rate characteristics: physiomarkers for detection of late-onset neonatal sepsis. *Clin Perinatol.* 2010;37(3):581-598. doi:10.1016/j.clp.2010.06.002.

111. Fairchild KD. Predictive monitoring for early detection of sepsis in neonatal ICU patients. *Curr Opin Pediatr.* 2013;25(2):172-179. doi:10.1097/MOP.0b013e32835e8fe6.

112. Pinsky MR. Functional haemodynamic monitoring. *Curr Opin Crit Care.* 2014;20(3):288-293. doi:10.1097/MCC.0000000000000090.

113. Creteur J, Carollo T, Soldati G, Buchele G, De Backer D, Vincent JL. The prognostic value of muscle StO2 in septic patients. *Intensive Care Med.* 2007;33(9):1549-1556. doi:10.1007/s00134-007-0739-3.

114. Mesquida J, Espinal C, Gruartmoner G, et al. Prognostic implications of tissue oxygen saturation in human septic shock. *Intensive Care Med.* 2012;38(4):592-597. doi:10.1007/s00134-012-2491-6.

115. Michard F, Boussat S, Chemla D, et al. Relation between respiratory changes in arterial pulse pressure and fluid responsiveness in septic patients with acute circulatory failure. *Am J Respir Crit Care Med.* 2000;162(1):134-138. doi:10.1164/ajrccm.162.1.9903035.

116. Berkenstadt H, Margalit N, Hadani M, et al. Stroke volume variation as a predictor of fluid responsiveness in patients undergoing brain surgery. *Anesth Analg.* 2001;92(4):984-989. doi:10.1097/00000539-200104000-00034.

117. Lanspa MJ, Grissom CK, Hirshberg EL, Jones JP, Brown SM. Applying dynamic parameters to predict hemodynamic response to volume expansion in spontaneously breathing patients with septic shock. *Shock.* 2013;39(2):155-160. doi:10.1097/SHK.0b013e31827f1c6a.

118. Garcia MI, Romero MG, Cano AG, et al. Dynamic arterial elastance as a predictor of arterial pressure response to fluid administration: a validation study. *Crit Care.* 2014;18(6):626. doi:10.1186/s13054-014-0626-6.

119. Foughty ZC, Tavaslioglu O, Rhee CJ, et al. Novel Method of calculating pulse pressure variation to predict fluid responsiveness to transfusion in very low birth weight infants. *J Pediatr.* 2021;234:265-268.e1. doi:10.1016/j.jpeds.2021.04.012.

120. Heskamp L, Lansdorp B, Hopman J, Lemson J, de Boode WP. Ventilator-induced pulse pressure variation in neonates. *Physiol Rep.* 2016;4(4):e12716. doi:10.14814/phy2.12716.

121. Neal ML. *Patient-Specific Modeling of the Cardiovascular System. Patient-Specific Modeling for Critical Care.* New York, NY; Springer; 2010.

122. Ivanova O, Khoo MK. Simulation of spontaneous cardiovascular variability using PNEUMA. *Conf Proc IEEE Eng Med Biol Soc.* 2004;2004:3901-3904. doi:10.1109/IEMBS.2004.1404091.

123. Clyman RI, Mauray F, Heymann MA, Roman C. Cardiovascular effects of patent ductus arteriosus in preterm lambs with respiratory distress. *J Pediatrics.* 1987;111(4):579-587.

124. Lien R, Hsu KH, Chu JJ, Chang YS. Hemodynamic alterations recorded by electrical cardiometry during ligation of ductus arteriosus in preterm infants. *Eur J Pediatr.* 2015;174(4):543-550. doi:10.1007/s00431-014-2437-9.

125. Weisz DE, Jain A, Ting J, McNamara PJ, El-Khuffash A. Non-invasive cardiac output monitoring in preterm infants undergoing patent ductus arteriosus ligation: a comparison with echocardiography. *Neonatology.* 2014;106(4):330-336. doi:10.1159/000365278.

126. Soleymani S, Khoo MC, Noori S, Seri I. Modeling of neonatal hemodynamics during PDA closure. *Conf Proc IEEE Eng Med Biol Soc.* 2015;2015:1886-1889. doi:10.1109/EMBC.2015.7318750.

127. Azhibekov T, Soleymani S, Lee BH, Noori S, Seri I. Hemodynamic monitoring of the critically ill neonate: An eye on the future. *Semin Fetal Neonatal Med.* 2015;20(4):246-254. doi:10.1016/j.siny.2015.03.003.

128. International Consortium for Blood Pressure Genome-Wide Association S, Ehret GB, Munroe PB, et al. Genetic variants in novel pathways influence blood pressure and cardiovascular disease risk. *Nature.* 2011;478(7367):103-109. doi:10.1038/nature10405.

129. Eijgelsheim M, Newton-Cheh C, Sotoodehnia N, et al. Genome-wide association analysis identifies multiple loci related to resting heart rate. *Hum Mol Genet.* 2010;19(19):3885-3894. doi:10.1093/hmg/ddq303.

130. Mezzavilla M, Iorio A, Bobbo M, et al. Insight into genetic determinants of resting heart rate. *Gene.* 2014;545(1):170-174. doi:10.1016/j.gene.2014.03.045.

131. Newton-Cheh C, Guo CY, Wang TJ, O'Donnell CJ, Levy D, Larson MG. Genome-wide association study of electrocardiographic and heart rate variability traits: the Framingham Heart Study. *BMC Med Genet.* 2007;8 Suppl 1(suppl 1):S7. doi:10.1186/1471-2350-8-S1-S7.

132. Vasan RS, Glazer NL, Felix JF, et al. Genetic variants associated with cardiac structure and function: a meta-analysis and replication of genome-wide association data. *JAMA.* 2009;302(2):168-178. doi:10.1001/jama.2009.978-a.

133. Turner ST, Bailey KR, Schwartz GL, Chapman AB, Chai HS, Boerwinkle E. Genomic association analysis identifies multiple loci influencing antihypertensive response to an angiotensin II receptor blocker. *Hypertension*. 2012;59(6):1204-1211. doi:10.1161/HYP.0b013e31825b30f8.
134. Turner ST, Boerwinkle E, O'Connell JR, et al. Genomic association analysis of common variants influencing antihypertensive response to hydrochlorothiazide. *Hypertension*. 2013;62(2):391-397. doi:10.1161/HYPERTENSIONAHA.111.00436.
135. Treszl A, Szabo M, Dunai G, et al. Angiotensin II type 1 receptor A1166C polymorphism and prophylactic indomethacin treatment induced ductus arteriosus closure in very low birth weight neonates. *Pediatr Res*. 2003;54(5):753-755. doi:10.1203/01.PDR.0000088016.67117.39.
136. Dagle JM, Lepp NT, Cooper ME, et al. Determination of genetic predisposition to patent ductus arteriosus in preterm infants. *Pediatrics*. 2009;123(4):1116-1123. doi:10.1542/peds.2008-0313.
137. Obermeyer Z, Emanuel EJ. Predicting the future – big data, machine learning, and clinical medicine. *N Engl J Med*. 2016;375(13):1216-1219. doi:10.1056/NEJMp1606181.
138. de Boode WP. Cardiac output monitoring in newborns. *Early Hum Dev*. 2010;86(3):143-148. doi:10.1016/j.earlhumdev.2010.01.032.
139. Nusmeier A, van der Hoeven JG, Lemson J. Cardiac output monitoring in pediatric patients. *Expert Rev Med Devices*. 2010;7(4):503-517. doi:10.1586/erd.10.19.
140. Peyton PJ, Chong SW. Minimally invasive measurement of cardiac output during surgery and critical care: a meta-analysis of accuracy and precision. *Anesthesiology*. 2010;113(5):1220-1235. doi:10.1097/ALN.0b013e3181ee3130.
141. de Boode WP. Clinical monitoring of systemic hemodynamics in critically ill newborns. *Early Hum Dev*. 2010;86(3):137-141. doi:10.1016/j.earlhumdev.2010.01.031.
142. Rennie JM, Chorley G, Boylan GB, Pressler R, Nguyen Y, Hooper R. Non-expert use of the cerebral function monitor for neonatal seizure detection. *Arch Dis Child Fetal Neonatal Ed*. 2004;89(1):F37-F40.
143. Toet MC, Lemmers PM. Brain monitoring in neonates. *Early Hum Dev*. 2009;85(2):77-84. doi:10.1016/j.earlhumdev.2008.11.007.

# Chapter 15

# Clinical Applications of Near-Infrared Spectroscopy in Neonates

Petra Lemmers, Suresh Victor, Michael Weindling, Laura Dix, Frank van Bel, and Gunnar Naulaers

## Key Points

- The status of cerebral oxygenation is not always represented appropriately by systemic arterial oxygenation, especially when there are changes in cerebral blood flow or cardiac output. Oxygenation monitoring of the brain by near-infrared spectroscopy (NIRS) is therefore an important
  additive measure in neonatal intensive care.
- Monitoring cerebral oxygenation by NIRS, in addition to arterial saturation monitoring by pulse
  oximetry, blood pressure, and brain function by aEEG, can help to prevent brain damage as well as prevent unnecessary treatment of the neonate.
- Cerebral oxygenation can be stabilized in the neonate using a dedicated treatment guideline in combination with cerebral oxygenation monitoring by NIRS.

## Introduction

Survival of the extremely preterm infant has greatly improved over the past decades. However, perinatal brain damage with adverse neurodevelopmental outcome continues to affect a considerable number of these infants.[1-12] Although the etiology of brain damage is multi-factorial and partly unknown (see Chapter 7), hypoxia, hyperoxia, specific and non-specific inflammation, and hemodynamic instability during the first days of postnatal life play an important role.[13-19] It is clear that further advances in survival and improvements in neurodevelopmental outcome can only be achieved if we learn more about the underlying pathophysiology so that more effective treatment modalities can be established. The first step in this direction is to develop the capability to continuously monitor clinically relevant hemodynamic variables and, if possible, treat the underlying condition at an early stage. Continuous monitoring of physiological parameters such as heart rate, blood pressure, arterial oxygen saturation ($SaO_2$), temperature, and, with increasing frequency, electrical activity of the brain using amplitude-integrated EEG (aEEG) have been integrated into the monitoring practices of neonatal intensive care units (NICUs). aEEG has been introduced into neonatal intensive care as a novel monitoring technique to continuously assess cerebral electric activity. Both the aEEG background patterns and the analysis of the raw EEG signal have been used for the evaluation of neurological function. The fewer channels compared to the classic full EEG improves its applicability, and the use of aEEG has increased.[20,21] Other, novel techniques used to continuously monitor additional hemodynamic parameters, such as cardiac output, are discussed in Chapters 9–11 in detail.

Intermittent tools to assess cerebral health, such as cranial ultrasound, Doppler flow velocity measurements, and (advanced) magnetic resonance imaging (MRI), have also been integrated into the care of the sick neonate (see Chapters 11–13 for details). These techniques, however, do not provide continuous information on the perfusion and oxygenation of the neonatal brain.

Therefore we need a reliable and practical clinical tool that monitors oxygenation of the neonatal brain noninvasively and continuously so that conditions potentially leading to brain injury can be recognized in a timely manner. An increasingly clinically used method is monitoring cerebral oxygenation by NIRS.[22-26]

# Principles of Near-Infrared Spectroscopy

Near-infrared (NIR) spectroscopy technology utilizes light in the near-infrared range (700–1000 nm). NIR spectroscopy instrumentation consists of fiber optic bundles or optodes placed either on opposite sides of the tissue being interrogated (usually a limb or the head of a baby) to measure transmitted light or close together to measure reflected light. NIR-light (laser or, more frequently, LED light) enters through one optode and a fraction of the photons are captured by a second optode and conveyed to a measuring device.

Jöbsis first introduced the use of NIR spectrophotometers for human tissue in 1977.[27] Human tissues contain a variety of substances whose absorption spectra at NIR wavelengths are well defined. They are present in sufficient quantities to contribute significant attenuation to measurements of transmitted light. The concentration of some absorbers such as water, melanin, and bilirubin remains virtually constant with time. However, the concentrations of some absorbing compounds, such as oxygenated hemoglobin ($HbO_2$) and deoxyhemoglobin (HbR), vary with tissue oxygenation. Therefore changes in light absorption can be related to changes in the concentrations of these compounds.

The absorption properties of hemoglobin alter when it changes from its oxygenated to its deoxygenated form. In the NIR region of the spectrum the absorption of the hemoglobin chromophores (HbR and $HbO_2$) decreases significantly compared to that observed in the visible region. The major part of the NIR spectroscopy signal is derived from hemoglobin, but other hemoglobin compounds, such as carboxyhemoglobin, also absorb light in the NIR region. However, the combined error due to ignoring these compounds in the measurement of the total hemoglobin signal is probably less than 1% in normal blood.

## NEAR-INFRARED SPECTROPHOTOMETERS

Three different methods of using NIR light for monitoring tissue oxygenation are currently used: continuous wave,[28-30] time-of-flight (also known as time-domain or time-resolved),[31] and the frequency domain methods.[30] For an extensive overview of the methods, we refer the reader to Wolf et al.[32] The *continuous wave method* has a very fast response but registers relative change only, and it is therefore not possible to make

absolute measurements using this technique. The *time-of-flight method* needs extensive data processing but provides more accurate measurements. It enables one to explore different information provided by the measured signals and has the potential to become a valuable tool in research and clinical environments. The *third approach*, which uses frequency domain or phase modulation technology, has a lower resolution than that of the time-of-flight method but has the potential to provide estimates of oxygen delivery sufficiently quickly for clinical purposes. Thus *frequency domain or phase modulation technology is potentially the best candidate* in the NICU and for bedside usage. Nevertheless, the continuous wave method devices have been widely used for research studies.[25,33-39]

## Continuous Wave Spectroscopy

In continuous wave spectroscopy changes in tissue chromophore concentrations from the baseline value can be obtained from the modified Beer-Lambert law[28]. However, the application of the Beer-Lambert law in its original form has limitations. Its linearity is limited by deviation in the absorption coefficient at high concentrations, scattering of light due to particulate matter in the sample, and ambient light.

Thus for light passing through a highly scattering medium, the Beer-Lambert law has been modified to include an additive term, $K$, due to scattering losses, and a multiplier to account for the increased optical pathlength due to scattering.[40-42]

The modified Beer-Lambert law is expressed as $A = P \times L \times E \times C + K$, where $A$ is absorbance, $P$ is the pathlength factor, $L$ is the path length, $E$ is the extinction coefficient, $C$ is the concentration of the compound, and $K$ is a constant. The differential pathlength factor describes the actual distance traveled by light. As it is dependent on the amount of scattering in the medium, its measurement is not straightforward. Examples of instruments using continuous wave technology are the NIRO 500 and NIRO 100, made by Hamamatsu Photonic, Hamamatsu, Japan.

## Spatially Resolved Spectroscopy

In spatially resolved spectroscopy multiple optodes, operating simultaneously, are placed around the head. This allows for a pathlength correction, assuming that tissue being interrogated is homogeneous, the so-called spatially resolved spectroscopy.[43,44] Spatially resolved spectroscopy measures hemoglobin oxygen saturation. The NIRO 300 (Hamamatsu Photonics, Hamamatsu City, Japan) and the INVOS 5100 (Somanetics, Troy, MI, United States) both measure cerebral hemoglobin oxygen saturation but use different terminology: tissue oxygenation index (TOI) from the NIRO 300 and regional cerebral oxygen saturation ($rSO_2$) from the INVOS 5100. This technique gives absolute values. A light detector measures tissue oxygenation index with three sensors at different distances from the light source. Tissue oxygenation index (TOI) is calculated according to the diffusion equation as follows: TOI (%) = $K_{HbO_2}$/($K_{HbO_2} + K_{HbR}$), where K is the constant scattering contribution and $HbO_2$ and $HbR$ are the oxygenated and deoxygenated hemoglobin, respectively. A similar concept is used in calculating regional oxygen saturation ($rSO_2$). There was good agreement for sensor-exchange experiments (removing and reapplying the sensor at same position); simultaneous left-to-right forehead measurements and sensors at different positions revealed acceptable and insignificant differences.[24,45] Quaresima and colleagues concluded that TOI reflected mainly the saturation of the intracranial venous compartment of circulation.[46] Variation in the results of studies were likely due to assumptions made about the distribution of cerebral blood between arterial and venous compartments.[47,48] Several other commercial instruments are on the market now, most of them using the same physical principles, although using different distances, algorithms, and probes. There are now several commercial monitors in use in the NICU.[49] Although different terms are used (TOI, $StO_2$, $rSO_2$), we will use $rSO_2$ further in the text when we talk about cerebral oxygenation.

### Time-of-Flight Instruments

This time-resolved technique consists of emitting a very short laser pulse into an absorbing tissue and recording the temporal response (time-of-flight) of the photons at some distance from the laser source.[31] There have only been a few reports on the use of time-of-flight instruments in neonates.[44,50,51]

### Frequency Domain Instruments

The frequency domain method is based on the modulation of a laser light at given frequencies.[30] Frequency domain instruments determine the absorption coefficient

and reduce the scattering coefficient of the tissue. Problems include noise and leakage associated with the high-frequency signal, but the devices are very compact and appropriate for bedside/incubator use. Frequency domain NIRS allows the absolute quantification of cerebral hemoglobin oxygen saturation and cerebral blood volume.[52-54] Using concurrent frequency domain measures of cerebral hemoglobin oxygen saturation and diffuse correlation spectroscopy measures of CBFi, cerebral oxygen consumption can be calculated.[55-57]

## Near-Infrared Spectroscopy in Clinical Care

The introduction of spatially resolved spectroscopy made it possible to use a new approach to monitoring cerebral oxygenation in the clinical setting. It measures the status of cerebral oxygenation by using regional cerebral oxygen saturation ($rScO_2$). Despite the different approaches, the measures of cerebral oxygenation reflect mixed tissue oxygen saturation by assuming that the contribution to the perfusion of the tissue interrogated is 25%, 5%, and 70% by the arteries, capillaries, and veins, respectively. The value is provided as an absolute number that can be measured continuously and over prolonged periods of time.[27]

For most of the instruments, a good correlation with jugular venous $O_2$ saturation has been documented.[58,59] The values are not identical, though primarily because TOI and $rScO_2$ reflect the changes in oxygenation in the arterial, capillary, *and* venous compartments. A comparison between the different monitoring techniques in adults during changes in oxygenation and changes in partial pressure of arterial $CO_2$ ($PaCO_2$) also yielded a good correlation between the TOI and $rScO_2$.[47,48] In addition, when comparing the left and right sides of the brain, the Bland-Altman limits of agreement for $rScO_2$ were −8.5 to + 9.5%, with even smaller limits during stable $SaO_2$ values between 85 and 97%.[45] However, due to the limitations of the technology, it is obvious that these measurements are better used for trend measurements rather than precise tissue oxygenation values.

Clinical monitoring of cerebral oxygenation by NIRS has already become routine in pediatric and adult intensive care and during cardiac surgical procedures in all age groups.[47,60-62] However, although information concerning brain tissue oxygenation may be important when considering the type and timing of an intervention and when assessing its impact on outcome, the use of NIRS has not yet been universally implemented in the daily care of neonates in the NICU, but the use in NICU's in Europe and the United States is increasing. Although the accumulating evidence supporting the use of NIRS in clinical practice is encouraging, more research is necessary to further consolidate its clinical importance.

In addition to $rScO_2$, cerebral fractional tissue oxygen extraction (cFTOE) is another important NIRS parameter. Cerebral fractional tissue oxygen extraction is derived from $rScO_2$ and $SaO_2$ based on the formula: $SaO_2 - rScO_2/SaO_2$. Thus cFTOE is a surrogate indicator of the actual cerebral fractional oxygen extraction, which can be measured with the validated jugular venous occlusion technique.[59,63] Naulaers et al. reported a positive correlation between NIRS-calculated cFTOE and actual fractional oxygen extraction of the brain in a newborn piglet model.[64] Because cFTOE is a ratio of two variables, an increase might either indicate reduced oxygen delivery to the brain with constant oxygen consumption or increased cerebral oxygen consumption not satisfied by oxygen delivery. The opposite is true in the case of a decrease in the cFTOE, reflecting either a decrease in oxygen extraction because of decreased oxygen utilization or an increase in oxygen delivery to the brain while cerebral oxygen consumption has remained unchanged. Obviously, either parameter might change at the same time, although relatively rapid changes in cerebral oxygen utilization are less common. Although NIRS-derived cFTOE is a less accurate parameter compared to fractional oxygen extraction determined by the jugular occlusion technique, the advantage of NIRS-derived cFTOE is that cerebral oxygen extraction can be continuously assessed.[38,65]

## Feasibility of NIRS-Monitored Cerebral Oxygenation and Extraction in Neonatal Clinical Care

Cerebral oxygenation and extraction can be monitored by NIRS-derived $rScO_2$ and cFTOE, respectively. In order to assess the utility of NIRS-monitored $rScO_2$

in clinical practice, it is essential to also obtain data on the signal-to-noise ratio and the inter- and intra-patient variability. When compared to pulse oximetry monitored $SaO_2$, it is a reliable and accepted trend monitor for systemic arterial oxygenation, but the signal-to-noise ratio is larger for NIRS-measured $rScO_2$.[24] However, when averaging the signal over a longer period, for example, over 30–60 seconds, a reliable NIRS signal can be obtained with an acceptable signal-to-noise ratio.[24] With respect to intra-patient variability, differences of up to 7% or more have been reported when performed with repeated placement of the NIRS sensor.[63] The limits of agreement after sensor replacement are in the $-17\%$ to $+17\%$ range.[24,66,67] These values are more than double that of the limits of agreement for $SaO_2$.[63] On the other hand, Menke et al reported a good reproducibility of NIRS-measured $rScO_2$ with an inter-measurement variance only slightly higher than the physiological baseline variation.[68] When comparing values during simultaneous monitoring of the left and right frontoparietal regions of the brain, limits of agreement of 7–9% have been reported.[45] Moreover, it appears that the experience of the investigator also plays an important role in the quality of the information obtained.

Reference values of $rScO_2$ or TOI during normal arterial oxygen saturations have been reported in several studies including preterm neonates. Of note is the fact that not all studies incorporated postnatal age or the clinical status of the infant when reporting their findings. Mean values ($\pm$ SD) of $rScO_2$ or TOI ranged between 61 and 75% ($\pm7$ to $\pm12\%$). These values are comparable to those obtained in adults (Table 15.1).[45,48,66,67,69-76]

Over the past decade or so, more and more NIRS devices with neonatal or pediatric sensors and algorithms have become available. Before interpreting the absolute values, though, attention must be paid to the differences between the adult and new neonatal sensors. Indeed, studies have shown that the newer, smaller neonatal sensors may measure at up to 10–15% higher values compared to the previously used adult sensors in neonates.[74,77] Therefore reference values for the neonatal or pediatric sensors in preterm and term neonates are necessary before their implementation in clinical practice. Indeed, a large study by Alderliesten et al. on 999 preterm infants has recently provided reference values for $rScO_2$ and cFTOE for different

**TABLE 15.1    Reference Values (Mean ([± SD]) of Regional Cerebral Oxygen Saturation (rScO₂)/Tissue Oxygen Index (TOI) (%) in Adults and Term and Preterm Neonates**

| Adults | | 67% (±8) | $n = 94^{69}$ |
|---|---|---|---|
| | | 66% (±8) | $n = 19$ (rScO$_2$/TOI)[48] |
| | | 68–76% | $n = 9$ (rScO$_2$)[76] |
| | | 61.5 (±6.1) | $n = 14$ (rScO$_2$)[73] |
| Term Neonates/Infants | Day 12 (0–365) | 61% (±12) | $n = 155$ (TOI)[70] |
| | Day 4.5 (0–190) | 63% (±12) | $n = 20$ (TOI)[67] |
| | 8 min after birth | 68% (IQR 55–80%) | $n = 20^{74}$ |
| Preterm Neonates | Day 1 | 57% (54–66) | $n = 15$ (TOI)[26] |
| (GA< 32 weeks) | Day 2 | 66% (62–82) | |
| | Day 3 | 76% (68–80) | |
| | NA | 75% (±10.2) | $n = 253$ (TOI)[71] |
| | >Day 7 | 66% (±8.8) | $n = 40$ (rScO$_2$)[72] |
| | Day 1 | 70% (±7.4) | $n = 38$ (rScO$_2$)[78] |
| | Day 2 | 71% (±8.8) | |
| | Day 3 | 70% (±7.8) | |
| | Days 1–3 | 62–71% (±7) | $n = 999$ (rScO$_2$)[75] |

The inter-patient variance of TOI/rScO$_2$ in these studies was larger than for pulse oximetry–measured oxygen saturation. Reference values for preterm infants are within the same range as the reference values of adults, infants, and term neonates. See text for details.

types of sensors.[75,78] Graphs of reference value curves allow for bedside interpretation of NIRS-monitored cerebral oxygenation (Table 15.1). These reference values can then be used for comparison with values obtained during conditions that may affect cerebral oxygenation (see below).

Another important use of cerebral oxygenation measurement is to avoid cerebral hypoxia. Therefore the threshold for cerebral hypoxia needs to be determined.

Several animal studies in newborn piglets and one human study in neonates with hypoplastic left heart syndrome who underwent open heart surgery have reported that rScO$_2$ values lower than 35–45% for more than 30–90 minutes are associated with functional (mitochondrial dysfunction or energy failure) and/or histological damage, especially in the hippocampus (a brain region very vulnerable to hypoxia in the perinatal period).[79-81] Moreover, a number of studies, mostly performed in adult cardiac intensive care units, have reported that a 20% decrease from the baseline or an absolute rScO$_2$ value of <50% before intervention is associated with hypoxic-ischemic brain lesions.[82] Thus these findings suggest that rScO$_2$ values below 45–50% for a prolonged period of time should be avoided if possible. A large international randomized controlled clinical trial has investigated if it is possible to detect and prevent cerebral oxygenation outside the assumed normal limits of 55–85% with NIRS monitoring (measured with the adult sensor) to prevent neurological injury and improve neurodevelopmental outcome.[83] The SafeBoosC II trial (safeguarding the brains of our smallest children) randomized infants to either visible or shielded NIRS recording of cerebral oxygenation and then compared the burden of hypoxia and hyperoxia between the two groups.[84] Infants with visible NIRS tracings spent a shorter time outside the normal range, mainly due to a reduction in the hypoxic burden due to clinical interventions. These findings indicate that unfavorable cerebral oxygen saturations can be detected by NIRS and prevented by timely interventions.[84] Because different monitors have different values, a liquid phantom was used to compare the absolute values and to define hypoxia thresholds for the different monitors.[49] In this way the hypoxia threshold for every monitor is defined (Figure 15.1).

Similar to the bedside detection and prevention of prolonged cerebral *hypoxia*, continuous monitoring of rScO$_2$ can also contribute to the prevention of prolonged cerebral *hyperoxia*, especially in the extremely

| Lower treshold values of neonatal sensors corresponding to: *Lower treshold (55%) of small adult sensor INVOS 5100c* | | |
|---|---|---|
| NIRS device/type of sensor | Lower treshold (%) | Δ from AS % |
| *Invos* neo-sensor | 63% | 8% |
| **FORESIGHT** small | 66% | 11% |
| **FORESIGHT** non-adhesive small | 67% | 12% |
| **NIRO** small | 61% | 6% |
| **NIRO** small re-usable | 63% | 8% |
| **NIRO** large | 62% | 7% |
| **NIRO** large re-usable | 62% | 7% |
| SenSmart neo 8004CB-NA | 66% | 11% |
| Oxyprem 1.4 reusable | 48% | |
| O3 Pediatric | 64% | |
| O3 Neonatal | 64% | |
| **Egos** | 56% | |

**Fig. 15.1 Lower threshold values of neonatal sensors as measured in lipid phantom.**[49] (Courtesy of SafeBoosC, Rigshospitalet.)

preterm infant who is particularly prone to oxygen toxicity. The importance of avoiding hyperoxia has been increasingly recognized, as an association between normal oxygen saturations and improved long-term neurodevelopmental outcome in extremely preterm infants has been documented.[19,85,86] With these considerations and the presented data in mind, NIRS-monitored rScO$_2$ and NIRS-derived cFTOE are likely to play an important role in monitoring and improving cerebral oxygenation in sick neonates in the future.

## Clinical Applications

### APPLICATION OF THE SENSOR AND ITS PITFALLS

The most important issue regarding the clinical application of noninvasive monitoring of cerebral oxygenation by NIRS is the ability to perform reliable, long-term monitoring in the most immature and unstable neonate without disturbing the infant. A critical part of initiating the process is the application of the sensor to the head. With appropriate placement, the sensor will allow reliable monitoring of the rScO$_2$ for a number of days without damaging the vulnerable skin, particularly of the very preterm infant. In addition, the sensor in place should not limit access to

performing ultrasound studies of the brain, placement of electrodes for aEEG monitoring, and attachment of CPAP devices. In our experience, application of the NIRS sensor with a soft dark elastic bandage to the frontoparietal region of the head provides protection from ambient light and doesn't irritate or damage the skin of even the smallest infants, while allowing reliable monitoring of rScO$_2$ for extended periods of time. Figure 15.2 shows an example of the application of the NIRS sensor used in all of our clinical studies.[22] Alternatively, application of sensors using the original adhesive tape on the skin is possible and this method is advocated by the manufacturers for most commercially available sensors (Figure 15.2).

Introduction of the system with structured theoretical courses and practical training for nurses and medical staff is a very important prerequisite for the successful use of this monitoring method in clinical practice. In addition, staff education about the potential benefits and risks of using NIRS is of great importance. In gaining experience nursing staff in the authors' institutions have been able to recognize inappropriate transducer placement, improper transducer fixation, or insufficient transducer shielding. In our experience this resulted in extended periods of uninterrupted and reliable rScO$_2$ monitoring, even in the smallest infants, and is comparable to SaO$_2$ monitoring. When interpreting the values in daily clinical practice, one has to be aware of several pitfalls. We have already discussed the importance of proper sensor application to prevent movement artifacts and the effect of ambient light. Yet, despite these precautionary measures, phototherapy light will sometimes cause disturbances in rScO$_2$ monitoring. Accordingly, covering the sensor with an additional dark sheet during periods of phototherapy is recommended to ensure more reliable signal acquisition. Other factors such as dislocation of the NIRS sensor, presence of hair, hematoma or edema, and/or other materials such as the plasters of the aEEG electrodes on the head can also cause disturbances of the NIRS signal. Interestingly, the influence of the curvature of the skull and head circumference seems negligible.[75]

### RELATION TO OTHER MONITORING DEVICES

NIRS-monitored changes in brain oxygenation, represented by rScO$_2$ (or TOI) and cFTOE, generate important continuous information in addition to data from

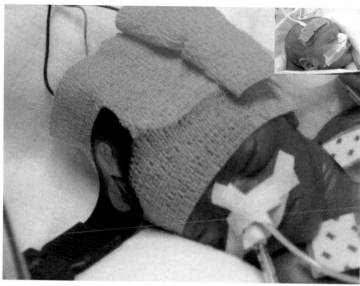

**Fig. 15.2 Application of the near-infrared sensor to the head of a preterm infant in the frontoparietal position using an elastic bandage.** The *inlay* shows the application of the sensor with an adhesive tape (published with parental permission). See text for details.

other monitoring devices such as pulse oximetry–monitored $SaO_2$, indwelling blood pressure monitoring, and heart rate and electrical brain activity monitors. Monitoring $SaO_2$ is necessary to calculate cFTOE as described earlier. The relationship between blood pressure and $rScO_2$ may provide information about the presence or lack of cerebral blood flow autoregulation (see below and Chapter 2).[87-90] As for the use of aEEG in combination with NIRS, our group has reported that persistent and unusually high $rScO_2$ values in term infants with severe perinatal asphyxia are probably due to profound vasodilation with or without vasoparalysis of the cerebral vascular bed. A decreased utilization of oxygen is also strongly associated with an abnormal aEEG pattern after the first postnatal day and adverse neurodevelopmental outcome at 2 years of age.[91,92] These findings indicate that monitoring cerebral oxygenation and oxygen extraction with NIRS along with other parameters reveals conditions at an early stage that might be associated with poor long-term outcomes.[84] The combination of the different parameters monitored can also be used in pharmacodynamic research. Medications given to neonates often have effects on both cerebral metabolism and hemodynamics, so using the combination of NIRS, aEEG, and hemodynamic parameters like blood pressure and heart rate will provide additional valuable information. An

example is the use of propofol, which has direct effects on both blood pressure and cerebral metabolism.[93-95] Further research in neurovascular coupling in preterm infants is ongoing.[96,97] Finally, efforts to develop a comprehensive, real-time cardiorespiratory and neurocritical care monitoring system are described in Chapter 14.

## CLINICAL CONDITIONS ASSOCIATED WITH LOW RSCO$_2$

Clinical conditions and treatment guidelines were well described in the SafeboosC II and III study.[98]

Low $rScO_2$ can be caused by low oxygen levels in the blood (hypoxic hypoxia), anemia (anemic hypoxia), or low cerebral blood flow (ischemic hypoxia).

*Hypoxic hypoxia* is the most frequent cause, as was shown in the SafeboosC II study.[99] This is evident as a decrease in oxygen saturation immediately causes a decrease in cerebral oxygenation.[72] First-line approach to treatment should focus on optimizing pulmonary blood flow and lung recruitment using $FiO_2$ or altering mechanical ventilation strategy.

*Anemic hypoxia* is a less frequent cause of cerebral hypoxia. Anemia may have an even more profound effect on cerebral oxygen delivery in neonates with hypotension receiving mechanical ventilation with high mean airway pressures. Studies have shown an improvement in cerebral oxygenation following red blood cell transfusion, with the strongest effect in infants with the lowest pre-transfusion cerebral oxygen saturation.[100] Van Hoften et al. have documented normalization of $rScO_2$ following packed red blood cell transfusions in 33 preterm infants and concluded that cerebral oxygenation in these infants may be at risk of hemoglobin (Hb) concentrations of <6 mmol/L (9.7 g/dL).[101] As discussed earlier, increased cFTOE (>0.4) is indicative of an imbalance between oxygen supply and demand, which may also improve with red blood cell transfusions.[102] This suggests a potential role for NIRS monitoring to identify infants with high cFTOE (and low $rScO_2$) who might benefit from red blood cell transfusions.[103,104]

*Ischemic hypoxia* is the most important reason to use NIRS as a diagnostic tool. A decrease in cerebral blood flow cannot be detected by the arterial saturation monitor. In this way a decrease in cerebral oxygenation with a normal arterial oxygen saturation, resulting in an increased FTOE, can be an important sign of low cerebral blood flow. There are several different but important causes of low cerebral blood flow in neonates.

As alluded to earlier, $PaCO_2$ is another important parameter and the most powerful one that influences brain perfusion (Chapter 2). Indeed, changes in $PaCO_2$ cause more robust changes in cerebral blood flow than changes in blood pressure outside the autoregulatory range (Chapter 2). Hypocapnia directly decreases cerebral blood flow by inducing vasoconstriction, thus reducing $rScO_2$ and increasing cFTOE, whereas hypercapnia induces vasodilatation, with increased $rScO_2$ and reduced cFTOE values. Accordingly, even small changes in $PaCO_2$ within the normal range may affect the neonatal brain.[105] Therefore monitoring $rScO_2$ and cFTOE together can be used as a noninvasive approach to identify changes in $PaCO_2$, provided that cerebral metabolic rate and the proportion of arterial and venous blood flow in the brain remain constant and hemoglobin concentration and $SaO_2$ don't change during the period of interrogation.[106] Figure 15.3A shows an example of a preterm infant with low $PaCO_2$ and $rScO_2$ values. Only when $PaCO_2$ increased to >30 mmHg did $rScO_2$ recover.

Perlman et al reported first that ductal steal has an impact on cerebral perfusion and is a risk factor for cerebral damage in the preterm infant.[107] Thus a hemodynamically significant patent ductus arteriosus (PDA) is a condition potentially associated with decreased oxygen delivery to the brain due to the impact

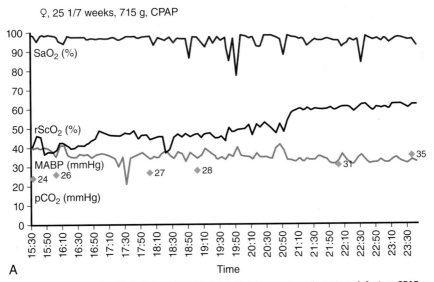

**Fig. 15.3A Patterns of SaO2** (*red line*), **rScO2** (*black line*), **and MABP** (*pink line*) **in an extremely preterm infant on CPAP on the first postnatal day.** Despite normal blood pressure values and arterial saturations, $rScO_2$ was very low (<50%). Although this infant was breathing spontaneously, she hyperventilated on CPAP to very low $PaCO_2$ values (*gray rhomboids*). Only when $pCO_2$ increased to >30 mmHg did $rScO_2$ normalize, suggesting the resolution of cerebral hypoperfusion caused by the hypocapnia-induced cerebral vasoconstriction. See text for details.

of the diastolic run-off in the cerebral vessels and the associated changes in perfusion pressure on cerebral oxygen delivery throughout the entire cardiac cycle. Several recent reports using NIRS-monitored $rScO_2$ found a substantial decrease in cerebral oxygenation to sometimes critically low values in the presence of a hemodynamically significant PDA, with recovery to normal values after successful ductal closure[108-111] (Figure 15.3B). The ductal diameter is the echocardiographic ductal characteristic that is best related to $rScO_2$, with the largest diameter resulting in the lowest $rScO_2$ values.[109] It appears that infants with a hemodynamically significant PDA unresponsive to pharmacologic closure with cyclo-oxygenase (COX) inhibitors are especially at risk before and during surgical ligation. Indeed, in a study of 20 infants we found extremely low $rScO_2$ and high cFTOE values before and during ligation.[112] Infants undergoing surgical ligation of the ductus are often exposed to low $rScO_2$ values for a prolonged period of time, which may adversely affect brain development.[113] It was shown that the $rScO_2$ values before ductal closure are significantly associated with cerebellar growth as measured by MRI, with

potential negative implications for neurodevelopment.[114] Moreover, early ductal screening and treatment seems to reduce in-hospital mortality.[115]

Another frequently encountered condition often related to low $rScO_2$ values is systemic hypotension. Hypotension can arise from various conditions, including but not restricted to hypovolemia, myocardial dysfunction, the presence of a hemodynamically significant PDA, and specific (sepsis) or non-specific inflammation or immaturity associated inability of the vascular bed to maintain an appropriate peripheral vascular resistance (also see Chapters 1, 20, and 21). Although blood pressure is one of the most frequently measured hemodynamic variables in neonatal intensive care, the lower limits of the gestational- and postnatal-age-dependent normal blood pressure range are not known (see Chapter 3) and depend on a number of additional factors such as the underlying pathology, the ability of the individual patient to compensate with increasing blood flow to the vital organs, and maintenance of a proper autoregulatory capacity of the cerebrovascular bed. Accordingly, evidence is emerging that a simple cut-off value based on gestational age is insufficient in establishing

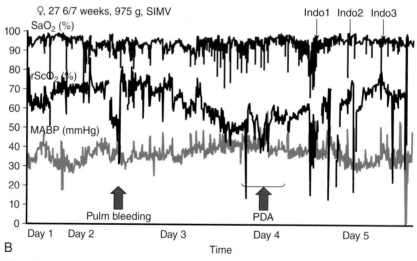

**Fig. 15.3B Representative patterns including measurements of arterial oxygen saturation ($SaO_2$; *red line*), regional cerebral oxygen saturation ($rScO_2$; *black line*), and mean arterial blood pressure (MABP; *pink line*) in a male preterm neonate of 27^6/7 weeks' gestation with severe respiratory distress syndrome during the first 5 postnatal days.** The infant received exogenous surfactant and was mechanically ventilated. The patient's course was complicated by pulmonary hemorrhage on day 2 (*arrow*). Although the pulmonary hemorrhage could have been an early indication of pulmonary overcirculation due to a patent ductus arteriosus (PDA), the infant only developed a hemodynamically significant PDA on day 4 (*arrow*) closed by indomethacin (Indo) (*arrows*). Note the decrease of $rScO_2$ (starting on day 3) to values below 50% at the time of the diagnosis of the hemodynamically significant PDA and the recovery of $rScO_2$ after the ductus closed on day 5. See text for details.

the diagnosis of hypotension (decreased perfusion pressure and blood flow in the vital organs along with decreased oxygen delivery) in an individual patient. The term "permissive hypotension" has been increasingly used to describe low blood pressure values without signs of impaired perfusion (Chapter 3).[116-119] Accordingly, the ability to assess cerebral oxygenation is an important tool to evaluate the status of end-organ perfusion. If cerebral oxygenation and extraction are within the normal range in an otherwise hemodynamically stable infant, the presence of a low blood pressure might call for further observation instead of initiation of treatment (see Chapters 3 and 20). However, more information is needed before we can safely identify which neonates with low blood pressure might benefit from which treatment, and large trials are currently being conducted to answer these questions (Chapters 3, 21, and 22). Recently it was shown that hypotension in combination with cerebral hypoxia is related to increased incidence of early intraventricular hemorrhage or death and impaired cerebral autoregulation.[120,121]

Prematurity is a risk factor for impaired or absent autoregulatory ability of the cerebral vascular bed, and critically ill infants seem to be even more affected (Chapter 2).[122,123] Impaired autoregulation is a risk for adverse neurodevelopmental outcome (Chapters 2 and 20) and might be one of the causes of insufficient oxygen delivery to the immature brain.[90,124] Cerebral autoregulation can be calculated with NIRS-monitored $rScO_2$ combined with simultaneously monitored mean arterial blood pressure (MABP).[88-90,125] This approach assumes that cerebral metabolic rate, hemoglobin concentration, and the proportion of arterial and venous blood perfusing the brain remain constant and that $SaO_2$ doesn't change. Accordingly, when a change in blood pressure is not associated with changes in cerebral oxygenation as assessed by $rScO_2$, cerebral autoregulation is presumed to be present. However, when there is an impairment or total lack of cerebral autoregulation, changes in blood pressure will have an immediate effect on cerebral oxygenation and thus on $rScO_2$. Indeed, the findings of Tsuji et al and Wong et al suggest that infants lacking cerebral blood flow autoregulation assessed by NIRS compared to gestational-age-matched infants with intact cerebral autoregulation have impaired short- and long-term central nervous system outcomes.[90,122] Several approaches are currently being tested for the continuous and real-time assessment of cerebral blood flow autoregulation.[88,125,126] Figure 15.3C shows an example of

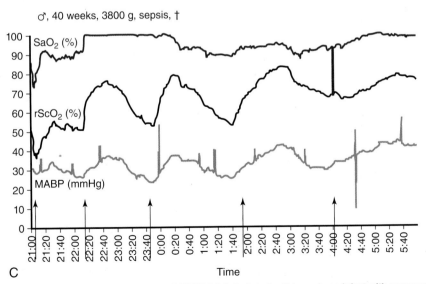

**Fig. 15.3C** Patterns of $SaO_2$ (*red line*), $rScO_2$ (*black line*), and MABP (*pink line*) during 8 hours in an infant with severe sepsis and systemic hypotension. Hypotension was treated with volume expansion and vasopressor-inotropes (*arrows*). Changes in $rScO_2$ mirrored the changes in blood pressure, suggesting a pressure-passive cerebral circulation with lack of autoregulation of cerebral blood flow. See text for details.

the use of NIRS-monitored $rScO_2$ to assess the autoregulatory ability of the cerebral vascular bed. The main concern using this approach is that the NIRS signal is also influenced by parameters other than blood pressure (see above) and that changes in $PaCO_2$ directly affect cerebral perfusion. Therefore, in addition to understanding the complexity of assessing the changes in cerebral perfusion by NIRS, appropriate monitoring and correction are necessary.

Of note is the fact that recent findings suggest that the use of NIRS to monitor $rScO_2$ during the first 12 postnatal hours may identify very preterm neonates at higher risk for the development of P/IVH during the second and third postnatal days (see Chapter 7).[127]

Preterm infants with severe respiratory distress syndrome often require ventilator support, sometimes utilizing high mean, inspiratory, and/or end-expiratory pressures on conventional ventilators or high-frequency oscillatory ventilation. The associated increase in intrathoracic pressure might decrease preload and thus cardiac output, resulting in a negative impact on cerebral hemodynamics with impaired cerebral oxygenation (see Chapter 4).[128] Indeed, monitoring of $rScO_2$ has revealed this association in real time and its use might contribute to early recognition and introduction of corrective measures to prevent such complications (Figure 15.3D).[129]

Infants with congenital cyanotic heart disease are at particularly high risk of compromised cerebral circulation. Most of these infants have baseline $rScO_2$ values below 55%, with $SaO_2$ values in the 70–85% range. Of note is the fact that an $rScO_2$ value of 55% is below the 2 SD of "normal" values defined by our data for preterm neonates. Thus neonates with congenital heart disease, even if it is a non-cyanotic but duct-dependent lesion, are at risk for cerebral damage. This is especially the case in combination with the risk factors discussed above including low systemic perfusion, hypotension, and/or abnormal $PaCO_2$ values.

Infants with cardiac and non-cardiac anomalies may require surgery shortly after birth. Neonatal surgery is also related to adverse neurodevelopmental outcome, including both the procedure itself and the anesthesia.[130,131] Importantly, peri- and postoperative NIRS monitoring of $rScO_2$ is useful to detect deteriorations and has the potential to improve the stability of cerebral oxygenation and is predictive for cerebral injury.[132-135] Indeed, by using cerebral NIRS monitoring, we can detect episodes of hypoxia in an even more reliable fashion than with $SaO_2$ monitoring by pulse-oximetry during the surgical procedure.[136,137]

Table 15.2 summarizes the clinical conditions associated with low $rScO_2$ values.

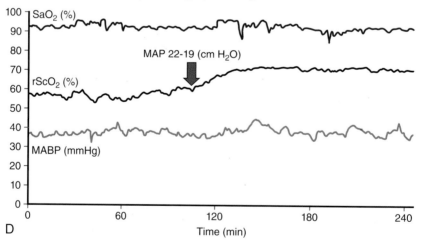

**Fig. 15.3D** Patterns of $SaO_2$ (*red line*), $rScO_2$ (*black line*), and MABP (*pink line*) in an infant with hypoplastic lungs following prolonged premature rupture of the membranes. The patient was ventilated with high-frequency oscillatory ventilation (*HFOV*) with very high mean airway pressures (MAPs; 22 cm $H_2O$). Note the increase in $rScO_2$ after decreasing MAP from 22 to 19 cm $H_2O$ indicating that the MAP before was likely inappropriately high and negatively affected preload and thus cardiac output. See text for details.

| TABLE 15.2 Conditions With Low or High Regional Cerebral Oxygen Saturation (rScO$_2$) | |
| --- | --- |
| **Low rScO$_2$** | **High rScO$_2$** |
| Hypoxia | Oxygen therapy: |
| Anemia | • PPHN |
| Hypocapnia | • Pneumothorax |
| PDA | • Apnea |
| During PDA ligation | Perinatal asphyxia |
| Hypotension | Hypercapnia |
| Lack of cerebral autoregulation | SGA |
| High mean airway pressure | |

The most important clinical conditions associated with low rScO$_2$ (<−2 SD) and high rScO$_2$ values (>2 SD) in the preterm infant. *PDA,* Patent ductus arteriosus; *PPHN,* persistent pulmonary hypertension of the neonate; *SGA,* small for GA.

## CLINICAL CONDITIONS ASSOCIATED WITH HIGH RSCO$_2$ VALUES

NIRS-monitored rScO$_2$ may also be helpful to detect hyperoxemia, which has been increasingly linked to adverse long-term outcomes, especially in the extremely preterm neonate.[15,18,19]

Oxygen supplementation is the major cause of periods of hyperoxemia. Spontaneously breathing preterm infants are often treated with additional oxygen supplementation to accelerate normalization of partial arterial oxygen pressure and SaO$_2$. Brief but repetitive episodes of hyperoxemia occur relatively frequently during recovery from apnea and bradycardia episodes in these infants, as well as when additional oxygen is provided before routine care or endotracheal intubation (Figure 15.3E). In addition, hyperoxemia often occurs in preterm or term neonates receiving prolonged oxygen therapy for severe respiratory distress syndrome, pulmonary hypertension of the newborn, pneumothorax, or severe bronchopulmonary dysplasia. Hyperoxia still occurs frequently despite the increased awareness that oxygen therapy for some of these conditions is obsolete and harmful and that uncontrolled oxygen administration in itself is harmful under any circumstances unless the SaO$_2$ is successfully maintained in a gestational and postnatal age-appropriate range. Furthermore, even if oxygen saturation is carefully monitored, oxygen supplementation during episodes of apnea of prematurity can still result in hyperoxemia. One of the reasons for our inability to curtail the occurrence of hyperoxemia is that pulse oximetry–measured SaO$_2$ is not sensitive enough when SaO$_2$ is above 95%. In such cases concomitant monitoring of cerebral oxygenation may, at least in part, be helpful to minimize the occurrence of potentially harmful hyperoxic episodes.

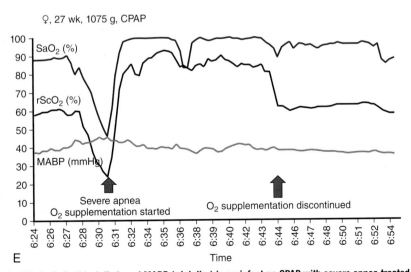

♀, 27 wk, 1075 g, CPAP

**Fig. 15.3E  Patterns of SaO$_2$ (*red line*), rScO$_2$ (*black line*), and MABP (*pink line*) in an infant on CPAP with severe apnea treated with stimulation and supplemental oxygen administration.** The rScO$_2$ increased to very high values and only decreased to baseline after the patient had been weaned off of supplemental oxygen. See text for details.

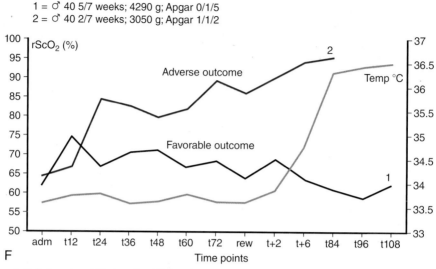

**Fig. 15.3F** Patterns of $rScO_2$ (*numbered black and red line*) and central temperature (*pink line*) in two term infants with hypoxic ischemic encephalopathy after severe perinatal asphyxia treated with moderate total body cooling (33.5°C) during the first 72 postnatal hours. Infant #1 had a normal MRI after having been rewarmed on day 5 and subsequently was found to have a favorable neurodevelopmental outcome. Infant #2 had an adverse outcome with severe abnormalities on MRI on day 5. Infant #1 showed normal $rScO_2$ values during hypothermia (time points: admission [adm] until rewarming [rew]) and also during and after rewarming (time points t +2 [2 hours after starting the process of rewarming]) until t108 (108 postnatal hours). Infant #2 had normal $rScO_2$ values on admission, increasing to high $rScO_2$ values at 24 hours of age (t24) and beyond. Persistently high $rScO_2$ values after 24 hours of age have been shown to be independently associated with adverse neurodevelopmental outcome in infants with hypoxic-ischemic encephalopathy following severe perinatal asphyxia. It is thought to be due to decreased utilization of oxygen and the inappropriately high oxygen delivery secondary to vasodilation/vasoparalysis. See text for details.

Episodes of hypercapnia cause an increase in brain perfusion and thus can contribute to cerebral hyperoxemia, especially in infants ventilated with additional oxygen supplementation. Again, NIRS-monitored $rScO_2$ may be used as an adjunct monitoring technique to aid in appropriately adjusting the oxygen therapy or to initiate $CO_2$ evaluation. Preterm infants who are born small for gestational age (SGA) show higher cerebral oxygenation after birth, compared to their appropriately grown peers.[138] Intrauterine growth restriction prompts the redistribution of blood in the fetus to the vital organs, including the brain, resulting in higher cerebral oxygen saturation, which persists after birth. Clinicians should be aware of this when interpreting the NIRS-monitored cerebral oxygenation in SGA infants.[139]

In addition to its use as a diagnostic tool to assess cerebral oxygen delivery and extraction, NIRS-monitored $rScO_2$ has been shown to be useful in predicting long-term prognosis in infants with hypoxic-ischemic encephalopathy following perinatal asphyxia. Our group has reported that abnormally high values of $rScO_2$ (>85–90%) in these infants during the first 24 postnatal hours are strongly and independently associated with adverse neurodevelopmental outcome at 2 years of age.[134] The high $rScO_2$ values are thought to be caused by low oxygen extraction due to a decrease in the metabolic activity of the injured brain, the inappropriately high cerebral oxygen delivery due to cerebral vasodilatation, and vasoparalysis along with the potential loss of cerebral autoregulation. Even when neonates with hypoxic-ischemic encephalopathy are treated with therapeutic hypothermia to prevent secondary injury associated with the ischemia-reperfusion cycle, the pattern of $rScO_2$ changes but keeps its prognostic value in relation to long-term neurodevelopmental outcome (Figure 15.3F)[140] (100). Conditions related to high $rScO_2$ values are also summarized in Table 15.2.

## Conclusion

Recent data indicate that NIRS-monitored cerebral oxygen saturation and extraction as measured by rScO$_2$ (or TOI) and cFTOE are of great value and have been increasingly incorporated into the standard clinical monitoring regimen in neonatal intensive care. Its noninvasive and bedside nature and the possibility to monitor the brain continuously and directly are among its attractive features. However, the inter- and intra-patient variability of the measurements and the fact that NIRS is a trend monitor rather than a technique capable of directly monitoring cerebral perfusion in absolute values remain obstacles to overcome. Substantial changes in the NIRS-monitored rScO$_2$, that is, in cerebral oxygenation, can alert the caregiver that potentially harmful changes in brain oxygenation are occurring, thus providing opportunities for intervention. NIRS monitoring has shown its usefulness in several clinical conditions, and reliable reference values are now available that increase its clinical applicability. Finally, the information provided by the use of this technology has improved our understanding of the limitations of our knowledge and led to the initiation of appropriately designed observational and interventional trials so that the interventions used in the clinical practice can be critically tested.

## REFERENCES

1. Younge N, Goldstein RF, Bann CM, et al. Survival and neurodevelopmental outcomes among periviable infants. *N Engl J Med.* 2017;376(7):617-628.
2. Anderson PJ, Doyle LW. Cognitive and educational deficits in children born extremely preterm. *Semin Perinatol.* 2008;32(1):51-58.
3. Wood NS, Costeloe K, Gibson AT, et al. The EPICure study: associations and antecedents of neurological and developmental disability at 30 months of age following extremely preterm birth. *Arch Dis Child Fetal Neonatal Ed.* 2005;90(2):F134-F140.
4. Wilson-Costello D, Friedman H, Minich N, Fanaroff AA, Hack M. Improved survival rates with increased neurodevelopmental disability for extremely low birth weight infants in the 1990s. *Pediatrics.* 2005;115(4):997-1003.
5. Wilson-Costello D, Friedman H, Minich N, et al. Improved neurodevelopmental outcomes for extremely low birth weight infants in 2000–2002. *Pediatrics.* 2007;119(1):37-45.
6. Samara M, Marlow N, Wolke D, Group EPS. Pervasive behavior problems at 6 years of age in a total-population sample of children born at </= 25 weeks of gestation. *Pediatrics.* 2008; 122(3):562-573.
7. Wolke D, Samara M, Bracewell M, Marlow N, Group EPS. Specific language difficulties and school achievement in children born at 25 weeks of gestation or less. *J Pediatr.* 2008;152(2):256-262.
8. Soderstrom F, Normann E, Jonsson M, Agren J. Outcomes of a uniformly active approach to infants born at 22–24 weeks of gestation. *Arch Dis Child Fetal Neonatal Ed.* 2021;106(4):413-417.
9. Marlow N, Ni Y, Lancaster R, et al. No change in neurodevelopment at 11 years after extremely preterm birth. *Arch Dis Child Fetal Neonatal Ed.* 2021;106(4):418-424.
10. Linsell L, Johnson S, Wolke D, et al. Cognitive trajectories from infancy to early adulthood following birth before 26 weeks of gestation: a prospective, population-based cohort study. *Arch Dis Child.* 2018;103(4):363-370.
11. Pascal A, Govaert P, Oostra A, Naulaers G, Ortibus E, Van den Broeck C. Neurodevelopmental outcome in very preterm and very-low-birthweight infants born over the past decade: a meta-analytic review. *Dev Med Child Neurol.* 2018;60(4):342-355.
12. Dai DWT, Franke N, Wouldes TA, et al. The contributions of intelligence and executive function to behaviour problems in school-age children born very preterm. *Acta Paediatr.* 2021; 110(6):1827-1834.
13. Logitharajah P, Rutherford MA, Cowan FM. Hypoxic-ischemic encephalopathy in preterm infants: antecedent factors, brain imaging, and outcome. *Pediatr Res.* 2009;66(2):222-229.
14. Dammann O, Allred EN, Kuban KC, et al. Systemic hypotension and white-matter damage in preterm infants. *Dev Med Child Neurol.* 2002;44(2):82-90.
15. Deulofeut R, Critz A, Adams-Chapman I, Sola A. Avoiding hyperoxia in infants < or = 1250 g is associated with improved short- and long-term outcomes. *J Perinatol.* 2006;26(11):700-705.
16. Perlman JM, McMenamin JB, Volpe JJ. Fluctuating cerebral blood-flow velocity in respiratory-distress syndrome. Relation to the development of intraventricular hemorrhage. *N Engl J Med.* 1983;309(4):204-209.
17. Van Bel F, Van de Bor M, Stijnen T, Baan J, Ruys JH. Aetiological role of cerebral blood-flow alterations in development and extension of peri-intraventricular haemorrhage. *Dev Med Child Neurol.* 1987;29(5):601-614.
18. Klinger G, Beyene J, Shah P, Perlman M. Do hyperoxaemia and hypocapnia add to the risk of brain injury after intrapartum asphyxia? *Arch Dis Child Fetal Neonatal Ed.* 2005;90(1):F49-F52.
19. Gerstner B, DeSilva TM, Genz K, et al. Hyperoxia causes maturation-dependent cell death in the developing white matter. *J Neurosci.* 2008;28(5):1236-1245.
20. Shah NA, Van Meurs KP, Davis AS. Amplitude-integrated electroencephalography: a survey of practices in the United States. *Am J Perinatol.* 2015;32(8):755-760.
21. Appendino JP, McNamara PJ, Keyzers M, Stephens D, Hahn CD. The impact of amplitude-integrated electroencephalography on NICU practice. *Can J Neurol Sci.* 2012;39(3):355-360.
22. van Bel F, Lemmers P, Naulaers G. Monitoring neonatal regional cerebral oxygen saturation in clinical practice: value and pitfalls. *Neonatology.* 2008;94(4):237-244.
23. Dix LM, van Bel F, Lemmers PM. Monitoring cerebral oxygenation in neonates: an update. *Front Pediatr.* 2017;5:46.
24. Greisen G. Is near-infrared spectroscopy living up to its promises? *Semin Fetal Neonatal Med.* 2006;11(6):498-502.
25. Kissack CM, Garr R, Wardle SP, Weindling AM. Cerebral fractional oxygen extraction in very low birth weight infants is high when there is low left ventricular output and hypocarbia but is unaffected by hypotension. *Pediatr Res.* 2004;55(3):400-405.
26. Naulaers G, Morren G, Van HS, Casaer P, Devlieger H. Cerebral tissue oxygenation index in very premature infants. *Arch Dis Child Fetal Neonatal Ed.* 2002;87(3):F189-F192.
27. Jobsis FF. Noninvasive, infrared monitoring of cerebral and myocardial oxygen sufficiency and circulatory parameters. *Science.* 1977;198(4323):1264-1267.

28. Stankovic MR, Maulik D, Rosenfeld W, et al. Role of frequency domain optical spectroscopy in the detection of neonatal brain hemorrhage – a newborn piglet study. *J Matern Fetal Med.* 2000;9(2):142-149.

29. Tsuji M, duPlessis A, Taylor G, Crocker R, Volpe JJ. Near infrared spectroscopy detects cerebral ischemia during hypotension in piglets. *Pediatr Res.* 1998;44(4):591-595.

30. Fantini S, Hueber D, Franceschini MA, et al. Non-invasive optical monitoring of the newborn piglet brain using continuous-wave and frequency-domain spectroscopy. *Phys Med Biol.* 1999;44(6):1543-1563.

31. Alfano RR, Demos SG, Galland P, et al. Time-resolved and nonlinear optical imaging for medical applications. *Ann N Y Acad Sci.* 1998;838:14-28.

32. Wolf M, Naulaers G, Van Bel F, Kleiser S, Greisen G. A review of near infrared spectroscopy for term and preterm newborns. *J Near Infrared Spectrosc.* 2012;20(1):43-55.

33. Meek JH, Tyszczuk L, Elwell CE, Wyatt JS. Cerebral blood flow increases over the first three days of life in extremely preterm neonates. *Arch Dis Child Fetal Neonatal Ed.* 1998;78(1):F33-F37.

34. Meek JH, Tyszczuk L, Elwell CE, Wyatt JS. Low cerebral blood flow is a risk factor for severe intraventricular haemorrhage. *Arch Dis Child Fetal Neonatal Ed.* 1999;81(1):F15-F18.

35. Urlesberger B, Pichler G, Gradnitzer E, Reiterer F, Zobel G, Muller W. Changes in cerebral blood volume and cerebral oxygenation during periodic breathing in term infants. *Neuropediatrics.* 2000;31(2):75-81.

36. Kissack CM, Garr R, Wardle SP, Weindling AM. Postnatal changes in cerebral oxygen extraction in the preterm infant are associated with intraventricular hemorrhage and hemorrhagic parenchymal infarction but not periventricular leukomalacia. *Pediatr Res.* 2004;56(1):111-116.

37. Wardle SP, Yoxall CW, Crawley E, Weindling AM. Peripheral oxygenation and anemia in preterm babies. *Pediatr Res.* 1998;44(1):125-131.

38. Wardle SP, Yoxall CW, Weindling AM. Cerebral oxygenation during cardiopulmonary bypass. *Arch Dis Child.* 1998;78(1):26-32.

39. Wardle SP, Yoxall CW, Weindling AM. Peripheral oxygenation in hypotensive preterm babies. *Pediatr Res.* 1999;45(3):343-349.

40. van der Zee P, Arridge SR, Cope M, Delpy DT. The effect of optode positioning on optical pathlength in near infrared spectroscopy of brain. *Adv Exp Med Biol.* 1990;277:79-84.

41. Delpy DT, Cope M, van der Zee P, Arridge S, Wray S, Wyatt J. Estimation of optical pathlength through tissue from direct time of flight measurement. *Phys Med Biol.* 1988;33(12):1433-1442.

42. Wyatt JS, Cope M, Delpy DT, et al. Measurement of optical path length for cerebral near-infrared spectroscopy in newborn infants. *Dev Neurosci.* 1990;12(2):140-144.

43. Matcher SJ, Cooper CE. Absolute quantification of deoxyhaemoglobin concentration in tissue near infrared spectroscopy. *Phys Med Biol.* 1994;39(8):1295-1312.

44. Fujisaka SI, Ozaki T, Suzuki T, et al. A clinical tissue oximeter using NIR time-resolved spectroscopy. *Adv Exp Med Biol.* 2016;876:427-433.

45. Lemmers PM, van Bel F. Left-to-right differences of regional cerebral oxygen saturation and oxygen extraction in preterm infants during the first days of life. *Pediatr Res.* 2009;65(2):226-230.

46. Quaresima V, Sacco S, Totaro R, Ferrari M. Noninvasive measurement of cerebral hemoglobin oxygen saturation using two near infrared spectroscopy approaches. *J Biomed Opt.* 2000;5(2):201-205.

47. Thavasothy M, Broadhead M, Elwell C, Peters M, Smith M. A comparison of cerebral oxygenation as measured by the NIRO 300 and the INVOS 5100 near-infrared spectrophotometers. *Anaesthesia.* 2002;57(10):999-1006.

48. Yoshitani K, Kawaguchi M, Tatsumi K, Kitaguchi K, Furuya H. A comparison of the INVOS 4100 and the NIRO 300 near-infrared spectrophotometers. *Anesth Analg.* 2002;94(3):586-590.

49. Kleiser S, Ostojic D, Andresen B, et al. Comparison of tissue oximeters on a liquid phantom with adjustable optical properties: an extension. *Biomed Opt Express.* 2018;9(1):86-101.

50. Ijichi S, Kusaka T, Isobe K, et al. Developmental changes of optical properties in neonates determined by near-infrared time-resolved spectroscopy. *Pediatr Res.* 2005;58(3):568-573.

51. Jelzow A, Wabnitz H, Tachtsidis I, Kirilina E, Bruhl R, Macdonald R. Separation of superficial and cerebral hemodynamics using a single distance time-domain NIRS measurement. *Biomed Opt Express.* 2014;5(5):1465-1482.

52. Zhao J, Ding HS, Hou XL, Zhou CL, Chance B. In vivo determination of the optical properties of infant brain using frequency-domain near-infrared spectroscopy. *J Biomed Opt.* 2005;10(2):024028.

53. Roche-Labarbe N, Carp SA, Surova A, et al. Noninvasive optical measures of CBV, StO(2), CBF index, and rCMRO(2) in human premature neonates' brains in the first six weeks of life. *Hum Brain Mapp.* 2010;31(3):341-352.

54. Choi J, Wolf M, Toronov V, et al. Noninvasive determination of the optical properties of adult brain: near-infrared spectroscopy approach. *J Biomed Opt.* 2004;9(1):221-229.

55. Roche-Labarbe N, Fenoglio A, Radhakrishnan H, et al. Somatosensory evoked changes in cerebral oxygen consumption measured non-invasively in premature neonates. *Neuroimage.* 2014;85(Pt 1):279-286.

56. Yoxall CW, Weindling AM. Measurement of cerebral oxygen consumption in the human neonate using near infrared spectroscopy: cerebral oxygen consumption increases with advancing gestational age. *Pediatr Res.* 1998;44(3):283-290.

57. Winter JD, Tichauer KM, Gelman N, Thompson RT, Lee TY, St Lawrence K. Changes in cerebral oxygen consumption and high-energy phosphates during early recovery in hypoxic-ischemic piglets: a combined near-infrared and magnetic resonance spectroscopy study. *Pediatr Res.* 2009;65(2):181-187.

58. Nagdyman N, Fleck T, Schubert S, et al. Comparison between cerebral tissue oxygenation index measured by near-infrared spectroscopy and venous jugular bulb saturation in children. *Intensive Care Med.* 2005;31(6):846-850.

59. Yoxall CW, Weindling AM, Dawani NH, Peart I. Measurement of cerebral venous oxyhemoglobin saturation in children by near-infrared spectroscopy and partial jugular venous occlusion. *Pediatr Res.* 1995;38(3):319-323.

60. Murkin JM. NIRS: a standard of care for CPB vs. an evolving standard for selective cerebral perfusion? *J Extra Corpor Technol.* 2009;41(1):P11-P14.

61. Hoffman GM. Neurologic monitoring on cardiopulmonary bypass: what are we obligated to do? *Ann Thorac Surg.* 2006;81(6):S2373-S2380.

62. Williams GD, Ramamoorthy C. Brain monitoring and protection during pediatric cardiac surgery. *Semin Cardiothorac Vasc Anesth.* 2007;11(1):23-33.

63. Yoxall CW, Weindling AM. The measurement of peripheral venous oxyhemoglobin saturation in newborn infants by near infrared spectroscopy with venous occlusion. *Pediatr Res.* 1996;39(6):1103-1106.

64. Naulaers G, Meyns B, Miserez M, et al. Use of tissue oxygenation index and fractional tissue oxygen extraction as noninvasive parameters for cerebral oxygenation. A validation study in piglets. *Neonatology.* 2007;92(2):120-126.

65. Wardle SP, Yoxall CW, Weindling AM. Determinants of cerebral fractional oxygen extraction using near infrared spectroscopy in preterm neonates. *J Cereb Blood Flow Metab.* 2000;20(2):272-279.

66. Naulaers G, Morren G, Van Huffel S, Casaer P, Devlieger H. Cerebral tissue oxygenation index in very premature infants. *Arch Dis Child Fetal Neonatal Ed.* 2002;87(3):F189-F192.

67. Dullenkopf A, Kolarova A, Schulz G, Frey B, Baenziger O, Weiss M. Reproducibility of cerebral oxygenation measurement in neonates and infants in the clinical setting using the NIRO 300 oximeter. *Pediatr Crit Care Med.* 2005;6(3):344-347.

68. Menke J, Voss U, Moller G, Jorch G. Reproducibility of cerebral near infrared spectroscopy in neonates. *Biol Neonate.* 2003;83(1):6-11.

69. Misra M, Stark J, Dujovny M, Widman R, Ausman JI. Transcranial cerebral oximetry in random normal subjects. *Neurol Res.* 1998;20(2):137-141.

70. Weiss M, Dullenkopf A, Kolarova A, Schulz G, Frey B, Baenziger O. Near-infrared spectroscopic cerebral oxygenation reading in neonates and infants is associated with central venous oxygen saturation. *Paediatr Anaesth.* 2005;15(2):102-109.

71. Sorensen LC, Greisen G. Precision of measurement of cerebral tissue oxygenation index using near-infrared spectroscopy in preterm neonates. *J Biomed Opt.* 2006;11(5):054005.

72. Petrova A, Mehta R. Near-infrared spectroscopy in the detection of regional tissue oxygenation during hypoxic events in preterm infants undergoing critical care. *Pediatr Crit Care Med.* 2006;7(5):449-454.

73. Olopade CO, Mensah E, Gupta R, et al. Noninvasive determination of brain tissue oxygenation during sleep in obstructive sleep apnea: a near-infrared spectroscopic approach. *Sleep.* 2007; 30(12):1747-1755.

74. Fauchere JC, Schulz G, Haensse D, et al. Near-infrared spectroscopy measurements of cerebral oxygenation in newborns during immediate postnatal adaptation. *J Pediatr.* 2010;156(3):372-376.

75. Alderliesten T, Dix L, Baerts W, et al. Reference values of regional cerebral oxygen saturation during the first 3 days of life in preterm neonates. *Pediatr Res.* 2016;79(1-1):55-64.

76. Macleod D, Vacchiano C. Simultaneous comparison of Foresight and INVOS cerebral oximeters to jugular bulb and arterial co-oximetry measurements in healthy volunteers. *SCA Suppl.* 2009;108:101-104.

77. Dix LM, van Bel F, Baerts W, Lemmers PM. Comparing near-infrared spectroscopy devices and their sensors for monitoring regional cerebral oxygen saturation in the neonate. *Pediatr Res.* 2013;74(5):557-563.

78. Lemmers PM, Toet M, van Schelven LJ, van Bel F. Cerebral oxygenation and cerebral oxygen extraction in the preterm infant: the impact of respiratory distress syndrome. *Exp Brain Res.* 2006;173(3):458-467.

79. Hou X, Ding H, Teng Y, et al. Research on the relationship between brain anoxia at different regional oxygen saturations and brain damage using near-infrared spectroscopy. *Physiol Meas.* 2007;28(10):1251-1265.

80. Kurth CD, Levy WJ, McCann J. Near-infrared spectroscopy cerebral oxygen saturation thresholds for hypoxia-ischemia in piglets. *J Cereb Blood Flow Metab.* 2002;22(3):335-341.

81. Dent CL, Spaeth JP, Jones BV, et al. Brain magnetic resonance imaging abnormalities after the Norwood procedure using regional cerebral perfusion. *J Thorac Cardiovasc Surg.* 2006;131(1):190-197.

82. Sakamoto T, Hatsuoka S, Stock UA, et al. Prediction of safe duration of hypothermic circulatory arrest by near-infrared spectroscopy. *J Thorac Cardiovasc Surg.* 2001;122(2):339-350.

83. Hyttel-Sorensen S, Austin T, van Bel F, et al. Clinical use of cerebral oximetry in extremely preterm infants is feasible. *Dan Med J.* 2013;60(1):A4533.

84. Hyttel-Sorensen S, Pellicer A, Alderliesten T, et al. Cerebral near infrared spectroscopy oximetry in extremely preterm infants: phase II randomised clinical trial. *BMJ.* 2015;350:g7635.

85. Tin W. Optimal oxygen saturation for preterm babies. Do we really know? *Biol Neonate.* 2004;85(4):319-325.

86. Chow LC, Wright KW, Sola A, Group COAS. Can changes in clinical practice decrease the incidence of severe retinopathy of prematurity in very low birth weight infants? *Pediatrics.* 2003;111(2):339-345.

87. De Smet D, Vanderhaegen J, Naulaers G, Van Huffel S. New measurements for assessment of impaired cerebral autoregulation using near-infrared spectroscopy. *Adv Exp Med Biol.* 2009; 645:273-278.

88. Brady KM, Mytar JO, Lee JK, et al. Monitoring cerebral blood flow pressure autoregulation in pediatric patients during cardiac surgery. *Stroke.* 2010;41(9):1957-1962.

89. Brady KM, Lee JK, Kibler KK, et al. Continuous time-domain analysis of cerebrovascular autoregulation using near-infrared spectroscopy. *Stroke.* 2007;38(10):2818-2825.

90. Wong FY, Leung TS, Austin T, et al. Impaired autoregulation in preterm infants identified by using spatially resolved spectroscopy. *Pediatrics.* 2008;121(3):e604-e611.

91. Toet MC, Lemmers PM, van Schelven LJ, van Bel F. Cerebral oxygenation and electrical activity after birth asphyxia: their relation to outcome. *Pediatrics.* 2006;117(2):333-339.

92. Szakmar E, Smith J, Yang E, Volpe JJ, Inder T, El-Dib M. Association between cerebral oxygen saturation and brain injury in neonates receiving therapeutic hypothermia for neonatal encephalopathy. *J Perinatol.* 2021;41(2):269-277.

93. Smits A, Thewissen L, Caicedo A, Naulaers G, Allegaert K. Propofol dose-finding to reach optimal effect for (semi-)elective intubation in neonates. *J Pediatr.* 2016;179:54-60.e9.

94. Smits A, Thewissen L, Dereymaeker A, Dempsey E, Caicedo A, Naulaers G. The use of hemodynamic and cerebral monitoring to study pharmacodynamics in neonates. *Curr Pharm Des.* 2017;23(38):5955-5963.

95. Thewissen L, Caicedo A, Dereymaeker A, et al. Cerebral autoregulation and activity after propofol for endotracheal intubation in preterm neonates. *Pediatr Res.* 2018;84(5):719-725.

96. Kozberg MG, Ma Y, Shaik MA, Kim SH, Hillman EM. Rapid postnatal expansion of neural networks occurs in an environment of altered neurovascular and neurometabolic coupling. *J Neurosci.* 2016;36(25):6704-6717.

97. Hendrikx D, Smits A, Lavanga M, et al. Measurement of neurovascular coupling in neonates. *Front Physiol.* 2019;10:65.

98. Pellicer A, Greisen G, Benders M, et al. The SafeBoosC phase II randomised clinical trial: a treatment guideline for targeted near-infrared-derived cerebral tissue oxygenation versus standard treatment in extremely preterm infants. *Neonatology.* 2013;104(3):171-178.

99. Riera J, Hyttel-Sorensen S, Bravo MC, et al. The SafeBoosC phase II clinical trial: an analysis of the interventions related with the oximeter readings. *Arch Dis Child Fetal Neonatal Ed.* 2016;101(4):F333-F338.

100. Seidel D, Blaser A, Gebauer C, Pulzer F, Thome U, Knupfer M. Changes in regional tissue oxygenation saturation and

100. desaturations after red blood cell transfusion in preterm infants. *J Perinatol.* 2013;33(4):282-287.

101. van Hoften JC, Verhagen EA, Keating P, ter Horst HJ, Bos AF. Cerebral tissue oxygen saturation and extraction in preterm infants before and after blood transfusion. *Arch Dis Child Fetal Neonatal Ed.* 2010;95(5):F352-F358.

102. Andersen CC, Karayil SM, Hodyl NA, Stark MJ. Early red cell transfusion favourably alters cerebral oxygen extraction in very preterm newborns. *Arch Dis Child Fetal Neonatal Ed.* 2015;100(5):F433-F435.

103. Banerjee J, Aladangady N. Biomarkers to decide red blood cell transfusion in newborn infants. *Transfusion.* 2014;54(10):2574-2582.

104. Mintzer JP, Parvez B, Chelala M, Alpan G, LaGamma EF. Monitoring regional tissue oxygen extraction in neonates ,1250 g helps identify transfusion thresholds independent of hematocrit. *J Neonatal Perinatal Med.* 2014;7(2):89-100.

105. Dix LML, Weeke LC, de Vries LS, et al. Carbon dioxide fluctuations are associated with changes in cerebral oxygenation and electrical activity in infants born preterm. *J Pediatr.* 2017;187:66-72.e1.

106. Vanderhaegen J, Naulaers G, Vanhole C, et al. The effect of changes in tPCO$_2$ on the fractional tissue oxygen extraction – as measured by near-infrared spectroscopy – in neonates during the first days of life. *Eur J Paediatr Neurol.* 2009;13(2):128-134.

107. Perlman JM, Hill A, Volpe JJ. The effect of patent ductus arteriosus on flow velocity in the anterior cerebral arteries: ductal steal in the premature newborn infant. *J Pediatr.* 1981;99(5):767-771.

108. Lemmers PM, Toet MC, van Bel F. Impact of patent ductus arteriosus and subsequent therapy with indomethacin on cerebral oxygenation in preterm infants. *Pediatrics.* 2008;121(1):142-147.

109. Dix L, Molenschot M, Breur J, et al. Cerebral oxygenation and echocardiographic parameters in preterm neonates with a patent ductus arteriosus: an observational study. *Arch Dis Child Fetal Neonatal Ed.* 2016;101(6):F520-F526.

110. Underwood MA, Milstein JM, Sherman MP. Near-infrared spectroscopy as a screening tool for patent ductus arteriosus in extremely low birth weight infants. *Neonatology.* 2007;91(2):134-139.

111. Variane GFT, Chock VY, Netto A, Pietrobom RFR, Van Meurs KP. Simultaneous Near-Infrared Spectroscopy (NIRS) and Amplitude-Integrated Electroencephalography (aEEG): dual use of brain monitoring techniques improves our understanding of physiology. *Front Pediatr.* 2019;7:560.

112. Lemmers PM, Molenschot MC, Evens J, Toet MC, van BF. Is cerebral oxygen supply compromised in preterm infants undergoing surgical closure for patent ductus arteriosus? *Arch Dis Child Fetal Neonatal Ed.* 2010;95(6):F429-F434.

113. Weisz DE, More K, McNamara PJ, Shah PS. PDA ligation and health outcomes: a meta-analysis. *Pediatrics.* 2014;133(4):e1024-e1046.

114. Lemmers PM, Benders MJ, D'Ascenzo R, et al. Patent ductus arteriosus and brain volume. *Pediatrics.* 2016;137(4):e20153090.

115. Roze JC, Cambonie G, Marchand-Martin L, et al. Association between early screening for patent ductus arteriosus and in-hospital mortality among extremely preterm infants. *JAMA.* 2015;313(24):2441-2448.

116. Dempsey EM, Barrington KJ. Evaluation and treatment of hypotension in the preterm infant. *Clin Perinatol.* 2009;36(1):75-85.

117. Dempsey EM. What should we do about low blood pressure in preterm infants. *Neonatology.* 2017;111(4):402-407.

118. Noori S, Seri I. Evidence-based versus pathophysiology-based approach to diagnosis and treatment of neonatal cardiovascular compromise. *Semin Fetal Neonatal Med.* 2015;20(4):238-245.

119. Alderliesten T, Lemmers PM, van Haastert IC, et al. Hypotension in preterm neonates: low blood pressure alone does not affect neurodevelopmental outcome. *J Pediatr.* 2014;164(5):986-991.

120. Thewissen L, Naulaers G, Hendrikx D, et al. Cerebral oxygen saturation and autoregulation during hypotension in extremely preterm infants. *Pediatr Res.* 2021;90(2):373-380.

121. Chock VY, Kwon SH, Ambalavanan N, et al. Cerebral oxygenation and autoregulation in preterm infants (early NIRS study). *J Pediatr.* 2020;227:94-100.e1.

122. Tsuji M, Saul JP, du PA, et al. Cerebral intravascular oxygenation correlates with mean arterial pressure in critically ill premature infants. *Pediatrics.* 2000;106(4):625-632.

123. Wong FY, Silas R, Hew S, Samarasinghe T, Walker AM. Cerebral oxygenation is highly sensitive to blood pressure variability in sick preterm infants. *PLoS One.* 2012;7(8):e43165.

124. Soul JS, Hammer PE, Tsuji M, et al. Fluctuating pressure-passivity is common in the cerebral circulation of sick premature infants. *Pediatr Res.* 2007;61(4):467-473.

125. Caicedo A, De Smet D, Naulaers G, et al. Cerebral tissue oxygenation and regional oxygen saturation can be used to study cerebral autoregulation in prematurely born infants. *Pediatr Res.* 2011;69(6):548-553.

126. Caicedo A, Alderliesten T, Naulaers G, Lemmers P, van Bel F, Van Huffel S. A new framework for the assessment of cerebral hemodynamics regulation in neonates using NIRS. *Adv Exp Med Biol.* 2016;876:501-509.

127. Wu TW, Lien RI, Seri I, Noori S. Changes in cardiac output and cerebral oxygenation during prone and supine sleep positioning in healthy term infants. *Arch Dis Child Fetal Neonatal Ed.* 2017;102(6):F483-F489.

128. Milan A, Freato F, Vanzo V, Chiandetti L, Zaramella P. Influence of ventilation mode on neonatal cerebral blood flow and volume. *Early Hum Dev.* 2009;85(7):415-419.

129. Hellstrom-Westas L, Rosen I, Svenningsen NW. Cerebral function monitoring during the first week of life in extremely small low birthweight (ESLBW) infants. *Neuropediatrics.* 1991;22(1):27-32.

130. Stolwijk LJ, Lemmers PM, Harmsen M, et al. Neurodevelopmental outcomes after neonatal surgery for major noncardiac anomalies. *Pediatrics.* 2016;137(2):e20151728.

131. Morriss Jr FH, Saha S, Bell EF, et al. Surgery and neurodevelopmental outcome of very low-birth-weight infants. *JAMA Pediatr.* 2014;168(8):746-754.

132. Costerus SA, van Hoorn CE, Hendrikx D, et al. Towards integrative neuromonitoring of the surgical newborn: A systematic review. *Eur J Anaesthesiol.* 2020;37(8):701-712.

133. Durandy Y, Rubatti M, Couturier R. Near infrared spectroscopy during pediatric cardiac surgery: errors and pitfalls. *Perfusion.* 2011;26(5):441-446.

134. Toet MC, Flinterman A, Laar I, et al. Cerebral oxygen saturation and electrical brain activity before, during, and up to 36 hours after arterial switch procedure in neonates without preexisting brain damage: its relationship to neurodevelopmental outcome. *Exp Brain Res.* 2005;165(3):343-350.

135. Costerus SA, Hendrikx D, Ijsselmuiden J, et al. Cerebral oxygenation and activity during surgical repair of neonates with

congenital diaphragmatic hernia: a center comparison analysis. *Front Pediatr*. 2021;9:798952.

136. Cruz SM, Akinkuotu AC, Rusin CG, et al. A novel multimodal computational system using near-infrared spectroscopy to monitor cerebral oxygenation during assisted ventilation in CDH patients. *J Pediatr Surg*. 2016;51(1):38-43.

137. Koch HW, Hansen TG. Perioperative use of cerebral and renal near-infrared spectroscopy in neonates: a 24-h observational study. *Paediatr Anaesth*. 2016;26(2):190-198.

138. Cohen E, Baerts W, Alderliesten T, Derks J, Lemmers P, van Bel F. Growth restriction and gender influence cerebral oxygenation in preterm neonates. *Arch Dis Child Fetal Neonatal Ed*. 2016; 101(2):F156-F161.

139. Cohen E, Baerts W, van Bel F. Brain-sparing in intrauterine growth restriction: considerations for the neonatologist. *Neonatology*. 2015;108(4):269-276.

140. Lemmers PM, Zwanenburg RJ, Benders MJ, et al. Cerebral oxygenation and brain activity after perinatal asphyxia: does hypothermia change their prognostic value? *Pediatr Res*. 2013; 74(2):180-185.

# Common Hemodynamic Dilemmas in the Neonate

# PATHOPHYSIOLOGY AND TREATMENT OF PATENT DUCTUS ARTERIOSUS

# Chapter 16

# Diagnosis, Evaluation, and Monitoring of Patent Ductus Arteriosus in the Very Preterm Infant

Audrey Hébert, Afif Faisal El-Khuffash, Shahab Noori, and Patrick J. McNamara

## Key Points

- Although presence of a patent ductus arteriosus (PDA) can easily be confirmed with echocardiography, diagnosis of a hemodynamically significant PDA is more challenging and not standardized.

- Evaluation of hemodynamic and clinical significance of a PDA should include assessment of the size of the PDA, magnitude of shunt volume, the ability of the heart to accommodate and compensate for the shunt, and the impact of the shunt on the pulmonary and systemic circulations.

- Clinical characteristics such as gestational and chronologic age, extent of cardiopulmonary support, and presence of other variables that may either enhance or mitigate the potential detrimental effects of a PDA may be useful in the evaluation of the hemodynamic and clinical significance of a PDA.

- Scoring systems based on clinical characteristics, echocardiography measurements, and other technologies such as near-infrared spectroscopy may be useful in evaluation and monitoring of a PDA in the future.

## Introduction

The diagnosis and management of a patent ductus arteriosus (PDA) with cardiorespiratory, and thus clinical, relevance in preterm neonates poses a major challenge in neonatal medicine. It is the most common cardiovascular abnormality in premature infants. Most (~70%) infants born at a gestational age (GA) of less than 29 weeks will have a persistent PDA by the end of the first postnatal week.[1] PDA is associated with several morbidities and mortality; however, a cause-and-effect relationship between the presence of a PDA and important short- and long-term clinical outcomes has not been definitively established. In addition, there are limitations due to study design of randomized control trials and the retrospective nature of cohort studies reporting clinical outcomes and the impact of various approaches to treatment (conservative, medical, device and surgical). More than 50% have a high rate of open-label treatment in the control arm and high treatment failure rate in the intervention arm.[2] There is considerable heterogeneity in infants included in PDA trials due to lack of a standardized definition of hemodynamic significance, resulting in inclusion of patients who may not benefit from PDA treatment.[3] As a result, the impact of PDA treatment on outcomes and treatment strategies (particularly modality and timing) varies between centers.[4] Finally, there continues to be a lack of physician equipoise such that the most vulnerable infants, potentially at greatest risk of PDA-attributable morbidity, are not always enrolled in clinical trials.[5]

## Developmental Role of the Ductus Arteriosus

The ductus arteriosus (DA) connects the main pulmonary artery to the descending aorta and is necessary for fetal survival. In the fetus the left ventricle (LV) receives oxygenated blood, returning from the placenta via the inferior vena cava and through the foramen ovale, and delivers it mainly to the upper part of the body. The right ventricle (RV) receives most blood

**303**

draining from the superior vena cava (SVC) and a proportionately lower amount of oxygenated blood from the umbilical venous system. Due to high pulmonary vascular resistance (PVR), most (80% to 90% depending on the gestational age of the fetus) of right ventricular output flows from the pulmonary artery to the descending aorta across the DA; hence the DA modulates flow to the lower part of the body. Similarly, the patent foramen ovale (PFO) is the route that modulates the delivery of oxygenated blood to the head and neck. After birth, LV afterload rises suddenly due to loss of the low resistance placental circulation. This is accompanied by lung aeration, which promotes a fall in PVR and an increase in pulmonary blood flow. This results in a change in the organ of gas exchange from the placenta to the lungs. The DA eventually closes (first functionally and then anatomically) over the subsequent days in term infants. However, in preterm infants the DA can remain patent for a prolonged period of time for a variety of reasons.

## Regulation of Ductal Tone and Constriction

In term infants closure of the PDA occurs within the first 48 hours after birth. Closure of the DA occurs in two phases. The *first phase* (within the first hours after birth), termed "functional closure," involves narrowing of the lumen by smooth muscle constriction. The *second phase*, termed "anatomic remodeling", consists of occlusion of the residual lumen by extensive neointimal thickening and loss of muscle media smooth muscle over the next few days.

The rate and degree of initial "functional" closure are determined by the balance between factors (mediators, second messengers and channels, among others) that favor constriction (oxygen, endothelin, calcium channels, catecholamines, and Rho kinase) and those that oppose it (intraluminal pressure, prostaglandins [PGs], nitric oxide [NO], carbon monoxide, potassium channels, cyclic adenosine monophosphate [AMP], and cyclic guanosine monophosphate). PGs play a key role in the regulation of ductal tone, especially during the first few postnatal weeks. Of these, $PGE_2$ is the most important factor in the regulation of DA tone during fetal development and acts on G protein–coupled E-prostanoid receptors to maintain ductal patency. It is generated from arachidonic acid

by cyclooxygenase-1 (COX-1) and COX-2, the COX component of $PG-H_2$ synthase, followed by peroxidation by the same enzyme complex and, finally, by the action of PGE synthase (see Chapter 5). COX-2 plays a major role in maintaining ductal patency during fetal life.[6] The current approach to medical therapy exploits this mechanism by the use of nonselective COX inhibitors (such as indomethacin and ibuprofen) and also by the use of acetaminophen, a peroxidase inhibitor, to close the DA postnatally.

Low oxygen tension in the fetus is another important factor for maintaining ductal patency.[7] Following birth, the rise in oxygen tension promotes an oxygen-mediated constriction that is facilitated by the inhibition of the potassium voltage channels ($K_V$ channels) present on the ductal smooth muscle cells and function to keep the cells in a hyperpolarized state.[8] The presence of oxygen leads to depolarization, which in turn activates L-type calcium channels, allowing an influx of calcium into the smooth muscle cells causing constriction. A counter-mechanism via the mitochondrial electron transport chain serves as the intrinsic oxygen-sensing mechanism that regulates this constrictive effect via formation of reactive oxygen radicals, which inhibit $K_V$ channels.[9] Interestingly, in vitro studies using rings of human DA tissue incubated in relatively low oxygen tension conditions (to mimic conditions of prematurity) for several days selectively fail to constrict in response to oxygen. This may explain, at least in part, failure of the DA to close in preterm infants.

The fall in PG levels following birth (due to the loss of placental PG production and increase in its removal by the lungs), accompanied by the rise in oxygen tension, promotes functional closure of the DA over the first 24–48 postnatal hours. After functional DA closure is achieved, the smooth muscle cells migrate from the media to the subendothelial layer, leading to neointimal formation.[10] Expansion of the neointima forms protrusions, or mounds, that permanently occlude the already constricted lumen.[11,12] This process results in an interruption of the blood supply to the innermost cellular layer, resulting in hypoxia and cell death.[13] The presence of intramural vasa vasorum is essential to ensure adequate provision of oxygen and nutrition to the thicker wall of the DA at term. During postnatal constriction, the intramural tissue pressure obliterates vasa vasorum flow in the muscle media. The ensuing ischemic and hypoxic insult inhibits local $PGE_2$ and NO production, induces local production of hypoxia-inducible factors (HIF) like HIF-1$\alpha$ and vascular endothelial growth factor (VEGF), and produces smooth muscle apoptosis in the muscle media. In addition, monocytes/macrophages adhere to the ductus wall and appear to be necessary for ductus remodeling.[14]

## RESISTANCE TO DUCTAL CLOSURE IN PREMATURE INFANTS

In contrast, in preterm infants the DA frequently fails to constrict or undergo anatomic remodeling after birth. In fact, a study by Semberova et al showed that the median time to PDA closure was 71 days in infants <26 weeks' gestation.[15] There is, however, little information regarding the biological mechanisms that contribute to late spontaneous closure. The incidence of persistent PDA is inversely related to gestational age due to several mechanisms.[16] The intrinsic tone of the extremely immature ductus (<70% of gestation) is decreased compared with the ductus at term.[17] This may be due to the presence of immature smooth muscle myosin isoforms, with a weaker contractile capacity,[18-21] and to decreased Rho kinase expression and activity.[22-24] Calcium entry through L-type calcium channels also appears to be impaired in the immature ductus.[23-25] In addition, the potassium channels, which inhibit ductus contraction, change during gestation from $K_{Ca}$ channels not regulated by oxygen tension to $K_V$ channels, which can be inhibited by increased oxygen concentrations.[26-28] The reduced expression and function of the putative oxygen-sensing $K_V$ channels in the immature ductus appear to contribute to ductus patency in several animal species.[24,26,28]

In most mammalian species the major factor that prevents the preterm ductus from constricting after birth is its increased sensitivity to the vasodilating effects of $PGE_2$ and NO.[29] The increased sensitivity of the preterm ductus to $PGE_2$ is due to increased cyclic AMP signaling. There is both increased cyclic AMP production, due to enhanced PG receptor coupling with adenylyl cyclase, and decreased cyclic AMP degradation by phosphodiesterase in the preterm ductus.[30,31] As a result, inhibitors of PG production (e.g., indomethacin, ibuprofen, mefenamic acid, paracetamol) are usually effective agents in promoting

ductus closure in the premature infant. Premature infants also have elevated circulating concentrations of $PGE_2$ due to the decreased ability of the premature lung to clear circulating $PGE_2$.[32] In the preterm newborn circulating concentrations of $PGE_2$ can reach the pharmacologic range during episodes of bacteremia and necrotizing enterocolitis and are often associated with reopening of a previously constricted DA.[33]

Little is known about the factors responsible for the changes that occur with advanced gestation. A recent study showed gene expression in pathways involved with oxygen-induced constriction, contractile protein maturation, tissue remodeling, and PG and NO signaling alter according to advancing GA.[34] Prenatal administration of glucocorticoids reduces the incidence of PDA in premature humans and animals.[35-40] Although postnatal glucocorticoid or corticosteroid administration also reduces the incidence of PDA, it is not clear whether this is a direct effect on ductal biology or an indirect effect on ambient conditions which promote ongoing ductal patency. In addition, it is important to recognize that glucocorticoid (dexamethasone) or corticosteroid (hydrocortisone) treatment, especially if it is given in the immediate postnatal period or combined with administration of COX inhibitors, respectively, has been associated with increased incidence of several other neonatal morbidities.[41,42] The patient's genetic background also seems to play a significant role in determining persistent ductus patency. Several single nucleotide polymorphisms in candidate genes have been identified that are associated with PDA in preterm infants: angiotensin receptor (ATR) type 1,[43] interferon-gamma (IFN-$\gamma$),[44] estrogen receptor-alpha PvuII,[45] transcription factor AP-2B (TFAP2B), PGI synthase, and TRAF1.[46] Studies suggest that an interaction between preterm birth and TFAP2B may be responsible for the PDAs that occur in some preterm infants: TFAP2B is uniquely expressed in ductus smooth muscle and regulates other genes that are important in ductus smooth muscle development.[47] Mutations in TFAP2B result in patency of the DA in mice and humans[48] and TFAP2B polymorphisms are associated with the PDA in preterm infants (especially those that are unresponsive to indomethacin).[49] Expression of *SLCO2A1* and *NOS3* genes (involved with PG reuptake/metabolism and NO production, respectively) is decreased in the

DA from non-Caucasians.[34] This may lead to an increase in PG and decrease in NO concentrations, thereby making ductal patency more PG dependent and possibly explaining the clinical finding of a better response to indomethacin in non-Caucasians.[34,49,50] Recently, an association was shown between two single nucleotide polymorphisms in *CYP2C9*, rs2153628, and rs1799853, and indomethacin response for the treatment of PDA. Findings suggest that response to indomethacin in the closure of PDA may be influenced by polymorphisms associated with altered indomethacin metabolism.[51] There is, however, little data on the genetic determinants of acetaminophen response.

Neointimal mounds are less well developed and often fail to occlude the lumen in preterm infants (especially those born before 28 weeks' gestation). The preterm ductus is a much thinner vessel than the full-term ductus; therefore there is no need for vasa vasorum because the vessel wall is nourished with oxygen via diffusion through luminal blood flow (vasa vasorum first appear in the outer ductus wall after 28 weeks' gestation). As a result, unless the ductus lumen is completely obliterated, the preterm ductus is less likely to develop profound hypoxia as it constricts after birth. Without a strong hypoxic signal, neointimal expansion is markedly diminished, resulting in mounds that fail to occlude the residual lumen[11,14,52,53]

## PATHOPHYSIOLOGIC CONTINUUM OF THE DUCTAL SHUNT IN PRETERM INFANTS

During fetal life, low systemic vascular resistance (SVR) due to the low resistance placenta, combined with elevated PVR, results in pulmonary artery–to-aorta ("right-to-left") flow across the DA. During normal neonatal transition, increased SVR associated with umbilical cord clamping occurs in parallel to a longitudinal decrease in PVR precipitated by ventilation of the lungs and an increase in pulmonary blood flow. The degree of right-to-left ductal shunt is approximately 50% within 5 minutes of birth, becoming mostly left to right by 10 to 20 minutes, and is entirely left to right by 24 hours of age in most healthy neonates.[54,55]

In preterm neonates the size and direction of the ductal shunt will have a variable impact on pulmonary and systemic hemodynamics. The role of the PDA shunt may be conceptualized within a physiologic continuum that extends from a life-sustaining conduit, neutral bystander, to a pathologic entity. In infants with critical congenital heart disease patency of the DA may be necessary to support pulmonary (e.g., tricuspid atresia) or systemic (e.g., critical aortic stenosis) blood flow. In acute pulmonary hypertension (aPH) of the newborn postnatal failure of pulmonary arterioles to relax (e.g., due to asphyxia, respiratory distress syndrome) results in high PVR and persistence of a right-to-left ductal shunt. The latter shunt may reduce right ventricular afterload and support post-ductal systemic blood flow, albeit with deoxygenated blood. PDA closure in this setting will negatively impact RV function and the adequacy of systemic blood flow. A bidirectional shunt in milder cases of aPH may play a neutral role, merely permitting the noninvasive estimation of the systemic-pulmonary pressure gradient.

If the DA remains patent after birth, preterm infants who experience the expected fall in PVR may be susceptible to the effects of a large systemic-to-pulmonary (left-to-right) shunt. Blood flows across the PDA continuously in systole and diastole, resulting in volume overload of the pulmonary artery, pulmonary veins, and left heart. Shunt volume ($Q$) is directly proportional to the fourth power of the ductal radius ($r$) and the aortopulmonary pressure gradient and is inversely proportional to the ductal length ($L$) and blood viscosity ($n$). It is important to consider the relative contributions of each component to shunt volume.

Increased pulmonary blood flow (termed pulmonary overcirculation) may lead to alveolar edema, reduced pulmonary compliance, and increased need for respiratory support.[56] Increased blood flow to the left heart results in dilatation and increased end-diastolic pressures in the left ventricle and atrium. In preterm infants with intrinsic immaturity of LV compliance and diastolic function, the increase in end-diastolic pressure may contribute to the evolution of pulmonary venous hypertension and pulmonary hemorrhage. The increase in pulmonary blood flow, due to a large left-to-right shunt, occurs at the expense of systemic blood flow (referred to as ductal steal), which may result in end-organ hypoperfusion and consequential morbidities (e.g. necrotizing enterocolitis, acute tubular necrosis).[57] In addition, ductal steal from the descending aorta, shorter diastolic and coronary perfusion times due to tachycardia, and increased myocardial oxygen demand may result in subendocardial ischemia. This pathophysiologic cascade is thought to explain, at least in part, the relation between a PDA and adverse outcomes.

## Myocardial Adaptation in Preterm Infants to Patent Ductus Arteriosus

Cardiac output is the result of the interactions between preload, afterload, intrinsic myocardial contractility, and heart rate. Under normal conditions, and in the absence of a PDA, LV output (LVO) in a neonate is in the range of 150–300 mL/min/kg. The presence of a PDA results in increased pulmonary blood flow and both left atrial (LA) and LV volume loading. In a prospective observational study, using two-dimensional speckle tracking echocardiography, most infants with a PDA displayed signs of LA dysfunction due to increased volume load. PDA diameter was found to be an independent contributor to poor LA contraction.[58] Studies have consistently shown a higher LV end-diastolic volume (preload) when the DA is open with a predominantly left-to-right shunting pattern. According to the Starling curve, the increase in myocardial muscle fiber stretch from higher preload augments stroke volume. Indeed, most studies have demonstrated increased LVO in the presence of a PDA with a predominant left-to-right shunt.[59-68] In the presence of a PDA the low-resistance pulmonary vascular bed is in parallel with the systemic vascular bed. This results in a reduction of LV afterload, which, in combination with the increased preload, enhances the myocardium's ability to increase its stroke volume. Traditionally, the presence of a PFO was thought to alter the effects of a PDA on LV stroke volume by exclusively decompressing the left atrium.[69] Interestingly, a recent study has shown that larger atrial communication in the first week of life may be a surrogate marker of hemodynamically significant PDA rather than shunt volume modulator. The presence of a large atrial communication may in fact increase the risk of ventilator requirement and composite outcome of death or CLD.[70]

There are important differences in both the structure and function of the myocardium between preterm and term neonates, and older children and adults. These differences place the immature myocardium at a disadvantage as far as contractility is concerned.[71] Furthermore, because coronary blood flow takes place primarily during diastole, myocardial performance might be adversely affected if diastolic blood pressure is low in the presence of a high-volume PDA shunt. Previous studies have suggested that myocardial ischemia may occur in the presence of a hemodynamically significant PDA (hsPDA).[72] More recently, studies have demonstrated compromised coronary artery perfusion and the presence of high cardiac-specific troponin levels (indicative of myocardial damage) in the presence of a PDA, suggesting a detrimental effect on myocardial perfusion and potential ischemia.[73,74] As premature infants have a less compliant myocardium than term infants, ventricular filling becomes dependent on the late diastolic phase of atrial contraction. In the setting of higher LV preload impaired diastolic function can lead to an increase in LA pressure and secondary pulmonary venous hypertension, potentially creating the biologic milieu that increases the risk of hemorrhagic pulmonary edema.

Some authors have suggested that because higher preload is associated with a greater stretch of myocardial fibers[75]; therefore myocardial contractility should increase in the presence of a PDA concurrent with the increased LVO. On the contrary, the lack of change in myocardial contractility, in the presence of a PDA, could also suggest a relative deterioration of myocardial function based on increased demands. However, using a relatively load-independent measure of myocardial contractility, Barlow et al. showed that hsPDA had no effect on contractility.[76] More recent studies, using more advanced functional parameters such as strain analyses, have also failed to demonstrate worsening function in the presence of the PDA.[77-79] Preservation of LV function occurs despite major changes in LV morphology over the first 4 postnatal weeks. This includes an increase in LA volume, LV end-diastolic volume, sphericity index (indicating a more globular heart), and filling pressure.[80]

The potential impact of a PDA on RV function remains poorly understood. Changes seen in the LV are typically a consequence of pulmonary overcirculation, as described previously. Conversely, systemic hypoperfusion may result in a reduction in RV preload even in the presence of a left-to-right PFO shunt. In addition, prolonged exposure to increased pulmonary blood flow may promote an increase in PVR and a resultant increase in RV afterload. Recent studies have demonstrated reduced RV function as early as day 7 in infants with a large PDA.[81] The clinical relevance of these changes to heart function and morphology and their potential impact on the evolution of PDA-associated morbidities is currently unknown.

## Effects of Patent Ductus Arteriosus on Blood Pressure

Blood pressure (BP) is the product of the interaction between cardiac output and peripheral vascular resistance (see Chapter 3). In general, systolic BP is primarily affected by changes in stroke volume, whereas diastolic BP is mainly reflective of changes in peripheral vascular resistance. Traditionally, low diastolic BP has been considered the hallmark of an hsPDA, and many studies have supported this notion.[66,77] Studies that specifically looked at the relationship between BP and PDA have shown similar decreases in both systolic and diastolic BP (and therefore no change in the pulse pressure), at least during the first postnatal week.[82,83] However, differences in BP and pulse pressure may be influenced by the location of BP measurements, pre- vs post-ductal. Typically, BP is measured from the umbilical arterial catheter (thus post-ductal) in the first postnatal week. Pre-ductal systolic BP is likely to be reflective of the increase in LV preload and higher than post-ductal values in patients with high-volume run-off through the PDA. This may generate discordance in systolic BP measurements, although this physiological hypothesis has yet to be confirmed in clinical trials. Older infants born at weights between 1000 and 1500 g with a PDA have slight, but clinically nonsignificant, decreases in systolic, diastolic, and mean BP. In contrast, infants born at less than 1000 g and with a PDA have both clinically and statistically lower systolic, diastolic, and mean BP but no change in pulse pressure.[83] Because stroke volume increases and vascular resistance decreases in the presence of a PDA, one might expect that systolic BP would be maintained despite the decrease in diastolic pressure. As mentioned previously, the recorded systolic BP in most studies to date is post-ductal, which

is not likely to reflect shunt-driven increases in LVO. In addition, cardiac output, ductal shunt volume, and peripheral resistance were not measured in any of these studies, making it difficult to accurately characterize the pulse pressure changes in the pre- vs post-ductal circulation. Therefore the lack of a discordance in pulse pressure from BP measured through an umbilical arterial line (post-ductal) could be used to exclude the presence of a high-volume PDA shunt. In immature animals a decrease in the diastolic and mean BP occurs even when the shunt is small, whereas a significant decrease in systolic BP occurs only when the PDA shunt is moderate or large.[61] In a more recent cohort of 141 preterm infants, born less than 29 weeks' gestation, systolic BP in infants with a PDA by the first postnatal week was only slightly lower than those without a PDA. It is not clear, however, if the location of BP measurement (pre- vs post-ductal) was consistent. On the contrary, diastolic and mean blood pressure was lower by the end of the first postnatal week, which translates into a higher pulse pressure (Figure 16.1).[1] In this group LVO was higher and diastolic flow in systemic vessels was lower, possibly explaining those findings (Figure 16.2). PDA may also contribute to the development of hypotension, even during the transitional period, in patients with rapid drop in pulmonary vascular resistance. A study found evidence for a possible role of a moderate-large PDA in vasopressor-dependent hypotension.[84] Similarly, PDA is reported to be an independent risk factor for refractory hypotension.[85]

## Effects of a Hemodynamically Significant Patent Ductus Arteriosus on Organ Perfusion

Despite the ability of the LV to increase its output in the face of a left-to-right PDA shunt, organ blood flow distribution is significantly altered. Interestingly, redistribution of systemic blood flow occurs even with small shunts.[61] Blood flow to the skin, bone, and skeletal muscle is most likely to be affected first by the left-to-right shunt. The organs affected thereafter are the gastrointestinal tract and kidneys, due to a combination of decreased perfusion pressure (ductal steal) and localized vasoconstriction (compensatory measure). Indeed, mesenteric blood flow is decreased in

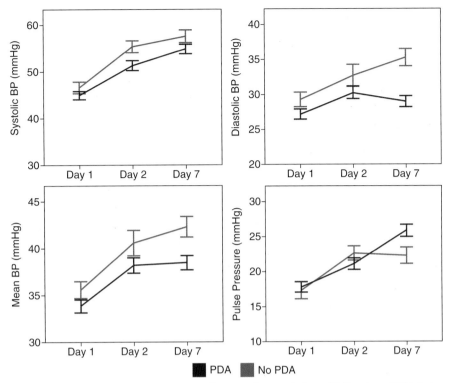

**Fig. 16.1 Changes in systolic, diastolic, mean, and pulse pressure in patent ductus arteriosus (PDA) and non-PDA infants over the first week of age.** PDA infants represent those with a PDA greater than 1.5 mm on day 7 of age. Data represent means and standard error. *BP*, Blood pressure. (Data modified from El-Khuffash A, James AT, Corcoran JD, et al. A patent ductus arteriosus severity score predicts chronic lung disease or death before discharge. *J Pediatr.* 2015;167[6]:1354–1361.)

both fasting and fed states in the presence of a PDA.[86] Clinically important decreases in blood flow to these organs may occur before there are signs of LV compromise.[65,66] In addition, treatment strategies used to facilitate closure of the PDA, such as indomethacin, may have an effect on organ blood flow independent of the hemodynamic changes associated with the presence of an hsPDA.[87] Data from a large national database, however, showed that the risk of necrotizing enterocolitis (NEC) was lower in patients with a PDA who received indomethacin vs those who remained untreated.[88]

Although cerebral blood flow (CBF) has also been assessed by near-infrared spectroscopy (NIRS) and magnetic resonance imaging (MRI) (see later and Chapter 13), blood flow velocity, measured by the Doppler technique, has been the most frequently used technique to assess changes in organ blood flow in the human neonate. In animal experimental models

organ blood flow has also been measured by the microsphere technique or direct flow measurements. As discussed in Chapter 12 in detail, each of these techniques has significant limitations. Unfortunately, it is not currently feasible to continuously measure absolute blood flow to different organs in human neonates.

Using the Doppler technique with ultrasonography, the amount of blood flowing through a vessel is a function of both the vessel diameter and mean blood flow velocity. Because of the small size of the neonatal blood vessels (e.g., anterior cerebral artery [ACA] or middle cerebral artery [MCA]), accurate measurement of vessel diameter is not possible. In addition, the Doppler technique assumes that the diameter of the vessel remains constant during the cardiac cycle, a notion that has been repeatedly challenged. Despite these limitations, Doppler velocity measurements and velocity-derived indices have been shown to have

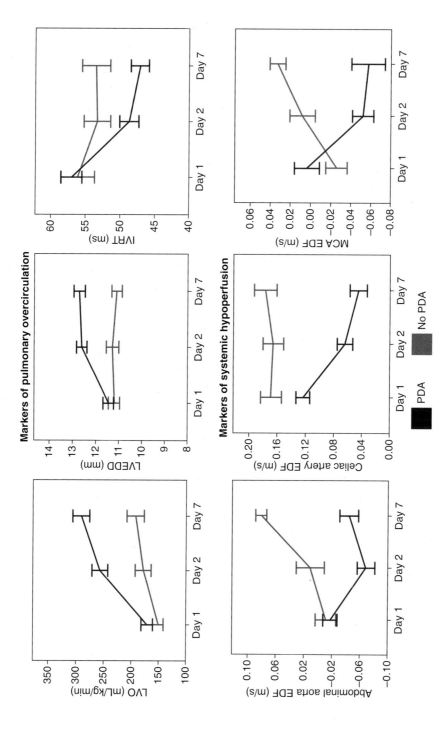

**Fig. 16.2 Patterns of echocardiography markers in infants with and without a patent ductus arteriosus (*PDA*) over the first week of age.** Divergence in echocardiography parameters becomes apparent within the first 48 hours following birth. "PDA infants" represents those with a PDA of greater than 1.5 mm on day 7 of age. Data represent means and standard error. *EDF*, End-diastolic frames; *IVRT*, isovolumic relaxation time; *LVEDD*, left ventricle end-diastolic dimension; *LVO*, left ventricular output; *MCA*, middle cerebral artery. (Data modified from El-Khuffash A, James AT, Corcoran JD, et al. A patent ductus arteriosus severity score predicts chronic lung disease or death before discharge. *J Pediatr.* 2015;167[6]:1354–1361.)

acceptable correlations with more invasive measures of organ blood flow.[89-91] The most commonly used Doppler indicators of organ blood flow are systolic, diastolic, and mean blood flow velocities; velocity time integral; pulsatility index (PI); and resistive index (RI). Because the PI and RI are inversely related to flow, and directly related to vascular resistance, an increase in the PI or RI indicates a reduction in organ blood flow and/or an increase in the vascular resistance of the organ.

## IMPACT ON CEREBRAL BLOOD FLOW

Although some studies suggest that CBF is maintained in the presence of an hsPDA,[60,66] most studies have shown a decrease in flow and a disturbance in cerebral hemodynamics.[61] Furthermore, indomethacin, one of the drugs used for pharmacologic closure of the PDA, has a direct, albeit transient, vasoconstrictive effect on the cerebral circulation, which is likely independent of the drug's effect on the COX enzyme.[92,93] Using the Doppler technique, Perlman et al. demonstrated a decrease in diastolic blood flow velocity in the ACA of preterm infants in the presence of hsPDA.[94] Similarly, Lemmers et al. reported that an hsPDA had a negative impact on cerebral oxygenation that resolved after treatment with indomethacin.[95] Investigators have also observed retrograde diastolic flow and increased PI in the ACA in the presence of a PDA.[96] In contrast, Shortland et al. found no difference in ACA CBF velocity between infants with and without a PDA[97]; however, they did report a higher incidence of periventricular leukomalacia (PVL) in the subgroup of infants with retrograde blood flow in the ACA.[97] One additional study showed progressive reduction in MCA end-diastolic flow velocity during the first postnatal week in extremely preterm infants.[98] These changes contrast sharply to those without a PDA in whom the velocity progressively increased. Correlations between a hsPDA and both end-diastolic velocity and RI in the ACA have also been made in very-low-birth-weight (VLBW) infants.[99] These data suggest that CBF progressively decreases as left-to-right shunts across the PDA become larger. An alternative hypothesis is that, in the face of sustained exposure to a high-volume PDA shunt, the consequential increase in preductal cardiac output (hence cerebral perfusion) leads to remodeling of cerebral arterioles. Theoretically,

the consequential increase in cerebral vascular resistance may limit the effective cerebral tissue perfusion; this hypothesis remains unproven. In preterm lambs[60] and humans[66] CBF is maintained at a constant level in the presence of a PDA, as long as LVO is increased. It appears that the increase in cardiac output, at least to a certain point, ensures adequate cerebral perfusion (albeit with an altered pattern) in patients with a PDA. Indeed, Baylen et al. reported a decrease in CBF when cardiac output was compromised in preterm lambs with a PDA.[67] However, there is no clear evidence to support the association of abnormal RI or other Doppler parameters in the cerebral arteries with brain injury and long-term neurodevelopmental outcome in the preterm infant.[100]

Furthermore, a hemodynamically significant PDA is an independent predictor of low SVC flow (a surrogate for systemic blood flow and perhaps CBF) in preterm infants.[101] This effect on SVC flow appears isolated to the first 12 hours after birth. Even in the term neonate during the first few minutes after birth, the rapid change in ductal shunting to a left-to-right pattern may affect CBF, as suggested by the strong inverse relationship between net left-to-right ductal shunting and MCA mean velocity.[54] This finding supports the notion that absence of a compensatory increase in cardiac output may be, at least in part, responsible for the low CBF associated with a PDA in preterm neonates.

## IMPACT ON SUPERIOR MESENTERIC AND CELIAC ARTERY BLOOD FLOW

Intestinal hypoperfusion is a known risk factor for NEC. Studies evaluating blood flow to the abdominal organs in general, and to the superior mesenteric artery (SMA) in particular, have uniformly demonstrated a decrease in blood flow in the presence of an hsPDA. Diastolic flow reversal in the descending aorta has been reported as early as 4 hours after birth; specifically, flow reversal can be seen in 34% and 46% of very preterm infants with a large PDA, at 12 and 24 hours after birth, respectively.[102] In addition, administration of indomethacin appears to directly reduce not only CBF but also intestinal blood flow.

Observational studies of preterm lambs, performed during the first 10 hours after delivery,[61] demonstrate that even small ductal shunts (those <40% of the

LVO) cause major reductions in blood flow to the abdominal organs. The decrease in organ blood flow occurs despite an increase in cardiac output and is due to the combined effects of decreased perfusion pressure and localized vasoconstriction. Similar findings were also reported by other investigators.[67] In premature primates mesenteric blood flow is decreased in both fasting and fed states in the presence of a PDA.[86] Despite the changes in blood flow, oxygen consumption in the terminal ileum appears to be unaffected by the presence of a PDA in preterm lambs.[65]

Similar findings have been reported in premature human infants. Martin et al. reported retrograde diastolic flow in the descending aorta of preterm infants with a large PDA, which resolved after closure of the DA.[96] Similarly, Deeg et al.[103] and Coombs et al.[104] demonstrated a decrease in both the systolic and diastolic blood flow velocities in the SMA and celiac artery in preterm infants with a PDA. The diastolic blood flow abnormalities appeared to be greater in the SMA.[104] Using ultrasound, Shimada et al. assessed LVO and abdominal aortic blood flow in VLBW infants before and after ductal closure and compared the findings with those obtained in patients without a

PDA (Figure 16.3).[66] Despite a higher LVO, postductal aortic flow was lower in the PDA group than in the controls. A marked increase in abdominal aortic blood flow was noted after PDA closure. These changes in intestinal perfusion have led to concerns when feeding infants with a PDA. Moreover, a recent prospective echocardiography study investigated the impact of red blood cell transfusion on PVR, systemic vascular resistance, myocardial function, and cerebral/splanchnic tissue oxygenation using NIRS in premature babies with and without a PDA. Infants in the PDA group had lower splanchnic oxygen saturations at baseline compared to the PDA closed group, which persisted over the study period and were unaltered by transfusion.[105]

As mentioned earlier, indomethacin also affects mesenteric blood flow[104,106] and compromises the premature intestine's ability to autoregulate its oxygen consumption.[65] On the other hand, ibuprofen, another nonselective COX inhibitor, mediates PDA closure without affecting mesenteric blood flow.[107] A recent meta-analysis comparing ibuprofen treatment of a PDA with indomethacin treatment suggests that ibuprofen may be associated with a lower incidence

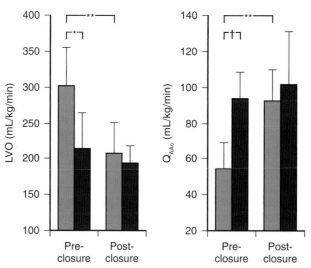

**Fig. 16.3 Left ventricular output (LVO) and blood flow volume of the abdominal aorta ($Q_{AAo}$) before and after closure of ductus arteriosus by mefenamic acid.** *Light red bars* represent the values for hemodynamically significant patent ductus arteriosus (hsPDA) group; *dark red bars* represent the values for group without hsPDA. Values are expressed as mean ± SD. *P < 0.002; **P < 0.001; †P < 0.0001. (From Shimada S, Kasai T, Konishi M, Fujiwara T. Effects of patent ductus arteriosus on left ventricular output and organ blood flows in preterm infants with respiratory distress syndrome treated with surfactant. *J Pediatr.* 1994;125:270–277.)

of NEC while being equally effective in producing PDA closure.[87]

## IMPACT ON PULMONARY BLOOD FLOW

The decreased ability of the preterm infant to maintain active pulmonary vasoconstriction[108] may be responsible, at least in part, for the pulmonary consequences of a "large" left-to-right PDA shunt in preterm infants relatively early after delivery.[109,110] Therapeutic maneuvers, such as surfactant replacement or inhaled nitric oxide, or prenatal conditions, such as intrauterine growth retardation, that lead to or are associated with an accelerated postnatal decrease in PVR can exacerbate the amount of left-to-right shunt and might result in an increased incidence of pulmonary hemorrhage.[111-113]

In premature animals a wide-open PDA increases the hydraulic pressures in the pulmonary vasculature, which in turn increases the rate of fluid transudation into the pulmonary interstitium.[114] Any increase in pulmonary microvascular perfusion pressure in premature infants with respiratory distress syndrome may also increase interstitial and alveolar lung fluid because of their low plasma oncotic pressures and increased capillary permeability. Leakage of plasma proteins into the developing lungs inhibits surfactant function and increases surface tension in the immature air sacs,[115] which are already compromised by surfactant deficiency. The increased fraction of inspired oxygen ($FiO_2$) and mean airway pressures required to overcome these early changes in compliance may contribute to the development of chronic lung disease.[116-118] Depending on the GA, and the species examined, changes in pulmonary mechanics may occur as early as 1 day after birth or not before several days of exposure to the left-to-right PDA shunt.[119,120]

Although it is true that preterm animals with a PDA have increased fluid and protein clearance into the lung interstitium, due to an increase in pulmonary microvascular filtration pressure, a simultaneous increase in lung lymph flow appears to eliminate the excess fluid and protein from the lungs.[114] This compensatory increase in lung lymph flow acts as an "edema safety factor," inhibiting fluid accumulation in the lungs. As a result, there is no net increase in water or protein accumulation in the lungs and there is no change in pulmonary mechanics.[118,120-123] This

delicate balance between PDA-induced fluid filtration and lymphatic reabsorption is consistent with the observation, made in human infants, that closure of the DA within the first 24 hours after birth has no effect on the course of hyaline membrane disease. However, if lung lymphatic drainage is impaired, alveolar epithelial permeability is altered, and the likelihood of pulmonary and alveolar edema increases dramatically. After several days of mechanical ventilation, the residual functioning lymphatics are more easily overwhelmed by the same size ductus shunt that is well accommodated on the first day after delivery. As a result, it is not uncommon for infants with a persistent PDA to develop pulmonary edema and alterations in pulmonary mechanics at 7 to 10 days after birth. In these infants improvement in lung compliance occurs following closure of the PDA.[118,124-128]

Not all of the changes associated with a PDA are necessarily detrimental to the immature infant with respiratory distress. The recirculation of oxygenated arterial blood through lungs that are not fully expanded can lead to improved levels of arterial partial pressure of oxygen ($PaO_2$).[61,129] Conversely, decreases in systemic arterial $O_2$ content have been observed following PDA closure, despite the absence of any alterations in pulmonary mechanics.

### Impact on Pulmonary Vascular Resistance

A persistent increase in pulmonary blood flow over a prolonged period delays the normal maturation of pulmonary blood vessels, which may lead to proliferation and hypertrophy of smooth muscle and the development of pulmonary vascular disease. In addition to abnormal shear stress and circumferential wall stretch to the pulmonary vasculature, there is endothelial cell dysfunction and an imbalance in the vasoactive mediators such as endothelin-1, prostacyclin, and nitric oxide that cause vasoconstriction. There is also increased intracellular matrix deposition and vascular remodeling involving smooth muscle hypertrophy and proliferation due to abnormal expression of fibroblast and vascular endothelial growth factors.[130] Animal studies have shown that the pulmonary overcirculation model leads to increased mean pulmonary arterial pressure and thickening of the pulmonary artery media similar to that seen in premature infants with pulmonary hypertension.[131]

Preterm infants with significant left-to-right shunt due to PDA might be at risk of pulmonary vascular remodeling, which may lead to RV dysfunction. Evidence from hemodynamic evaluation via cardiac catheterization, performed at the time of percutaneous device closure, revealed that infants referred for intervention at a postnatal age >8 weeks compared to <4 weeks postnatal age had higher PVR.[132] Evidence from pediatric literature has shown that persistence of an hsPDA beyond a year leads to intimal thickening and that beyond 2 years to fibrosis. In at least 50% of patients with a chronic large untreated hsPDA, irreversible pulmonary vascular changes may occur by 2 years of age.[133] Moreover, it is unclear if late spontaneous closure occurs through normal postnatal developmental mechanisms or secondary to pulmonary vascular remodeling due to pulmonary overcirculation. A recent study has shown that a nonintervention PDA treatment policy was associated with an increased occurrence of chronic pulmonary hypertension in infants with bronchopulmonary dysplasia (BPD).[134]

### Associations of PDA to Mortality and Morbidities

Persistence of PDA has been associated with numerous adverse outcomes, although a definitive causal link between these associations has yet to be demonstrated.[135] Associations with adverse outcomes are reported in observational studies. Noori et al and Sellmer et al showed that failure of ductal closure was associated with an increase in mortality in very preterm infants.[136,137] Many reports have linked PDA with an increased risk of BPD. El-Khuffash and colleagues have demonstrated that markers of increased PDA shunt volume on postnatal day 2 can reliably predict later occurrence of death/BPD in extremely preterm infants.[138] In an Italian cohort each week of a hemodynamically significant PDA represented an added risk for BPD, while the duration of a nonsignificant PDA did not. In patients who received ligation later intervention and prolonged PDA exposure were the only factors associated with BPD or death.[139] PDA was shown to be an independent risk factor for the development of necrotizing enterocolitis in VLBW infants.[88] Some studies have reported an increased risk of intraventricular hemorrhage[137]; however, many reports have

failed to show an effect of PDA on incidence of abnormal cranial ultrasound.[140,141]

## Clinical and Radiologic Diagnosis of Patent Ductus Arteriosus

The emergence of detectable clinical signs of PDA occurs when PVR declines and both left heart volume loading and systemic arterial diastolic "steal" ensue. Cardiomegaly and tachycardia result in an active precordium, and diastolic hypotension leads to a wide pulse pressure and bounding central pulses and easily palpable peripheral pulses (e.g., palmar pulses).[142] A holosystolic murmur of irregular intensity is typically audible at the upper left sternal border. Pulmonary overcirculation manifests as radiographic engorgement, increased need for supplemental oxygen, and increased work of breathing. The clinical signs of PDA are generally apparent beyond the first postnatal week but lag behind the echocardiography diagnosis of an hsPDA by several days.[143]

A large left-to-right ductal shunt results in pulmonary overcirculation and left heart enlargement, which projects as LA and ventricular dilatation and increased pulmonary vascular markings on chest radiographs (Figure 16.4). The electrocardiogram may demonstrate sinus tachycardia, LA enlargement, and left ventricular hypertrophy. Smaller shunts may be associated with a normal radiograph and electrocardiogram. Of note, the electrocardiogram is not a reliable screening tool to identify an hsPDA.[144]

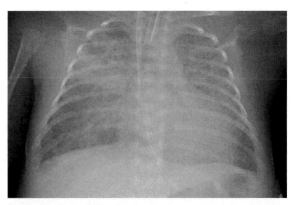

**Fig. 16.4 Chest radiograph in a ventilated preterm infant with a large patent ductus arteriosus.** Note the *large heart shadow* and the *increased lung markings* representing pulmonary overcirculation.

# Echocardiographic Diagnosis and Assessment of a Patent Ductus Arteriosus

Ultrasound is the most reliable method of evaluating a PDA and has become the mainstay for diagnosis, disease staging, and treatment response monitoring. Evaluation and staging of DA shunt severity requires assessment of ductal size, transductal Doppler flow pattern, indices of pulmonary overcirculation and left heart volume loading, and surrogate markers of systemic hypoperfusion. Traditional assessments of the hemodynamic significance of a PDA have relied substantially on ductal diameter alone. Although ductal diameter is one of the most important determinants of ductal shunt volume (owing to the exponential relationship between ductal radius and flow), the use of ductal diameter, in isolation, to determine the hemodynamic significance of the ductal shunt should be avoided due to the potential for measurement error and the poor outcome-predictive ability of diameter alone. A comprehensive echocardiographic evaluation provides a more holistic picture, with redundancies to mitigate measurement error within the individual echo parameters (Tables 16.1 and 16.2).

## DUCTUS ARTERIOSUS SIZE AND TRANSDUCTAL DOPPLER FLOW PATTERN

Ductal diameter on two-dimensional echocardiography ≥1.5 mm on the first day after birth predicts the development of a clinically symptomatic PDA.[145] Ductal size indexed for body weight may be more predictive of hsPDA compared to absolute value of ductal size.[146] An hsPDA is characterized by an unrestrictive or arterial left-to-right flow pattern, with a very low diastolic velocity. Peak systolic velocity (PSV) of less than 1.5 m/s has been traditionally described as "unrestrictive." On the other hand, clinicians should

## TABLE 16.1 Echocardiography Parameters of PDA Hemodynamic Significance in Extremely Preterm Infants (<29 Weeks' Gestation) After the First Postnatal Day

| Parameter[a] | HEMODYNAMIC SIGNIFICANCE | | |
| --- | --- | --- | --- |
| | Mild | Moderate | Severe |
| **PDA Diameter** | | | |
| 2D diameter (mm) | <1.5 | 1.5–3 | >3 |
| PDA to LPA ratio | <0.5 | 0.5–1 | >1 |
| **PDA Doppler** | | | |
| Vmax (m/s) | >2.5 | 1.5–2.5 | <1.5 |
| Systolic to diastolic velocity ratio | <2 | 2–4 | >4 |
| LV chamber dilatation (Z score) | <+2.0 | +2.0 to +3.0 | >+3.0 |
| **Pulmonary Overcirculation** | | | |
| LA to Ao ratio | <1.5 | 1.5–2.0 | >2.0 |
| Mitral valve E to A ratio | <1 | <1 | >1 |
| IVRT (milliseconds) | >40 | 30–40 | <30 |
| LPA Vmax diastole (m/s) | <0.3 | 0.3–0.5 | >0.5 |
| LVO (mL/kg/min) | <200 | 200–300 | >300 |
| PV D wave (m/s) | <0.35 | 0.35–0.45 | >0.45 |
| **Systemic Hypoperfusion** | | | |
| Abdominal Ao diastolic flow | Forward | Reversed | Reversed |
| Celiac artery diastolic flow | Forward | Absent | Reversed |
| MCA diastolic flow | Forward | Forward | Absent/Reversed |

*2D*, Two-dimensional; *Ao*, aorta; *IVRT*, isovolumic relaxation time; *LA*, left atrium; *LPA*, left pulmonary artery; *LV*, left ventricle; *LVO*, left ventricular output; *MCA*, middle cerebral artery; *PDA*, patent ductus arteriosus; *PV*, pulmonary vein; *Vmax*, maximum velocity.
[a]Applies beyond the first 48 hours.

**TABLE 16.2 Interobserver Variability for Echocardiography Parameters**

| Parameter | Correlation Coefficient |
|---|---|
| Ductal diameter | 0.85 (0.68–0.94)[a] |
| Left pulmonary artery diameter | 0.62 (0.34–0.80)[a] |
| E to A ratio | 0.90 (0.77–0.95)[a] |
| IVRT | 0.84 (0.63–0.93)[a] |
| Aortic diameter | 0.99 (0.80–0.95)[a] |
| Aortic velocity time index | 0.79 (0.63–0.90)[a] |
| Left ventricular output | 0.97 (0.94–0.99)[a] |
| LV end-diastolic diameter | 0.93 (0.86–0.97)[a] |
| LA to Ao ratio | 0.65 (0.44–0.82)[a] |
| Descending aorta diastolic flow | 0.75 (0.43–1.00)[a] |
| Celiac diastolic flow | 0.88 (0.65–1.00)[a] |

*Ao*, Aorta; *IVRT*, isovolumic relaxation time; *LA*, left atrium; *LV*, left ventricle.
[a]Lin's concordance correlation coefficient.
[b]Kappa coefficient.

recall that PSV may be elevated (>2.0 m/s) either in the setting of a restrictive ductal shunt or due to a very high-volume shunt promoted by low PVR. Peak PDA systolic velocity should be interpreted in tandem with the "pulsatility" of the PDA Doppler pattern, which can be quantified using the ratio of the PDA PSV to minimum diastolic velocity (MDV).[147] The Doppler profile of a *restrictive PDA* is characterized by a high-velocity shunt throughout systole and diastole and a low PSV to MDV ratio (Figure 16.5). In addition, transductal velocity ratio (PSV ratio of the pulmonary end over the aortic end of the ductus) has been shown to correlate with other indices of hemodynamic significance of PDA and has been proposed as a measure of the degree of ductal constriction.[148]

## PULMONARY OVERCIRCULATION AND LEFT HEART LOADING

Pulmonary artery Doppler patterns and left heart inflow, dilatation, and output are surrogate markers of the pulmonary–to–systemic blood flow ratio (Qp to Qs). Left pulmonary artery antegrade diastolic velocity greater than 0.3 m/s correlates with a moderate PDA.[149] LVO of greater than 300 mL/kg/min on the first day after delivery predicts a later symptomatic PDA.[145] Subsequently, infants with a symptomatic PDA have significantly higher LVO (419 [305 to 562] mL/kg/min)

than infants without PDA (221 ± 56 mL/kg/min), and LVO returns to normal after surgical ligation (246 [191–292] mL/kg/min).[150,151]

LV end-diastolic dimension (LVEDD), a surrogate for LV end-diastolic volume, is increased in infants with PDA and has been correlated with the need for medical and surgical treatment.[152] LVEDD increases with patient weight and may be compared with normative data from extremely preterm infants, although LVEDD greater than 15 mm/kg approximates the upper limit of normal.[152] In infants with a left-to-right shunt across the PDA LA dilatation occurs due to volume loading from excessive pulmonary venous return. The LA to aortic root ratio (LA:Ao) is a commonly used echocardiographic index of LA dilatation. A recent study of preterm infants less than 30 weeks' gestation showed ductal size >2.0 mm and LA:Ao >1.4, especially in combination, which are associated with a greater risk of abnormal organ blood flows.[153] Indeed, an LA:Ao ratio greater than 1.5 has high sensitivity for a symptomatic PDA but is poorly predictive on the first postnatal day and may be unreliable in the presence of a large transatrial shunt that may unload the left heart (Figure 16.6).[154] Recent echocardiography data has shown that atrial communication >1 mm in patients with a PDA ≥1.5 mm, during the first postnatal week, may be a marker of a more pathologic hsPDA and may have consequences to left heart volume loading in premature infants.[70] Another marker of left heart volume, pulmonary vein wave velocity, can be measured in the presence of PDA. The flow pattern of pulmonary veins, systolic (S wave), diastolic (D wave), and atrial contraction (A wave), can be obtained by applying a pulsed wave Doppler. Although there is currently limited data for this variable, a peak velocity cut-off of 0.5 m/s for the D wave may be present with moderate to severe shunt.[155,156] An important caveat is that peak velocity may fall as the vein dilates with progressive increases in pulmonary blood flow. The early phase of filling (E wave) in preterm infants has a lower velocity than the late phase (A wave), resulting in an E to A wave ratio of less than 1. This relates to developmental immaturity of the preterm myocardium and impaired diastolic performance, therein limiting early diastolic flow. LA pressure loading occurs due to progressive LV diastolic dysfunction associated with very large

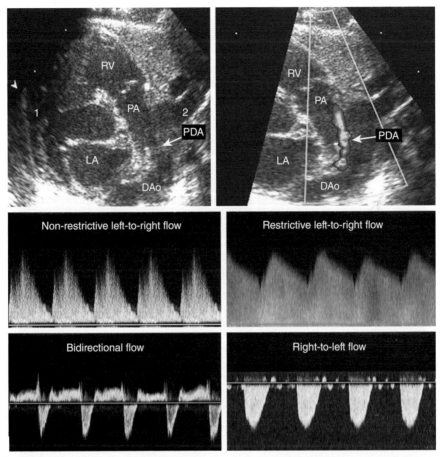

**Fig. 16.5  Patent ductus arteriosus (*PDA*) two-dimensional (*2D*), color Doppler image, and Doppler flow patterns.** The *top panel* demonstrates the PDA in 2D and color Doppler. *Pulsatile or nonrestrictive pattern:* characterized by a left-to-right shunt with an arterial waveform and high peak systolic velocity to end-diastolic velocity ratio. *Restrictive pattern:* characterized by high systolic and diastolic velocity and low peak systolic velocity to end-diastolic velocity ratio. *Bidirectional pattern:* elevated pulmonary pressures equal to or near systemic pressures; *Right-to-left flow pattern:* suprasystemic pulmonary pressures. *DAo,* descending aorta; *LA,* left atrium; *RV,* right ventricle; *PA,* pulmonary artery.

volume PDA shunts and drives early passive diastolic LV filling, resulting in a mitral E to A wave ratio greater than 1.[157] In addition, earlier mitral valve opening in the presence of higher left atrial pressure results in a shortened isovolumic relaxation time (<40 ms). (Figure 16.7).[158]

## SYSTEMIC ARTERIAL DIASTOLIC FLOW REVERSAL

Ultrasound can be used to provide an estimate of systemic hypoperfusion by assessing Doppler flow patterns in certain blood vessels that are affected by ductal steal, namely, the abdominal aorta, the celiac trunk, and the MCA. Diastolic flow reversal in the abdominal aorta is the measurement that best correlates with cardiac MRI estimates of ductal shunt volume.[102] Reduced celiac artery flow (CAF), quantified as a CAF to LVO ratio of less than 0.1, correlates well with conventional echocardiography indices of the hemodynamic significance of the PDA.[159] Aberrant diastolic flows in the SMA and MCA have been associated with a PDA shunt and improve after PDA ligation. However, their relevance to neonatal and neurodevelopmental outcomes is presently unknown.[160]

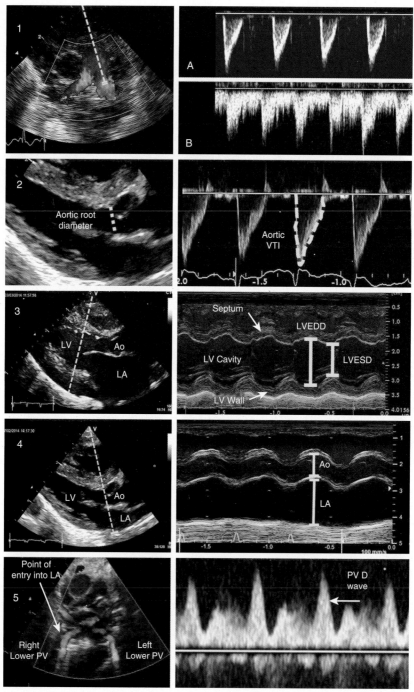

**Fig. 16.6  Assessment of pulmonary overcirculation.** (1) Measurement of diastolic flow in the left pulmonary artery. *Panel (B)* illustrates forward diastolic flow in the presence of significant left-to-right ductal flow. (2) Measurement of left ventricular output (*LVO*): increased LVO in the setting of a PDA indicates increased pulmonary venous return. (3) Measurement of LV diameter in diastole: increased LV diameter is another surrogate marker for increased LV end-diastolic volume. (4) LA to Ao ratio: atrial enlargement can be indexed to a relatively fixed aortic root diameter to further estimate the degree of increased LA volume. *Ao,* Aorta; *LA,* left atrium; *LV,* left ventricle; *LVEDD,* left ventricle end-diastolic dimension; *LVESD,* left ventricle end-systolic dimension; *PDA,* patent ductus arteriosus; *PV,* pulmonary vein; *VTI,* velocity time integral.

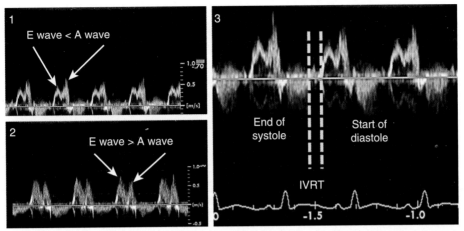

Fig. 16.7 **Pulsed wave Doppler of left ventricular inflow across the mitral valve, demonstrating the early ("E") and late ("A," during atrial contraction) ventricular filling velocities.** Transmitral valve left ventricle (LV) filling in normal-term infants is characterized by a predominance of early diastolic ("E") filling, with limited late LV filling occurring during atrial contraction ("A"), resulting in an E to A ratio greater than 1.0. (1) Healthy preterm infants without a patent ductus arteriosus (*PDA*) have intrinsically decreased LV diastolic function, relying more on late atrial filling, and E to A ratio less than 1.0. (2 and 3) Preterm infants with a large PDA have increased left atrial pressure, which results in earlier mitral valve opening and drives early passive filling, leading to shortened isovolumetric relaxation time (<40 ms) and a "pseudonormalized" E to A ratio greater than 1.0. *IVRT*, Isovolumic relaxation time.

## The Use of Biomarkers in Patent Ductus Arteriosus Assessment: Brain Natriuretic Peptide and N-Terminal Pro–Brain Natriuretic Peptide

In response to volume and pressure loading, myocytes in the left and right ventricles cleave pro–brain natriuretic peptide (BNP) into the biologically active BNP and the inactive amino-terminal pro-BNP (NT-pBNP). BNP promotes natriuresis and diuresis to counteract the effects of LV volume loading secondary to a significant PDA. Studies have evaluated the reliability of BNP and NTpBNP measurements in various potential roles in clinical care, including the replacement of echocardiography for the diagnosis of PDA, the assessment of treatment response, the triage of patients for early targeted PDA screening, or as an add-on to echocardiography. The interpretation and integration of BNP and NTpBNP measurements into clinical care is hampered by the availability of multiple testing kits, each with a discrete reference range and published results, in observational studies correlating these biomarkers with the development of a PDA.

## BRAIN NATRIURETIC PEPTIDE/N-TERMINAL PRO–BRAIN NATRIURETIC PEPTIDE AND THE DIAGNOSIS OF PRESYMPTOMATIC PATENT DUCTUS ARTERIOSUS

The early identification of asymptomatic ductal shunting would be clinically useful in centers seeking to administer targeted indomethacin prophylaxis but who have limited access to echocardiography. Umbilical cord concentrations of BNP are positively correlated with the subsequent postnatal development of symptomatic PDA.[161] In addition, NTpBNP concentrations on day 1 are inversely proportional to decreasing GA but are nonspecific for the diagnosis of PDA.[162] These findings suggest that factors other than PDA contribute to in utero and early postnatal changes in BNP/NTpBNP (such as elevated pulmonary pressures).

Both BNP and NTpBNP are predictive of an hsPDA after the second postnatal day and may be used to triage patients for echocardiography evaluation or empiric therapy. Several cutoffs exist in the literature for both BNP and NTpBNP for the identification of a PDA. However, translation to clinical use is hampered by heterogeneity of the studies, the variety of cutoffs used based on the analytic method or exact timing of sampling, and the increasing availability of echocardiography in many neonatal intensive care units (NICUs).[163-165] In addition, infants with a PDA who respond to indomethacin treatment have greater absolute and relative decreases in BNP and NTpBNP than non-responders. However, there is significant overlap in the serum concentrations of these biomarkers among responders and non-responders, meaning that echocardiography follow-up cannot be reliably replaced.

## Near-Infrared Spectroscopy and Patent Ductus Arteriosus Assessment

NIRS offers the ability to perform noninvasive assessments of target organ blood flow, in particular, the brain and splanchnic circulation.[166] The ability to assess cerebral and mesenteric perfusion in real time may offer the ability to better appraise the hemodynamic impact a PDA has on these organs. This may also provide an enhanced insight into the pathologic basis for the associations between the PDA and important morbidities, aid in triaging PDAs into pathologic versus innocent bystanders, and help to determine which patients warrant treatment. NIRS may also enable the treating physician to monitor treatment response.

Studies using NIRS in infants with a PDA have, however, yielded mixed results. Early evidence of the application of NIRS in PDA assessment, from a pilot study of 29 infants, suggested that infants with a PDA necessitating treatment had lower pretreatment renal and skeletal muscle regional saturations. Following treatment, regional saturations "increased toward the range seen in patients who did not require treatment of a PDA."[167] Consistent with this finding, another study found lower cerebral oxygen saturation and higher extraction in the presence of PDA, with normalization of these values 24 hours after starting indomethacin.[83] A recent study of 380 infants, born less than 32 weeks' GA, demonstrated that regional cerebral oxygen saturations were inversely related to PDA diameter, suggesting that a larger ductal diameter may be associated with lower CBF.[168] A prospective study of infants <32 weeks' gestation with hsPDA investigated cerebral NIRS after the first dose of either paracetamol (15 mg/kg) or ibuprofen (10 mg/kg).

Cerebral regional oxygenation and fractional oxygen extraction ratio were not altered in both treatment groups, but resistance index decreased in the ibuprofen group.[169] Another study by van der Laan et al. also failed to demonstrate an association between renal or cerebral regional oxygenation and a hemodynamically significant PDA.[170] On the other hand, a small study found low renal but not cerebral regional oxygen saturation to be associated with a hemodynamically significant DA.[171] The differing results between these studies likely stem from the heterogeneity of the study participants, the timing of assessments, the consistency of adjudication of hemodynamic significance of the PDA, comorbidities, and the positioning of the sensors. Studies to date have not investigated the relationship between PDA shunt volume and changes in regional tissue oxygenation, nor have they investigated the relationship between disturbed regional tissue oxygenation and important PDA-related morbidities.

## Comprehensive Appraisal of the Hemodynamic Significance of the Patent Ductus Arteriosus

A cause-and-effect relationship between a PDA and adverse short- and long-term outcomes has been difficult to elucidate. This may either stem from the possibility that no actual relationship exists or, more likely, the failure (to date) to accurately appraise and identify hemodynamically significant shunts of sufficient *magnitude* and *duration* of exposure to impact end-organ health in a biologically meaningful manner. A multiparametric approach to determination of hemodynamic significance should integrate surrogate measures of the magnitude of shunt volume, the ability of the heart to accommodate and compensate for the shunt, the impact of the shunt on the pulmonary and systemic circulations, and important clinical characteristics that may either enhance or mitigate the potential detrimental effects of a PDA (Figure 16.8). The ability to accurately risk-stratify PDA shunts into those that are innocent bystanders and those likely to be pathologic is greatly enhanced if echocardiographic measurements of ductal characteristics, markers of pulmonary overcirculation, and markers of systemic hypoperfusion are integrated with the clinical status

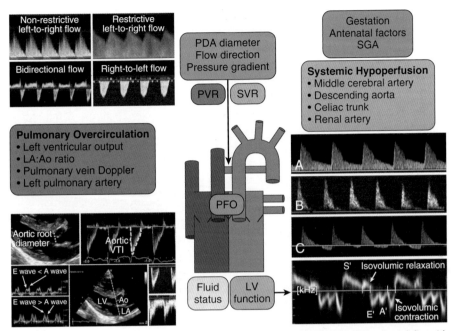

**Fig. 16.8 Determinants of hemodynamic significance of a patent ductus arteriosus (PDA).** Volume of the shunt, left ventricular function, and clinical parameters are all important in determining treatment. *Ao*, Aorta; *LA*, left atrium; *LV*, left ventricle; *PFO*, patent foramen ovale; *PVR*, pulmonary vascular resistance; *SGA*, small for gestational age; *SVR*, systemic vascular resistance; *VTI*, velocity time integral.

to provide a comprehensive picture of the infants' well-being. In addition, each echocardiography measurement is prone to operator and/or equipment-related measurement error, which may be superseded by a multiparametric approach. Surrogate measures of shunt volume, degree of cardiac adaptation to the shunt, pulmonary overcirculation, and systemic hypoperfusion may distinguish hemodynamically significant shunts in the transitional period.[172] In the presence of an open ductus, as PVR falls and shunt volume increases during the first few postnatal days, these echocardiography markers become increasingly more useful in determining the hemodynamic significance of the PDA (Figure 16.9). However, delaying assessment could lead to a prolonged exposure to the potential detrimental effects of a PDA and mitigate the presumed benefits of early treatment.

Gestational age plays an independent role in the evolution of morbidities, and therefore it should be considered an important factor in determining PDA significance. Infants in the lower GA brackets (≤26 weeks) are more likely to be predisposed to the

effects of the pathophysiologic consequences of the PDA. In addition, important antenatal events (such as the administration of steroids, growth restriction, uteroplacental insufficiency) and maternal illness (such as preeclampsia and diabetes) can independently modulate the risk of adverse events in the setting of a PDA. The role of left heart function, in particular diastolic function, is rarely considered. As discussed, shunting into the pulmonary circulation in association with a PDA leads to increased pulmonary venous return and increased LV preload. Left heart diastolic function plays a key role in handling this increased blood volume returning to the heart. Compromised diastolic function secondary to the stiff immature myocardium may contribute to increased pulmonary venous pressure because it cannot accommodate the increased blood return to the left atrium, therefore worsening the effect of increased pulmonary blood flow. Impaired diastolic function in the setting of increased pulmonary venous return will lead to higher LA pressure and eventual pulmonary venous congestion. Therefore, assessment of systolic

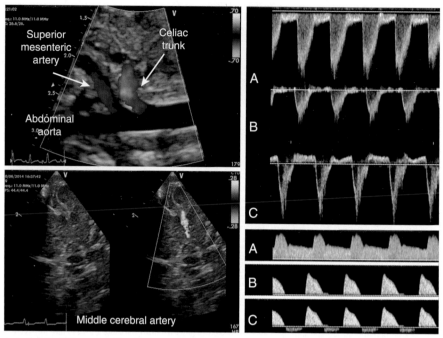

**Fig. 16.9  Assessment of systemic hypoperfusion.** Measurement of pulsed wave Doppler pattern in the celiac trunk, the abdominal aorta, and the middle cerebral artery can highlight the effect of left-to-right shunting across the patent ductus arteriosus. In the *top Doppler panel*, three abdominal aortic Doppler waveforms are illustrated demonstrating normal forward diastolic flow (A), absent diastolic flow (B), and reversed diastolic flow (C). A similar pattern can be seen in the *lower Doppler panel*, which is representative of celiac and middle cerebral arteries.

and diastolic function of LV can provide valuable information on the significance of a PDA. In addition to ultrasound, biomarkers and NIRS may also be used in the future to provide a comprehensive approach to the management of PDA.

There have been recent attempts to devise a comprehensive PDA appraisal approach by relating early PDA characteristics and integrating them with important clinical features to facilitate the prediction of the evolution of PDA-associated morbidities, particularly respiratory morbidities such as BPD. Recent observational studies have demonstrated that a multiparametric echocardiography assessment, applied at 24–48 hours of age, using several separate scoring systems can identify infants with a PDA that went on to develop severe periventricular/intraventricular hemorrhage, BPD, or death.[1,139,173,174] In addition, these markers may be able to predict poor neurodevelopmental outcome associated with a PDA.[175] It is plausible that applying a staging system for ductal disease severity at an earlier time point may facilitate

better-targeted treatment. The predictive value of PDA severity score (PDAsc) based on integration of clinical and echocardiography (36–48 hours) parameters was studied in a recent multicenter prospective observational study of 141 infants born at $26 \pm 1.4$ weeks' GA.[138] GA at birth, PDA diameter and flow velocity, LVO, and LV left diastolic wave (LV A' wave) were independently associated with the composite outcome of death or BPD on multiple logistic regression analysis. PDAsc ranged from 0 (low risk) to 13 (high risk). A cutoff PDAsc of 5.0 had an area under the curve of 0.92 for the ability to predict BPD/death. A PDAsc cutoff of 5.0 has a sensitivity and specificity of 92% and 87%, respectively, and positive and negative predictive values of 92% and 82%, respectively. The use of a PDA score, based on echocardiography parameters, demonstrated that a high composite score correlated with higher incidence of chronic lung disease.[139,176] Other scoring systems are currently being investigated and are summarized in Table 16.3.[177]

## TABLE 16.3  PDA Scoring Systems

| PDA Score | Population | Echocardiography Parameters | Association to Outcomes |
|---|---|---|---|
| McNamara et al.[178] | | Transductal diameter<br>Transductal Flow<br>LA:Ao ratio<br>Mitral regurgitant jet<br>E:A ratio<br>IVRT<br>Diastolic flow in superior mesenteric artery, middle cerebral artery or renal artery | See Sehgal et al. |
| Sehgal et al.[176] | <32 weeks preterm infants | Transductal diameter<br>Ductal velocity<br>PDA:LPA diameter<br>Antegrade PA diastolic flow<br>Antegrade LPA diastolic flow<br>LA:Ao ratio<br>LV:Ao ratio<br>LVO:SVC flow ratio<br>E wave:A wave ratio<br>IVRT | Higher composite scores were associated with increased risk of developing CLD |
| El-Khuffash et al.[138] | <29 weeks preterm infants | PDA diameter<br>Maximum velocity across the PDA shunt<br>LVO<br>LV diastolic function LV free wall: a′ wave using TDI | PDA score on day 2 can predict the later occurrence of CLD/death |
| Rios et al. (Iowa PDA score)[70] | <32 weeks preterm infants | Mitral valve E wave velocity<br>IVRT<br>PV D wave velocity<br>LA:Ao<br>LVO<br>Diastolic flow in descending aorta and/or celiac/ middle cerebral artery<br>Ductal diameter / weight | Increased risk of ventilator requirement and composite outcome of death or CLD |
| SZMC PDA severity score[177] | <29 weeks preterm infants | Ductal diameter<br>LA:Ao ratio<br>Retrograde diastolic flow in the abdominal aorta<br>Ductus arteriosus shunt flow pattern | Associated with composite outcome of CLD/death and with periventricular leukomalacia |
| Elsayed Y et al.[141] | <31 weeks preterm infants | Ductal diameter<br>Peak PDA flow velocity<br>LA:Ao ratio<br>Mitral E:A ratio<br>LVO<br>LVEDD<br>Diastolic aortic flow | PDA score associated with increased odds of survival with any adverse outcome |

*CLD*, Chronic lung disease *IVRT*, isovolumic relaxation time; *LA:Ao*, left atrium diameter to aortic root diameter; *LPA*, left pulmonary artery; *LV*, left ventricle; *LVEDD*, left ventricular end-diastolic dimension; *LVO*, Left ventricular output; *PA*, pulmonary artery; *PV*, pulmonary vein; *SVC*, superior vena cava.

## Summary

PDA is a common problem in VLBW infants. The shunt across the PDA is primarily left to right in the immediate hours after birth. If the DA remains open, it results in a progressive increase in pulmonary overcirculation and left-sided cardiac volume overload, with accompanying systemic hypoperfusion. Despite the immaturity of the myocardium, the heart is capable of augmenting cardiac output even in VLBW neonates. The increase in cardiac output is a result of an increase in stroke volume without a meaningful change in heart rate. Because of the diversion of blood from the aorta to the pulmonary artery, the decrease in post-ductal systolic, diastolic, and mean BP, and the vasoconstriction that occurs in selected vascular beds is such that the increase in LVO does not lead to an increase or even maintenance of *effective* systemic blood flow. Both animal and human studies show compromised organ blood flow patterns, especially to organs supplied by the aorta distal to the PDA. Further research should focus on comprehensive adjudication of hemodynamic significance, the use of newer diagnostic modalities, and the selection of infants with hemodynamically significant shunts of a magnitude such that spontaneous closure is less likely but who would most likely benefit from targeted and effective treatment.

## REFERENCES

1. El-Khuffash A, James AT, Corcoran JD, et al. A patent ductus arteriosus severity score predicts chronic lung disease or death before discharge. *J Pediatr.* 2015;167(6):1354-1361.e2.
2. Hundscheid T, Onland W, van Overmeire B, et al. Early treatment versus expectative management of patent ductus arteriosus in preterm infants: a multicentre, randomised, non-inferiority trial in Europe (BeNeDuctus trial). *BMC Pediatr.* 2018;18:262.
3. Bussmann N, Smith A, Breatnach CR, et al. Patent ductus arteriosus shunt elimination results in a reduction in adverse outcomes: a post hoc analysis of the PDA RCT cohort. *J Perinatol.* 2021; 41:1134-1141.
4. El-Khuffash A, Weisz DE, McNamara PJ. Reflections of the changes in patent ductus arteriosus management during the last 10 years. *Arch Dis Child Fetal Neonatal Ed.* 2016;101(5):F474-F478.
5. Liebowitz M, Katheria A, Sauberan J, et al. PDA-TOLERATE (PDA: TO LEave it alone or respond and treat early) trial investigators. Lack of equipoise in the PDA-TOLERATE Trial: a comparison of eligible infants enrolled in the trial and those treated outside the trial. *J Pediatr.* 2019;213:222-226.
6. Guerguerian AM, Hardy P, Bhattacharya M, et al. Expression of cyclooxygenases in ductus arteriosus of fetal and newborn pigs. *Am J Obstet Gynecol.* 1998;179(6 Pt 1):1618-1626.
7. Hermes-DeSantis ER, Clyman RI. Patent ductus arteriosus: pathophysiology and management. *J Perinatol.* 2006;26(suppl 1): S14-S18.
8. Weir EK, Lopez-Barneo J, Buckler KJ, et al. Acute oxygen-sensing mechanisms. *N Engl J Med.* 2005;353(19):2042-2055.
9. Michelakis ED, Rebeyka I, Wu X, et al. O2 sensing in the human ductus arteriosus: regulation of voltage-gated K+ channels in smooth muscle cells by a mitochondrial redox sensor. *Circ Res.* 2002;91(6):478-486.
10. Francalanci P, Camassei FD, Orzalesi M, et al. CD44-v6 expression in smooth muscle cells in the postnatal remodeling process of ductus arteriosus. *Am J Cardiol.* 2006;97(7):1056-1059.
11. Clyman RI. Mechanisms regulating the ductus arteriosus. *Biol Neonate.* 2006;89(4):330-335.
12. Silver MM, Freedom RM, Silver MD, et al. The morphology of the human newborn ductus arteriosus: a reappraisal of its structure and closure with special reference to prostaglandin E1 therapy. *Hum Pathol.* 1981;12(12):1123-1136.
13. Clyman RI, Chan CY, Mauray F, et al. Permanent anatomic closure of the ductus arteriosus in newborn baboons: the roles of postnatal constriction, hypoxia, and gestation. *Pediatr Res.* 1999;45(1):19-29.
14. Waleh N, Seidner S, McCurnin D, et al. The role of monocyte-derived cells and inflammation in baboon ductus arteriosus remodeling. *Pediatr Res.* 2005;57(2):254-262.
15. Semberova J, Sirc J, Miletin J, et al. Spontaneous closure of patent ductus arteriosus in infants ≤1500 g. *Pediatrics.* 2017;140(2): e20164258.
16. Reller MD, Rice MJ, McDonald RW. Review of studies evaluating ductal patency in the premature infant. *J Pediatr.* 1993; 122(6):S59-S62.
17. Kajino H, Chen YQ, Seidner SR, et al. Factors that increase the contractile tone of the Ductus Arteriosus also regulate its anatomic remodeling. *Am J Physiol Regul Integr Comp Physiol.* 2001;281:R291-R301.
18. Brown S, Liu XT, Ramaekers F, Rosenfeld C. Differential maturation in ductus arteriosus and umbilical artery smooth muscle during ovine development. *Pediatr Res.* 2002;51:34A.
19. Sakurai H, Matsuoka R, Furutani Y, et al. Expression of four myosin heavy chain genes in developing blood vessels and other smooth muscle organs in rabbits. *Eur J Cell Biol.* 1996; 69(2):166-172.
20. Colbert MC, Kirby ML, Robbins J. Endogenous retinoic acid signaling colocalizes with advanced expression of the adult smooth muscle myosin heavy chain isoform during development of the ductus arteriosus. *Circ Res.* 1996;78(5):790-798.
21. Reeve H, Tolarova S, Cornfield D, et al. Developmental changes in K+ channel expression may determine the O2 response of the ductus arteriosus. *FASEB J.* 1997;11:420A.
22. Kajimoto H, Hashimoto K, Bonnet SN, et al. Oxygen activates the Rho/Rho-Kinase pathway and induces RhoB and ROCK-1 expression in human and rabbit ductus arteriosus by increasing mitochondria-derived reactive oxygen species. A newly recognized mechanism for sustaining ductal constriction. *Circulation.* 2007;115:1777-1788.
23. Clyman RI, Waleh NS, Kajino H, et al. Calcium-dependent and calcium-sensitizing pathways in the mature and immature ductus arteriosus. *Am J Physiol Regul Integr Comp Physiol.* 2007; 293(4):R1650-R1656.
24. Cogolludo AL, Moral-Sanz J, Van der Sterren S, et al. Maturation of O2 sensing and signalling in the chicken ductus arteriosus. *Am J Physiol Lung Cell Mol Physiol.* 2009;297(4):L619-L630.

25. Thebaud B, Wu XC, Kajimoto H, et al. Developmental absence of the O2 sensitivity of L-type calcium channels in preterm ductus arteriosus smooth muscle cells impairs O2 constriction contributing to patent ductus arteriosus. *Pediatr Res.* 2008; 63(2):176-181.

26. Waleh N, Reese J, Kajino H, et al. Oxygen-induced tension in the sheep ductus arteriosus: effects of gestation on potassium and calcium channel regulation. *Pediatr Res.* 2009;65(3):285-290.

27. Wu C, Hayama E, Imamura S, et al. Developmental changes in the expression of voltage-gated potassium channels in the ductus arteriosus of the fetal rat. *Heart Vessels.* 2007;22(1):34-40.

28. Thebaud B, Michelakis ED, Wu XC, et al. Oxygen-sensitive Kv channel gene transfer confers oxygen responsiveness to preterm rabbit and remodeled human ductus arteriosus: implications for infants with patent ductus arteriosus. *Circulation.* 2004;110(11):1372-1379.

29. Clyman RI, Waleh N, Black SM, et al. Regulation of ductus arteriosus patency by nitric oxide in fetal lambs. The role of gestation, oxygen tension and vasa vasorum. *Pediatr Res.* 1998; 43:633-644.

30. Waleh N, Kajino H, Marrache AM, et al. Prostaglandin E2–mediated relaxation of the ductus arteriosus: effects of gestational age on g protein-coupled receptor expression, signaling, and vasomotor control. *Circulation.* 2004;110(16):2326-2332.

31. Liu H, Manganiello VC, Clyman RI. Expression, activity and function of cAMP and cGMP phosphodiesterases in the mature and immature ductus arteriosus. *Pediatr Res.* 2008;64:477-481.

32. Clyman RI, Mauray F, Heymann MA, et al. Effect of gestational age on pulmonary metabolism of prostaglandin E1 & E2. *Prostaglandins.* 1981;21(3):505-513.

33. Gonzalez A, Sosenko IR, Chandar J, et al. Influence of infection on patent ductus arteriosus and chronic lung disease in premature infants weighing 1000 grams or less. *J Pediatr.* 1996; 128(4):470-478.

34. Waleh N, Barrette AM, Dagle JM, et al. Effects of advancing gestation and non-caucasian race on ductus arteriosus gene expression. *J Pediatr.* 2015;167(5):1033-1041.e2.

35. Collaborative Group on Antenatal Steroid Therapy. *Prevention of Respiratory Distress Syndrome: Effect of Antenatal Dexamethasone Administration,* Publication No 85-2695. Washington DC: National Institutes of Health; 1985:44.

36. Clyman RI, Ballard PL, Sniderman S, et al. Prenatal administration of betamethasone for prevention of patent ductus arteriosus. *J Pediatr.* 1981;98:123-126.

37. Clyman RI, Mauray F, Roman C, et al. Effects of antenatal glucocorticoid administration on the ductus arteriosus of preterm lambs. *Am J Physiol.* 1981;241:H415-H420.

38. Momma K, Mishihara S, Ota Y. Constriction of the fetal ductus arteriosus by glucocorticoid hormones. *Pediatr Res.* 1981; 15:19-21.

39. Thibeault DW, Emmanouilides GC, Dodge ME. Pulmonary and circulatory function in preterm lambs treated with hydrocortisone in utero. *Biol Neonate.* 1978;34:238-247.

40. Waffarn F, Siassi B, Cabal L, et al. Effect of antenatal glucocorticoids on clinical closure of the ductus arteriosus. *Am J Dis Child.* 1983;137:336-338.

41. Watterberg KL, Gerdes JS, Cole CH, et al. Prophylaxis of early adrenal insufficiency to prevent bronchopulmonary dysplasia: a multicenter trial. *Pediatrics.* 2004;114(6):1649-1657.

42. Group VONSS. Early postnatal dexamethasone therapy for the prevention of chronic lung disease. *Pediatrics.* 2001;108(3): 741-748.

43. Treszl A, Szabo M, Dunai G, et al. Angiotensin II type 1 receptor A1166C polymorphism and prophylactic indomethacin treatment induced ductus arteriosus closure in very low birth weight neonates. *Pediatr Res.* 2003;54(5):753-755.

44. Bokodi G, Derzbach L, Banyasz I, et al. Association of interferon gamma T+874A and interleukin 12 p40 promoter CTC-TAA/GC polymorphism with the need for respiratory support and perinatal complications in low birthweight neonates. *Arch Dis Child Fetal Neonatal Ed.* 2007;92(1):F25-F29.

45. Derzbach L, Treszl A, Balogh A, et al. Gender dependent association between perinatal morbidity and estrogen receptor-alpha Pvull polymorphism. *J Perinat Med.* 2005;33(5):461-462.

46. Dagle JM, Lepp NT, Cooper ME, et al. Determination of genetic predisposition to patent ductus arteriosus in preterm infants. *Pediatrics.* 2009;123(4):1116-1123.

47. Ivey KN, Sutcliffe D, Richardson J, et al. Transcriptional regulation during development of the ductus arteriosus. *Circ Res.* 2008;103(4):388-395.

48. Zhao F, Weismann CG, Satoda M, et al. Novel TFAP2B mutations that cause Char syndrome provide a genotype-phenotype correlation. *Am J Hum Genet.* 2001;69(4):695-703.

49. Cotton RB, Haywood JL, FitzGerald GA. Symptomatic patent ductus arteriosus following prophylactic indomethacin. A clinical and biochemical appraisal. *Biol Neonate.* 1991;60(5):273-282.

50. Chorne N, Jegatheesan P, Lin E, et al. Risk factors for persistent ductus arteriosus patency during indomethacin treatment. *J Pediatr.* 2007;151(6):629-634.

51. Smith CJ, Ryckman KK, Bahr TM, Dagle JM. Polymorphisms in CYP2C9 are associated with response to indomethacin among neonates with patent ductus arteriosus. *Pediatr Res.* 2017; 82(5):776-780.

52. Clyman RI, Seidner SR, Kajino H, et al. VEGF regulates remodeling during permanent anatomic closure of the ductus arteriosus. *Am J Physiol.* 2002;282(1):R199-R206.

53. Kajino H, Goldbarg S, Roman C, et al. Vasa vasorum hypoperfusion is responsible for medial hypoxia and anatomic remodeling in the newborn lamb ductus arteriosus. *Pediatr Res.* 2002; 51(2):228-235.

54. Noori S, Wlodaver A, Gottipati V, et al. Transitional changes in cardiac and cerebral hemodynamics in term neonates at birth. *J Pediatr.* 2012;160(6):943-948.

55. van Vonderen JJ, te Pas AB, Kolster-Bijdevaate C, et al. Noninvasive measurements of ductus arteriosus flow directly after birth. *Arch Dis Child Fetal Neonatal Ed.* 2014;99(5):F408-F412.

56. Lakshminrusimha S. The pulmonary circulation in neonatal respiratory failure. *Clin Perinatol.* 2012;39(3):655-683.

57. Rios DR, Bhattacharya S, Levy PT, McNamara PJ. Circulatory insufficiency and hypotension related to the ductus arteriosus in neonates. *Front Pediatr.* 2018;6:62.

58. de Waal K, Phad N, Boyle A. Left atrium function and deformation in very preterm infants with and without volume load. *Echocardiography.* 2018;35(11):1818-1826.

59. Alverson DC, Eldridge MW, Johnson JD, et al. Effect of patent ductus arteriosus on left ventricular output in premature infants. *J Pediatr.* 1983;102:754-757.

60. Baylen BG, Ogata H, Oguchi K, et al. The contractility and performance of the preterm left ventricle before and after early patent ductus arteriosus occlusion in surfactant-treated lambs. *Pediatr Res.* 1985;19(10):1053-1058.

61. Clyman RI, Mauray F, Heymann MA, et al. Cardiovascular effects of a patent ductus arteriosus in preterm lambs with respiratory distress. *J Pediatr.* 1987;111:579-587.

62. Clyman RI, Roman C, Heymann MA, et al. How a patent ductus arteriosus effects the premature lamb's ability to handle additional volume loads. *Pediatr Res.* 1987;22:531-535.

63. Walther FJ, Kim DH, Ebrahimi M, et al. Pulsed Doppler measurement of left ventricular output as early predictor of symptomatic patent ductus arteriosus in very preterm infants. *Biol Neonate.* 1989;56(3):121-128.

64. Lindner W, Seidel M, Versmold HJ, et al. Stroke volume and left ventricular output in preterm infants with patent ductus arteriosus. *Pediatr Res.* 1990;27:278-281.

65. Meyers RL, Alpan G, Lin E, et al. Patent ductus arteriosus, indomethacin, and intestinal distension: effects on intestinal blood flow and oxygen consumption. *Pediatr Res.* 1991;29:569-574.

66. Shimada S, Kasai T, Konishi M, et al. Effects of patent ductus arteriosus on left ventricular output and organ blood flows in preterm infants with respiratory distress syndrome treated with surfactant. *J Pediatr.* 1994;125(2):270-277.

67. Baylen BG, Ogata H, Ikegami M, et al. Left ventricular performance and regional blood flows before and after ductus arteriosus occlusion in premature lambs treated with surfactant. *Circulation.* 1983;67(4):837-843.

68. Tamura M, Harada K, Takahashi Y, et al. Changes in left ventricular diastolic filling patterns before and after the closure of the ductus arteriosus in very-low-birth weight infants. *Tohoku J Exp Med.* 1997;182(4):337-346.

69. Evans N, Iyer P. Assessment of ductus arteriosus shunt in preterm infants supported by mechanical ventilation: effect of interatrial shunting. *J Pediatr.* 1994;125(5 Pt 1):778-785.

70. Rios DR, de Freitas Martin F, El-Khuffash A, et al. Early role of the atrial-level communication in premature infants with patent ductus arteriosus. *J Am Soc Echocardiogr.* 2021;4(4):423-432.e1.

71. Noori S, Seri I. Pathophysiology of newborn hypotension outside the transitional period. *Early Hum Dev.* 2005;81(5):399-404.

72. Way GL, Pierce JR, Wolf RR, et al. ST depression suggesting subendocardial ischemia in neonates with respiratory distress syndrome and patent ductus arteriosus. *J Pediatr.* 1979;95:609-611.

73. Arvind Sehgal PJM. Coronary Artery Hypo-perfusion Is Associated with Impaired Diastolic Dysfunction in Preterm Infants after Patent Ductus Arteriosus PDA Ligation [abstract]. Toronto, Canada: Pediatric Academic Societies; 2007.

74. El-Khuffash AF, Molloy EJ. Influence of a patent ductus arteriosus on cardiac troponin T levels in preterm infants. *J Pediatr.* 2008;153(3):350-353.

75. Haizlip KM, Bupha-Intr T, Biesiadecki BJ, Janssen PML. Effects of increased preload on the force-frequency response and contractile kinetics in early stage of cardiac muscle hypertrophy. *Am J Physiol Heart Circ Physio.* 2021;302(12):H2509-H2517.

76. Barlow AJ, Ward C, Webber SA, et al. Myocardial contractility in premature neonates with and without patent ductus arteriosus. *Pediatr Cardiol.* 2004;25(2):102-107.

77. James AT, Corcoran JD, Breatnach CR, et al. Longitudinal assessment of left and right myocardial function in preterm infants using strain and strain rate imaging. *Neonatology.* 2016;109(1):69-75.

78. Czernik C, Rhode S, Helfer S, et al. Development of left ventricular longitudinal speckle tracking echocardiography in very low birth weight infants with and without bronchopulmonary dysplasia during the neonatal period. *PLoS One.* 2014;9(9):e106504.

79. Helfer S, Schmitz L, Buhrer C, et al. Tissue doppler-derived strain and strain rate during the first 28 days of life in very low birth weight infants. *Echocardiography.* 2013;31(6):765-772.

80. de Waal K, Phad N, Lakkundi A, et al. Cardiac function after the immediate transitional period in very preterm infants using speckle tracking analysis. *Pediatr Cardiol.* 2016;37(2):295-303.

81. James AT, Corcoran JD, Franklin O, et al. Clinical utility of right ventricular fractional area change in preterm infants. *Early Hum Dev.* 2016;92:19-23.

82. Ratner I, Perelmuter B, Toews W, et al. Association of low systolic and diastolic blood pressure with significant patent ductus arteriosus in the very low birth weight infant. *Crit Care Med.* 1985;13(6):497-500.

83. Evans N, Moorcraft J. Effect of patency of the ductus arteriosus on blood pressure in very preterm infants. *Arch Dis Child.* 1992;67(10 Spec No):1169-1173.

84. Liebowitz M, Koo J, Wickremasinghe A, et al. Effects of prophylactic indomethacin on vasopressor-dependent hypotension in extremely preterm infants. *J Pediatr.* 2017;182:21-27.e2.

85. Sarkar S, Dechert R, Schumacher RE, et al. Is refractory hypotension in preterm infants a manifestation of early ductal shunting? *J Perinatol.* 2007;27(6):353-358.

86. McCurnin D, Clyman RI. Effects of a patent ductus arteriosus on postprandial mesenteric perfusion in premature baboons. *Pediatrics.* 2008;122(6):e1262-e1267.

87. Ohlsson A, Walia R, Shah S. Ibuprofen for the treatment of patent ductus arteriosus in preterm and/or low birth weight infants. *Cochrane Database Syst Rev.* 2003;(2):CD003481. doi:10.1002/14651858.CD003481.

88. Dollberg S, Lusky A, Reichman B, et al. Ductus arteriosus, indomethacin and necrotizing enterocolitis in very low birth weight infants: a population-based study. *J Ped Gast Nutr*, 2005;40:184-188.

89. Raju TN. Cerebral Doppler studies in the fetus and newborn infant. *J Pediatr.* 1991;119(2):165-174.

90. Greisen G, Johansen K, Ellison PH, et al. Cerebral blood flow in the newborn infant: comparison of Doppler ultrasound and 133xenon clearance. *J Pediatr.* 1984;104(3):411-418.

91. Hansen NB, Stonestreet BS, Rosenkrantz TS, et al. Validity of Doppler measurements of anterior cerebral artery blood flow velocity: correlation with brain blood flow in piglets. *Pediatrics.* 1983;72(4):526-531.

92. Chemtob S, Beharry K, Rex J, et al. Prostanoids determine the range of cerebral blood flow autoregulation of newborn piglets. *Stroke.* 1990;21(5):777-784.

93. Laudignon N, Chemtob S, Bard H, et al. Effect of indomethacin on cerebral blood flow velocity of premature newborns. *Biol Neonate.* 1988;54(5):254-262.

94. Perlman JM, Hill A, Volpe JJ. The effect of patent ductus arteriosus on flow velocity in the anterior cerebral arteries: ductal steal in the premature newborn infant. *J Pediatr.* 1981;99:767-771.

95. Lemmers PM, Toet MC, van Bel F. Impact of patent ductus arteriosus and subsequent therapy with indomethacin on cerebral oxygenation in preterm infants. *Pediatrics.* 2008;121(1):142-147.

96. Martin CG, Snider AR, Katz SM, et al. Abnormal cerebral blood flow patterns in preterm infants with a large patent ductus arteriosus. *J Pediatr.* 1982;101:587-593.

97. Shortland DB, Gibson NA, Levene MI, et al. Patent ductus arteriosus and cerebral circulation in preterm infants. *Dev Med Child Neurol.* 1990;32(5):386-393.

98. Breatnach CR, Franklin O, McCallion N, et al. The effect of a significant patent ductus arteriosus on doppler flow patterns of preductal vessels: an assessment of the brachiocephalic artery. *J Pediatr*. 2017;180:279-281.e1.

99. Jim WT, Chiu NC, Chen MR, et al. Cerebral hemodynamic change and intraventricular hemorrhage in very low birth weight infants with patent ductus arteriosus. *Ultrasound Med Biol*. 2005;31(2):197-202.

100. Camfferman FA, de Goederen R, Govaert P, et al. Diagnostic and predictive value of Doppler ultrasound for evaluation of the brain circulation in preterm infants: a systematic review. *Pediatr Res*. 2020;87(suppl 1):50-58.

101. Kluckow M, Evans N. Low superior vena cava flow and intraventricular haemorrhage in preterm infants. *Arch Dis Child Fetal Neonatal Ed*. 2000;82(3):F188-F194.

102. Groves AM, Kuschel CA, Knight DB, et al. Does retrograde diastolic flow in the descending aorta signify impaired systemic perfusion in preterm infants? *Pediatr Res*. 2008;63(1):89-94.

103. Deeg KH, Gerstner R, Brandl U, et al. Doppler sonographic flow parameter of the anterior cerebral artery in patent ductus arteriosus of the newborn infant compared to a healthy control sample. *Klin Padiatr*. 1986;198(6):463-470.

104. Coombs RC, Morgan MEI, Durin GM, et al. Gut blood flow velocities in the newborn: effects of patent ductus arteriosus and parenteral indomethacin. *Arch Dis Child*. 1990;65:1067-1071.

105. Smith A, Armstrong S, Dempsey E, El-Khuffash A. The impact of a PDA on tissue oxygenation and haemodynamics following a blood transfusion in preterm infants. *Pediatr Res*. 2023;93(5):1314-1320. doi:10.1038/s41390-022-01967-3.

106. Yanowitz TD, Yao AC, Werner JC, et al. Effects of prophylactic low-dose indomethacin on hemodynamics in very low birth weight infants. *J Pediatr*. 1998;132(1):28-34.

107. Pezzati M, Vangi V, Biagiotti R, et al. Effects of indomethacin and ibuprofen on mesenteric and renal blood flow in preterm infants with patent ductus arteriosus. *J Pediatr*. 1999;135(6):733-738.

108. Lewis AB, Heymann MA, Rudolph AM. Gestational changes in pulmonary vascular responses in fetal lambs in utero. *Circ Res*. 1976;39:536-541.

109. Jacob J, Gluck G, DiSessa T, et al. The contribution of PDA in the neonate with severe RDS. *J Pediatr*. 1980;96(1):79-87.

110. Gersony WM, Peckham GJ, Ellison RC, et al. Effects of indomethacin in premature infants with patent ductus arteriosus: results of a national collaborative study. *J Pediatr*. 1983;102:895-906.

111. Raju TNK, Langenberg P. Pulmonary hemorrhage and exogenous surfactant therapy – a metaanalysis. *J Pediatr*. 1993;123(4):603-610.

112. Alpan G, Clyman RI. Cardiovascular effects of surfactant replacement with special reference to the patent ductus arteriosus. In: Robertson B, Taeusch HW, eds. *Surfactant Therapy for Lung Disease: Lung Biology in Health and Disease*. 84. Marcel Dekker, Inc; 1995:531-545.

113. Rakza T, Magnenant E, Klosowski S, et al. Early hemodynamic consequences of patent ductus arteriosus in preterm infants with intrauterine growth restriction. *J Pediatr*. 2007;151(6):624-628.

114. Alpan G, Scheerer R, Bland RD, et al. Patent ductus arteriosus increases lung fluid filtration in preterm lambs. *Pediatr Res*. 1991;30:616-621.

115. Ikegami M, Jacobs H, Jobe A. Surfactant function in respiratory distress syndrome. *J Pediatr*. 1983;102:443-447.

116. Brown E. Increased risk of bronchopulmonary dysplasia in infants with patent ductus arteriosus. *J Pediatr*. 1979;95:865-866.

117. Cotton RB, Stahlman MT, Berder HW, et al. Randomized trial of early closure of symptomatic patent ductus arteriosus in small preterm infants. *J Pediatr*. 1978;93:647-651.

118. Clyman RI. Commentary: recommendations for the postnatal use of indomethacin. An analysis of four separate treatment strategies. *J Pediatr*. 1996;128:601-607.

119. McCurnin D, Seidner S, Chang LY, et al. Ibuprofen-induced patent ductus arteriosus closure: physiologic, histologic, and biochemical effects on the premature lung. *Pediatrics*. 2008;121(5):945-956.

120. Perez Fontan JJ, Clyman RI, Mauray F, et al. Respiratory effects of a patent ductus arteriosus in premature newborn lambs. *J Appl Physiol*. 1987;63(6):2315-2324.

121. Shimada S, Raju TNK, Bhat R, et al. Treatment of patent ductus arteriosus after exogenous surfactant in baboons with hyaline membrane disease. *Pediatr Res*. 1989;26:565-569.

122. Krauss AN, Fatica N, Lewis BS, et al. Pulmonary function in preterm infants following treatment with intravenous indomethacin. *Am J Dis Child*. 1989;143:78-81.

123. Alpan G, Mauray F, Clyman RI. Effect of patent ductus arteriosus on water accumulation and protein permeability in the premature lungs of mechanically ventilated premature lambs. *Pediatr Res*. 1989;26:570-575.

124. Gerhardt T, Bancalari E. Lung compliance in newborns with patent ductus arteriosus before and after surgical ligation. *Biol Neonate*. 1980;38:96-105.

125. Naulty CM, Horn S, Conry J, et al. Improved lung compliance after ligation of patent ductus arteriosus in hyaline membrane disease. *J Pediatr*. 1978;93:682-684.

126. Stefano JL, Abbasi S, Pearlman SA, et al. Closure of the ductus arteriosus with indomethacin in ventilated neonates with respiratory distress syndrome. Effects of pulmonary compliance and ventilation. *Am Rev Respir Dis*. 1991;143(2):236-239.

127. Yeh TF, Thalji A, Luken L, et al. Improved lung compliance following indomethacin therapy in premature infants with persistent ductus arteriosus. *Chest*. 1981;80(6):698-700.

128. Szymankiewicz M, Hodgman JE, Siassi B, et al. Mechanics of breathing after surgical ligation of patent ductus arteriosus in newborns with respiratory distress syndrome. *Biol Neonate*. 2004;85(1):32-36.

129. Dawes GS, Mott JC, Widdicombe JG. The patency of the ductus arteriosus in newborn lambs and its physiological consequences. *J Physiol*. 1955;128:361-383.

130. Adatia I, Kothari SS, Feinstein JA. Pulmonary hypertension associated with congenital heart disease: pulmonary vascular disease: the global perspective. *Chest*. 2010;137(6):52S-61S.

131. Rondelet B, Kerbaul F, Van Beneden R, et al. Prevention of pulmonary vascular remodeling and of decreased BMPR-2 expression by losartan therapy in shunt-induced pulmonary hypertension. *Am J Physio Heart Circ Physiol*. 2005;289:H2319-H2324.

132. Phillip R, Rush Waller B, Chilakala S, et al. Hemodynamic and clinical consequences of early versus delayed closure of patent ductus arteriosus in extremely low birth weight infants. *J Perinatol*. 2021;41:100-108.

133. Rosenzweig EB, Barst RJ. Congenital heart disease and pulmonary hypertension: pharmacology and feasibility of late surgery. *Prog Cardiovasc Dis*. 2012;55(2):128-133.

134. Hébert A, De Carvalho Nunes G, Maltais-Bilodeau C, et al. *Non-Interventional Approach to PDA in Preterm Infants: Time to Look at the Chronic Pulmonary Hypertension Outcome (Abstract).* Baltimore: Pediatric Academic Society; 2022.

135. Benitz WE. Treatment of persistent patent ductus arteriosus in preterm infants: time to accept the null hypothesis? *J Perinatol.* 2010;30(4):241-252.

136. Noori S, McCoy M, Friedlich P, et al. Failure of ductus arteriosus closure is associated with increased mortality in preterm infants. *Pediatrics.* 2009;123:e138-e144.

137. Sellmer A, Bjerre JV, Schmidt MR, et al. Morbidity and mortality in preterm neonates with patent ductus arteriosus on day 3. *Arch Dis Child Fetal Neonatal Ed.* 2013;98(6):F505-F510.

138. El-Khuffash A, James AT, Corcoran JD, et al. A patent ductus arteriosus severity score predicts chronic lung disease or death before discharge. *J Pediatr.* 2015;167(6):1354-1361.e2.

139. Schena F, Francescato G, Cappelleri A, et al. Association between hemodynamically significant patent ductus arteriosus and bronchopulmonary dysplasia. *J Pediatr.* 2015;166(6):1488-1492.

140. Kluckow M, Jeffery M, Gill A, Evans N. A randomised placebo-controlled trial of early treatment of the patent ductus arteriosus. *Arch Dis Child Fetal Neonatal Ed.* 2014;99(2):F99-F104.

141. Elsayed Y, Seshia M, Soni R, et al. Pre-symptomatic prediction of morbidities in preterm infants with patent ductus arteriosus by targeted neonatal echocardiography and brain-type natriuretic peptide. *J Pediatr Neonat Individual Med.* 2016;5(2):e050210.

142. Stuckey D. Palmar pulsation: a physical sign of patent ductus arteriosus in infancy. *Med J Aust.* 1957;44(19):681-682.

143. Skelton R, Evans N, Smythe J. A blinded comparison of clinical and echocardiographic evaluation of the preterm infant for patent ductus arteriosus. *J Paediatr Child Health.* 1994;30(5):406-411.

144. Shipton SE, van der Merwe PL, Nel ED. Diagnosis of haemodynamically significant patent ductus arteriosus in neonates – is the ECG of diagnostic help? *Cardiovasc J S Afr.* 2001;12(5):264-267.

145. Kluckow M, Evans N. Early echocardiographic prediction of symptomatic patent ductus arteriosus in preterm infants undergoing mechanical ventilation. *J Pediatr.* 1995;127(5):774-779.

146. D'Amato G, Errico G, Franco C, et al. Ductal size indexed to weight and body surface area correlates with morbidities in preterm infants ≤32 weeks. *J Matern Fetal Neonatal Med.* 2021;34(19):3133-3139.

147. Smith A, Maguire M, Livingstone V, et al. Peak systolic to end diastolic flow velocity ratio is associated with ductal patency in infants below 32 weeks of gestation. *Arch Dis Child Fetal Neonatal Ed.* 2015;100(2):F132-F136.

148. Davies MW, Betheras FR, Swaminathan M. A preliminary study of the application of the transductal velocity ratio for assessing persistent ductus arteriosus. *Arch Dis Child Fetal Neonatal Ed.* 2000;82(3):F195-F199.

149. Hiraishi S, Horiguchi Y, Misawa H, et al. Noninvasive Doppler echocardiographic evaluation of shunt flow dynamics of the ductus arteriosus. *Circulation.* 1987;75(6):1146-1153.

150. Lindner W, Seidel M, Versmold HT, et al. Stroke volume and left ventricular output in preterm infants with patent ductus arteriosus. *Pediatr Res.* 1990;27(3):278-281.

151. Alverson DC, Eldridge MW, Johnson JD, et al. Effect of patent ductus arteriosus on left ventricular output in premature infants. *J Pediatr.* 1983;102(5):754-757.

152. Zecca E, Romagnoli C, Vento G, et al. Left ventricle dimensions in preterm infants during the first month of life. *Eur J Pediatr.* 2001;160(4):227-230.

153. Hsu KH, Nguyen J, Dekom S, Ramanathan R, Noori S. Effects of patent ductus arteriosus on organ blood flow in infants born very preterm: a prospective study with serial echocardiography. *J Pediatr.* 2020;216:95-100.e2.

154. Harling S, Hansen-Pupp I, Baigi A, et al. Echocardiographic prediction of patent ductus arteriosus in need of therapeutic intervention. *Acta Paediatr.* 2011;100(2):231-235.

155. Martins F, Jain A, Javed H, McNamara PJ. *Echocardiographic Markers of Hemodynamic Significance of Persistent Ductus Arteriosus (PDA): Beyond Ductal Size (Abstract).* San Diego, California: Pediatric Academic Societies; 2015.

156. Jasani B, Martins FF, Weisz DE, et al. Patent ductus arteriosus shunt volume in preterm neonates using pulmonary vein diastolic velocity. *Pediatr Res.* 2022;91(1):4-7.

157. Sehgal A, McNamara PJ. Does echocardiography facilitate determination of hemodynamic significance attributable to the ductus arteriosus? *Eur J Pediatr.* 2009;168(8):907-914.

158. Schmitz L, Stiller B, Koch H, et al. Diastolic left ventricular function in preterm infants with a patent ductus arteriosus: A serial Doppler echocardiography study. *Early Hum. Dev.* 2004;76(2):91-100.

159. El-Khuffash A, Higgins M, Walsh K, et al. Quantitative assessment of the degree of ductal steal using celiac artery blood flow to left ventricular output ratio in preterm infants. *Neonatology.* 2008;93(3):206-212.

160. Hoodbhoy SA, Cutting HA, Seddon JA, et al. Cerebral and splanchnic hemodynamics after duct ligation in very low birth weight infants. *J Pediatr.* 2009;154(2):196-200.

161. Mannarino S, Garofoli F, Cerbo RM, et al. Cord blood, perinatal BNP values in term and preterm newborns. *Arch Dis Child Fetal Neonatal Ed.* 2010;95(1):F74.

162. Farombi-Oghuvbu I, Matthews T, Mayne PD, et al. N-terminal pro-B-type natriuretic peptide: a measure of significant patent ductus arteriosus. *Arch Dis Child Fetal Neonatal Ed.* 2008;93(4):F257-F260.

163. Chen S, Tacy T, Clyman R. How useful are B-type natriuretic peptide measurements for monitoring changes in patent ductus arteriosus shunt magnitude? *J Perinatol.* 2010;30(12):780-785.

164. El-Khuffash A, Molloy EJ. Are B-type natriuretic peptide (BNP) and N-terminal-pro-BNP useful in neonates? *Arch Dis Child Fetal Neonatal Ed.* 2007;92(4):F320-F324.

165. Martinovici D, Vanden Eijnden S, Unger P, et al. Early NT-proBNP is able to predict spontaneous closure of patent ductus arteriosus in preterm neonates, but not the need of its treatment. *Pediatr Cardiol.* 2011;32(7):953-957.

166. Murkin JM, Arango M. Near-infrared spectroscopy as an index of brain and tissue oxygenation. *Br J Anaesth.* 2009;103(suppl 1):i3-i13.

167. Underwood MA, Milstein JM, Sherman MP. Near-infrared spectroscopy as a screening tool for patent ductus arteriosus in extremely low birth weight infants. *Neonatology.* 2007;91(2):134-139.

168. Dix L, Molenschot M, Breur J, et al. Cerebral oxygenation and echocardiographic parameters in preterm neonates with a patent ductus arteriosus: an observational study. *Arch Dis Child Fetal Neonatal Ed.* 2016;101(6):F520-F526.

169. Dani C, Poggi C, Cianchi I, et al. Effect on cerebral oxygenation of paracetamol for patent ductus arteriosus in preterm infants. *Eur J Pediatr.* 2018;177(4):533-539.

170. van der Laan ME, Roofthooft MT, Fries MW, et al. A hemodynamically significant patent ductus arteriosus does not affect cerebral or renal tissue oxygenation in preterm infants. *Neonatology*. 2016;110(2):141-147.

171. Chock VY, Rose LA, Mante JV, et al. Near-infrared spectroscopy for detection of a significant patent ductus arteriosus. *Pediatr Res*. 2016;80(5):675-680.

172. EL-Khuffash A, Bussmann N, Breatnach CR, et al. A pilot randomized controlled trial of early targeted patent ductus arteriosus treatment using a risk based severity score (The PDA RCT). *J Pediatr*. 2021;229:127-133.

173. El-Khuffash A, Barry D, Walsh K, et al. Biochemical markers may identify preterm infants with a patent ductus arteriosus at high risk of death or severe intraventricular haemorrhage. *Arch Dis Child Fetal Neonatal Ed*. 2008;93(6):F407-F412.

174. Gursoy T, Hayran M, Derin H, et al. A clinical scoring system to predict the development of bronchopulmonary dysplasia. *Am J Perinatol*. 2015;32(7):659-666.

175. El-Khuffash AF, Slevin M, McNamara PJ, et al. N-terminal pro natriuretic peptide and a patent ductus arteriosus scoring system predict death before discharge or neurodevelopmental outcome at 2 years in preterm infants. *Arch Dis Child Fetal Neonatal Ed*. 2011;96(2):F133-F137.

176. Sehgal A, Paul E, Menahem S. Functional echocardiography in staging for ductal disease severity. *Eur J of Pediatr*. 2012; 172(2):179-184.

177. Fink D, El-Khuffash A, McNamara PJ, et al. Tale of two patent ductus arteriosus severity scores: similarities and differences. *Am J Perinatol*. 2017;35(1):55-58.

178. McNamara PJ, Sehgal A. Towards rational management of the patent ductus arteriosus: the need for disease staging. *Arch Dis Child Fetal Neonatal Ed*. 2007;92(6):F424-F427.

# Chapter 17

# Pharmacological Management of Patent Ductus Arteriosus in the Very Preterm Neonate

## Souvik Mitra and Prakesh S. Shah

## Key Points

- The pharmacological management of PDA in the very preterm neonate remains a controversial topic, as the risks and benefits of the pharmacotherapeutic options remain unclear.

- NSAIDs (indomethacin and ibuprofen) and acetaminophen are the most common and effective pharmacological agents used for PDA closure.

- No major differences in the efficacy between the three agents have been established in comparative effectiveness trials. However, choice of therapy may be guided by their respective adverse effect profiles.

- Wide variations in the timing, dosage, and type of pharmacological agent have been reported internationally.

- Future research should attempt to tease out the interaction between patient characteristics; the timing of treatment; choice, route, and dosage of the medication; and degree of hemodynamic significance of the PDA.

## Introduction

This chapter reviews the epidemiology and current state of pharmacological management (prophylactic and therapeutic) of the patent ductus arteriosus (PDA) in the very preterm neonate. Until now, the optimal management of PDA has been controversial in the scientific community, with no clear consensus or generally accepted guidelines for management. Most of the dispute stems from several sources: the natural history of PDA, the hemodynamic significance of PDA, especially concerning its impact on end-organ perfusion and its potential long-term consequences on neurodevelopment,

variable efficacy of the available treatments, unpredictable side effects of pharmacological and surgical therapy, and the lack of information on patient-important clinical outcomes and long-term neurodevelopmental outcomes associated with treatment. The wide variations in PDA management reported worldwide reflect our poor understanding of these uncertainties. While efforts are underway to expand our current understanding of the condition, clinicians should continue to weigh the risks and benefits of different treatment options when deciding the correct clinical course of action.

Apart from pharmacological therapy, conservative management and mechanical closure (surgical and percutaneous transcatheter route) of PDA are employed in the management of PDA. Conservative management approaches may range from watchful waiting to non-pharmacological shunt modulation strategies such as increasing the positive end-expiratory pressure. In contrast, pharmaceutical agents for PDA therapy are specifically used to stimulate ductal closure. Pharmacological agents stimulate PDA closure via inhibition of prostaglandin production, which play a significant role in maintaining ductal patency in utero and during the first 1–2 postnatal weeks. These agents are specifically designed to target either cyclooxygenase (COX) or peroxidase (POX), the second and third enzymes in the process of prostaglandin synthesis, respectively. These agents include the COX inhibitors indomethacin and ibuprofen and the POX inhibitor acetaminophen (paracetamol) (Figure 17.1).[1] Adding to the complexity of pharmacological management is the question of when to treat, which may include

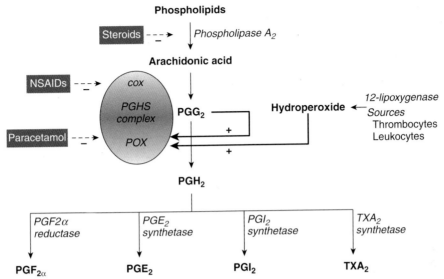

**Fig. 17.1 The figure depicts arachidonic acid metabolism along with the inhibitory effects of medications and the stimulatory actions of endogenous substances on the enzymes of the pathway**[1] **See text for details.** (Allegaert K, Anderson B, Simons S, van Overmeire B. Paracetamol to induce ductus arteriosus closure: is it valid?. *Arch Dis Child*. 2013;98(6):462–466. Copyright: BMJ Publishing Group Ltd & Royal College of Paediatrics and Child Health.)

prophylactic (treat all without assessing), early asymptomatic (detect and treat early before PDA becomes significant during first week after birth), and symptomatic (treat when PDA becomes clinically and hemodynamically significant) treatment.

## Epidemiology of PDA Treatment

Variations in the management of PDA in very preterm and very-low-birth-weight infants have been well reported in North America, Europe, Australia, and Asia. These differences have been described for all aspects of treatment, including if, when, and how to treat PDA. Surveys conducted over the past 20 years regarding the practitioner's approach to treatment of PDA have yielded consistently variable results. In North America a survey of 100 Canadian neonatologists in 1998 revealed a wide variation in practices regarding management of PDA both within and between centers.[2] Fluid restriction and indomethacin were used for treatment by 89% of neonatologists surveyed, while surgery was reserved for patients unresponsive to pharmacological agents or had contraindications. Use of echocardiography for diagnosis of PDA also varied among clinicians. Almost a decade later, 56 fellowship program directors in the United

States were surveyed regarding the management of PDA.[3] A quarter of respondents were using prophylactic indomethacin for prevention of interventricular hemorrhage (IVH) and 9% used indomethacin to treat asymptomatic PDA. In cases of persistent PDA three-quarters of respondents indicated use of more than one course of indomethacin, with nearly half reporting usage of two courses and half reporting three courses, if needed. Most respondents were keen on administering indomethacin below 2 weeks of age and used echocardiography criteria to determine PDA treatment.

Hoellering and Cooke also surveyed neonatologists from Australia and New Zealand in 2007 for management of PDA in neonates of 28 weeks' gestation or less or birth weights less than 1000 g.[4] Expectant (or conservative) management of PDA was favored by 35% of clinicians, while 32% used echocardiographic-targeted prophylaxis, 16% used pre-symptomatic treatment, and 17% used a prophylactic approach; however, nearly half of participating units reported using more than one approach, often depending upon the preference of the individual practitioner. Interestingly, 86% of physicians used long courses of indomethacin and nearly one-quarter of respondents indicated that their approach was not influenced by published literature.

This raises important questions regarding the level of effect that individual units or practitioners have on the outcomes of neonates with PDA.

In a survey of 24 European Societies of Neonatology and Perinatology, Guimaraes and colleagues reported data on 45 responses from 19 countries.[5] Most neonatal units used intravenous indomethacin (71%), followed by intravenous ibuprofen (36%) and oral ibuprofen (29%); some units reported use of multiple agents. Approximately half of the centers used a second course and one-quarter of them used a third course of pharmacotherapy in the event of persistent ductus. Nearly all (96%) units treated hemodynamically significant PDA (hsPDA), but a quarter also treated non-hsPDA. Only one neonatal unit preferred surgical ligation as the first-line therapy. In France nearly three-quarters of the 49 neonatal units surveyed between 2007 and 2008 reported the use of both clinical and echocardiography criteria to decide on treatment for PDA, whereas the remaining relied on echocardiography criteria alone.[6] Most units also used echocardiography to diagnose PDA, but the criteria used to describe hsPDA differed. All units used ibuprofen to treat PDA, with most units using a standard course (see Section 3.2 on Ibuprofen below). Between one-half and two-thirds of centers indicated a tendency to use a second course when either the first course failed or if the duct reopened after successful closure. In the event of contraindications to medical treatment or ductal malformation, 39% of units considered surgery as the primary treatment.

Irmesi et al. recently collated information from published randomized trials of PDA management around the world.[7] They identified that treatment with indomethacin and ibuprofen was more prevalent in the United States and Canada, whereas ibuprofen was the most common agent used in Europe. Worldwide variations were further exposed in a recent international survey of investigators from 335 neonatal units in 11 high-income countries.[8] The results indicated that Japan, Sweden, Finland, and the Tuscany region of Italy routinely perform echocardiogram screening for PDA. Treatment rates of pre-symptomatic PDA based on routine echocardiography results alone, regardless of a patient's clinical status, was in the range of 6–85% (6% of units in Canada; 7% in Illinois;19% in Israel; 50% in Sweden; 40% in Spain; 27% in Switzerland; 50% in Australia and New Zealand; 40% in Finland; 75% in Tuscany, Italy; and 85% in Japan) among those who conduct echocardiography screening.[8]

Apart from the survey data described above, reports of actual practices in the management of PDA have recently been published. A recent cohort study from the iNEO (International Network for Evaluating Outcomes of Neonates) collaboration that included 39,096 infants born between 24 and 28 weeks' gestation from across 6 countries (139 NICUs) demonstrated a wide variation in PDA treatment practices. While the overall PDA treatment rate was 45% in this cohort (13–77% by NICU), the observed to expected PDA treatment ratio ranged from 0.30 to 2.14.[9] It was further noted that the relationship between the observed to expected PDA treatment ratio and primary composite outcome of death and severe neurological injury followed a U-shaped curve, suggesting that both low and high PDA treatment rates were associated with worse clinical outcomes.[9] In another study Hagadorn and colleagues examined trends in the management of PDA in 19 US children's hospitals between 2005 and 2014 and linked the data to neonatal outcomes.[10] Approximately three-quarters of infants with PDA were treated with pharmacological management or surgery, with wide variation noted among hospitals. There was a steady decline in the number of neonates treated over the years, with the odds of treatment decreasing by 11% in each year of the study period. The trend of reducing treatment was temporally associated with a decline in mortality; however, bronchopulmonary dysplasia (BPD), periventricular leukomalacia, retinopathy of prematurity (ROP), and acute renal failure increased. In a population-based cohort study Edstedt Bonamy et al. evaluated regional variations and their relationship with outcomes in PDA management across 19 regions in 11 European countries between 2011 and 2012.[11] The proportion of neonates ≤31 weeks' gestation who received PDA treatment varied from 10% to 39% between units, and it was independent of perinatal characteristics of patients. Variations in PDA treatment rate were not associated with neonatal outcomes.

In Canada conservative management of PDA in neonates between 23 and 32 weeks' gestation increased from 14 to 38% between 2006 and 2012, while using pharmacotherapy alone and surgical treatment alone decreased from 58 to 49% and 7.1 to 2.5%, respectively, and both pharmacotherapy and surgical ligation dropped from 21 to 10% (all $P <$ 0.01) during the same time period.[12] With an increase in conservative management, there was a reduction in the composite outcome of mortality or major morbidity between 2009 and 2012 compared to 2006 and 2008; however, there remains the possibility of confounding by indication. Slaughter et al. attempted to adjust for residual confounding parameters by incorporating clinician preference-based variation in practice as an instrument in their analyses.[13] They reported that though an infant's chance of receiving pharmacotherapy increased by 0.84% for each 1% increase in the hospital's annual pharmacotherapy rate for treatment of PDA, there was no association between pharmacotherapy and mortality and mortality or BPD in neonates of ≤28 weeks' gestation. This finding suggests that conservative management of PDA may be a rational approach for a subset of preterm infants with PDA. However, more work needs to be done to identify the right patient population who would benefit from treatment of the PDA (Chapter 19).

In a prospective cohort from France Rozé et al. evaluated the role of early screening (before day 3 of postnatal life) in neonates <29 weeks' gestation.[14] The authors determined that screened infants were more likely to be treated for PDA than unexposed infants (55% vs. 43%; odds ratio [OR] 1.62, 95% confidence interval [CI] 1.32–2.00). Screened neonates were at lower odds of mortality (OR 0.73, 95% CI 0.54–0.98) and pulmonary hemorrhage (OR 0.60, 95% CI 0.38–0.95). However, when instrumental variable analyses using unit preference for early screening were conducted, there was no statistically significant association between early screening and mortality (OR 0.62, 95% CI 0.37–1.04), suggesting that questions about screening, prophylaxis, and treatment could only best be answered in well-designed randomized trials. The variations reported above in both survey designs and in studies comparing the evolution of approaches and their relationship with outcomes indicate that the management of PDA is widely variable within neonatal units and at regional, national, and international levels.

## Pharmacological Interventions

Pharmacological interventions for PDA can be divided into two groups: agents used for symptomatic treatment (i.e. management of pulmonary edema and heart failure) and agents that induce PDA closure. Based on symptoms associated with pulmonary hyperperfusion and heart failure, diuretics such as furosemide have been used to reduce overall fluid overload. Use of furosemide in the context of PDA management remains controversial. Animal studies suggest furosemide may stimulate renal production of prostaglandin E2, thereby contributing to ductal patency.[15] Further, three randomized controlled trials (RCTs) exploring the role of furosemide in indomethacin-treated infants for symptomatic PDA have failed to demonstrate any benefit.[16] In addition, loop diuretics, such as furosemide, are associated with various side effects, including electrolyte imbalance, nephrocalcinosis, and hearing impairment.[17] However, a recent large observational study of 43,576 infants demonstrated that exposure to furosemide for any indication was associated with reduced odds of PDA treatment (adjusted odds ratio = 0.72, 95% CI 0.65–0.79).[18] Therefore controversy remains on the role of furosemide in the management of symptomatic PDA. While the Canadian Pediatric Society suggests considering the use of furosemide for conservative management of symptomatic PDA, further research is required to strongly recommend its use.[19]

As previously mentioned, the three main pharmacological agents used to induce PDA closure are indomethacin, ibuprofen, and acetaminophen (paracetamol), each of which is described below. More than 80 RCTs have been conducted over the past 40 years exploring different dosages, duration, and routes of administration of these drugs. The complexity of management of PDA is summarized in Figure 17.2, where strategies that have been tested in randomized trials are delineated.[20]

### INDOMETHACIN
#### Mechanism of Action

Indomethacin is a potent and non-selective inhibitor of the COX enzyme and promotes PDA closure by inhibiting the synthesis of prostaglandins, including prostaglandin E2.[21] The half-life of indomethacin is 4–5 hours

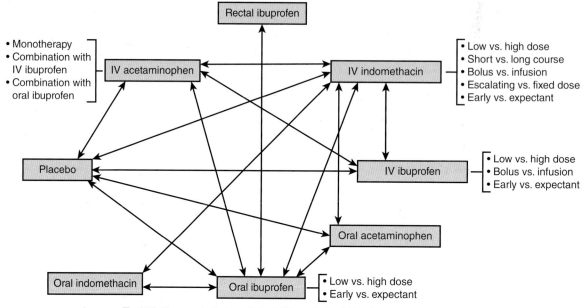

Fig. 17.2 Pharmacological agents tested in randomized trials for management of PDA.

longer on average in preterm neonates <32 weeks' gestation compared to those >32 weeks' gestation (17.2 ± 0.8 vs. 12.5 ± 0.5 hours) and thus prolonged accumulation can occur in very preterm neonates.[22]

### Dose, Route, and Frequency

Intravenous indomethacin has been used in various dosing regimens.[21] Initial animal studies demonstrated that intravenous indomethacin in doses of 0.2–0.4 mg/kg substantially reduced PDA diameter in fetal lambs.[23] Most RCTs conducted in preterm neonates have used three doses of 0.1–0.2 mg/kg/dose every 12–24 hours apart; however, many modifications of this strategy have been carried out. In one study dose escalation of indomethacin starting from 0.2 mg/kg and increasing to 1 mg/kg in non-responders resulted in a 98.5% PDA closure rate.[24] It should be noted that higher doses are typically associated with increased risk of side effects. In another study a high-dose (0.2–0.5 mg/kg/dose) and low-dose (0.1 mg/kg/dose) regimen of indomethacin were compared in cases of persistent PDA following conventional treatment with the three conventional doses.[25] Although the authors reported no difference in PDA closure rates (55% vs. 48%, respectively), the infants exposed to the higher

dosage displayed increased rates of renal compromise and moderate to severe retinopathy.[25]

Though the most common route of administration of indomethacin is intravenous, it has been used orally, rectally, and intra-arterially. Six studies of oral use (ranging between 9 and 74 neonates) have reported PDA closure rates of 66–67%. Intra-arterial use in 26 neonates was successful in 76% of cases, whereas a 66% closure rate was observed in a small group of neonates treated either orally (n = 1) or rectally (n = 5).[21] Both of these routes have not been widely used due to concerns of damage to mucosal layers from local direct effects of indomethacin, as well as the effects on prostaglandin synthesis inhibition affecting mucosal integrity of the gastrointestinal tract, especially the ileum.

The usual duration for one course of indomethacin treatment is 48–72 hours. For some neonates, ductal closure can be a lengthy remodeling process and may need prolonged treatment. Five randomized trials compared PDA closure rates in neonates treated with a prolonged course of indomethacin versus routine treatment using a three-dose course and reported no difference in PDA closure rates but identified that an increased risk of necrotizing enterocolitis (NEC) was associated with longer indomethacin exposure (relative risk [RR] 1.87, 95% CI 1.07–3.27).[26] Some practitioners advocate for an echocardiogram to be performed after the last dose (third dose of a routine course) and to continue treatment until the duct closes. However, based on concerns of adverse effects, a prolonged course is not recommended by most.

Typically, indomethacin is administered as a slow infusion to avoid rapidly rising concentrations characteristic of bolus infusions. The potential impact of indomethacin concentration on cerebral, renal, and splanchnic blood flow has led to recommendations for infusion to be administered over a 20- to 30-minute period. Studies have reported reduced blood flow,[27] and similar[28] or higher closure rates (81% vs. 43%; $P = 0.03$),[29] with bolus infusion compared with continuous infusion. However, as suggested by a previous systematic review, the evidence may be too limited to draw a conclusion regarding the superiority of either approach.[30] Pharmacokinetic data from a small series of neonates suggest that in neonates who had lower plasma levels, faster clearance, and shorter half-life, the drug was less effective. In addition, there was a 20-fold variation in the plasma levels 24 hours after indomethacin administration among neonates.[31]

### Efficacy

Indomethacin is a potent medication for PDA closure, with historically proven rates of ductal closure. Closure rates following an initial course vary from 48 to 98.5% depending on dose, duration, and method of administration.[21,32,33] However, it is important to keep in mind that the majority of the placebo-controlled RCTs on indomethacin efficacy were conducted in the 1980s and 1990s and included more mature preterm infants with high spontaneous PDA closure rates. Therefore these numbers stated above may not be reflective of the PDA closure efficacy of indomethacin in extremely-low-gestational-age infants. Many times a repeat course is provided when either a PDA fails to close following the first course or reopens after initial closure. The reported success rates with a second course are approximately 40–50%.[32] Very rarely is a third course of indomethacin attempted, as exposure to more than two courses has been associated with periventricular leukomalacia.[34] It is unclear what pathological mechanisms play a role in this association but the indomethacin-induced prolonged

decrease in cerebral blood flow might contribute to this phenomenon. The efficacy of indomethacin declines with decreasing gestational age and increasing postnatal age.[35] Data regarding efficacy of indomethacin beyond 2 months of age suggest its ineffectiveness at this age.[21] Similarly, it is unclear whether indomethacin is as useful in the treatment of periviable neonates of 22 and 23 weeks' gestation as the efficacy decreases with decreasing gestational age.

### Timing of Administration

Indomethacin is used for prophylactic, early asymptomatic, and symptomatic treatment. Prophylactic use is employed in the first 24 hours after birth, irrespective of the presence of a PDA. Since most (85%) PDAs in VLBW infants have been shown to close spontaneously before hospital discharge, this strategy predisposes many neonates to overtreatment.[36] The underlying basis of prophylactic administration is to reduce the incidence and/or severity of peri/intraventricular hemorrhage (P/IVH) through modulation of the PDA shunt effect in addition to lowering cerebral perfusion via mechanisms independent of its effect on prostaglandin synthesis. A systematic review and meta-analysis of 19 studies identified a significant reduction in the incidence of symptomatic PDA (RR 0.44; 95% CI 0.38–0.50) and need for surgical ligation of a PDA (RR 0.51; 95% CI 0.37–0.71) with prophylactic use compared to placebo.[37] Indomethacin use was also associated with reduced rates of any P/IVH (RR 0.88; 95% CI 0.80–0.98) and severe P/IVH (RR 0.66; 95% CI 0.53–0.82). However, there was no improvement in neurodevelopmental outcomes during early childhood despite a reduction in the severity of P/IVH.[37,38] This has created diverse opinions and practices regarding the use of prophylactic indomethacin in routine clinical settings. Certain subgroups, such as male sex, lack of antenatal corticosteroids, and extremely-low-gestational-age neonates, especially those born <27 weeks' gestation, have been identified as potential candidates for prophylactic indomethacin. In addition, units with a higher underlying rate of P/IVH might use this approach as, in this situation; the benefits may outweigh the risks of prophylactic indomethacin administration.

Using indomethacin during the "early asymptomatic phase" significantly lowers the number of patients exposed to the drug compared to prophylactic measures described above, yet several patients who would have had a spontaneous closure will still be exposed. A systematic review of three RCTs reported a reduction in symptomatic PDA (RR 0.36, 95% CI 0.19–0.68) and duration of oxygen therapy following indomethacin use in the early asymptomatic phase; however, there was no difference in any other neonatal complications and no assessment of long-term neurodevelopmental outcomes.[39] A recent RCT compared treatment with indomethacin and a placebo within the first 12 hours after delivery in infants who positively screened for a "large" PDA, irrespective of their effects on hemodynamic status.[40] The trial was stopped prematurely due to unavailability of indomethacin. There was a significant reduction in pulmonary hemorrhage (2% vs. 21%), early P/IVH (4.5% vs. 12.5%), and need for later medical treatment of PDA (20% vs. 40%) with early asymptomatic treatment. However, there was no difference in the primary outcome of death or abnormal head ultrasound findings.[40]

Another approach is to treat PDA when it becomes symptomatic or hemodynamically significant. This method prevents unnecessary exposure to indomethacin as far as the PDA is concerned. Early treatment is used to describe the administration of the medication within the first 5–7 postnatal days, while late treatment is considered to occur in the second week after birth. A meta-analysis of four trials conducted between 1980 and 1990 revealed a significant reduction in BPD (OR 0.39; 95% CI 0.21–0.76) and duration of mechanical ventilation in infants receiving early versus late symptomatic treatment.[41] Furthermore, higher PDA closure rates by day 6 (73% vs. 44%; $P < 0.001$) and day 9 (91% vs. 78%; $P < 0.05$) in early versus late treatment groups were shown in a randomized controlled trial.[42] Infants treated early were more susceptible to side effects, such as lower urine output and higher creatinine levels, and experienced more severe adverse events. A recent systematic review of early treatment versus expectant management of the hemodynamically significant PDA showed that very early (defined as treatment initiated <3 days of age) or early treatment (defined as treatment initiated <7 days) with indomethacin was not associated with improvement in any clinically meaningful outcomes such as death, BPD, NEC, or need for PDA ligation, but it was associated with increased exposure to NSAIDs.[43] Of

note, a before-after observational study also showed that delayed initiation of treatment is feasible and may reduce exposure to pharmacologic agents; however, this approach may result in an increase in the combined outcome of death or BPD.[44]

### Side Effects

Indomethacin produces alterations in cerebral, renal, and splanchnic blood flow in a concentration-dependent manner and thus can lead to side effects including cerebral ischemia, renal dysfunction, and gut ischemia, and it also impairs platelet aggregation. Reduction of blood flow in the renal arteries occurs within the first 30 minutes of indomethacin administration and continues for 2 hours.[45] This can lead to elevations in urea and creatinine levels and even renal failure. Mucosal injury associated with indomethacin is secondary to effects on prostaglandin synthesis. Prophylactic indomethacin has been associated with increased odds of spontaneous intestinal perforation (SIP) independent of early feeding, in a Canadian cohort of extremely preterm infants ($n = 4268$; adjusted OR [aOR] 2.43, 95% CI 1.41–4.19).[46] A recent individual patient data meta-analysis of RCTs further suggests that prophylactic indomethacin increases the risk of SIP when given concomitantly with prophylactic hydrocortisone.[47] The risk of SIP may further be increased in extremely preterm infants who received antenatal corticosteroids within 7 days before birth (aOR 1.67, 95% CI 1.15–2.43).[48] The association of indomethacin with NEC, on the contrary, is a subject of debate, since the occurrence of NEC could be due to the disturbance of blood flow in the presence of a hemodynamically significant PDA rather than indomethacin alone.[27] Still, indomethacin is also known to reduce splanchnic blood flow during its administration, and therefore this cause-and-effect relationship remains unclear.[27] Because of concerns regarding intestinal blood flow, feeding is either discontinued, held, or sustained depending upon the attending medical team's preference; however, similar outcomes have been reported with each approach.[49]

### Take-Home Message

Overall, there is high certainty of evidence from RCTs to demonstrate that indomethacin is effective in closing a symptomatic PDA compared to no treatment in preterm infants.[50] Rate of successful PDA closure is approximately 70% with the first course and 50% with a repeat course. However, evidence is insufficient regarding the effects of indomethacin on other clinically relevant outcomes and medication-related adverse effects.[50] Recommended use includes a routine course of three doses after excluding contraindications, followed by repeat use for persistent PDA, if clinically indicated. Varying side effects, concerns over the impact of oral use on immature gastric mucosa, and the availability of potentially safer alternatives have led to a decrease in indomethacin use for treatment of PDA. Finally, the decrease in the rate of P/IVH with the use of prophylactic indomethacin might serve as an indication of its use in a selected group of patients with higher risk of P/IVH (see Chapter 6).

## IBUPROFEN

### Mechanism of Action

Ibuprofen is a non-selective COX inhibitor that does not alter cerebral perfusion and has a reduced effect on renal and gut perfusion. Ibuprofen inhibits COX-1 and COX-2 enzymes in a rapid and reversible manner. It is metabolized in the liver and excreted in urine, and thus physiological impairment of hepatic or renal function may lead to adverse reactions.

### Dose, Route, and Frequency

The usual dose is 10 mg/kg on day 1, followed by two doses of 5 mg/kg 24 hours apart. This dosage, which was based on a small ($n = 34$) phase I study of early (within 3 hours of birth) administration of intravenous ibuprofen lysine, has since remained the most commonly used dosage regimen in clinical and research settings irrespective of the gestational and postnatal age.[51] It has been demonstrated in a dose-finding study that the standard 10-5-5 mg/kg dosing regimen had a very low probability of success in extremely preterm infants born <27 weeks of gestation (30.6%, 95% [Credible intervals] CrIs 13–56%).[52] Pharmacokinetic studies have also suggested that to achieve therapeutic serum concentrations, higher doses may be required with increasing postnatal age (15-7.5-7.5 mg/kg for postnatal ages of 3–5 days and 20-10-10 mg/kg for postnatal ages >5 days), further emphasizing the importance of postnatal age–dependent dosing.[43] This

could partly explain why the efficacy of ibuprofen for PDA closure (around 71–74%) demonstrated in RCTs of early therapy (median age of start of ibuprofen: 3 days) have not been replicated in clinical practice where therapy is usually delayed (median age 6 days) with a primary pharmacotherapy failure rate of around 40–50%.[53,54] In fact, meta-analyses of RCTs demonstrate a reduced rate of failure to close the PDA with high doses of ibuprofen compared with standard doses (RR 0.37, 95% CI 0.22–0.61).[55] Adaptive dosing in the form of continued doses of ibuprofen (up to 6 doses if PDA was not closed) was associated with an 88% closure rate (similar to indomethacin).[56] Doubling of the doses during the second course was associated with 60% closure rates compared to 10% in infants receiving the same dose when a consecutive treatment protocol was used, underscoring the need for further studies on ibuprofen dosing, pharmacokinetics, and pharmacodynamics.[57]

Ibuprofen can be given orally or intravenously. A comparison of oral and intravenous ibuprofen pharmacokinetics demonstrated that the peak serum levels are reached earlier with intravenous delivery; however, the elimination is slower after enteral administration, resulting in a higher area under the curve (AUC) for serum ibuprofen concentration with the latter ($AUC_{0-24}$, 618 μg/mL·h for enteral vs. 462 μg/mL·h for intravenous).[58] Several trials have also compared the efficacy of routes of administration. A systematic review of oral versus intravenous ibuprofen indicated a lower risk of failure to close a PDA with oral ibuprofen use (RR 0.38, 95% CI 0.26–0.56).[55] Furthermore, higher rates of sustained closure have been observed after continuous infusion compared to bolus infusion (closure after one or two courses 86% in continuous infusion group versus 68% after one or two courses in intermittent infusion group; $P = 0.02$).[59]

Intravenous ibuprofen is available in two preparations, ibuprofen lysine and ibuprofen-tris-hydroxymethyl-aminomethane (THAM). In one retrospective study from Italy it was identified that ibuprofen lysine was more effective than ibuprofen THAM in reducing the need for PDA ligation (73% vs. 51%, $P = 0.002$) when used prophylactically in neonates of ≤28 weeks' gestation.[60] There is ongoing controversy on whether the efficacy significantly varies between the two formulations. A systematic review and network meta-analysis of existing RCTs is currently underway to address this question.[61]

## Efficacy

Similar to indomethacin, ibuprofen is also an effective agent for closure of the PDA. The response rate for the first and second courses mimics that of indomethacin, with approximate closure rates of 70% and 50%, respectively. A detailed systematic review of studies evaluating the therapeutic use of ibuprofen revealed that both oral (RR 0.26, 95% CI 0.11–0.62) and intravenous (RR 0.62, 95% CI 0.44–0.86) ibuprofen reduces failure of PDA closure in comparison to placebo treatment.[55] Ibuprofen has been compared to indomethacin in several RCTs. A systematic review of these trials indicated that ibuprofen and indomethacin (both oral and intravenous) are similar in terms of their efficacy in ductal closure (RR 1.07, 95% CI 0.92–1.24), rates of PDA reopening after the first course (RR 1.57, 95% CI 0.83, 2.99), and need for surgical ligation (RR 1.06, 95% CI 0.81, 1.39).[55] In addition, ibuprofen was associated with a lower incidence of renal dysfunction (as indicated by its effect on urine output and serum creatinine), shorter duration of mechanical ventilation (−2.4 days, 95% CI −3.7 days to −1.0 day), and lower incidence of NEC (RR 0.68, 95% CI 0.49–0.94). There were no differences in P/IVH, ROP, and survival or neurodevelopmental outcomes between the two agents.[55]

## Timing of Administration

Similar to indomethacin, ibuprofen has also been used for prophylactic, asymptomatic, and symptomatic PDA management. Prophylactic ibuprofen may marginally reduce the risk of severe P/IVH (RR 0.67, 95% CI 0.45–1.00).[62] Use of prophylactic oral or intravenous ibuprofen reduces the incidence of PDA on postnatal day 3 or 4 (RR 0.39, 95% CI 0.31–0.48), need for rescue treatment with cyclooxygenase inhibitors (RR 0.17, 95% CI 0.11–0.26), and need for surgical PDA ligation (RR 0.46, 95% CI 0.22–0.96) compared with placebo or no treatment, but it has no benefit on any other patient-important clinical outcomes.[62]

Yoo et al. evaluated mortality and neonatal complications following the use of ibuprofen in two groups of neonates, including 14 (15.4%) preterm infants of <28 weeks' gestation with clinical symptoms of hsPDA

and 77 (84.6%) asymptomatic neonates with no evidence of hsPDA.[63] Infants in the symptomatic group were of younger gestation (by 1 week) and lower birth weight (by 225 g) and had higher severity of illness scores. They also received more courses of ibuprofen. In a logistic regression analysis after adjustment for severity of illness, birth weight, birth year, and invasive ventilator care ≤2 postnatal days, there were no significant differences in mortality, frequency of secondary ligation, NEC, P/IVH, BPD, or death between the two groups. The authors concluded that treatment of asymptomatic or non-hsPDA may not be warranted.

A recent systematic review on early treatment versus expectant management of the hemodynamically significant PDA showed that very early treatment with ibuprofen (defined as treatment initiated <3 days of age) may reduce the incidence of BPD (RR 0.54, 95% CI 0.35–0.83).[43] The review failed to demonstrate benefit of early (defined as treatment initiated <7 days) or very early therapy for any other clinical outcomes, while both approaches were associated with increased exposure to NSAIDs compared to expectant management.[43]

## Side Effects

Major side effects of ibuprofen include oliguria, high bilirubin levels, gastrointestinal hemorrhage, and pulmonary hypertension. The use of ibuprofen-THAM has been associated with higher rates of gastrointestinal complications, as well as pulmonary hypertension.[64] The association of ibuprofen use with pulmonary hypertension was initially thought to be specific with the ibuprofen-THAM preparation, possibly related to acidification of ibuprofen solution by the use of normal saline flush, subsequently causing precipitation and embolism.[65] However, there are similar reports of pulmonary hypertension with early use of ibuprofen lysine preparation as well.[66,67] In a recent cohort of 144 neonates who received ibuprofen treatment for PDA, 10 cases developed pulmonary arterial hypertension, of which 7 occurred in the intravenous ibuprofen-THAM group (n = 100), 2 in the oral ibuprofen group (n = 40), and 1 in those who received intravenous ibuprofen lysine preparation (n = 4).[66] Risk factors for the development of pulmonary arterial hypertension were noted to be small for gestational age, maternal hypertension, and oligohydramnios.[66]

## Take-Home Message

Several studies have confirmed that ibuprofen has similar potency for PDA closure as indomethacin but carries a lower profile of side effects. Therefore ibuprofen should be considered the pharmacotherapy of choice for a symptomatic PDA over indomethacin. Higher-dose ibuprofen may be considered, especially for preterm infants beyond the first 3–5 days of age. However, caution should be exercised when treating extremely preterm infants with high-dose ibuprofen due to limited safety and efficacy data. Given that oral ibuprofen is as effective as intravenous ibuprofen and is likely to result in reduced side effects, it may be the preferred route for ductal closure in infants who are receiving enteral feeds.

## ACETAMINOPHEN (PARACETAMOL)

### Mechanism of Action

Acetaminophen, also known as paracetamol, acts on PDA closure through the inhibition of POX-mediated conversion of prostaglandin $G_2$ to prostaglandin $H_2$. In addition, there is some evidence that acetaminophen may have a substantial inhibitory effect on the COX-2 enzyme.[68] There has been a growing interest in the use of acetaminophen as a potential pharmacotherapy for PDA in extremely preterm infants given its relatively better safety profile compared to indomethacin or ibuprofen.

### Dose, Route, and Frequency

The compound's pharmacokinetics, including the dose and route of administration, have not been well-studied compared to indomethacin and ibuprofen. The potential effect of acetaminophen in closing the PDA was first reported in a case series of 5 preterm infants (GA 26–32 weeks; postnatal age 3–35 days) where the index case was administered oral acetaminophen at a dose of 15 mg/kg per dose every 6 hours orally for 7 days incidentally for an unrelated reason.[69] Since then, the same dosage of 15 mg/kg dose every 6 hours for 2–7 days has been used in clinical trials and clinical practice with little exploration of dose-dependent effects.[69,70] A recent study that explored the pharmacokinetic profile of acetaminophen administered at a dose of 20 mg/kg loading within 24 hours of birth followed by 7.5 mg/kg every 6 hours for 4 days in preterm infants born <32 weeks' gestation as a part of the Preterm Infants' Paracetamol Study (PreParaS trial) demonstrated that the efficacy of acetaminophen for ductal closure was substantially reduced with each week of gestation below 27 weeks. This highlights the need for optimal dose finding studies, especially in extremely preterm infants at the highest risk of PDA-attributable morbidity.[71]

The most commonly used route of acetaminophen administration is oral. The increased availability of the intravenous formulation presents an attractive option for clinicians, especially for preterm infants who are unable to tolerate feeds and have contraindications to NSAIDs. However, an RCT of 86 VLBW infants showed that indomethacin was more effective in closing a PDA (55% vs. 6%) and preventing procedural closure (15% vs. 47%) versus intravenous acetaminophen.[72] Another RCT of 101 VLBW infants demonstrated that standard dose ibuprofen was more effective in closing a PDA (78% vs. 52%; $P = 0.026$) as compared to intravenous acetaminophen. These findings call into question the efficacy of the intravenous formulation in the highest-risk population of very preterm infants.[73]

### Efficacy

There have been 27 published RCTs on the use of acetaminophen for treatment of PDA. These include comparisons with placebo, indomethacin, and ibuprofen, as well as combination therapy with ibuprofen.[74] In addition, 24 ongoing trials have been identified, which are expected to add to the current body of evidence. The overall efficacy of acetaminophen is approximately 70% when compared to both ibuprofen (18 RCTs, 1535 infants) and indomethacin (4 RCTs, 380 infants). There was moderate certainty of evidence to suggest that acetaminophen is as effective as ibuprofen and low certainty of evidence to suggest that acetaminophen is as effective as indomethacin in closing a PDA.[74] There were no differences in any other patient-important clinical outcomes with acetaminophen when compared with ibuprofen or indomethacin. Efficacy in the subgroup of infants <32 weeks' gestation ranged from 67 to 76%.[74] However, there remains paucity of data in the extremely preterm population born <28 weeks' gestation.

Combination therapy using acetaminophen and ibuprofen has been explored with variable success.[75]

Meta-analysis of two small RCTs (111 infants) failed to demonstrate any significant difference in failure of PDA closure when compared to ibuprofen alone (RR 0.77, 95% CI 0.43–1.36).[74] However, failure of PDA closure may be marginally lower after two courses of combination therapy compared to ibuprofen monotherapy (RR 0.28, 95% CI 0.08–0.99). Given the relative safety of acetaminophen, this is an area that will benefit from future large trials.

### Timing of Administration

Most clinical trials have explored the use of acetaminophen for symptomatic PDA treatment; few have explored its prophylactic use. A meta-analysis of three RCTs showed that although prophylactic acetaminophen was effective in closing a PDA (RR 3.70, 95% CI 2.38–5.56), this higher efficacy failed to translate into a significant improvement for any other clinical outcome.[74]

Given the paucity of good-quality pharmacokinetic data, it is uncertain if acetaminophen efficacy is a function of postnatal age, similar to ibuprofen, and whether dose adjustments are required for later treatment. A recent systematic review suggests early acetaminophen use (initiated within 14 days after birth) was associated with a large reduction in failure to close a PDA (2 RCTs, 127 infants, RR 0.35, 95% CI 0.23–0.53), while a similar effect was not observed with later initiation of acetaminophen (1 RCT, 55 infants, RR 0.85, 95% CI 0.72–1.01).[74] However, given the better safety profile, some clinicians may still choose to use a third course of pharmacotherapy using acetaminophen, following two initial failed courses of NSAIDs, while contemplating procedural PDA closure. This practice requires further interrogation as a recent retrospective observational study did show that extremely preterm infants with a persistent symptomatic PDA who were treated with a 3- to 7-day course of oral acetaminophen following two failed courses with indomethacin or ibuprofen had reduced rates of surgical ligation but increased rates of CLD.[76]

### Side Effects

Acetaminophen is generally well tolerated, with substantially lower short-term adverse effects as compared to indomethacin and ibuprofen. A meta-analysis of RCTs suggests acetaminophen is associated with lower rates of NEC (4 RCTs, 384 infants, RR 0.42, 95% CI 0.19–0.96) and gastrointestinal bleeds (7 RCTs, 693 infants, RR 0.37, 95% CI 0.19–0.73) as compared to indomethacin and ibuprofen, respectively.[74] Other side effects may include hepatotoxicity, as well as hemodynamic and thermodynamic effects. Therapeutic doses of acetaminophen used for analgesic purposes have not been shown to be associated with acute side effects. The oral preparation of acetaminophen is often diluted significantly prior to administration due to concerns about the solution's high osmolality and the potential associated risk for the subsequent development of NEC.

There is limited data on the effect of acetaminophen on neurodevelopmental outcomes. Viberg et al[77] showed that exposure to acetaminophen during a critical period of brain development can induce long-lasting effects on cognitive function in mice and alter the adult response to acetaminophen. Moreover, acute neonatal exposure in mice also led to altered locomotor activity and affected spatial learning in adulthood. Avella-Garcia et al.[78] followed children of 1 year and 5 years of age who were exposed to maternal intake of acetaminophen before 32 weeks' gestation. The authors found that prenatal exposure to acetaminophen may alter attention function at 5 years of age while affecting males and females differently. However, this study suffers from issues of inexact delineation of the quantity, timing, and duration of maternal acetaminophen intake. Through analyzing data from a population-based cohort in Denmark, Liew et al.[79] reported that prenatal use of acetaminophen was associated with a higher risk of hyperkinetic disorder (hazard ratio 1.37; 95% CI 1.19–1.59), need for attention deficit hyperactivity disorder treatment (hazard ratio 1.29; 95% CI 1.15–1.44), and attention deficit hyperactivity disorder–like behaviors at 7 years of age (RR 1.13; 95% CI 1.01–1.27). There was also some evidence for a dose-response relationship. Finally, in an ecological analysis Bauer and Kriebel[80] reported that country-level autism was correlated with rates of circumcision. Given that this procedure is often accompanied by the use of acetaminophen for pain management, the possibility of an associative link has been entertained. Further data on both the side effects and the impact of acetaminophen on neurodevelopmental outcomes are clearly needed.

## Take-Home Message

Acetaminophen appears to be as effective as ibuprofen and indomethacin in closing a PDA while having a favorable short-term safety profile. Future efforts should address issues around optimal dosage (as monotherapy or in conjunction with other NSAIDs), route, duration of therapy, and its effectiveness in extremely preterm neonates, who are the most likely candidates for treatment. In addition, potential long-term effects of neonatal acetaminophen administration on neurodevelopment need to be examined.

## Comparison of the Three Pharmacological Agents

All three agents have been tested against one another in various combinations (Figure 17.1) with no major differences observed for any of the patient and family important clinical outcomes, with the exception of the effect of prophylactic indomethacin on decreasing the rates of P/IVH.

There is currently no RCT that has evaluated all the three agents (acetaminophen, ibuprofen, and indomethacin) as prophylactic therapies in the same trial. A recent Bayesian network meta-analysis (28 RCTs, 3999 infants) evaluated the comparative effectiveness and safety of all prophylactic therapies versus 'no prophylaxis' in preterm infants.[81] The authors concluded that prophylactic indomethacin probably results in a small reduction in severe IVH (network RR 0.66, 95% credible intervals [CrI] 0.49 to 0.87; absolute risk difference [ARD] 43 fewer [95% CrI, 65 fewer to 16 fewer] per 1000; median rank 2; moderate certainty), a moderate reduction in mortality (network RR 0.85, 95% CrI 0.64–1.1; ARD 24 fewer [95% CrI, 58 fewer to 16 more] per 1000; median rank 2; moderate certainty), and surgical PDA closure (network RR 0.40, 95% CrI 0.14–0.66; ARD 52 fewer [95% CrI, 75 fewer to 30 fewer] per 1000; median rank 2; moderate certainty), but it may result in a small increase in CLD (network RR 1.10, 95% CrI 0.93–1.3; ARD 36 more [95% CrI, 25 fewer to 108 more] per 1000; low certainty). Prophylactic ibuprofen probably results in a small reduction in severe IVH (network RR 0.69, 95% CrI 0.41–1.14; ARD 39 fewer [95% CrI, 75 fewer to 18 more] per 1000; median rank 2; moderate certainty) and moderate reduction in surgical PDA closure (network RR 0.24, 95% CrI 0.06–0.64; ARD 66 fewer [95% CrI, from 82 fewer to 31 fewer] per 1000; median rank 1; moderate certainty) and may result in a moderate reduction in mortality (network RR 0.83, 95% CrI 0.57–1.2; ARD 27 fewer [95% CrI, from 69 fewer to 32 more] per 1000; median rank 2; low certainty). For acetaminophen, the estimate of effects was very uncertain for any of the clinically relevant outcomes.

With regards to management of symptomatic PDA, to date, only one randomized study has evaluated all three agents (acetaminophen, ibuprofen, and indomethacin) relative to each other.[82] In this prospective study preterm neonates, born at a gestational age less than 28 weeks' or weight of <1500 g, who were diagnosed with hsPDA by echocardiography and clinical examination were randomized to one of the three intervention groups (100 in each arm). Patients received a second course of the same treatment regimen if the PDA failed to close. Overall, there was no difference in the rate of ductal closure after the first (80% vs. 77% vs. 81%) or second course (88% vs. 83% vs. 87%) of acetaminophen, ibuprofen, and indomethacin, respectively. There was also no difference in neonatal complications and side effects between all groups, with the exception of a higher occurrence of intestinal bleeding in the indomethacin- and ibuprofen-treated patients ($P < 0.05$).[82] A Bayesian network meta-analysis of 68 RCTs (4802 infants) showed that high-dose oral ibuprofen was associated with a significantly higher odds of PDA closure versus intravenous formulations of standard dose ibuprofen (OR 3.59; 95% CrI 1.64–8.17) or indomethacin (OR 2.35; 95% CrI 1.08–5.31).[20] However, data was insufficient to draw meaningful conclusions on clinically important outcomes such as CLD, NEC, and IVH.

## Conclusions and Implications for Practice and Research

Despite a large body of evidence from RCTs, pharmacotherapy of the PDA in preterm infants remains controversial. In summary, ibuprofen has replaced indomethacin as the gold standard in infants where medical management is sought, whereas acetaminophen has emerged as a potentially less toxic alternative, with similar efficacy to the NSAIDs. Clinicians are increasingly considering the use of higher doses of ibuprofen, preferably using enteral formulations, especially for delayed treatment.[19] However, the safety of such approaches in the most vulnerable preterm population is yet to be firmly established. From a pharmacoprophylaxis perspective, clinicians have generally moved away from using NSAIDs in all extremely preterm infants. However, with increased survival of infants at the limits of viability, some clinicians have reconsidered the use of selective pharmacoprophylaxis using indomethacin, especially in infants at the highest risk of P/IVH and mortality, while there is a growing interest in exploring the use of prophylactic or early selective use of acetaminophen in extremely-low-gestational-age infants given its favorable short term safety profile. The effects of such approaches on long-term neurodevelopmental, cardiovascular, and renal health are yet to be determined.

It is important to recognize that most trials of PDA pharmacotherapy were designed to examine whether pharmacotherapy was effective in closing a PDA. Most of the RCTs were not designed or powered to explore whether pharmacotherapy for PDA improved clinically relevant outcomes. Hence most trials had a backup treatment option had the PDA remained open following the initial intervention, as evidenced by the significantly higher rate of open-label treatment in the placebo group.[83] Therefore caution should be exercised while assessing the benefits and harms of pharmacotherapy in light of patient-important outcomes. Further, with regard to patient-important outcomes, it is important to highlight the over-emphasis on BPD as the primary clinical endpoint in many of the previous trials. BPD, commonly defined in previous RCTs as oxygen requirement at 36 weeks postmenstrual age, may not be the most important clinical outcome from a parent's perspective, as compared to other respiratory morbidities, such as need for mechanical ventilation at 36 weeks postmenstrual age (severe BPD) or chronic severe pulmonary hypertension. Therefore future trials should be adequately powered for outcomes that are clinically meaningful for patients and their families.

The diagnosis of a hemodynamically significant PDA remains a challenge in clinical trials. Although echocardiography characteristics have been identified, they are not reliable enough to effectively identify the right population who would benefit from early effective closure of the ductus (these concepts are further discussed in Chapters 16 and 19). Even in cases where perturbation of blood flow to splanchnic organs has been identified, its clinical significance remains uncertain. This has led to a growing skepticism around the management of ductus in preterm infants, with some clinicians/centers advocating in favor of abandoning PDA evaluation and treatment altogether.

To better guide clinicians in the management of PDA, further understanding of the physiologic changes caused by the condition is required. The identification of biochemical or imaging biomarkers that signal affected organ blood flow arising from the systematic diversion of blood to the lungs by a significant PDA may complement current diagnostic tools. Furthermore, the identification of mechanisms by which higher pulmonary vascular flow secondary to hsPDA affects the developing lungs and pulmonary blood flow regulation may help guide the development of new therapies, as not all neonates with higher flow result in pulmonary edema and hemorrhage.[84] Pharmacokinetics and pharmacodynamics of all three agents are poorly studied and future studies should build that component in their design so that such questions can be answered simultaneously rather than as afterthoughts. Ideally, randomized controlled studies would be the preferred approach to evaluate the impact of diagnostic tests or therapeutic interventions. However, large cohorts could also be studied with careful selection of analytical techniques that incorporate as many residual confounding variables as possible (propensity score methods, instrumental variable analyses) and answer two critical biases associated with the assessment of long-term outcomes of PDA, confounding by indication or contraindication and survival bias.[85] Future studies will need to try to account for these biases when assessing the impact of therapies on survival free of neurodevelopmental impairment. In the meantime, clinicians will continue debating the risks and benefits of various treatment options until enough evidence is available to establish generally accepted guidelines for the management of PDA in the preterm neonate. Finally, utilizing comprehensive, real-time monitoring and data acquisition systems along with mathematical modeling and machine learning (Chapter 14), differences among individual patients affecting PDA rates, rates of spontaneous closure, and the patient's response to the different treatment approaches could also be recognized and modeled to the phenotypic profile of the given patient, providing a precision medicine approach to the pharmacological management of the PDA.

## REFERENCES

1. Allegaert K, Anderson B, Simons S, van Overmeire B. Paracetamol to induce ductus arteriosus closure: is it valid? *Arch Dis Child.* 2013;98(6):462-466. doi:10.1136/archdischild-2013-303688.
2. Lai LS, McCrindle BW. Variation in the diagnosis and management of patent ductus arteriosus in premature infants. *Paediatr Child Health.* 1998;3(6):405-410. doi:10.1093/pch/3.6.405.
3. Amin SB, Handley C, Carter-Pokras O. Indomethacin use for the management of patent ductus arteriosus in preterms: a web-based survey of practice attitudes among neonatal fellowship program directors in the United States. *Pediatr Cardiol.* 2007;28(3):193-200. doi:10.1007/s00246-006-0093-1.
4. Hoellering AB, Cooke L. The management of patent ductus arteriosus in Australia and New Zealand. *J Paediatr Child Health.* 2009;45(4):204-209. doi:10.1111/j.1440-1754.2008.01461.x.
5. Guimarães H, Rocha G, Tomé T, Anatolitou F, Sarafidis K, Fanos V. Non-steroid anti-inflammatory drugs in the treatment of patent ductus arteriosus in European newborns. *J Matern Fetal Neonatal Med.* 2009;22(suppl 3):77-80. doi:10.1080/14767050903198314.
6. Brissaud O, Guichoux J. Patent ductus arteriosus in the preterm infant: a survey of clinical practices in French neonatal intensive care units. *Pediatr Cardiol.* 2011;32(5):607-614. doi:10.1007/s00246-011-9925-8.
7. Irmesi R, Marcialis MA, Anker JVD, Fanos V. Non-steroidal anti-inflammatory drugs (NSAIDs) in the management of patent ductus arteriosus (PDA) in preterm infants and variations in attitude in clinical practice: a flight around the world. *Curr Med Chem.* 2014;21(27):3132-3152. doi:10.2174/0929867321666140304095434.
8. Isayama T, Kusuda S, Adams M, et al. International variation in the management of patent ductus arteriosus and its association with infant outcomes: a survey and linked cohort study. *J Pediatr.* 2022;244:24-29.e7. doi:10.1016/j.jpeds.2021.12.071.
9. Isayama T, Kusuda S, Reichman B, et al. Neonatal intensive care unit-level patent ductus arteriosus treatment rates and outcomes in infants born extremely preterm. *J Pediatr.* 2020;220:34-39.e5. doi:10.1016/j.jpeds.2020.01.069.
10. Hagadorn JI, Brownell EA, Trzaski JM, et al. Trends and variation in management and outcomes of very low-birth-weight infants with patent ductus arteriosus. *Pediatr Res.* 2016;80(6):785-792. doi:10.1038/pr.2016.166.
11. Edstedt Bonamy AK, Gudmundsdottir A, Maier RF, et al. Patent ductus arteriosus treatment in very preterm infants: a European Population-Based Cohort Study (EPICE) on variation and outcomes. *Neonatology.* 2017;111(4):367-375. doi:10.1159/000454798.
12. Lokku A, Mirea L, Lee SK, Shah PS, Canadian Neonatal Network. Trends and outcomes of patent ductus arteriosus treatment in very preterm infants in Canada. *Am J Perinatol.* 2017;34(5):441-450. doi:10.1055/s-0036-1593351.
13. Slaughter JL, Reagan PB, Newman TB, Klebanoff MA. Comparative effectiveness of nonsteroidal anti-inflammatory drug treatment vs no treatment for patent ductus arteriosus in preterm infants. *JAMA Pediatr.* 2017;171(3):e164354. doi:10.1001/jamapediatrics.2016.4354.
14. Rozé JC, Cambonie G, Marchand-Martin L, et al. Association between early screening for patent ductus arteriosus and in-hospital mortality among extremely preterm infants. *JAMA.* 2015;313(24):2441-2448. doi:10.1001/jama.2015.6734.
15. Toyoshima K, Momma K, Nakanishi T. In vivo dilatation of the ductus arteriosus induced by furosemide in the rat. *Pediatr Res.* 2010;67(2):173-176. doi:10.1203/PDR.0b013e3181c2df30.
16. Brion LP, Campbell DE. Furosemide for symptomatic patent ductus arteriosus in indomethacin-treated infants. *Cochrane Database Syst Rev.* 2001;(3):CD001148. doi:10.1002/14651858.CD001148.
17. Lee BS, Byun SY, Chung ML, et al. Effect of furosemide on ductal closure and renal function in indomethacin-treated preterm infants during the early neonatal period. *Neonatology.* 2010;98(2):191-199. doi:10.1159/000289206.
18. Thompson EJ, Greenberg RG, Kumar K, et al. Association between furosemide exposure and patent ductus arteriosus in hospitalized very low birth weight infants. *J Pediatr.* 2018;199:231-236. doi:10.1016/j.jpeds.2018.03.067.
19. Mitra S, Weisz D, Jain A, Jong G't. Management of the patent ductus arteriosus in preterm infants. *Paediatr Child Health.* 2022;27(1):63-64. doi:10.1093/pch/pxab085.
20. Mitra S, Florez ID, Tamayo ME, et al. Association of placebo, indomethacin, ibuprofen, and acetaminophen with closure of hemodynamically significant patent ductus arteriosus in preterm infants. *JAMA.* 2018;319(12):1221-1238. doi:10.1001/jama.2018.1896.
21. Pacifici GM. Clinical pharmacology of indomethacin in preterm infants: implications in patent ductus arteriosus closure. *Paediatr Drugs.* 2013;15(5):363-376. doi:10.1007/s40272-013-0031-7.
22. Bhat R, Vidyasagar D, Fisher E, et al. Pharmacokinetics of oral and intravenous indomethacin in preterm infants. *Dev Pharmacol Ther.* 1980;1(2-3):101-110.
23. Friedman WF. Physiology and pharmacology of the ductus arteriosus: studies of the responses of the ductus arteriosus. In: *Proceedings of the 75th Ross Conference on Pediatric Research;* 1977.
24. Sperandio M, Beedgen B, Feneberg R, et al. Effectiveness and side effects of an escalating, stepwise approach to indomethacin treatment for symptomatic patent ductus arteriosus in premature infants below 33 weeks of gestation. *Pediatrics.* 2005;116(6):1361-1366. doi:10.1542/peds.2005-0293.
25. Jegatheesan P, Ianus V, Buchh B, et al. Increased indomethacin dosing for persistent patent ductus arteriosus in preterm infants: a multicenter, randomized, controlled trial. *J Pediatr.* 2008;153(2):183-189. doi:10.1016/j.jpeds.2008.01.031.
26. Herrera C, Holberton J, Davis P. Prolonged versus short course of indomethacin for the treatment of patent ductus arteriosus in preterm infants. *Cochrane Database Syst Rev.* 2007;(2):CD003480. doi:10.1002/14651858.CD003480.pub3.
27. Christmann V, Liem KD, Semmekrot BA, van de Bor M. Changes in cerebral, renal and mesenteric blood flow velocity during continuous and bolus infusion of indomethacin. *Acta Paediatr.* 2002;91(4):440-446. doi:10.1080/080352502317371698.
28. Hammerman C, Glaser J, Schimmel MS, Ferber B, Kaplan M, Eidelman AI. Continuous versus multiple rapid infusions of indomethacin: effects on cerebral blood flow velocity. *Pediatrics.* 1995;95(2):244-248.
29. de Vries NKS, Jagroep FK, Jaarsma AS, Elzenga NJ, Bos AF. Continuous indomethacin infusion may be less effective than bolus infusions for ductal closure in very low birth weight infants. *Am J Perinatol.* 2005;22(2):71-75. doi:10.1055/s-2005-837273.
30. Görk AS, Ehrenkranz RA, Bracken MB. Continuous infusion versus intermittent bolus doses of indomethacin for patent ductus

arteriosus closure in symptomatic preterm infants. *Cochrane Database Syst Rev.* 2008;(1):CD006071. doi:10.1002/14651858. CD006071.pub2.

31. Brash AR, Hickey DE, Graham TP, Stahlman MT, Oates JA, Cotton RB. Pharmacokinetics of indomethacin in the neonate. Relation of plasma indomethacin levels to response of the ductus arteriosus. *N Engl J Med.* 1981;305(2):67-72. doi:10.1056/NEJM198107093050203.

32. Godambe S, Newby B, Shah V, Shah PS. Effect of indomethacin on closure of ductus arteriosus in very-low-birthweight neonates. *Acta Paediatr.* 2006;95(11):1389-1393. doi:10.1080/08035250600615150.

33. Gersony WM, Peckham GJ, Ellison RC, Miettinen OS, Nadas AS. Effects of indomethacin in premature infants with patent ductus arteriosus: results of a national collaborative study. *J Pediatr.* 1983;102(6):895-906. doi:10.1016/s0022-3476(83)80022-5.

34. Sangem M, Asthana S, Amin S. Multiple courses of indomethacin and neonatal outcomes in premature infants. *Pediatr Cardiol.* 2008;29(5):878-884. doi:10.1007/s00246-007-9166-z.

35. Achanti B, Yeh TF, Pildes RS. Indomethacin therapy in infants with advanced postnatal age and patent ductus arteriosus. *Clin Invest Med.* 1986;9(4):250-253.

36. Semberova J, Sirc J, Miletin J, et al. Spontaneous closure of patent ductus arteriosus in infants ≤1500 g. *Pediatrics.* 2017;140(2):e20164258. doi:10.1542/peds.2016-4258.

37. Fowlie PW, Davis PG, McGuire W. Prophylactic intravenous indomethacin for preventing mortality and morbidity in preterm infants. *Cochrane Database Syst Rev.* 2010;(7):CD000174. doi:10.1002/14651858.CD000174.pub2.

38. Schmidt B, Roberts RS, Fanaroff A, et al. Indomethacin prophylaxis, patent ductus arteriosus, and the risk of bronchopulmonary dysplasia: further analyses from the Trial of Indomethacin Prophylaxis in Preterms (TIPP). *J Pediatr.* 2006;148(6):730-734. doi:10.1016/j.jpeds.2006.01.047.

39. Cooke L, Steer P, Woodgate P. Indomethacin for asymptomatic patent ductus arteriosus in preterm infants. *Cochrane Database Syst Rev.* 2003;(2):CD003745. doi:10.1002/14651858.CD003745.

40. Kluckow M, Jeffery M, Gill A, Evans N. A randomised placebo-controlled trial of early treatment of the patent ductus arteriosus. *Arch Dis Child Fetal Neonatal Ed.* 2014;99(2):F99-F104. doi:10.1136/archdischild-2013-304695.

41. Clyman RI. Recommendations for the postnatal use of indomethacin: an analysis of four separate treatment strategies. *J Pediatr.* 1996;128(5 Pt 1):601-607. doi:10.1016/s0022-3476(96)80123-5.

42. Van Overmeire B, Van de Broek H, Van Laer P, Weyler J, Vanhaesebrouck P. Early versus late indomethacin treatment for patent ductus arteriosus in premature infants with respiratory distress syndrome. *J Pediatr.* 2001;138(2):205-211. doi:10.1067/mpd.2001.110528.

43. Mitra S, Scrivens A, von Kursell AM, Disher T. Early treatment versus expectant management of hemodynamically significant patent ductus arteriosus for preterm infants. *Cochrane Database Syst Rev.* 2020;12:CD013278. doi:10.1002/14651858.CD013278.pub2.

44. Kaempf JW, Wu YX, Kaempf AJ, Kaempf AM, Wang L, Grunkemeier G. What happens when the patent ductus arteriosus is treated less aggressively in very low birth weight infants? *J Perinatol.* 2012;32(5):344-348. doi:10.1038/jp.2011.102.

45. Pezzati M, Vangi V, Biagiotti R, Bertini G, Cianciulli D, Rubaltelli FF. Effects of indomethacin and ibuprofen on mesenteric and renal blood flow in preterm infants with patent ductus arteriosus. *J Pediatr.* 1999;135(6):733-738. doi:10.1016/s0022-3476(99)70093-4.

46. Stavel M, Wong J, Cieslak Z, Sherlock R, Claveau M, Shah PS. Effect of prophylactic indomethacin administration and early feeding on spontaneous intestinal perforation in extremely low-birth-weight infants. *J Perinatol.* 2017;37(2):188-193. doi:10.1038/jp.2016.196.

47. Shaffer ML, Baud O, Lacaze-Masmonteil T, Peltoniemi OM, Bonsante F, Watterberg KL. Effect of prophylaxis for early adrenal insufficiency using low-dose hydrocortisone in very preterm infants: an individual patient data meta-analysis. *J Pediatr.* 2019;207:136-142.e5. doi:10.1016/j.jpeds.2018.10.004.

48. Kandraju H, Kanungo J, Lee KS, et al. Association of co-exposure of antenatal steroid and prophylactic indomethacin with spontaneous intestinal perforation. *J Pediatr.* 2021;235:34-41.e1. doi:10.1016/j.jpeds.2021.03.012.

49. Louis D, Torgalkar R, Shah J, Shah PS, Jain A. Enteral feeding during indomethacin treatment for patent ductus arteriosus: association with gastrointestinal outcomes. *J Perinatol.* 2016;36(7):544-548. doi:10.1038/jp.2016.11.

50. Evans P, O'Reilly D, Flyer JN, Soll R, Mitra S. Indomethacin for symptomatic patent ductus arteriosus in preterm infants. *Cochrane Database Syst Rev.* 2021;1:CD013133. doi:10.1002/14651858.CD013133.pub2.

51. Varvarigou A, Bardin CL, Beharry K, Chemtob S, Papageorgiou A, Aranda JV. Early ibuprofen administration to prevent patent ductus arteriosus in premature newborn infants. *JAMA.* 1996;275(7):539-544.

52. Desfrere L, Zohar S, Morville P, et al. Dose-finding study of ibuprofen in patent ductus arteriosus using the continual reassessment method. *J Clin Pharm Ther.* 2005;30(2):121-132. doi:10.1111/j.1365-2710.2005.00630.x.

53. Dersch-Mills D, Alshaikh B, Soraisham AS, Akierman A, Yusuf K. Effectiveness of injectable ibuprofen salts and indomethacin to treat patent ductus arteriosus in preterm infants: observational cohort study. *Can J Hosp Pharm.* 2018;71(1):22-28.

54. Mitra S, McNamara PJ. Patent ductus arteriosus-time for a definitive trial. *Clin Perinatol.* 2020;47(3):617-639. doi:10.1016/j.clp.2020.05.007.

55. Ohlsson A, Walia R, Shah SS. Ibuprofen for the treatment of patent ductus arteriosus in preterm or low birth weight (or both) infants. *Cochrane Database Syst Rev.* 2020;2:CD003481. doi:10.1002/14651858.CD003481.pub8.

56. Su BH, Lin HC, Chiu HY, Hsieh HY, Chen HH, Tsai YC. Comparison of ibuprofen and indometacin for early-targeted treatment of patent ductus arteriosus in extremely premature infants: a randomised controlled trial. *Arch Dis Child Fetal Neonatal Ed.* 2008;93(2):F94-F99. doi:10.1136/adc.2007.120584.

57. Decobert F, Kampf F, Durrmeyer X. Efficiency of a double-dosed second ibuprofen course for the closure of patent ductus arteriosus in extremely premature infants. E-PAS. 2008;5842.4.

58. Barzilay B, Youngster I, Batash D, et al. Pharmacokinetics of oral ibuprofen for patent ductus arteriosus closure in preterm infants. *Arch Dis Child Fetal Neonatal Ed.* 2012;97(2):F116-F119. doi:10.1136/adc.2011.215160.

59. Lago P, Salvadori S, Opocher F, Ricato S, Chiandetti L, Frigo AC. Continuous infusion of ibuprofen for treatment of patent ductus arteriosus in very low birth weight infants. *Neonatology.* 2014;105(1):46-54. doi:10.1159/000355679.

60. De Carolis MP, Bersani I, De Rosa G, Cota F, Romagnoli C. Ibuprofen lysinate and sodium ibuprofen for prophylaxis of patent ductus arteriosus in preterm neonates. *Indian Pediatr.* 2012;49(1):47-49. doi:10.1007/s13312-012-0006-8.

61. Mitra S, Robart T. *Comparative Effectiveness and Safety of Intravenous Ibuprofen lysine Salt Versus Ibuprofen Tromethamine Salt for*

*Patent Ductus Arteriosus Closure in Preterm Infants: A Systematic Review and Network Meta-Analysis.* Accessed March 17, 2022. Available at: https://www.crd.york.ac.uk/prospero/display_record.php?RecordID=273018.

62. Ohlsson A, Shah SS. Ibuprofen for the prevention of patent ductus arteriosus in preterm and/or low birth weight infants. *Cochrane Database Syst Rev.* 2020;1:CD004213. doi:10.1002/14651858. CD004213.pub5.

63. Yoo H, Lee JA, Oh S, et al. Comparison of the mortality and in-hospital outcomes of preterm infants treated with ibuprofen for patent ductus arteriosus with or without clinical symptoms attributable to the patent ductus arteriosus at the time of ibuprofen treatment. *J Korean Med Sci.* 2017;32(1):115-123. doi:10.3346/jkms.2017.32.1.115.

64. Gournay V, Roze JC, Kuster A, et al. Prophylactic ibuprofen versus placebo in very premature infants: a randomised, double-blind, placebo-controlled trial. *Lancet.* 2004;364(9449):1939-1944. doi:10.1016/S0140-6736(04)17476-X.

65. Sehgal A, Kumarshingri PSN. Pulmonary hypertension in an infant treated with ibuprofen. *Indian J Pediatr.* 2013;80(8):697-699. doi:10.1007/s12098-012-0829-2.

66. Kim SY, Shin SH, Kim HS, Jung YH, Kim EK, Choi JH. Pulmonary arterial hypertension after ibuprofen treatment for patent ductus arteriosus in very low birth weight infants. *J Pediatr.* 2016;179:49-53.e1. doi:10.1016/j.jpeds.2016.08.103.

67. Bellini C, Campone F, Serra G. Pulmonary hypertension following L-lysine ibuprofen therapy in a preterm infant with patent ductus arteriosus. *CMAJ.* 2006;174(13):1843-1844. doi:10.1503/cmaj.051446.

68. Hinz B, Cheremina O, Brune K. Acetaminophen (paracetamol) is a selective cyclooxygenase-2 inhibitor in man. *FASEB J.* 2008;22(2):383-390. doi:10.1096/fj.07-8506com.

69. Hammerman C, Bin-Nun A, Markovitch E, Schimmel MS, Kaplan M, Fink D. Ductal closure with paracetamol: a surprising new approach to patent ductus arteriosus treatment. *Pediatrics.* 2011;128(6):e1618-e1621. doi:10.1542/peds.2011-0359.

70. El-Khuffash A, Jain A, Corcoran D, et al. Efficacy of paracetamol on patent ductus arteriosus closure may be dose dependent: evidence from human and murine studies. *Pediatr Res.* 2014;76(3):238-244. doi:10.1038/pr.2014.82.

71. Bouazza N, Treluyer JM, Foissac F, et al. Pharmacokinetics of intravenous paracetamol (acetaminophen) and ductus arteriosus closure after premature birth. *Clin Pharmacol Ther.* 2021;110(4):1087-1095. doi:10.1002/cpt.2380.

72. Davidson JM, Ferguson J, Ivey E, Philip R, Weems MF, Talati AJ. A randomized trial of intravenous acetaminophen versus indomethacin for treatment of hemodynamically significant PDAs in VLBW infants. *J Perinatol.* 2021;41(1):93-99. doi:10.1038/s41372-020-0694-1.

73. Dani C, Lista G, Bianchi S, et al. Intravenous paracetamol in comparison with ibuprofen for the treatment of patent ductus arteriosus in preterm infants: a randomized controlled trial. *Eur J Pediatr.* 2021;180(3):807-816. doi:10.1007/s00431-020-03780-8.

74. Ohlsson A, Shah PS. Paracetamol (acetaminophen) for patent ductus arteriosus in preterm or low birth weight infants. *Cochrane Database Syst Rev.* 2020;1:CD010061. doi:10.1002/14651858. CD010061.pub4.

75. Kimani S, Surak A, Miller M, Bhattacharya S. Use of combination therapy with acetaminophen and ibuprofen for closure of the patent ductus arteriosus in preterm neonates. *Paediatr Child Health.* 2021;26(4):e177-e183. doi:10.1093/pch/pxaa057.

76. Mashally S, Nield LE, McNamara PJ, et al. Late oral acetaminophen versus immediate surgical ligation in preterm infants with persistent large patent ductus arteriosus. *J Thorac Cardiovasc Surg.* 2018;156(5):1937-1944. doi:10.1016/j.jtcvs.2018.05.098.

77. Viberg H, Eriksson P, Gordh T, Fredriksson A. Paracetamol (acetaminophen) administration during neonatal brain development affects cognitive function and alters its analgesic and anxiolytic response in adult male mice. *Toxicol Sci.* 2014;138(1):139-147. doi:10.1093/toxsci/kft329.

78. Avella-Garcia CB, Julvez J, Fortuny J, et al. Acetaminophen use in pregnancy and neurodevelopment: attention function and autism spectrum symptoms. *Int J Epidemiol.* 2016;45(6):1987-1996. doi:10.1093/ije/dyw115.

79. Liew Z, Ritz B, Rebordosa C, Lee PC, Olsen J. Acetaminophen use during pregnancy, behavioral problems, and hyperkinetic disorders. *JAMA Pediatr.* 2014;168(4):313-320. doi:10.1001/jamapediatrics.2013.4914.

80. Bauer AZ, Kriebel D. Prenatal and perinatal analgesic exposure and autism: an ecological link. *Environ Health.* 2013;12:41. doi:10.1186/1476-069X-12-41.

81. Mitra S, Gardner CE, MacLellan A, et al. Prophylactic cyclooxygenase inhibitor drugs for the prevention of morbidity and mortality in preterm infants: a network meta-analysis. *Cochrane Database Syst Rev.* 2022;4(4):CD013846. doi:10.1002/14651858. CD013846.pub2.

82. El-Mashad AER, El-Mahdy H, El Amrousy D, Elgendy M. Comparative study of the efficacy and safety of paracetamol, ibuprofen, and indomethacin in closure of patent ductus arteriosus in preterm neonates. *Eur J Pediatr.* 2017;176(2):233-240. doi:10.1007/s00431-016-2830-7.

83. Hundscheid T, Onland W, van Overmeire B, et al. Early treatment versus expectative management of patent ductus arteriosus in preterm infants: a multicentre, randomised, non-inferiority trial in Europe (BeNeDuctus trial). *BMC Pediatr.* 2018;18(1):262. doi:10.1186/s12887-018-1215-7.

84. El-Khuffash A, Weisz DE, McNamara PJ. Reflections of the changes in patent ductus arteriosus management during the last 10 years. *Arch Dis Child Fetal Neonatal Ed.* 2016;101(5):F474-F478. doi:10.1136/archdischild-2014-306214.

85. Weisz DE, More K, McNamara PJ, Shah PS. PDA ligation and health outcomes: a meta-analysis. *Pediatrics.* 2014;133(4):e1024-e1046. doi:10.1542/peds.2013-3431.

# Chapter 18

# Interventional Management of the Patent Ductus Arteriosus

Adrianne Rahde Bischoff, Carl Backes, Dany E. Weisz, Bassel Mohammad Nijres, and Patrick J. McNamara

## Key Points

- Percutaneous (or transcatheter) PDA closure is an emerging technique that has gained popularity in the most recent years and is being performed in progressively smaller and younger patients. Advancements in the technique, the launch of devices that are more appropriate for the preterm ductal morphology, and increased experience have expanded the use of percutaneous closure with high rates of technical success and few major adverse events.

- Post-closure cardiorespiratory instability is characterized by oxygenation and/or ventilation failure and systolic hypotension with or without the need for inotropes. The onset of symptoms is typically 6–12 hours post-closure, is common in preterm infants, and is likely related to increased left ventricular afterload.

- Early targeted administration of intravenous milrinone to preterm infants with low cardiac output in the immediate post-closure period may ameliorate symptoms of post-closure cardiorespiratory instability.

- Respiratory instability is likely secondary to increased LV filling pressures and pulmonary venous hypertension, which may be secondary to ventricular stiffening and myocardium properties related to diastolic function.

## Introduction

The decision for definitive closure of a patent ductus arteriosus (PDA) remains one of the biggest controversies in neonatology. Importantly, there is marked center-to-center variation in the incidence of ligation among extremely-low-birth-weight (ELBW) infants, and overall rates of surgical ligation reported by international neonatal networks are decreasing.[1,2] The reasons behind this secular trend are likely multifactorial, but in many centers surgical ligation is being substituted, and even superseded, by the practice of percutaneous closure.[3] Percutaneous (or transcatheter) PDA closure is an emerging technique that has gained popularity in the most recent years and is being performed in progressively smaller and younger patients. Advancements in the technique with decreased fluoroscopy time, venous retrograde approach, the launch of devices that are more appropriate for the preterm ductal morphology, and increased experience have expanded the use of percutaneous closure, with high rates of technical success and few major adverse events.[4]

Observational studies have associated PDA surgery with adverse neonatal outcomes and neurodevelopmental impairment (NDI) in early childhood, although bias due to residual confounding threatens the validity of these studies. Infants treated with surgical ligation undergo major rapid changes in systemic hemodynamics, which commonly lead to postoperative cardiorespiratory instability. In addition, given that dependence on mechanical ventilation is the *sine qua non* of referring an infant for definitive PDA closure, the increasing availability and use of advanced noninvasive methods of ventilation may permit earlier endotracheal extubation of extremely preterm infants. Consequently, clinician perceptions of the merits of a definitive intervention may differ, prompting them to avoid interventional PDA closure, with the hope of spontaneous ductal closure.

It's important to note though that, specifically in ELBW, the rate of spontaneous closure is poor; more than 50% of infants born <750 g still have a PDA around day 50.[5] Additionally, the impact of chronic pulmonary overcirculation on the pulmonary parenchyma and on pulmonary vasculature remodeling must be appreciated. Despite several controversies in the literature regarding the impact of PDA closure on different neonatal outcomes, there is increasing evidence of a correlation between prolonged shunt exposure and the development of bronchopulmonary dysplasia (BPD). Although the TIPP trial showed no decrease in the incidence of BPD with the use of prophylactic indomethacin,[6] one recent study reported that a change toward a strict nonintervention approach to PDA resulted in an absolute increase of 31% in BPD in infants born less than 26 weeks.[7] Prolonged exposure to shunts also has a detrimental impact on pulmonary vascular development, and the presence of an untreated large PDA in the first 2 years of life may result in pulmonary vascular disease in as many as 50% of patients.[8,9] Philip et al. demonstrated that exposure to a PDA beyond 8 weeks of life is associated with an elevation in pulmonary vascular resistance (PVR) index, greater respiratory severity score, and prolonged use of mechanical ventilation.[10] In preterm infants, who have a smaller cross-sectional area of pulmonary vessels and several other inflammatory risk factors, the elevation in PVR occurs more frequently and at an earlier age,[9,11,12] while prolonged PDA exposure is also a potential contributor in the development of pulmonary vein stenosis. Figure 18.1 summarizes the multiple contributors to the pathophysiology of PDA shunt-related pulmonary hypertension.

Although the risks of prolonged shunts are relatively well established, the timing and indication for definitive closure have not been rigorously evaluated. Simultaneously, although the percutaneous approach is deemed to be less invasive and with less adverse events, the evidence regarding appropriate timing and indication for referral remain unknown. As a result, contemporary practice is dominated by considerable uncertainty regarding the role of definitive closure. In this chapter we review the evidence regarding the benefits and risks of PDA interventional closure in very preterm neonates and provide a pathophysiology-based management paradigm to guide peri-closure care in these high-risk infants.

## Definitive PDA Closure: Timing, Patient Selection, and Staging

In contemporary practice the "definitive PDA closure decision" remains an enduring controversy for clinicians. There is currently a paucity of knowledge regarding the clinical and echocardiography characteristics of infants with persistent PDA who may benefit from definitive closure. The relative risks and benefits of interventional closure compared with conservative management are unknown. Although dependence on mechanical ventilation remains the primary criterion for definitive closure referral, the relative independent contribution of the PDA to ongoing respiratory insufficiency is, at present, difficult to quantify. Infants with similar echocardiography indices of PDA hemodynamic significance may have varying degrees of respiratory failure (none to severe) owing to differences in nascent lung disease of prematurity, pulmonary arterial pressure, and tolerance of the increased pulmonary blood flow from the ductal shunt.

Limited evidence from clinical trials and careful reflection on contemporary treatment practices provides some boundaries for surgical treatment, mostly by limiting the use of ligation in the first postnatal week. Although the trial by Cassady et al. reported reduced necrotizing enterocolitis (NEC) rates with prophylactic surgical ligation on the first postnatal day in ELBW infants, several factors render this practice now untenable.[13] *First*, prophylactic indomethacin has both relatively high efficacy for early closure and reduces all grades of intraventricular hemorrhage (IVH), providing a therapeutic alternative with additional benefit. *Second*, early PDA ligation may result in increased right ventricular (RV) afterload, so early ligation may be harmful in preterm infants with increased pulmonary artery pressure, a common finding in severe respiratory distress syndrome. *Finally*, the natural history of ductal closure has been described, with many infants experiencing early spontaneous closure. Exposing all infants to the risks of interventional closure is therefore inappropriate.[14]

Persistent ductal shunt may be considered a chronic, consistent contributor to impaired pulmonary compliance. Infants with a persistent PDA may be considered for interventional closure when the clinical and echocardiography evaluations identify a

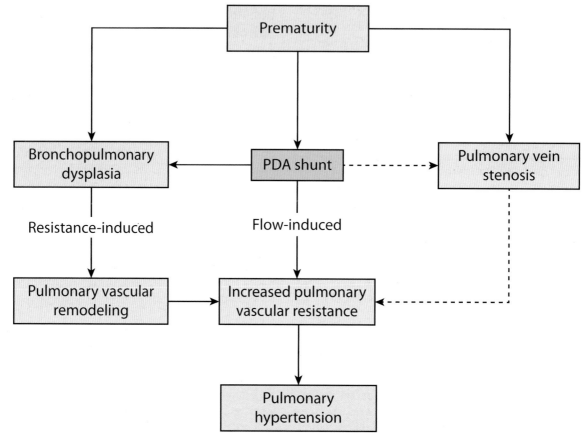

Fig. 18.1 **Different contributors of pulmonary hypertension in the setting of patent ductus arteriosus shunt.**

shunt of sufficient volume that may be actively contributing to respiratory insufficiency. Echocardiography markers of ductal significance may include measurements of left heart volume loading (i.e., pulmonary vein D wave velocity, mitral E wave velocity, left atrium to aorta ratio and isovolumic relaxation time), estimates of Qp:Qs (left-to-right ventricular output ratio) and of systemic hypoperfusion (diastolic flow reversal in the descending aorta and/or systemic vessels such as celiac and middle cerebral artery).[15,16] Persistent dependence on invasive or noninvasive ventilation in combination with moderate-severe echocardiography indicators of hemodynamic significance suggests an impaired ability to compensate for the ductal shunt. It is, however, important to consider preterm infants who have clinical features of chronic end-organ hypoperfusion (systemic hypotension, renal failure, feeding

intolerance) in the absence of an acute etiology (e.g., sepsis, NEC) accompanied by echocardiographic indices of a large ductal shunt. In these infants echocardiography indices are often in the "severe" range across all parameters, although there are little data regarding the direct clinical relevance of these deviations from normal. Early interventional closure after failure of medical therapy may be indicated for this subgroup of infants as well as a strategy to prevent BPD and pulmonary vascular remodeling in the most immature high-risk patients.

## Impact of Definitive PDA Closure

### SURGICAL PDA LIGATION AND OUTCOMES

The clinical decision to treat a preterm neonate with surgical PDA ligation is controversial, owing to uncertainty regarding the impact of PDA surgery on neonatal and neurodevelopmental outcomes. A limited number of randomized clinical trials, all conducted more than 3 decades ago, have evaluated the impact of surgical ligation in preterm infants on neonatal outcomes.[17-19] A common salient feature of these studies is a lack of external validity to permit their interpretation within modern neonatal intensive care; these trials were either performed prior to the availability of pharmacological PDA treatment, identified "hemodynamically significant" PDA based on clinical exam rather than echocardiography, and/or enrolled relatively mature preterm neonates, and thus bear minimal resemblance to care provided to the micropremature neonates being considered for PDA surgery in contemporary practice.

In lieu, observational studies have contributed most prominently to the evidence of the potential effect of PDA ligation on clinical outcomes. Large retrospective cohort studies have associated PDA ligation with increased neonatal morbidity and NDI in early childhood.[20-25] A meta-analysis of randomized trials and adjusted observational studies demonstrated that, compared with medically treated infants, ligated infants were more likely to develop moderate-severe BPD, severe retinopathy of prematurity, and moderate-severe NDI, although with improved survival.[26] In light of concerns regarding NDI and neonatal morbidities, the safety of PDA ligation has been questioned.[27] These concerns have been associated with a secular trend toward a reduction in infants being treated with surgical ligation in North American centers.[1,2]

However, residual confounding bias threatens the validity of observational studies that have associated PDA ligation with increased neonatal morbidity and NDI compared with medical management alone. Most studies only adjusted for antenatal and perinatal confounders (e.g., gestational age). Because ligation typically occurs several weeks after birth, such studies likely inadequately addressed confounding by indication – those infants referred for ligation may have been more "ill" and/or have larger ductal shunts at the time of the decision to treat with surgery, compared with infants who are treated with medical management alone. Illness severity, characterized by postnatal pre-ligation morbidities such as

intraventricular hemorrhage and sepsis, and intensive care parameters such as dependence on mechanical ventilation, are important confounders as they are associated with both the decision to treat with PDA ligation and also with neonatal morbidity and NDI. The potential effect of residual confounding bias in past studies was highlighted in a recent large multicenter cohort study of extremely preterm neonates with PDA, where after adjustment for postnatal pre-ligation confounders, ligation was no longer associated with adverse outcomes.[28] These findings have direct clinical relevance; specifically, neonatologists and pediatric cardiac surgeons may now consider to no longer prioritize the risk of adverse neonatal and neurodevelopmental outcomes as a reason to avoid surgical PDA ligation.

## PERCUTANEOUS PDA CLOSURE AND OUTCOMES
### Improving Risk/Benefit Profiles

Traditionally, technical success in percutaneous PDA closure is defined as placement of the device in the catheterization laboratory. Alternatively, technical failure is defined as the inability to place a device (or device placement, but subsequent need for removal due to malposition).[29] In a meta-analysis that synthesized studies (1994–2016), 635 infants <6 kg undergoing percutaneous PDA closure were identified.[30] Among that cohort, the authors observed a technical success rate of 92% (95% confidence interval [CI] 88.8–95.0]; rates of *any* complications and *clinically significant* complications were 23.3% (95% CI 6.5–30.8) and 10.1% (95% CI 7.8–12.5), respectively.[30] Using similar definitions, a more contemporary meta-analysis (2021) from Bischoff et al. investigated the technical success and safety profile of percutaneous closure among 373 infants <1.5 kg.[4] Interestingly, the authors observed procedural success rates of 96% (95% CI 93–98%), while rates of any complications and clinically significant complications were 27% (95% CI 17–38%) and 8% (95% CI 5–10%), respectively.[4] To further increase rates of technical success and minimize adverse events, a leadership panel of pediatric interventional cardiologists recently published consensus-based guidelines that address pre-, intra-, and post-procedural considerations of percutaneous PDA closure in lower-weight infants.[31] Thus risk-benefit profiles for the procedure are expected to continue to improve over the next decade.[32] However, in the absence of direct comparison of percutaneous closure versus alternative treatments, available risk/benefit profiles for the procedure lack the requisite context to guide evidence-based clinical practice.

## Novel Percutaneous PDA Closure Devices

Despite high rates of technical success with "off-label" use of various devices,[4,30,33] the need for percutaneous PDA closure devices that address the unique ductal morphology and profile of preterm infants was clear.[30,34-38] Accordingly, over the past decade, in the spirit of collaboration and innovation, the pediatric cardiology community and private industry have partnered to design PDA closure devices specifically tailored for the preterm infant.[39,40] For example, the Amplatzer Piccolo Occluder was modified (short-length, low-profile delivery system) to make it suitable for use in preterm infants.[41] In fact, following successful execution of a multicenter, non-randomized clinical trial, the Amplatzer Piccolo Occluder (or Amplatzer Duct Occluder II Additional Sizes, ADO-II AS; Abbott, Chicago, Illinois) was approved (2019) by the Food and Drug Administration (FDA) for percutaneous PDA closure in preterm infants >3 postnatal days and weighing >700 g.[41,42] Of note, the Amplatzer Piccolo Occluder is FDA approved for PDAs ≤4 mm in diameter; thus off-label use of alternative devices remains common.[39] For example, leading investigators recently reported that the Microvascular Plug 7Q is safe and feasible among premature infants with PDAs >4 mm in diameter.[43] Although the ductus in preterm infants is typically long and tubular, marked variability in ductal length demands that a variety of device modalities be available.[32,44] In the absence of comparative studies the optimal device to close the PDA remains at the discretion of the interventional cardiologist and various institution and individual providers.[33]

## Treatments for Definitive Ductal Closure

Surgical PDA ligation via thoracotomy was the traditional method of procedural PDA closure.[45] However, over the last 2 decades, associations between surgical ligation and adverse outcomes, including neurodevelopmental delays, have emerged.[46,47] These observations have led to growing interest among the pediatric health care community in percutaneous PDA closure as a treatment to achieve definitive ductal closure. A recent study using the Pediatric Health Information System (PHIS) database compared short-term outcomes among infants undergoing definitive ductal closure, including percutaneous ($n = 175$) or surgical PDA closure. Although infants undergoing percutaneous ductal closure were older (0.53 vs. 0.1 years, $P < 0.001$) and less premature (20% vs. 60%; $P < 0.001$), the authors observed that those undergoing percutaneous closure had lower mortality (0% vs. 1.7%, $P = 0.02$) and reduced hospital length of stay (difference in 3 days; 95% CI 1.1–4.9 days; $P = 0.002$) than those undergoing surgical ligation.[48] Other investigators have observed similar rates of safety and feasibility between percutaneous PDA closure versus surgical ligation.[49] In the absence of contemporary randomized controlled trials (RCTs) comparing percutaneous closure versus surgical ligation, fundamental questions on the best approach to achieve definitive ductal closure will remain unanswered.[33]

## Fundamental Need for Contemporary Randomized Controlled Trial

In view of the lack of comparative data, a multidisciplinary leadership panel convened and developed research priorities for the use of percutaneous PDA closure.[50,51] The need for a multicenter RCT of percutaneous PDA closure, with well-defined inclusion/exclusion criteria, rigorously applied treatment protocols, consideration of potentially harmful exposures (e.g., cardiac anesthesia), and longer-term neurodevelopmental assessments, was emphasized.[51] Consistent with US trends in surgical PDA ligation rates,[45] the panel did not have interest or equipoise for a comparison of percutaneous closure versus surgical ligation. In fact, in view of widespread acceptance in the health care community, conservative management ("watchful waiting," diuretics, fluid restriction) was determined to be the best comparative treatment modality.[52] Following iterative discussions, an National Institute of Health (NIH)–funded study comparing percutaneous PDA closure versus conservative treatment ("PIVOTAL: Percutaneous Intervention Versus

Observational Trial of Arterial Ductus in Lower Gestational Age Infants") is planned to begin recruitment in 2023 (NCT #03982342).[53]

## PDA Closure Periprocedural Management

Pre-closure evaluation is aimed at verifying ongoing suitability for PDA closure, optimizing stability to improve procedural tolerance, and identifying neonates at modifiable risk of post-closure morbidity. Repeat echocardiography should be performed within 48 hours of definitive closure to confirm PDA severity and rule out the development of spontaneous ductal closure or constriction, which occurs in a small but important minority of extremely preterm neonates after referral for ligation.[54] Baseline hemoglobin, platelet count, and prothrombin time should be obtained for correction of anemia and verification of normal coagulation function. Adrenocorticotropin stimulation testing can be performed preoperatively to assess adrenal cortex responsiveness, which may be impaired in preterm infants with PDA.[55] Preoperative serum cortisol ≤750 nmol/L (≤17 μg/dL) after adrenocorticotropic hormone (ACTH) stimulation is associated with increased postoperative hypotension and respiratory failure.[51] On the other hand, routine preoperative stress-dose hydrocortisone has not been associated with improved cardiovascular stability, regardless of gestational age.[56] Maintenance of euvolemia pre-closure is recommended, given that aggressive fluid restriction and use of diuretics may further exacerbate decreased systemic blood flow to post-ductal organs and have no impact on shunt volume.[57] On the contrary, additional volume loading does not prevent post-closure cardiovascular instability.[58] Lastly, during the procedure (ligation or percutaneous closure), neonates typically receive mechanical ventilatory support. Use of a volume-targeted, pressure-limited mode (when on conventional ventilation) may reduce the risk of baro- and volutrauma resulting from rapid changes in pulmonary compliance after interruption of the PDA shunt.[59] While there are no specific respiratory strategies recommended, high-frequency modes have equivalent success to conventional mechanical ventilation in experienced centers.[60] Detailed technical information about percutaneous PDA closure can be found in the Appendix 18A.

## Care of the Preterm Infant After Definitive PDA Closure

### PHYSIOLOGIC CHANGES AFTER CLOSURE: DECREASE IN LEFT VENTRICULAR PRELOAD, INCREASE IN AFTERLOAD, AND DECREASE IN LEFT VENTRICULAR OUTPUT

PDA closure results in significant changes in loading conditions to the left ventricle (LV). Specifically, there is an instantaneous drop in LV and left atrium preload due to decreased pulmonary blood flow return, with a proportional reduction in LV output.[61-64] Given that most patients are above the critical filling volume and go from a state of "high" to "normal" preload, the impact on LV contractility dictated by the Frank-Starling law is limited. In addition, the normalization of pulmonary blood flow leads to improved lung compliance and function.[59,65] With the removal of the low resistance circuit of the pulmonary vasculature, the LV is exposed exclusively to systemic vascular resistance (SVR), with resultant increase in LV afterload.[63] Using noninvasive electrical cardiometry to monitor hemodynamic changes intraoperatively, Lien et al. demonstrated that there was a significant decline in LV output and surge in SVR upon sudden termination of ductal shunting.[66] The deterioration in LV output was associated with a decrease in stroke volume rather than heart rate, and the magnitude of the reduction was particularly pronounced among ELBW infants.[66,67] The changes in loading conditions were also demonstrated after percutaneous PDA closure, with a decrease in end-diastolic and end-systolic volume, an increase in arterial and end-systolic elastance, and a decrease in LV output subsequent to the procedure.[68]

### MYOCARDIAL DYSFUNCTION

PDA ligation in premature baboons resulted in impaired LV systolic performance and ventilation failure, coinciding with an increase in SVR.[69] LV fractional shortening (FS) deteriorates 6–12 hours after surgical ligation,[69] whereas in humans there is an immediate decrease in LV FS as well as mean velocity of circumferential fiber shortening (mVCFc) that persists after 24 hours.[64] Similar findings have been confirmed with modern echocardiographic analysis in preterm infants, mostly in the past 15 years.[61,70] The LV myocardial performance index, which incorporates the isovolumetric contraction and relaxation times and adjusts, at least in theory, for preload by accounting for the ejection time, deteriorated acutely after ligation, mimicking the changes in LV output.[63] LV efficiency, defined as the ratio of stroke volume to pressure-volume area, transiently deteriorates within 1–24 hours after ligation and then recovers to preoperative levels by 2–4 days after ligation.[68,70]

In a cohort of 19 very preterm infants evaluated with tissue Doppler imaging and myocardial deformation techniques after PDA ligation, systolic and diastolic LV tissue Doppler velocities and global LV longitudinal strain decreased immediately after ligation.[71] The former remained lower than the preoperative levels at 18 hours, whereas the latter improved 18 hours after the procedure.[71] These findings were replicated in a cohort of extremely preterm infants undergoing percutaneous PDA closure, where targeted neonatal echocardiography 1 hour after closure showed a significant decrease in global longitudinal strain, as well as myocardial work index and work efficiency.[68] Notably, these longitudinal changes can be affected, to a certain extent, by the acute changes in loading conditions rather than solely myocardial performance alone.[72] Saida et al. demonstrated that a larger preoperative LV internal dimension in diastole was predictive of a decrease in postoperative FS of the LV.[73] Traditional echocardiography markers of LV systolic performance, such as ejection fraction, are load dependent and cannot be interpreted as an isolated index of contractility. However, there is evidence to suggest that PDA closure leads to an inverse stress-velocity relationship: a preload-independent afterload-adjusted method of assessing LV contractility.[64]

Preterm infants have decreased sarcoplasmic reticulum and a poorly developed or absent T-tubule system in their myocytes; thus they have less mature excitation-contraction and relaxation mechanisms.[74] As a result, the ability of the myocardium of premature neonates to respond to a sudden surge in SVR is limited compared with that of term neonates.[75] The risk of impaired LV systolic performance and associated clinical deterioration appears to be greater in more immature infants after PDA closure.[64,75]

## HEMODYNAMIC CHANGES IN MESENTERIC AND CEREBRAL CIRCULATIONS

Doppler evaluation of systemic arteries, such as the celiac, superior mesenteric, renal, and cerebral arteries, demonstrates significant postoperative changes after surgical ligation.[73] Hoodbhoy et al. reported an increase in average velocities in both the celiac and superior mesenteric arteries within 3 hours post-PDA ligation, but such a phenomenon was not found in the middle cerebral artery until 24 hours after surgery.[76] The normalization of Doppler estimates of diastolic flow after PDA ligation strongly implicates the PDA as the cause of abnormal preoperative diastolic flow in systemic arteries. However, the utility of these sonographic changes in managing post-closure care is unknown.

The reported association of PDA ligation and neurodevelopmental impairment has led to concerns regarding the effect of postoperative myocardial dysfunction and systemic hypotension on cerebral perfusion, especially in extremely preterm infants with reduced capacity for cerebrovascular autoregulation.[77] Leslie et al. evaluated cerebral electrical activity changes after ligation using amplitude-integrated electroencephalography and found a decrease in the lower trace margin and proportion of patients with trace continuity after surgery, independent of cardiac output status.[78] However, other studies that have used near-infrared spectroscopy to assess changes in regional cerebral oxygen saturation and cerebral blood flow have shown conflicting results.[77] There are no studies to date evaluating the effect of percutaneous PDA closure on cerebral perfusion and/or electrical activity. The relationship of post-closure brain perfusion and later neurosensory impairment requires further evaluation.

## Post-Closure Cardiorespiratory Instability and Milrinone Prophylaxis

The post-closure course may be complicated by acute cardiorespiratory instability. Traditional post-ligation cardiac syndrome (PLCS) occurs in up to half of infants undergoing surgical PDA ligation and typically occurs between 6 and 12 hours after surgery.[63,72,79,80] The true incidence of cardiorespiratory instability has not been described after percutaneous closure,[81] although in one study of patients who received targeted milrinone prophylaxis, approximately 50% of the infants developed predominant respiratory instability which unlike PDA surgery was most commonly seen in hypertensive patients.[68] The two components of instability included are ventilation and/or oxygenation impairment with or without cardiovascular compromise, which may include systolic hypotension and/or need to start/increase inotropic support.[63,79,82-84] Data suggests that increased LV afterload is a greater contributor to the pathophysiology of post-closure instability rather than reduced preload. Impairment in indices of LV systolic function and peak measures of LV afterload coincide with the clinical onset of instability at approximately 8 hours post-operatively.[64] In contrast, the effects of reduced LV preload, such as low LV output, are echocardiographically evident as early as 1 hour after surgery when the patient is clinically asymptomatic.[68,85] Reduced preload may limit the immature myocardium's ability to maintain cardiac output under conditions of increased afterload and may be clinically important in select infants with coexisting severe acute inflammatory lesions (e.g., NEC) where capillary leak may reduce intravascular volume.

The risk for vasopressor-inotrope use after surgical PDA ligation relates to lower birth weight, earlier gestational age, or higher ventilatory support.[72] Retrospective studies have failed to identify any relationship between surgical technique, anesthetic approach, or intraoperative fluid management and the development of hypotension.[58,84] Jain et al. reported that an LV output of less than 200 mL/kg/min estimated by echocardiography 1 hour after PDA ligation was a sensitive predictor of systolic hypotension and the need for inotropes.[79] Reduced tissue Doppler systolic indices (LV basal lateral peak systolic annular velocity [S'], basal septal S' and basal RV S') at 1 hour postoperatively correlate strongly with early low LV output, potentially providing an additional echocardiography indicator of infants at higher risk for cardiovascular instability.[85]

Milrinone, a selective phosphodiesterase III inhibitor, is a systemic vasodilator with lusitropic and positive inotropic effects (see Chapter 5, *Neonatal Hemodynamic Pharmacology*)[80] that can be used as a prophylactic agent in a selective population. Jain et al. demonstrated that early postoperative administration of milrinone in infants with low cardiac output (<200 mL/kg/min) was associated with a significant reduction in ventilation failure (from 48% to 15%), need for inotropes (from 56% to 19%), and the incidence of overall PLCS (from 44% to 11%).[79] Milrinone treatment was also associated with longitudinal improvement in tissue Doppler imaging and speckle-tracking echocardiography–derived indicators of systolic function within 18 hours, likely due to the effects of afterload reduction and improvement in myocardial systolic performance.[85] This practice is supported by a randomized placebo-controlled trial of universal prophylactic milrinone after open congenital heart disease surgery in a pediatric population, which demonstrated a 64% relative risk reduction in death or low cardiac output syndrome in the first 36 hours postoperatively in the milrinone group (26.7% vs. 9.6%, $P = 0.007$).[86] Post-closure milrinone treatment has not been evaluated in a randomized trial in preterm infants after interventional PDA closure.

## Isolated Post-Closure Respiratory Instability

Postoperatively, ligation of the PDA has been shown to improve pulmonary dynamic compliance, tidal volume, and minute ventilation.[65] However, not all patients exhibit immediate improvement; specifically, a subset develop early (4–12 hours after surgery) oxygenation or ventilation failure, requiring an escalation of respiratory support.[64,79] In preterm baboons PDA ligation was found to produce a significant increase in the expression of genes involved in pulmonary inflammation (COX-2, tumor necrosis factor [TNF]-α, and CD14) and a significant decrease in α-epithelial sodium channel (ENaC) expression, resulting in a decrease in the rate of alveolar fluid clearance.[87] This deleterious inflammatory response to the surgical procedure may, at least in part, mediate deterioration in lung function in preterm infants.[88]

Ting et al. reported that the incidence of oxygenation or ventilation failure remained high (51.2%) in preterm infants undergoing PDA ligation, despite the implementation of an early targeted milrinone prophylaxis approach for infants with early echocardiography evidence of low cardiac output.[84] A similar incidence occurred in a high-risk population of infants <2 kg at the time of percutaneous PDA closure, where despite a targeted milrinone prophylaxis approach, 43% of the infants developed respiratory instability in the first 24 hours.[68] Postoperative LV diastolic dysfunction, manifested by prolonged isovolumic relaxation time (IVRT) on early echocardiography, was associated with subsequent respiratory instability.[84] This may be related to the inability of the premature LV, with an *a priori* diastolic dysfunction, to adapt to the acute post-closure increase in LV afterload, leading to further augmentation in LV filling pressures, secondary to pulmonary venous hypertension and oxygenation failure.[84] In a more contemporary study infants who developed respiratory instability had higher end-systolic elastance both prior to and after percutaneous PDA closure. Since ventricular stiffening is associated with higher changes in pressure even in small loading perturbations, it is possible that intrinsic myocardium properties related to diastolic function may provide a basis for an increased vulnerability to changes in loading conditions.[68] The subpopulation of infants with respiratory instability and LV diastolic dysfunction after percutaneous PDA closure are more likely to be hypertensive. Therefore, infants with LV diastolic dysfunction may benefit from a higher dose of milrinone to exert its lusitropic effects, although an adequately powered prospective study is needed to address this hypothesis.[89]

## Hypothalamic-Pituitary-Adrenal (HPA) Gland Axis and Post-Closure Cardiovascular Instability

The HPA axis is crucial in regulating organ maturational events, especially the increased concentration of β-adrenergic receptors in tissues, and effective cardiovascular responsiveness to endogenous and pharmacologic vasoactive agents.[90] Preterm infants are prone to life-threatening hypotension secondary to HPA axis immaturity, resulting from adrenocortical insufficiency.[91] Under stress, the premature adrenal gland may not respond appropriately to elevated ACTH, producing only a blunted cortisol response.[91-93] Adrenal hypoperfusion secondary to chronic ductal "steal" has been postulated to be another contributory mechanism in infants with persistent PDA.[56] The combination of developmental immaturity of the HPA axis with chronic adrenal hypoperfusion is a potential contributor to early cardiovascular instability and catecholamine-resistant hypotension.[56,94,95] Widespread use of stress dose hydrocortisone has not been associated with improved outcomes,[96] while postoperative cortisol measurements may delay initiation of therapy. Pre-closure assessment of adrenal performance with an adrenocorticotropic hormone (ACTH) stimulation test, however, can guide early administration to appropriately selected patients.[62] Therefore stress dose hydrocortisone may be indicated for patients who were receiving chronic steroid therapy preoperatively, as well as those who become symptomatic, particularly if accompanied by a failed pre-ligation ACTH stimulation test.[97] The use of steroids for definitive closure has not been studied today and merits prospective evaluation.

## Surgical and Percutaneous Closure Complications

### SURGICAL COMPLICATIONS

Table 18.1 describes the most common complications of surgical PDA closure.

### PERCUTANEOUS CLOSURE COMPLICATIONS

Many difficulties surround PDA device closure in premature infants, including small patient and vessel sizes, small cardiac structures, thin cardiac walls, and associated comorbidities. Their overall tenuous status puts them at increased risk of complications. Complications could arise before, during, and after the procedure. Some of the most common complications of percutaneous PDA closure include:

1. *Hypothermia:* premature infants have a relatively larger body surface area, putting them at risk of heat loss. This can be mitigated by covering the patients with a plastic sheet, handling them underneath the sheet whenever possible, using a heat source (heating lamp and/or forced air warmer, etc.), increasing ambient temperature in the catheterization lab to 75–76°F, and avoiding use of cold fluids. Placement of an esophageal temperature probe allows monitoring of the patient's temperature and can be used as a landmark to guide device placement.[39,98,99]
2. *Access site complications:* thrombosis, dissection, or hematoma can be encountered. The risk can be minimized by obtaining access under ultrasound guidance, gentle wire advancement, avoiding wire and sheath mismatch, and flushing the sheath with heparinized saline.[98,100]
3. *Cardiac injuries:* this includes tricuspid valve regurgitation, cardiac perforation/tamponade, and PDA dissection. The risk can be minimized

**TABLE 18 1    Surgical Complications of Patent Ductus Arteriosus Ligation**

| Complication | Incidence | Pathophysiology, Risk Factors, and Diagnosis | Management and Association with Outcomes |
|---|---|---|---|
| Vocal cord paresis | 9% (all preterm neonates)[102] 23% (extremely preterm neonates) | Occurs due to injury to the left recurrent laryngeal nerve, which courses adjacent to PDA prior to innervating left vocal fold Risk factors[103]: Lower GA Surgical technique (more common with vascular clip than ligation)[104] | Associated with[105]: Prolonged ventilator dependency Severe BPD Prolonged tube feeding and gastrostomy tube placement Increased length of stay Dysphonia, which may persist into adulthood[106] |
| Pneumothorax | 1.6–5.4%[107,108] | Occurs due to intrapleural accumulation of air either through the thoracotomy site or alveolar rupture from mechanical ventilation | Thoracostomy tube or drain |
| Chylothorax | Rare (<1%) | Occurs due to traumatic disruption of the thoracic duct or adjacent lymphatic channels[108] | High mortality Thoracostomy tube, nil-per-os, octreotide |
| Phrenic nerve paralysis | Rare (<1%) | Occurs due to traumatic injury to phrenic nerve | Associated with[109]: Prolonged ventilator dependency Increased BPD Management[110]: Prediction of spontaneous recovery uncertain Diaphragmatic plication used in select patients |
| Injury/ligation of adjacent structures | Rare (<1%) | Large PDA size may result in misidentification of the transverse aortic arch, left mainstem bronchus, or left pulmonary artery as the PDA[111-114] | High mortality Surgical correction required |
| PDA rupture or major bleeding | 1% | PDA tissue is friable in extremely preterm neonates[112]; rapid onset of hemodynamic compromise and radio-dense lesion on CXR | High mortality Surgical correction required |

by careful equipment manipulation. All manipulation should be performed under fluoroscopy guidance, avoiding jerky forceful wire/catheter advancement. If pericardial effusion develops, supportive care, pericardial drainage, and blood transfusion are used as needed. The cardiac surgery team should be immediately contacted to decide whether surgical intervention is feasible and warranted.[98]

4. *Iatrogenic left pulmonary artery stenosis or aortic coarctation*: if this is identified prior to releasing the device (the device is deployed but it is still connected to the delivery wire), the device should be retrieved and repositioned or a different-sized device should be placed. If it is identified after device release, treatment options will be based on the severity of stenosis, time of identification, and associated comorbidities.[32,98,100]

5. *Air or thrombus embolism*: air embolism can be easily prevented by de-airing and flushing the sheath and all catheters prior to their use. There is no consensus on whether heparin should be given to prevent thrombosis. Many interventionalists tend to complete the procedure without heparin administration as they believe heparinized saline used to flush sheath and catheters is sufficient.

6. *Device embolization:* the device may embolize to the systemic or pulmonary circulations. It usually can be snared out via the transcatheter approach. Sometimes surgical removal is needed.[39,98,100]

7. *Contrast-induced renal dysfunction:* the risk can be minimized by judicious use of contrast. Usually, 1 mL of contrast is enough to delineate the anatomy. If the patient has pre-existing renal dysfunction, closure under fluoroscopy and echo guidance without contrast injection may be considered.

8. *Blood loss:* Although uncommon, blood transfusion sometimes is required, as a small amount of blood loss could be significant in small infants.[98]

9. *Death:* the mortality rate of PDA device closure is low, with an estimation of approximately 2%. It usually results from cardiac perforation.[81]

## Immediate Post-Procedural Management

Immediate post-closure care should be directed at ruling out urgent surgical/percutaneous complications, such as pneumothorax, bleeding, and device embolization. A chest radiograph should be performed to confirm endotracheal tube placement and identify air leak or pulmonary overdistension. Preterm infants should remain invasively ventilated in the immediate post-closure period and the mean airway pressure and tidal volume adjusted to optimize lung inflation and compliance. Infants may experience a rapid improvement in pulmonary compliance after ligation, owing to the rapid decrease in pulmonary capillary hydrostatic pressure. Failure to anticipate a need for reduction in positive end-expiratory pressure may lead to lung overdistension with resultant impairment in systemic and pulmonary venous return, systemic hypotension and/or low cardiac output state, and the potential for the development of a pneumothorax or hypotension.

Most preterm infants are hemodynamically stable in the immediate (<2 hours) post-closure period but demonstrate an abrupt increase in diastolic blood pressure due to loss of the pulmonary vascular bed and increase in resting pressure against the systemic vessels. The presence of early (<4 hours) diastolic or combined (systolic and diastolic) hypotension is atypical and should prompt investigation for hemorrhage, obstruction to LV output (e.g., pneumothorax), severe pulmonary arterial hypertension (if hypoxemic), and

causes of decreased SVR (e.g., adrenal insufficiency, sepsis). Intravascular volume expansion and intravenous stress-dose hydrocortisone can be considered. Vasoconstricting agents should be avoided in these infants in lieu of agents that improve LV systolic function and reduce afterload, such as dobutamine or milrinone. However, refractory and/or isolated diastolic hypotension after fluid resuscitation may be treated with judicious use of an intravenous infusion of vasopressors (i.e., dopamine, norepinephrine, or vasopressin). In these cases hydrocortisone treatment should be strongly considered.

The immediate increase in diastolic blood pressure (and resultant rise in mean blood pressure) may mask a diminished post-closure systolic blood pressure indicative of acutely decreased LV systolic function. Systolic and diastolic blood pressures should therefore be distinctly measured, recorded, and evaluated in the post-closure period. The gradual development of isolated systolic hypotension and/or low cardiac output state, with or without echocardiographic confirmation of LV systolic dysfunction, may be managed with an intravenous infusion of dobutamine (5–10 mcg/kg/min) or epinephrine (0.03–0.1 mcg/kg/min).

Targeted neonatal echocardiography, if available, should be performed at 1 hour after PDA closure to identify markers associated with higher risk for cardiorespiratory instability. At the University of Iowa NICU, a threshold LV output of less than 170 mL/min/kg is an indication to start prophylaxis with milrinone infusion, especially in high-risk patients (<1 kg, <3 weeks of life) and those with systemic hypertension and/or with other echocardiographic signs of LV systolic and/or diastolic dysfunction (i.e., ejection fraction <55%, isovolumic relaxation time >60 ms, etc.).[79] For infants with borderline LVO (170–200 mL/kg/min), other indices of LV systolic/diastolic performance are considered, including tissue Doppler imaging and longitudinal strain.[62] Milrinone infusion is initiated at 0.33 mcg/kg/min (0.2 mcg/kg/min if <1 kg) accompanied by a normal saline bolus (10 mL/kg) during the first hour to augment preload and offset the decrease in SVR associated with milrinone. Milrinone is contraindicated in the setting of diastolic hypotension (less than third percentile for gestational age) due to its vasodilator properties and potential for worsening hypotension. Milrinone is typically continued for 24–48 hours, although patients with systemic hypertension and/or cardiorespiratory instability occasionally require dose escalation or treatment for a longer period.

In cases of respiratory instability in the post-procedural period, the mean airway pressure should be adjusted. If the blood pressure is normal/high in addition to respiratory instability, increased milrinone dosage (rescue milrinone for those who did not receive prophylaxis) and/or diuretics may be considered as a strategy to improve pulmonary venous hypertension and pulmonary edema. In centers without access to timely postoperative echocardiography, the administration of prophylactic intravenous milrinone to infants based on pre-closure risk factors may be considered.[86] Care must be taken to ensure that milrinone is administered only to clinically stable infants demonstrating the expected postoperative hemodynamic effects, namely stable respiratory status and a rise in postoperative diastolic blood pressure and normal-to-increased systolic blood pressure.

## Future Directions

A recently completed single-arm, prospective, nonrandomized study provides additional evidence on the reasonable safety profile of the Amplatzer Piccolo Occluder for PDA closure, including infants ≥700 g. Not surprisingly, the US FDA's endorsement of the Amplatzer TM Piccolo Occluder has led to growing interest in the device among health care providers to achieve definitive ductal closure.[101] However, in view of the lack of comparative trials using percutaneous PDA closure, fundamental questions on optimal treatments for preterm infants warranting definitive ductal closure remain unanswered.[36] Thus a multidisciplinary leadership panel convened and developed research priorities for the use of percutaneous PDA closure.[50,51] The need for a multicenter RCT of percutaneous PDA closure, with well-defined inclusion/exclusion criteria, rigorously applied treatment protocols, consideration of potentially harmful exposures (e.g., cardiac anesthesia), and longer-term neurodevelopmental assessments, was emphasized.[51] Consistent with US trends in surgical PDA ligation rates,[45] the panel did not have interest or equipoise for a comparison of percutaneous closure versus surgical ligation. In fact, in view of widespread acceptance in the health care community, conservative management ("watchful waiting," diuretics, fluid restriction) was determined to be the best comparative treatment modality.[52]

To that end, as mentioned, the National Institute of Health (NIH) has recently funded a multicenter (26-site) study comparing percutaneous PDA closure versus conservative treatment ("PIVOTAL: Percutaneous Intervention Versus Observational Trial of Arterial Ductus in Lower Gestational Age Infants"), which will begin recruitment in 2023 (NCT #03982342).[53]

## Summary: The PDA Closure Decision and Post-Procedural Management

Definitive PDA closure has evolved over the past several years from a predominant surgical approach to a more contemporary less invasive percutaneous approach. While definitive indications and benefits of interventional closure remain to be validated, high-risk infants may benefit from closure in order to prevent morbidities such as BPD and pulmonary vascular disease. Definitive closure, whether surgical or percutaneous, is associated with significant changes in loading conditions of the LV. Understanding the underlying physiological changes may help in the identification of infants who are more likely to develop post-closure cardiorespiratory instability.

## APPENDIX 18A
## Percutaneous PDA Closure
### AVAILABLE DEVICES

The Amplatzer Piccolo Occluder (Abbott, Plymouth, MN) is the only device that has been specifically designed to close the patent ductus arteriosus (PDA) in small infants. In January 2019 it gained FDA approval for PDA closure in infants weighing more than 700 g. Since then, it has been adopted as the first line for PDA closure in small infants by many programs. Other devices that have been used (off-label) are Microvascular Plug (Medtronic, Minneapolis, MN), Amplatzer Vascular Plug II (AVP II) (Abbott, Plymouth, MN), different brands of coils, and KA Micro Plug (KA Medical, Minneapolis, MN).[32,39,98,100,115-118]

The Piccolo device is made of a nitinol mesh of thin wires. It has two retention discs (proximal and distal) and a central cylindrical waist. The device is packaged and connected with its own delivery wire through a micro-screw. It comes in three different waist sizes, namely 3, 4, and 5 mm, and three different lengths, that is, 2, 4, and 6 mm (Figure 18.2). Choosing the

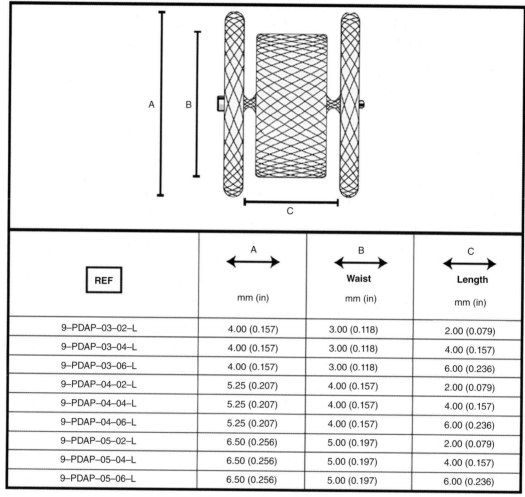

| REF | A mm (in) | B Waist mm (in) | C Length mm (in) |
|---|---|---|---|
| 9–PDAP–03–02–L | 4.00 (0.157) | 3.00 (0.118) | 2.00 (0.079) |
| 9–PDAP–03–04–L | 4.00 (0.157) | 3.00 (0.118) | 4.00 (0.157) |
| 9–PDAP–03–06–L | 4.00 (0.157) | 3.00 (0.118) | 6.00 (0.236) |
| 9–PDAP–04–02–L | 5.25 (0.207) | 4.00 (0.157) | 2.00 (0.079) |
| 9–PDAP–04–04–L | 5.25 (0.207) | 4.00 (0.157) | 4.00 (0.157) |
| 9–PDAP–04–06–L | 5.25 (0.207) | 4.00 (0.157) | 6.00 (0.236) |
| 9–PDAP–05–02–L | 6.50 (0.256) | 5.00 (0.197) | 2.00 (0.079) |
| 9–PDAP–05–04–L | 6.50 (0.256) | 5.00 (0.197) | 4.00 (0.157) |
| 9–PDAP–05–06–L | 6.50 (0.256) | 5.00 (0.197) | 6.00 (0.236) |

**Fig. 18.2 Available Piccolo device sizes.**

appropriate device is based on the patient's weight and PDA dimensions. This device is delivered through a special 4-Fr catheter, i.e., Amplatzer TorqVue LP catheter (Abbott, Plymouth, MN).[98]

## VASCULAR ACCESS

Historically, percutaneous PDA closure required the placement of femoral venous and arterial sheaths. Nevertheless, due to the high risk of arterial access complications in young infants, especially those weighing less than 2 kg, PDA closure has been tailored to avoid the placement of an arterial sheath. To compensate for the lack of arterial access, an intraprocedural echocardiogram is being heavily relied upon to guide the procedure.[32,98,100] Accessing the femoral vessel should be below the inguinal ligament ideally under ultrasound guidance. Wire positioning should be confirmed by fluoroscopy prior to sheath advancement. The wire should be seen at the right of the spine, indicating the position inside the inferior vena cava. The needle is removed, and a short 4-Fr sheath is inserted over the wire. The authors use a 4-Fr 7 cm prelude ideal (Merit Medical Systems, South Jordan, UT) sheath as it has the smallest outer diameter compared with the other commercially available sheaths.[119] The wire and dilator are removed, and the sheath is flushed with heparinized saline.

## CROSSING THE PATENT DUCTUS ARTERIOSUS

Various combinations of wires and catheters can be used to cross the tricuspid valve and PDA. Most interventionalists use a combination of a 4-Fr angled glide catheter (Terumo, Japan) and a soft floppy end 0.035″ wire, such as the Wholey wire (Medtronic, Minneapolis, MN). After advancing the combination of wire and catheter inside the right atrium, the catheter is rotated toward the expected location of the tricuspid valve (pointing anteriorly and leftward). With meticulous wire manipulation, the wire is advanced crossing the tricuspid valve, pulmonary valve, and PDA into the descending aorta. After confirming wire positioning in the descending aorta, the catheter is advanced over the wire inside the aorta and the wire is removed. Slowly and carefully, the catheter is pulled back inside the PDA and an angiogram is obtained by hand injection of a small amount of contrast to delineate the anatomy.

## DEVICE PLACEMENT

An angled glide catheter is exchanged over the wire for the TorqVue LP delivery catheter. The chosen device is prepped, inserted inside the delivery catheter, and advanced until it reaches the tip of the delivery catheter. The delivery catheter is slowly pulled back inside the PDA. The device discs and central waist are delivered sequentially inside the PDA. The aim is to place the device entirely inside the PDA without protruding into the aorta or main pulmonary artery. An instrument inserted inside the esophagus, such as a feeding tube or temperature probe, can be used as a landmark (Figure 18.3A). If the device is entirely intraductal, it is usually situated to the left of the instrument and the endotracheal tube in

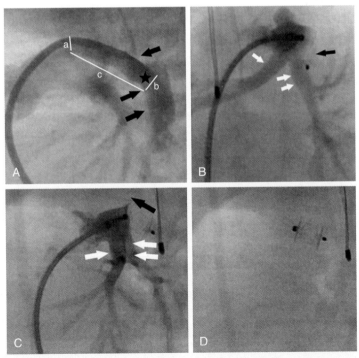

**Fig. 18.3 Steps of patent ductus arteriosus (PDA) device closure in premature infants.** (A) PDA angiogram in the straight lateral projection, a. pulmonic end, b. aortic end (ampulla), c. length. The feeding tube (*black arrows*) aligns well with the PDA ampulla (*star*). (B) Pulmonary artery angiogram through the TorqVue LP catheter after deploying the Piccolo device (*black arrow*) in the frontal projection with 20° caudal and 20° left anterior oblique angulation. The right pulmonary artery (*single white arrow*) and left pulmonary artery (*two white arrows*) have good flow with no stenosis. (C) Same angiogram in B obtained in the lateral projection with 15° caudal angulation shows favorable device position (anterior to the temperature probe and oriented superiorly at its anterior portion, pointing at 10 o'clock [*black arrow*]). (D) Lateral chest x-ray after device release shows the device continues to have favorable position as described in "C".

the frontal projection (Figure 18.3B) and anterior to it in the lateral projection (Figures 18.3C and D). The ideal device configuration is to be oriented more superiorly at its anterior portion (Figures 18.3C and D). After deploying the device and prior to release, a targeted transthoracic echocardiogram is performed, with special attention to the device position, presence of residual shunt, and flow across the left pulmonary artery (LPA) and aortic arch. If the position of the device is suboptimal, the device is recaptured inside the delivery catheter and redeployed in the appropriate position. After confirming an adequate device position, the device is released by counterclockwise rotation of the delivery wire. As soon as the wire is detached from the device, it should be pulled back inside the delivery catheter and the entire system is removed outside the body. Straight biplane chest X-ray is obtained (single frame cine) to be used for future comparison. A detailed echocardiogram is performed to assess the device position and residual shunt and rule out pericardial effusion. The sheath is removed, and manual pressure is held until hemostasis is achieved.

## REFERENCES

1. Lokku A, Mirea L, Lee SK, Shah PS. Trends and outcomes of patent ductus arteriosus treatment in very preterm infants in Canada. *Am J Perinatol.* 2017;34(5):441-450. doi:10.1055/s-0036-1593351.
2. Hagadorn JI, Brownell EA, Trzaski JM, et al. Trends and variation in management and outcomes of very-low-birth-weight infants with patent ductus arteriosus. *Pediatr Res.* 2016;80(6):785-792. doi:10.1038/pr.2016.166.
3. Apalodimas L, Waller Iii BR, Philip R, Crawford J, Cunningham J, Sathanandam S. A comprehensive program for preterm infants with patent ductus arteriosus. *Congenit Heart Dis.* 2019;14(1):90-94. doi:10.1111/chd.12705.
4. Bischoff AR, Jasani B, Sathanandam SK, Backes C, Weisz DE, McNamara PJ. Percutaneous closure of patent ductus arteriosus in infants 1.5 kg or less: a meta-analysis. *J Pediatr.* 2021;230:84-92.e14. doi:10.1016/j.jpeds.2020.10.035.
5. Semberova J, Sirc J, Miletin J, et al. Spontaneous closure of patent ductus arteriosus in infants </=1500 g. *Pediatrics.* 2017;140(2):e20164258. doi:10.1542/peds.2016-4258.
6. Schmidt B, Roberts RS, Fanaroff A, et al. Indomethacin prophylaxis, patent ductus arteriosus, and the risk of bronchopulmonary dysplasia: further analyses from the Trial of Indomethacin Prophylaxis in Preterms (TIPP). *J Pediatr.* 2006;148(6):730-734. doi:10.1016/j.jpeds.2006.01.047.
7. Altit G, Saeed S, Beltempo M, Claveau M, Lapointe A, Basso O. Outcomes of extremely premature infants comparing patent ductus arteriosus management approaches. *J Pediatr.* 2021;235:49-57.e2. doi:10.1016/j.jpeds.2021.04.014.
8. Rosenzweig EB, Barst RJ. Congenital heart disease and pulmonary hypertension: pharmacology and feasibility of late surgery. *Prog Cardiovasc Dis.* 2012;55(2):128-133. doi:10.1016/j.pcad.2012.07.004.
9. Bischoff AR, Moronta SC, McNamara PJ. Going home with a patent ductus arteriosus: is it benign? *J Pediatr.* 2021;240:10-13. doi:10.1016/j.jpeds.2021.09.009.
10. Philip R, Waller BR, Chilakala S, et al. Hemodynamic and clinical consequences of early versus delayed closure of patent ductus arteriosus in extremely low birth weight infants. *J Perinatol.* 2021;41(1):100-108. doi:10.1038/s41372-020-00772-2.
11. Philip R, Lamba V, Talati A, Sathanandam S. Pulmonary hypertension with prolonged patency of the ductus arteriosus in preterm infants. *Children (Basel).* 2020;7(9):139. doi:10.3390/children7090139.
12. Philip R, Nathaniel Johnson J, Naik R, et al. Effect of patent ductus arteriosus on pulmonary vascular disease. *Congenit Heart Dis.* 2019;14(1):37-41. doi:10.1111/chd.12702.
13. Cassady G, Crouse DT, Kirklin JW, et al. A randomized, controlled trial of very early prophylactic ligation of the ductus arteriosus in babies who weighed 1000 g or less at birth. *N Engl J Med.* 1989;320(23):1511-1516. doi:10.1056/nejm198906083202302.
14. Rolland A, Shankar-Aguilera S, Diomandé D, Zupan-Simunek V, Boileau P. Natural evolution of patent ductus arteriosus in the extremely preterm infant. *Arch Dis Child Fetal Neonatal Ed.* 2015;100(1):F55-F58. doi:10.1136/archdischild-2014-306339.
15. Rios DR, Martins FF, El-Khuffash A, Weisz DE, Giesinger RE, McNamara PJ. Early role of the atrial-level communication in premature infants with patent ductus arteriosus. *J Am Soc Echocardiogr.* 2021;34(4):423-432.e1. doi:10.1016/j.echo.2020.11.008.
16. Martins FF, Bassani DG, Rios DI, et al. Relationship of patent ductus arteriosus echocardiographic markers with descending aorta diastolic flow. *J Ultrasound Med.* 2021;40(8):1505-1514. doi:10.1002/jum.15528.
17. Cotton RB, Stahlman MT, Bender HW, Graham TP, Catterton WZ, Kovar I. Randomized trial of early closure of symptomatic patent ductus arteriosus in small preterm infants. *J Pediatr.* 1978;93(4):647-651. doi:10.1016/s0022-3476(78)80910-x.
18. Levitsky S, Fisher E, Vidyasagar D, et al. Interruption of patent ductus arteriosus in premature infants with respiratory distress syndrome. *Ann Thorac Surg.* 1976;22(2):131-137. doi:10.1016/s0003-4975(10)63973-2.
19. Gersony WM, Peckham GJ, Ellison RC, Miettinen OS, Nadas AS. Effects of indomethacin in premature infants with patent ductus arteriosus: results of a national collaborative study. *J Pediatr.* 1983;102(6):895-906. doi:10.1016/s0022-3476(83)80022-5.
20. Mirea L, Sankaran K, Seshia M, et al. Treatment of patent ductus arteriosus and neonatal mortality/morbidities: adjustment for treatment selection bias. *J Pediatr.* 2012;161(4):689-694.e1. doi:10.1016/j.jpeds.2012.05.007.
21. Chorne N, Leonard C, Piecuch R, Clyman RI. Patent ductus arteriosus and its treatment as risk factors for neonatal and neurodevelopmental morbidity. *Pediatrics.* 2007;119(6):1165-1174. doi:10.1542/peds.2006-3124.
22. Kabra NS, Schmidt B, Roberts RS, et al. Neurosensory impairment after surgical closure of patent ductus arteriosus in extremely low birth weight infants: results from the Trial of Indomethacin Prophylaxis in Preterms. *J Pediatr.* 2007;150(3):229-234.e1. doi:10.1016/j.jpeds.2006.11.039.
23. Madan JC, Kendrick D, Hagadorn JI, Frantz ID, III. Patent ductus arteriosus therapy: impact on neonatal and 18-month outcome. *Pediatrics.* 2009;123(2):674-681. doi:10.1542/peds.2007-2781.
24. Bourgoin L, Cipierre C, Hauet Q, et al. Neurodevelopmental outcome at 2 years of age according to patent ductus arteriosus management in very preterm infants. *Neonatology.* 2016;109(2):139-146. doi:10.1159/000442278.

25. Janz-Robinson EM, Badawi N, Walker K, Bajuk B, Abdel-Latif ME. Neurodevelopmental outcomes of premature infants treated for patent ductus arteriosus: a population-based cohort study. *J Pediatr*. 2015;167(5):1025-1032.e3. doi:10.1016/j.jpeds.2015.06.054.

26. Weisz DE, More K, McNamara PJ, Shah PS. PDA ligation and health outcomes: a meta-analysis. *Pediatrics*. 2014;133(4):e1024-e1046. doi:10.1542/peds.2013-3431.

27. Clyman RI. Surgical ligation of the patent ductus arteriosus: treatment or morbidity? *J Pediatr*. 2012;161(4):583-584. doi:10.1016/j.jpeds.2012.05.066.

28. Weisz DE, Mirea L, Rosenberg E, et al. Association of patent ductus arteriosus ligation with death or neurodevelopmental impairment among extremely preterm infants. *JAMA Pediatr*. 2017;171(5):443-449. doi:10.1001/jamapediatrics.2016.5143.

29. El-Said HG, Bratincsak A, Foerster SR, et al. Safety of percutaneous patent ductus arteriosus closure: an unselected multicenter population experience. *J Am Heart Assoc*. 2013;2(6):e000424. doi:10.1161/JAHA.113.000424.

30. Backes CH, Rivera BK, Bridge JA, et al. Percutaneous Patent Ductus Arteriosus (PDA) closure during infancy: a meta-analysis. *Pediatrics*. 2017;139(2):e20162927. doi:10.1542/peds.2016-2927.

31. Sathanandam S, Gutfinger D, Morray B, et al. Consensus guidelines for the prevention and management of periprocedural complications of transcatheter patent ductus arteriosus closure with the Amplatzer Piccolo Occluder in extremely low birth weight infants. *Pediatr Cardiol*. 2021;42(6):1258-1274. doi:10.1007/s00246-021-02665-3.

32. Zahn EM, Peck D, Phillips A, et al. Transcatheter closure of patent ductus arteriosus in extremely premature newborns: early results and midterm follow-up. *JACC Cardiovasc Interv*. 2016;9(23):2429-2437. doi:10.1016/j.jcin.2016.09.019.

33. Backes CH, Kennedy KF, Locke M, et al. Transcatheter occlusion of the patent ductus arteriosus in 747 infants <6 kg: insights from the NCDR IMPACT registry. *JACC Cardiovasc Interv*. 2017;10(17):1729-1737. doi:10.1016/j.jcin.2017.05.018.

34. Morville P, Akhavi A. Transcatheter closure of hemodynamic significant patent ductus arteriosus in 32 premature infants by Amplatzer ductal Occluder additional size-ADOIIAS. *Catheter Cardiovasc Interv*. 2017;90(4):612-617. doi:10.1002/ccd.27091.

35. Morville P, Douchin S, Bouvaist H, Dauphin C. Transcatheter occlusion of the patent ductus arteriosus in premature infants weighing less than 1200 g. *Arch Dis Child Fetal Neonatal Ed*. 2018;103(3):F198-F201. doi:10.1136/archdischild-2016-312582.

36. Narin N, Pamukcu O, Baykan A, et al. Transcatheter closure of PDA in premature babies less than 2 kg. *Anatol J Cardiol*. 2017;17(2):147-153. doi:10.14744/AnatolJCardiol.2016.6847.

37. Narin N, Pamukcu O, Baykan A, Sunkak S, Ulgey A, Uzum K. Percutaneous PDA closure in extremely low birth weight babies. *J Interv Cardiol*. 2016;29(6):654-660. doi:10.1111/joic.12352.

38. Rodriguez Ogando A, Ballesteros Tejerizo F, Blanco Bravo D, Sanchez Luna M, Zunzunegui Martinez JL. Transcatheter occlusion of patent ductus arteriosus in preterm infants weighing less than 2 kg with the Amplatzer Duct Occluder II additional sizes device. *Rev Esp Cardiol (Engl Ed)*. 2018;71(10):865-866. doi:10.1016/j.rec.2017.08.014.

39. Agrawal H, Waller BR III, Surendan S, Sathanandam S. New patent ductus arteriosus closure devices and techniques. *Interv Cardiol Clin*. 2019;8(1):23-32. doi:10.1016/j.iccl.2018.08.004.

40. Philip R, Tailor N, Johnson JN, et al. Single-center experience of 100 consecutive percutaneous patent ductus arteriosus closures in infants </= 1000 grams. *Circ Cardiovasc Interv*. 2021;14(6):e010600. doi:10.1161/CIRCINTERVENTIONS.121.010600.

41. Sathanandam SK, Gutfinger D, O'Brien L, et al. Amplatzer Piccolo Occluder clinical trial for percutaneous closure of the patent ductus arteriosus in patients >/=700 grams. *Catheter Cardiovasc Interv*. 2020;96(6):1266-1276. doi:10.1002/ccd.28973.

42. P020042 Supplemental Premarket Approval (PMA) of the AMPLATZER Piccolo Occluder (2019).

43. Nasef MA, Sullivan DO, Ng LY, et al. Use of the Medtronic Microvascular Plug 7Q for transcatheter closure of large patent ductus arteriosus in infants weighing less than 2.5 kg. *Catheter Cardiovasc Interv*. 2022;99(5):1545-1550. doi:10.1002/ccd.30105.

44. Zahn EM, Nevin P, Simmons C, Garg R. A novel technique for transcatheter patent ductus arteriosus closure in extremely preterm infants using commercially available technology. *Catheter Cardiovasc Interv*. 2015;85(2):240-248. doi:10.1002/ccd.25534.

45. Bixler GM, Powers GC, Clark RH, Walker MW, Tolia VN. Changes in the diagnosis and management of patent ductus arteriosus from 2006 to 2015 in United States neonatal intensive care units. *J Pediatr*. 2017;189:105-112. doi:10.1016/j.jpeds.2017.05.024.

46. Ulrich TJB, Hansen TP, Reid KJ, Bingler MA, Olsen SL. Post-ligation cardiac syndrome is associated with increased morbidity in preterm infants. *J Perinatol*. 2018;38(5):537-542. doi:10.1038/s41372-018-0056-4.

47. Serrano RM, Madison M, Lorant D, Hoyer M, Alexy R. Comparison of "post-patent ductus arteriosus ligation syndrome" in premature infants after surgical ligation vs. percutaneous closure. *J Perinatol*. 2020;40(2):324-329. doi:10.1038/s41372-019-0513-8.

48. Kuntz MT, Staffa SJ, Graham D, et al. Trend and outcomes for surgical versus transcatheter patent ductus arteriosus closure in neonates and infants at US children's hospitals. *J Am Heart Assoc*. 2022;11(1):e022776. doi:10.1161/JAHA.121.022776.

49. Lenoir M, Wanert C, Bonnet D, et al. Anterior minithoracotomy vs. transcatheter closure of patent ductus arteriosus in very preterm infants. *Front Pediatr*. 2021;9:700284. doi:10.3389/fped.2021.700284.

50. Sathanandam S, Agrawal H, Chilakala S, et al. Can transcatheter PDA closure be performed in neonates ≤1000 grams? The Memphis experience. *Congenit Heart Dis*. 2019;14(1):79-84. doi:10.1111/chd.12700.

51. Mitchell CC, Rivera BK, Cooper JN, et al. Percutaneous closure of the patent ductus arteriosus: opportunities moving forward. *Congenit Heart Dis*. 2019;14(1):95-99. doi:10.1111/chd.12704.

52. Letshwiti JB, Semberova J, Pichova K, Dempsey EM, Franklin OM, Miletin J. A conservative treatment of patent ductus arteriosus in very low birth weight infants. *Early Hum Dev*. 2017;104:45-49. doi:10.1016/j.earlhumdev.2016.12.008.

53. ClinicalTrials.gov. *PIVOTAL: Percutaneous Intervention Versus Observational Trial of Arterial Ductus in Lower Gestational Age Infants*; 2022.]

54. Mashally S, Banihani R, Jasani B, et al. Is late treatment with acetaminophen safe and effective in avoiding surgical ligation among extremely preterm neonates with persistent patent ductus arteriosus? *J Perinatol*. 2021;41(10):2519-2525. doi:10.1038/s41372-021-01194-4.

55. Watterberg KL, Scott SM, Backstrom C, Gifford KL, Cook KL. Links between early adrenal function and respiratory outcome in preterm infants: airway inflammation and patent ductus

arteriosus. *Pediatrics.* 2000;105(2):320-324. doi:10.1542/peds.105.2.320.

56. El-Khuffash A, McNamara PJ, Lapointe A, Jain A. Adrenal function in preterm infants undergoing patent ductus arteriosus ligation. *Neonatology.* 2013;104(1):28-33. doi:10.1159/000350017.

57. De Buyst J, Rakza T, Pennaforte T, Johansson AB, Storme L. Hemodynamic effects of fluid restriction in preterm infants with significant patent ductus arteriosus. *J Pediatr.* 2012;161(3):404-408. doi:10.1016/j.jpeds.2012.03.012.

58. Lemyre B, Liu L, Moore GP, Lawrence SL, Barrowman NJ. Do intra-operative fluids influence the need for post-operative cardiotropic support after a PDA ligation? *Zhongguo Dang Dai Er Ke Za Zhi.* 2011;13(1):1-7.

59. Gerhardt T, Bancalari E. Lung compliance in newborns with patent ductus arteriosus before and after surgical ligation. *Biol Neonate.* 1980;38(1-2):96-105. doi:10.1159/000241348.

60. Noonan M, Turek JW, Dagle JM, McElroy SJ. Intraoperative high-frequency jet ventilation is equivalent to conventional ventilation during patent ductus arteriosus ligation. *World J Pediatr Congenit Heart Surg.* 2017;8(5):570-574. doi:10.1177/2150135117717974.

61. El-Khuffash AF, Jain A, McNamara PJ. Ligation of the patent ductus arteriosus in preterm infants: understanding the physiology. *J Pediatr.* 2013;162(6):1100-1106. doi:10.1016/j.jpeds.2012.12.094.

62. Giesinger RE, Bischoff AR, McNamara PJ. Anticipatory perioperative management for patent ductus arteriosus surgery: understanding postligation cardiac syndrome. *Congenit Heart Dis.* 2019;14(2):311-316. doi:10.1111/chd.12738.

63. Noori S, Friedlich P, Seri I, Wong P. Changes in myocardial function and hemodynamics after ligation of the ductus arteriosus in preterm infants. *J Pediatr.* 2007;150(6):597-602. doi:10.1016/j.jpeds.2007.01.035.

64. McNamara PJ, Stewart L, Shivananda SP, Stephens D, Sehgal A. Patent ductus arteriosus ligation is associated with impaired left ventricular systolic performance in premature infants weighing less than 1000 g. *J Thorac Cardiovasc Surg.* 2010;140(1):150-157. doi:10.1016/j.jtcvs.2010.01.011.

65. Szymankiewicz M, Hodgman JE, Siassi B, Gadzinowski J. Mechanics of breathing after surgical ligation of patent ductus arteriosus in newborns with respiratory distress syndrome. *Biol Neonate.* 2004;85(1):32-36. doi:10.1159/000074955.

66. Lien R, Hsu KH, Chu JJ, Chang YS. Hemodynamic alterations recorded by electrical cardiometry during ligation of ductus arteriosus in preterm infants. *Eur J Pediatr.* 2015;174(4):543-550. doi:10.1007/s00431-014-2437-9.

67. Lindner W, Seidel M, Versmold HT, Döhlemann C, Riegel KP. Stroke volume and left ventricular output in preterm infants with patent ductus arteriosus. *Pediatr Res.* 1990;27(3):278-281. doi:10.1203/00006450-199003000-00015.

68. Bischoff AR, Stanford AH, McNamara PJ. Short-term ventriculo-arterial coupling and myocardial work efficiency in preterm infants undergoing percutaneous patent ductus arteriosus closure. *Physiol Rep.* 2021;9(22):e15108. doi:10.14814/phy2.15108.

69. Taylor AF, Morrow WR, Lally KP, Kinsella JP, Gerstmann DR, deLemos RA. Left ventricular dysfunction following ligation of the ductus arteriosus in the preterm baboon. *J Surg Res.* 1990;48(6):590-596.

70. Nagata H, Ihara K, Yamamura K, et al. Left ventricular efficiency after ligation of patent ductus arteriosus for premature infants. *J Thorac Cardiovasc Surg.* 2013;146(6):1353-1358. doi:10.1016/j.jtcvs.2013.02.019.

71. El-Khuffash AF, Jain A, Dragulescu A, McNamara PJ, Mertens L. Acute changes in myocardial systolic function in preterm infants undergoing patent ductus arteriosus ligation: a tissue Doppler and myocardial deformation study. *J Am Soc Echocardiogr.* 2012;25(10):1058-1067. doi:10.1016/j.echo.2012.07.016.

72. Moin F, Kennedy KA, Moya FR. Risk factors predicting vasopressor use after patent ductus arteriosus ligation. *Am J Perinatol.* 2003;20(6):313-320. doi:10.1055/s-2003-42693.

73. Saida K, Nakamura T, Hiroma T, Takigiku K, Yasukochi S. Preoperative left ventricular internal dimension in end-diastole as earlier identification of early patent ductus arteriosus operation and postoperative intensive care in very low birth weight infants. *Early Hum Dev.* 2013;89(10):821-823. doi:10.1016/j.earlhumdev.2013.07.011.

74. McNamara PJ, Weisz DE, Giesinger RE, Jain A. Hemodynamics. In: MacDonald MG MMKS, eds. *Avery's Neonatology: Pathophysiology and Management of the Newborn.* Philadelphia: Wolters Kluwer; 2016:457-486.

75. Rowland DG, Gutgesell HP. Noninvasive assessment of myocardial contractility, preload, and afterload in healthy newborn infants. *Am J Cardiol.* 1995;75(12):818-821.

76. Hoodbhoy SA, Cutting HA, Seddon JA, Campbell ME. Cerebral and splanchnic hemodynamics after duct ligation in very low birth weight infants. *J Pediatr.* 2009;154(2):196-200. doi:10.1016/j.jpeds.2008.07.051.

77. Noori S. Pros and cons of patent ductus arteriosus ligation: hemodynamic changes and other morbidities after patent ductus arteriosus ligation. *Semin Perinatol.* 2012;36(2):139-145. doi:10.1053/j.semperi.2011.09.024.

78. Leslie AT, Jain A, El-Khuffash A, Keyzers M, Rogerson S, McNamara PJ. Evaluation of cerebral electrical activity and cardiac output after patent ductus arteriosus ligation in preterm infants. *J Perinatol.* 2013;33(11):861-866. doi:10.1038/jp.2013.85.

79. Jain A, Sahni M, El-Khuffash A, Khadawardi E, Sehgal A, McNamara PJ. Use of targeted neonatal echocardiography to prevent postoperative cardiorespiratory instability after patent ductus arteriosus ligation. *J Pediatr.* 2012;160(4):584-589.e1. doi:10.1016/j.jpeds.2011.09.027.

80. Kimball TR, Ralston MA, Khoury P, Crump RG, Cho FS, Reuter JH. Effect of ligation of patent ductus arteriosus on left ventricular performance and its determinants in premature neonates. *J Am Coll Cardiol.* 1996;27(1):193-197. doi:10.1016/0735-1097(95)00452-1.

81. Bischoff AR, Jasani B, Sathanandam SK, Backes C, Weisz DE, McNamara PJ. Percutaneous closure of patent ductus arteriosus in infants </=1.5 kg: a meta-analysis. *J Pediatr.* 2021;230:84-92.e14. doi:10.1016/j.jpeds.2020.10.035.

82. Teixeira LS, Shivananda SP, Stephens D, Van Arsdell G, McNamara PJ. Postoperative cardiorespiratory instability following ligation of the preterm ductus arteriosus is related to early need for intervention. *J Perinatol.* 2008;28(12):803-810. doi:10.1038/jp.2008.101.

83. Harting MT, Blakely ML, Cox Jr CS, Lantin-Hermoso R, Andrassy RJ, Lally KP. Acute hemodynamic decompensation following patent ductus arteriosus ligation in premature infants. *J Invest Surg.* 2008;21(3):133-138. doi:10.1080/08941930802046469.

84. Ting JY, Resende M, More K, et al. Predictors of respiratory instability in neonates undergoing patent ductus arteriosus ligation after the introduction of targeted milrinone treatment. *J Thorac Cardiovasc Surg.* 2016;152(2):498-504. doi:10.1016/j.jtcvs.2016.03.085.

85. El-Khuffash AF, Jain A, Weisz D, Mertens L, McNamara PJ. Assessment and treatment of post patent ductus arteriosus ligation syndrome. *J Pediatr*. 2014;165(1):46-52.e1. doi:10.1016/j.jpeds.2014.03.048.

86. Hoffman TM, Wernovsky G, Atz AM, et al. Efficacy and safety of milrinone in preventing low cardiac output syndrome in infants and children after corrective surgery for congenital heart disease. *Circulation*. 2003;107(7):996-1002. doi:10.1161/01.cir.0000051365.81920.28.

87. Waleh N, McCurnin DC, Yoder BA, Shaul PW, Clyman RI. Patent ductus arteriosus ligation alters pulmonary gene expression in preterm baboons. *Pediatr Res*. 2011;69(3):212-216. doi:10.1203/PDR.0b013e3182084f8d.

88. Noori S, McCoy M, Anderson MP, Ramji F, Seri I. Changes in cardiac function and cerebral blood flow in relation to peri/intraventricular hemorrhage in extremely preterm infants. *J Pediatr*. 2014;164(2):264-270.e1-3. doi:10.1016/j.jpeds.2013.09.045.

89. Kalfa D, Krishnamurthy G, Cheung E. Patent ductus arteriosus surgical ligation: still a lot to understand. *J Thorac Cardiovasc Surg*. 2016;152(2):505-506. doi:10.1016/j.jtcvs.2016.04.013.

90. Liggins GC. The role of cortisol in preparing the fetus for birth. *Reprod Fertil Dev*. 1994;6(2):141-150. doi:10.1071/rd9940141.

91. Ng PC, Lam CW, Fok TF, et al. Refractory hypotension in preterm infants with adrenocortical insufficiency. *Arch Dis Child Fetal Neonatal Ed*. 2001;84(2):F122-F124. doi:10.1136/fn.84.2.f122.

92. Hochwald O, Holsti L, Osiovich H. The use of an early ACTH test to identify hypoadrenalism-related hypotension in low birth weight infants. *J Perinatol*. 2012;32(6):412-417. doi:10.1038/jp.2012.16.

93. Masumoto K, Kusuda S, Aoyagi H, et al. Comparison of serum cortisol concentrations in preterm infants with or without late-onset circulatory collapse due to adrenal insufficiency of prematurity. *Pediatr Res*. 2008;63(6):686-690. doi:10.1203/PDR.0b013e31816c8fcc.

94. Clyman RI, Wickremasinghe A, Merritt TA, et al. Hypotension following patent ductus arteriosus ligation: the role of adrenal hormones. *J Pediatr*. 2014;164(6):1449-1455.e1. doi:10.1016/j.jpeds.2014.01.058.

95. Quintos JB, Boney CM. Transient adrenal insufficiency in the premature newborn. *Curr Opin Endocrinol Diabetes Obes*. 2010;17(1):8-12. doi:10.1097/MED.0b013e32833363cc.

96. Satpute MD, Donohue PK, Vricella L, Aucott SW. Cardiovascular instability after patent ductus arteriosus ligation in preterm infants: the role of hydrocortisone. *J Perinatol*. 2012;32(9):685-689. doi:10.1038/jp.2011.166.

97. Weisz DE, Giesinger RE. Surgical management of a patent ductus arteriosus: Is this still an option? *Semin Fetal Neonatal Med*. 2018;23(4):255-266. doi:10.1016/j.siny.2018.03.003.

98. Sathanandam SK, Gutfinger D, O'Brien L, et al. Amplatzer Piccolo Occluder clinical trial for percutaneous closure of the patent ductus arteriosus in patients >/=700 grams. *Catheter Cardiovasc Interv*. 2020;96(6):1266-1276. doi:10.1002/ccd.28973.

99. Willis A, Pereiras L, Head T, et al. Transport of extremely low birth weight neonates for persistent ductus arteriosus closure in the catheterization lab. *Congenit Heart Dis*. 2019;14(1):69-73. doi:10.1111/chd.12706.

100. Backes CH, Cheatham SL, Deyo GM, et al. Percutaneous Patent Ductus Arteriosus (PDA) closure in very preterm infants: feasibility and complications. *J Am Heart Assoc*. 2016;5(2):e002923. doi:10.1161/JAHA.115.002923.

101. Backes CH, Giesinger RE, Rivera BK, et al. Percutaneous closure of the patent ductus arteriosus in very low weight infants: considerations following US food and drug administration approval of a novel device. *J Pediatr*. 2019;213:218-221. doi:10.1016/j.jpeds.2019.05.062.

102. Engeseth MS, Olsen NR, Maeland S, Halvorsen T, Goode A, Røksund OD. Left vocal cord paralysis after patent ductus arteriosus ligation: a systematic review. *Paediatr Respir Rev*. 2018;27:74-85. doi:10.1016/j.prrv.2017.11.001.

103. Rukholm G, Farrokhyar F, Reid D. Vocal cord paralysis post patent ductus arteriosus ligation surgery: risks and co-morbidities. *Int J Pediatr Otorhinolaryngol*. 2012;76(11):1637-1641. doi:10.1016/j.ijporl.2012.07.036.

104. Spanos WC, Brookes JT, Smith MC, Burkhart HM, Bell EF, Smith RJ. Unilateral vocal fold paralysis in premature infants after ligation of patent ductus arteriosus: vascular clip versus suture ligature. *Ann Otol Rhinol Laryngol*. 2009;118(10):750-753. doi:10.1177/000348940911801011.

105. Benjamin JR, Smith PB, Cotten CM, Jaggers J, Goldstein RF, Malcolm WF. Long-term morbidities associated with vocal cord paralysis after surgical closure of a patent ductus arteriosus in extremely low birth weight infants. *J Perinatol*. 2010;30(6):408-413. doi:10.1038/jp.2009.124.

106. Engan M, Engeset MS, Sandvik L, et al. Left vocal cord paralysis, lung function and exercise capacity in young adults born extremely preterm with a history of neonatal patent ductus arteriosus surgery – a national cohort study. *Front Pediatr*. 2021;9:780045. doi:10.3389/fped.2021.780045.

107. Heuchan AM, Hunter L, Young D. Outcomes following the surgical ligation of the patent ductus arteriosus in premature infants in Scotland. *Arch Dis Child Fetal Neonatal Ed*. 2012;97(1):F39-F44. doi:10.1136/adc.2010.206052.

108. Kang SL, Samsudin S, Kuruvilla M, Dhelaria A, Kent S, Kelsall WA. Outcome of patent ductus arteriosus ligation in premature infants in the East of England: a prospective cohort study. *Cardiol Young*. 2013;23(5):711-716. doi:10.1017/s1047951112001795.

109. Hsu KH, Chiang MC, Lien R, et al. Diaphragmatic paralysis among very low birth weight infants following ligation for patent ductus arteriosus. *Eur J Pediatr*. 2012;171(11):1639-1644. doi:10.1007/s00431-012-1787-4.

110. Smith BM, Ezeokoli NJ, Kipps AK, Azakie A, Meadows JJ. Course, predictors of diaphragm recovery after phrenic nerve injury during pediatric cardiac surgery. *Ann Thorac Surg*. 2013;96(3):938-942. doi:10.1016/j.athoracsur.2013.05.057.

111. Fleming WH, Sarafian LB, Kugler JD, Nelson Jr RM. Ligation of patent ductus arteriosus in premature infants: importance of accurate anatomic definition. *Pediatrics*. 1983;71(3):373-375.

112. Chang AC, Wells W. Shunt lesions. In: Chang AC, Hanley FL, Wernovsky G, Wessel DL, eds. *Pediatric cardiac intensive care*. Baltimore: Wessel Williams & Wilkins; 1998.

113. Harris LL, Krishnamurthy R, Browne LP, Morales DL, Friedman EM. Left main bronchus obstruction after patent ductus arteriosus ligation: an unusual complication. *Int J Pediatr Otorhinolaryngol*. 2012;76(12):1855-1856. doi:10.1016/j.ijporl.2012.09.002.

114. Kim D, Kim SW, Shin HJ, Hong JM, Lee JH, Han HS. Unintended pulmonary artery ligation during PDA ligation. *Heart Surg Forum*. 2016;19(4):E187-E188. doi:10.1532/hsf.1449.

115. Baspinar O, Sahin DA, Sulu A, et al. Transcatheter closure of patent ductus arteriosus in under 6 kg and premature infants. *J Interv Cardiol*. 2015;28(2):180-189. doi:10.1111/joic.12196.

116. Roberts P, Adwani S, Archer N, Wilson N. Catheter closure of the arterial duct in preterm infants. *Arch Dis Child Fetal Neonatal Ed.* 2007;92(4):F248-F250. doi:10.1136/adc.2005.078600.

117. Heyden CM, El-Said HG, Moore JW, Guyon Jr PW, Katheria AC, Ratnayaka K. Early experience with the Micro Plug Set for preterm patent ductus arteriosus closure. *Catheter Cardiovasc Interv.* 2020;96(7):1439-1444. doi:10.1002/ccd.29298.

118. Francis E, Singhi AK, Lakshmivenkateshaiah S, Kumar RK. Transcatheter occlusion of patent ductus arteriosus in pre-term infants. *JACC Cardiovasc Interv.* 2010;3(5):550-555. doi:10.1016/j.jcin.2010.01.016.

119. Mathis C, Romans R, Divekar A. Variation in the outer diameter of vascular sheaths commonly used in infant cardiac catheterization. *Catheter Cardiovasc Interv.* 2020;96(3):620-625. doi:10.1002/ccd.28825.

# Chapter 19

# Pathophysiology-Based Management of the Hemodynamically Significant Patent Ductus Arteriosus in the Very Preterm Neonate

Stephanie M. Boyd, Elizabeth Rachel Fisher, and Martin Kluckow

## Key Points

- The simplistic "treat all or treat none" approach to management of a patent ductus arteriosus (PDA) has been increasingly challenged in recent years as the variation in clinical and hemodynamic presentation has been realized.

- Spontaneous closure rates, poor efficacy of medical treatment, and a combination of selection bias, high open-label treatment rates, and inappropriate outcome measures in clinical trials are among the major factors that have resulted in a lack of confidence in the usefulness of treating a PDA.

- Definition and adjudication of hemodynamic significance in clinical trials of PDA therapy has been inconsistent, resulting in groups of infants with heterogeneous underlying physiologies receiving the same pharmacologic therapy.

- The era of personalized medicine, whereby the individual characteristics of the patient (genetics, physiology/pathophysiology, biochemistry, clinical variables) are taken into consideration when deciding on a clinical care pathway, is ideally suited to many of the neonatal hemodynamic treatment dilemmas, including PDA management.

- Understanding the clinical and hemodynamic variability of an individual patient's PDA may allow more specific decision-making around "when" to treat, "whom" to treat, and "with what" treatment approach. In this regard, better evaluation tools and development of multi-parameter scoring systems and treatment algorithms based on patient characteristics are likely to be increasingly important.

- Essential to decision-making around PDA management is a detailed cardiovascular assessment that determines hemodynamic significance of the ductus for the individual patient in their clinical context.

## Introduction

Historically, the default position of most neonatologists has been to treat the patent ductus arteriosus (PDA), particularly in the very-low-birth-weight (VLBW) infant (<1500 g). More recently, as our intensive care practices have evolved and outcomes continue to improve for the smallest, most vulnerable infants, the need for medical treatment, particularly with non-steroidal anti-inflammatory drugs (NSAIDs), has been increasingly questioned. This uncertainty has been driven by a number of factors, including our inability to identify infants who would most benefit from treatment, high spontaneous closure rates in infants >1000 g, variable efficacy of the medications available, balancing the risks of side effects, and the failure of trials of treatment to show clear short- or long-term benefits. However, it is not likely that an "all or none" solution is applicable – there are likely to be a subset of newborns with a PDA who should be treated at an appropriate time in order to avoid possible deleterious effects from a hemodynamically significant left-to-right shunt. Identification of these infants with a hemodynamically significant PDA (hsPDA) in whom treatment is more likely to be beneficial has become a priority. This is essential in seeking to avoid unnecessary therapies and undesirable side effects, balanced with minimizing the potential risks of exposure to adverse PDA physiology. A necessary prerequisite for appropriate patient selection for PDA treatment is an in-depth understanding of individual pathophysiology; specifically, the effects will be dependent on a number of underlying elements – the gestational age of the infant, the magnitude of any left-to-right transductal shunt (which is governed by the Poiseuille law of fluid dynamics), and associated degrees of systemic hypoperfusion and pulmonary over-circulation, as well as myocardial performance. Systemic hypoperfusion, due to the effects of circulatory "steal" on the systemic circulation, is manifested through alterations in systemic arterial pressure and perfusion to the brain, kidney, and gut. Pulmonary over-circulation, or excessive pulmonary blood flow, can result in higher respiratory support needs and pulmonary hemorrhage, as well as contribute to risks of subsequent bronchopulmonary dysplasia (BPD) and chronic pulmonary hypertension. Clinician-performed ultrasound (CPU) of the heart in the neonatal intensive care unit (NICU) by the clinician caring for the baby in a longitudinal setting is an important adjunct to clinical assessment when defining the hemodynamic profile of an infant with a PDA. Understanding how to assess the underlying elements of the pathophysiological scenario allows a more individualized decision to be made regarding the need for treatment, in order to both maximize potential benefit and minimize risks of treatment-related harm.

## Pathophysiology of Patent Ductus Arteriosus

The tendency of the ductus arteriosus (DA) to remain patent in preterm infants is thought to be related to developmental immaturity of ductal anatomy,[1] as well as altered prostaglandin responsiveness[2] and metabolism (see also Chapter 16).[3] Not all PDAs are pathological, however, even in the preterm population. It is important to consider the PDA in the context of the clinical picture and associated hemodynamic state of the patient. For example, a PDA may be considered supportive in the setting of critically low pulmonary blood flow (either due to right ventricular outflow tract obstruction or severe pulmonary hypertension), left ventricular (LV) dysfunction, or left heart obstruction (e.g., coarctation of the aorta). A PDA is considered hemodynamically significant, and potentially pathological, when there are clinical and/or echocardiographic markers of a moderate or large volume left-to-right (systemic-to-pulmonary) shunt.

Flow through the DA is determined by the Poiseuille law ($Q = \Delta P \pi r^4 / 8L\mu$), where $Q$ denotes flow, $\Delta P$ is the pressure gradient across the ductus, $L$ is the ductal length, and $\mu$ is the viscosity (see Chapter 16). This has important implications for understanding factors that modulate ductal flow. The pressure difference in the systemic and pulmonary circulations is an important determinant of transductal shunt, particularly during the postnatal transition. The high systemic vascular resistance (SVR) and declining pulmonary vascular resistance (PVR) state of the transitioning preterm neonate creates a unique physiological vulnerability to high-volume left-to-right ductal shunting. The inherent diastolic "dysfunction" of the preterm myocardium and poor adaptive ability in the face of adverse loading conditions further compounds this risk. Physiologically, the negative consequences of an hsPDA can be considered complications relating to one or more among pulmonary over-circulation, systemic hypoperfusion, and/or hypoperfusion-reperfusion, which arise as a result of a significant left-to-right transductal shunt. Retrograde diastolic blood flow (ductal "steal") diverts blood flow from post-ductal organs, such as the kidneys and gut, resulting in hypoperfusion. Conversely, the increased left ventricular output (LVO) secondary to left-to-right ductal shunting increases blood flow to pre-ductal organs, such as the brain. The latter is a potential mechanism for both peri-/intraventricular hemorrhage (P/IVH) associated with reperfusion, and white matter injury.[4] As is evident from the Poiseuille equation, blood viscosity, and specifically red cell mass, blood platelet levels, and intravascular volume status, also have the potential to modulate flow across the PDA and should not be disregarded when considering factors contributing to the ductal flow pattern. Although PDA size is frequently ascertained as part of a comprehensive hemodynamic assessment, ductal morphology is less commonly evaluated. Several different anatomical subtypes of

PDA exist,[5] which may contribute to the limitations of using PDA size as a single marker from which to estimate shunt volume. The several factors regulating PDA flow highlight the importance of a comprehensive hemodynamic assessment when appraising the ductus and embarking on treatment-related decisions. The concept of hsPDA involves complex interactions between intrinsic, patient-related conditions, the anatomy of the PDA itself, and the medical therapies used as part of newborn intensive care practice. In summary, relevant considerations include:

- Clinical factors, including gestational and chronological age, birth weight, the likelihood of spontaneous closure, respiratory support, gastrointestinal health, and cardiocirculatory status (systolic and diastolic blood pressure, serum lactate, urine output, etc.).
- Nature of the PDA, i.e., pathological versus physiological or supportive.
- An estimation of transductal shunt volume, including markers of systemic hypoperfusion, pulmonary over-circulation, and myocardial function.

## Factors to Consider in PDA Clinical Decision-Making

Although the relative contribution of the preterm patent ductus to important neonatal morbidities has been studied extensively and evidence of association is strong, the role and merits of treatment remain controversial. The argument that the PDA is an innocent bystander with high likelihood of spontaneous closure, rather than a pathologic condition, is becoming increasingly prevalent in neonatology.[6] As a result, there is a secular trend toward a conservative or non-intervention approach to PDA. Opting for non-treatment and awaiting spontaneous closure implies acceptance of any short- and long-term consequences of a PDA, which are in part related to the timing of intervention. The adverse effects of hsPDA relate to the duration and magnitude of exposure to a left-to-right shunt, inherent circulatory adaptive mechanisms,[4] and interplay of important clinical factors (e.g., gestational age, comorbidities, chronological age, end-organ function). Prolonged patency is associated with numerous adverse outcomes, including

prolongation of assisted ventilation and higher rates of BPD, pulmonary hemorrhage, P/IVH, periventricular leukomalacia (PVL), renal impairment, necrotizing enterocolitis (NEC), systemic hypotension, and death.[7,32] The key issue is whether intervention at a particular time point prevents some or all of these complications with minimal side-effects related to treatment. Importantly, for *each individual infant*, there will be a different risk/benefit equation.

## Consequences of a Patent Ductus Arteriosus

In most newborn infants, even in the first postnatal hours, the ductal shunt is completely left-to-right or bidirectional with a dominant left-to-right component, illustrating that pulmonary pressures are usually sub-systemic shortly after birth. Using superior vena cava (SVC) flow as a surrogate measure of systemic blood flow, a negative association has been observed between duct diameter and SVC flow at 5 hours of age, but this association was not significant in subsequent studies at 12, 24, and 48 hours.[8] The association between the early low systemic blood flow and development of P/IVH and later necrotizing enterocolitis (NEC) suggests a possible mechanism by which PDA shunting contributes to the pathophysiology of these conditions.[8] There is also mounting evidence to suggest a PDA may cause pulmonary hemorrhage in preterm neonates because of overload of the pulmonary circulation in the presence of a low resistance pulmonary vasculature and that early ductal treatment may prevent this.[9-11]

A pathological PDA causes high left-to-right shunt volumes, which may flood the lungs and cause pulmonary edema. Pulmonary edema reduces lung compliance, resulting in increased ventilator and oxygen requirements. All these factors together might contribute to the development of BPD, known to be associated with the persistence of an hsPDA. Each week of exposure to a hemodynamically significant DA represented an added risk for BPD (odds ratio 1.7).[12] A higher incidence of BPD has also been observed in extremely preterm infants receiving conservative management of PDA, compared with infants without PDA.[13] There is emerging but not unequivocal[14] evidence that a tolerant approach to PDA may be associated with a higher incidence of BPD, particularly if treatment is delayed until after the first postnatal week.[13,15,16] Use of multiparameter scoring systems may also be predictive of future BPD and death – a high PDA severity score on day 2 is associated with these outcomes.[17]

A PDA may cause hemodynamic disturbances, resulting in "steal" of blood from the systemic circulation, including the mesenteric arteries, with consequences of decreased oxygen delivery to the gut and the potential for tissue injury and NEC. Even a low-volume PDA shunt can reduce mesenteric artery flow and decrease the expected postprandial increase in blood flow.[18] Because reduced intestinal blood flow is a contributor to the development of NEC, hsPDA may be a causative factor for NEC.[19] In a study involving a relatively large number of neonates, presence of a PDA was an independent risk factor for the development of NEC in VLBW infants.[20]

There is ample evidence on the basis of Doppler and near-infrared spectroscopy (NIRS) studies to suggest that cerebral blood flow is reduced in the presence of a PDA.[18] In a recent study using NIRS, cerebral tissue oxygen saturation was lowest in a group of newborns just prior to the surgical closure of PDA. Magnetic resonance imaging (MRI)–measured global and regional cerebral (and cerebellar) volumes were lower in the subgroup of infants that met criteria for surgical ligation compared with patients treated medically and those without a PDA. The surgical group also had a lower cerebellar volume compared with other groups. The authors speculated that prolonged exposure to left-to-right shunting, based on the amount of time elapsed between the diagnosis of PDA and actual surgical closure, was contributary.[21] Although hsPDA has an effect on cerebral hemodynamics, whether it is causative for P/IVH is a question that remains unanswered. Cerebral autoregulation is likely to play some role, particularly in immature infants, in protecting against P/IVH (see Chapter 7 for pathophysiology of P/IVH). Intact autoregulation is variable in immature infants,[22] and one of the risk factors for impaired autoregulation may be a PDA-attributable reduction in cerebral blood flow. Early (in particular prophylactic) treatment with indomethacin results in both closure of the PDA and decreased risk of severe P/IVH. However, many clinicians are not convinced

that prophylactic or early targeted treatment of the PDA is helpful because of the lack of demonstration of improved neuro developmental outcomes.[42] PDA is also a risk factor for development of PVL.[23] Finally, PDA is associated with a higher mortality rate.[7,32] In a retrospective study, after adjustment for perinatal factors, level of maturity, disease severity, and morbid pathologies, the hazard risk for death in neonates with a PDA was eightfold higher than in those with a closed ductus.[24] Exclusion of patients who died during the first 2 weeks or inclusion of those who underwent ductal ligation did not alter the findings. In neonates born prior to 28 weeks of gestation a PDA diameter $\geq 1.5$ mm on postnatal day 3 was associated with greater odds of mortality.[25]

What about spontaneous closure of a PDA – is it possible to do nothing and just wait?

## Spontaneous Closure

Due to reduced spontaneous ductal closure rates coupled with significant pulmonary-systemic pressure differences and immature cardiovascular adaptive responses, extremely preterm infants (<28 weeks' gestation) are at higher risk of complications from hsPDA. These risks exist both in the early postnatal period, with susceptibility to pulmonary flooding and systemic hypoperfusion and their consequences, as well as on a more chronic basis due to effects of prolonged left-to-right shunting on the developing heart, brain, kidneys, intestines, and lungs. A PDA in a relatively mature preterm neonate is of less concern, as the left-to-right shunt appears to be better tolerated and the cardiovascular system and cerebral autoregulation protective mechanisms are more developed. Despite this, previous systematic meta-analyses regarding PDA treatment include many trials more than 20 years old and those that focused on larger, more mature infants of up to 33–34 weeks' gestation, where spontaneous closure in the first few days is almost inevitable.[26] Inclusion of both extremely preterm and relatively mature neonates in the same studies makes it difficult to understand the efficacy of treatment versus the effects of spontaneous closure. The protagonists of no treatment argue on the basis of these studies, despite inclusion of a wide mix of gestational age groups, poor diagnostic criteria for PDA, including limited and inconsistent assessment of hemodynamic significance, high rates of open-label treatment in control groups, small sample sizes, selection bias, and/or lack of objective enrolment criteria at randomization. Importantly, spontaneous closure in the placebo control arm of the randomized controlled trials, as well as high levels of open-label treatment in both trial arms (from 30 to 70%),[27] make the interpretation of outcomes in many of the PDA trials difficult at best. In fact, much of the efficacy of our current treatment drugs may be ascribed more to high spontaneous closure rates, particularly in more mature infants, rather than the treatments themselves. The real natural course of PDA in treatment-naïve extremely preterm neonates and the true efficacy of the medications used for treatment are not well understood, although literature on outcomes of non-intervention has evolved in more recent years.

Interest in the role of non-treatment or conservative management of the PDA has prompted a number of studies attempting to address these questions. In a study of the natural evolution of PDA in extremely-low-birth-weight (ELBW) neonates,[5] the authors observed a 73% spontaneous DA closure rate in newborns born at less than 28 weeks. However, deaths (both early and late), undiagnosed probable PDAs, and infants discharged home with persistent PDAs were excluded from the study. In the end, 41% of potentially eligible neonates were excluded, many with morbidity and mortality potentially attributable to or contributed to by the PDA, including pulmonary hemorrhage, severe P/IVH, and hypoxic respiratory failure. This significantly impacts upon our ability to draw conclusions about the potential risks of non-treatment based on this study, noting also that a high incidence of pulmonary hemorrhage (25%) was observed.[28] Similarly, Koch et al. reported a 34% permanent closure rate of PDA in ELBW neonates.[29] Of note, around one-quarter of potentially eligible infants were omitted as a result of either death or provision of comfort care, and there was no use of cardiac ultrasound (US) to adjudicate hemodynamic significance. Despite these shortcomings, the observation that for each week of increase in gestational age above 23 weeks, the odds of spontaneous PDA closure increased by a ratio of 1.5 is noteworthy. This is consistent with the known direct relationship between gestational age,

birth weight, and persistence of the PDA.[24] Spontaneous closure rates of 21–31% among infants with 23–27 weeks of gestation have been reported historically, with lowest rates in the most immature infants.[30,31] It is important to note that these earlier studies were undertaken prior to the widespread adoption of non-invasive ventilation for extremely preterm newborns and preceding the higher survival rates currently achieved at <25 weeks of gestation.

Two larger observational studies of minimal/no treatment of the PDA have been published from the same group. The first study[14] compares three different PDA management approaches in 138 VLBW infants. Infants received either symptomatic, early targeted (during the first 48 hours), or conservative treatment. The authors found no short-term differences between the groups and a decreased rate of BPD in the conservative treatment group. The second, more contemporaneous study[32] is a retrospective cohort study in two European units that enrolled 297 VLBW infants, of whom 280 received conservative PDA management. The authors documented a median time to PDA closure of 71 days for infants born at <26 weeks, compared with 8 days at 28–29 weeks and just 6 days for infants born at or above 30 weeks.[32] Despite closure rates at hospital discharge of 85% for the overall cohort, spontaneous closure rates <750 g were particularly low, with a substantial proportion of these infants experiencing a prolonged period of exposure to ductal shunting.[32] Detailed assessment of PDA hemodynamic significance was not provided; however, it can be assumed that a subset of patients, perhaps 30–50%,[33] would have had a moderate or large volume left-to-right shunt. In addition, of 26 infants who died, 16 had a cause of death potentially related to PDA. In 2022, among a large cohort of infants discharged home with a PDA after preterm birth, lower rates of spontaneous closure than previously observed (47–58%) were reported in the first 12–18 months after birth.[34] There were also three infant deaths in this group, of whom two had documented evidence of pulmonary hypertension, which was progressive.[34] A greater likelihood of BPD and death has also been reported elsewhere with non-treatment,[35,36] with an increase in BPD rates of 31% in one study in an era of non-intervention.[37] Pulmonary vascular remodeling as a result of chronic pulmonary over-circulation has been postulated as a mechanism for some of these observations, as well as a potential driver of preterm ductal closure.[38] Elevations in pulmonary arterial pressure are initially due to increased pulmonary blood flow (PBF) in the setting of hsPDA, which chronically may relate to pulmonary vascular remodeling and altered vasoreactivity.[39,40] Increases in PVR may eventually be substantial enough to lead to PDA shunt reversal in some patients.[39,40] These studies highlight that non-intervention of PDA is not necessarily benign, even if early morbidities such as P/IVH and pulmonary hemorrhage are avoided. They also serve to emphasize the importance of considering individual patient factors, such as gestational age and PDA hemodynamic significance, in clinical decision-making. Notwithstanding the limitations of the literature, it is clear that spontaneous closure rates are lowest among the smallest, most preterm infants, who are also the most vulnerable to PDA-related morbidities.

## Role of Conservative Management

The role of conservative management of PDA is an important area of research, although there are no data focusing on the impact in the most extremely preterm infants with prolonged exposure to moderate-high volume shunts. A systematic review and meta-analysis on outcomes of conservative management of PDA, which encompassed 12 cohort studies and 4 randomized controlled trials (RCTs), was recently published.[41] Findings of cohort studies included a higher risk for mortality (risk ratio 1.34) and a lower risk of BPD, P/IVH, NEC, and retinopathy of prematurity with conservative management.[41] Reductions in prematurity complications may be contributed to by survival bias, however. In a subgroup analysis of two cohort studies where echocardiographic criteria for PDA were used, a lower risk of BPD in the group receiving conservative treatment, with no difference in mortality or other morbidities between the two groups, was noted. Meta-analyses of the RCTs showed no difference in outcome with conservative management when compared with intervention (pharmacological or surgical).[41] This is consistent with findings from a network meta-analysis of all major treatment options for PDA, including placebo or non-treatment,[42] although relatively high rates of open-label treatment in the "no

treatment" arms were observed in included studies. Two recent trials documented lower rates of open-label treatment and may offer a more accurate assessment of the effects of true conservative PDA management. One was a small pilot trial of 72 infants receiving either intravenous NSAID treatment or placebo in the first 72 hours after birth, with no difference in secondary outcomes.[43] The second randomized 142 infants to oral ibuprofen or placebo between postnatal days 6 and 14[44] and, although no differences were identified in clinical outcomes, the authors noted low efficacy of NSAIDs, particularly in the most preterm infants. Although these are small studies, they provide a starting point for design of larger trials investigating conservative management without a requirement for high rates of open-label NSAID treatments as "rescue".

Lastly, it is worth drawing a distinction between non-treatment and "conservative treatment" that involves shunt modulation strategies to attempt to reduce ductal flow or treatments to improve heart failure symptoms, without the use of medications or surgery for PDA closure. These include fluid restriction, use of diuretics, positive end-expiratory pressure (PEEP), postnatal corticosteroids, targeted hematocrit, hemoglobin level or platelet thresholds, and increased caloric intake. There are limited data available on the efficacy of these supportive care measures, and documentation of how strategies such as these are utilized in clinical trials of pharmacological PDA treatment is variable. In general, judicious fluid management is suggested, in part based on evidence that excessive fluid intake in the first week after birth is associated with an increased incidence of both hsPDA and NEC.[45] There is not strong evidence for fluid restriction, however, and an overly restricted fluid intake has been associated with a greater risk of acute kidney injury[44] as well as concerns about inadequate nutritional intake. In addition, theoretically, reducing overall circulating fluid volume without any effect on the proportion of cardiac output that is directed toward the lungs may risk exacerbating post-ductal hypoperfusion from hsPDA. Cerebral hypoperfusion is an additional risk, with a small prospective multicenter study demonstrating a significant reduction in SVC flow with fluid restriction for PDA.[46]

Furosemide, a loop diuretic, is commonly used for treatment of congestive cardiac failure, including in neonates. The role of frusemide in modulating ductal shunt has not been well studied due to historical concerns, including prostaglandin-mediated dilatation of ductus arteriosus vessels in an animal model[47] and an increased incidence of PDA in an RCT where the drug was used.[48] There is also considerable overlap in symptomatology between longstanding hsPDA with pulmonary congestion, and BPD, which makes the role of diuretics in this setting difficult to study. More evidence is needed, particularly in infants with pulmonary venous congestion due to diastolic dysfunction, to ascertain the role of diuretics in supportive care of infants with PDA. Appraisal of diastolic function has therefore been suggested as a means of more carefully selecting patients for a trial of diuretic therapy from a research perspective.[43]

Increasing PVR through use of PEEP, generally through use of continuous positive airway pressure (CPAP) for respiratory support, has been implemented but has not been shown to produce changes in lung function (from reduced pulmonary congestion),[49] although there is a suggestion ductal flow may be reduced.[50] Physiologically, higher hematocrit, and hence greater blood viscosity, has the potential to limit shunt volume. However, clinical trials of targeted hematocrit to date – either by delayed cord clamping or liberal blood transfusion thresholds – have not shown a reduction in NSAID exposure or surgical ligation for PDA treatment.[51,52] A more liberal approach to platelet transfusion has similarly not translated into meaningful clinical benefit in the trial setting[53] and is not presently routinely recommended.

## Treatment Approaches for hsPDA

Overall, there are clear limitations of PDA management, driven in large part by the considerable variation in PDA pathophysiology among individual patients. Therefore, one of the aims of contemporary PDA management could be to identify and target a population that would be most likely to benefit from PDA treatment while avoiding unnecessary treatment in others. To achieve this aim, we need to address three key questions:
- *When* to treat?
- *Which* PDA to treat?
- *How* to treat a PDA?

## WHEN TO TREAT A PDA?

There are a number of time points at which the PDA can be treated. These are:
- *Prophylactic* treatment: given to "all comers" based on gestational age and/or weight criteria within the first 24 hours after birth, without utilizing an assessment of hemodynamic significance of the shunt.
- *Early targeted* (within the first 6–24 hours after birth) treatment: based on cardiac US criteria of hemodynamic significance, prior to the onset of clinical features of PDA.
- *Pre-symptomatic* (at 24–72 hours of age) treatment: based on PDA assessment prior to onset of symptoms, but slightly later than typical early targeted treatment. Treatment during this window has not been shown to reduce the risk of pulmonary hemorrhage or P/IVH.
- *Early symptomatic* (in the first 3–7 days after birth) treatment: after onset of clinical symptoms. This is a common time point for treatment; however, treatment at this stage has not been shown to reduce the risks of pulmonary hemorrhage or P/IVH. Symptoms arise due to the hemodynamic effects of left-to-right ductal shunting and may become clinically apparent during this time period.
- *Late symptomatic* (after postnatal day 7) treatment: after onset of clinical symptoms. The ductus may be less amenable to pharmacological closure at this stage.

The time frame of treatment is one determinant of the likely outcomes. P/IVH and pulmonary hemorrhage are early complications of a PDA, usually developing during the first 3–7 postnatal days. There is reasonably good evidence that prophylactic or early targeted treatment of the PDA, mainly with indomethacin, can prevent both P/IVH and pulmonary hemorrhage,[9,54] with treatment given prior to entering the peak risk period (days 2–7) for these complications. Of note, indomethacin, unlike ibuprofen, transiently decreases cerebral blood flow and improves cerebral blood flow autoregulation, at least in part independently of its inhibitory effect on prostaglandin synthesis.[55] Therefore the effect of prophylactic indomethacin on decreasing the rate of P/IVH[42] or white matter injury[56] is thought to be not only related to a direct effect on ductal shunting.

Assessing whether PDA treatment can prevent later complications such as NEC or BPD, which have a multifactorial etiology and a longer development phase, is more difficult. There are some animal data to support prevention of BPD by early ductal closure with indomethacin.[57,58] Demonstrating this in the human infant is more difficult, partly due to the multifactorial etiology, but also because in most clinical trials there is no true placebo group. High open-label rates of treatment mean that many infants enrolled in PDA treatment trials still receive NSAIDs – just at a later time point.

Clinical symptoms of an hsPDA, such as a murmur, active precordium, high volume pulses, poor growth, and increased work of breathing, are nonspecific and may become evident later in the clinical course.[59,60] Signs of cardiac failure usually do not develop until the second or third postnatal week. Most randomized controlled trials have not been designed to address the question of whether a symptomatic PDA should be treated during the neonatal period; rather, they were designed to assess the relationship between timing of treatment and efficiency of PDA closure. Symptomatic treatment trials are scarce, and results have not shown any major advantage in terms of prevention of adverse effects from the PDA.[61] By the time of PDA clinical symptomatology, it may already be too late and the PDA may already have contributed to the development of one or more of the complications of prematurity. Studies from the pre-surfactant and antenatal steroid era suggest early symptomatic treatment may reduce the duration of mechanical ventilation and BPD compared to late symptomatic treatment.[62]

The efficacy of NSAIDs commonly used for the treatment of PDA decreases with increasing postnatal age. Up to 85% of PDAs would close if the first dose of indomethacin was administered within 24 hours after birth, whereas the rate decreases to 48% if started at or beyond 72 hours.[63] Earlier treatment, prior to a sustained period of systemic hypoperfusion, is associated with a reduced rate of gastrointestinal side-effects, such as spontaneous intestinal perforation (SIP) and NEC. The absence of an increased rate of gut-associated side effects in the prophylactic treatment studies[9,64,65] supports this pathophysiology.

### Prophylactic and Early Targeted Treatment

Prophylactic and early targeted treatment, which are typically instituted within the first 24 hours after birth, are the most widely studied and probably most effective modes of PDA treatment. A Cochrane analysis including 19 trials comprising 2872 infants[54] concluded that prophylactic treatment with indomethacin has a number of immediate benefits, in particular, a reduction in symptomatic PDA, the need for ductal ligation, and a decreased rate of P/IVH, particularly severe P/IVH. There was also a borderline decrease in PVL, ventriculomegaly, and other white matter abnormalities, with a trend toward a decrease in pulmonary hemorrhage. The large trial of Indomethacin Prophylaxis in Preterm infants (TIPP)[64] did not show a statistically significant decrease in pulmonary hemorrhage, although re-analysis demonstrated a reduction in the rate of *early serious* pulmonary hemorrhage.[66] This is consistent with the findings of a double-blinded RCT demonstrating a reduction in *early* pulmonary hemorrhage with cardiac US-targeted treatment.[9] In addition, screening echocardiography before postnatal day 3, in a national population–based cohort of extremely preterm infants, was associated with lower in-hospital mortality and likelihood of pulmonary hemorrhage, though not with differences in NEC, severe BPD, or severe cerebral lesions.[67]

Although prophylactic indomethacin decreases severe forms of P/IVH, a significant benefit in terms of long-term effect on neurodevelopmental outcomes has not been demonstrated. There continues to be debate regarding the role of remote long-term outcomes in adjudicating the benefit of PDA treatment – this is particularly pertinent when considering the lack of assessment of hemodynamic significance in a large number of PDA treatment trials. Regarding NEC, there is little evidence to support or refute the role of PDA. The only study showing a decreased incidence of NEC with PDA treatment is an older study in infants <1000 g after early prophylactic PDA ligation.[68] Research has consistently shown a reduction in intestinal blood flow in the presence of a PDA, providing biological plausibility for an association with gut injury and NEC. Superior mesenteric artery flow usually increases after feeding; however, this physiological phenomenon is blunted in the presence of an hsPDA.[69-72] Certainly the pathophysiology of hsPDA can result in disturbances of post-ductal arterial blood flow, providing a basis for concern regarding the risk of NEC with untreated hsPDA. It is likely that the magnitude and duration of left-to-right shunt, together with individual patient factors, modify the risk profile for preterm infants at risk of NEC and that treatment of carefully selected patients might be expected to reduce this risk.

Although prophylactic treatment has several important benefits, it also results in unnecessary treatment of infants in whom a PDA might have closed spontaneously without significant end-organ effects of left-to-right shunting. If prophylactic or early targeted treatment is desired, indomethacin is currently the drug of choice, as ibuprofen has not as yet been shown to have similar short-term benefits. On the other hand, high-dose oral ibuprofen has recently been shown to be the most effective agent overall for achieving closure of hsPDA.[42] If gastrointestinal status permits, high-dose oral ibuprofen is increasingly preferred for treatment of an hsPDA outside the window

for prophylactic or early targeted treatment, i.e. for treatment of PDA once symptomatic. There is little evidence, however, to suggest that treating a PDA when it becomes symptomatic is helpful in the long term[73]; rather, we may lose an opportunity to prevent significant early complications.[9,64] Identification and targeting of a particular subset of the population who are least likely to undergo spontaneous PDA closure and are most vulnerable to complications are therefore priorities. Cardiac US is an obvious way to aid in identifying this subgroup of patients and it is in this area that significant research efforts in neonatal hemodynamics have been focused. The potential timings of interventions for PDA, along with their advantages and disadvantages based on pathophysiology, are shown in Table 19.1.

**TABLE 19.1  Summary of Advantages and Disadvantages of Different PDA Treatment Time Points**

| Treatment Type | Advantages | Disadvantages |
|---|---|---|
| Prophylactic (within 6–24 hours after birth, preferably within the first 12 hours) | Most widely studied<br>Decreased P/IVH and pulmonary hemorrhage<br>Excellent closure rates | Due to frequency of spontaneous closure, exposes a large number of infants to the side effects of NSAID treatment; many unnecessarily |
| Early targeted (within 6–24 hours after birth, preferably within the first 12 hours) | Decreased P/IVH and pulmonary hemorrhage<br>Targets treatment to most significant shunts<br>Excellent closure rates | Exposes infants to treatment prior to onset of clinical symptoms; in some of these infants the PDA may spontaneously close without sequelae |
| Pre-symptomatic (usually by days 3–7 on the basis of ultrasound) | Exposes fewer babies to the risks of treatment<br>Targets treatment to most significant shunts<br>Very good closure rates | Few studies<br>Often outside window to prevent P/IVH and pulmonary hemorrhage |
| Early symptomatic (usually postnatal days 3–7) | Exposes fewer babies to the risks of treatment | Increases the chance of PDA-related morbidity and mortality (compared with earlier treatment)<br>Closure rate is lower<br>Few studies |
| Late symptomatic (after postnatal day 7) | Exposes fewest babies to the risks of treatment | Increases the chance of PDA related morbidity and mortality<br>Reduced closure rates<br>Unproven usefulness and safety profile<br>Non-standardized approach |
| Conservative (no medication or surgery) | No initial exposure to medication but risk of need for later treatment | Increases the likelihood of PDA-related morbidity and mortality<br>Risks of long-standing hsPDA, including late morbidity post-discharge |

## HOW TO TREAT A PDA?

First-line treatment for hsPDA is generally medical, with NSAIDs, namely indomethacin or ibuprofen. Success rates for hsPDA closure with indomethacin are around 60–80%,[74] with similar results reported using ibuprofen.[75] Indomethacin is generally preferred for prophylactic or early targeted treatment due to a demonstrated reduction in P/IVH and pulmonary hemorrhage rates. Paracetamol is increasingly being used for PDA closure,[42,76,77] with advantages that include a more favorable side-effect profile[42] and similar efficacy to indomethacin or ibuprofen.[76] There are, however, a paucity of long-term follow-up data among infants receiving paracetamol,[76] with a limited population studied to date[78] and insufficient controlled trial data involving extremely preterm neonates <26 weeks.[74] There is limited evidence to support use of paracetamol as a "rescue" treatment after NSAID therapy has failed,[79] and clinicians sometimes opt to use paracetamol where NSAIDs are contraindicated. Detailed discussion of pharmacotherapy for PDA is available in Chapter 17.

Surgical closure of a PDA, either by ligation or transcatheter device closure (TCDC), is largely employed as a "rescue" therapy for infants who have failed medical management, or occasionally where NSAIDs are contraindicated. There has been a secular move away from early surgical closure following unsuccessful medical management due to concern regarding associations between PDA ligation and adverse outcomes in large studies of preterm infants,[80-84] including an increased risk of neurodevelopmental impairment.[80,81,83] However, these studies have a number of limitations, including a lack of adjustment for the duration of ductal shunting, an important modifier of sequelae associated with hsPDA. One retrospective study of 754 extremely preterm infants, which accounted for neonatal comorbidities prior to PDA ligation, demonstrated improved survival without increased risk of neurodevelopmental impairment with ligation.[85] TCDC is becoming an increasingly available option as interventional cardiologists become more skilled in the procedure for small, premature infants. Long-term follow-up data after TCDC are awaited. A detailed discussion of interventional management of PDA is available in Chapter 18.

## WHICH PDA TO TREAT: HOW TO DETERMINE HEMODYNAMIC SIGNIFICANCE?

From the available evidence, early targeted treatment for a specific population is probably the best approach we can presently offer for management of the PDA. This is in view of the need to balance the risk of treatment side-effects in a vulnerable population with the adverse pathophysiology and potential consequences of persistent, large-volume left-to-right shunting. Parameters to take into consideration when making a decision regarding whether to treat the PDA include gestational age, postnatal age, level of respiratory support, existing comorbidities, clinical and US features of PDA, and possibly cardiac biochemical markers and additional measures of tissue oxygenation. The definition of hsPDA varies between clinicians and centers, as well as between trials of PDA management.[26] Investigators have used cardiac US alone or in combination with physical examination findings, cardiac biochemical markers, and/or other hemodynamic assessment tools in an attempt to more objectively define an hsPDA. A number of scoring systems have been developed to try to provide some uniformity.[86,87] Infants with a high composite score on a staging system by Sehgal et al. were noted to have a higher incidence of subsequent CLD.[88] A more complex PDA scoring system has been published using five factors that were independently associated with CLD/death (gestation at birth, PDA diameter, maximum flow velocity, LV output, and LV a' wave). This PDA score had a range from 0 (low risk) to 13 (high risk). Infants who developed CLD/death had a higher score than those who did not.[17]

Irrespective of whether formal scoring systems are used, bedside cardiac clinician-performed ultrasound (CPU), also referred to as targeted neonatal echocardiography (TnECHO), plays an important role in the management of PDA in preterm neonates in many units globally. A number of training programs for neonatal clinicians have been developed in recognition of the role of CPU in enhancing decision-making at the bedside.[89] Given the lag of clinical features of PDA behind US markers by a mean of 2 days,[59] CPU in the early postnatal period can facilitate identification of an hsPDA in the pre-symptomatic period. The details of techniques for echocardiography measurements used in PDA assessment are discussed in Chapter 16.

In this chapter we shall discuss the clinical utility of these parameters in identifying hsPDA. Broadly, PDA evaluation should incorporate assessment of the following[1]:

- Characteristics of the PDA: diameter, direction of flow, systolic and diastolic flow velocities, and their ratio (including flow pattern).
- Markers of pulmonary over-circulation: left ventricular output (LVO) and at least one marker of left heart volume loading (left atrial to aortic root ratio [LA:Ao], left ventricular end-diastolic dimension [LVEDD], left pulmonary artery end-diastolic velocity [LPA EDV], pulmonary vein d wave velocity) or left heart pressure loading (isovolumic relaxation time [IVRT], mitral valve E:A).
- Indices of systemic shunt effect (systemic hypoperfusion): Doppler flow patterns in the postductal arterial circulation – descending aorta and celiac trunk, and in the middle cerebral artery.

Foremost, it should be remembered that the magnitude of ductal shunting is determined by a complex interplay between systemic and pulmonary pressure/impedance, myocardial function, and size of the DA (length and radius), as well as viscosity of the blood and morphology of the ductus. It must also be remembered that the PDA is dynamic – alterations in cardiorespiratory status and medical therapies, as well as longitudinal changes in cardiovascular physiology with age, can all impact ductal flow from one hemodynamic assessment to the next. This highlights the importance of serial, longitudinal clinical, and US interrogation of the neonatal cardiovascular system, including the PDA. Comprehensive assessment, repeated as often as is necessary and with any relevant clinical treatment or change, enables appreciation of the effects of ductal shunting for the individual infant in their clinical context.

The ideal way to measure a PDA shunt would be to quantify transductal flow or the total volume of shunt. A variable diameter across the course of the ductus, variation in ductal anatomy, and the non-laminar nature of its flow make this difficult, however. In addition, systolic and diastolic cardiac function and the ability of the preterm myocardium to adapt to the additional preload imposed by left-to-right PDA shunting, as well as comorbidities (e.g., sepsis, perinatal

events) are important modifiers of shunt effect. Ductal shunting cannot be simply estimated from a single ductal diameter measurement alone – this would be an oversimplification of complex physiology. Additionally, reliance on a single measurement in isolation makes errors in interpretation of hemodynamic significance more likely. The sensitivity, specificity, and reproducibility of many of these measurements vary substantially.[1] When clinical decisions are being made based on hemodynamic assessments, it is important to consider a multiparametric approach due intrinsic reliability issue of individual markers. The PDA may be best thought of as a physiologic continuum, from low- to high-volume shunts, rather than a dichotomous entity (present or absent), with hemodynamic assessment designed to allow the clinician to ascertain where on that continuum the PDA lies for an individual patient at a specific time point.

## Characteristics of the PDA

Absolute diameter is the most commonly used marker in a PDA assessment, although reports on accuracy of ductal diameter for prediction of hemodynamic significance have been inconsistent. Indeed, transductal pressure may be a more important determinant of shunt volume than PDA size (diameter). There may be minimal shunting of blood in a "large" duct if the pulmonary systolic pressure is similar to or higher than the systemic systolic pressure. Nonetheless, a diameter cut-off of $\geq 1.5$ mm in the first 24 hours has been shown to be moderately predictive of a subsequently treated hsPDA,[90] and a diameter of $\geq 2.0$ mm (on days 3 and 7) has been shown to be highly predictive of hsPDA.[91] It is important to note, however, that many infants with a PDA of $\geq 1.5$ mm in the early postnatal period do not subsequently require treatment.[90,92,93] Assessment using diameter in isolation does not take into consideration the non-cylindrical nature of many PDAs, the weight of the infant (and hence relative size of the vasculature), and myocardial function, nor the other factors governing ductal flow. The PDA to left pulmonary artery (PDA:LPA) ratio is sometimes used as an alternative marker of PDA size and indirectly of shunt volume, though this has a variable predictive value for hsPDA. A ratio of $\geq 1$ has been used to define a large PDA, $\geq 0.5$ to $\leq 1$ a moderate PDA, and $\leq 0.5$ a small

PDA.[94] PDA size relative to infant weight has also been used, with a PDA size of >2 mm/kg at 72 hours found to be predictive of hsPDA.[92] When combined with other markers of hemodynamic significance, ductal diameter becomes more useful. Preterm infants with a PDA diameter of >1.5 mm, when associated with preceding low SVC flow (<40 mL/kg/min) on the first postnatal day, a left-to-right shunt and elevated RVO or LPA flow velocity, are considered to be at risk of pulmonary hemorrhage.[9,95] An infant with these characteristics may be considered a good candidate for early targeted treatment to reduce this risk. In addition to assessment of ductal diameter, attention should be paid to the Doppler pattern. The peak velocity at the end of diastole is usually zero or very low and implies an almost equal pulmonary and systolic pressure in diastole. Peak systolic flow velocity is usually less than 1.5 m/s, and if it increases above this, there is usually constriction of the DA. An hsPDA will

have a "pulsatile" flow pattern and an unrestrictive left-to-right flow.[92] A "pulsatile" PDA pattern is a descriptor used for a PDA with systolic to diastolic ratio of ≥2 and is highly suggestive of hsPDA.[91,96] A bidirectional (>30% right-to-left) or pure right-to-left shunt suggests elevated pulmonary pressure, LV dysfunction, or duct-dependent congenital heart disease and is not consistent with a pathological hsPDA. In the setting of pulmonary hypertension, the ductus may serve as a "pop-off" valve for an RV exposed to high afterload. Closure of the PDA in this instance can precipitate worsening RV dysfunction and should be avoided. The size, Doppler characteristics, and other cardiac US markers suggestive of hsPDA are outlined in Table 19.2.

### Markers of Pulmonary Over-Circulation

In the newborn, where atrial and ductal shunts are present, the left ventricular output (LVO) represents

---

**TABLE 19.2   Cardiac Ultrasound Markers of Hemodynamic Significance of PDA[1,4]**

| Echocardiographic Measure | Moderate hsPDA | Large hsPDA | Limitations |
|---|---|---|---|
| **PDA Size** | | | |
| Absolute diameter (mm) Can also be indexed to patient body weight | 1.5–3.0 mm | >3.0 mm | Location of measurement (in 2D at narrowest end, usually pulmonary) Does not consider ductal morphology |
| PDA to LPA ratio | 0.5–1 | >1 | |
| **PDA Doppler** | | | |
| Doppler pattern | Unrestrictive pulsatile ductal flow | Unrestrictive pulsatile ductal flow | Chronic high-volume PDA shunts can present with high peak systolic velocity |
| Systolic to diastolic velocity ratio | 2.0–4.0 | >4.0 | |
| PDA Vmax (m/s) | 1.5–2.5 | <1.5 | |
| **Pulmonary Overcirculation** | | | |
| LVO (mL/kg/min) | 200–300 | >300 | Can be falsely low if myocardial systolic function impaired and/or in presence of hypovolemia |
| LA to Ao ratio | 1.5–2.0 | >2.0 | Affected by atrial shunt |
| LVEDD (cm) | 0.2–0.5 | >0.5 | Influenced by atrial shunt and LV dysfunction |
| LPA EDV (m/s) | 0.3–0.5 | >0.5 | LPA dilatation commonly occurs in association with high-volume shunt |
| Pulmonary vein d wave velocity (m/s) | 0.35–0.45 | >0.45 | Velocity may fall as pulmonary vein becomes dilated with sustained exposure to large shunts |
| Mitral valve E:A | <1 | >1 | Not reliable if severe MR |
| IVRT (ms) | 30–40 | <30 | |

## TABLE 19.2 Cardiac Ultrasound Markers of Hemodynamic Significance of PDA—cont'd

| Echocardiographic Measure | Moderate hsPDA | Large hsPDA | Limitations |
|---|---|---|---|
| **Systemic Hypoperfusion ("Steal")** | | | |
| Descending aorta diastolic flow | Reversed | Reversed | Dependent on location of measurement |
| MCA diastolic flow | Forward | Absent or reversed | Dependent on location of measurement |
| Celiac artery diastolic flow | Absent | Reversed | Dependent on location of measurement |

2D, two-dimensional; aPH, acute pulmonary hypertension; APH, antepartum hemorrhage; BPD, bronchopulmonary dysplasia; CXR, chest X-ray; DBP, diastolic blood pressure; desc. Ao, descending aorta; E:A, E:A ratio; ELBW, extremely low birth weight; HPA, hypothalamic-pituitary-adrenal; HR, heart rate; hsPDA, hemodynamically significant patent ductus arteriosus; IV, intravenous; IVRT, isovolumic relaxation time; LA, left atrium; LA:Ao, left atrial to aortic root ratio; LPA, left pulmonary artery; LPA EDV, left pulmonary artery end-diastolic velocity; L-R, left-to-right; LV, left ventricle; LVO, left ventricular output; MCA, middle cerebral artery; NEC, necrotizing enterocolitis; NSAID, non-steroidal anti-inflammatory drug; P/IVH, peri-/intraventricular hemorrhage; PBF, pulmonary blood flow; PDA, patent ductus arteriosus; PHTN, pulmonary hypertension; PPROM, preterm premature rupture of membranes; pulm. d wave, pulmonary vein d wave; PVR, pulmonary vascular resistance; R-L, right-to-left; SBF, systemic blood flow; Rx: treatment; SBP, systolic blood pressure; SpO$_2$, oxygen saturation; TCDC, transcatheter device closure; US, ultrasound; Vmax, maximum velocity.

the systemic blood flow plus the PDA shunt. A large left-to-right shunt results in an increased LVO (>300 mL/kg/min). If there are other markers suggestive of hsPDA, but the LVO is normal, this should raise concerns regarding LV failure (and inability of the immature myocardium to cope with the demand of the added preload from left-to-right ductal shunting), hypovolemia, and/or significant shunting at atrial level. The LVO:SVC flow ratio may be a more reliable estimation of the ductal flow because it is unaffected by the transatrial flow, unlike other markers. The LVO:SVC ratio has been shown to correlate well with ductal size and is independent of transatrial shunt.[97-100] A recent study demonstrated, however, that although LVO:SVC ratio was higher in infants with a left-to-right PDA shunt, this was related to increased LVO rather than differences in SVC flow.[101] SVC flow was maintained irrespective of increased (pre-ductal) cardiac output in these patients. Additional studies, such as with MRI, may help validate these measurements further.

Pulmonary artery flow is considered to be a surrogate marker of significant shunting and increases as the right ventricular output is combined with the left-to-right ductal shunt. An LPA end-diastolic flow of greater than 0.2 m/s correlates with a hsPDA, although its impact on clinical outcome is unknown.[102] Visually, flow appears turbulent with an increased velocity at end-diastole. Pulsatility index (PI) refers

to a variable reflecting the downstream resistance to blood flow in the vascular bed; therefore the PI of the LPA provides insight into right ventricular contractility, preload, and afterload.[100] Left heart size and flow are useful surrogates of increased pulmonary blood flow and provide useful insight into the magnitude of transductal flow. The left atrial to aortic root ratio (LA:Ao) can be used to estimate the increase in effective pulmonary blood flow. An LA:Ao >1.4 is commonly used to ascertain ductal significance, although this lacks sensitivity and specificity as measurement of a three-dimensional structure in two dimensions may be error prone. In addition, significant transatrial shunting may reduce the size of the LA by decompressing it, thereby giving a falsely low LA:Ao ratio even in the presence of significant pulmonary overload. The left atrium takes time to dilate and may not be a useful parameter to assess ductal significance in the first few postnatal days.[103] Attention should also be paid to the size of the atrial communication (AC) – an hsPDA will lead to increased left-to-right shunting via the patent foramen ovale/atrial septal defect and eventually tends to lead to stretching of the AC. A recent retrospective study demonstrated an association between the size of AC in the first postnatal week in infants with PDA diameter ≥1.5 mm and other markers of PDA shunt volume, as well as with the composite outcome of chronic lung disease or death before discharge.[104] The role of early identification and treatment of patients with high-volume PDAs in association with larger ACs is yet to be fully evaluated.

In addition to assessment of left heart volume loading, isovolumic relaxation time (IVRT) and mitral valve E/A ratio may provide some insight into left heart pressure loading. In healthy-term infants, LV filling across the mitral valve is characterized by predominantly early diastolic ("E" wave) filling, with limited LV filling during atrial contraction ("A" wave) in late diastole. This results in an E/A ratio of >1. Healthy preterm infants without a PDA rely on late atrial ("A" wave) filling to a greater degree due to inherently reduced diastolic function (resulting in a lesser degree of relaxation and filling in early diastole). Presence of a large PDA in preterm infants increases left atrial pressure due to increased pulmonary venous return. This results in earlier mitral valve opening and increased early passive filling. This in turn causes the IVRT to be shortened (<40 ms) and results in "pseudonormalization" of the E/A ratio to >1. An E/A ratio of >1 and/or IVRT <40 ms in a preterm infant with a PDA should prompt consideration of left heart pressure loading and is a marker suggesting hemodynamic significance of the duct. Volume/pressure loading of the left heart can also result in mitral valve regurgitation (MR) and stretching of the inter-atrial septum, which leads to an increase in the size of the atrial communication. In 2D imaging the LA and LV will appear dilated as a result of the increased pulmonary venous return to the LA. Visual qualitative assessment of LA/LV dilatation requires significant experience in interpreting neonatal cardiac US images, including exposure to a sufficient number of scans of healthy newborns to understand normal cardiac appearances.

### Indices of Systemic Shunt Effect

Ductal shunting away from the systemic circulation becomes more pronounced in diastole. This can manifest as absence or reversal of diastolic flow in the descending aorta or other post-ductal arterial circulation, such as the celiac or mesenteric arteries, despite an increase in LVO. This phenomenon is sometimes known as "ductal steal", which puts the infant at risk of hypoperfusion in the brain, splanchnic, and renal vessels. Diastolic flow reversal in the middle cerebral

artery (MCA) generally only occurs in large PDA shunts. In preterm infants less than 31 weeks' gestation with a ductal diameter of greater than 1.7 mm, descending aortic diastolic reversal has been associated with a 35% decrease in descending aorta flow volume.[105] However, the authors did not find any reduction in SVC flow and concluded that preterm infants with high-volume ductal shunt may have preserved upper body perfusion but reduced lower body perfusion. Greater than 50% diastolic flow reversal is more likely to be associated with hsPDA.[72] An MRI validation study found that reversed diastolic flow in the (post-ductal) descending aorta on echocardiography was the best predictor of a high-volume left-to-right ductal shunt.[106]

## Risk-Benefit Assessment and Individualized Therapy

In the age of personalized medicine, we have the capacity to treat each patient as an individual. This is likely to be most important when there is a group of patients with heterogeneous physiology, such as in the setting of PDA. Among a group of preterm infants with PDA, there are likely to be a subset of patients for whom treatment of PDA is beneficial, perhaps some for whom treatment offers more closely balanced risks and benefits, and some for whom treatment is more likely to be harmful. Age, comorbidities, likelihood of spontaneous closure, and clinical and cardiac US markers of hemodynamic significance are all important considerations. Detailed hemodynamic assessment can help delineate these groups and enable the clinician to make a more informed therapeutic decision. Table 19.3 summarizes some of the common clinical scenarios involving PDA management in the neonatal intensive care unit setting and offers some pathophysiology-based guidance to aid decision-making. The following case studies illustrate how pathophysiology-based management of the PDA can be utilized in individual patients. There may be more than one approach that is suitable, and given the limitations of the literature, some flexibility is to be expected. The case examples discuss an approach to understanding hemodynamic significance and outline some of the common principles of contemporary PDA management.

**TABLE 19.3  Hemodynamic Scenarios in Assessment of PDA and Suggested Management Approaches**

| Hemodynamics | Clinical Scenario | Clinical Features | Cardiac US Findings | Management |
|---|---|---|---|---|
| [1]<br>Early hsPDA + Low SBF<br>Increased cardiac preload from L-R PDA shunt<br>Reduced ability of preterm myocardium to adapt to ↑LV preload from PDA shunt and ↑LV afterload of transitional circulation (high resting peripheral tone, removal of placenta); immature HPA axis | ELBW infant in first 12 h, inadequate antenatal steroid coverage, preceding low flow state and systemic hypotension<br>+/− preceding APH<br>+/− perinatal hypoxia-ischemia<br>+/− growth restriction | hsPDA generally clinically silent; however, infant may have systemic hypotension related to low SBF<br>Mechanically ventilated | PDA > 1.5 mm<br>Growing or pulsatile pattern (PDA Vmax < 2 m/s, systolic to diastolic ratio > 2)<br>L-R shunt<br>Reversed diastolic flow in desc. Ao<br>Features of pulmonary over-circulation and left heart volume loading, e.g.,<br>• LVO > 300 due to steal from hsPDA<br>• ↑ LPA EDV and/or pulm. d wave velocity due to increased PBF | Indomethacin if platelet count and renal function satisfactory<br>Re-evaluation:<br>• Early to reassess SBF<br>• After second dose indomethacin (may not require third dose)<br>• After treatment course to assess transductal shunt |
| [2]<br>aPH With Supportive PDA<br>↓ perfusion in post-ductal arterial circulation<br>↑ PBF<br>↓ → ↑ DBP from PDA run-off<br>↑ SBP from increased preload (↓ SBP if impaired myocardial systolic function) | Preterm infant<br>+/− history of PPROM/oligohydramnios<br>+/− features of sepsis | Labile oxygenation, pre- and post-ductal SpO$_2$ differential, issues with oxygenation > ventilation | PDA with ≥30% R-L shunt<br>Bidirectional shunt at atrial level<br>+/− features of myocardial dysfunction<br>No features of ↑ PBF (+/− features of ↓ PBF depending on aPH severity) | Supportive treatment of aPH<br>Avoid ductal closure<br>Serial hemodynamic assessment – risk of L-R shunt causing hsPDA as PVR falls |
| [3]<br>Early Symptomatic hsPDA | Preterm infant in the first 7 days after birth | Symptoms and signs may include:<br>• Low DBP, normal or high SBP (unless LV systolic dysfunction)<br>• +/− ↑ HR<br>• Renal impairment<br>• Feed intolerance/NEC<br>• P/IVH<br>• Pulmonary hemorrhage<br>• Metabolic acidosis | PDA > 2.0 mm<br>Pulsatile pattern<br>L-R shunt<br>Reversed diastolic flow in desc. Ao<br>Features of pulmonary over-circulation and left heart volume loading, e.g.,<br>• LVO > 300 due to steal from hsPDA<br>• ↑ LPA EDV and/or pulm. d wave velocity<br>• E:A > 1 due to increased LA pressure<br>+/− LA/LV dilatation | Treatment options:<br>• High-dose oral ibuprofen (if tolerating enteral feeds)<br>• IV ibuprofen (if not tolerating enteral feeds)<br>• IV indomethacin (in first 48–72 h)<br>• Acetaminophen (generally not first line; consider if active bleeding OR reassess bleeding risk and NSAID Rx in 24–48 h)<br>• Conservative with shunt modulation strategies |

*Continued on following page*

**TABLE 19.3    Hemodynamic Scenarios in Assessment of PDA and Suggested Management Approaches—cont'd**

| Hemodynamics | Clinical Scenario | Clinical Features | Cardiac US Findings | Management |
|---|---|---|---|---|
| [4]<br>Late Symptomatic PDA<br>Subacute or chronic L-R shunt<br>↑ PBF<br>Cardiac dilatation from increased pulmonary venous return, +/− MR<br>↓ perfusion in post-ductal arterial circulation<br>↓ DBP from PDA run-off<br>↑ SBP from increased preload<br>(↓ SBP if impaired myocardial systolic function)<br>+/− pulmonary venous hypertension from chronic L-R shunt<br>+/− myocardial dysfunction | Postnatal age 1–12 weeks or more | Symptoms and signs may include:<br>• Low DBP, normal or high SBP (unless LV systolic dysfunction)<br>• +/− ↑ HR<br>• Dependence on respiratory support (mechanical or long-term non-invasive)<br>• CXR changes (cardiomegaly, pulmonary plethora)<br>• Renal impairment<br>• Feed intolerance/NEC<br>• Metabolic acidosis | PDA > 2.0 mm<br>L-R shunt<br>Reversed diastolic flow in desc. Ao<br>Features of pulmonary over-circulation with LA enlargement (unless offset by large atrial shunt), e.g.,<br>• LA:Ao > 1.4<br>• LVO > 300 due to steal from hsPDA<br>• IVRT < 40 due to ↑ LA pressure<br>LA/LV dilatation from increased pulmonary venous return<br>+/− Moderate or large atrial communication | Treatment options:<br>• High-dose oral ibuprofen (if tolerating enteral feeds)<br>• IV ibuprofen (if not tolerating enteral feeds)<br>• Acetaminophen (generally not first line; consider following NSAID course(s) or while awaiting surgical closure)<br>• Surgical closure (TCDC or ligation)<br>• Conservative with shunt modulation strategies |
| [5]<br>Non-hsPDA<br>Physiological PDA | Preterm infant stable on non-invasive respiratory support, tolerating enteral feeds<br>No hemodynamic instability | No specific clinical features of hsPDA<br>+/− cardiac murmur<br>No cardiomegaly or pulmonary plethora on CXR | Small-volume PDA shunt<br>Features may include:<br>• Diameter < 2.0 mm<br>• LA:Ao < 1.5<br>• LVO < 300<br>• IVRT > 40<br>• Mitral valve E:A < 1<br>• No ↑ LPA EDV or pulm. d wave velocity<br>• No left-sided cardiac dilatation | • Conservative, +/− shunt modulation strategies<br>• Regular clinical reassessment<br>• Full hemodynamic assessment if clinical change and non-urgent progress cardiac US |
| [6]<br>Long-Term PDA<br>Chronic L-R shunt<br>↑ PBF<br>+/− Cardiac dilatation from increased pulmonary venous return, +/− MR<br>+/− pulmonary venous hypertension from chronic L-R shunt<br>Risk of evolving chronic pulmonary hypertension over time | Present at discharge<br>Persistent PDA after non-treatment or prior unsuccessful treatment(s)<br>Increased risk of BPD[39,40]<br>Spontaneous closure rates 47-58% by 12-18 months of age[38]<br>Risk of shunt reversal if PHTN of sufficient severity and duration[43,44]<br>Risk of death associated with progressive PHTN[38] | Symptoms and signs may include:<br>• CXR changes (cardiomegaly, pulmonary plethora)<br>• Tachypnea, hepatomegaly (if large volume shunt – features of congestive cardiac failure)<br>• Poor weight gain/postnatal growth failure | PDA > 2.0 mm<br>L-R shunt<br>Features of pulmonary over-circulation with LA enlargement (unless offset by large atrial shunt), e.g.,<br>• LVO > 300 due to steal from hsPDA<br>• IVRT < 40 due to ↑ LA pressure<br>+/− LA/LV dilatation from increased pulmonary venous return<br>+/− Moderate or large atrial communication | Treatment options:<br>• Surgical closure (TCDC or ligation)<br>• Conservative with follow-up – including option for closure later in infancy/childhood<br>Cardiologist assessment pre-discharge and outpatient cardiology follow-up essential |

*hsPDA*, hemodynamically significant PDA; *SBF*, systemic blood flow; *L-R*, left-to-right; *PDA*, patent ductus arteriosus; *LV*, left ventricle; *HPA*, hypothalamic-pituitary-adrenal; *ELBW*, extremely low birth weight; *APH*, antepartum hemorrhage; *aPH*, acute pulmonary hypertension; *LVO*, left ventricular output; *LPA*, left pulmonary artery; *EDV*, end diastolic velocity; *pulm.*, pulmonary vein; *PBF*, pulmonary blood flow; *PVR*, pulmonary vascular resistance; *RV*, right ventricle; *PPROM*, prolonged premature rupture of membranes; *SpO2*, oxygen saturation; *R-L*, right-to-left; *Ao*, descending aorta; *DBP*, diastolic blood pressure; *SBP*, systolic blood pressure; *HR*, heart rate; *NEC*, necrotizing enterocolitis; *P/IVH*, periventricular/intraventricular hemorrhage desc; *E:A* - mitral valve, *E:A* ratio; *LA*, left atrial; *IV*, intravenous; *NSAID*, non-steroidal anti-inflammatory drug; *Rx*, treatment; *MR*, mitral regurgitation; *CXR*, chest x-ray; *LA:Ao*, left atrial to aortic root ratio; *IVRT*, Isovolumetric relaxation time; *TCDC*, transcutaneous device closure; *US*, ultrasound; *BPD*, bronchopulmonary dysplasia; *PHTN*, pulmonary hypertension

## Assessing Response to Treatment and Outcomes

Longitudinal, serial, and hemodynamic assessments are an important aspect of cardiovascular management of the PDA. This approach facilitates targeting the right treatment for the right patient at the right time. Sometimes complete cessation of the transductal shunt (or closed PDA – which is more of an anatomical pathological term than a clinical or US description) is not required for achievement of clinical improvement. The therapeutic goal should be to understand the effect of a PDA on a patient in their clinical context and identify and treat shunts that are thought to be pathological while avoiding treatment in the setting of a pathological or supportive ductus. This requires a detailed hemodynamic assessment, incorporating individual patient factors as well as the significance of the ductal shunt and design of an individualized plan of care. Frequent reassessment can enable the clinician to limit treatment-related toxicities by tailoring the duration of treatment to hemodynamic response. For example, many PDAs, particularly if treated early in the pre-symptomatic period, may show restriction after 1–2 doses of an NSAID medication, such that the full three-dose schedule is not required to achieve the desired outcome of reducing pathological ductal shunting and its sequelae. Serial examinations can also identify an evolving hsPDA amongst preterm infants with acute PH as pulmonary vascular resistance falls, or those with changing PDA physiology related to sepsis or NEC. PDA physiology is dynamic, and it is important to understand what is happening for the patient in real-time, as management strategies must evolve to meet the clinical need. Currently, long-term data do not support a dogmatic approach to PDA management or treatment in every case. Indeed, lack of careful patient selection exposes infants unnecessarily to risks of treatment-related harm, and time may increase the likelihood of complications of prematurity amongst untreated infants with the most pathological hemodynamics.

## Conclusions

Management of the PDA remains controversial, and there is marked variation in clinical approaches to this common condition affecting preterm infants. This is largely driven by the heterogeneity of infants enrolled in most PDA treatment trials, as well as a number of study design-related issues. The PDA may be considered a continuum from physiological, small-volume shunting during perinatal transition at the one end to a persistent, large-volume left-to-right shunt with significant disturbances in physiology at the other. Treatment of a group of patients based on clinical criteria or limited US markers, such as PDA diameter, has not been shown to improve outcomes. Treatment targeted to high-risk populations, such as extremely preterm infants with high-volume PDA shunts in the first few postnatal days, has demonstrated a reduction in the serious complications of P/IVH and pulmonary hemorrhage. Unfortunately, the neonatal hemodynamic literature has not reported on large numbers of infants selected for detailed PDA assessment and individualized treatment targeting only high-volume, pathological shunts. It is hoped that future clinical trials will entail a more nuanced approach, with careful selection of patients and a detailed understanding of their physiology, to enable a more solid evidence-base for decision-making. In the interim a drift toward non-treatment of the PDA[43] due to the lack of clinical evidence for an improvement in long-term outcomes is not recommended and is not without substantial risks. Conservative management has not been shown to result in an increase in some of the major morbidities of the preterm population; however, serious sequelae of untreated large-volume PDA shunts including death, BPD, and chronic PH have been documented. It is the authors' approach to screen the highest-risk infants for hsPDA with cardiac US in the first 24 hours after birth and treat those with large and probably pathological shunts. Although treatment of the PDA once symptomatic has not been broadly shown to be beneficial, it is likely that normalizing physiology of patients with large ductal shunts during a time period when they remain at risk of multisystem sequelae of prematurity is an appropriate strategy. Infants who are unable to be weaned from respiratory support or establish enteral feeding and who have not responded to multiple courses of medical treatment may be candidates for surgical closure. With the advent of transcatheter device PDA closure, the risk profile for an interventional strategy may be changing; however, this remains an area of active study. Ultimately, achieving a strong understanding of PDA hemodynamics and factors at play in an individual patient enables the clinician to make a more informed decision about how to approach the PDA. Individualization of therapy based on a detailed assessment and appreciation of patient-specific factors and real-time physiology is well suited to neonatal hemodynamic problems, of which the PDA remains a prime example.

## Case Studies

### Case 1

The first case is a 23-week GA female infant with a birth weight (BW) of 550 g, now 12 hours old. She was born vaginally and a single dose of steroid was administered prior to birth. She was intubated at delivery and mechanically ventilated on minimal ventilatory pressures with an $FiO_2$ of 0.3. She received two doses of surfactant. At 2 hours of age, hypotension was noted, which was stabilized with a dobutamine infusion of 10 mcg/kg/min. Post-treatment, there was a post-ductal noninvasive BP of 41 (MAP 28) mmHg, with a heart rate of 158 bpm. The serum lactate was 2.4 mmol/L and she was oliguric with normal renal function. Her platelet count was $160 \times 10^9$/L. A bedside head US shows no evidence of ventricular or parenchymal hemorrhage.

A clinician-performed ultrasound (CPU) was performed. (Figure 19.1), which showed a 2.2 mm PDA with a pulsatile flow pattern, shunting purely left to right with a peak velocity of 1.1 m/s. There was normal left ventricular systolic function and qualitatively mild to moderately reduced RV systolic function. The left pulmonary artery end-diastolic velocity (LPA EDV) was 0.27 m/s and there was diastolic flow reversal in the descending aorta, celiac trunk, and middle cerebral artery (MCA). There was a small PFO shunting left-to-right.

*Summary:* At 12 hours of age, there is a large-volume, hemodynamically significant PDA with US findings consistent with systemic hypoperfusion and pulmonary overcirculation.

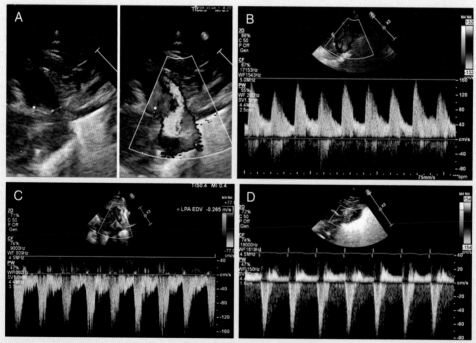

**Fig. 19.1 Findings in case study 1.** (A) 2D and color Doppler views of 2.2 mm PDA. (B) Pulse wave (PW) color Doppler profile showing a pulsatile, unrestrictive ductal flow pattern with pure left-to-right shunt. (C) Left pulmonary artery end-diastolic velocity of 0.27 m/s. (D) Reversed diastolic flow in the descending aorta.

## Case 1 (Continued)

### CASE 1 OUTCOME

Cardiac CPU confirmed a large volume, hemodynamically significant PDA shunt in an extremely preterm infant at significant risk of early complications. Although the left ventricular output (LVO) is in the normal range, this is likely due to reduced systolic function in combination with the large left-to-right shunt. The LVO was more than 1.5 times the right ventricular output (RVO), which is an additional clue to presence of a significant left-to-right shunt at ductal level. The infant received early targeted treatment with indomethacin, with good effect. Her follow-up ductal scan after three doses showed a very small, constricting PDA that was no longer hemodynamically significant.

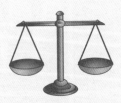

**Benefits of treatment**
1. Prevention of intraventricular and pulmonary hemorrhage
2. Optimal window for efficacy
3. Prevention of long-term effects of high-volume shunt on developing kidneys, gut, lungs, and brain

**Risks of treatment**
1. Unnecessary treatment in some infants (spontaneous ductal closure in ~30%)
2. Potential adverse effects on the gastrointestinal tract, kidneys, and platelet count
3. Loss of RV offload by the duct may exacerbate RV dysfunction

## Case 2

The second case is a 24-week GA male infant with a BW of 770 g, now 18 hours old. There was chorioamnionitis and spontaneous vaginal delivery following cervical cerclage at 20 weeks. Conventional mechanical ventilation was commenced at pressures of 18/5 cmH$_2$O in FiO$_2$ 0.35. Three doses of surfactant were administered with some response; however, oxygenation remained labile. The heart rate was 147 bpm and pre-ductal BP 35/28 (MAP 31) mmHg unsupported with a serum lactate of 1.1 mmol/L. There was an elevated CRP of 82 mg/L and mild thrombocytopenia (119 × 10$^9$/L). Cranial US showed bilateral germinal matrix hemorrhage with intraventricular extension (Grade II IVH).

A CPU was performed (Figure 19.2), which demonstrated a 1.5 mm PDA with bidirectional Doppler profile, shunting right-to-left 32% of the time. There was a tricuspid regurgitation (TR) jet with an estimated pulmonary gradient of 28 mmHg. There was also a reduced time to peak velocity:right ventricular ejection time (TPV:RVET) ratio of 0.28 and a flat interventricular septum. The LV ejection fraction was 64%, with an LV output of 186 mL/kg/min (normal = 150–300 mL/kg/min).

Tricuspid annular plane systolic excursion (TAPSE) was 0.45 cm and RV output was 164 mL/kg/min. Note that the mean TAPSE at 26 weeks' gestation is 0.44 cm (normative values have been published for preterm infants from 26 weeks).[107] There was antegrade diastolic flow in the descending aorta and celiac trunk and a small PFO shunting bidirectionally.

*Summary*: There is a small PDA with significant right-to-left shunt in the context of pulmonary hypertension. Biventricular systolic function appears good. There was coexistent bilateral intraventricular hemorrhage.

*Continued on following page*

**Case 2** (*Continued*)

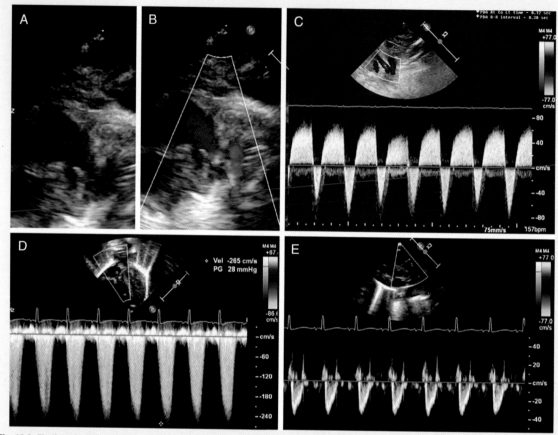

**Fig. 19.2   Findings in Case Study 2.** (A) 2D view of 1.5 mm PDA. (B) Color Doppler image showing right-to-left ductal flow. (C) Bidirectional PDA PW Doppler profile, 32% right to left. (D) Tricuspid regurgitation; estimated pulmonary gradient of 28 mmHg + right atrial pressure. (E) Reduced time to peak velocity:right ventricular ejection time (TPV:RVET) ratio of 0.28.

### CASE 2 OUTCOME

Cardiac CPU shows a small volume PDA shunt with features of acute pulmonary hypertension (bidirectional ductal/atrial shunting, reduced pulmonary artery acceleration time and elevated pulmonary gradient from TR jet). Measures of pulmonary over-circulation, systemic perfusion, and left heart volume and pressure loading did not suggest a significant left-to-right ductal shunt. Therefore there was no indication for PDA treatment, given the role of the ductus in offloading the right ventricle in the setting of elevated pulmonary arterial pressure, and due to the lack of a hemodynamically significant left-to-right shunt. Hesitancy should still exist

regarding ductal treatment even if there is larger volume of left-to-right shunt in this infant due to elevated pulmonary pressure. In the setting of acute hemorrhage and concomitant sepsis there would be concern about further bleeding with NSAID treatment.

Serial assessment of clinical findings, laboratory markers of sepsis, and US progress of the existing IVH are important for this infant. He remains at risk of development of a significant left-to-right ductal shunt as pulmonary pressures fall, especially after use of selective pulmonary vasodilators such as inhaled nitric oxide. There is also concern regarding hemodynamic changes in association with potential sepsis and possible progression of IVH.

## Case 2 (Continued)

**Benefits of treatment**

1. Nil, based on current echocardiographic features
2. If, on serial assessment, ductal shunt became larger and predominantly left-to-right with a fall in PVR and concomitant sepsis, the role of treatment should be re-evaluated at that time

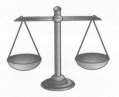

**Risks of treatment**

1. Note the supportive role of a PDA in acute pulmonary hypertension – PDA closure may increase RV afterload and result in impairment of RV function and clinical deterioration
2. There are risks of side-effects from unnecessary ductal treatment

## Case 3

The third case is a 25-week GA male infant, steroid covered, with a BW of 850 g on day 3. He was receiving respiratory support with CPAP 7 cmH$_2$O in FiO$_2$ 0.28. He received a single dose of surfactant at 3 hours of age. Following this, there was a widening pulse pressure, with down-trending diastolic pressure with a BP of 49/21 (MAP 30) mmHg, and a heart rate of 143 bpm and serum lactate 1.3 mmol/L.

There were easily palpable femoral pulses. There was feed intolerance with non-bilious vomiting on trophic enteral feeds of 1 mL every 4 hours and normal urine output, renal function, and platelet count. There was no evidence of peri-/intraventricular hemorrhage on head US.

A CPU was performed (Figure 19.3), which demonstrated a 2.7 mm PDA with a pulsatile Doppler pattern,

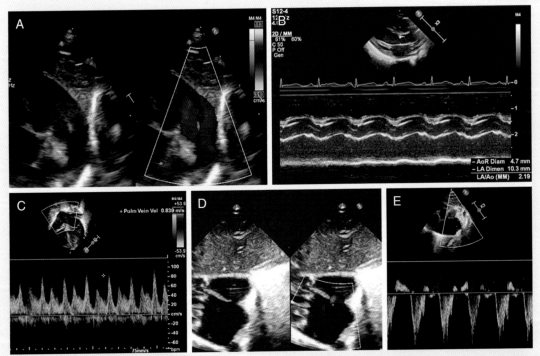

**Fig. 19.3  Findings in Case Study 3.** (A) 2D and color Doppler views of 2.7 mm PDA. (B) Enlarged left atrial:aortic root ratio of 2.2. (C) Pulmonary vein D wave velocity of 84 cm/s. (D) PFO of 1.9 mm, shunting left to right. (E) Flow reversal throughout diastole in descending aorta.

*Continued on following page*

shunting purely left-to-right. The LV output was 463 mL/kg/min with a left pulmonary artery end-diastolic velocity (LPA EDV) of 0.28 m/s and an enlarged left atrial:aortic root (LA:Ao) ratio of 2.2. There was qualitative left atrial and ventricular volume loading and a PFO of 1.9 mm, shunting left to right. Diastolic flow was reversed in the superior mesenteric artery and absent in the middle cerebral artery.

*Summary*: There is a moderate-severe hemodynamically significant PDA with features of pulmonary over-circulation, systemic hypoperfusion, and evidence of left heart volume and pressure loading despite shunting through the PFO.

### CASE 3 OUTCOME

A CPU was performed in view of this infant's prematurity, respiratory distress, wide pulse pressure, and feed intolerance, with the latter two being suggestive of ductal systemic hypoperfusion. The CPU showed evidence of a hemodynamically significant PDA. The LVO was elevated; however, the moderate atrial shunt may have offset this, leading to

a lower calculated LVO than is reflective of PDA shunt volume.

The infant received early symptomatic ductal treatment with intravenous ibuprofen. Indomethacin could also have been used; however, after 48–72 hours, ibuprofen may be preferred due to pre-existing exposure of the preterm mesenteric circulation to an hsPDA and possible increased risk of gastrointestinal side effects in this setting. The route of administration was intravenous rather than oral due to poor feed tolerance. Repeat CPU after two doses of ibuprofen showed no transductal shunt, normalization of left heart dilatation, and forward diastolic flow in the descending aorta on US, correlating with clinical improvements in ventilation and feeding.

Serial hemodynamic assessment enabled treatment to be limited to two doses of the planned three-dose course of ibuprofen, minimizing exposure to potential medication side effects.

**Benefits of treatment**

1. Limit sequelae from systemic hypoperfusion (cerebral, GI, and renal)
2. Limit pulmonary over-circulation
3. Good window for efficacy

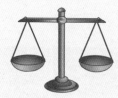

**Risks of treatment**

1. Adverse effect profile
2. Limited efficacy
3. Potential spontaneous ductal closure in due course without treatment

### Case 4

The fourth case was a 26-week GA male infant with a BW of 825 g delivered via emergency cesarean section for severe maternal preeclampsia. He was intubated at 2 hours for surfactant administration, then extubated back to CPAP 7 cmH₂O in FiO₂ 0.25. There was acute hypoxemia at 36 hours of age due to a small-volume pulmonary hemorrhage. He was re-intubated and transitioned quickly to high-frequency oscillatory ventilation (HFOV). A bedside head US shows no evidence of intraventricular or parenchymal hemorrhage.

A CPU was performed (Figure 19.4), which demonstrated a 2.0 mm PDA with bidirectional blood flow (29% right-to-left flow). The LVEF was 57% and LV output was measured at 198 mL/kg/min and RV output was 155 mL/kg/min. There was an LPA EDV of 0.09 m/s and a left atrial:aortic root (LA:Ao) ratio of 1.5. There was forward diastolic flow in the descending aorta.

*Summary*: There was a small to moderate PDA without other features of hemodynamic significance. Since the ductal shunt was balanced without evidence of pulmonary over-circulation, systemic hypoperfusion, or left heart volume or pressure loading, a conservative management approach was taken and serial reassessment performed. The infant continued to have recurrent episodes of small pulmonary hemorrhage over the next 24 hours, despite high mean airway pressures on HFOV and transfusion of fresh frozen plasma. He had normal renal function and a mild thrombocytopenia of $78 \times 10^9$/L.

A repeat CPU was performed on day 4 (Figure 19.5). The additional findings included a 3.0 mm PDA with pulsatile, now entirely left-to-right flow. The LPA EDV had increased to 0.29 m/s with an LA:Ao ratio of 1.6 and an LV output of 387 mL/kg/min.

*Summary*: The PDA was now moderate to large and hemodynamically significant and pharmacological treatment was indicated.

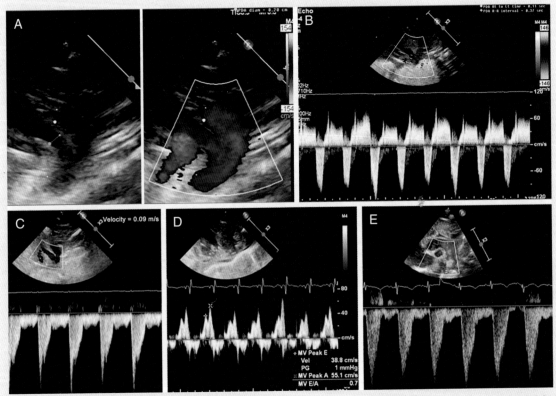

**Fig. 19.4 Findings in Case Study 4 (first CPU).** (A) 2.0 mm PDA on 2D view, with right-to-left flow on color Doppler. (B) Bidirectional ductal flow pattern, 30% right to left. (C) Left pulmonary artery end-diastolic velocity of 0.09 m/s. (D) Mitral valve E:A ratio of 0.7. (E) Forward diastolic flow in descending aorta.

*Continued on following page*

**Case 4** (*Continued*)

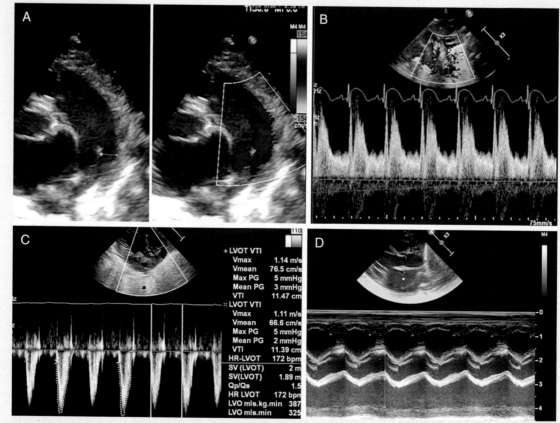

**Fig. 19.5 Findings in Case Study 4 (second CPU).** (A) 3.0 mm PDA on 2D view; flow now left to right on color Doppler. (B) Pulsatile ductal pattern on PW Doppler. (C) Increased left ventricular output of 387 mL/kg/min. The VTI measurements appear slightly over-estimated in this image. (D) Left atrial:aortic root ratio of 1.6.

## CASE 4 OUTCOME

This is an extremely preterm infant with persistent pulmonary hemorrhage likely contributed to by a hemodynamically significant PDA. There was evidence of pulmonary over-circulation from an hsPDA potentially causing increased pulmonary capillary pressure. Healthy term and preterm newborns experience a physiological decline in pulmonary vascular resistance (PVR) with increasing postnatal age, which may be more prominent in the setting of weaning mean airway pressure as respiratory support is reduced. This set of physiological and pathophysiological changes creates a hemodynamic state predisposing to pulmonary hemorrhage. CPU demonstrated an increased LVO and LA:Ao ratio and pulsatile Doppler pattern, suggestive of a hemodynamically significant PDA. Absent diastolic flow in the descending aorta may be consistent with altered

systemic perfusion from diastolic run-off into the PDA; however, it is a less robust predictor of high-volume PDA shunt than reversed flow. Absent diastolic flow in the descending aorta can also be seen in well infants with a closed duct. This case emphasizes the dynamic nature of the neonatal cardiovascular system and importance of serial assessments.

The clinician elected to treat the PDA with a 5-day course of acetaminophen (paracetamol) following the second CPU, given the relatively lower risk of worsening thrombocytopenia and exacerbating bleeding compared with NSAID treatment. This comes at the cost of potentially lower efficacy and limited long-term outcome data for infants at this gestation treated with acetaminophen. The patient received a 5-day course of oral acetaminophen (paracetamol). On repeat CPU at completion, there was no transductal flow seen.

## Case 4 *(Continued)*

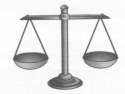

**Benefits of treatment**

1. Improvement or resolution of pulmonary hemorrhage
2. Facilitate weaning of ventilation and extubation

**Risks of treatment**

1. Risks of exacerbating bleeding from suppressive effects on platelets
2. Outside optimal window to prevent pulmonary hemorrhage
3. Risk of gastrointestinal side effects

## Case 5

The fifth case was that of a 27-week GA female infant with a BW of 905 g, now postnatal day 10. She was born in the setting of preterm premature rupture of membranes (PPROM) and clinical chorioamnionitis. She was stable in the first week on CPAP for respiratory support, slowly establishing enteral feeds. On day 10, there was increasing respiratory distress and rising $FiO_2$. The PEEP was increased to 7 $cmH_2O$ in $FiO_2$ 0.32. The BP was 46/19 (MAP 28) mmHg, HR 152 bpm, and serum lactate 1.6 mmol/L. There was a continuous murmur audible with hyperdynamic precordium and bounding femoral pulses. There was normal renal function and platelet count, and she was enterally fed at 150 mL/kg/day.

A CPU was performed (Figure 19.6), which demonstrated a 2.6 mm PDA with an unrestrictive pulse wave

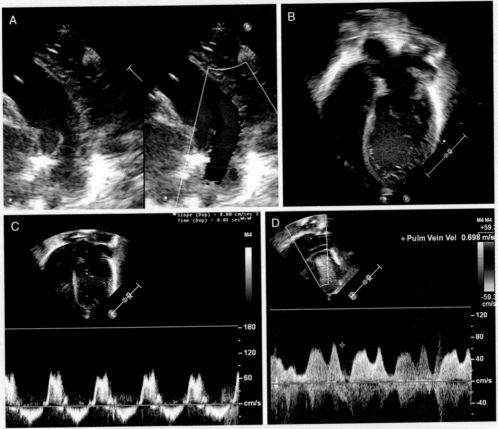

**Fig. 19.6 Findings in Case Study 5.** (A) 2.6 mm PDA with left-to-right flow on 2D and color Doppler views. (B) Apical four-chamber image showing left atrial and ventricular dilatation. (C) Isovolumetric relaxation time of 30 ms. (D) Elevated pulmonary vein D wave velocity of 0.70 m/s.

*Continued on following page*

## Case 5 (Continued)

Doppler pattern with left-to-right flow. There was a high LVO of 547 mL/kg/min and a dilated left atrium (LA: Ao ratio 2.4) and a left pulmonary artery end-diastolic velocity (LPA EDV) of 0.33 m/s. There was reversal of diastolic flow in the descending aorta and intermittent reversal in the celiac artery.

*Summary:* There is a large volume PDA shunt with evidence of pulmonary over-circulation, left heart volume, and pressure loading with systemic hypoperfusion.

### CASE 5 OUTCOME

The infant was treated with three doses of oral ibuprofen (20 mg/kg, 10 mg/kg, 10 mg/kg). Follow-up CPU at completion showed the duct to be constricting and 1.4 mm in

diameter, with normalization of markers of hemodynamic significance. No acute complications of treatment were observed. Selection of pharmacotherapy for ductal closure after the first postnatal week is less straightforward. A recent network meta-analysis[76] found high-dose oral ibuprofen to result in a higher likelihood of closure of hsPDA, when compared with intravenous ibuprofen (standard dose) or intravenous indomethacin. The increased effectiveness of oral ibuprofen compared with the intravenous formulation may relate to the longer half-life and duration of contact with the PDA[108] and/or a greater "area under the curve"[109] from a pharmacokinetic viewpoint.

**Benefits of treatment**

1. Potential to improve respiratory status with ductal constriction or closure
2. May facilitate ductal closure and limit long-term exposure to high-volume left-to-right shunt

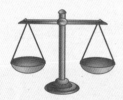

**Risks of treatment**

1. Adverse effect profile – potentially greater risk of gastrointestinal effects following prolonged exposure of the gut to high-volume left-to-right shunt
2. Reduced efficacy
3. Less robust consensus regarding first-line medication

## Case 6

The sixth case was that of a 27-week GA female infant with a BW of 865 g, now postnatal day 3.

She was a dichorionic diamniotic (DCDA) twin born by emergency cesarean section for PPROM and preterm labor. She was initially on CPAP 6 cmH₂O in FiO₂ 0.21 .A single dose of surfactant was given at 4 hours of age. A murmur is heard on routine assessment with otherwise normal cardiac examination. There was no evidence of peri-/intraventricular hemorrhage on head US.

A CPU was performed (Figure 19.7), which demonstrated a 2.1 mm PDA with a high-velocity waveform and closing pattern. The LA:Ao ratio was 1.4 and LVO 238 mL/kg/min. The LPA EDV was 0.11 m/s and there was antegrade diastolic flow in the descending aorta and superior mesenteric artery (SMA).

*Summary:* There was a small-to-moderate volume PDA without features of hemodynamic significance, with a continuous flow pattern suggesting further constriction is likely.

**Case 6** (*Continued*)

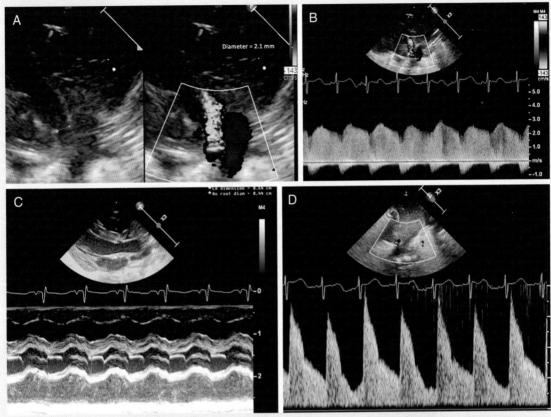

**Fig. 19.7 Findings in Case Study 6.** (A) 2D and color Doppler views demonstrating a 2.1 mm PDA with turbulent left-to-right flow. (B) High-velocity, continuous (closing) ductal pattern on PW Doppler. (C) Left atrial:aortic root ratio of 1.4, not suggestive of significant left heart volume loading. (D) Forward diastolic flow in the superior mesenteric artery.

### CASE 6 OUTCOME

This infant was managed conservatively, with appropriate CPAP support, judicious fluid management, and early enteral nutrition establishment. Meta-analyses of conservative PDA management have not demonstrated greater risks of mortality, P/IVH, or NEC.[75] This is reassuring and provides a basis for non-treatment. However, heterogeneity of patient groups in clinical trials has a substantial impact on the quality of evidence for PDA management.

This highlights the importance of individualized decision-making, for which cardiac US is well placed to assist. Although a murmur is present in both this infant and in the previous case (Case 5), the hemodynamic effects of the PDA differ markedly between patients.

It is likely that for infants such as this one, with a PDA that is not hemodynamically significant, the benefits of treatment are outweighed by risks of potential harm.

**Benefits of treatment**
1. Facilitates early ductal closure

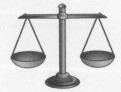

**Risks of treatment**
1. Unnecessary exposure to treatment and its potential side effects
2. PDA likely to close spontaneously

## Case 7

The seventh case was that of a 29-week GA male infant with a BW of 1250 g who is now 3 weeks old. He was born out of hospital via a vaginal delivery without antenatal steroid coverage. He was ventilated for 4 days, including reintubation on day 2 for a large pulmonary hemorrhage. At 3 weeks of age, he is requiring CPAP at 7 cmH$_2$O in FiO$_2$ 0.26. He is enterally fed with several recent episodes of blood-stained gastric aspirates. There is a loud continuous systolic murmur and bounding femoral pulses on examination.

A CPU was performed, which shows a hemodynamically significant PDA that is 2.5 mm in diameter with a pulsatile flow pattern and additional features of a large-volume left-to-right shunt.

He received 5 days of oral paracetamol, selected instead of ibuprofen to avoid the risk of gastrointestinal hemorrhage. There was a poor response to treatment, with ductal reassessment thereafter showing a 2.6 mm PDA with features of both pulmonary over-circulation (LPA EDV of 0.4 m/s), systemic hypoperfusion (reversed diastolic flow in the descending aorta), and signs of intracardiac shunting and dilatation (LA:Ao ratio of 1.8, a large PFO with significant left-to-right shunt, and increased LVO of 766 mL/kg/min). He was subsequently treated with a 3-day course of oral ibuprofen. The PDA was largely unchanged on

assessment following ibuprofen treatment. Thereafter he was managed conservatively with a combination of hydrochlorothiazide and spironolactone therapy and a restricted fluid intake and high PEEP.

At 6 weeks of age, he was dependent upon respiratory support and diuretics and has persistent tachypnea and increased work of breathing, with associated postnatal growth failure. He had an ongoing continuous murmur and hyperdynamic precordium. There was progressive cardiomegaly and pulmonary congestion on chest x-ray with background features of evolving chronic lung disease (Figure 19.8).

A CPU was repeated (Figure 19.9), which demonstrated a 3.8 mm PDA with pulsatile ductal pattern with turbulent left-to-right flow. There was an LPA EDV of 0.37 m/s, an LVEF of 51%, and an LVO of 829 mL/kg/min. The LA:Ao ratio was 2.2 and there was diastolic flow reversal in the descending aorta and SMA.

*Summary*: There was a large-volume, hemodynamically significant PDA with evidence of left heart volume and pressure loading, pulmonary over-circulation, and systemic hypoperfusion.

The infant was referred to pediatric cardiology for assessment and consideration of surgical ductal closure (ligation or transcatheter device closure).

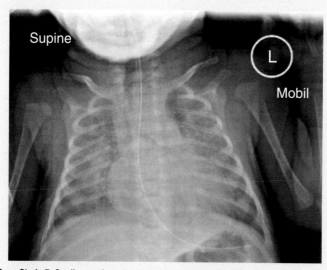

**Fig. 19.8 Chest X-ray in Case Study 7.** Cardiomegaly and pulmonary edema are noted, together with features of chronic lung disease.

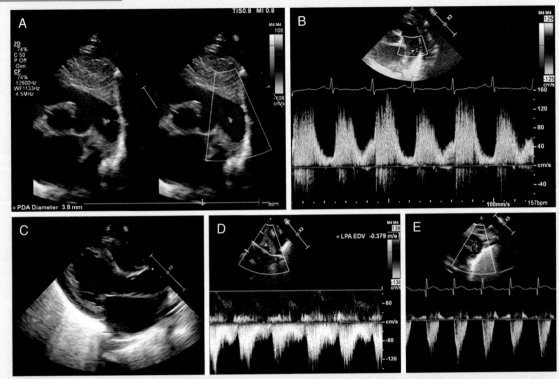

**Fig. 19.9 Findings for Case Study 7 (CPU at 6 weeks).** (A) 2D and color Doppler views demonstrating a large 3.8 mm PDA with left-to-right flow. (B) Pulsatile ductal pattern on PW Doppler (peak systolic velocity ~140 cm/s, diastolic velocity ~20 cm/s). (C) Parasternal long-axis view demonstrating moderate dilatation of left atrium and left ventricle. (D) Left pulmonary artery end-diastolic velocity of 0.38 m/s. (E) Reversed flow throughout diastole in the descending aorta.

## CASE 7 OUTCOME

The infant was transferred to the quaternary children's hospital and underwent transcatheter device closure (TCDC) of his PDA at 8 weeks of age. This was uncomplicated, with a postoperative echocardiogram demonstrating no transductal shunt. He was transferred back to the referring NICU 24 hours later. After 3–4 weeks of age, the likelihood of successful pharmacological closure of PDA is slim. In this patient there were clinical and US features of a hemodynamically significant PDA with high-volume left-to-right shunt. The ongoing dependence on respiratory support and

diuretics and postnatal growth failure were of concern. Repeat CPU assessment confirmed the clinical features of congestive cardiac failure secondary to a large left-to-right shunt. Options for this infant were to either continue to await spontaneous ductal closure, without clinical or US features suggesting this is likely to occur in the short term, or to refer for consideration of surgical PDA closure. Interventional PDA closure may either be with TCDC or ligation, with the latter being the traditional method. TCDC is increasingly preferred, however, due to the avoidance of risks associated with thoracotomy (Chapter 18).

*Continued on following page*

## Case 7 *(Continued)*

**Benefits of treatment**

1. Definitive ductal closure
2. Facilitate weaning off respiratory support
3. Support growth and reversal of postnatal growth failure
4. Prevent further deleterious effects of pulmonary overcirculation and systemic hypoperfusion on the lungs and brain, respectively
5. Possible reduced mortality risk

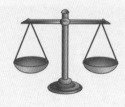

**Risks of treatment**

1. Procedural complications
2. Transient instability related to post-ligation cardiac syndrome (refer to Chapter 18)
3. Risks associated with medical retrieval to pediatric cardiac center
4. Concern regarding neurodevelopmental impact of surgical PDA closure (refer to Chapter 18)

## REFERENCES

1. Van Laere D, van Overmeire B, Gupta S, et al. Application of NPE in the assessment of a patent ductus arteriosus. *Pediatr Res.* 2018;84:46-56.
2. Clyman RI, Campbell D, Heymann MA, Mauray F. Persistent responsiveness of the neonatal ductus arteriosus in immature lambs: a possible cause for reopening of patent ductus arteriosus after indomethacin-induced closure. *Circulation.* 1985; 71:141-145.
3. Gournay V. The ductus arteriosus: physiology, regulation, and functional and congenital anomalies. *Arch Cardiovasc Dis.* 2011;104:578-585.
4. Ruoss J, Bazacliu C, Giesinger RE, McNamara PJ. Patent ductus arteriosus and cerebral, cardiac, and gut hemodynamics in premature neonates. *Semin Fetal Neonatal Med.* 2020;25(5): 101120.
5. Krichenko A, Benson LN, Burrows P, Moes CAF, Mclaughlin P, Freedom RM. Angiographic classification of the isolated, persistently patent ductus arteriosus and implications for percutaneous catheter occlusion. *Am J Cardiol.* 1989;63:877-880.
6. Benitz WE. Learning to live with patency of the ductus arteriosus in preterm infants. *J Perinatol.* 2011;31(suppl 1):S42-S48.
7. Brooks JM, Travadi JN, Patole SK, Doherty DA, Simmer K. Is surgical ligation of patent ductus arteriosus necessary? The Western Australian experience of conservative management. *Arch Dis Child Fetal Neonatal Ed.* 2005;90(3):F235-F239.
8. Kluckow M, Evans N. Low superior vena cava flow and intraventricular haemorrhage in preterm infants. *Arch Dis Child Fetal Neonatal Ed.* 2000;82:188-194.
9. Kluckow M, Jeffery M, Gill A, Evans N. A randomised placebo-controlled trial of early treatment of the patent ductus arteriosus. *Arch Dis Child Fetal Neonatal Ed.* 2014;99(2):F99-F104.
10. Garland J, Buck R, Weinberg M. Pulmonary hemorrhage risk in infants with a clinically diagnosed patent ductus arteriosus: a retrospective cohort study. *Pediatrics.* 1994;94(5):719-723.
11. Lewis MJ, McKeever PK, Rutty GN. Patent ductus arteriosus as a natural cause of pulmonary hemorrhage in infants: a medicolegal dilemma. *Am J Forensic Med Pathol.* 2004;25(3): 200-204.
12. Schena F, Francescato G, Cappelleri A, et al. Association between hemodynamically significant patent ductus arteriosus and bronchopulmonary dysplasia. *J Pediatr.* 2015;166(6): 1488-1492.
13. Chen HL, Yang RC, Lee WT, et al. Lung function in very preterm infants with patent ductus arteriosus under conservative management: an observational study. *BMC Pediatr.* 2015; 15:167.
14. Letshwiti JB, Semberova J, Pichova K, Dempsey EM, Franklin OM, Miletin J. A conservative treatment of patent ductus arteriosus in very low birth weight infants. *Early Hum Dev.* 2017; 104:45-49.
15. Sadeck LS, Leone CR, Procianoy RS, et al. Effects of therapeutic approach on the neonatal evolution of very low birth weight infants with patent ductus arteriosus. *J Pediatr (Rio J).* 2014;90(6):616-623.
16. Clyman RI, Liebowitz M. Treatment and nontreatment of the patent ductus arteriosus: Identifying their roles in neonatal morbidity. *J Pediatr.* 2017;189:13-17.
17. El-Khuffash A, James AT, Corcoran JD, et al. A patent ductus arteriosus severity score predicts chronic lung disease or death before discharge. *J Pediatr.* 2015;167(6):1354-1361.e2.
18. Noori S. Patent ductus arteriosus in the preterm infant: to treat or not to treat? *J Perinatol.* 2010;30(suppl):S31-S37.
19. Jhaveri N, Moon-Grady A, Clyman RI. Early surgical ligation versus a conservative approach for management of patent ductus arteriosus that fails to close after indomethacin treatment. *J Pediatr.* 2010;157(3):381-387.
20. Dollberg S, Lusky A, Reichman B, Network IN. Patent ductus arteriosus, indomethacin and necrotizing enterocolitis in very low birth weight infants: a population-based study. *J Pediatr Gastroenterol Nutr.* 2005;40(2):184-188.
21. Lemmers PM, Benders MJ, D'Ascenzo R, et al. Patent ductus arteriosus and brain volume. *Pediatrics.* 2016;137(4):e20153090.
22. Wong FY, Barfield CP, Campbell L, Brodecky VA, Walker AM. Validation of cerebral venous oxygenation measured using near-infrared spectroscopy and partial jugular venous occlusion in the newborn lamb. *J Cereb Blood Flow Metab.* 2008;28(1):74-80.
23. Chung MY, Fang PC, Chung CH, Huang CB, Ou Yang MH, Chen CC. Risk factors for hemodynamically-unrelated cystic periventricular leukomalacia in very low birth weight premature infants. *J Formos Med Assoc.* 2005;104(8):571-577.
24. Noori S, McCoy M, Friedlich P, et al. Failure of ductus arteriosus closure is associated with increased mortality in preterm infants. *Pediatrics.* 2009;123(1):e138-e144.
25. Sellmer A, Bjerre JV, Schmidt MR, et al. Morbidity and mortality in preterm neonates with patent ductus arteriosus on day 3. *Arch Dis Child Fetal Neonatal Ed.* 2013;98(6):F505-F510.

26. Zonnenberg I, de WK. The definition of a haemodynamic significant duct in randomized controlled trials: a systematic literature review review. *Acta Paediatrica*. 2012;101(3):247-251.

27. Evans N. Preterm patent ductus arteriosus: a continuing conundrum for the neonatologist? *Semin Fetal Neonatal Med*. 2015;20(4):272-277.

28. Rolland A, Shankar-Aguilera S, Diomande D, Zupan-Simunek V, Boileau P. Natural evolution of patent ductus arteriosus in the extremely preterm infant. *Arch Dis Child Fetal Neonatal Ed*. 2015;100(1):F55-F58.

29. Koch J, Hensley G, Roy L, Brown S, Ramaciotti C, Rosenfeld CR. Prevalence of spontaneous closure of the ductus arteriosus in neonates at a birth weight of 1000 grams or less. *Pediatrics*. 2006;117(4):1113-1121.

30. Narayanan M, Cooper B, Weiss H, Clyman RI. Prophylactic indomethacin: factors determining permanent ductus arteriosus closure. *J Pediatr*. 2000;136(3):330-337.

31. Dani C, Bertini G, Corsini I, et al. The fate of ductus arteriosus in infants at 23–27 weeks of gestation: from spontaneous closure to ibuprofen resistance. *Acta Paediatr*. 2008;97(9):1176-1180.

32. Semberova J, Sirc J, Miletin J, et al. Spontaneous closure of patent ductus arteriosus in infants </=1500 g. *Pediatrics*. 2017;140(2):e20164258.

33. de Waal K, Phad N, Collins N, Boyle A. Cardiac remodeling in preterm infants with prolonged exposure to a patent ductus arteriosus. *Congenit Heart Dis*. 2017;12(3):364-372.

34. Tolia V, Powers GC, Kelleher AS, et al. Low rate of spontaneous closure in premature infants discharged with a patent ductus arteriosus: a multicenter prospective study. *J Pediatr*. 2022;240:31-36.

35. Relangi D, Somashekar S, Jain D, et al. Changes in patent ductus arteriosus treatment strategy and respiratory outcomes in premature infants. *J Pediatr*. 2021;235:58-62.

36. Hagadorn J, Bennett MV, Brownell EA, Payton KSE, Benitz WE, Lee HC. Covariation of neonatal intensive care unit-level patent ductus arteriosus management and in-neonatal intensive care unit outcomes following preterm birth. *J Pediatr*. 2018;203:225-233.

37. Altit G, Saeed S, Beltempo M, Claveau M, Lapointe A, Basso O. Outcomes of extremely premature infants comparing patent ductus arteriosus management approaches. *J Pediatr*. 2021;235:49-57.

38. Rahde Bischoff A, Cavallaro Moronta S, McNamara PJ. Going home with a patent ductus arteriosus: is it benign? *J Pediatr*. 2021;240:10-13.

39. Philip R, Nathaniel Johnson J, Naik R, et al. Effect of patent ductus arteriosus on pulmonary vascular disease. *Congenit Heart Dis*. 2019;14:37-41.

40. Philip R, Lamba V, Talati A, Sathanandam S. Pulmonary hypertension with prolonged patency of the ductus arteriosus in preterm infants. *Children (Basel)*. 2020;7:139.

41. Hundscheid T, Jansen EJS, Onland W, Kooi EMW, Andriessen P, de Boode WP. Conservative management of patent ductus arteriosus in preterm infants – a systematic review and meta-analyses assessing differences in outcome measures between randomized controlled trials and cohort studies. *Front Pediatr*. 2021;9:626261.

42. Mitra S, Florez ID, Tamayo ME, et al. Association of placebo, indomethacin, ibuprofen, and acetaminophen with closure of hemodynamically significant patent ductus arteriosus in preterm infants. *JAMA*. 2018;319(12):1221-1238.

43. De Waal K, Prasad R, Kluckow M. Patent ductus arteriosus management and the drift towards therapeutic nihilism – What is the evidence? *Semin Fetal Neonatal Med*. 2021;26(2):101219.

44. Sung S, Lee MH, Ahn Sy, Chang YS, Park WS. Effect of nonintervention vs oral ibuprofen in patent ductus arteriosus in preterm infants: a randomized clinical trial. *JAMA Pediatr*. 2020;174(8):755-763.

45. Bell E, Acarregui MJ. Restricted versus liberal water intake for preventing morbidity and mortality in preterm infants. *Cochrane Database Syst Rev*. 2014;2014;CD000503.

46. De Buyst J, Rakza T, Pennaforte T, Johansson AB, Storme L. Hemodynamic effects of fluid restriction in preterm infants with significant patent ductus arteriosus. *J Pediatr* 2012;161(3):404-408.

47. Toyoshima K, Momma K, Nakanishi T. In vivo dilatation of the ductus arteriosus induced by furosemide in the rat. *Pediatr Res*. 2010;67:173-176.

48. Green T, Thompson TR, Johnson DE, Lock JE. Furosemide promotes patent ductus arteriosus in premature infants with the respiratory distress syndrome. *N Engl J Med*. 1983;308:743-748.

49. Chen H, Yang RC, Lee WT, et al. Lung function in very preterm infants with patent ductus arteriosus under conservative management: an observational study. *BMC Pediatr*. 2015;15:167.

50. Fajardo M, Claure N, Swaminathan S, et al. Effect of positive end-expiratory pressure on ductal shunting and systemic blood flow in preterm infants with patent ductus arteriosus. *Neonatology*. 2014;105(1):9-13.

51. Fogarty M, Osborn DA, Askie L, et al. Delayed vs early umbilical cord clamping for preterm infants: a systematic review and metaanalysis. *Am J Obstet Gynecol*. 2018;218(1):1-18.

52. Franz A, Engel C, Bassler D, et al. Effects of liberal vs restrictive transfusion thresholds on survival and neurocognitive outcomes in extremely low-birth-weight infants: the ETTNO randomized clinical trial. *JAMA*. 2020;324(6):560-570.

53. Ding R, Zhang Q, Duan Y, Wang D, Sun Q, Shan R. The relationship between platelet indices and patent ductus arteriosus in preterm infants: a systematic review and meta-analysis. *Eur J Pediatr*. 2021;180(3):699-708.

54. Fowlie PW, Davis PG, McGuire W. Prophylactic intravenous indomethacin for preventing mortality and morbidity in preterm infants. [Update of Cochrane Database Syst Rev. 2002;(3):CD000174; PMID: 12137607]. *Cochrane Database Syst Rev*. 2010;2010(7):CD000174.

55. Chock VY, Ramamoorthy C, Van Meurs KP. Cerebral autoregulation in neonates with a hemodynamically significant patent ductus arteriosus. *J Pediatr*. 2012;160(6):936-942.

56. Miller SP, Mayer EE, Clyman RI, Glidden DV, Hamrick SE, Barkovich AJ. Prolonged indomethacin exposure is associated with decreased white matter injury detected with magnetic resonance imaging in premature newborns at 24 to 28 weeks' gestation at birth. *Pediatrics*. 2006;117(5):1626-1631.

57. McCurnin DC, Yoder BA, Coalson J, et al. Effect of ductus ligation on cardiopulmonary function in premature baboons. *Am J Respir Crit Care Med*. 2005;172(12):1569-1574.

58. Chang LY, McCurnin D, Yoder B, Shaul PW, Clyman RI. Ductus arteriosus ligation and alveolar growth in preterm baboons with a patent ductus arteriosus. *Pediatr Res*. 2008;63(3):299-302.

59. Skelton R, Evans N, Smythe J. A blinded comparison of clinical and echocardiographic evaluation of the preterm infant for patent ductus arteriosus. *J Paediatr Child Health*. 1994;30:406-411.

60. Alagarsamy S, Chhabra M, Gudavalli M, Nadroo AM, Sutija VG, Yugrakh D. Comparison of clinical criteria with echocardiographic findings in diagnosing PDA in preterm infants. *J Perinat Med.* 2005;33(2):161-164.

61. Gersony WM, Peckham GJ, Ellison RC, Miettinen OS, Nadas AS. Effects of indomethacin in premature infants with patent ductus arteriosus: results of a national collaborative study. *J Pediatr.* 1983;102(6):895-906.

62. Clyman RI. Recommendations for the postnatal use of indomethacin: an analysis of four separate treatment strategies. *J Pediatr.* 1996;128(5 Pt 1):601-607.

63. Yang CZ, Lee J. Factors affecting successful closure of hemodynamically significant patent ductus arteriosus with indomethacin in extremely low birth weight infants. *World J Pediatr.* 2008; 4(2):91-96.

64. Schmidt B, Davis P, Moddemann D, et al. Long-term effects of indomethacin prophylaxis in extremely-low-birth-weight infants. *New Engl J Med.* 2001;344(26):1966-1972.

65. Wadhawan R, Oh W, Vohr BR, et al. Spontaneous intestinal perforation in extremely low birth weight infants: association with indometacin therapy and effects on neurodevelopmental outcomes at 18–22 months corrected age. *Arch Dis Child Fetal Neonatal Ed.* 2013;98(2):F127-F132.

66. Alfaleh K, Smyth JA, Roberts RS, et al. Prevention and 18-month outcomes of serious pulmonary hemorrhage in extremely low birth weight infants: results from the trial of indomethacin prophylaxis in preterms. *Pediatrics.* 2008;121(2): e233-e238.

67. Rozé JC, Cambonie G, Marchand-Martin L, et al. Association between early screening for patent ductus arteriosus and in-hospital mortality among extremely preterm infants. *JAMA.* 2015;313(24):2441-2448.

68. Cassady G, Crouse DT, Kirklin JW, et al. A randomized, controlled trial of very early prophylactic ligation of the ductus arteriosus in babies who weighed 1000 g or less at birth. *N Engl J Med.* 1989;320(23):1511-1516.

69. McCurnin D, Clyman RI. Effects of a patent ductus arteriosus on postprandial mesenteric perfusion in premature baboons. *Pediatrics.* 2008;122(6):e1262-e1267.

70. Shimada S, Kasai T, Hoshi A, Murata A, Chida S. Cardiocirculatory effects of patent ductus arteriosus in extremely low-birth-weight infants with respiratory distress syndrome. *Pediatr Int.* 2003;45(3):255-262.

71. Coombs RC, Morgan ME, Durbin GM, Booth IW, McNeish AS. Gut blood flow velocities in the newborn: effects of patent ductus arteriosus and parenteral indomethacin. *Arch Dis Child.* 1990;65:1067-1071.

72. Freeman-Ladd M, Cohen JB, Carver JD, Huhta JC. The hemodynamic effects of neonatal patent ductus arteriosus shunting on superior mesenteric artery blood flow. *J Perinatol.* 2005; 25(7):459-462.

73. Benitz WE. Treatment of persistent patent ductus arteriosus in preterm infants: time to accept the null hypothesis? *J Perinatol.* 2010;30(4):241-252.

74. Giesinger R, Bischoff AR, Boyd SM, Stanford AH, McNamara PJ. Neonatal cardiovascular pharmacology. In: Aranda JV, van den Anker JN, eds. *Yaffe and Aranda's Neonatal and Pediatric Pharmacology: Therapeutic Principles in Practice.* 5th ed. Lippincott Williams & Wilkins; 2021:14.

75. Ohlsson A, Walia R, Shah SS. Ibuprofen for the treatment of patent ductus arteriosus in preterm or low birth weight (or both) infants. *Cochrane Database Syst Rev.* 2020;2(2):CD003481.

76. Ohlsson A, Shah PS. Paracetamol (acetaminophen) for patent ductus arteriosus in preterm or low birth weight infants. *Cochrane Database Syst Rev.* 2020;1(1):CD010061.

77. Terrin G, Conte F, Oncel MY, et al. Paracetamol for the treatment of patent ductus arteriosus in preterm neonates: a systematic review and meta-analysis. *Arch Dis Child Fetal Neonatal Ed.* 2016;101(2):F127-F136.

78. Hundscheid T, Onland W, van Overmeire B, et al. Early treatment versus expectative management of patent ductus arteriosus in preterm infants: a multicentre, randomised, non-inferiority trial in Europe (BeNeDuctus trial). *BMC Pediatr.* 2018;18(1):261.

79. Jasani B, Weisz DE, McNamara PJ. Evidence-based use of acetaminophen for hemodynamically significant ductus arteriosus in preterm infants. *Semin Perinatol.* 2018;42:243-252.

80. Kabra NS, Schmidt B, Roberts RS, et al. Neurosensory impairment after surgical closure of patent ductus arteriosus in extremely low birth weight infants: results from the Trial of Indomethacin Prophylaxis in Preterms. *J Pediatr.* 2007;150(3): 229-234.

81. Madan JC, Kendrick D, Hagadorn JI, Frantz ID III, National Institute of Child Health, Human Development Neonatal Research Network. Patent ductus arteriosus therapy: impact on neonatal and 18-month outcome. *Pediatrics.* 2009;123(2): 674-681.

82. Mirea L, Sankaran K, Seshia M, et al. Treatment of patent ductus arteriosus and neonatal mortality/morbidities: adjustment for treatment selection bias. *J Pediatr.* 2012;161:689-694.

83. Weisz D, More K, McNamara PJ, Shah PS. PDA ligation and health outcomes: a meta-analysis. *Pediatrics.* 2014;133: e1024-e1046.

84. Weisz D, Mirea L, Resende MHF, et al. Outcomes of surgical ligation after unsuccessful pharmacotherapy for patent ductus arteriosus in neonates born extremely preterm. *J Pediatr.* 2018; 195:292-296.

85. Weisz D, Mirea L, Rosenberg E, et al. Association of patent ductus arteriosus ligation with death or neurodevelopmental impairment among extremely preterm infants. *JAMA Pediatr.* 2017;171(5):443-448.

86. McNamara PJ, Sehgal A. Towards rational management of the patent ductus arteriosus: the need for disease staging. *Arch Dis Child Fetal Neonatal Ed.* 2007;92(6):F424-F427.

87. Fink D, El-Khuffash A, McNamara PJ, Nitzan I, Hammerman C. Tale of two patent ductus arteriosus severity scores: similarities and differences. *Am J Perinatol.* 2018;35(1):55-58.

88. Sehgal A, Paul E, Menahem S. Functional echocardiography in staging for ductal disease severity: role in predicting outcomes. *Eur J Pediatr.* 2013;172(2):179-184.

89. Hébert A, Lavoie PM, Giesinger RE, et al. Evolution of training guidelines for echocardiography performed by the neonatologist: toward hemodynamic consultation. *J Am Soc Echocardiogr.* 2019;32(6):785-790.

90. Kluckow M, Evans N. Early echocardiographic prediction of symptomatic patent ductus arteriosus in preterm infants undergoing mechanical ventilation. *J Pediatr.* 1995;127(5):774-779.

91. Yum S, Moon CJ, Youn YA, Lee JY, Sung IK. Echocardiographic assessment of patent ductus arteriosus in very low birthweight infants over time: prospective observational study. *J Matern Fetal Neonatal Med.* 2018;31:164-172.

92. Harling S, Hansen-Pupp I, Baigi A, Pesonen E. Echocardiographic prediction of patent ductus arteriosus in need of therapeutic intervention. *Acta Paediatr.* 2011;100(2):231-235.

93. De Waal K, Phad N, Stubbs M, Chen Y, Kluckow M. A randomised placebo-controlled pilot trial of early targeted non-steroidal anti-inflammatory drugs in preterm infants with a patent ducts arteriosus. *J Pediatr.* 2021;228:82–86.e2.

94. Wald RM, Adatia I, Van Arsdell GS, Hornberger LK. Relation of limiting ductal patency to survival in neonatal Ebstein's anomaly. *Am J Cardiol.* 2005;96(6):851-856.

95. Kluckow M, Evans N. Ductal shunting, high pulmonary blood flow, and pulmonary hemorrhage. *J Pediatr.* 2000; 137(1):68-72.

96. Su BH, Watanabe T, Shimizu M, Yanagisawa M. Echocardiographic assessment of patent ductus arteriosus shunt flow pattern in premature infants. *Arch Dis Child Fetal Neonatal Ed.* 1997;77(1):F36-F40.

97. Sehgal A, Menahem S. Interparametric correlation between echocardiographic markers in preterm infants with patent ductus arteriosus. *Pediatr Cardiol.* 2013;34(5):1212-1217.

98. El Hajjar M, Vaksmann G, Rakza T, Kongolo G, Storme L. Severity of the ductal shunt: a comparison of different markers. *Arch Dis Child Fetal Neonatal Ed.* 2005;90(5):F419-F422.

99. Phillipos EZ, Robertson MA, Byrne PJ. Serial assessment of ductus arteriosus hemodynamics in hyaline membrane disease. *Pediatrics.* 1996;98(6 Pt 1):1149-1153.

100. Engur D, Deveci M, Turkmen MK. Early signs that predict later haemodynamically significant patent ductus arteriosus. *Cardiol Young.* 2016;26(3):439-445.

101. Rahde Bischoff A, Giesinger RE, Stanford AH, Ashwath R, McNamara PJ. Assessment of superior vena cava flow and cardiac output in different patterns of patent ductus arteriosus shunt. *Echocardiography.* 2021;38:1524-1533.

102. Hirsimaki H, Kero P, Wanne O. Doppler ultrasound and clinical evaluation in detection and grading of patent ductus arteriosus in neonates. *Critical Care Medicine.* 1990;18:490-493.

103. Iyer P, Evans N. Re-evaluation of the left atrial to aortic root ratio as a marker of patent ductus arteriosus. *Arch Dis Child.* 1994;70:F112-F117.

104. Rios D, de Freitas Martins F, El-Khuffash A, Weisz DE, Giesinger RE, McNamara PJ. Early role of the atrial-level communication in premature infants with patent ductus arteriosus. *J Am Soc Echocardiogr.* 2021;34(4):423-432.

105. Groves AM, Kuschel CA, Knight DB, Skinner JR. Does retrograde diastolic flow in the descending aorta signify impaired systemic perfusion in preterm infants? *Pediatr Res.* 2008; 63(1):89-94.

106. Broadhouse K, Price AN, Durighel G, et al. Assessment of PDA shunt and systemic blood flow in newborns using cardiac MRI. *NMR Biomed.* 2013;26:1135-1141.

107. Koestenberger M, Nagel B, Ravekes W, et al. Systolic right ventricular function in preterm and term neonates: Reference values of the tricuspid annular plane systolic excursion (TAPSE) in 258 patients and calculation of Z-score values. *Neonatology.* 2011;100(1):85-92.

108. Dani C, Vangi V, Bertini G, et al. High-dose ibuprofen for patent ductus arteriosus in extremely preterm infants: a randomized controlled study. *Clinical Pharmacol Ther.* 2012; 91(4):590-596.

109. Barzilay B, Youngster I, Batash D, et al. Pharmacokinetics of oral ibuprofen for patent ductus arteriosus closure in preterm infants. *Arch Dis Child Fetal Neonatal Ed.* 2012;97(2): F116-F119.

# PATHOPHYSIOLOGY AND TREATMENT OF NEONATAL SHOCK

# Chapter 20

# Cardiovascular Compromise in the Preterm Infant During the First Postnatal Day

## Martin Kluckow and Istvan Seri

## Key Points

- The very-low-birth-weight infant is hemodynamically vulnerable due to a unique set of risk factors, which include an immature myocardium with poor response to volume load and afterload, immature autonomic vasoregulation, and thus ineffective cardiovascular compensatory mechanisms, a propensity to develop specific or non-specific inflammatory responses, the imposition of positive airway pressure, systemic-to-pulmonary shunts, and variability in the degree of placental restoration of blood volume according to cord clamp timing.

- In part due to the immaturity of cerebral autoregulation and the limited range of cerebral perfusion pressure in preterm neonates, the low cardiac output, state that may occur is associated with adverse outcomes, including neurological injury and potential long-term developmental impairment.

- Assessment of the degree of hemodynamic impairment is difficult, with reliance on standard hemodynamic assessment tools such as capillary refill time, acidosis, and blood pressure all having limitations, especially when used in isolation.

- Awareness of the risks of hemodynamic instability with appropriate treatment response may decrease the risk of some of the severe complications of prematurity.

- Clinician performed cardiac ultrasound (CPU) can assist in recognizing hemodynamic compromise and allow targeted management of the underlying problems.

## Introduction

The birth of a very-low-birth-weight (VLBW) infant creates a unique set of circumstances that can adversely affect the cardiovascular system, resulting in cardiovascular compromise. The cardiovascular system of the fetus is adapted to an in utero environment that is constant and stable. The determinants of cardiac output, such as preload and afterload, are maintained in equilibrium without interference from the external factors that may affect a neonate born prematurely. Postnatal factors that can affect the cardiovascular function of the VLBW infant include perinatal asphyxia, sepsis, positive pressure respiratory support, unnecessary exposure to high oxygen concentration, and cord clamp time. During the immediate transitional period, these factors may alter preload and change afterload at a time of rapid transition from the fetal circulation, characterized by low systemic vascular resistance, to the postnatal neonatal circulation with higher peripheral vascular resistance. The predominantly systemic to pulmonary shunts at the atrial and ductal level through persisting fetal channels can further reduce potential systemic blood flow (Figure 20.1).

The situation is made more complex by the difficulty in assessing the adequacy of the cardiovascular system in the VLBW infant. The small size of the infant and the frequent presence of shunting at both ductal and atrial levels preclude the use of many of the routine cardiovascular assessment techniques used in children and adults to determine cardiac output. As a result, clinicians are forced to fall back on more easily measured parameters such as the blood pressure. However, blood pressure is the dependent measure among the three determinants of systemic circulation, with cardiac output and systemic vascular resistance being the independent determinants. Accordingly, changes in blood pressure do not necessarily reflect

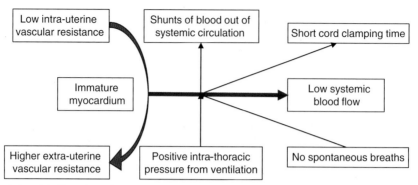

**Fig. 20.1 Suggested model of how the various external and internal influences on the cardiovascular system of the VLBW infant can result in low systemic blood flow.**

changes in the cardiac output and subsequent changes in organ blood flow and tissue oxygen delivery (see Chapters 2 and 15).

Hypotension occurs in up to 30% of VLBW infants, with 16% to 52% of these infants receiving treatment with volume expansion and up to 39% receiving vasopressors (see Chapter 3 for details).[1] More recent surveys of the management of extremely-low-birth-weight (ELBW) infants have demonstrated treatment (fluid bolus or vasopressor administration) rates for hypotension up to 93% at 23 weeks' gestational age (GA) and up to 73% of infants at 27 weeks' GA.[2-4] Most treatment was commenced in the first 24 hours of postnatal life. Similarly, low systemic blood flow in the first 24 hours is seen in up to 35% of VLBW infants, but not all of these infants will have hypotension initially, though many will develop it.[5] Recent studies of the incidence of low superior vena cava (SVC) flow show a reduced incidence (5–21% of ELBW infants), possibly reflecting changes in obstetric and delivery room management, respiratory care, and perhaps fluid management of the neonate.[6-8] There is a wide variation in the assessment and management of cardiovascular compromise both among institutions and individual clinicians.[1,9] As with many other areas in medicine where there is variation in practice with multiple treatment options, the lack of good evidence for both when to treat cardiovascular compromise and whether treatment benefits the long-term outcome of infants underlies this uncertainty. This chapter explores the importance of the unique changes involved in the transitional circulation during the first postnatal day and how they impact the presentation, assessment, and management of neonatal cardiovascular compromise.

## Definition of Hypotension and Its Relationship to Low Systemic Perfusion

The definition of normal blood pressure and hypotension is discussed in detail in Chapter 3. This chapter will focus on the relevance of these definitions to the VLBW infant. Hypotension can be defined as the blood pressure value where vital organ (brain) blood flow autoregulation is lost. If effective treatment is not initiated at this point, blood pressure may further decrease and reach a "functional threshold" when neuronal function is impaired, and then the "ischemic threshold" resulting in tissue ischemia with likely permanent organ damage.[10] Neither the blood pressure causing loss of autoregulation nor the critical blood pressure resulting in direct tissue damage has been clearly defined for the VLBW neonate in the immediate postnatal period.[11] The distinction between the three levels of hypotension is important because, although loss of autoregulation and cellular function *may* predispose to brain injury, reaching the ischemic threshold of hypotension by definition *is associated with direct tissue damage*. Finally, these thresholds may be affected by several factors, including gestational and postmenstrual age, the duration of hypotension, and the presence of acidosis and/or infection. Furthermore, these thresholds are thought to be specific to the individual patient and are affected by the neonate's ability to compensate in order to maintain adequate oxygen delivery to the organs (see Chapters 1 and 7).

Although the normal autoregulatory blood pressure range in the VLBW infant is not known, in clinical practice there are generally two definitions of early hypotension in widespread use:

- Mean blood pressure less than 30 mmHg in any gestation infant in the first postnatal days. This definition is based on pathophysiologic associations between cerebral injury (white matter damage or intraventricular hemorrhage) and mean blood pressure less than 30 mmHg[12,13] and to a lesser degree on more recent data looking at maintenance of cerebral blood flow (CBF) measured by near-infrared spectroscopy (NIRS)[14-17] and single-photon emission computed tomography(SPECT)[18] over a range of blood pressures, suggesting a reduction in CBF when a particular (28–30 mmHg) mean blood pressure threshold is reached. It is important to note that although the 10th centile for infants of all gestational ages is at or above 30 mmHg by the third postnatal day, in more immature infants the 10th centile of mean blood pressure is lower than 30 mmHg during the first 3 days.[19] Additionally, there are very few infants with GA <25 weeks included in these studies. Therefore it is too simplistic to use a single cut-off value for blood pressure across a range of gestation and postnatal ages.
- Mean blood pressure less than the gestational age in weeks during the first postnatal days, which roughly correlates with the 10th centile for age in tables of normative data.[12,20] This statistical definition has also been supported by professional body guidelines such as the Joint Working Group of the British Association of Perinatal Medicine.[21] Again this rule of thumb applies mainly in the first 24–48 hours of extrauterine life; after this time, there is a gradual increase in the expected mean blood pressure such that most premature infants have a mean blood pressure greater than 30 mmHg and thus above gestational age by postnatal day 3 (Chapter 3).[20]

The current definitions are not related to physiologic endpoints such as maintenance of organ blood flow or tissue oxygen delivery. However, most but not all studies using [133]Xe clearance, SPECT, or NIRS to assess changes in CBF found that the lower limit of the autoregulatory blood pressure range may be around 30 mmHg even in the 1-day-old ELBW neonate.[15,18,22-24] Again there is little data published for infants <25 weeks' GA. Indeed, preterm neonates with a mean blood pressure at or above 30 mmHg appear to have an intact static autoregulation of their CBF during the first postnatal day.[25] It is reasonable to assume that, although the gestational age–equivalent blood pressure value is below the CBF autoregulatory range, this value is still higher than the suspected ischemic blood pressure threshold for the VLBW patient population.[24]

A confounding finding to the straightforward-appearing blood pressure-CBF relationship has been provided by a series of studies using superior vena cava (SVC) flow measurements to indirectly assess brain perfusion in the VLBW neonate with a focus on the ELBW infant in the immediate postnatal period.[5,26] The findings of these studies suggest that, in the ELBW neonate, blood pressure in the normal range may not always guarantee normal vital organ (brain) blood flow. Although, caution is needed when interpreting these findings as only approximately 30% of the blood in the SVC represents the blood coming back from the brain, in the preterm neonate (Chapter 2), animal and additional human data support this notion (see Chapter 7). In the compensated phase of shock redistribution of blood flow from the non-vital organs (e.g., muscle, skin, kidneys, intestine, etc.) to the vital organs (brain, heart, adrenals), as well as neuroendocrine compensatory and local vascular mechanisms ensure that blood pressure and organ blood flow to the vital organs are maintained within the normal range. With progression of the condition, shock enters its uncompensated phase, and blood pressure, vital organ perfusion, and oxygen delivery also decrease. Since the immature myocardium of the ELBW neonate may not be able to compensate for the sudden increase in peripheral vascular resistance (LV afterload) immediately following delivery, cardiac output may fall.[26,27] Yet, despite the decrease in cardiac output, many ELBW neonates maintain their blood pressure in the normal range by redistributing blood flow to the organs that are vital at that particular developmental stage (see Chapter 7). As referred to earlier, data suggest that the rapidly developing cerebral cortex and white matter of the ELBW neonate have not yet reached vital organ assignments with appropriately developed vasodilatory responses when perfusion falls.[23,26,27] However, by the second to third postnatal days, forebrain vascular response matures and normal blood pressure is more likely to be associated with normal brain and systemic blood flow.[26,27] The molecular mechanisms by which the vasculature of the cerebral cortex and white matter of the ELBW neonate mature rapidly and become "high-priority" vascular beds soon after delivery are unknown.[27,28]

## The Transitional Circulation in the VLBW Infant

The traditional understanding of the changes occurring in the transitional circulation of the preterm infant suggests that atrial and ductal shunts in the first postnatal hours are of little significance and are bidirectional or primarily right to left in direction as a result of the higher pulmonary vascular resistance expected in the newborn premature infant.[29] In contrast to this understanding, longitudinal studies using bedside noninvasive ultrasound show significant variability in the time taken for the preterm infant to transition from the in utero right ventricle (RV)–dominant, low-resistance circulation to the bi-ventricular, higher-resistance postnatal circulation. Shortly after delivery, the severing of the umbilical vessels, the inflation of the lungs with air, and the associated changes in oxygenation lead to a sudden increase in the resistance in the systemic circulation and a lowering of resistance in the pulmonary circulation. Cardiac output now passes in a parallel fashion through the pulmonary and the systemic circulation except for the blood flow shunting through the closing fetal channels. The role of placental transfusion and the timing of cord clamp and how this affects transitional hemodynamics are discussed in Chapter 6.

In healthy-term infants the ductus arteriosus is functionally closed by the second postnatal day and the right ventricular pressure usually falls to adult levels by about 2–3 days after birth.[30,31] This constriction and functional closure of the ductus arteriosus is then followed by anatomical closure over the next 2–3 weeks. In contrast, in the VLBW infant there is frequently a failure of complete closure of both the foramen ovale and the ductus arteriosus in the expected time frame, probably due to structural

immaturity and the immaturity of the mechanisms involved.[32,33] The persistence of the fetal channels in the setting of decreasing pulmonary pressures leads to blood flowing preferentially from the aorta to the pulmonary artery, resulting in a relative loss of blood from the systemic circulation and pulmonary circulatory overload. Contrary to traditional understanding, this systemic to pulmonary shunting can occur as early as the first postnatal hours, with recirculation of 50% or more of the normal cardiac output back into the lungs.[34] The myocardium subsequently attempts to compensate by increasing the total cardiac output. There can be up to a twofold increase in the left ventricular (LV) output by 1 hour of age, resulting primarily from an increased stroke volume rather than increased heart rate.[35] A significant proportion of this increased blood flow is likely to be passing through the ductus arteriosus.[36] There is a wide range of early ductal constriction, with some infants able to effectively close or minimize the size of the ductus arteriosus within a few hours of birth while others achieve an initial constriction, followed by an increase in size of the ductus and yet another group having a persistent large ductus arteriosus with no evidence of early constriction and subsequent limitation of shunt size.[37] Pulmonary blood flow can be more than twice the systemic blood flow as early as the first few postnatal hours, which may be enough to cause clinical effects, such as reduced systemic blood pressure and blood flow, increases in ventilatory requirements, or even pulmonary hemorrhagic edema.[37]

In utero, the fetal communications of the foramen ovale and ductus arteriosus result in a lack of separation between the left and right ventricular outputs, making it difficult to quantitate their individual contributions. In addition to heart rate, ventricular systolic function is determined by the physiologic principles of preload (distension of the ventricle by blood prior to contraction), contractility (the intrinsic ability of the myocardial fibers to contract), and afterload (the combined resistance of the blood, the ventricular walls, and the vascular beds). The myocardium of the VLBW infant is less mature than that of a term infant, with fewer mitochondria and less energy stores. This results in a limitation in the ability to respond to changes in the determinants of the cardiac output, in particular, the afterload.[38,39] Consequently the myocardium of the VLBW infant, just like the fetal myocardium, is likely to be less able to respond to stresses that occur in the postnatal period, such as increased peripheral vascular resistance with the resultant increase in afterload. There is a significant difference in the influence of determinants of cardiac output in the newborn premature infant with a dramatically increased afterload and changes in the preload caused by the inflation of the lungs. Furthermore, the effect of lung inflation on preload is different when lung inflation occurs by positive pressure ventilation rather than by the negative intrathoracic pressures generated by spontaneous breathing. The newborn ventricle is more sensitive to changes in the afterload, such that small changes can have large effects, especially if the preload and contractility are not optimized.[38]

Failure of the normal transitional changes to occur in a timely manner can result in impairment of cardiac function leading to low cardiac output states and hypotension in the VLBW infant. As oxygen delivery is primarily related to oxygen-carrying capacity and the oxygen content of blood and volume of blood flow to the organ, delivery of oxygen to vital organs may be impaired where there is cardiovascular impairment.[40] Therefore the timely identification and appropriate management of early low cardiac output states and hypotension are of vital importance in the overall care of the VLBW infant.

## Physiologic Determinants of the Blood Pressure in the VLBW Infant

The product of cardiac output and peripheral vascular resistance determines arterial blood pressure. The main influences on the cardiac output are the preload or blood volume and myocardial contractility. Peripheral vascular resistance is determined by vascular tone, which in the presence of an unconstricted ductus arteriosus may not only be the systemic peripheral vascular resistance but is also contributed to by the pulmonary vascular resistance. Myocardial contractility is difficult to assess in the newborn as the accepted measures of contractility in the adult, such as the echocardiographic measure of fractional shortening, are adversely influenced by the asymmetry of the

ventricles caused by the in utero right ventricular dominance. In this regard, use of load-independent measures of cardiac contractility, such as mean velocity of fractional shortening or LV wall stress indices, may provide more useful information (Chapters 9 and 10; Figure 20.2).[41] Some studies have found a relationship between myocardial dysfunction and hypotension in the preterm infant, while others have not, even though a similar measurement method was used. Blood volume correlates poorly with blood pressure in hypotensive neonates.[42-45] Due to the unique characteristics of the newborn cardiovascular system discussed earlier, systemic blood pressure is closely related to changes in the systemic vascular resistance. As systemic vascular resistance cannot be measured directly, the measurement of cardiac output or systemic blood flow becomes an essential element in understanding the dynamic changes occurring in the cardiovascular system of the VLBW infant.

In the absence of simple techniques to measure cardiac output and systemic vascular resistance (Chapter 14), clinicians have tended to rely on blood pressure as the sole assessment of circulatory compromise. However, in the VLBW neonate with a closed ductus arteriosus during the first 24–48 hours, there is only a weak relationship between mean blood pressure and cardiac output (Figure 20.3).[43] Relying on measurements of blood pressure alone can lead the clinician to make assumptions about the underlying physiology of the cardiovascular system that may be incorrect, especially during the period of early transition with the fetal channels open (Chapter 3). Indeed, many hypotensive preterm infants potentially have a normal or high left ventricular output.[43,46,47] One of the reasons for this apparent paradox relates to the presence of a hemodynamically significant ductus arteriosus, which causes an increase in left ventricular output while also causing a reduction in the overall systemic vascular resistance. In addition, variations in the peripheral vascular resistance may cause a change in the underlying cardiac output that does not affect the blood pressure. This phenomenon makes it possible for two infants with the same blood pressure to have markedly different cardiac outputs. Thus the physiologic determinants of blood pressure may affect the blood pressure in multiple ways – acting via an

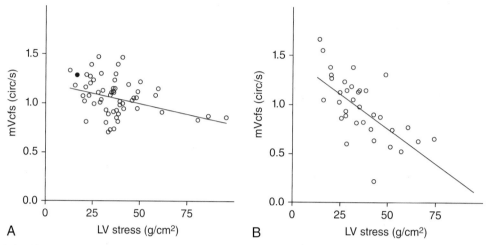

**Fig. 20.2** Relationship between mean velocity of circumferential fractional shortening (mVcfs) of the left ventricle (LV) and LV wall stress (a measure of LV contractility) at 3 hours post birth in infants who had normal (Panel A) and low (Panel B) SVC flows in the first 24 hours. Infants who developed low SVC flow had reduced LV contractility (*P* 0.02). (Reproduced with permission from Takahashi Y, Harada K, Kishkurno S, et al. Postnatal left ventricular contractility in very low birth weight infants. *Pediatr Cardiol.* 1997;18(2):112-117.[39])

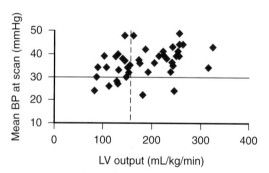

**Fig. 20.3** The weak relationship between mean systemic blood pressure and simultaneously measured left ventricular (*LV*) output. Some infants with a mean blood pressure (*BP*) greater than 30 mmHg have critically low cardiac output (<150 mL/kg/min), and conversely, some infants with normal LV output have low mean blood pressure (<30 mmHg).[43]

effect on cardiac performance and thus cardiac output, altering the vascular resistance, or sometimes altering both. The site where blood pressure is measured can also cause variation with a discordance between blood pressure measured via the commonly used post-ductal umbilical artery and the left ventricular output.

## Clinical Determinants of Blood Pressure in the VLBW Infant

### GESTATIONAL AGE AND POSTNATAL AGE

Both GA and postnatal age are major determinants of the systemic blood pressure, as can be seen by examining nomograms and tables of normal blood pressure data (see Chapter 3). Generally, blood pressure is higher in more mature infants and progressively increases with advancing postnatal age. The reasons why blood pressure increases with postnatal age are unclear but are probably related to changes in the underlying vascular tone mediated by various humoral regulators and possibly up-regulation of receptors involved in myocardial responses. Simultaneously, there are temporal physical changes in the transitional circulation, such as closure of the ductus arteriosus, which will affect both blood pressure and blood flow.

### USE OF ANTENATAL GLUCOCORTICOID THERAPY

There is evidence that sick VLBW infants have relative adrenal insufficiency and that this condition may be one of the underlying causes of cardiovascular dysfunction, with the propensity to inflammation in these patients contributing to the pathogenesis of clinical conditions such as bronchopulmonary dysplasia.[48-50] Low cortisol levels have been documented in hypotensive infants requiring cardiovascular support.[51] The use of antenatal glucocorticoids to assist in fetal lung maturation may therefore have an additional effect of improving neonatal blood pressure. Likely mechanisms for this effect include acceleration of adrenergic receptor expression and maturation of myocardial structure and function. The enhanced adrenergic receptor expression also increases the sensitivity of the myocardium and peripheral vasculature to endogenous catecholamines.[52] Randomized controlled trials of the use of antenatal glucocorticoids have shown variable effects on the neonatal blood pressure. In some trials there was an increase in mean blood pressure of VLBW infants in the treated group with a decreased need for cardiovascular support, while others have shown little difference between the mean blood pressures of infants whose mothers did and did not receive antenatal steroids.[53-56]

## BLOOD LOSS

Acute blood loss in the VLBW infant is unusual and can result from *prenatal events* (such as feto-maternal hemorrhage, antepartum hemorrhage or twin-twin transfusion syndrome) or *intrapartum events* (such as a tight nuchal cord resulting in an imbalance between blood flow to and from the fetus or postnatally from a large subgaleal hematoma or hemorrhage into an organ such as the liver or brain). Acute blood loss can result in significant hypotension, but due to the immediate compensatory mechanisms of the cardiovascular system, this effect may be delayed. Similarly, a drop in the infant's hemoglobin level can also be delayed following significant acute hemorrhage.

## TIMING OF UMBILICAL CORD CLAMP

Both the volume of placental transfusion and the normal sequence of the transition can be affected by the timing of clamping of the umbilical cord, with later clamping being associated with a smoother hemodynamic transition (at least in an animal model),[57] increased systemic blood pressure, and decreased need for cardiovascular support and blood transfusions.[58] An emerging concept of placental blood volume restoration is intriguing, whereby the perceived placental transfusion of "extra" blood is actually a rebalancing of the plasma volume lost due to the physiologically increased capillary permeability during labor, the blood volume lost into the placenta during labor and delivery, and the effect of immediate cord clamping on the "rebalancing" process itself. Indeed, immediate clamping of the cord can deprive the preterm infant of the placental transfusion and thus of the return to normal blood volume, potentially rendering the infant hemodynamically vulnerable (see Chapter 6 for details).

## POSITIVE PRESSURE VENTILATION

Many VLBW infants are exposed to positive pressure respiratory support in the first postnatal days. Positive end-expiratory pressure (PEEP) or nasal continuous positive airway pressure (CPAP) is often utilized to reduce the atelectasis resulting from collapse of unstable alveoli when surfactant is lacking, particularly in more immature infants. Although surfactant deficiency is the main reason for provision of positive pressure support in preterm neonates, other conditions such as sepsis, pneumonia, and immaturity of the lungs without surfactant deficiency also benefit from positive pressure support. The use of excessive ventilation pressures in the premature infant, especially with improving lung compliance, can result in secondary interference with cardiac function and pulmonary vascular resistance. Heart function can be impaired by a reduction in the preload from reduced systemic or pulmonary venous return and/or direct compression of cardiac chambers also resulting in a reduced stroke volume or an increase in afterload. This latter scenario is particularly concerning for the right ventricle (RV) and may reduce cardiac output.[59] As the right and left sides of the heart are connected in series, a reduction in the RV output will in turn result in a reduction in the LV cardiac output.

Studies in VLBW infants have shown a fall-off in the systemic oxygen delivery if the PEEP was greater than 6 cm of water and a reduction in the cardiac output at a PEEP level of 9 cm of water in mechanically ventilated infants.[60] However, as these findings were not normalized for lung compliance, their generalizability requires caution. A study of VLBW infants (mean GA 29 weeks) before and during treatment with mechanical ventilation for severe respiratory distress syndrome demonstrated a reduction in LV dimensions and filling rate, with a resultant decrease in the cardiac output by about 40% compared with control values. The addition of a packed cell blood transfusion prevented the decrease in ventricular size and reduction in cardiac output.[61] Blood pressure did not change significantly in the group where cardiac output dropped. In longitudinal clinical studies of blood pressure and blood flow, mean airway pressure has a consistently negative influence on both mean blood pressure and systemic blood flow.[26,43,62,63] Consequently careful titration of the positive pressure to the underlying respiratory pathology is essential; however, more recent clinical studies have failed to demonstrate clinically relevant decreases in blood flow in the conventional range of pressure support.[64,65]

## PATENT DUCTUS ARTERIOSUS (SEE CHAPTER 16)

A patent ductus arteriosus (PDA) may not be recognized clinically in the first days after delivery as the flow through it is generally not turbulent and therefore no murmur is audible.[66] Despite this, the flow is almost always left to right or bidirectional with a predominantly left-to-right pattern.[34] A PDA is usually thought to be associated with a low diastolic blood pressure, but some data suggest that it can be associated with both low diastolic and systolic blood pressure, making a PDA one of the possible causes of systemic hypotension.[67] As clinical detection of a PDA in the first postnatal days is difficult, cardiac ultrasound is required for early diagnosis.[66] The classic clinical signs of a murmur, bounding pulses and a hyperdynamic precordium, usually become evident only after the third postnatal day, making clinical detection much more accurate at that time.[66]

## CALCULATED SYSTEMIC VASCULAR RESISTANCE

There is a reciprocal relationship between the systemic vascular resistance and cardiac output in the healthy term, preterm, and sick ventilated infant.[68] This relationship is particularly important when considering the use of vasopressor-inotropes such as dopamine in preterm infants, where an increase in the peripheral vascular resistance can increase the

blood pressure but have no impact on, or even decrease, the cardiac output.[69] The peripheral resistance varies markedly in the preterm infant and can be affected by numerous factors, including environmental temperature; carbon dioxide level; the maturity of the sympathoadrenal system; patency of the ductus arteriosus; presence of vasoactive substances such as catecholamines, prostacyclin, and nitric oxide; and sepsis.[37,68,70] It is important to note that, in patients with a PDA, both the left and right ventricles are exposed to the combined pulmonary and systemic vascular resistance. The potential variability of the peripheral resistance in VLBW infants means that significant changes in cardiac output or blood flow cannot be identified by measurement of the systemic blood pressure alone.

## Assessment of Cardiovascular Compromise in the Shocked VLBW Infant

Because of the wide variation in blood pressure levels at varying gestations and postnatal ages, some authors have cautioned against the simplicity of just treating low BP alone but suggest that the clinician should look for some other evidence of hypoperfusion, such as decreased capillary return, oliguria, or metabolic acidosis.[71,72] The assessment of cardiovascular adequacy (i.e., tissue oxygen delivery in the VLBW infant) is more of a challenge than in older children and adults. Measures of cardiovascular function used in these groups, such as pulmonary wedge pressure, central venous pressure, and cardiac output measured via thermodilution, are impractical in the preterm infant due to their size and fragility and the frequent presence of cardiac shunting. Assessment usually consists of a mainly clinical appraisal of the perfusion via capillary refill time (CRT) and urine output and the documentation of the pulse rate and blood pressure. The acid-base balance and evidence of lactic acidosis are further important adjuncts to this assessment, but unless serum lactate levels are serially monitored, monitoring changes in pH and base deficit may be misleading due to the increased bicarbonate losses through the immature kidney. Indeed, the use of all of these parameters has specific limitations in the newborn, and particularly in the VLBW infant.

## CAPILLARY REFILL TIME

CRT is a widely utilized proxy of both cardiac output and peripheral resistance in neonates, and normal values have been documented for this group of infants.[73] A number of confounding factors lead to the CRT being potentially inaccurate, and these include the different techniques used (sites tested and pressing time), interobserver variability, ambient temperature, medications, and maturity of skin blood flow control mechanisms.[74] In addition, even in older children receiving intensive care, there is only a weak relationship between the CRT and other hemodynamic measures, such as the stroke volume index.[75] A study investigating the relationship between a measure of systemic blood flow (SVC flow) and CRT in VLBW infants showed that a CRT of ≥3 seconds had only 55% sensitivity and 81% specificity for predicting low systemic blood flow. However, a markedly increased CRT of 4 seconds or more was more closely correlated with low blood flow states.[76]

## URINE OUTPUT

Monitoring urine output is useful in the assessment of cardiovascular well-being in the adult; however, the immature renal tubule in VLBW infants is inefficient at concentrating the urine and therefore has an impaired capacity to appropriately adjust urine osmolality and flow in the face of high serum osmolality.[77] As a result, even if the glomerular filtration rate is decreased markedly, there can be little change in urine output. In addition, the significant physiological decrease in urine output immediately after delivery further compromises our ability to appropriately assess the adequacy of urine output in the neonate. Finally, accurate measurement of urine output is not easy in VLBW infants, generally requiring collection via a urinary catheter or via a collection bag, both techniques being invasive with significant potential complications and thus infrequently done in regular clinical practice.

## PULSE RATE

A rising pulse rate is usually indicative of hypovolemia in the adult. The mechanism relies on a mature autonomic nervous system, with detection of reduced blood volume and then blood pressure via baroreceptors and subsequent increase in the heart rate in an attempt to sustain appropriate cardiac output. Neonates, especially preterm infants, have a faster baseline heart rate and immature myocardium and autonomic nervous system affecting the cardiovascular response to hypovolemia. There are many other influences on the heart rate in the immediate postnatal period, so it cannot be relied upon as an accurate assessment of cardiovascular status.

## METABOLIC ACIDOSIS/LACTIC ACIDOSIS

After exhaustion of all compensatory mechanisms (Chapter 2), tissue hypoxia due to low arterial oxygen tension, inadequate systemic and organ blood flow, or a combination of these two factors results in a switch to anaerobic metabolism at the cellular level. Reduced systemic blood flow may therefore result in an increase in the serum lactate. A combined lactate value of more than 4 mmol with prolonged capillary refill time of more than 4 seconds predicts low SVC flow with 97% specificity.[78] Serum lactate levels have been correlated with illness severity and mortality in critically ill adults and in ventilated neonates with respiratory distress syndrome.[79-86] The normal lactate level in this group of infants is less than 2.5 mmol/L, and there is an association with mortality as the serum lactate level increases above this threshold.[84,85]

## BLOOD PRESSURE (SEE ALSO CHAPTER 3)

Invasive measurement of the arterial blood pressure using a fluid-filled catheter and pressure transducer is usually performed either via an indwelling umbilical artery catheter in the descending aorta or a peripherally placed arterial catheter. There is a strong correlation between blood pressure obtained via a peripheral artery catheter and that obtained via the umbilical artery.[87] The agreement between direct and indirect (noninvasive) measures of blood pressure is generally also good.[88-93] However, the noninvasive technique is more problematic in the VLBW infant as it is more dependent on choice of the appropriate cuff size and is non-continuous.[94] In the newborn a cuff width-to-arm ratio between 0.45 and 0.55 increases the accuracy of indirect blood pressure measurements when compared with direct measures.[19,95] Accuracy of the invasive blood pressure measurement is dependent on proper use of the equipment, including accurate placement of the transducer at the level of the heart; proper calibration of the system; and avoidance of blockages, air bubbles, or blood clots in the catheter line. With the increased use of noninvasive respiratory support even in the smallest infants, access to invasive blood pressure is becoming less common, resulting in the need for other ways to assess perfusion and cardiovascular adequacy.

## CARDIAC OUTPUT (SEE ALSO CHAPTER 12)

Invasive hemodynamic measures such as pulmonary artery thermodilution and mixed venous oxygen saturation monitoring are commonly used in adult intensive care to allow accurate and continuous assessment of the cardiovascular system. The size of both term and preterm infants with the associated difficulty of placing intracardiac catheters has precluded the use of such measures, especially in the group of infants less than 30 weeks' gestation. Another issue specific to premature infants is the potential inaccuracy of the dye dilution and thermodilution method in the presence of intra-cardiac shunts through the ductus arteriosus and the foramen ovale. Noninvasive methods of measuring cardiac output, particularly Doppler ultrasound, have become more popular, aided by improvements in picture resolution and reductions in ultrasound transducer size. Doppler ultrasound was first used to noninvasively measure the cardiac output in neonates in 1982, and subsequently has been validated against more invasive techniques in children, neonates, and VLBW infants.[96,97] The expected coefficient of variation using Doppler compares favorably to that of indicator-dilution and thermodilution. Chapter 12 reviews other novel approaches, such as impedance electrical cardiometry for the continuous beat-to-beat assessment of stroke volume and cardiac output in detail. Finally, another newer modality for measuring cardiac output is functional cardiac magnetic resonance imaging (MRI), which is envisaged to be predominantly a research tool at present (Chapter 13).[98]

## MONITORING OF PERIPHERAL AND MUCOSAL BLOOD FLOW

Laser Doppler and visible light technology (T-Stat) are techniques currently being assessed for usefulness in directly assessing systemic vascular resistance in neonates.[99,100]

## PULSE OXIMETER–DERIVED PERFUSION INDEX

The perfusion index is derived from the plethysmographic signal of a pulse oximeter, using a ratio of the pulsatile component (arterial) and the non-pulsatile components of the light reaching the detector. The perfusion index is measured noninvasively, displayed continuously, and subsequently has potential as a marker of low systemic blood flow. Several studies have validated the perfusion index against other measures of systemic blood flow, including SVC flow, and found it to be reasonably predictive of low flow states.[101] More recently, statistical analysis methods have been used to more carefully assess the quantitative features of the perfusion index signal in the first 24 postnatal hours and relate these to adverse outcomes.[102]

## SYSTEMIC BLOOD FLOW

As discussed earlier, normal mean blood pressure does not guarantee normal LV output or CBF in preterm infants, even in the subgroup in whom the ductus arteriosus has closed (Figure 20.3).[27,43,47] Further problems arise in assessing systemic blood flow in the preterm infant as a result of failure or delay of the normal circulatory transition and closure of the fetal channels. Indeed, the assumption that the LV and RV outputs are identical is often incorrect in the VLBW infant. As also discussed earlier, increased blood flowing through the PDA (ductal shunt) will be reflected in an increased LV output and the blood flowing left to right through a patent foramen ovale (atrial shunt) will be reflected in an increased RV output (Figure 20.4).[37]

Systemic blood flow falls dramatically in many extremely premature infants in the first hours after delivery, and this reduction in flow is usually associated with an increase in peripheral vascular resistance. A substantial proportion of these infants will initially have a "normal" blood pressure (i.e., they are in "compensated shock"; see Chapter 1). Of the VLBW infants who initially develop low systemic blood flow, about 80% will subsequently develop systemic hypotension. Accordingly, utilizing hypotension to direct cardiovascular interventions results in a considerable delay in

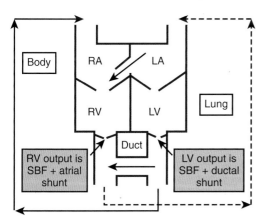

**Fig. 20.4 Diagram demonstrating the points where right and left ventricular output is measured using Doppler ultrasound.** The RV output will consist of the combined systemic venous return and any left-to-right shunting across the foramen ovale. The LV output will consist of the total pulmonary venous return and the blood destined to cross the ductus arteriosus.[37])

infants with low systemic blood flow and the lack of recognition of a low systemic blood flow in patients with normal or high BP. Hypotension may also be associated with normal or even a high systemic blood flow, as frequently occurs in the preterm infant with persisting hypotension after the first postnatal days or those with "hyperdynamic" sepsis.[103] These infants generally have low systemic vascular resistance with peripheral vasodilation.

## Short- and Long-Term Effects of Cardiovascular Compromise/Shock in the VLBW Infant

An important aim of intensive care management in VLBW infants is the maintenance of tissue oxygenation and avoidance of impaired cerebral perfusion. Cerebral blood flow (CBF), which is an important determinant of cerebral oxygen delivery, is determined by the relationship of cerebral perfusion pressure, systemic blood flow, and the vascular resistance of the cerebral circulation. The process of cerebral autoregulation allows maintenance of a constant CBF in the face of variations in the blood pressure, systemic blood flow, and resistance within the autoregulatory range of mean blood pressure (see Chapter 2

for details). There is evidence that sick preterm infants may have impaired or lost CBF autoregulation, resulting in a pressure-passive cerebral circulation mirroring fluctuations in blood pressure.[104] Accordingly, CBF is often low when there is systemic hypotension.[104] However, we do not know where the blood pressure lower elbow of the CBF autoregulatory curve is in preterm neonates (Chapter 2). It is also unclear at what level of hypotension ischemic tissue damage occurs. Interestingly, cerebral fractional oxygen extraction is not related to blood pressure until very low levels (<20 mmHg) of mean blood pressure, suggesting that sufficient oxygen to meet cerebral demand can be delivered, even in the presence of hypotension (Chapters 2, 7, and 8).[27,40,105,106] This finding supports the concept that there is a difference between the autoregulatory and ischemic threshold of blood pressure, with the latter being reached only when increasing fractional cerebral oxygen extraction cannot compensate for the decreased oxygen delivery anymore. However, because of the differences among infants in their ability to compensate for the decreases in perfusion pressure and/or systemic blood flow, a single blood pressure value cannot be used to define the ischemic threshold for preterm infants even with the same gestational and postnatal age (Chapters 2 and 20).

Several studies have suggested that autoregulation is intact in many preterm babies but appears to be compromised in a subgroup who seem to be at particularly high risk of peri-/intraventricular hemorrhage (P/IVH).[107,108] High coherence between mean arterial blood pressure and measures of CBF/oxygenation indicates impaired cerebral autoregulation and is associated with a subgroup of preterm infants at high risk of adverse outcome.[109] It has been suggested that infants with severe P/IVH are more likely to have blood pressure passive changes in CBF and oxygenation in the first postnatal days.[12-15,108]

### PERI-/INTRAVENTRICULAR HEMORRHAGE (SEE CHAPTERS 3 AND 7)

A number of studies have described associations between low mean blood pressure and subsequent P/IVH and neurological injury.[12,13,110-113] It was these observations of an association between systemic blood pressure and cerebral injury that led to current recommendations for treatment of blood pressure. However, a large population-based study has not found systemic hypotension to be an independent risk factor for P/IVH in VLBW infants.[114] Importantly, there is no evidence from appropriately designed, prospective, controlled clinical trials that treatment of hypotension decreases the incidence of P/IVH and neurological injury. Two RCTs with a no-treatment arm designed to establish or refute causation have so far been published.[115,116] Because of difficulties in obtaining informed consent or refusal of enrollment by the clinician, Batton et al. concluded that such studies are not feasible.[115] The other trial randomized hypotensive preterm neonates to dopamine or placebo for 2 hours after enrollment. If mean blood pressure in mmHg remained less than the gestational age in weeks by more than 5 points and/or a combination of systemic hypotension and criteria for poor perfusion were noted, another vasopressor/inotrope or inotrope could be added. Due to difficulties in enrolling subjects, this trial was also terminated early, with only 7% of the target sample recruited. While the investigators found that the need for another vasopressor/inotrope was significantly higher in the placebo arm (66% vs. 38%), the study remained severely underpowered for the primary outcome of survival without significant brain injury to be addressed.[116] The failed efforts of these two well-designed RCTs are of significant concern for future trials planned to establish or refute causation between treatment of hypotension and improved outcomes.

## PERIVENTRICULAR LEUKOMALACIA

The potential relationship between low CBF and white matter injury due to the specific vulnerability of the periventricular white matter in the preterm infant has led to concerns that hypotension may be a precursor of white matter injury. Observational data again have shown a relationship between hypotension (often mean arterial blood pressure below 30 mmHg) and adverse cranial ultrasound findings.[13] However, as with P/IVH, larger population-based studies have failed to identify systemic hypotension as an independent risk factor for white matter injury.[117,118] It is conceivable that the pathogenesis of periventricular leukomalacia, just like that of P/IVH, is multifactorial

and, in addition to changes in cerebral perfusion pressure, factors such as specific or non-specific inflammation and oxidant injury play a significant role in its development. The relationship between hemodynamics and brain injury is further explored in Chapters 7 and 8.

## LONG-TERM NEURODEVELOPMENTAL OUTCOME (SEE ALSO CHAPTER 3)

Hypotension in VLBW infants has been correlated with longer-term adverse neurodevelopmental outcome.[112,113,119,120] There are no prospective studies evaluating the effect of untreated hypotension on any important long-term outcomes; however, there is a prospective study showing that hypotensive preterm infants had an increased risk of adverse neurodevelopmental outcome at term.[121] Several retrospective studies have raised the possibility that preterm infants treated for hypotension may have a worse outcome than untreated infants – it is unclear whether the effect is due to the treatment or other factors associated with hypotension.[72,113,122] Of note is that assessing all hypotensive patients as one group, regardless of their initial underlying physiology or response to treatment, is a significant further limitation of the retrospective studies. Interestingly, the findings of the only prospective randomized clinical trial addressing this issue revealed that hypotensive preterm VLBW neonates had a higher rate of severe P/IVH compared with non-hypotensive controls.[122] However, the outcome of the hypotensive preterm neonates who responded to dopamine or epinephrine with an increase in blood pressure during the first postnatal day was the same as in the controls. Furthermore, there was no association between abnormal ultrasound findings and the use of vasopressors/inotropes. Finally, at 2- to 3-year follow-up, there was no difference in the rate of abnormal neurological outcome between survivors of the hypotensive and control groups. Although these findings provide some reassurance about the safety and potential benefits of vasopressors/inotropes for the treatment of early hypotension in VLBW neonates, the small sample size and the lack of an "untreated hypotensive group" limit the generalizability of the findings of this study.[122] In support of the latter findings a retrospective multicenter study (EPIPAGE 2) found that antihypotensive treatment was associated with higher survival without major morbidity and a lower incidence of central nervous system abnormalities compared to untreated matched controls.[123]

A study of systemic blood flow in VLBW infants demonstrated an independent relationship between low systemic blood flow (particularly the duration of the insult) and adverse neurodevelopmental outcome at 3 years of age.[124]

## Treatment Options in the Management of Cardiovascular Compromise/Shock in the VLBW Infant

The appropriate management of cardiovascular compromise/shock in the VLBW infant will vary according to the underlying physiology. The clinician must consider a number of possible factors, including the infant's GA, postnatal age, measures of cardiovascular adequacy (such as cardiac output or systemic blood flow if available), and associated pathologic conditions. An early cardiac ultrasound can assist greatly in the diagnostic process by providing information about the presence, size, and direction of the ductus arteriosus shunt; presence of pulmonary hypertension; assessment of cardiac contractility; adequacy of venous filling; and measurement of cardiac output or systemic blood flow (Chapter 10).

Before instituting specific treatment for hypotension, potentially reversible causes such as a measurement error (transducer height in comparison to patient's right atrium, calibration of the transducer, air bubble, or blood clot in the measurement catheter), PDA, hypovolemia from blood or fluid loss, pneumothorax, use of excessive mean airway pressure, sepsis, and adrenal insufficiency should be considered and managed appropriately. Therapeutic options that have a cardiovascular physiologic basis for efficacy and have been subjected to clinical trial include volume loading (with crystalloid or colloid), vasopressor/inotropes and inotropic agents, hydrocortisone, and other glucocorticoids. Further details regarding the hemodynamically based management of circulatory compromise and shock in the ELBW infant are reviewed in Chapter 24.

Finally, secular movement toward less aggressive treatment of hypotension has provided an insight into the potential effects of sustained hypotension without clinical evidence of poor perfusion (i.e., "permissive" or "isolated hypotension").[125] A prospective population-based cohort study matched 119 extremely preterm infants untreated for "isolated" hypotension to 119 neonates having received antihypotensive treatment without clinical evidence of poor perfusion.[123] The investigators used the most common clinical definition of hypotension (mean blood pressure less than the gestational age in week during the first 72 hours after delivery). The authors found that subjects treated for "isolated hypotension" had a higher rate of survival without severe morbidity and a lower rate of severe P/IVH and cerebral injury. In addition, the association between treatment and better outcome was stronger when hypotension was defined as mean blood pressure in mmHg less than gestational age in weeks by more than 5 points. While the dose-effect relationship theoretically strengthens the possibility of causality, firm conclusions can only be drawn when and if appropriate RCTs are performed to address this specific question.

## Conclusion

The appropriate assessment and treatment of the VLBW infant with cardiovascular impairment or shock requires the clinician to obtain adequate information about the etiology and underlying physiologic determinants of the condition. The clinician should be aware of the physiologic changes that occur in areas such as myocardial function and vital organ blood flow allocation in the first postnatal days. An understanding of the actions of the therapeutic options available and the specific effects of these treatments on the circulation of the VLBW infant is also important. The addition of cardiac ultrasound to the assessment process provides information about the size and shunt direction of the ductus arteriosus and the function of the myocardium and its filling as well as about the cardiac output and calculated peripheral vascular resistance. Figure 20.5 summarizes the approach to management of hypotension in the ELBW infant using the additional information provided by ultrasound (shaded in pink in the diagram below) and NIRS.

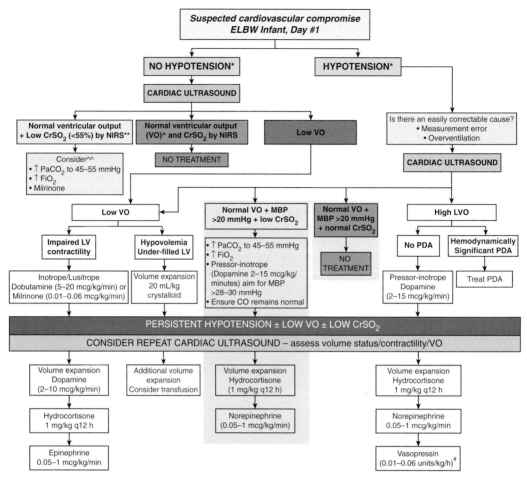

**Fig. 20.5** Treatment of cardiovascular compromise based on assessment of blood pressure, cardiac ultrasound, and near-infrared spectroscopy (NIRS). *Definition of hypotension per agreed-upon criteria.
**Using NIRS with proposed cut-off value below which brain injury is more frequent.[126]
^Use left VO in the absence of significant left-to-right PDA shunting; use right VO if significant left-to-right PDA shunting and insignificant foramen ovale shunting is present.
^^Consideration based on recent data to be confirmed.[127,128] Vasopressin dose recommendation per Rios and Kaiser.[129]
*CO*, cardiac output; *CrSO₂*, cerebral tissue O₂ saturation; *ELBW*, extremely low birth weight; *FiO₂*, fraction of expired oxygen; *h*, hour; *LV*, left ventricle; *LVO*, Left ventricular output; *MBP*, mean blood pressure; *PaCO₂*, arterial partial pressure of CO₂; *PDA*, patent ductus arteriosus; *VO*, ventricular output. (Structure originally adapted from Subhedar NV.[130])
As the pharmacodynamic response and not the pharmacokinetic data are to be used to guide the dose-escalation of the vasopressor-inotropes (dopamine, epinephrine, norepinephrine), the dose needed to elicit the required hemodynamic response may exceed the maximum doses given in parenthesis.

## REFERENCES

1. Al Aweel I, Pursley DM, Rubin LP, Shah B, Weisberger S, Richardson DK. Variations in prevalence of hypotension, hypertension, and vasopressor use in NICUs. *J Perinatol.* 2001;21(5):272-278.
2. Laughon M, Bose C, Clark R. Treatment strategies to prevent or close a patent ductus arteriosus in preterm infants and outcomes. *J Perinatol.* 2007;27(3):164-170.
3. Rios DR, Moffett BS, Kaiser JR. Trends in pharmacotherapy for neonatal hypotension. *J Pediatr.* 2014;165(4):697-701.e1.
4. Stranak Z, Semberova J, Barrington K, et al. International survey on diagnosis and management of hypotension in extremely preterm babies. *Eur J Pediatr.* 2014;173(6):793-798.
5. Kluckow M, Evans N. Superior vena cava flow in newborn infants: a novel marker of systemic blood flow. *Arch Dis Child Fetal Neonatal Ed.* 2000;82(3):F182-F187.
6. Miletin J, Dempsey EM, Miletin J, Dempsey EM. Low superior vena cava flow on day 1 and adverse outcome in the very low birthweight infant. *Arch Dis Child Fetal Neonatal Ed.* 2008;93(5):F368-F371.

7. Paradisis M, Evans N, Kluckow M, et al. Randomized trial of milrinone versus placebo for prevention of low systemic blood flow in very preterm infants. *J Pediatr.* 2009;154(2):189-195.

8. de Waal K, Kluckow M. Superior vena cava flow: role, assessment and controversies in the management of perinatal perfusion. *Semin Fetal Neonatal Med.* 2020;25(5):101122.

9. Laughon M, Bose C, Allred E, et al. Factors associated with treatment for hypotension in extremely low gestational age newborns during the first postnatal week. *Pediatrics.* 2007; 119(2):273-280.

10. McLean CW, Noori, S, Cayabyab, R, Seri, I. Cerebral circulation and hypotension in the premature infant – diagnosis and treatment. In: Perlman JM, ed. *Questions and Controversies in Neonatology – Neurology.* 2nd ed. Philadelphia: Saunders/Elsevier; 2011:3-27.

11. Seri I. Circulatory support of the sick preterm infant. *Semin Neonatol.* 2001;6(1):85-95.

12. Watkins AM, West CR, Cooke RW. Blood pressure and cerebral haemorrhage and ischaemia in very low birthweight infants. *Early Hum Dev.* 1989;19(2):103-110.

13. Miall-Allen VM, de Vries LS, Whitelaw AG. Mean arterial blood pressure and neonatal cerebral lesions. *Arch Dis Child.* 1987;62(10):1068-1069.

14. Tsuji M, Saul JP, du PA, et al. Cerebral intravascular oxygenation correlates with mean arterial pressure in critically ill premature infants. *Pediatrics.* 2000;106(4):625-632.

15. Munro MJ, Walker AM, Barfield CP. Hypotensive extremely low birth weight infants have reduced cerebral blood flow. *Pediatrics.* 2004;114(6):1591-1596.

16. Austin NC, Pairaudeau PW, Hames TK, Hall MA. Regional cerebral blood flow velocity changes after indomethacin infusion in preterm infants. *Arch Dis Child.* 1992;67:851-854.

17. da Costa CS, Czosnyka M, Smielewski P, Austin T. Optimal mean arterial blood pressure in extremely preterm infants within the first 24 hours of life. *J Pediatr.* 2018;203:242-248.

18. Borch K, Lou HC, Greisen G. Cerebral white matter blood flow and arterial blood pressure in preterm infants. *Acta Paediatr.* 2010;99(10):1489-1492.

19. Nuntnarumit P, Yang W, Bada-Ellzey HS. Blood pressure measurements in the newborn. *Clin Perinatol.* 1999;26(4):981-996.

20. Hegyi T, Carbone MT, Anwar M, et al. Blood pressure ranges in premature infants. i. the first hours of life. *J Pediatr.* 1994; 124(4):627-633.

21. Development of audit measures and guidelines for good practice in the management of neonatal respiratory distress syndrome: Report of a joint working group of the British Association of Perinatal Medicine and the research unit of the Royal College of Physicians. *Arch Dis Child.* 1992;67(10):1221-1227.

22. Greisen G, Borch K. White matter injury in the preterm neonate: the role of perfusion. *Dev Neurosci.* 2001;23(3):209-212.

23. Greisen G. Autoregulation of cerebral blood flow in newborn babies. *Early Hum Dev.* 2005;81(5):423-428.

24. Tyszczuk L, Meek J, Elwell C, Wyatt JS. Cerebral blood flow is independent of mean arterial blood pressure in preterm infants undergoing intensive care. *Pediatrics.* 1998;102(2 Pt 1):337-341.

25. Seri I, Abbasi S, Wood DC, Gerdes JS. Regional hemodynamic effects of dopamine in the sick preterm neonate. *J Pediatr.* 1998;133(6):728-734.

26. Kluckow M, Evans N. Low superior vena cava flow and intraventricular haemorrhage in preterm infants. *Arch Dis Child Fetal Neonatal Ed.* 2000;82:188-194.

27. Kissack CM, Garr R, Wardle SP, Weindling AM. Cerebral fractional oxygen extraction in very low birth weight infants is

high when there is low left ventricular output and hypocarbia but is unaffected by hypotension. *Pediatr Res.* 2004;55(3): 400-405.

28. Seri I. Hemodynamics during the first two postnatal days and neurodevelopment in preterm neonates. *J Pediatr.* 2004;145: 573-575.

29. Friedman AH, Fahey JT. The transition from fetal to neonatal circulation: normal responses and implications for infants with heart disease. *Semin Perinatol.* 1993;17:106-121.

30. Mahoney LT, Coryell KG, Lauer RM. The newborn transitional circulation: a two-dimensional Doppler echocardiographic study. *J Am Coll Cardiol.* 1985;6(3):623-629.

31. Gentile R, Stevenson G, Dooley T, Franklin D, Kawabori I, Pearlman A. Pulsed Doppler echocardiographic determination of time of ductal closure in normal newborn infants. *J Pediatr.* 1981;98(3):443-448.

32. Evans N, Iyer P. Longitudinal changes in the diameter of the ductus arteriosus in ventilated preterm infants: correlation with respiratory outcomes. *Arch Dis Child Fetal Neonatal Ed.* 1995;72(3):F156-F161.

33. Seidner SR, Chen YQ, Oprysko PR, et al. Combined prostaglandin and nitric oxide inhibition produces anatomic remodeling and closure of the ductus arteriosus in the premature newborn baboon. *Pediatr Res.* 2001;50(3):365-373.

34. Evans N, Iyer P. Assessment of ductus arteriosus shunt in preterm infants supported by mechanical ventilation: effects of interatrial shunting. *J Pediatr.* 1994;125:778-785.

35. Agata Y, Hiraishi S, Oguchi K, et al. Changes in left ventricular output from fetal to early neonatal life. *J Pediatr.* 1991;119: 441-445.

36. Drayton MR, Skidmore R. Ductus arteriosus blood flow during first 48 hours of life. *Arch Dis Child.* 1987;62(10):1030-1034.

37. Kluckow M, Evans N. Low systemic blood flow in the preterm infant. *Semin Neonatol.* 2001;6(1):75-84.

38. Teitel DF. Physiologic development of the cardiovascular system in the fetus. In: Polin RA, Fox WW, eds. *Fetal and Neonatal Physiology.* Vol 2. Philadelphia: W.B. Saunders Company; 1998: 827-836.

39. Takahashi Y, Harada K, Kishkurno S, Arai, Ishida A, Takada G. Postnatal left ventricular contractility in very low birth weight infants. *Pediatr Cardiol.* 1997;18(2):112-117.

40. Weindling AM, Kissack CM. Blood pressure and tissue oxygenation in the newborn baby at risk of brain damage. *Biol Neonate.* 2001;79(3-4):241-245.

41. Osborn D, Evans N, Kluckow M. Diagnosis and treatment of low systemic blood flow in preterm infants. *NeoReviews.* 2004;5(3):e109-e121.

42. Gill AB, Weindling AM. Echocardiographic assessment of cardiac function in shocked very low birthweight infants. *Arch Dis Child.* 1993;68:17-21.

43. Kluckow M, Evans N. Relationship between blood pressure and cardiac output in preterm infants requiring mechanical ventilation. *J Pediatr.* 1996;129(4):506-512.

44. Bauer K, Linderkamp O, Versmold HT. Systolic blood pressure and blood volume in preterm infants. *Arch Dis Child.* 1993;69 (5 Spec No):521-522.

45. Barr PA, Bailey PE, Sumners J, Cassady G. Relation between arterial blood pressure and blood volume and effect of infused albumin in sick preterm infants. *Pediatrics.* 1977;60(3):282-289.

46. Lopez SL, Leighton JO, Walther FJ. Supranormal cardiac output in the dopamine- and dobutamine-dependent preterm infant. *Pediatr Cardiol.* 1997;18(4):292-296.

47. Pladys P, Wodey E, Beuchee A, Branger B, Betremieux P. Left ventricle output and mean arterial blood pressure in preterm infants during the 1st day of life. *Eur J Pediatr.* 1999;158(10):817-824.

48. Ng PC, Lam CW, Fok TF, et al. Refractory hypotension in preterm infants with adrenocortical insufficiency. *Arch Dis Child Fetal Neonatal Ed.* 2001;84(2):F122-F124.

49. Watterberg KL. Adrenal insufficiency and cardiac dysfunction in the preterm infant. *Pediatr Res.* 2002;51(4):422-424.

50. Hanna CE, Jett PL, Laird MR, Mandel SH, Lafranchi SH, Reynolds JW. Corticosteroid binding globulin, total serum cortisol, and stress in extremely low-birth-weight infants. *Am J Perinatol.* 1997;14(4):201-204.

51. Scott SM, Watterberg KL. Effect of gestational age, postnatal age, and illness on plasma cortisol concentrations in premature infants. *Pediatr Res.* 1995;37(1):112-116.

52. Sasidharan P. Role of corticosteroids in neonatal blood pressure homeostasis. *Clin Perinatol.* 1998;25(3):723-740.

53. Moise AA, Wearden ME, Kozinetz CA, Gest AL, Welty SE, Hansen TN. Antenatal steroids are associated with less need for blood pressure support in extremely premature infants. *Pediatrics.* 1995;95(6):845-850.

54. Demarini S, Dollberg S, Hoath SB, Ho M, Donovan EF. Effects of antenatal corticosteroids on blood pressure in very low birth weight infants during the first 24 hours of life. *J Perinatol.* 1999;19(6 Pt 1):419-425.

55. LeFlore JL, Engle WD, Rosenfeld CR. Determinants of blood pressure in very low birth weight neonates: lack of effect of antenatal steroids. *Early Hum Dev.* 2000;59(1):37-50.

56. Leviton A, Kuban KC, Pagano M, Allred EN, Van-Marter L. Antenatal corticosteroids appear to reduce the risk of postnatal germinal matrix hemorrhage in intubated low birth weight newborns. *Pediatrics.* 1993;91(6):1083-1088.

57. Bhatt S, Polglase GR, Wallace EM, Te Pas AB, Hooper SB. Ventilation before umbilical cord clamping improves the physiological transition at birth. *Front Pediatr.* 2014;2:113.

58. Rabe H, Diaz-Rossello JL, Duley L, Dowswell T. Effect of timing of umbilical cord clamping and other strategies to influence placental transfusion at preterm birth on maternal and infant outcomes. *Cochrane Database Syst Rev.* 2012;8:CD003248.

59. Cheifetz IM. Cardiorespiratory interactions: the relationship between mechanical ventilation and hemodynamics. *Respir Care.* 2014;59(12):1937-1945.

60. Trang TT, Tibballs J, Mercier JC, Beaufils F. Optimization of oxygen transport in mechanically ventilated newborns using oximetry and pulsed Doppler-derived cardiac output. *Crit Care Med.* 1988;16:1094-1097.

61. Maayan C, Eyal F, Mandelberg A, Sapoznikov D, Lewis B. Effect of mechanical ventilation and volume loading on left ventricular performance in premature infants with respiratory distress syndrome. *Crit Care Med.* 1986;14(10):858-860.

62. Skinner JR, Boys RJ, Hunter S, Hey EN. Pulmonary and systemic arterial pressure in hyaline membrane disease. *Arch Dis Child.* 1992;67(4):366-373.

63. Evans N, Kluckow M. Early determinants of right and left ventricular output in ventilated preterm infants. *Arch Dis Child Fetal Neonatal Ed.* 1996;74(2):F88-F94.

64. Chang HY, Cheng KS, Lung HL, et al. Hemodynamic effects of nasal intermittent positive pressure ventilation in preterm infants. *Medicine (Baltimore).* 2016;95(6):e2780.

65. Beker F, Rogerson SR, Hooper SB, Wong C, Davis PG. The effects of nasal continuous positive airway pressure on cardiac function in premature infants with minimal lung disease: a crossover randomized trial. *J Pediatr.* 2014;164(4):726-729.

66. Skelton R, Evans N, Smythe J. A blinded comparison of clinical and echocardiographic evaluation of the preterm infant for patent ductus arteriosus. *J Paediatr Child Health.* 1994;30:406-411.

67. Evans N, Moorcraft J. Effect of patency of the ductus arteriosus on blood pressure in very preterm infants. *Arch Dis Child.* 1992;67:1169-1173.

68. Fenton AC, Woods KL, Leanage R, et al. Cardiovascular effects of carbon dioxide in ventilated preterm infants. *Acta Paediatr.* 1992;81:498-503.

69. Roze JC, Tohier C, Maingueneau C, Lefevre M, Mouzard A. Response to dobutamine and dopamine in the hypotensive very preterm infant. *Arch Dis Child.* 1993;69:59-63.

70. Seri I, Rudas G, Bors Z, Kanyicska B, Tulassay T. Effects of low-dose dopamine infusion on cardiovascular and renal functions, cerebral blood flow, and plasma catecholamine levels in sick preterm neonates. *Pediatr Res.* 1993;34(6):742-749.

71. Versmold HT, Kitterman JA, Phibbs RH, Gregory GA, Tooley WH. Aortic blood pressure during the first 12 hours of life in infants with birth weight 610 to 4,220 grams. *Pediatrics.* 1981;67(5):607-613.

72. Dempsey EM, Al Hazzani F, Barrington KJ, Dempsey EM, Al Hazzani F, Barrington KJ. Permissive hypotension in the extremely low birthweight infant with signs of good perfusion. *Arch Dis Child Fetal Neonatal Ed.* 2009;94(4):F241-F244.

73. Strozik KS, Pieper CH, Roller J. Capillary refilling time in newborn babies: normal values. *Arch Dis Child Fetal Neonatal Ed.* 1997;76(3):F193-F196.

74. Schriger DL, Baraff L. Defining normal capillary refill: variation with age, sex, and temperature. *Ann Emerg Med.* 1988;17(9):932-935.

75. Tibby SM, Hatherill M, Murdoch IA. Capillary refill and core-peripheral temperature gap as indicators of haemodynamic status in paediatric intensive care patients. *Arch Dis Child.* 1999;80(2):163-166.

76. Osborn DA, Evans N, Kluckow M. Clinical detection of low upper body blood flow in very premature infants using blood pressure, capillary refill time, and central-peripheral temperature difference. *Arch Dis Child Fetal Neonatal Ed.* 2004;89(2):F168-F173.

77. Linshaw MA. Concentration of the urine. In: Polin RA, Fox WW, eds. *Fetal and Neonatal Physiology.* Vol 2. Philadelphia: W.B. Saunders Company; 1998:1634-1653.

78. Miletin J, Pichova K, Dempsey EM, Miletin J, Pichova K, Dempsey EM. Bedside detection of low systemic flow in the very low birth weight infant on day 1 of life. *Eur J Pediatr.* 2009;168(7):809-813.

79. Cady Jr LD, Weil MH, Afifi AA, Michaels SF, Liu VY, Shubin H. Quantitation of severity of critical illness with special reference to blood lactate. *Crit Care Med.* 1973;1(2):75-80.

80. Peretz DI, Scott HM, Duff J, Dossetor JB, MacLean LD, McGregor M. The significance of lacticacidemia in the shock syndrome. *Ann N Y Acad Sci.* 1965;119(3):1133-1141.

81. Rashkin MC, Bosken C, Baughman RP. Oxygen delivery in critically ill patients. Relationship to blood lactate and survival. *Chest.* 1985;87(5):580-584.

82. Vincent JL, Dufaye P, Berre J, Leeman M, Degaute JP, Kahn RJ. Serial lactate determinations during circulatory shock. *Crit Care Med.* 1983;11(6):449-451.

83. Weil MH, Afifi AA. Experimental and clinical studies on lactate and pyruvate as indicators of the severity of acute circulatory failure (shock). *Circulation*. 1970;41(6):989-1001.

84. Beca JP, Scopes JW. Serial determinations of blood lactate in respiratory distress syndrome. *Arch Dis Child*. 1972;47(254):550-557.

85. Deshpande SA, Platt MP. Association between blood lactate and acid-base status and mortality in ventilated babies. *Arch Dis Child Fetal Neonatal Ed*. 1997;76(1):F15-F20.

86. Graven SN, Criscuolo D, Holcomb TM. Blood lactate in the respiratory distress syndrome: significance in prognosis. *Am J Dis Child*. 1965;110(6):614-617.

87. Butt WW, Whyte HW. Blood pressure monitoring in neonates: comparison of umbilical and peripheral artery measurements. *J Pediatr*. 1984;105:630-632.

88. Colan SD, Fujii A, Borow KM, MacPherson D, Sanders SP. Noninvasive determination of systolic, diastolic and end-systolic blood pressure in neonates, infants and young children: comparison with central aortic pressure measurements. *Am J Cardiol*. 1983;52(7):867-870.

89. Emery EF, Greenough A. Non-invasive blood pressure monitoring in preterm infants receiving intensive care. *Eur J Pediatr*. 1992;151(2):136-139.

90. Kimble KJ, Darnall RA, Jr., Yelderman M, Ariagno RL, Ream AK. An automated oscillometric technique for estimating mean arterial pressure in critically ill newborns. *Anesthesiology*. 1981;54(5):423-425.

91. Lui K, Doyle PE, Buchanan N. Oscillometric and intra-arterial blood pressure measurements in the neonate: a comparison of methods. *Aust Paediat J*. 1982;18(1):32-34.

92. Park MK, Menard SM. Accuracy of blood pressure measurement by the Dinamap monitor in infants and children. *Pediatrics*. 1987;79(6):907-914.

93. O'Shea J, Dempsey EM, O'Shea J, Dempsey EM. A comparison of blood pressure measurements in newborns. *Am J Perinatol*. 2009;26(2):113-116.

94. Dannevig I, Dale HC, Liestol K, Lindemann R. Blood pressure in the neonate: three non-invasive oscillometric pressure monitors compared with invasively measured blood pressure. *Acta Paediatr*. 2005;94(2):191-196.

95. Dionne JM, Bremner SA, Baygani SK, et al. Method of blood pressure measurement in neonates and infants: a systematic review and analysis. *J Pediatr*. 2020;221:23-31.e5.

96. Alverson DC, Eldridge M, Dillon T, Yabek SM, Berman Jr W. Noninvasive pulsed Doppler determination of cardiac output in neonates and children. *J Pediatr*. 1982;101:46-50.

97. Walther FJ, Siassi B, Ramadan NA, Ananda AK, Wu PY. Pulsed Doppler determinations of cardiac output in neonates: normal standards for clinical use. *Pediatrics*. 1985;76:829-833.

98. Groves AM, Groves AM. Cardiac magnetic resonance in the study of neonatal haemodynamics. *Semin Fetal Neonatal Med*. 2011;16(1):36-41.

99. Stark MJ, Clifton VL, Wright IM, Stark MJ, Clifton VL, Wright IMR. Microvascular flow, clinical illness severity and cardiovascular function in the preterm infant. *Arch Dis Child Fetal Neonatal Ed*. 2008;93(4):F271-F274.

100. Amir G, Ramamoorthy C, Riemer RK, et al. Visual light spectroscopy reflects flow-related changes in brain oxygenation during regional low-flow perfusion and deep hypothermic circulatory arrest. *J Thorac Cardiovasc Surg*. 2006;132(6):1307-1313.

101. Takahashi S, Kakiuchi S, Nanba Y, et al. The perfusion index derived from a pulse oximeter for predicting low superior vena cava flow in very low birth weight infants. *J Perinatol*. 2010;30(4):265-269.

102. Van Laere D, O'Toole JM, Voeten M, McKiernan J, Boylan GB, Dempsey E. Decreased variability and low values of perfusion index on day one are associated with adverse outcome in extremely preterm infants. *J Pediatr*. 2016;178:119-124.e111.

103. de Waal K, Evans N. Hemodynamics in preterm infants with late-onset sepsis. *J Pediatr*. 2010;156(6):918-922.e1.

104. Lou HC, Lassen NA, Friis-Hansen B. Impaired autoregulation of cerebral blood flow in the distressed newborn infant. *J Pediatr*. 1979;94(1):118-121.

105. Victor S, Marson AG, Appleton RE, Beirne M, Weindling AM. Relationship between blood pressure, cerebral electrical activity, cerebral fractional oxygen extraction, and peripheral blood flow in very low birth weight newborn infants. *Pediatr Res*. 2006;59:314-319.

106. Wardle SP, Yoxall CW, Weindling AM. Peripheral oxygenation in hypotensive preterm babies. *Pediatr Res*. 1999;45(3):343-349.

107. Perlman JM, McMenamin JB, Volpe JJ. Fluctuating cerebral blood-flow velocity in respiratory-distress syndrome. Relation to the development of intraventricular hemorrhage. *N Engl J Med*. 1983;309(4):204-209.

108. Pryds O, Greisen G, Lou H, Friis-Hansen B. Heterogeneity of cerebral vasoreactivity in preterm infants supported by mechanical ventilation. *J Pediatr*. 1989;115(4):638-645.

109. Wong FY, Leung TS, Austin T, et al. Impaired autoregulation in preterm infants identified by using spatially resolved spectroscopy. *Pediatrics*. 2008;121(3):e604-e611.

110. Bada HS, Korones SB, Perry EH, et al. Mean arterial blood pressure changes in premature infants and those at risk for intraventricular hemorrhage. *J Pediatr*. 1990;117(4):607-614.

111. Cunningham S, Symon AG, Elton RA, Zhu C, McIntosh N. Intra-arterial blood pressure reference ranges, death and morbidity in very low birthweight infants during the first seven days of life. *Early Hum Dev*. 1999;56(2-3):151-165.

112. Grether JK, Nelson KB, Emery ES, Cummins SK. Prenatal and perinatal factors and cerebral palsy in very low birth weight infants. *J Pediatr*. 1996;128:407-411.

113. Fanaroff JM, Wilson-Costello DE, Newman NS, Montpetite MM, Fanaroff AA. Treated hypotension is associated with neonatal morbidity and hearing loss in extremely low birth weight infants. *Pediatrics*. 2006;117:1131-1135.

114. Heuchan AM, Evans N, Henderson Smart DJ, Simpson JM. Perinatal risk factors for major intraventricular haemorrhage in the Australian and New Zealand Neonatal Network, 1995–1997. *Arch Dis Child Fetal Neonatal Ed*. 2002;86(2):F86-F90.

115. Batton BJ, Li L, Newman NS, et al. Feasibility study of early blood pressure management in extremely preterm infants. *J Pediatr*. 2012;161(1):65-69.e1.

116. Dempsey EM, Barrington KJ, Marlow N, et al. Hypotension in Preterm Infants (HIP) randomised trial. *Arch Dis Child Fetal Neonatal Ed*. 2021;106(4):398-403.

117. de Vries LS, Regev R, Dubowitz LM, Whitelaw A, Aber VR. Perinatal risk factors for the development of extensive cystic leukomalacia. *Am J Dis Child*. 1988;142(7):732-735.

118. Perlman JM, Risser R, Broyles RS. Bilateral cystic periventricular leukomalacia in the premature infant: associated risk factors. *Pediatrics*. 1996;97(6 Pt 1):822-827.

119. Goldstein RF, Thompson RJ, Jr., Oehler JM, Brazy JE. Influence of acidosis, hypoxemia, and hypotension on neurodevelopmental

outcome in very low birth weight infants. *Pediatrics.* 1995;95(2): 238-243.

120. Low JA, Froese AB, Galbraith RS, Smith JT, Sauerbrei EE, Derrick EJ. The association between preterm newborn hypotension and hypoxemia and outcome during the first year. *Acta Paediatr.* 1993;82(5):433-437.

121. Martens SE, Rijken M, Stoelhorst GM, et al. Is hypotension a major risk factor for neurological morbidity at term age in very preterm infants? *Early Hum Dev.* 2003;75(1–2):79-89.

122. Pellicer A, Bravo MC, Madero R, et al. Early systemic hypotension and vasopressor support in low birth weight infants: impact on neurodevelopment. *Pediatrics.* 2009;123(5):1369-1376.

123. Durrmeyer X, Marchand-Martin L, Porcher R, et al. Abstention or intervention for isolated hypotension in the first 3 days of life in extremely preterm infants: association with short-term outcomes in the EPIPAGE 2 cohort study. *Arch Dis Child Fetal Neonatal Ed.* 2017;102(6):490-496.

124. Hunt RW, Evans N, Rieger I, Kluckow M. Low superior vena cava flow and neurodevelopment at 3 years in very preterm infants. *J Pediatr.* 2004;145(5):588-592.

125. Miller LE, Laughon MM, Clark RH, et al. Vasoactive medications in extremely low gestational age neonates during the first postnatal week. *J Perinatol.* 2021;41(9):2330-2336.

126. Plomgaard AM, van Oeveren W, Petersen TH, et al. The Safe-BoosC II randomized trial: treatment guided by near-infrared spectroscopy reduces cerebral hypoxia without changing early biomarkers of brain injury. *Pediatr Res.* 2016;79(4):528-535.

127. Pellicer A, Greisen G, Benders M, et al. The SafeBoosC phase II randomised clinical trial: a treatment guideline for targeted near-infrared-derived cerebral tissue oxygenation versus standard treatment in extremely preterm infants. *Neonatology.* 2013;104(3):171-178.

128. Noori S, Anderson M, Soleymani S, Seri I. Effect of carbon dioxide on cerebral blood flow velocity in preterm infants during postnatal transition. *Acta Paediatr.* 2014;103(8):e334-339.

129. Rios DR, Kaiser JR. Vasopressin versus dopamine for treatment of hypotension in extremely low birth weight infants: a randomized, blinded pilot study. *J Pediatr.* 2015;166(4):850-855.

130. Subhedar NV. Treatment of hypotension in newborns. *Semin Neonatol.* 2003;8(6):413-423.

# Chapter 21

# Assessment and Management of Septic Shock and Hypovolemia

Koert de Waal and Istvan Seri

## Key Points

- Sepsis can progress rapidly from mild clinical signs to full-blown septic shock with high morbidity and mortality.
- The clinical recognition of the onset of sepsis and the onset of neonatal septic shock can be challenging.
- In conjunction with the use of comprehensive cardiorespiratory monitoring, early and serial assessment with ultrasound aids in the recognition of the type of septic shock and in the following of the hemodynamic response to treatment.
- Septic shock in neonates usually presents with high cardiac output and low systemic vascular resistance (i.e., warm shock) and can be accompanied by pulmonary hypertension and diastolic dysfunction.
- Any significant decrease in blood pressure (compared to the blood pressure before the infant became unwell) should be considered hypotension which potentially heralds the onset of the uncompensated phase of septic shock.
- First-line treatment should be targeting vasodilatory shock with carefully individualized volume support and the use of vasoactive agents.
- The earlier commencement of appropriately titrated vasopressor-inotrope therapy may have several potential beneficial effects and should be prioritized in newborns with clinical or ultrasound evidence of progression to full-blown septic shock.
- True hypovolemic shock is rare in newborns.

## Introduction

Sepsis remains a leading cause of morbidity and mortality in the neonatal population. There is a strong inverse relationship between the incidence of sepsis, gestational age, and birth weight. The incidence and mortality in term or late preterm infants with sepsis has slowly decreased over time, but the incidence and case-fatality rate remain high in very-low-birth-weight (VLBW) infants.[1-5] This chapter addresses the clinical and hemodynamic presentation and cardiovascular and antibiotic management of neonates, with sepsis caused by bacterial infection. Primarily because of scant hemodynamic data, the clinical and cardiovascular presentation of neonates with sepsis caused by viral (herpes virus, enteroviruses, etc.) or fungal infection might be somewhat different.

Currently, there is no unified consensus definition of neonatal sepsis.[6,7] Definitions of neonatal sepsis in the literature emphasize microbiological evidence of infection, without consideration for potential organ dysfunction, and include general clinical practice items such as treatment duration with antibiotics. The last pediatric consensus definition was presented in 2005 and incorporated the presence of evidence for a systemic inflammatory response.[8] However, this definition is not applicable to the newborn population as many neonates with septic shock would not qualify, similar to what was found in adults.[9,10] The "Sepsis-3 Group" has recently defined sepsis in adults as a life-threatening organ dysfunction caused by a dysregulated host response to infection, and septic shock is defined as a subset of sepsis in which underlying circulatory and cellular/metabolic abnormalities are profound enough to significantly increase mortality.[10]

It would not be unreasonable to use a similar but adapted version for septic shock in newborns, but some questions still remain. *First*, the host response of newborns is different from that of adults. The fetus lives in a unique environment where protection against infection is paramount. Yet, the fetus also must avoid the development of harmful, dysregulated inflammatory immune responses that could lead to preterm birth. Birth is the transition from the intra-uterine environment with low-grade presence of maternal bacteria essential for the development of, among others, the immune system to a new environment abundant in foreign antigens and pathogens requiring a balanced immunological response. Much remains to be understood about the newborn's immune response to infection, and whether these biochemical processes can be used in the early detection of a dysregulated immune response and/or to guide treatment of neonatal infections.[11,12]

*Second*, there is no consensus on the definition of a life-threatening organ dysfunction in newborns. Newborn illness score systems with a focus on acute physiology like the SNAPPE or CRIB scores have generally placed much emphasis on risk assessment on the first postnatal day and have not been validated for use thereafter.[13] Sepsis-specific scores like the NEOMOD have been tested and modified for performance but are infrequently used and reported in the literature.[14] Pediatric organ dysfunction scores have shown increased mortality for the same scoring range in newborns and older infants, but newborns showed different primary organ involvement with acute illness.[15] The neonatal sequential organ failure assessment score (nSOFA) uses parameters of respiratory support, oxygenation, cardiovascular support, and platelet count.[16] When applied to preterm infants with late-onset sepsis, the maximum nSOFA score at 6 hours after the clinical diagnosis was established showed a strong association with mortality and thus could be proposed as an operational definition of organ dysfunction in this population.[17] Although the nSOFA score has an excellent diagnostic accuracy for mortality due to sepsis and all-cause mortality, its validity is highly dependent on local guidelines for the use of systemic steroids and criteria for intubation. A subsequent study revealed a wide variance between centers in all-cause mortality of preterm infants with high nSOFA scores, questioning its generalizability.[18]

*Finally*, the ability of translating the "Sepsis-3" definition and its tools to the newborn population also depends on data regarding sepsis mortality. However, wide ranges of mortality have been reported for sepsis

in newborns. Recent epidemiological data from research networks showed that mortality from early-onset sepsis (EOS) and late-onset sepsis (LOS) in very-low-birth-weight (VLBW) infants was in the range of 12–33% and 4–16%, respectively.[3,5,19,20] Risk factors for developing EOS and LOS in VLBW infants have been amply described, but limited data are available on risk factors for death due to sepsis. Decreasing gestational age, birth weight, and the presence of gram-negative organisms are associated with higher risk of mortality due to sepsis, but more data are required to better understand the risk factors involved in the progression from sepsis to septic shock.[21,22] The "Sepsis-3" definition defines septic shock as a circulatory and cellular/metabolic abnormality profound enough to increase mortality. In the neonatal literature and for logistical reasons septic shock is often defined as sepsis with hypotension requiring catecholamines. The rate of infants who progress from sepsis to septic shock is reported as 26% for EOS and between 9 and 22% for LOS and depends on the infective agent.[3,23,24] Most studies did not report case fatality separately for infants with septic shock. Gorantiwar et al. presented a decade's worth of data from a single center in Australia and reported a mortality rate of 40% in preterm infants with LOS *and* sepsis shock, suggesting that mortality is significantly higher when shock develops. In a yet unpublished retrospective study of similar design our group found a 33% mortality rate for preterm infants with EOS. However, the rate increased to 67% in infants who progressed from sepsis to septic shock.[25] Data on other aspects commonly associated with mortality, such as lactate levels and lactate clearance, fluid load, fluid accumulation, and multi-organ dysfunction, have been sparsely reported for the neonatal population with sepsis.[26,27] Phenotyping of neonatal sepsis might be possible with accurate documentation of timing of treatments, biochemical profiles, or reporting of progression from sepsis to septic shock.[28,29] In summary, there is a need to develop a better understanding of the clinical, phenotypic, and even genotypic factors associated with progression from sepsis to septic shock in neonates with EOS or LOS, before we can appropriately define mortality and/or describe the appropriateness and efficacy of treatment modalities and short- and long-term outcome in the affected patient population.

# Hemodynamics in Sepsis

## HEMODYNAMIC RESPONSE TO SEPSIS IN ADULTS

Sepsis starts with a disruption of the finely tuned immunological balance of inflammation and anti-inflammation, driving the vascular response to sepsis and leading to ineffective tissue oxygen delivery and extraction due to inappropriate vasodilatation with preserved or increased cardiac output. This hemodynamic effect, along with the infectious agent– and/or its toxin-induced direct cellular metabolic derangement, is also responsible for the loss of the cellular oxygen demand-delivery coupling. The increased capillary leak and generalized vasodilation result in an absolute and relative decrease in effective circulating blood volume, respectively, resulting in load-driven alterations in left and right ventricular function. The decrease in effective circulating blood volume leads to a decrease in circulatory filling pressure (reduced preload), while the inappropriate vasodilatation with low systemic vascular resistance leads to reduced afterload and lower organ perfusion pressure.[30]

Although the cascade of inflammatory activation often leads to cardiomyocyte dysfunction with reduced myocardial contractility, the initial phase of sepsis is often described as a patient with high systemic blood flow, i.e., warm shock.[31] The pressure-volume curve of the heart is operating at lower pressures but with larger stroke volume due to the vascular changes affecting the preload and afterload (Figure 21.1). The interaction between the left ventricle and the arterial system, known as ventriculo-arterial coupling (VAC), is one of the main determinants of cardiovascular function during sepsis and can be used as a marker to target treatment in adults.[32,33]

Other hemodynamic changes during sepsis in adults include diastolic dysfunction, combined left and right ventricular dysfunction, and pulmonary hypertension. Of note, pulmonary hypertension and, in particular, diastolic dysfunction are significantly associated with increased mortality and warrant thorough investigation in the newborn population as well.[34-37] In summary, vasodilatation and the associated relative hypovolemia and altered ventriculo-arterial interactions are key

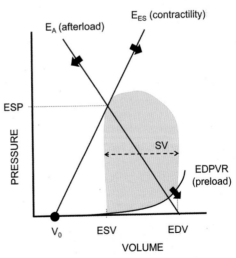

**Fig. 21.1 Schematic representation of ventriculo-arterial coupling (*VAC*) in sepsis.** Schematic representation of VAC in the pressure-volume loop of the left ventricle (*LV*). Left ventricular elastance (*EES*) is the slope of the line running from end-systolic pressure (*ESP*) to V₀ (•) and represents contractility. Arterial elastance (*EA*) is the slope of the line running from the end-diastolic volume (*EDV*) to the ESP and represents the afterload at end-systole. Filling of the left ventricle is depicted with the end-diastolic pressure-volume relationship (EDPVR) and represents preload at end-diastole. The area in grey depicts cardiac stroke work. During the initial phase of sepsis, the LV operates at lower ESP and lower preload, resulting in a higher stroke volume.

hemodynamic factors in adults with sepsis, especially in the early phases. Stroke volume is initially high, and cardiac dysfunction (systolic and/or diastolic) and pulmonary hypertension are common.

## HEMODYNAMIC RESPONSE TO SEPSIS IN NEWBORNS

Although early studies in newborns showed that septic shock presented with reduced cardiac output and increased systemic and pulmonary vascular resistance (i.e., "cold shock" with PPHN), the generalizability of this concept has been challenged by the findings of recent studies. Acknowledging the maturational differences of the structure of all three layers of the vascular wall and the myocardium, newborns, and especially preterm infants, are often in a pro-inflammatory state following delivery. Accordingly, one might expect to see the same hemodynamic pathophysiology in sepsis as found in adults. Kharrat et al. recently summarized papers describing hemodynamics in the neonatal population with sepsis.[38] The definition of sepsis

varied per studies and some even included infants without a positive blood culture. In addition, most studies were performed in countries with a relatively high perinatal sepsis rate and the oldest study reviewed was published only 12 years ago. An additional confounding variable to be considered when interpreting the findings was the fact that the timing of the ultrasound assessment after the onset of sepsis was not always reported. A summary of the 14 studies included is presented in Table 21.1.[25,39-50] Systemic blood flow was predominantly high, assessed through either ventricular output (the Vti method) or volumetric changes (ejection fraction, stroke volume). Most studies commented on the presence of cardiac dysfunction (systolic, diastolic, and/or global cardiac function) and some reported the presence of pulmonary hypertension. Overall, the findings support the assumption that newborns with sepsis mostly present with a hemodynamic pattern characteristic of warm shock and added cardiac dysfunction and pulmonary

**TABLE 21.1  Selected Hemodynamic Data in Preterm and Term Infants with Sepsis. Systemic Blood Flow Represents the Interaction Between the Ventricle and the Arterial System and was Assessed with the VTI Method (Right or Left Ventricular Output, Superior Vena Cava Flow) and/or M Mode or Method of Disks (Stroke Volume, Ejection Fraction). Cardiac Dysfunction was Assessed with Tissue Doppler Velocities, Myocardial Performance Index, E:A Ratio, E:e´ Ratio, and/or Tricuspid Annular Plane Systolic or Tricuspid Regurgitation Jet Velocity. Los, Late-Onset Sepsis; EOS, Early-onset Sepsis. For Further Details Regarding Assessment of Cardiovascular Dysfunction Utilizing Ultrasound, See Chapter 10**

| Study | Year | n With Sepsis | Gestational Age | Time | High Systemic Blood Flow | Cardiac Dysfunction | Mortality |
|---|---|---|---|---|---|---|---|
| de Waal et al. | 2010 | 20 | Preterm | LOS | + | | 25% |
| Abdel-Hady et al. | 2012 | 20 | Term | LOS | + | + | 30% |
| Tomerak et al. | 2012 | 30 | Preterm/term | LOS | + | + | 37% |
| Saini et al. | 2014 | 52 | Preterm | LOS | + | + | 81% |
| Ramadhina et al. | 2015 | 30 | Preterm | EOS/LOS | + | + | 13% |
| Awany et al. | 2016 | 40 | Term | LOS | | + | |
| Alzahrani et al. | 2017 | 30 | Term | | + | + | |
| Deshpande et al. | 2017 | 31 | Preterm/term | LOS | + | | |
| Fahmey et al. | 2020 | 50 | Term | EOS/LOS | = | + | 38% |
| Saini et al. | 2021 | 23 | Preterm | EOS | + | | 70% |
| Yengkhom et al. | 2021 | 67 | Preterm | LOS | +/= | + | |
| Deshpande et al. | 2021 | 33 | Preterm/term | LOS | | + | |
| Gorantiwar et al. | 2021 | 25 | Preterm | LOS | + | | 40% |
| Johnston et al. | 2022 | 27 | Preterm | EOS | +/= | + | 33% |

hypertension, similar to that found in adults. Only two studies presented longitudinal hemodynamic data in their cohorts. de Waal et al. described a cohort of 20 preterm infants (median gestational age of 27 weeks) with LOS and at least two clinical signs of cardiovascular compromise. The infants underwent echocardiography within 2 hours of presentation, which was then repeated every 12 hours until clinical recovery or death.[39] All infants presented with high systemic blood flow, suggesting warm shock as the main hemodynamic presentation. Of note is that early and remarkable hemodynamic changes took place in the infants who died; specifically, their hemodynamic presentation changed from warm shock to cold shock, with a sudden decline in cardiac output and increase in systemic vascular resistance. This change occurred in most cases within 12 hours of the onset of sepsis, also highlighting the importance of serial echocardiographic assessments of infants with septic shock. Only systemic blood flow was assessed in this study, so no data could be presented on cardiac dysfunction or pulmonary hypertension.

Saini et al. investigated 52 preterm infants (median gestational age of 31 weeks) with fluid-resistant septic shock around postnatal day 4.[42] Half of the patients presented with a positive blood culture, while the others had clinically diagnosed sepsis. Nine infants (17%) sustained blood pressure in the normal range, while the others (83%) progressed to septic shock. Both left and right ventricular output were elevated at baseline, and the patients had a shortened isovolumetric relaxation time suggesting diastolic dysfunction. Repeat measurements 30–40 minutes after start of dopamine or dobutamine showed surprisingly little changes in hemodynamics. This may relate either to the repeat measures being taken too early, lack of appropriate titration of the drugs, incorrect physiologic choice (vasopressor preferred circulation, e.g., epinephrine, norepinephrine, or vasopressin), or – although less likely – shock had already progressed to the point of no return in this cohort, with a very high (81%) mortality rate.

In summary, more data and trials with a more sophisticated design are needed. In the ideal study all infants with suspected sepsis would be followed using a comprehensive hemodynamic monitoring system and interrogated with echocardiography and vascular ultrasound every 6 hours until resolution of the clinical signs that triggered the sepsis evaluation. In addition, careful volume resuscitation and testing for the use of the most appropriate vasopressor-inotrope are needed.[51] Data collection should include clinical and hemodynamic response to each treatment in culture-positive patients. This huge undertaking is unlikely to occur as it is likely impossible to be performed as a single-center study. An alternative approach would be development of an international multicenter patient registry until a well-designed and executed multicenter study is performed.

## Management of Neonates With Bacterial Sepsis

The basic steps in the management of neonates with bacterial sepsis include clinical recognition, microbiological evaluation, starting appropriately chosen antibiotics tailored according to the sensitivity of the identified bacterium, and appropriate cardiorespiratory support if the condition progresses to septic shock. Sepsis can present with a wide range of clinical signs and symptoms.[7] Increased respiratory support, apnea, lethargy, the presence of a central line, and capillary refill time >2 seconds were common in preterm infants with LOS.[52] Yet these clinical signs and presentations were not universally seen. Due to the non-specific nature of clinical signs and symptoms at the start of sepsis, it can take the clinical team 5–12 hours to recognize the need for antibiotics.[24] Various biomarkers are available to help the clinician (C-reactive protein, procalcitonin, cell surface antigens, cytokines), but their diagnostic advantage in preterm infants with LOS remains controversial.[53,54] The utilization of heart rate characteristic monitoring tools has shown promise in earlier detection and initiation of antibiotic treatment, resulting in decreased sepsis-associated mortality in preterm neonates.[53]

Blood pressure, and especially changes in blood pressure, can be used to signify the start of the uncompensated phase of septic shock. Zhu et al. described blood pressure changes in a cohort of 147 preterm infants with culture-positive (excluding coagulase-negative staphylococcus) LOS. They found a decrease (up to 47%) in mean blood pressure in the infants who died and minimal blood pressure changes in the infants who survived. Changes were seen in both systolic (−24%) and diastolic (−21%) blood pressure in the first 12 hours after sepsis work-up was completed. Importantly, baseline mean blood pressure value in mmHg before the infants became sick, as well as shortly thereafter, was well above the number of corrected gestational age in weeks. Thus the fairly controversial rule-of-thumb of utilizing the mean blood pressure value in mmHg less than gestational age in weeks to initiate treatment should not be used in neonates with LOS, but rather use the change in blood pressure.

Bedside cardiac ultrasound is the most commonly used hemodynamic monitoring tool in sepsis in adults, children, and newborns, as it can provide information on systemic blood flow (high or low), myocardial function, and the presence of intracardiac and extracardiac shunts and acute pulmonary hypertension. Furthermore, with longitudinal scans, the clinical team can diagnose hemodynamic changes from warm shock to cold shock at an early stage and modify the treatment from vasopressor-inotrope to inotrope/lusitrope treatment where needed.[55] Training, guidelines, and accreditation of bedside clinicians using this monitoring technique are available, as the value of bedside neonatal cardiac ultrasound has been increasingly recognized in the last decade.[56]

As described earlier, the hemodynamic abnormalities in septic shock are inappropriate and dysregulated vasodilation, a relative and, later in the course, also an absolute decrease in circulating blood volume and increased systemic blood flow with impaired myocardial contractility. Fluid therapy is used as a first step to counteract this pathophysiology. However, the efficacy of fluid resuscitation in septic shock has been called into question.[57] We have shown that a single fluid bolus in infants with septic shock had variable responses, as was found in other studies.[24,42,48] This can be explained by the fact that at high pre-existing preload, a fluid bolus will not increase stroke volume but might cause harm due to accumulation of fluid in the lungs. (Figure 21.2)

There are strong and consistent negative associations between fluid overload and adverse clinical outcomes in the pediatric and adult literature, so new strategies are needed to determine fluid responsiveness in neonates with sepsis or suspected hypovolemia.

Ultrasound-guided fluid management in neonatology is still in its developmental phase. Accordingly, several ultrasound measures have been explored. The

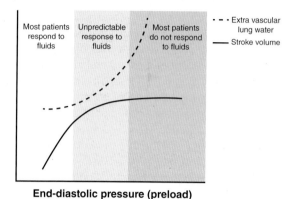

**Fig. 21.2 Schematic representation of the relationship between preload, stroke volume, and extravascular lung water.** Schematic representation of the relationship between preload and stroke volume (Frank-Starling curve, *solid line*) and between preload and extravascular lung water (Marik-Phillips curve, *dotted line*). At low preload, most patients will respond to a fluid bolus with increased stroke volume. Further up the curve, fluid responsiveness becomes unpredictable. Finally, at high pre-existing preload, stroke volume will not increase with a fluid bolus and excessive volume may cause harm. Sepsis shifts the Marik-Phillips curve to the left and fluid will earlier accumulate in the lungs as extravascular lung water.

diameter of the inferior vena cava and its collapsibility can be used to estimate preload but, like in adults, this has a limited ability to identify the magnitude of changes in right atrial pressure.[58-60] Furthermore, interpretation during spontaneous breathing with mechanical ventilation and especially during high-frequency ventilation is limited, as positive pressure ventilation increases the size of the right atrium and inferior vena cava even without increased right atrial pressure.[61] Assessing fluid responsiveness, i.e., the increase in preload with a fluid bolus, is probably more helpful in sepsis compared to estimating preload. Stroke volume or peak velocity of the aortic blood flow can be measured before and after a fluid bolus in spontaneous breathing infants (with or without mechanical ventilation), as well as peak velocity variation within the respiratory cycle in infants on mechanical ventilation without spontaneous breaths. A more than 15% increase in peak velocity after a fluid bolus or over 15% difference in peak velocity with respiratory variation is generally considered to be indicative of fluid responsiveness in adults and children. A further fluid bolus can be given in fluid-responsive patients, and this process is then repeated until no fluid response is seen.[62,63] We have adopted an approach for preterm infants with suspected LOS by giving a fluid bolus of 5 mL/kg over 5 minutes and found that in most cases no further fluid response was seen after just one bolus (de Waal, unpublished data) (Figure 21.3).

The second step in hemodynamic septic shock management is the start of cardiovascular medications. In warm shock (high blood flow on cardiac ultrasound) a vasopressor-inotrope (norepinephrine, epinephrine or dopamine) or vasopressor (vasopressin) is preferred. In cold shock (low blood flow) an inotrope (dobutamine, epinephrine) or lusitrope (milrinone) is the first line of management. In patients with cold shock receiving inotrope/lusitrope treatment a low-dose vasopressor/inotrope may be added to keep perfusion pressure in the perceived normal range. There are no randomized trials specifically

addressing the treatment of newborns with septic shock, and there is minimal observational data on treatment of septic shock in this population available. Historically, dopamine is most used in the neonatal setting. Dopamine has several unwanted effects including significantly increasing pulmonary vascular resistance; hence many clinicians have now replaced dopamine with norepinephrine as vasopressor/inotrope in sepsis as many patients also have sepsis-associated pulmonary hypertension. Vasopressin can be used as first line of treatment in neonates with warm shock without evidence of myocardial compromise, i.e., with relative normal cardiac contractility. In cold shock the use of dopamine is associated with increased mortality when compared to epinephrine. Choice of medications, their mechanisms of action, and dosing for neonates in shock, including septic shock, is discussed in Chapter 5.

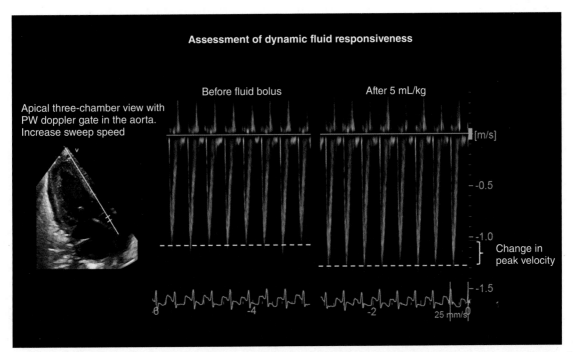

**Fig. 21.3 Assessment of dynamic fluid responsiveness with transthoracic echocardiography.** Assessment of dynamic fluid responsiveness with transthoracic echocardiography. The apical three-chamber view with pulse wave Doppler and increased sweep speed was used to acquire peak aortic blood flow velocity. A 5 mL/kg fluid bolus was administered in 5 minutes, and the measurement was repeated. If the peak velocity increased by 15% or more, the infant was classified as fluid responsive. This process was repeated until the peak velocity no longer increased by >15%. It is important to avoid making clinical changes during the assessment and preferred to perform the study during steady or minimal spontaneous respiratory effort. In mechanically ventilated infants without spontaneous breathing, assessment of the variation in peak velocity within the respiratory cycle can also predict fluid responsiveness. Note the reduced respiratory variation in peak velocity after the fluid bolus in this example.

A new concept has emerged in adult medicine related to the timing and initiation of vasopressor treatment in warm shock. The time lapse between obtaining a blood culture and giving the first fluid bolus and/or starting a vasopressor/inotrope can be substantial. In our cohort 3 and 12 hours usually passed after the blood culture had been obtained and the first fluid bolus and vasopressor/inotrope treatment was initiated respectively. By this time, significant systemic hypotension had developed in most cases.[24,27] Stabilizing systemic blood pressure as soon as possible is of utmost importance to re-establish organ perfusion pressure in patients with septic shock. We speculate that earlier initiation of fluid and especially vasopressor/inotrope might improve outcomes. Findings of observational and randomized studies in adults showed that early norepinephrine use can prevent severe prolonged hypotension, increase cardiac output, improve microcirculation, prevent fluid overload, and improve clinical outcomes including mortality.[64-66] Ranjit et al. concluded that norepinephrine may be considered the first-choice vasopressor/inotrope treatment after careful administration of fluid bolus(es) in vasodilatory shock in a pediatric intensive care setting.[67] Starting norepinephrine in a neonatal setting comes with several hurdles, including the need for a central line and an arterial line placement, but in a disease where mortality easily reaches 40% or more, this clinical approach warrants attention. One needs to be aware of the potentially enhanced alpha-adrenergic effects of norepinephrine in the neonatal patient population, even in sepsis, despite the expected critical illness associated with adrenergic receptor downregulation. Therefore starting the drug at low doses and carefully titrating it to the target hemodynamic response is of paramount importance in an attempt to avoid significant swings in arterial blood pressure and thus cerebral blood flow. This is especially important in preterm neonates with sepsis who are at high risk for intracranial complications.

In neonates with septic shock and evidence for pulmonary hypertension, inhaled nitric oxide administration, along with provision of appropriate respiratory support, is of great importance. Desphande et al. found that in 33 mostly preterm neonates with culture-proven LOS almost half of the patients had evidence of pulmonary hypertension on echocardiography. Most patients had a mild (pulmonary artery pressure at 36–45 mmHg) or moderate (pulmonary artery pressure at 46–55 mmHg) elevation in pulmonary artery pressures. However, 3% developed severe pulmonary hypertension. Using the principles of cardiovascular physiology (pressure = flow × resistance + left atrium pressure), the elevated pulmonary arterial pressure in EOS can be a mix of raised pulmonary vascular resistance and increased left atrial pressure. However, in neonates with LOS it might be predominantly driven by increased pulmonary blood flow and raised left atrial pressure. This may explain why inhaled nitric oxide can be effective in EOS but not in preterm infants with LOS.[68,69] Inhaled nitric oxide is currently the treatment of choice in sepsis-induced pulmonary hypertension during the transitional period, especially when pulmonary blood flow is low, but caution must be applied when using iNO in patients with LOS and high pulmonary blood flow. An echocardiographic study examining the status of the systemic and pulmonary circulation should always be performed if administration of inhaled nitric oxide is entertained, especially in neonates with LOS.

## Hemodynamic Compromise in Viral Infections

Not much is known about the hemodynamic effects of (fulminant) viral infections in newborns. The condition is rare, and a recent overview of case reports of neonatal enterovirus infections described respiratory symptoms, poor perfusion, arrhythmias, and cardiogenic shock as clinical characteristics.[70] Findings on cardiac ultrasound include left ventricular dysfunction or bi-ventricular dysfunction, with or without cardiac remodeling, suggestive of myocarditis. Progression to cardiac collapse is possible with need for ECMO therapy. Unlike bacterial shock with cardiac involvement, recovery of cardiac function can be prolonged (typically 6 months is expected) and the differential diagnosis includes a myocardial infarct, another rare diagnosis in newborns.[71] In adults speckle tracking imaging can help differentiate between global or segmental myocardial dysfunction and thus the diagnosis of myocarditis versus myocardial infarction.[72] Immunomodulation with IVIG can help improve cardiac function in children, but its effect in newborns is less promising unless given early in the disease process.[73] Further treatments should focus on heart failure during the recovery phase.

## Hypovolemic Shock in Neonates

True hypovolemic shock is rare in neonates and is mostly seen early after birth. Causes include peripartum bleeding from the fetal side of the placenta, feto-maternal hemorrhage, feto-fetal hemorrhage, or a postpartum hemorrhage of the neonate. With ongoing bleeding, the autonomic sympathetic system is activated with inhibition of the parasympathetic system leading to increased heart rate, cardiac contractility, and arterial and venous tone. Blood volume from the non-vital organs and the venous system will be recruited to help preserve blood flow to the brain, heart, and adrenal glands. The decreased perfusion pressure and increased sympathetic tone-associated epinephrine and norepinephrine release activates the renin-angiotensin-aldosterone system in the juxtaglomerular apparatus of the kidneys. If the bleeding cannot be stopped, severe hypovolemia will finally lead to severe acidosis and myocardial dysfunction, organ failure, and death.

The optimal approach to hemorrhagic hypovolemia in neonates has not been well studied. Most of what is known about physiology and management has been extrapolated from animal and adult data. First-line resuscitation of hemorrhagic shock starts with volume, and the limited available clinical evidence would suggest isotonic saline.[74] A second step would be replacing the type of volume lost, in this case, blood. Neonates with severe bleeding or anemia may require a massive transfusion with blood products. The definition of a massive transfusion in pediatric patients varies. According to one suggestion, a transfusion of >50% of total blood volume in 3 hours, replacement of >100% total blood volume in 24 hours, or transfusion to replace an ongoing blood loss of >10% of the total blood volume per minute would qualify as a massive transfusion.[75] Most massive transfusion protocols for adults employ a physiological 1:1:1 transfusion ratio of red blood cells, plasma, and platelets, but there is limited neonatal data to make recommendations. Importantly, the availability of an institute-specific massive transfusion protocol has the potential to improve outcomes. Neonates in particular are at risk for metabolic derangements and/or coagulopathy after a massive transfusion and should be monitored closely for hypocalcemia, hypomagnesemia, and fluctuations in potassium, glucose, and pH, as well as for signs of oozing or bleeding.[76]

There has been a paradigm shift in the approach toward major bleeding in adults. Observational data showed that aggressive fluid resuscitation increases the risk of mortality, probably by promoting dilution coagulopathy and delayed clot formation due, at least in part, to increased arterial pressure. The current recommended approach is low-volume fluid resuscitation while maintaining an acceptable level of tissue perfusion with permissive hypotension.[77] Noradrenaline is the first line of vasopressor-inotrope used in adults as it induces significant venoconstriction, particularly at the level of the splanchnic circulation. This increases the pressure in capacitance vessels and actively shifts splanchnic blood volume to the systemic circulation. The effect of dopamine on the splanchnic circulation is complex, and the information in the literature is controversial. However, in newborn animal models dopamine was the most effective vasoactive drug in increasing gut blood flow and might be an alternative to norepinephrine.[78] The effect of catecholamines administered during hypovolemia depends, to a large extent, on the volume of blood in the splanchnic reservoir. When hypovolemia is severe, the physiologic responses to maintain volume and pressure may have already emptied the splanchnic reservoir. The use of exogenous catecholamines should thus be limited to a brief period and should not be viewed as a substitute for the immediate replacement of blood volume.

The use of vasopressin may be beneficial in the management of fluid- and transfusion-resistant uncontrolled bleeding. Vasopressin does not only restore the depleted intrinsic vasopressin production but seems to be also more effective in maintaining vascular tone compared to catecholamines in a hypovolemic and acidotic environment.[79] However, data on the addition of terlipressin during hypovolemia and resuscitation is inconsistent.[80,81]

Finally, the effects of physiologic cord clamping on hemodynamic transition and the volume status of the neonate are discussed in Chapter 6.

## Summary

Sepsis remains a common complication in neonates and is associated with significant morbidity and mortality, especially in very preterm infants. Approximately 1 in 5 preterm infants who develop sepsis will progress to septic shock, which increases mortality threefold. Consensus is needed for a clinically appropriate definition of sepsis and septic shock in neonates, and an adapted version of the adult Sepsis-3 definition and the nSOFA score would be good starting points. More data is needed on risk factors for progression to septic shock, what hemodynamics are most prevalent, and how hemodynamic support treatments can reduce mortality. Data thus far has shown that understanding the systemic and pulmonary blood flows can assist in determining first-line hemodynamic treatment. Further data is needed on ultrasound-guided fluid management and earlier initiation of appropriate vasopressor-inotrope treatment in neonatal septic shock.

## REFERENCES

1. Stoll BJ, Hansen N. Infections in VLBW infants: studies from the NICHD Neonatal Research Network. *Semin Perinatol.* 2003;27(4):293-301. doi:10.1016/s0146-0005(03)00046-6.
2. Braye K, Foureur M, de Waal K, Jones M, Putt E, Ferguson J. Epidemiology of neonatal early-onset sepsis in a geographically diverse Australian health district 2006-2016. *PLoS One.* 2019;14(4):e0214298. doi:10.1371/journal.pone.0214298.
3. Giannoni E, Agyeman PKA, Stocker M, et al. Neonatal sepsis of early onset, and hospital-acquired and community-acquired late onset: a prospective population-based cohort study. *J Pediatr.* 2018;201:106-114.e4. doi:10.1016/j.jpeds.2018.05.048.
4. Greenberg RG, Kandefer S, Do BT, et al. Late-onset sepsis in extremely premature infants: 2000-2011. *Pediatr Infect Dis J.* 2017;36(8):774-779. doi:10.1097/inf.0000000000001570.
5. Köstlin-Gille N, Härtel C, Haug C, et al. Epidemiology of early and late onset neonatal sepsis in very low birthweight infants: data from the German neonatal network. *Pediatr Infect Dis J.* 2021;40(3):255-259. doi:10.1097/inf.0000000000002976.
6. McGovern M, Giannoni E, Kuester H, et al. Challenges in developing a consensus definition of neonatal sepsis. *Pediatr Res.* 2020;88(1):14-26. doi:10.1038/s41390-020-0785-x.
7. Hayes R, Hartnett J, Semova G, et al., Infection, Inflammation, Immunology and Immunisation (I4) section of the European Society for Paediatric Research (ESPR). Neonatal sepsis definitions from randomised clinical trials. *Pediatr Res.* 2023;93(5):1141-1148.
8. Goldstein B, Giroir B, Randolph A. International pediatric sepsis consensus conference: definitions for sepsis and organ dysfunction in pediatrics. *Pediatr Crit Care Med.* 2005;6(1):2-8. doi:10.1097/01.pcc.0000149131.72248.e6.
9. Wynn JL, Wong HR, Shanley TP, Bizzarro MJ, Saiman L, Polin RA. Time for a neonatal-specific consensus definition for sepsis. *Pediatr Crit Care Med.* 2014;15(6):523-528. doi:10.1097/pcc.0000000000000157.
10. Singer M, Deutschman CS, Seymour CW, et al. The third international consensus definitions for sepsis and septic shock (Sepsis–3). *JAMA.* 2016;315(8):801-810. doi:10.1001/jama.2016.0287.
11. Clapp DW. Developmental regulation of the immune system. *Semin Perinatol.* 2006;30(2):69-72. doi:10.1053/j.semperi.2006.02.004.
12. Collins A, Weitkamp JH, Wynn JL. Why are preterm newborns at increased risk of infection? *Arch Dis Child Fetal Neonatal Ed.* 2018;103(4):F391-F394. doi:10.1136/archdischild-2017-313595.
13. Tarnow-Mordi WO. What is the role of neonatal organ dysfunction and illness severity scores in therapeutic studies in sepsis? *Pediatr Crit Care Med.* 2005;6(suppl 3):S135-S137. doi:10.1097/01.pcc.0000161581.42668.5e.
14. Cetinkaya M, Köksal N, Özkan H. A new scoring system for evaluation of multiple organ dysfunction syndrome in premature infants. *Am J Crit Care.* 2012;21(5):328-337. doi:10.4037/ajcc2012312.
15. Bestati N, Leteurtre S, Duhamel A, et al. Differences in organ dysfunctions between neonates and older children: a prospective, observational, multicenter study. *Crit Care.* 2010;14(6):R202. doi:10.1186/cc9323.
16. Wynn JL, Polin RA. A neonatal sequential organ failure assessment score predicts mortality to late-onset sepsis in preterm very low birth weight infants. *Pediatr Res.* 2020;88(1):85-90. doi:10.1038/s41390-019-0517-2.
17. Fleiss N, Coggins SA, Lewis AN, et al. Evaluation of the neonatal sequential organ failure assessment and mortality risk in preterm infants with late-onset infection. *JAMA Netw Open.* 2021;4(2):e2036518. doi:10.1001/jamanetworkopen.2020.36518.
18. Wynn JL, Mayampurath A, Carey K, Slattery S, Andrews B, Sanchez-Pinto LN. Multicenter validation of the neonatal sequential organ failure assessment score for prognosis in the neonatal intensive care unit. *J Pediatr.* 2021;236:297-300.e1. doi:10.1016/j.jpeds.2021.05.037.
19. Flannery DD, Edwards EM, Puopolo KM, Horbar JD. Early-onset sepsis among very preterm infants. *Pediatrics.* 2021;148(4):e2021052456. doi:10.1542/peds.2021-052456.
20. Lee SM, Chang M, Kim KS. Blood culture proven early onset sepsis and late onset sepsis in very-low-birth-weight infants in Korea. *J Korean Med Sci.* 2015;30(suppl 1):S67-S74. doi:10.3346/jkms.2015.30.S1.S67.
21. Hornik CP, Fort P, Clark RH, et al. Early and late onset sepsis in very-low-birth-weight infants from a large group of neonatal intensive care units. *Early Hum Dev.* 2012;88(suppl 2):S69-S74. doi:10.1016/s0378-3782(12)70019-1.
22. Lim WH, Lien R, Huang YC, et al. Prevalence and pathogen distribution of neonatal sepsis among very-low-birth-weight infants. *Pediatr Neonatol.* 2012;53(4):228-234. doi:10.1016/j.pedneo.2012.06.003.
23. Berardi A, Sforza F, Baroni L, et al. Epidemiology and complications of late-onset sepsis: an Italian area-based study. *PLoS One.* 2019;14(11):e0225407. doi:10.1371/journal.pone.0225407.
24. Gorantiwar S, de Waal K. Progression from sepsis to septic shock and time to treatments in preterm infants with late-onset sepsis. *J Paediatr Child Health.* 2021;57(12):1905-1911. doi:10.1111/jpc.15606.

25. Johnston N, de Waal K. Clinical and hemodynamic characteristics of preterm infants with early onset sepsis. Presented at Children's Hospital Showcase; Newcastle, Australia; 2022.

26. Baczynski M, Kharrat A, Zhu F, et al. Bloodstream infections in preterm neonates and mortality-associated risk factors. *J Pediatr.* 2021;237:206-212.e1. doi:10.1016/j.jpeds.2021.06.031.

27. Zhu F, Baczynski M, Kharrat A, Ye XY, Weisz D, Jain A. Blood pressure, organ dysfunction, and mortality in preterm neonates with late-onset sepsis. *Pediatr Res.* 2022;92(2):498-504. doi:10.1038/s41390-021-01768-0.

28. Sanchez-Pinto LN, Stroup EK, Pendergrast T, Pinto N, Luo Y. Derivation and validation of novel phenotypes of multiple organ dysfunction syndrome in critically ill children. *JAMA Netw Open.* 2020;3(8):e209271. doi:10.1001/jamanetworkopen.2020.9271.

29. Gordon SM, Srinivasan L, Taylor DM, et al. Derivation of a metabolic signature associated with bacterial meningitis in infants. *Pediatr Res.* 2020;88(2):184-191. doi:10.1038/s41390-020-0816-7.

30. Casserly B, Read R, Levy MM. Hemodynamic monitoring in sepsis. *Crit Care Clin.* 2009;25(4):803-823, ix. doi:10.1016/j.ccc.2009.08.006.

31. Greer J. Pathophysiology of cardiovascular dysfunction in sepsis. *BJA Education.* 2015;15(6):316-321. doi:10.1093/bjaceaccp/mkv003.

32. Guarracino F, Bertini P, Pinsky MR. Cardiovascular determinants of resuscitation from sepsis and septic shock. *Crit Care.* 2019;23(1):118. doi:10.1186/s13054-019-2414-9.

33. Pinsky MR, Guarracino F. How to assess ventriculoarterial coupling in sepsis. *Curr Opin Crit Care.* 2020;26(3):313-318. doi:10.1097/mcc.0000000000000721.

34. Sanfilippo F, Corredor C, Fletcher N, et al. Diastolic dysfunction and mortality in septic patients: a systematic review and meta-analysis. *Intensive Care Med.* 2015;41(6):1004-1013. doi:10.1007/s00134-015-3748-7.

35. Sanfilippo F, Corredor C, Fletcher N, et al. Left ventricular systolic function evaluated by strain echocardiography and relationship with mortality in patients with severe sepsis or septic shock: a systematic review and meta-analysis. *Crit Care.* 2018;22(1):183. doi:10.1186/s13054-018-2113-y.

36. Vallabhajosyula S, Gillespie SM, Barbara DW, Anavekar NS, Pulido JN. Impact of new-onset left ventricular dysfunction on outcomes in mechanically ventilated patients with severe sepsis and septic shock. *J Intensive Care Med.* 2018;33(12):680-686. doi:10.1177/0885066616684774.

37. Vallabhajosyula S, Geske JB, Kumar M, Kashyap R, Kashani K, Jentzer JC. Doppler-defined pulmonary hypertension in sepsis and septic shock. *J Crit Care.* 2019;50:201-206. doi:10.1016/j.jcrc.2018.12.008.

38. Kharrat A, Jain A. Hemodynamic dysfunction in neonatal sepsis. *Pediatr Res.* 2022;91(2):413-424. doi:10.1038/s41390-021-01855-2.

39. de Waal K, Evans N. Hemodynamics in preterm infants with late-onset sepsis. *J Pediatr.* 2010;156(6):918-922.e1. doi:10.1016/j.jpeds.2009.12.026.

40. Abdel-Hady HE, Matter MK, El-Arman MM. Myocardial dysfunction in neonatal sepsis: a tissue Doppler imaging study. *Pediatr Crit Care Med.* 2012;13(3):318-323. doi:10.1097/PCC.0b013e3182257b6b.

41. Tomerak RH, El-Badawy AA, Hussein G, Kamel NR, Razak AR. Echocardiogram done early in neonatal sepsis: what does it add? *J Investig Med.* 2012;60(4):680-684. doi:10.2310/JIM.0b013e318249fc95.

42. Saini SS, Kumar P, Kumar RM. Hemodynamic changes in preterm neonates with septic shock: a prospective observational study*. *Pediatr Crit Care Med.* 2014;15(5):443-450. doi:10.1097/pcc.0000000000000115.

43. Ramadhina N, Sukardi R, Advani N, Rohsiswatmo R, Putra ST, Djer MM. Ventricular function and high-sensitivity cardiac troponin T in preterm infants with neonatal sepsis. *Paediatr Indones.* 2015;55(4):5.

44. Awany M, Tolba O, Al-Biltagi M, Al-Asy H, El-Mahdy H. Cardiac functions by tissue doppler and speckle tracking echocardiography in neonatal sepsis and its correlation with sepsis markers and cardiac troponin-T. *J Pediatr Neonatal Care.* 2016;5(3):6.

45. Alzahrani A. Cardiac function affection in infants with neonatal sepsis. *J Clin Trial.* 2017;7(5):4.

46. Deshpande S, Suryawanshi P, Chaudhary N, Maheshwari R. Cardiac output in late onset neonatal sepsis. *J Clin Diagnostic Res.* 2017;11(11):4.

47. Fahmey SS, Hodeib M, Refaat K, Mohammed W. Evaluation of myocardial function in neonatal sepsis using tissue Doppler imaging. *J Matern Fetal Neonatal Med.* 2020;33(22):3752-3756. doi:10.1080/14767058.2019.1583739.

48. Saini SS, Sundaram V, Kumar P, Rohit MK. Functional echocardiographic preload markers in neonatal septic shock. *J Matern Fetal Neonatal Med.* 2022;35(25):6815-6822. doi:10.1080/14767058.2021.1926447.

49. Yengkhom R, Suryawanshi P, Murugkar R, Gupta B, Deshpande S, Singh Y. Point of care neonatal ultrasound in late-onset neonatal sepsis. *J Neonatol.* 2021;35(2):4.

50. Deshpande S, Suryawanshi P, Holkar S, et al. Pulmonary hypertension in late onset neonatal sepsis using functional echocardiography: a prospective study. *J Ultrasound.* 2022;25(2):233-239. doi:10.1007/s40477-021-00590-y.

51. Azhibekov T, Soleymani S, Lee BH, Noori S, Seri I. Hemodynamic monitoring of the critically ill neonate: an eye on the future. *Semin Fetal Neonatal Med.* 2015;20(4):246-254. doi:10.1016/j.siny.2015.03.003.

52. Bekhof J, Reitsma JB, Kok JH, Van Straaten IH. Clinical signs to identify late-onset sepsis in preterm infants. *Eur J Pediatr.* 2013;172(4):501-508. doi:10.1007/s00431-012-1910-6.

53. Eschborn S, Weitkamp JH. Procalcitonin versus C-reactive protein: review of kinetics and performance for diagnosis of neonatal sepsis. *J Perinatol.* 2019;39(7):893-903. doi:10.1038/s41372-019-0363-4.

54. Sullivan BA, Fairchild KD. Predictive monitoring for sepsis and necrotizing enterocolitis to prevent shock. *Semin Fetal Neonatal Med.* 2015;20(4):255-261. doi:10.1016/j.siny.2015.03.006.

55. de Boode WP. Individualized hemodynamic management in newborns. *Front Pediatr.* 2020;8:580470. doi:10.3389/fped.2020.580470.

56. Boyd S, Kluckow M. Point of care ultrasound in the neonatal unit: applications, training and accreditation. *Early Hum Dev.* 2019;138:104847. doi:10.1016/j.earlhumdev.2019.104847.

57. Marik PE, Byrne L, van Haren F. Fluid resuscitation in sepsis: the great 30 mL per kg hoax. *J Thorac Dis.* 2020;12(suppl 1):S37-S47. doi:10.21037/jtd.2019.12.84.

58. Beigel R, Cercek B, Luo H, Siegel RJ. Noninvasive evaluation of right atrial pressure. *J Am Soc Echocardiogr.* 2013;26(9):1033-1042. doi:10.1016/j.echo.2013.06.004.

59. Sato Y, Kawataki M, Hirakawa A, et al. The diameter of the inferior vena cava provides a noninvasive way of calculating central venous pressure in neonates. *Acta Paediatr.* 2013;102(6):e241-e246. doi:10.1111/apa.12247.

60. Patel SG, Woolman P, Li L, Craft M, Danford DA, Kutty S. Relation of right atrial volume, systemic venous dimensions, and flow patterns to right atrial pressure in infants and children. *Am J Cardiol.* 2017;119(9):1473-1478. doi:10.1016/j.amjcard.2017.01.013.

61. Hruda J, Rothuis EG, van Elburg RM, Sobotka-Plojhar MA, Fetter WP. Echocardiographic assessment of preload conditions does not help at the neonatal intensive care unit. *Am J Perinatol.* 2003;20(6):297-303. doi:10.1055/s-2003-42771.

62. Desai N, Garry D. Assessing dynamic fluid-responsiveness using transthoracic echocardiography in intensive care. *BJA Educ.* 2018;18(7):218-226. doi:10.1016/j.bjae.2018.03.005.

63. Desgranges FP, Desebbe O, Pereira de Souza Neto E, Raphael D, Chassard D. Respiratory variation in aortic blood flow peak velocity to predict fluid responsiveness in mechanically ventilated children: a systematic review and meta-analysis. *Paediatr Anaesth.* 2016;26(1):37-47. doi:10.1111/pan.12803.

64. Scheeren TWL, Bakker J, Kaufmann T, et al. Current use of inotropes in circulatory shock. *Ann Intensive Care.* 2021;11(1):21. doi:10.1186/s13613-021-00806-8.

65. Hamzaoui O, Shi R. Early norepinephrine use in septic shock. *J Thorac Dis.* 2020;12(suppl 1):S72-S77. doi:10.21037/jtd.2019.12.50.

66. Permpikul C, Tongyoo S, Viarasilpa T, Trainarongsakul T, Chakorn T, Udompanturak S. Early Use of Norepinephrine in Septic Shock Resuscitation (CENSER). A randomized trial. *Am J Respir Crit Care Med.* 2019;199(9):1097-1105. doi:10.1164/rccm.201806-1034OC.

67. Ranjit S, Natraj R, Kandath SK, Kissoon N, Ramakrishnan B, Marik PE. Early norepinephrine decreases fluid and ventilatory requirements in pediatric vasodilatory septic shock. *Indian J Crit Care Med.* 2016;20(10):561-569. doi:10.4103/0972-5229.192036.

68. Mercier JC, Lacaze T, Storme L, Rozé JC, Dinh-Xuan AT, Dehan M. Disease-related response to inhaled nitric oxide in newborns with severe hypoxaemic respiratory failure. French Paediatric Study Group of Inhaled NO. *Eur J Pediatr.* 1998;157(9):747-752. doi:10.1007/s004310050928.

69. Baczynski M, Ginty S, Weisz DE, et al. Short-term and long-term outcomes of preterm neonates with acute severe pulmonary hypertension following rescue treatment with inhaled nitric oxide. *Arch Dis Child Fetal Neonatal Ed.* 2017;102(6):F508-F514. doi:10.1136/archdischild-2016-312409.

70. Zhang M, Wang H, Tang J, et al. Clinical characteristics of severe neonatal enterovirus infection: a systematic review. *BMC Pediatr.* 2021;21(1):127. doi:10.1186/s12887-021-02599-y.

71. de Vetten L, Bergman KA, Elzenga NJ, van Melle JP, Timmer A, Bartelds B. Neonatal myocardial infarction or myocarditis? *Pediatr Cardiol.* 2011;32(4):492-497. doi:10.1007/s00246-010-9865-8.

72. Fung G, Luo H, Qiu Y, Yang D, McManus B. Myocarditis. *Circ Res.* 2016;118(3):496-514. doi:10.1161/circresaha.115.306573.

73. Chuang YY, Huang YC. Enteroviral infection in neonates. *J Microbiol Immunol Infect.* 2019;52(6):851-857. doi:10.1016/j.jmii.2019.08.018.

74. Keir AK, Karam O, Hodyl N, et al. International, multicentre, observational study of fluid bolus therapy in neonates. *J Paediatr Child Health.* 2019;55(6):632-639. doi:10.1111/jpc.14260.

75. Diab YA, Wong EC, Luban NL. Massive transfusion in children and neonates. *Br J Haematol.* 2013;161(1):15-26. doi:10.1111/bjh.12247.

76. Goel R, Josephson CD. Recent advances in transfusions in neonates/infants. *F1000Res.* 2018;7:F1000. doi:10.12688/f1000research.13979.1.

77. Spahn DR, Bouillon B, Cerny V, et al. The European guideline on management of major bleeding and coagulopathy following trauma: fifth edition. *Crit Care.* 2019;23(1):98. doi:10.1186/s13054-019-2347-3.

78. Nachar RA, Booth EA, Friedlich P, et al. Dose-dependent hemodynamic and metabolic effects of vasoactive medications in normotensive, anesthetized neonatal piglets. *Pediatr Res.* 2011;70(5):473-479. doi:10.1203/PDR.0b013e31822e178e.

79. Anand T, Skinner R. Arginine vasopressin: the future of pressure-support resuscitation in hemorrhagic shock. *J Surg Res.* 2012;178(1):321-329. doi:10.1016/j.jss.2012.02.062.

80. Urbano J, González R, López J, et al. Comparison of normal saline, hypertonic saline albumin and terlipressin plus hypertonic saline albumin in an infant animal model of hypovolemic shock. *PLoS One.* 2015;10(3):e0121678. doi:10.1371/journal.pone.0121678.

81. Gil-Anton J, Mielgo VE, Rey-Santano C, et al. Addition of terlipressin to initial volume resuscitation in a pediatric model of hemorrhagic shock improves hemodynamics and cerebral perfusion. *PLoS One.* 2020;15(7):e0235084. doi:10.1371/journal.pone.0235084.

# Chapter 22

# Hemodynamics of the Neonate Following Perinatal Hypoxic-Ischemia and the Effects of Therapeutic Hypothermia

Regan Giesinger[†], Samir Gupta,* and Yogen Singh

## Introduction

Globally, neonatal encephalopathy precipitated by perinatal hypoxia-ischemia remains a common cause of brain injury. The incidence varies from 1 to 3 per 1000 to up to 25 per 1000 in developed and developing countries, respectively.[1] Therapeutic hypothermia has been demonstrated to improve both survival and neurological morbidity[2]; however, there remains a significant burden of mortality and long-term neurological sequelae among survivors.[3-7] Birth asphyxia, defined as a lack of blood flow or gas exchange to or from the fetus in the period immediately before, during, or after delivery,[8] accounts for approximately 1 million deaths per year,[6,7] making it a leading cause of infant mortality. In addition, the approximately 1 million children who survive birth asphyxia yearly do so with chronic neuro-developmental morbidities, including cerebral palsy and intellectual and learning disabilities.[9] Although the cellular and metabolic contributors to brain injury are complex, abnormal cerebral blood flow is an essential contributor to brain injury by this mechanism (Figure 22.1). In this chapter we will review the interrelationship between the cardiovascular system and the brain, the impact of therapeutic hypothermia on hemodynamics, and management considerations specific to this patient population.

## Fetal Cardiovascular Adaptation to Hypoxia-Ischemia

The primary determinants of fetal cerebral blood flow are cardiac output, arterial oxygen content, and blood pressure, as has been shown in a fetal lamb model.[10,11] Over the range of cerebral autoregulation, the fetal lamb maintains a constant cerebral blood flow despite a wide range of experimentally varied cardiac output (200–700 mL/min/kg).[10] Adaptation to low cardiac output involves a complex mechanism that begins with a surge of catecholamines and an associated increase in systemic blood pressure.[11,12] This increase in blood pressure is associated with a redistribution of systemic blood flow to the brain.[10] Simultaneously, there is an increase in pulmonary vascular resistance which acts to divert more blood from the lungs to essential organs, including the brain, coronary circulation, and adrenal glands. This is facilitated by an increase in right ventricular afterload, which diverts a greater proportion of placental flow from the right to left atrium, and therefore the brain and coronary circulation.[13-15] When these and other compensatory mechanisms fail, brain injury may occur.

## The Role of Cerebral Autoregulation

In healthy infants cerebral blood flow (CBF) remains constant over a relatively wide range of changes in systemic mean arterial blood pressure. In animal models the fetal autoregulatory curve differs from that of the

---

*Division Chief Neonatology, Sidra Medicine, AL Luqta Street, Education City North Campus, Qatar Foundation, PO Box 26999-Doha, Qatar; Email: sgupta@sidra.org

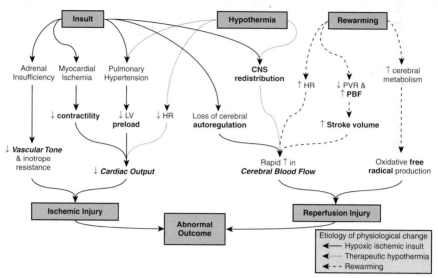

**Fig. 22.1** **The interrelationship between contributors to ischemia resulting from the initial insult, therapeutic hypothermia, and reperfusion injury on rewarming.** Both ischemia and reperfusion may impact the degree of brain injury by modifying cerebral blood flow and oxygen delivery, particularly in the presence of impaired cerebral autoregulation. Resumption of cellular activity after transient suppression is a putative source of potentially damaging oxidative radicals. *HR*, heart rate; *LV*, left ventricle; *PBF*, pulmonary blood flow; *PVR*, pulmonary vascular resistance; *RV*, right ventricle.[100]

adult.[16,17] The curve is narrower, particularly at the upper elbow of the curve, and importantly, the normal mean arterial blood pressure in the less mature animal is only marginally above the lower elbow of the autoregulatory curve. In human preterm and term infants the mean blood pressure value at the lower elbow of the autoregulatory curve, or the blood pressure threshold associated with neuronal dysfunction and then tissue injury are unknown.[18]

Autoregulation is disrupted by hypoxia, hyperoxia, hypocarbia, hypercarbia, and/or acidosis.[19] Severe disruption of autoregulation results in a pressure-passive cerebral circulation. In animal models the role of asphyxia-associated impaired CBF autoregulation in the pathogenesis of ischemic cerebral injury has been clearly described. If the same is true for humans, the clinical implications are of importance, as hypotension and decreased cardiac output result in decreases in CBF and thus secondary energy failure and neuronal injury.[20] As expected, this process is more pronounced in the more vulnerable regions of the brain, such as the parasagittal cortex or periventricular white matter.[17] However, in humans this link between cerebral ischemia and cardiovascular dysfunction is not yet clear, and thus it is not known whether appropriate cardiovascular support

and stabilization of CBF improve outcomes in asphyxiated infants.

## Cardiovascular Effects of Hypoxemia-Ischemia

The effects of HI insult on the cardiovascular system are complex, and it is important to understand the principles of developmental cardiovascular physiology and pathophysiology in these sick infants.

### IMPACT ON THE MYOCARDIUM

Both the primary insult and the ongoing redistribution of blood flow can lead to reduced myocardial perfusion, potentially resulting in myocardial ischemia, especially in the sub-endocardial tissue and papillary muscles. Echocardiography studies have consistently demonstrated differences in various measures of wventricular function between patients with HIE and healthy controls, particularly using advanced measurement techniques such as tissue Doppler imaging and speckle tracking.[21,22] Structural and metabolic characteristics of the neonatal myocardium confer a greater vulnerability to the effects of hypoxia-ischemia. Specifically, the antioxidant capacity remains underdeveloped at the time of birth, despite upregulation toward late gestation,[23] which primes the neonate for oxidative stress during postnatal resuscitation. In addition, ischemia interrupts the normal transition of cardiomyocytes from a glycolytic metabolic pathway utilizing lactic acid to the oxidation of fatty acids.[24] This transition is required for efficient energy utilization and adaptation to the oxygen-rich environment. Thus its interruption may confer added vulnerability. Myocardial ischemia may be further complicated by diminished preload, asphyxia-induced autonomic dysfunction, and/or vasoplegia.[25] Adequate coronary perfusion, which is often compromised due to hypotension following asphyxia, is critical for optimal cardiac function and may represent an additional metabolic disadvantage. Decreased myocardial contractility may also occur secondary to acidosis and hypoxia.[3,26-28]

Approximately 25% of neonates with myocardial necrosis on autopsy have a clinical history of asphyxia, making it the most common single cause of perinatal myocardial ischemia.[29,30] Transient myocardial ischemia, as diagnosed by electrocardiogram and other non-specific findings, occurs in two-thirds of asphyxiated infants.[26] Clinical features may or may not be externally evident[26]; however, both electrocardiography changes and abnormalities of cardiac enzymes have been linked to the severity of neurological outcomes.[3,26,31-33] This supports the importance of monitoring for transient myocardial ischemia, even among so-called "stable" patients. These patients are often normotensive until they are no longer able to compensate and may present with acute cardiovascular collapse. Several factors point to the central role of myocardial ischemia in the pathogenesis of shock among HIE patients. These include higher cardiac troponin T compared to healthy controls[32] and the association of elevation in this enzyme with low cardiac output and impaired coronary perfusion.[33] That the burden of brain injury is greater among patients with concurrent cardiac dysfunction has also been suggested using echocardiography,[34] and as modern evaluative tools become increasingly sophisticated, new associations will become relevant. This includes a recently reported relationship between right ventricular function at 24 hours postnatal age and both short- (i.e., death or abnormal brain magnetic resonance imaging)[35] and long-term (survival with neurological impairment)[36] outcomes.

## IMPACT ON PULMONARY VASCULAR RESISTANCE AND PULMONARY BLOOD FLOW

Although there are important effects of perinatal hypoxia-ischemia in the systemic circulation, the pulmonary vascular impact merits specific consideration. As previously mentioned, part of the fetal adaptive response to impaired CBF includes a redirection of pulmonary blood flow into essential systemic circulatory beds. This, coupled with the fact that neonatal resuscitation efforts are less effective at establishing functional residual capacity than a spontaneously breathing neonate, places the fetus with HIE at risk of failed postnatal transition. Additionally, hypoxia and acidosis are potent pulmonary vasoconstrictors. Finally, neonates with a hypoxic-ischemic injury often have associated morbidities such as meconium aspiration syndrome, lung parenchymal disease, and/or sepsis. These conditions negatively impact lung compliance and/or alter circulating inflammatory mediators, which may independently have a negative impact on cardiac function (Figure 22.2). Pulmonary vasoconstriction has several important downstream effects. *First*, it produces an afterload stress on the right ventricle, which may exacerbate pre-existing myocardial dysfunction. *Second*, heterometric adaptation, or dilation, of the right ventricle and septal flattening negatively impact left ventricular function due to ventricular-ventricular interaction. *Finally*, impaired pulmonary blood flow occurs due to high resistance, compromised right ventricular systolic function, and systemic recirculation of right ventricular output via right-to-left ductal shunt when the ductus is open. This results in compromised left ventricular filling, low left ventricular output, and therefore further impairment of coronary perfusion pressure.

## IMPACT OF ELEVATED PULMONARY ARTERY PRESSURE ON CARDIAC ADAPTATION

Although both ventricles may be affected by perinatal ischemic injury, the right ventricle is particularly vulnerable. There are several putative mechanisms for this. *First*, the right ventricle plays a dominant role in both fetal and transitional circulation. This results in a higher metabolic demand and therefore a greater requirement for perfusion, oxygen, and other substrate. *Second*, the conformation of the right ventricle produces a greater circumferential area-to-radius ratio, which results in a greater degree of wall stress for any given afterload compared to the left. *Third*, when pulmonary artery

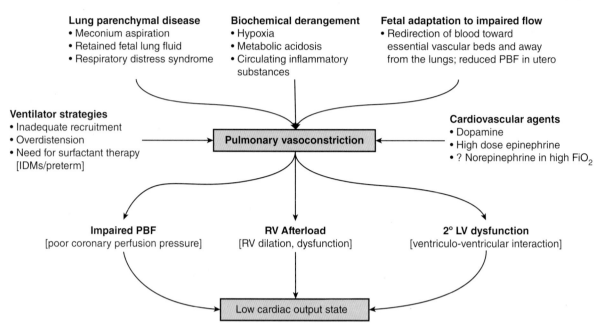

**Fig. 22.2 Biological and therapeutic contributors to pulmonary vasoconstriction and their downstream consequences.** Pulmonary vasoconstriction leads to low pulmonary blood flow and therefore reduced filling of the aortic sinus, which, in turn, contributes to impaired coronary blood flow. Right ventricular afterload, due to pulmonary vasoconstriction, causes dilation and progressive RV dysfunction, which further exacerbates the problem with low pulmonary blood flow. Finally, abnormal RV conformation leads to secondary LV dysfunction by compressing the LV cavity and impacting both systolic and diastolic performance. All of these combine to create a progressive low cardiac output state if not promptly treated. *IDM*, infant of diabetic mother; *PBF*, pulmonary blood flow; *RV*, right ventricle.

pressure is high due to elevated pulmonary vascular resistance, the right ventricle may fail to empty normally at the end of systole, leading to increased end-systolic ventricular pressure. When added to diastolic inflow, this gradually increases right ventricular and atrial cavity pressures and reduces the gradient to flow from the aortic root. Aortic root pressure may also be low due to impaired cardiac output. The combination of high right heart pressures and low aortic root pressure leads to impaired coronary blood flow to the right ventricle and impairs the balance of supply and demand of substrate for myocardial metabolism.

## ROLE OF ADRENAL INSUFFICIENCY

Perinatal hypoxic-ischemic injury is associated with adrenal insufficiency with or without adrenal hemorrhage. (See Chapter 23 for further details.) In a lamb asphyxia model both ACTH and cortisol are secreted during an asphyxial event as part of fetal compensation. Within 3–5 minutes of interrupted fetal blood flow, fetal adaptation begins to fail and even essential organs have compromised perfusion.[37] ACTH levels

return to normal with restoration of normal blood flow; however, serum cortisol may remain elevated for hours to days.[38,39] Human neonates demonstrate biochemical changes suggesting a shift in adrenal production toward the glucocorticoid pathway.[40] Although these studies suggest an intact stress response following asphyxia, a piglet model suggests a delayed response to ACTH stimulation despite high cortisol levels.[41] Adrenal hemorrhage and associated adrenal insufficiency have been associated with perinatal hypoxia-ischemia and may be a source of anemia.[42] The mechanism is thought to relate to a physical vulnerability to compression/trauma in the setting of a difficult delivery.[43] Centralized redistribution of blood to the adrenal glands may confer further vulnerability due to the need to rapidly accommodate a larger blood volume, and the risk of vascular congestion and endothelial damage may also contribute.[43] Most adrenal hemorrhages are right sided (70%), with bilateral disease in 10%.[43] Bilateral hemorrhages may particularly be associated with adrenal insufficiency. Even in the absence of adrenal insufficiency, postnatal glucocorticoid supplementation may improve dependence on vasoactive medications[44] and may play theoretically an important role in capillary leak.

## Cardiovascular Effects of Therapeutic Hypothermia/Rewarming

In the care of neonates with hypoxic-ischemic encephalopathy, it is essential to remember that therapeutic hypothermia is a post-resuscitation intervention. This is because reduction in core temperature results in predictable cardiovascular changes, which may have deleterious consequences. Both severe and moderate hypothermia have been associated with cardiovascular changes in animal models. In a neonatal lamb model a core temperature of 30°C was associated with a 50% increase in PAP, and even a temperature of 34–35°C has been linked to reduced cardiac output and left ventricular performance in neonatal piglets.[45,46] This increase in PVR at lower body temperature may relate to increased vascular tone, circulating catecholamines, and/or the rheological properties of blood, which increases in viscosity at lower temperatures.[47,48] Human clinical studies suggest that some neonates experience an increase in requirement for oxygen[49] and echocardiography evidence of an increase in PVR[50] during TH, which are reversed by rewarming. An increase in clinical pulmonary hypertension was not evident from pooled randomized trial analyses[51]; however, quantification of pulmonary artery pressure was not systematically performed and neonates with hypoxemic respiratory failure were largely excluded in these large studies.[2,52] These factors make it difficult to generalize trial results to the broader population as it relates to cardiovascular presentation.

Reduced cardiac output, which occurs in the context of sinus bradycardia due to prolonged ventricular repolarization, has been clearly shown.[53,54] It is typical for stroke volume to be relatively preserved.[55–57] Among patients with an otherwise healthy cardiovascular system, however, this is matched by lower metabolic rate and typically does not independently result in impaired tissue oxygen perfusion.[53] Lower superior vena cava (SVC) flow overall[53] with a redistribution of total systemic flow to the central nervous system, as reflected by a greater ratio of SVC:LVO, has been shown to be associated with abnormal MRI.[56] This may reflect abnormal cerebral autoregulation; however, clinical relevance

needs further exploration. It is reasonable to speculate, however, that relative bradycardia may be either protective or a response to lower cardiac metabolism and may be associated with the lower cardiac troponin I seen following TH in both neonatal animal and human studies.[58,59] Given that these changes reverse with rewarming, it may be meritorious to closely monitor systemic and cerebral hemodynamics as temperature is increased, particularly to avoid iatrogenic hypertension. In addition, rewarming affects metabolism and clearance of drugs, including cardiovascular medications.[60]

### POTENTIAL CARDIOPROTECTIVE ROLE OF THERAPEUTIC HYPOTHERMIA

The potential cardioprotective effects of therapeutic hypothermia are important to consider, in addition to its neuroprotective effects. In models of adult ischemic heart disease lower metabolism with preservation of energy has been suggested and there is some literature to support positive inotropy[61]. The isolated ischemic dog heart model has lower ATP consumption at 32–34°C and both rabbit and pig models demonstrate smaller infarct size and lesser post-ischemic LV dysfunction.[62–64] TH may also be used in the postoperative management of pediatric congenital heart disease.[65] Limitation of reactive oxygen species, inflammation modulation, and the possible mitigation of mitochondrial damage are other proposed mechanisms.[66] Given the differences in cardiac metabolism, myocardial composition, and mechanism of injury, neonatal data specific to HIE patients should be considered.

## Cardiovascular Assessment of Neonates With Hypoxic-Ischemic Encephalopathy

Cardiovascular dysfunction among patients with perinatal hypoxic-ischemic injury primarily presents with two phenotypes: with and without hypoxemic respiratory failure. Chapters 25–27 extensively review the evaluation and management of neonatal acute pulmonary hypertension; however, there are several nuances that are specific to the patient with HIE undergoing TH, which will be covered in the following sections. Neonates with HIE have a high intrinsic risk for neurological events, and seizures may present with isolated vital sign abnormalities. Thus brain electrical monitoring using either an amplitude-integrated or full montage electroencephalogram is highly recommended for all neonates, particularly those experiencing abnormal vital signs (e.g., hypoxemia, hypo/hypertension).

## CLINICAL EVALUATION

While heart rate may be useful in the pre-cooling phase, hypoxia-ischemia often leads to compensatory tachycardia or, in more advanced cases, bradycardia related to autonomic dysregulation. Due to the decreased metabolic demand and the direct effects of cooling itself, therapeutic hypothermia is typically associated with a decrease in heart rate in all infants such that a heart rate in the "normal range" may reflect an attempt at compensation for low cardiac output. The use of blood pressure as a metric of cardiovascular health may also be challenging. Therapeutic hypothermia is associated with a reduction in cardiac output.[35,67] The low systolic blood pressure, which is associated with reduced cardiac output, may therefore be adaptive. However, among patients with heart dysfunction, low systolic pressure may be an important early sign of cardiac compromise. At the same time, peripheral vasoconstriction may elevate diastolic pressure and mask low mean arterial pressure due to its greater temporal contribution to each beat of the cardiac cycle.[53] This is further emphasized by the lack of consensus on a definition of "normal blood pressure"[68] in this population and recent evidence that significant heart dysfunction may be present in spite of what would typically be considered normal by most clinicians.[69,70] While arterial pressure is an important trending tool, over-reliance may lead to over or under-treatment. As a practical matter, invasive blood pressure measurements are encouraged over noninvasive assessments, due to their suggested higher accuracy in critically ill patients (Chapter 3). If low systolic blood pressure is recorded, it should be correlated with the requirements for oxygen. Normal oxygenation with low systolic blood pressure primarily reflects cardiac systolic dysfunction. On the contrary, the finding of low systolic blood pressure and impaired oxygenation should alert the clinician to evaluate for acute pulmonary hypertension with or without heart dysfunction. Persistent low diastolic arterial pressure should alert the clinician to the potential for vasodilator shock, which may be due to sepsis, adrenal insufficiency, or poorly cleared vasodilating medications (e.g., morphine, milrinone).[71,72]

To add to the complexity, hypoxic-ischemic injury is often associated with multiorgan dysfunction.[4] This makes clinical evaluation of circulatory adequacy using end-organ performance as a surrogate marker challenging for many patients. Both lactate and base deficit have been shown to reflect the severity of the initial insult,[73] and rate of lactate decline has limited data showing no association with cardiac output as measured by noninvasive cardiac output monitoring.[55] Urine output, similarly, is commonly difficult to interpret. Up to 70% of neonates with hypoxic-ischemic injury are reported to experience acute kidney injury, of which approximately 30% may be classified as severe.[4,74] In addition, even among patients with healthy kidneys, therapeutic hypothermia is associated with a temperature-dependent reduction in urine output in a human adult model.[75] All things taken together, while clinical assessment is essential and patients should be considered their own controls, the early use of alternative monitoring techniques such as targeted neonatal echocardiography should be considered where feasible.

## ROLE OF ECHOCARDIOGRAPHY

Quantitative echocardiography with objective measures of both left and right ventricular function is recommended early in the disease course. Cardiac dysfunction is common and may be sub-clinical initially, presenting late with an unexpected acute decompensation. This is particularly true among patients with a low burden of associated lung disease. Pulmonary vasoconstriction due to failed transition, therapeutic hypothermia, or a combination of both is common, and in the absence of lung disease the pneumoconstriction occurs in the lungs to ensure that perfused areas are aerated maximally.[76] Thus substantial pulmonary vasoconstriction, and therefore high right ventricular afterload, may be present in the absence of clinically apparent pulmonary hypertension (Figure 22.3). Although many centers have integrated echocardiography into the assessment of neonates with HIE either as a screening or diagnostic tool, the majority report using objective measures of LV but not RV performance and CO remains uncommonly reported except in centers with access to TnECHO.[68]

Targeted neonatal echocardiography may be particularly valuable for integrating ambient physiology

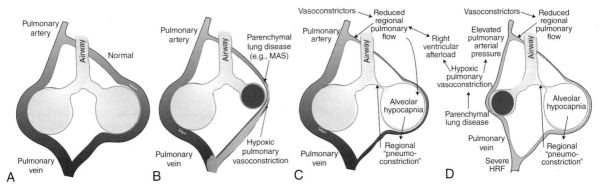

**Fig. 22.3 Ventilation perfusion changes associated with hypoxic-ischemic encephalopathy (*HIE*).** In normal patients and with mild HIE without lung disease, alveolar ventilation and pulmonary arterial pressure are normal with optimal lung perfusion (A). In parenchymal lung disease, such as meconium aspiration syndrome (*MAS*), asymmetric lung disease leads to alveolar hypoxia and constriction of adjacent pulmonary vasculature by hypoxic pulmonary vasoconstriction (B). In severe HIE without lung disease systemic vasoconstrictors (intrinsic such as endothelin and thromboxane or iatrogenic such as dopamine and therapeutic hypothermia) can lead to impaired regional pulmonary blood flow. Impaired gas exchange leads to alveolar hypocapnia and regional "pneumoconstriction" (C). A combination of severe HIE and parenchymal lung disease can lead to severe elevation of pulmonary arterial pressure and right ventricular afterload, causing dysfunction (D).[101]

into the clinical context and for serial evaluation over time and following intervention. Direct and indirect measures may be used to quantify the relative contribution of right and left ventricular dysfunction, objectify the systemic and pulmonary blood flow, and evaluate the role of shunts. Because of the potential complexity of the physiology in this patient population, it is essential that echocardiography be comprehensive and standardized and performed by trained experts. A detailed review of the evaluation of pulmonary hypertension/right heart performance may be found in Chapter 27; however, our minimum suggested components for a complete evaluation of the patient who has experienced hypoxic-ischemic injury may be found in Table 22.1. Given the prominence of RV disease and the association of abnormal function at 24 hours postnatal age with adverse outcome,[35] quantitative assessment of RV performance (Chapter 10) including TAPSE (Figure 22.4) and fractional area change (FAC) (Figure 22.5) should be measured.[35]

While it is the norm for patients to experience deranged pulmonary and/or systemic blood flow following a hypoxic-ischemic event, it is essential to remember that anatomic heart disease may concurrently be present. It is often assumed that placental failure or critical delivery events are the underlying cause of hypoxic-ischemic encephalopathy; however, postnatal cardiovascular collapse due to anatomic or severe

functional heart disease may rarely present in a similar fashion. All echocardiography performed in this patient population should collect images of sufficient quality to rule out critical anatomic heart disease, including anomalous pulmonary venous drainage, arch abnormalities, and other duct-dependent systemic and pulmonary blood flow disorders.

## Approach to Management of Cardiovascular Dysfunction

There are several overlapping themes with the management of acute pulmonary hypertension for patients with and without hypoxic-ischemic injury. The use of inhaled nitric oxide, optimization of lung parenchymal disease, and sedation may be important therapeutic modalities regardless of the presence of comorbid hypoxia-ischemia. There are, however, several important considerations that are unique to the infant with multiorgan dysfunction undergoing therapeutic hypothermia. These span the following categories: *first*, the approach to respiratory management; *second*, the nonhypoxic HIE patient; and *third*, pharmacological considerations.

### RESPIRATORY MANAGEMENT CONSIDERATIONS

Because many neonates with HIE do not have concurrent lung disease and instead fail to transition due to

**TABLE 22.1    Suggested Measurements for All Patients with Hypoxic-Ischemic Injury Undergoing Therapeutic Hypothermia[103]**

| Hemodynamic (Physiologic) Parameter | Clinical Utility | Advantages | Limitations |
|---|---|---|---|
| **Measures of Right Ventricular Function** | | | |
| RVO[104] Right ventricular output; mL/min/kg | Surrogate marker of pulmonary blood flow and RV function | Published normal data which is useful to objectify pulmonary blood flow. Serial evaluations can greatly aid in following disease progression | • Dependent on Doppler angle, position of sample volume, and precise measurement • May over-estimate if dilated RVOT (e.g., prolonged PH) |
| RV-FAC[102] Right ventricular fractional area change | Global measure of RV function | Published normal data for the transitional period. Ejection fraction assessment of RV | • Needs high-quality imaging for endocardial definition • Influenced by septal motion in apical four-chamber |
| TAPSE[105] Tricuspid annular plane systolic excursion; mm | Measure of longitudinal RV contractility | Published normal data • Feasible and easy to measure • Independent of shunts and heart rate | • Angle dependent and assumes no regional wall motion defects • Exaggerated by severe TR |
| **Measures of Pulmonary Pressure** | | | |
| **Physiologic Parameter** | **Clinical Utility** | **Advantages** | **Limitations** |
| RVSP[105] Right ventricular systolic pressure; mmHg; utilizes tricuspid regurgitant jet | Direct measure of RV systolic pressure | Validated against invasive cardiac catheterization | • Tricuspid valve damage may cause TR with normal RVSP • Angle dependent and requires complete envelope • Absence of TR is common despite severe aPH |
| Subjective assessment of septal curvature | Used to judge relative RV vs. LV pressure | Easy to measure; universally available | Subjective and low inter-rater reliability, particularly for mild-moderate disease |
| Eccentricity index[106] | | Reproducible, validated in neonates | Relative to LVSP, therefore may underestimate RVSP in systemic hypertension |
| PAP:AOP[105] Ratio of pulmonary artery to aortic pressure; utilizes Doppler of the ductus arteriosus | Direct comparison of pulmonary to systemic pressure | Useful to qualify RVSP as sub-systemic, supra-systemic, or equal systemic | • Not possible without PDA and may be unreliable if PDA is restrictive, tortuous, or S shaped • pH varies with ambient conditions (e.g., $SpO_2$, pH) |
| **Measures of Pulmonary Vascular Resistance** | | | |
| **Physiologic Parameter** | **Clinical Utility** | **Advantages** | **Limitations** |
| PAAT[107] Pulmonary artery acceleration time, ms | May be used to serially monitor changes in PVR with time or treatment | Easy to measure | Underestimated by RV dysfunction and unreliable in the presence of shunts. Single time-point measures. Limited evidence in neonates |
| RVET:PAAT[107] PAAT indexed to RV ejection time, ms Mid-systolic notching of PA Doppler waveform[108] | | | |

| TABLE 22.1 Suggested Measurements for All Patients with Hypoxic-Ischemic Injury Undergoing Therapeutic Hypothermia (Continued) | | | |
|---|---|---|---|
| **Measures of Systemic Blood Flow** | | | |
| **Physiologic Parameter** | **Clinical Utility** | **Advantages** | **Limitations** |
| LVO[104] Left ventricular output; mL/min/kg | Surrogate marker of systemic blood flow and LV function | Published normal data Serial evaluations can greatly aid in following disease progression | Dependent on Doppler angle and position of sample volume PDA shunt dependent |

*aPH*, acute pulmonary hypertension; *LV*, left ventricle; *LVSP*, left ventricular systolic pressure; *PDA*, patent ductus arteriosus; *PH*, pulmonary hypertension; *PVR*, pulmonary vascular resistance; *RV*, right ventricle; *RVOT*, right ventricular outflow tract; *SpO2*, oxygen saturation; *TR*, tricuspid regurgitant.

In Addition to these Functional Measures, all Echocardiograms should have Imaging of Sufficient Quality to Rule Out Anatomic Congenital Heart Disease.

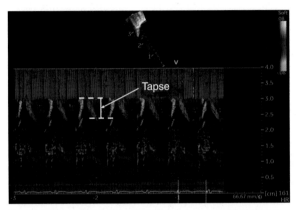

**Fig. 22.4 Tricuspid annulus plane systolic excursion (*TAPSE*) measurement.** With or without the tissue Doppler overlay, TAPSE is measured via M-mode with the cursor aligned from the apex of the RV to the lateral tricuspid annulus in a right ventricle–centered apical four-chamber view. TAPSE is a measure of displacement and is most reported in centimeters or millimeters. Normative data for term infants has been published.[102] (Data from Jain A, Mohamed A, El-Khuffash A, et al. A comprehensive echocardiographic protocol for assessing neonatal right ventricular dimensions and function in the transitional period: normative data and z scores. *J Am Soc Echocardiogr.* 2014;27(12):1293-1304. doi:10.1016/j.echo.2014.08.018.)

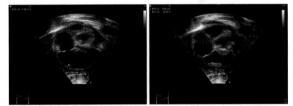

**Fig. 22.5 Right ventricular fractional area change (*RV-FAC*) measurement.** RV-FAC is a surrogate measurement for the RV ejection fraction that cannot be measured using echocardiography due to conformation of the RV. In a right ventricular three-chamber view in which the tricuspid, aorta, and pulmonary artery can all be seen opening, the maximal size in diastole is traced. The minimal size at the end of myocardial systole is then traced for the same beat. The RV-FAC is then calculated according to the following formula:

$$RV - FAC = \frac{(RV\ diastolic\ area - RV\ systolic\ area)}{RV\ diastolic\ area}$$

A change of at least 0.35 is typically considered normal.

acidosis and central apnea, it is essential for clinicians to remember the U-shaped relationship between pulmonary vascular resistance and lung volumes (Figure 22.6). At low lung volumes, below functional residual capacity, pulmonary vascular resistance is high due to a combination of hypoxic pulmonary vasoconstriction and tortuosity of small vessels which may collapse.[77] At high tidal volume, alveolar distension leads to impaired flow through the adjacent capillary bed and again produces a sharp increase in pulmonary vascular resistance.[78] The use of "open lung" ventilation strategy,[79] common in preterm respiratory distress syndrome management, presumes that the flow component of ventilation to perfusion matching is intact and should not be extrapolated to this patient population. Instead, optimal distending pressure should be evaluated using an assessment of lung compliance, being careful not to assume that a high oxygen requirement is equivalent to atelectasis.

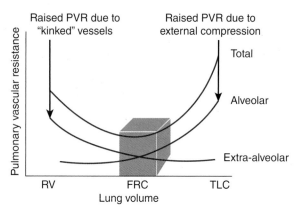

**Fig. 22.6 Relationship between lung volume and pulmonary vascular resistance.** At lung volumes below functional residual capacity, extra-alveolar pulmonary vessels are tortuous and therefore resistance to flow is high. Above functional residual capacity, as total lung volume is reached, alveolar vessels become compressed by airspace over-distension. The balance of optimal pulmonary vascular resistance exists when lung volume is within the central range described in this figure.[103]

Similarly, adjudication of the adequacy of carbon dioxide clearance requires alternative considerations in this population. Carbon dioxide and oxygen measurements may be impacted for a variety of reasons that do not relate to iatrogenic over-ventilation, including low metabolism/production, high ventilation to perfusion ratio, and low temperature. Thus care should be taken to evaluate other aspects of respiratory function such as neurological and cardiovascular status prior to extubation of patients with hypoxic-ischemic injury. *First*, hypocarbia and hypercarbia may both be influenced by pulmonary blood flow and temperature and thus do not necessarily reflect the adequacy of ventilation as is typical. Low pulmonary blood flow increases the ventilation to perfusion ratio; therefore more carbon dioxide is cleared for a given gas flow rate to the alveolus. *Second*, reduced temperature results in lower partial pressure of gas and increases solubility, assuming that the volume of the gas is constant.[80] During whole-body hypothermia, both $PaCO_2$ and $PaO_2$ decrease; hence blood gases are corrected for body temperature in most studies evaluating TH. The oxygen-hemoglobin dissociation curve shifts left as temperature falls. Pulse oximetry does not accurately predict corrected $PaO_2$ and might underestimate hypoxemia and increase the risk of pulmonary hypertension. *Finally*, positive pressure ventilation may have an important role in modulating cardiac loading conditions, including a favorable impact on the transmural pressure gradient of the left ventricular outflow tract. In situations of left ventricular dysfunction, intubation may be a positive modulator of forward flow.

Targeting $PaCO_2$ (temperature-corrected) in the mid-40s is thought to promote CBF, resulting in uniform brain cooling. End-tidal $CO_2$ correlates well with temperature-corrected $PaCO_2$ in infants undergoing whole-body TH.[81] Targeting $SpO_2$ in the 92–98% range results in a $PaO_2$ of 70 mmHg during normothermia but only a $PaO_2$ of 51 mmHg at 33.5°C.[81] Frequent arterial blood gas monitoring with a target of corrected $PaO_2$ 50–80 mmHg and preductal $SpO_2$ ≥92% is recommended.

## THE NON-HYPOXEMIC PATIENT WITH CARDIOVASCULAR INSUFFICIENCY

As previously discussed, cardiac dysfunction may be sub-clinical but highly relevant in both the likelihood of acute deterioration and prognosis. Thus it is important to have a high index of suspicion for deranged hemodynamics, even in the absence of significant hypoxemia. Although commonly used,[68] treatment of systemic hypotension with dopamine should be reconsidered in this population. Given the ambient physiological conditions of elevated pulmonary and systemic afterload and cardiac dysfunction, *dopamine*, which is both a systemic and pulmonary vasoconstrictor,[82,83] may not be biologically logical for most patients. Additionally, dopamine use has been associated with a greater risk of a composite of death/abnormal brain magnetic resonance imaging[84] and a more severe pattern of brain injury in some studies. It is typical for hypotension to present as systolic and relate to either or both cardiac dysfunction and impaired pulmonary blood flow. Agents with positive inotropic properties, such as *dobutamine*, which is a mixed alpha-1- and beta-agonist, or low-dose (<0.1 mcg/kg/min) *epinephrine*, which has more potent μ-binding properties, may be more logical first-line therapies. For critically unwell neonates, the pulmonary circulation may be pressure passive and *fluid boluses* may force the circulation to move while other, more long-lasting therapies are initiated. Consideration of blood products as a substitute for crystalloid may be reasonable but should not delay urgent resuscitative therapies. Early utilization of *prostaglandin E1* for patients with severe univentricular heart dysfunction may be lifesaving. For patients with severe uncoupled right ventricular disease, maintenance of left-to-right ductal shunt may support pulmonary blood flow. These patients typically manifest as non-hypoxic with impaired systemic hemodynamics. Similarly, for patients with severe left heart dysfunction, maintenance of right-to-left ductal shunt in a similar management strategy, as would be used with aortic coarctation (target SpO$_2$ 75–85%, avoidance of pulmonary vasodilation), may be crucial to attaining systemic blood flow. For the patient with diastolic hypotension in whom sepsis, adrenal insufficiency, or excessive vasodilating medications should be suspected, judicious use of systemic vasoconstrictors such as *norepinephrine* and/or *vasopressin* to maintain a diastolic in the normal range could be considered in addition to *glucocorticoid* supplementation (Figure 22.7). Avoidance of rapid fluctuations in preductal perfusion pressure and weaning during rewarming as physiological changes reverse are recommended. Although not scientifically proven, until more data is available to adjudicate their contribution to further brain injury, efforts to minimize the risk of postnatal ischemia-reperfusion brain injury may be prudent.

## PHARMACOLOGICAL CONSIDERATIONS

Polypharmacy is common in patients with hypoxia-ischemia for several anecdotal reasons. The first of these is that multi-system disease may necessitate treatment with medications that have unwanted side effects on the cardiovascular system. Phenobarbital and midazolam, commonly used as anticonvulsants, are potent systemic vasodilators. Morphine, which may be used as a sedative for patients with acute pulmonary hypertension, induces the release of histamine and may also be a source of systemic vasodilation, particularly among morphine naïve patients treated with high-dose infusions (>20 mcg/kg/h).[71]

Dexmedetomidine has early literature suggesting it to be a reasonable alternative sedative; however, the associated bradycardia may be problematic, and safety has yet to be established in large-scale trials.[85] The second reason for polypharmacy relates to patient complexity and the tendency for therapies to be increased in the face of little benefit. Declining patient condition may, in fact, be iatrogenic due to inaccurate physiological assumptions or drug side effects. Early and frequent quantitative echocardiography may improve pathophysiological clarity in both escalation and weaning of therapeutic agents.

*Finally*, it is important to consider pharmacokinetic differences which relate to both disease and temperature. In the first postnatal week neonates have altered PK parameters, including increased volume of distribution and decreased absorption, metabolism, and excretion.[86] Hypothermia further decreases metabolism and excretion of medications due to reduced hepatic activity[87] and decreased renal blood flow.[88] *Milrinone*, commonly used in the treatment of neonatal acute pulmonary hypertension, is excreted renally and has been associated with severe hypotension with a requirement for rapid escalation in vasopressor requirement in a population of cooled patients with concomitant pulmonary hypertension; its use should be considered cautiously.[72] PK differences modify medication safety profile, which is particularly important for sedatives and anticonvulsants for which high doses and combination therapy may frequently be required.[89] Although midazolam metabolism by CYP3A prevents excessive accumulation in neonates,[86] co-administration of phenobarbital results in increased clearance of midazolam.[90] Higher doses may be required with combined therapy and caution is advised to avoid toxicity when changing from phenobarbital to an alternative anticonvulsant while giving continuous midazolam. Though TH minimally affects phenobarbital PK,[89-91] severity of asphyxia is inversely related to phenobarbital clearance.[92] Oral topiramate, in contrast, has lower absorption, metabolism, and clearance during TH, but toxic levels have not been identified.[93,94] Alternative sedatives, such as dexmedetomidine, result in increased requirement for volume expansion, vasoactive agents, and higher incidence of hypotensive cardiac arrest in an animal model.[95]

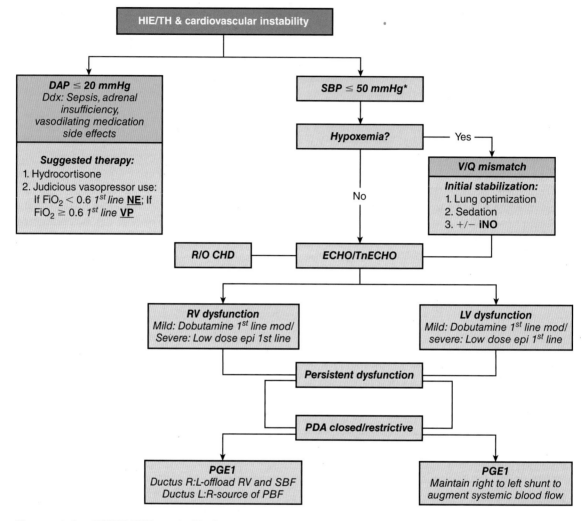

**Fig. 22.7 Suggested management algorithm of patients with hypoxic-ischemic injury undergoing therapeutic hypothermia who present with cardiovascular instability.** For patients with systolic hypotension or need for a cardiovascular agent, the primary physiological driver is typically heart dysfunction with or without impaired ventilation to perfusion matching. An approach focused on positive inotropy and maintenance of ductal shunt for refractory cases with judicious vasopressor use if significantly low diastolic arterial pressure is recommended. Echocardiography/targeted neonatal echocardiography screening is recommended for all patients with moderate-severe encephalopathy, and specific priority should be given to those treated with vasoactive medications regardless of blood pressure. *CHD*, congenital heart disease; *DAP*, diastolic arterial pressure; *ECHO*, echocardiogram; *epi*, epinephrine; *FiO2*, fraction of inspired oxygen; *iNO*, inhaled nitric oxide; *L:R*, left to right; *LV*, left ventricle; *NE*, norepinephrine; *PBF*, pulmonary blood flow; *R:L*, right to left; *R/O*, rule out; *RV*, right ventricle; *SBF*, systemic blood flow; *TnECHO*, targeted neonatal echocardiogram; *V/Q*, ventilation to perfusion; *VP*, vasopressin.

## THE USE OF EXTRACORPOREAL MEMBRANE OXYGENATION (ECMO)

For patients believed to have reversible lung/cardio-vascular disease and a good neurological prognosis, ECMO is offered in some institutions.[68] The study of ECMO in this patient population, however, is challenging due to low frequency and evolution of both medical care of HIE patients and ECMO technology. Although one would expect the outcomes for neonates who did versus did not receive respiratory ECMO for HIE to improve over time, the Extracorporeal Life Support Organization (ELSO) registry suggests no change over the time period of 2005–2013.[96] The publication of a more modern cohort may yield a different result, more applicable to today's population. If offered, several considerations are important. *First*, major changes in PK are likely following ECMO initiation due to a dramatic increase in volume of distribution and reduction in hepatic and renal clearance.[97] *Second*, side effects, particularly of bleeding, are important to consider. A single-center study reported a 30% risk of intracranial hemorrhage for HIE patients while on ECMO.[98] Similarly, a cohort of patients cooled for non-HIE indications between 2012 and 2014 demonstrated a >2-fold increase in intracranial bleeding than a comparable population of normothermic neonates[99]; however, these populations were different in several other important ways. In units where ECMO is not available or the side effects are not felt to outweigh the benefits, oxygenation may improve if cooling temperature is increased by 0.5°C first instead of immediately fully abandoning TH. This may allow for safer transfer to an ECMO center or enable some degree of relief from hypoxemia.

## Conclusions

Neonates with moderate to severe hypoxic insult often have right ventricular dysfunction and cardiovascular instability. Therapeutic hypothermia is a standard practice in the treatment of these patients in the developed world. Both TH and rewarming lead to significant hemodynamic changes that can be further affected by mechanical ventilation, use of inotropes, vasopressors, and other medications used in the treatment of infants with HIE, as well as by comorbidities, including pulmonary hypertension and sepsis. Conventional hemodynamic assessment only provides indirect markers of cardiovascular well-being that are plagued with confounders. Comprehensive or targeted neonatal echocardiography may provide enhanced physiological clarity and a guide to titration and weaning of cardiovascular agents. Finally, more research is needed to better understand the hemodynamic changes and the impact of interventions during the acute phases of the hypoxic-ischemic injury and

therapeutic hypothermia so that further improvements in short- and long-term neurodevelopmental outcomes can be achieved. In the meantime, an approach centered on avoidance of physiologic extremes using medications that target the known physiological contributors to disease is recommended.

## REFERENCES

1. Kurinczuk JJ, White-Koning M, Badawi N. Epidemiology of neonatal encephalopathy and hypoxic-ischaemic encephalopathy. *Early Hum Dev*. 2010;86(6):329-338. doi:10.1016/j.earlhumdev.2010.05.010.
2. Jacobs SE, Morley CJ, Inder TE, et al. Whole-body hypothermia for term and near-term newborns with hypoxic-ischemic encephalopathy: a randomized controlled trial. *Arch Pediatr Adolesc Med*. 2011;165(8):692-700. doi:10.1001/archpediatrics.2011.43.
3. Martin-Ancel A, Garcia-Alix A, Gaya F, Cabanas F, Burgueros M, Quero J. Multiple organ involvement in perinatal asphyxia. *J Pediatr*. 1995;127(5):786-793.
4. Shah P, Riphagen S, Beyene J, Perlman M. Multiorgan dysfunction in infants with post-asphyxial hypoxic-ischaemic encephalopathy. *Arch Dis Child Fetal Neonatal Ed*. 2004;89(2):F152-F155. doi:10.1136/adc.2002.023093.
5. Freeman JM, Nelson KB. Intrapartum asphyxia and cerebral palsy. *Pediatrics*. 1988;82(2):240-249.
6. Lawn JE, Cousens S, Zupan J. 4 million neonatal deaths: when? Where? Why? *Lancet*. 2005;365(9462):891-900. doi:10.1016/s0140-6736(05)71048-5.
7. Lawn JE, Manandhar A, Haws RA, Darmstadt GL. Reducing one million child deaths from birth asphyxia – a survey of health systems gaps and priorities. *Health Res Policy Syst*. 2007;5:4. doi:10.1186/1478-4505-5-4.
8. Gillam-Krakauer M, Gowen Jr CW. *Birth Asphyxia*. Tampa, FL: StatPearls. StatPearls Publishing LLC; 2020.
9. Organization WH. *World Health Report*. WHO. Accessed December 12, 2020. Available at: http://www.who.int/whr/2004/annex/en/index.html.
10. Ashwal S, Dale PS, Longo LD. Regional cerebral blood flow: studies in the fetal lamb during hypoxia, hypercapnia, acidosis, and hypotension. *Pediatr Res*. 1984;18(12):1309-1316. doi:10.1203/00006450-198412000-00018.
11. Johnson GN, Palahniuk RJ, Tweed WA, Jones MV, Wade JG. Regional cerebral blood flow changes during severe fetal asphyxia produced by slow partial umbilical cord compression. *Am J Obstet Gynecol*. 1979;135(1):48-52.
12. Giussani DA. The fetal brain sparing response to hypoxia: physiological mechanisms. *J Physiol*. 2016;594(5):1215-1230. doi:10.1113/jp271099.
13. Rudolph AM, Yuan S. Response of the pulmonary vasculature to hypoxia and H+ ion concentration changes. *J Clin Invest*. 1966;45(3):399-411. doi:10.1172/jci105355.
14. Rudolph AM, Heymann MA. The circulation of the fetus in utero. Methods for studying distribution of blood flow, cardiac output and organ blood flow. *Circ Res*. 1967;21(2):163-184. doi:10.1161/01.res.21.2.163.
15. Kara T, Narkiewicz K, Somers VK. Chemoreflexes – physiology and clinical implications. *Acta Physiol Scand*. 2003;177(3):377-384. doi:10.1046/j.1365-201X.2003.01083.x.

16. Goldaber KG, Gilstrap LC III, Leveno KJ, Dax JS, McIntire DD. Pathologic fetal acidemia. *Obstet Gynecol.* 1991;78(6):1103-1107.

17. Tweed A, Cote J, Lou H, Gregory G, Wade J. Impairment of cerebral blood flow autoregulation in the newborn lamb by hypoxia. *Pediatr Res.* 1986;20(6):516-519. doi:10.1203/00006450-198606000-00007.

18. McLean CW, Noori S, Cayabyab R, Seri I. Cerebral circulation and hypotension in the premature infant-diagnosis and treatment. In: Perlman JM, ed. *Questions and Controversies in Neonatology-Neurology.* Philadelphia: Saunders/Elsevier; 2011.

19. Kaiser JR, Gauss CH, Williams DK. The effects of hypercapnia on cerebral autoregulation in ventilated very low birth weight infants. *Pediatr Res.* 2005;58(5):931-935. doi:10.1203/01.pdr.0000182180.80645.0c.

20. Vannucci RC, Towfighi J, Vannucci SJ. Secondary energy failure after cerebral hypoxia-ischemia in the immature rat. *J Cereb Blood Flow Metab.* 2004;24(10):1090-1097. doi:10.1097/01.wcb.0000133250.03953.63.

21. Nestaas E, Stoylen A, Brunvand L, Fugelseth D. Longitudinal strain and strain rate by tissue Doppler are more sensitive indices than fractional shortening for assessing the reduced myocardial function in asphyxiated neonates. *Cardiol Young.* 2011;21(1):1-7. doi:10.1017/s1047951109991314.

22. Sobeih AA, El-Baz MS, El-Shemy DM, Abu El-Hamed WA. Tissue Doppler imaging versus conventional echocardiography in assessment of cardiac diastolic function in full term neonates with perinatal asphyxia. *J Matern-Fetal Neonatal Med.* 2021;34(23):3896-3901. doi:10.1080/14767058.2019.1702640.

23. Gill RS, Pelletier JS, LaBossiere J, Bigam DL, Cheung PY. Therapeutic strategies to protect the immature newborn myocardium during resuscitation following asphyxia. *Can J Physiol Pharmacol.* 2012;90(6):689-695. doi:10.1139/y2012-041.

24. Piquereau J, Ventura-Clapier R. Maturation of cardiac energy metabolism during perinatal development. *Front Physiol.* 2018;9:959. doi:10.3389/fphys.2018.00959.

25. Joynt C, Cheung PY. Cardiovascular supportive therapies for neonates with asphyxia – a literature review of pre-clinical and clinical studies. *Front Pediatr.* 2018;6:363. doi:10.3389/fped.2018.00363.

26. Armstrong K, Franklin O, Sweetman D, Molloy EJ. Cardiovascular dysfunction in infants with neonatal encephalopathy. Research support, non-U.S. Gov't review. *Arch Dis Child.* 2012;97(4):372-375. doi:10.1136/adc.2011.214205.

27. Benumof JL, Wahrenbrock EA. Dependency of hypoxic pulmonary vasoconstriction on temperature. *J Appl Physiol Respir Environ Exerc Physiol.* 1977;42(1):56-58.

28. Dattilo G, Tulino V, Tulino D, et al. Perinatal asphyxia and cardiac abnormalities. *Int J Cardiol.* 2011;147(2):e39-e40. doi:10.1016/j.ijcard.2009.01.032.

29. Bamber AR, Pryce J, Cook A, Ashworth M, Sebire NJ. Myocardial necrosis and infarction in newborns and infants. *Forensic Sci Med Pathol.* 2013;9(4):521-527. doi:10.1007/s12024-013-9472-0.

30. Setzer E, Ermocilla R, Tonkin I, John E, Sansa M, Cassady G. Papillary muscle necrosis in a neonatal autopsy population: incidence and associated clinical manifestations. *J Pediatr.* 1980;96(2):289-294.

31. Barberi I, Calabro MP, Cordaro S, et al. Myocardial ischemia in neonates with perinatal asphyxia: electrocardiographic, echocardiographic and enzymatic correlations. *Eur J Pediatr.* 1999;158:742-747.

32. Costa S, Zecca E, De Rosa G, et al. Is serum troponin T a useful marker of myocardial damage in newborn infants with perinatal asphyxia? *Acta Paediatr.* 2007;96(2):181-184.

33. Sehgal A, Wong F, Mehta S. Reduced cardiac output and its correlation with coronary blood flow and troponin in asphyxiated infants treated with therapeutic hypothermia. *Eur J Pediatr.* 2012;171(10):1511-1517. doi:10.1007/s00431-012-1764-y.

34. Liu J, Li J, Gu M. The correlation between myocardial function and cerebral hemodynamics in term infants with hypoxic-ischemic encephalopathy. *J Trop Pediatr.* 2007;53(1):44-48. doi:10.1093/tropej/fml053.

35. Giesinger RE, El Shahed AI, Castaldo MP, et al. Impaired right ventricular performance is associated with adverse outcome following hypoxic ischemic encephalopathy. *Am J Respir Crit Care Med.* 2019;200(10):1294-1305. doi:10.1164/rccm.201903-0583OC.

36. Giesinger RE, El Shahed AI, Castaldo MP, et al. Neurodevelopmental outcome following hypoxic ischaemic encephalopathy and therapeutic hypothermia is related to right ventricular performance at 24-hour postnatal age. *Arch Dis Child Fetal Neonatal Ed.* 2022;107(1):70-75. doi:10.1136/archdischild-2020-321463.

37. Hernandez-Andrade E, Hellström-Westas L, Thorngren-Jerneck K, et al. Perinatal adaptive response of the adrenal and carotid blood flow in sheep fetuses subjected to total cord occlusion. *J Matern Fetal Neonatal Med.* 2005;17(2):101-109. doi:10.1080/14767050500043509.

38. Davidson JO, Fraser M, Naylor AS, Roelfsema V, Gunn AJ, Bennet L. Effect of cerebral hypothermia on cortisol and adrenocorticotropic hormone responses after umbilical cord occlusion in preterm fetal sheep. *Pediatr Res.* 2008;63(1):51-55.

39. Gardner DS, Fletcher AJ, Fowden AL, Giussani DA. Plasma adrenocorticotropin and cortisol concentrations during acute hypoxemia after a reversible period of adverse intrauterine conditions in the ovine fetus during late gestation. *Endocrinology.* 2001;142(2):589-598. doi:10.1210/endo.142.2.7980.

40. Procianoy RS, Giacomini CB, Oliveira ML. Fetal and neonatal cortical adrenal function in birth asphyxia. *Acta Paediatr Scand.* 1988;77(5):671-674. doi:10.1111/j.1651-2227.1988.tb10728.x.

41. Chapados I, Chik CL, Cheung PY. Plasma cortisol response to ACTH challenge in hypoxic newborn piglets resuscitated with 21% and 100% oxygen. *Shock.* 2010;33(5):519-525. doi:10.1097/SHK.0b013e3181c99727.

42. Chein CL, Chen WP, Yang LY, Fu LS, Lin CY. Early detection of neonatal adrenal hemorrhage by ultrasonography. *Zhonghua Min Guo Xiao Er Ke Yi Xue Hui Za Zhi.* 1996;37(2):128-132.

43. Toti MS, Ghirri P, Bartoli A, et al. Adrenal hemorrhage in newborn: how, when and why- from case report to literature review. *Ital J Pediatr.* 2019;45(1):58. doi:10.1186/s13052-019-0651-9.

44. Kovacs K, Szakmar E, Meder U, et al. A randomized controlled study of low-dose hydrocortisone versus placebo in dopamine-treated hypotensive neonates undergoing hypothermia treatment for hypoxic-ischemic encephalopathy. *J Pediatr.* 2019;211:13-19.e3. doi:10.1016/j.jpeds.2019.04.008.

45. Toubas PL, Hof RP, Heymann MA, Rudolph AM. Effects of hypothermia and rewarming on the neonatal circulation. *Arch Fr Pediatr.* 1978;35(suppl 10):84-92.

46. Dudgeon DL, Randall PA, Hill RB, McAfee JG. Mild hypothermia: its effect on cardiac output and regional perfusion in the neonatal piglet. *J Pediatr Surg.* 1980;15(6):805-810. doi:10.1016/s0022-3468(80)80284-3.

47. Poulos ND, Mollitt DL. The nature and reversibility of hypothermia-induced alterations of blood viscosity. *J Trauma*. 1991;31(7):996-998; discussion 998-1000. doi:10.1097/00005373-199107000-00020.

48. Schubert A. Side effects of mild hypothermia. *J Neurosurg Anesthesiol*. 1995;7(2):139-147. doi:10.1097/00008506-199504000-00021.

49. Thoresen M, Whitelaw A. Cardiovascular changes during mild therapeutic hypothermia and rewarming in infants with hypoxic-ischemic encephalopathy. *Pediatrics*. 2000;106(1 Pt 1):92-99.

50. Sehgal A, Linduska N, Huynh C. Cardiac adaptation in asphyxiated infants treated with therapeutic hypothermia. *J Neonatal Perinatal Med*. 2019;12(2):117-125. doi:10.3233/npm-1853.

51. Thoresen M. Hypothermia after perinatal asphyxia: selection for treatment and cooling protocol. *J Pediatr*. 2011;158(suppl 2):e45-e49. doi:10.1016/j.jpeds.2010.11.013.

52. Simbruner G, Mittal RA, Rohlmann F, Muche R. Systemic hypothermia after neonatal encephalopathy: outcomes of neo. nEURO.network RCT. *Pediatrics*. 2010;126(4):e771-e778. doi:10.1542/peds.2009-2441.

53. Gebauer CM, Knuepfer M, Robel-Tillig E, Pulzer F, Vogtmann C. Hemodynamics among neonates with hypoxic-ischemic encephalopathy during whole-body hypothermia and passive rewarming. *Pediatrics*. 2006;117(3):843-850. doi:10.1542/peds.2004-1587.

54. Manabe M, Fujino M, Kusuki H, et al. Effect of hypothermia on myocardial depolarization and repolarization in neonates with hypoxic-ischemic encephalopathy due to asphyxia. *Pediatr Cardiol*. 2022;43(8):1792-1798. doi:10.1007/s00246-022-02916-x.

55. Eriksen VR, Trautner S, Hahn GH, Greisen G. Lactate acidosis and cardiac output during initial therapeutic cooling in asphyxiated newborn infants. *PLoS One*. 2019;14(3):e0213537. doi:10.1371/journal.pone.0213537.

56. Hochwald O, Jabr M, Osiovich H, Miller SP, McNamara PJ, Lavoie PM. Preferential cephalic redistribution of left ventricular cardiac output during therapeutic hypothermia for perinatal hypoxic-ischemic encephalopathy. Observational study research support, non-U.S. Gov't. *J Pediatr*. 2014;164(5):999-1004.e1. doi:10.1016/j.jpeds.2014.01.028.

57. More KS, Sakhuja P, Giesinger RE, et al. Cardiovascular associations with abnormal brain magnetic resonance imaging in neonates with hypoxic ischemic encephalopathy undergoing therapeutic hypothermia and rewarming. *Am J Perinatol*. 2018;35(10):979-989. doi:10.1055/s-0038-1629900.

58. Liu X, Chakkarapani E, Stone J, Thoresen M. Effect of cardiac compressions and hypothermia treatment on cardiac troponin I in newborns with perinatal asphyxia. *Resuscitation*. 2013;84(11):1562-1567. doi:10.1016/j.resuscitation.2013.07.003.

59. Liu X, Tooley J, Loberg EM, Suleiman MS, Thoresen M. Immediate hypothermia reduces cardiac troponin I after hypoxic-ischemic encephalopathy in newborn pigs. *Pediatr Res*. 2011;70(4):352-356. doi:10.1038/pr.2011.577.

60. Wood T, Thoresen M. Physiological responses to hypothermia. *Semin Fetal Neonatal Med*. 2015;20(2):87-96. doi:10.1016/j.siny.2014.10.005.

61. Weisser J, Martin J, Bisping E, et al. Influence of mild hypothermia on myocardial contractility and circulatory function. *Basic Res Cardiol*. 2001;96(2):198-205. doi:10.1007/s003950170071.

62. Jones RN, Reimer KA, Hill ML, Jennings RB. Effect of hypothermia on changes in high-energy phosphate production and utilization in total ischemia. *J Mol Cell Cardiol*. 1982;14(suppl 3):123-130. doi:10.1016/0022-2828(82)90140-7.

63. Darbera L, Chenoune M, Lidouren F, et al. Hypothermic liquid ventilation prevents early hemodynamic dysfunction and cardiovascular mortality after coronary artery occlusion complicated by cardiac arrest in rabbits. *Crit Care Med*. 2013;41(12):e457-e465. doi:10.1097/CCM.0b013e3182a63b5d.

64. Dae MW, Gao DW, Sessler DI, Chair K, Stillson CA. Effect of endovascular cooling on myocardial temperature, infarct size, and cardiac output in human-sized pigs. *Am J Physiol Heart Circ Physiol*. 2002;282(5):H1584-H1591. doi:10.1152/ajpheart.00980.2001.

65. Deakin CD, Knight H, Edwards JC, et al. Induced hypothermia in the postoperative management of refractory cardiac failure following paediatric cardiac surgery. *Anaesthesia*. 1998;53(9):848-853. doi:10.1046/j.1365-2044.1998.00563.x.

66. Kohlhauer M, Berdeaux A, Ghaleh B, Tissier R. Therapeutic hypothermia to protect the heart against acute myocardial infarction. *Arch Cardiovasc Dis*. 2016;109(12):716-722. doi:10.1016/j.acvd.2016.05.005.

67. Hochwald O, Jabr M, Osiovich H, Miller SP, McNamara PJ, Lavoie PM. Preferential cephalic redistribution of left ventricular cardiac output during therapeutic hypothermia for perinatal hypoxic-ischemic encephalopathy. *J Pediatr*. 2014;164(5):999-1004.e1. doi:10.1016/j.jpeds.2014.01.028.

68. Giesinger RE, Levy PT, Lauren Ruoss J, et al. Cardiovascular management following hypoxic-ischemic encephalopathy in North America: need for physiologic consideration. *Pediatr Res*. 2021;90(3):600-607. doi:10.1038/s41390-020-01205-8.

69. Bischoff AR, Giesinger RE, McNamara PJ. Subclinical left ventricular systolic dysfunction due to coronary arterial thrombosis in a neonate with hypoxic ischemic encephalopathy undergoing therapeutic hypothermia. *CASE (Phila)*. 2022;6(7):330-334. doi:10.1016/j.case.2022.04.008.

70. Giesinger RE, Castaldo MP, Breatnach CR, Mertens L, El-Khuffash A, McNamara PJ. Persistent right ventricular dysfunction despite inotrope use is associated with deranged cerebral hemodynamics among neonates with hypoxic-ischemic encephalopathy. E-PAS2019: 2840.332.

71. Alcaraz C, Bansinath M, Turndorf H, Puig MM. Cardiovascular effects of morphine during hypothermia. *Arch Int Pharmacodyn Ther*. 1989;297:133-147.

72. Bischoff AR, Habib S, McNamara PJ, Giesinger RE. Hemodynamic response to milrinone for refractory hypoxemia during therapeutic hypothermia for neonatal hypoxic ischemic encephalopathy. *J Perinatol*. 2021;41(9):2345-2354. doi:10.1038/s41372-021-01049-y.

73. Shah S, Tracy M, Smyth J. Postnatal lactate as an early predictor of short-term outcome after intrapartum asphyxia. *J Perinatol*. 2004;24(1):16-20. doi:10.1038/sj.jp.7211023.

74. Bozkurt O, Yucesoy E. Acute kidney injury in neonates with perinatal asphyxia receiving therapeutic hypothermia. *Am J Perinatol*. 2021;38(9):922-929. doi:10.1055/s-0039-1701024.

75. Guluma KZ, Liu L, Hemmen TM, et al. Therapeutic hypothermia is associated with a decrease in urine output in acute stroke patients. *Resuscitation*. 2010;81(12):1642-1647. doi:10.1016/j.resuscitation.2010.08.003.

76. Vidal Melo Marcos F, Harris RS, Layfield D, Musch G, Venegas Jose G. Changes in regional ventilation after autologous blood clot pulmonary embolism. *Anesthesiology*. 2002;97(3):671-681. doi:10.1097/00000542-200209000-00022.

77. Creamer KM, McCloud LL, Fisher LE, Ehrhart IC. Ventilation above closing volume reduces pulmonary vascular resistance hysteresis. *Am J Respir Crit Care Med*. 1998;158(4):1114-1119. doi:10.1164/ajrccm.158.4.9711081.

78. Jardin F, Vieillard-Baron A. Right ventricular function and positive pressure ventilation in clinical practice: from hemodynamic subsets to respirator settings. *Intensive Care Med.* 2003;29(9):1426-1434. doi:10.1007/s00134-003-1873-1.

79. De Jaegere A, van Veenendaal MB, Michiels A, van Kaam AH. Lung recruitment using oxygenation during open lung high-frequency ventilation in preterm infants. *Am J Respir Crit Care Med.* 2006;174(6):639-645. doi:10.1164/rccm.200603-351OC.

80. Chandan G, Cascella M. *Gas Laws and Clinical Application.* StatPearls. Tampa, FL: StatPearls Publishing LLC; 2020.

81. Afzal B, Chandrasekharan P, Tancredi DJ, Russell J, Steinhorn RH, Lakshminrusimha S. Monitoring gas exchange during hypothermia for hypoxic-ischemic encephalopathy. *Pediatr Crit Care Med.* 2019;20(2):166-171. doi:10.1097/pcc.0000000000001799.

82. Cheung PY, Barrington KJ, Pearson RJ, Bigam DL, Finer NN, Van Aerde JE. Systemic, pulmonary and mesenteric perfusion and oxygenation effects of dopamine and epinephrine. *Am J Respir Crit Care Med.* 1997;155(1):32-37. doi:10.1164/ajrccm.155.1.9001285.

83. Manouchehri N, Bigam DL, Churchill T, Rayner D, Joynt C, Cheung PY. A comparison of combination dopamine and epinephrine treatment with high-dose dopamine alone in asphyxiated newborn piglets after resuscitation. Comparative study research support, non-U.S. Gov't. *Pediatr Res.* 2013;73 (4 Pt 1):435-442. doi:10.1038/pr.2013.17.

84. Pazandak C, McPherson C, Abubakar M, Zanelli S, Fairchild K, Vesoulis Z. Blood pressure profiles in infants with Hypoxic Ischemic Encephalopathy (HIE), response to dopamine, and association with brain injury. *Front Pediatr.* 2020;8:512. doi:10.3389/fped.2020.00512.

85. Elliott M, Burnsed J, Heinan K, et al. Effect of dexmedetomidine on heart rate in neonates with hypoxic ischemic encephalopathy undergoing therapeutic hypothermia. *J Neonatal Perinatal Med.* 2022;15(1):47-54. doi:10.3233/npm-210737.

86. Kearns GL, Abdel-Rahman SM, Alander SW, Blowey DL, Leeder JS, Kauffman RE. Developmental pharmacology – drug disposition, action, and therapy in infants and children. *N Eng J Med.* 2003;349(12):1157-1167. doi:doi:10.1056/NEJMra035092.

87. Tortorici MA, Kochanek PM, Poloyac SM. Effects of hypothermia on drug disposition, metabolism, and response: A focus of hypothermia-mediated alterations on the cytochrome P450 enzyme system. *Crit Care Med.* 2007;35(9):2196-2204. doi:10.1097/01.ccm.0000281517.97507.6e.

88. Wilson TE. Renal sympathetic nerve, blood flow, and epithelial transport responses to thermal stress. *Auton Neurosci.* 2017;204:25-34. doi:10.1016/j.autneu.2016.12.007.

89. Pokorna P, Wildschut ED, Vobruba V, van den Anker JN, Tibboel D. The impact of hypothermia on the pharmacokinetics of drugs used in neonates and young infants. *Curr Pharm Des.* 2015;21(39):5705-5724. doi:10.2174/1381612821666150901110929.

90. Favié LMA, Groenendaal F, van den Broek MPH, et al. Phenobarbital, midazolam pharmacokinetics, effectiveness, and drug-drug interaction in asphyxiated neonates undergoing therapeutic hypothermia. *Neonatology.* 2019;116(2):154-162. doi:10.1159/000499330.

91. van den Broek MP, Groenendaal F, Toet MC, et al. Pharmacokinetics and clinical efficacy of phenobarbital in asphyxiated newborns treated with hypothermia: a thermopharmacological approach. *Clin Pharmacokinet.* 2012;51(10):671-679. doi:10.1007/s40262-012-0004-y.

92. Pokorná P, Posch L, Šíma M, et al. Severity of asphyxia is a covariate of phenobarbital clearance in newborns undergoing hypothermia. *J Matern Fetal Neonatal Med.* 2019;32(14):2302-2309. doi:10.1080/14767058.2018.1432039.

93. Filippi L, Poggi C, la Marca G, et al. Oral topiramate in neonates with hypoxic ischemic encephalopathy treated with hypothermia: a safety study. *J Pediatr.* 2010;157(3):361-366. doi:10.1016/j.jpeds.2010.04.019.

94. Filippi L, la Marca G, Fiorini P, et al. Topiramate concentrations in neonates treated with prolonged whole body hypothermia for hypoxic ischemic encephalopathy. *Epilepsia.* 2009;50(11):2355-2361. doi:10.1111/j.1528-1167.2009.02302.x.

95. Ezzati M, Kawano G, Rocha-Ferreira E, et al. Dexmedetomidine combined with therapeutic hypothermia is associated with cardiovascular instability and neurotoxicity in a piglet model of perinatal asphyxia. *Dev Neurosci.* 2017;39(1-4):156-170. doi:10.1159/000458438.

96. Cuevas Guaman M, Lucke AM, Hagan JL, Kaiser JR. Bleeding complications and mortality in neonates receiving therapeutic hypothermia and extracorporeal membrane oxygenation. *Am J Perinatol.* 2018;35(3):271-276. doi:10.1055/s-0037-1607197.

97. Wildschut ED, de Wildt SN, Mâthot RA, Reiss IK, Tibboel D, Van den Anker J. Effect of hypothermia and extracorporeal life support on drug disposition in neonates. *Semin Fetal Neonatal Med.* 2013;18(1):23-27. doi:10.1016/j.siny.2012.10.002.

98. Agarwal P, Altinok D, Desai J, Shanti C, Natarajan G. In-hospital outcomes of neonates with hypoxic-ischemic encephalopathy receiving extracorporeal membrane oxygenation. *J Perinatol.* 2019;39(5):661-665. doi:10.1038/s41372-019-0345-6.

99. Cashen K, Reeder RW, Shanti C, Dalton HJ, Dean JM, Meert KL. Is therapeutic hypothermia during neonatal extracorporeal membrane oxygenation associated with intracranial hemorrhage? *Perfusion.* 2018;33(5):354-362. doi:10.1177/0267659117747693.

100. Giesinger RE, Bailey LJ, Deshpande P, McNamara PJ. Hypoxic-ischemic encephalopathy and therapeutic hypothermia: the hemodynamic perspective. *J Pediatr.* 2017;180:22-30.e2. doi:10.1016/j.jpeds.2016.09.009.

101. Rios DR, Lapointe A, Schmolzer GM, et al. Hemodynamic optimization for neonates with neonatal encephalopathy caused by a hypoxic ischemic event: physiological and therapeutic considerations. *Semin Fetal Neonatal Med.* 2021;26(4):101277. doi:10.1016/j.siny.2021.101277.

102. Jain A, Mohamed A, El-Khuffash A, et al. A comprehensive echocardiographic protocol for assessing neonatal right ventricular dimensions and function in the transitional period: normative data and z scores. *J Am Soc Echocardiogr.* 2014;27(12):1293-1304. doi:10.1016/j.echo.2014.08.018.

103. Jain A, Giesinger RE, Dakshinamurti S, et al. Care of the critically ill neonate with hypoxemic respiratory failure and acute pulmonary hypertension: framework for practice based on consensus opinion of neonatal hemodynamics working group. *J Perinatol.* 2022;42(1):3-13. doi:10.1038/s41372-021-01296-z.

104. Slama M, Susic D, Varagic J, Ahn J, Frohlich ED. Echocardiographic measurement of cardiac output in rats. *Am J Physiol*

*Heart Circ Physiol.* 2003;284(2):H691-H697. doi:10.1152/ajpheart.00653.2002.

105. Badano LP, Ginghina C, Easaw J, et al. Right ventricle in pulmonary arterial hypertension: haemodynamics, structural changes, imaging, and proposal of a study protocol aimed to assess remodelling and treatment effects. *Eur J Echocardiogr.* 2010;11(1):27-37. doi:10.1093/ejechocard/jep152.

106. Ryan T, Petrovic O, Dillon JC, Feigenbaum H, Conley MJ, Armstrong WF. An echocardiographic index for separation of right ventricular volume and pressure overload. *J Am Coll Cardiol.* 1985;5(4):918-927.

107. Jain A, McNamara PJ. Persistent pulmonary hypertension of the newborn: advances in diagnosis and treatment. *Semin Fetal Neonatal Med.* 2015;20(4):262-271. doi:10.1016/j.siny.2015.03.001.

108. Giesinger RE, More K, Odame J, Jain A, Jankov RP, McNamara PJ. Controversies in the identification and management of acute pulmonary hypertension in preterm neonates. *Pediatr Res.* 2017;82(6):901-914. doi:10.1038/pr.2017.200.

# Chapter 23

# Glucocorticoids and Adrenal Function in Neonates With Hypotension

Erika F. Fernandez

## Key Points

1. Corticosteroids are increasingly used in the acutely ill newborn population to increase blood pressure and reduce inotrope exposure.

2. There are clinical and disease states in infants in which glucocorticoids have been studied and found to have potential benefit. Populations who may respond to corticosteroids include ill term and preterm infants with hypotension and infants with pulmonary hypertension, meconium aspiration syndrome, hypoxic-ischemic encephalopathy, sepsis, and congenital diaphragmatic hernia. Cortisol levels have varying clinical utility in these conditions.

3. Hydrocortisone is the most studied corticosteroid for the treatment of hypotension, and although doses have varied in studies, doses as low as 1 mg/kg/day are effective in stabilizing cardiovascular insufficiency.

4. Despite the growing literature on the benefits of hydrocortisone for the treatment of hypotension, there remains a lack of data on long-term outcomes. The administration of hydrocortisone in the short term has been associated with hyperglycemia, hypertrophic cardiomyopathy, hypertension, and sepsis.

5. Glucocorticoid therapy should be tailored for each patient and account for gestational age, condition, and response of the patient while limiting the exposure as much as possible and monitoring for known complications.

## Introduction

Since the last edition of this chapter, studies have continued to observe higher blood pressure and less inotrope need in infants given corticosteroids. However, despite the growing number of studies and the increasing utilization of corticosteroids in newborns,[1-5] there remains no consensus on a singular pathway for recognition, treatment, and the assessment of best practices and outcomes. This is in comparison to other populations whose societies or colleges have created unified guidelines. The American College of Critical Care Medicine updated their guidelines in 2017 on the hemodynamic support of pediatric and neonatal septic shock.[6] In the same year the Multispecialty Task Force for the Society of Critical Care Medicine and the European Society of Intensive Care Medicine updated their guidelines on critical illness–related corticosteroid insufficiency (CIRCI) in critically ill patients.[7] Since the initial publications of these guidelines, there has been ongoing testing of these guidelines resulting in ongoing changes and improvements.[8] In the newborn population there are no unified standards. The American Academy of Pediatrics (AAP) Committee on Fetus and Newborn (COFN), a leader in proposing standards of care in the United States, recently published its first clinical report in 2022, on the *Recognition and Management of Cardiovascular Insufficiency in the Very Low Birth Weight Newborn.*[9] However, the section on cardiovascular use of steroids is limited, with no clear trigger or strategy for initiating and administering steroids. The last *Cochrane Review on Treatment for Hypotension in Very Low Birth Weight Infants* was published in 2011, and corticosteroids were recognized to be as effective as dopamine in treating refractory hypotension but, because long-term safety and benefit data were lacking, they were not recommended for routine use.[10] Corticosteroid treatment in newborn infants for hypotension has been recommended by various experts in general article reviews.[11-14] In one of these reviews Dr Watterberg proposed one of the most detailed algorithms for use of hydrocortisone for hypotension and included suggested dosing and timing.[11] However, it remains that without a formally established consensus, it is difficult to assess the extent to which these recommendations have been utilized. There have been significant research efforts to better understand the use of corticosteroids in the newborn population; however, large randomized controlled trials (RCTs) designed to evaluate short and long-term effects of hydrocortisone for the treatment of cardiovascular insufficiency are very challenging to conduct and execute. The Neonatal Research Network has attempted to conduct RCTs on the hemodynamic effects of corticosteroids in sick preterm and term infants with hypotension in the past decade but was unable to complete the enrollment of patients.[15,16] Reasons for the low enrollment rates included fewer-than-anticipated infants with low blood pressure, difficulties in obtaining consent within the narrow study window, and lack of physician equipoise. In addition, many patients at the time of screening (within 2–12 hours of age or onset of presentation) have already been administered corticosteroids (up to 33% and higher).[16,17] The enrollment of preterm infants has also been hampered by high rates of early indomethacin administration. With the difficulty of conducting rigorous studies and given the use of steroids in the acutely ill newborn population, alternative approaches and creativity may be needed to answer the question of best clinical practices, long-term safety, and potential benefits.

There is a need to construct a clear and consensus-driven guideline directing a more standardized approach to the use of corticosteroids in the newborn infant. This should include: (1) triggers to aid recognition of infants who may be amenable to corticosteroids, including clinical presentation, disease states, and laboratory values; (2) a pathway for the administration of corticosteroids, including type, timing, dosing, and duration; and (3) a standardized assessment of performance of the pathway to evaluate safety and overall outcomes.

# Recognition of Potential Patients for the Administration of Corticosteroids

## CLINICAL PRESENTATION AND PATIENT CHARACTERISTICS

The *most common clinical presentation* in the newborn infant who may be responsive to corticosteroids is *hypotension* and, in particular, those with "vasopressor-resistant hypotension". Vasopressor-resistant hypotension is present when hypotension persists despite vasopressor administration. There are varying definitions of vasopressor-resistant hypotension based on varying inotrope levels but it is most often defined as when dopamine dose is at least >10 mcg/kg/min. Dopamine is usually considered the first line for treatment of hypotension because, despite the fact that small studies showed no difference between hydrocortisone and dopamine as first-line treatment in morbidity or mortality, it is the most studied.[18] Hypotension in the critically ill newborn has been associated with adrenal insufficiency. However, regardless of the presence of adrenal insufficiency, corticosteroids elevate systemic blood pressure, so it is important to understand the populations and disease states in which corticosteroids have been studied. Until there is more information on the effect of corticosteroids on developing organs and their safety, corticosteroids should be limited to those infants requiring "rescue" treatment for vasopressor-resistant hypotension versus prophylaxis. The clinical presentation of infants with adrenal insufficiency often includes hypotension but may also include other signs and symptoms of classic adrenal insufficiency, such as hypoglycemia, hyponatremia, hyperkalemia, acidosis, tachycardia, and weakness (Figure 23.1). However, these signs are often masked by the tightly controlled fluid, electrolyte, and temperature management of infants in the newborn intensive care unit.

### Adrenal Insufficiency

While this chapter focuses mainly on infants with transient medical conditions which may be responsive to short-course corticosteroids, the clinical presentation may look the same as for those infants with chronic conditions of adrenal insufficiency. An example of a chronic condition is congenital adrenal hyperplasia

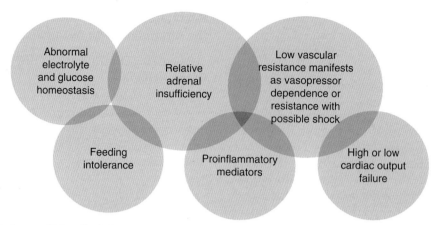

**Fig. 23.1  Clinical features and interaction between adrenal insufficiency and cardiovascular function.** Severe illness and cardiovascular instability are features of both relative adrenal insufficiency (RAI) and vasopressor-resistant hypotension. RAI may or may not be associated with vasopressor-resistant hypotension and vasopressor-resistant hypotension may or may not be associated with RAI.

which requires an extensive workup and will need long-term glucocorticoid replacement.[19,20] Fortunately, these chronic diseases are rare (10–15 per 100,000 for chronic primary adrenal insufficiencies and 150–280 per million for central adrenal insufficiencies). However, it is important not to miss these diagnoses and, when faced with a critically ill newborn with vasopressor-resistant hypotension, it may be prudent to obtain a cortisol level prior to initiating corticosteroids to help guide the potential future evaluation for these chronic conditions. Although a singular random cortisol value is often of limited use in these chronic conditions, a random cortisol value >18–22 mcg/dL most often rules out most chronic conditions of adrenal insufficiency, while those with cortisol values <5–7 mcg/dL in critical illness may prompt further evaluation including, at the minimum, an adrenocorticotrophin hormone stimulation test.

### Relative Adrenal Insufficiency

Relative adrenal insufficiency is characterized by its transience because most patients who recover will have normal HPA axis function and corticosteroid activity. *Relative adrenal insufficiency* is defined as a condition when there is inadequate corticosteroid activity compared with the level of illness in a critically ill patient[7,21-24] and may arise from inadequate cortisol levels resulting from problems anywhere along the

HPA axis from synthesis to function or tissue resistance to corticosteroids. Adrenal insufficiency in critically ill patients is also known as "functional adrenal insufficiency", "transient adrenocortical insufficiency of prematurity", or "critical illness-related corticosteroid insufficiency". For the purposes of this chapter, the term "relative adrenal insufficiency" is used interchangeably with these terms. The diagnosis of relative adrenal insufficiency in a critically ill patient should not make one complacent about, or underestimate, the potentially life-threatening nature of this type of adrenal insufficiency.[25] Since the 1980s, relative adrenal insufficiency has become increasingly recognized in sick premature and term neonates, infants, children, and adults.[7,14,26-51]

The **overall incidence of relative adrenal insufficiency** in *critically ill adult* patients is approximately 10–20% in general and around 60% in patients with severe sepsis, and septic shock in particular.[52,53] Reported proportions of *critically ill pediatric* patients with "inadequate" cortisol response vary widely, from as low as 2% often up to 87%.[43-45,54-56] Overall, in the *critically ill neonate* the incidence is less well understood because there is no consensus on the diagnostic criteria of relative adrenal insufficiency of the ill newborn.[40,43,46,57-68] However, it has been reported that almost 20% of ill, mechanically ventilated late preterm and term newborns and up to 33% of all extreme preterm newborns in the United States are receiving corticosteroids for cardiovascular insufficiency.[1,2]

*The timing of presentation of relative adrenal insufficiency* is most often reported in the first few postnatal days in critically ill newborn infants. There is some evidence from a Japanese cohort that adrenal insufficiency can also occur later in life (4–7 days of age) in ill newborn infants with respiratory distress or sepsis.[45] Surveys in Japan found that approximately 4–8% of VLBW infants are receiving postnatal corticosteroid therapy after 7 days of age, with symptoms suggestive of relative adrenal insufficiency, including hypotension and high cortisol precursors.[69,70]

*Postulated pathophysiologic mechanisms for relative adrenal insufficiency* in ill patients include adrenergic receptor insensitivity due to receptor downregulation (Figure 23.2), proinflammatory cytokine-mediated suppression of the function of the pituitary and adrenal glands, inadequate HPA axis response to stress, limited adrenal reserve, gestational age–associated immaturity of the adrenal gland, corticosteroid tissue resistance, and limited adrenal perfusion (Figure 23.3).[32,41,42,71-75]

*Prolonged exposure to inflammatory mediators* is one of the proposed mechanisms for both vasopressor-resistant hypotension manifesting via receptor downregulation and relative adrenal insufficiency presenting

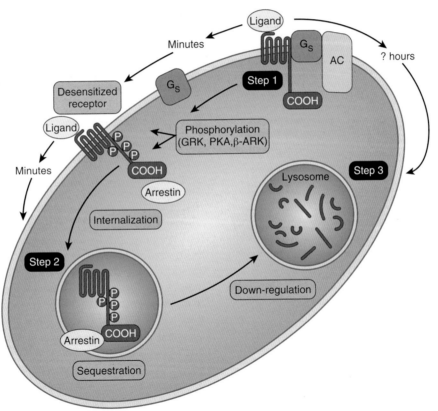

**Fig. 23.2 Cellular mechanisms of adrenergic receptor downregulation.** Following exposure to agonists, transmembrane $\beta_2$-adrenergic receptors coupling to the stimulatory guanine nucleotide-binding regulatory proteins ($G_s$) undergo rapid (minutes) and longer-term (hours) regulatory processes induced by the receptor-specific ligands. These processes result in attenuation of the adenylyl cyclase (*AC*) enzyme and cyclic adenosine monophosphate (*cAMP*) formation. The initial process includes phosphorylation-regulated functional desensitization due to phosphorylation of the intracellular loops at the carboxyl terminus of the adrenoreceptor by G protein–coupled receptor kinase (*GRK*), cAMP-dependent protein kinase A (*PKA*), and β-adrenergic receptor kinase (β-*ARK*) (*Step 1*). Phosphorylation (*P*) is followed by coupling of the receptor to arrestin and loss of hydrophilic ligand binding. Arrestin promotes internalization of the receptor, which is then targeted for sequestration (*Step 2*) into the cytosolic compartment. The final step, downregulation (*Step 3*), refers to the agonist-induced decrease in the number of the receptors following prolonged exposure to agonists and results in degradation of the receptor, presumably via a lysosomal pathway.

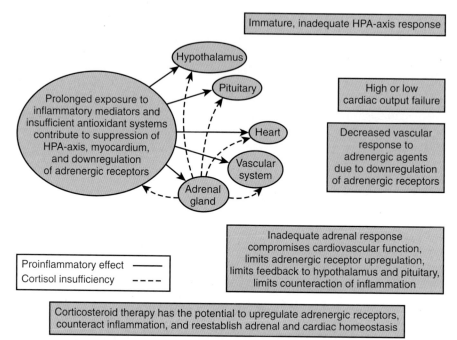

**Fig. 23.3 Interaction among the hypothalamus-pituitary-adrenal axis, cardiovascular function, and inflammation.** Corticosteroid therapy upregulates adrenergic receptor and adenylate cyclase expression and membrane assembly, counteracts inflammation, and re-establishes cardiovascular and adrenal homeostasis. *HPA axis*, hypothalamus-pituitary-adrenal axis.

with suppression of the function of the adrenal gland and/or HPA axis. Decreased vascular responsiveness to adrenergic agents is due to downregulation of adrenergic receptors.[76] Downregulation of adrenergic receptors in clinical conditions occurs within hours due to prolonged exposure to intrinsic (stress response) or extrinsic (vasopressor therapy) catecholamines and inflammatory mediators such as nitric oxide (NO), tumor necrosis factor, and other inflammatory cytokines (interleukin-1 [IL-1], IL-2, IL-6, interferon-gamma).[58,77] Thus production of proinflammatory cytokines also contributes to decreased vascular reactivity to catecholamines and thus to the development of vasopressor-resistant hypotension and has been described in patients with septic shock.[78] In the scenario in which severe illness promotes inflammation and concomitant cortisol insufficiency–associated decreased cardiovascular responsiveness to catecholamines, corticosteroid therapy re-establishes vascular responsiveness and counteracts inflammation.

Newborns, especially those born prematurely, have unique susceptibilities to relative adrenal insufficiency,

which is, at least in part, due to the *immaturity of their HPA axis* and especially the cortical function of the adrenal gland. In addition, the changes in adrenal cortical hormone production, especially cortisol during the transition to extrauterine life and the gestational age–dependent changes in placental 11β-hydroxysteroid dehydrogenase type 2 activity, and thus the effect of maternal corticosteroids on fetal corticosteroid production, pose special challenges for the newborn, especially the preterm neonate. Fetal adrenal glands begin to synthesize cortisol de novo at approximately 22–24 weeks' gestation, followed by a steady increase throughout the rest of the pregnancy.[79] Corticotrophin-releasing hormone (CRH) production by the placenta also increases through gestation, resulting in maternal and fetal serum CRH concentrations at term that are much higher than at any other time in life.[80] Placental CRH stimulates cortisol production in the fetal adrenal gland. At birth, the very high placental CRH production ceases to have an effect on the newborn. The pituitary gland of the newborn, which has been exposed to high concentrations of CRH during fetal life, may become transiently insensitive to the lower concentrations of CRH produced by the hypothalamus of the neonate. Therefore it may not be able to increase ACTH production to appropriately stimulate the adrenal gland for several days after delivery. Healthy term newborns tolerate this period of relative HPA insufficiency. However, this situation may predispose the newborn to the development of relative adrenal insufficiency in critical illness. Relative adrenal insufficiency could then contribute to the severity of systemic hypotension and attenuate the response of the cardiovascular system to treatment.

### Relative Adrenal Insufficiency in Preterm Infants

Relative adrenal insufficiency has been described in ill preterm infants who present with cardiovascular instability in addition to random and/or stimulated cortisol levels that are inadequate for the degree of illness severity and by rapid clinical and hemodynamic improvement following corticosteroid therapy.[23,46,51,52,54] In 1989, Ward and Colasurdo were the first to describe a small cohort of ventilated, sick, extremely premature infants who presented with signs consistent with adrenal insufficiency or "Addisonian crisis".[28] These infants had signs of relative adrenal insufficiency, including hypotension, oliguria, and hyponatremia and had cortisol values less than 15 mcg/dL (414 nmol/L).

Since this time, subsequent investigations have further elucidated the clinical and laboratory presentation of relative adrenal insufficiency in ill, hypotensive premature infants.[27-30,33,34,37,39,45,47,81-86] The study by Yoder and colleagues in very premature baboons has provided the most direct, albeit non-human, evidence that relative adrenal insufficiency, cardiovascular insufficiency, and prematurity are related.[87] In earlier studies, this group of investigators documented that most extremely premature baboons, delivered at approximately 67% of baboon gestation (around 26 weeks' human gestation), required volume expansion and vasopressor-inotrope therapy to treat the subjects' hypotension, oliguria, and acid-base imbalance. Many of the premature baboons (38%) also required hydrocortisone to successfully treat their hypotension despite receiving vasopressor-inotrope therapy.[88] This group of researchers also demonstrated that decreased urinary free cortisol excretion in the

first postnatal day correlated with decreased left ventricular function. Furthermore, hydrocortisone therapy (0.5–1.0 mg/kg/day for 1–2 days) corrected the hypotension and the left ventricular dysfunction, reduced vasopressor-inotrope requirement and mortality, and increased serum cortisol to levels comparable to those seen in baboons with no evidence of relative adrenal insufficiency or cardiovascular dysfunction.[87]

Investigators have documented two intriguing observations regarding cortisol levels in well and sick premature infants. Many *healthy premature infants*, with no signs of relative adrenal insufficiency, have random cortisol levels that are not detectable or less than 5 mcg/dL (138 nmol/L), a threshold considered to indicate adrenal insufficiency.[29,35,36,40,47,54,82,84-86,89-91] On the other hand, there is a population of *sick premature infants* with serum cortisol levels similar to or lower than cortisol levels in well preterm or term infants.[27-29,36,54,84,85,90,92,93] The finding that sick premature infants do not have the expected increase in random cortisol levels commensurate with their illness acuity is supportive of the presence of relative adrenal insufficiency in this population.

Relative adrenal insufficiency has been described more often in those ill preterm infants whose predominant clinical presentation is hypotension. *Blood pressure has been found to positively correlate with the cortisol* production rate,[94] where patients with low random or basal serum cortisol values were more likely to have low blood pressure. In an RCT of hydrocortisone administration in hypotensive preterm infants, the overall baseline (control) median serum cortisol concentrations were 3.3 and 4.1 mcg/dL in the treated and placebo groups, respectively.[54] These values are considered low for the degree of illness severity in preterm infants when compared to the 50th percentile of the serum cortisol values in ill infants (7.2 mcg/dL).[4] In 54 surfactant-treated, 1-day-old preterm infants of 24–36 weeks' gestation, serum cortisol values were lower in those with left ventricular output ≤180 mL/min/kg compared to those >180 mL/min/kg.[30,48,95]

Further support for relative adrenal insufficiency in the *preterm population* comes from studies that have found that adrenal insufficiency results from immature cortisol synthesis in the adrenal gland. Ng et al. reported normal pituitary response to CRH, but blunted adrenal response, in sick premature infants with vaso-pressor-resistant hypotension and low serum cortisol values. These findings led Ng et al. to speculate that, in preterm neonates, the adrenal gland was responsible for the adrenal insufficiency.[39] Findings from other investigators support this notion because sick premature infants have been found to have low random cortisol levels, elevated cortisol precursors, and blunted response to ACTH stimulation.[40,47,84,85,90,91,93,96] Watterberg et al. reported that, compared with term infants, sick premature infants had higher cortisol precursor concentrations (17α-OH pregnenolone, 17α-OH progesterone, and 11-deoxycortisol) and lower serum cortisol concentrations. In another small prospective study of infants born at less than 30 weeks' gestation, Huysman et al. demonstrated that critically ill, ventilated infants, compared with less sick, non-ventilated infants, had lower cortisol levels, elevated cortisol precursor levels of 17-hydroxyprogesterone, and insufficient cortisol response to ACTH (0.5 mcg/kg) stimulation.[82] Korte et al. also reported an abnormal adrenal response to cosyntropin (ACTH) in 51 ventilated, premature infants of less than 32 weeks' gestation who had baseline cortisol levels of less than 5 mcg/dL (138 nmol/L). Among the 51 infants, 64% and 37% had inadequate cortisol response (<9 mcg/dL) to stimulation with 0.1 and 0.2 mcg/kg cosyntropin, respectively.[40] Preterm infants, due to immaturity of the HPA axis, may be at unique risk for adrenal insufficiency and may be considered candidates for corticosteroids when not responsive to otherwise routine management, including volume and vasopressors.

## Relative Adrenal Insufficiency in Late Preterm and Term Infants

There is growing evidence that many ill term and late preterm infants also exhibit evidence of relative adrenal insufficiency.[44,45,56,89,97-99] In 1972, Gutai et al. were one of the first groups of authors to describe suboptimal cortisol responses to illness in a small number of stressed term newborn infants.[100] Indeed, there was no difference in the median random cortisol value between the 12 ill infants (5.2 mcg/dL) and 28 healthy newborns (4.1 mcg/dL) but all infants responded to 5 units of ACTH appropriately. A subsequent study by Thomas et al. found that 27% of ill term newborns studied had a basal cortisol of less

than 2 mcg/dL, and only 33% of these infants had an appropriate response to ACTH (>18 mcg/dL).[89] In the first study to investigate cardiovascular responses to dexamethasone in hypotensive term newborn infants, Tantivit et al. reported that five of the seven infants studied had cortisol values <10 mcg/dL.[55] All of these infants responded to dexamethasone administration with prompt hemodynamic stabilization. Soliman et al. found an overall increase in basal circulating cortisol concentrations by two- to threefold in neonates with sepsis and respiratory distress.[45] Yet, over 30% of these infants had cortisol values suggestive of relative adrenal insufficiency (<15 mcg/dL). Patients with lower basal cortisol levels and peak cortisol responses to ACTH had higher mortality. Recent reports also suggest that, similar to preterm infants, critically ill late preterm and term infants with hypotension may have problems with adrenal synthesis of cortisol, as higher cortisol precursor levels have also been documented in those presenting with vasopressor-resistant hypotension.[51,101] In a larger prospective observational study 35 sick late preterm and term infants on mechanical ventilation had a median random cortisol level of 4.6 mcg/dL, which is a value very low for the degree of illness.[56] These infants had relatively low ACTH values as well but demonstrated appropriate cortisol responses to ACTH stimulation (1 mcg/kg), suggesting this study population had secondary adrenal insufficiency.

Recognizing that acutely ill term and preterm infants may be at risk for adrenal insufficiency due to developmental reasons, including prematurity of the HPA axis at varying levels or due to poor/delayed transition of the HPA axis immediately after birth, may help guide recognition of infants who may be considered for steroid treatment. Subsets of these ill infants with acute pulmonary hypertension (aPH), meconium aspiration syndrome (MAS), hypoxic-ischemic encephalopathy (HIE), and sepsis have undergone further study with regard to their responsiveness to glucocorticoids and/or the presence of adrenal insufficiency.

## Acute Pulmonary Hypertension (aPH) of Newborn

There has been increasing attention on the effect of corticosteroids in those infants with aPH. Corticosteroids have been shown to improve oxygenation by decreasing phosphodiesterase-5 (PDE5) expression and activity and increasing cGMP, thereby promoting vascular dilatation of the lungs in animal models (lambs) with PH.[102] One small study enrolled newborns with aPH due to all causes and found that in 15 patients, those who received intravenous hydrocortisone had an increase in systemic blood pressure and an improvement in oxygenation measures.[5] Cortisol levels were not measured, so it was unclear if infants were responsive due to relative adrenal insufficiency or to the other basic physiologic effects of corticosteroids such as the effect on inflammation. In one of the largest observational cohort studies, 30% of the 2743 infants with aPH including those with MAS and congenital diaphragmatic hernia (CDH) had received hydrocortisone.[5,103] A comparison between the hydrocortisone-treated group and the non-treated group, however, showed no difference in outcomes of death, chronic lung disease (CLD), or oxygen at discharge. In a small subset of these infants with MAS there was lower oxygen use at discharge (odds ratio [OR] 0.56, 95% confidence interval [95% CI] 0.21–0.91). Cortisol values were not measured.

### Meconium Aspiration Syndrome

In infants with MAS, studies have more often focused on the administration of steroids for the effect on inflammation due to the presence of meconium in the lungs versus the presence of adrenal insufficiency or hypotension.[104] In a small study term infants born with meconium-stained amniotic fluid who presented with respiratory distress had lower ACTH and cortisol levels than did infants with meconium-stained amniotic fluid without respiratory distress.[105]

### Hypoxic-Ischemic Encephalopathy

There has been recent interest in infants undergoing hypothermia treatment for HIE with volume-resistant hypotension. An RCT of 35 infants randomized to receive hydrocortisone of 0.5 mg/kg/dose q 6 hours versus placebo had low cortisol values suggestive of adrenal insufficiency (median 3.5 mcg/dL in treatment group and 3.3 mcg/dL in placebo group). The infants who received hydrocortisone more often reached the target blood pressure in 2 hours after hydrocortisone (94 vs. 58%) and required less inotrope duration and dosage compared to the placebo group.[106] Another

similar study of 30 infants with HIE found similar cortisol levels between those with vasopressor-resistant hypotension versus those without, but higher DHEA levels in those with hypotension, suggesting adrenal insufficiency.[107]

### Sepsis

In pediatric patients with sepsis the debate continues whether corticosteroids should be administered mostly because of the lack of large RCTs to support the evidence. However, surveys show that 90% of clinicians already agree that there are certain septic patients (those with vasopressor-resistant hypotension) who may benefit from corticosteroids.[17]

Newborns may be at higher risk due to the immaturity of the HPA axis to synthesize cortisol soon after birth, in addition to the potential HPA axis changes due to inflammation from sepsis. Studies have shown there are lower-than-expected cortisol levels, elevated precursors to cortisol, and very high DHEA levels in septic newborn infants with therapy-resistant hypotension.[50,108] One of these studies by Bhat et al. showed that 17 of 30 infants (57%) with neonatal shock had cortisol values ≤15 mcg/dL with adequate rise (≥9 mg/dL) after ACTH, suggesting poor response to the illness and adequate response to ACTH, but with depressed baseline levels.[50]

### Congenital Diaphragmatic Hernia

In 2000 Pittinger et al. first described low cortisol values in sick infants with CDH and found that 79% had random cortisol levels of <7 mcg/dL.[99] Two of the four critically ill patients had an inappropriately low cortisol response to cosyntropin. However, a recent study in which up to 34% of infants received hydrocortisone found that infants exposed to a longer course of hydrocortisone had an increased risk of sepsis (OR 1.04, 95% CI 1.005–1.075, $P = 0.02$) and mortality (OR 1.11, 95% CI 1.02–1.2, $P = 0.02$).[109]

Investigators continue to explore the diseases and clinical presentations of infants who may benefit from corticosteroid treatment while continuing to assess for the potential complications of treatment.

## LABORATORY TRIGGERS (CORTISOL LEVELS)

Although there are newborn patients whose clinical presentation and disease suggest they may benefit from adjunctive corticosteroid administration, there is still not a reliable mechanism by which to identify these patients. Measuring adrenal function can be complex because acute illness may affect the HPA axis at varying levels and also varies with stage of development, age, disease state, and timing of the disease. The diagnosis of relative adrenal insufficiency is made by determining "inadequate" cortisol response or cortisol production and has been defined in various ways.

In other ill populations there are recommended guidelines for diagnosing relative adrenal insufficiency. The recommendation for critically ill adults was proposed in 2008 as a total serum cortisol level of less than 9 mcg/dL following 250 mcg of cosyntropin (ACTH) administration or a random total cortisol of less than 10 mcg/dL (276 nmol/L).[110] The updated guidelines in 2017, curiously, showed less enthusiasm for these thresholds but they remained the same.[7] In their most recent 2017 publication on clinical practice parameters for hemodynamic support of pediatric and neonatal septic shock, the American College of Critical Care Medicine has changed their stance from 2007. In 2007, it was stated that there was "equipoise on the question of adjunctive steroid therapy and thus the diagnosis of relative adrenal insufficiency for pediatric and newborn septic shock (outside of classic adrenal insufficiency) is pending further trials". In the new 2017 guidelines, the recommendation is to treat a subset of infants with septic shock and vasopressor-resistant hypotension with hydrocortisone who have absolute adrenal insufficiency as defined by peak cortisol <18 mcg/dL after ACTH or basal cortisol <4 mcg/dL or basal cortisol <18 mcg/dL with need for inotropic support.[6,68]

*Devising diagnostic criteria for* relative adrenal insufficiency *in infants* is particularly challenging because of the relatively little amount of available data.[111] Neonatal investigators most often report isolated, random serum cortisol levels or stimulated serum cortisol levels at specific time points following ACTH stimulation.

*Using random cortisol values* at the time of stress in VLBW infants, Korte et al. were some of the first investigators to define normal adrenal function as a random cortisol level of >15 mcg/dL (414 nmol/L) and an inadequate serum cortisol as a serum cortisol

level less than 5 mcg/dL (<138 nmol/L).[40] In critically ill term and late preterm infants Fernandez et al. showed that those with random cortisol values less than 15 mcg/dL had higher blood pressure within 24 hours after hydrocortisone administration than those with cortisol values >15 mcg/dL.[44] In addition, these infants demonstrated a decreased need for vasopressors and had a lower heart rate after hydrocortisone administration. In term and late preterm infants, a cut-off random cortisol value of 15 mcg/dL is often used, based on smaller studies and the pediatric and adult population, or 18 mcg/dL in the presence of vasopressor-resistant hypotension.[6,14] In his review, PC Ng published a mathematical model that further takes into account clinical variables that may change the percentile of the diagnostic serum cortisol for preterm infants. He suggested that a serum cortisol value of less than 200 nmol/L (7.25 mcg/dL) be used to diagnose relative (transient) adrenal insufficiency of prematurity. This value represents the 25th percentile of serum cortisol levels in well VLBW and the 50th percentile in vasopressor-dependent VLBW infants.[14] However, debate continues on the use of random cortisol values as a diagnostic tool because total plasma cortisol can have marked hourly variability in both adults and neonates.[53,112,113] In addition, random cortisol values may not correlate with outcome, response to therapy, or severity of illness.[56,112,114] However, a baseline random cortisol is often the most practical and easiest to obtain in the acute setting of the rapidly deteriorating newborn and may help to determine the need for further evaluation.

Of note is the fact that cortisol level thresholds may also change slightly based on the laboratory methods. Newer laboratory methods of mass spectrometry and platform methods (Elecsys Cortisol II, Roche Diagnostics, Mannheim, Germany) are more specific because they can detect lower cortisol concentrations than older standard immunoassays.[115] The newer methods tend to show lower cortisol values by 1–2 mcg/dL compared to the older ones.

To further test for relative adrenal insufficiency, investigators have more often used the *ACTH stimulation test* as opposed to CRH alone.[92,93,116] ACTH test is done by using the corticotropin analogs such as tetracosactrin (Synacthen) or cosyntropin (Cortrosyn). ACTH as the stimulating agent has been trialed with dosages ranging from 0.1 to 62.5 mcg/kg.[36,40,45,60,82,84,89,93,117-120] Adrenal stimulation with supraphysiologic ACTH doses can induce a compromised adrenal gland to produce an "adequate"-appearing serum cortisol response and thus miss the diagnosis of relative adrenal insufficiency.[40] Indeed, ACTH doses at 0.1–0.2 mcg/kg[40,60,117,118] and doses at 0.5–1.0 mcg/kg[60,82] are more likely to reveal "relative" adrenal insufficiency than higher ACTH doses. Yet, even within the dose range of 0.1–1.0 mcg/kg, the proportion of sick premature infants with "inadequate" cortisol response varies greatly. In a study of ventilated VLBW infants of less than 32 weeks' gestation and with random serum cortisol levels of less than 5 mcg/dL (138 nmol/L), Korte et al. reported that 64% and 37% of infants had inadequate cortisol response (less than 9 mcg/dL) to ACTH at doses of 0.1 and 0.2 mcg/dL, respectively.[40] In a trial of ventilated 3-week-old 25 weeks' gestation *preterm infants*, Watterberg et al. reported that 21% and 2% of infants had inadequate cortisol response to 0.1 and 1.0 mcg/kg ACTH, respectively.[60] In critically ill *term infants*, after giving 1 mcg/kg of ACTH, Fernandez et al. found no infants with a cortisol value of less than 18 mcg/dL, and all patients had increased serum cortisol by greater than 9 mcg/dL.[56] In addition, there was no association between ACTH-stimulated cortisol values and severity of illness, need for vasopressor-inotropes, or days on mechanical ventilation. In non-mechanically ventilated infants with sepsis, Soliman et al. found that when an ACTH stimulation dose of 250 mcg/1.73 m² was used, no patients met the criteria of having adrenal insufficiency, whereas 13% of the patients were diagnosed with adrenal insufficiency when 1 mcg/1.73 m² of ACTH was given.[45] Importantly, patients with lower stimulated cortisol values did have higher mortality. In 2012, Hochwald et al. reported that if an ACTH stimulation test using a dose of 1 mcg/kg is performed in premature infants of less than 29 weeks' gestation, with varying degrees of illness in the first 8 postnatal hours, the test could predict those with adrenal insufficiency using hypotension requiring vasopressor-inotrope treatment as a marker.[121] They determined that an ACTH-induced change in cortisol of less than 12% from baseline provided the highest sensitivity (75%) and specificity

(93%) for detecting the development of hypotension in this population. On the other hand, random basal cortisol levels did not predict hypotension with an area under the receiver operating characteristic curve (ROC) of 48%.[121]

The most recent standard for performing the ACTH stimulation test is to use a total dose of 1 mcg of ACTH (1 mL Cortrosyn diluted in 1- or 2-mL normal saline) and administer over 2 minutes, after which the IV is then flushed. Cortisol levels are measured at baseline and then at 30 minutes. Measuring cortisol levels additionally at 60 minutes after ACTH may reduce the risk of false-positives. Cortisol thresholds for a normal ACTH stimulation test are in the range of >15–19 mcg/dL, but most often it is >18 mcg/dL.[122,123]

Measuring ACTH, unless undergoing evaluation for chronic adrenal insufficiency, is not feasible in most institutions and there is usually not a sufficient turnaround time to have an impact on the acute management of the critically ill patient. During critical illness, plasma corticotropin levels have also been variably found to be low, normal, or high and likely follow a dynamic pattern over the course of the disease and vary with developmental age.[7]

*Free cortisol* and not protein-bound cortisol is responsible for the physiologic effects at the cellular level and was thought to potentially be a better diagnostic tool for adrenal insufficiency.[125] Yoder et al. found that urinary free cortisol levels were directly proportional to and highly correlated with plasma cortisol levels in premature baboon models.[124] Urinary free cortisol measurements may also avoid the potential fluctuations seen in serum cortisol levels and the need for frequent blood sampling.[87] Vezina et al. described unbound cortisol concentrations in critically ill newborns with hypotension requiring vasopressor-inotrope administration.[125] However, free cortisol levels have not been fully validated in the ill newborn populations. Additionally, recent reports suggest that free cortisol levels may also not be added information in ill children with septic shock.[126] In addition, free cortisol tests are not always widely available and the time to get results is often too long to impact decision-making.

The diagnosis of adrenal insufficiency in the preterm and term neonate, according to measurements of serum cortisol and the response to ACTH stimulation, may be influenced by the various procedures and the testing itself in acutely ill patients.[127] Thus the validity and interpretation of adrenal function tests, especially amid critical illness, is subject to an ongoing debate among adult, pediatric, and neonatal critical care physicians. However, there are general upper and lower threshold cortisol values that may help to guide decisions.

## Corticosteroid Administration

Sometimes, cortisol values may not help identify those patients who might benefit from corticosteroids as there are conflicting reports on the correlation of cortisol levels with response to therapy or outcomes. There are a number of reports that also show documented low cortisol values in neonates with vasopressor-resistant hypotension *responsive* to corticosteroid treatment.[27,28,30,33,39,54,83,128] However, other studies report a similar presentation of responsiveness to corticosteroids treatment without cortisol data or relation to cortisol data.[30,33,45,129,130]

### TYPE OF GLUCOCORTICOID

Hydrocortisone is by far the most widely used over dexamethasone, both clinically and in studies, likely due to its better safety profile and the additional mineralocorticoid activity. Studies of early use (<7 days of age) and higher-dose dexamethasone demonstrate an adverse effect on neurodevelopment in preterm neonates.[120,131] Supportive evidence from animal and laboratory studies indicates that unbalanced stimulation of glucocorticoid receptors in the brain induces apoptosis, which can be rescued by the addition of a mineralocorticoid.[132] This would explain why dexamethasone, especially when given early and in higher doses (0.5 mg/kg q 12 hours 3 times during the first 2 postnatal days),[133] is associated with significant cerebral pathology (white matter injury, decrease in brain volume, etc.), whereas hydrocortisone seems to be devoid of such effects.

### CLINICAL EFFECT

Hydrocortisone increases blood pressure and reduces vasopressor requirements in all populations. A meta-analysis in preterm neonates with hypotension and

vasopressor dependence found that hydrocortisone is effective in increasing blood pressure (seven studies, N = 144, r = 0.71, 95% CI 0.18–0.92) and reducing vasopressor requirement (five studies, N = 93, r = 0.74, 95% CI 0.0084–0.96). The study's findings were robust and found that by random effects meta-analysis, the numbers of new studies needed to cancel out the effects of hydrocortisone on blood pressure increase and the decrease in vasopressor requirement are 78 for blood pressure increase and 47 for reducing vasopressor requirement.[134]

### DOSING

Studies of vasopressor-dependent, critically ill newborn infants have used variable hydrocortisone dosing (1–3 mg/kg/day), and all have shown an increase in blood pressure, a decrease in volume and vasopressor-inotrope requirement, and a decrease in heart rate without confirmed increases in adverse events.[30,37,44,54,114,134,135] In preterm infants doses as low as 1 mg/kg/day of hydrocortisone have been shown to increase blood pressure significantly.[119] A recent study of 106 preterm infants with hypotension on inotropes showed no differences in efficacy between dosing of 4 mg/kg/day versus 1–3 mg/kg/day.[136] A planned systemic and meta-analysis has been proposed to study different doses of hydrocortisone on the effect of end organ perfusion in infants with hypotension: *low-dose* (initial dose of ≤1 mg/kg, followed by ≤2 mg/kg/day or cumulative daily dose of ≤3 mg/kg on the first day of treatment) versus *high-dose* (initial dose of >1 mg/kg, followed by >2 mg/kg/day or cumulative daily dose of >3 mg/kg on the first day of treatment).[137]

The *elimination half-life* of bound hydrocortisone in neonates is much longer than in adults. In adults the half-life of bound cortisol is reported to be 2 ± 0.3 hours[138] and, for free cortisol, 61 minutes.[139] In 1962 Reynolds et al. were the first to report pharmacokinetics in five term infants after a bolus of 5 mg/kg of hydrocortisone.[140] The mean peak serum concentration (30–80 minutes after dose) was 557 mcg/dL, and mean serum half-life was just under 4 hours (range 2.4–7.1 hours). In a recent study of unbound hydrocortisone concentrations in 62 preterm infants treated for vasopressor-resistant hypotension, the half-life of free cortisol was 2.9 hours.[125] This is three times longer than in the adult population and consistent with other reports on hydrocortisone pharmacokinetics in preterm infants as described in a recent review.[11] As illustrated in this review, high cortisol levels can result from administration of high or "stress" dosing of hydrocortisone because the longer half-life in preterm infants is often not appreciated. In a small pilot study of six infants hydrocortisone at 0.4–0.8 mg/kg/dose resulted in serum cortisol trough levels greater than 20 mcg/dL for 8 to 12 hours compared to the median endogenous serum cortisol value in sick extremely-low-birth-weight (ELBW) infants of 16 mcg/dL at less than 48 hours of age. Given this information, hydrocortisone should be given at no shorter interval than every 6 hours for late preterm and term infants and up to every 12 hours in extreme prematurity.

## ONSET OF ACTION

The *time to documented cardiovascular response to hydrocortisone* is often measured in hours in the ill newborn population. In *preterm infants*, Helbock reported an increase in blood pressure as early as 30 minutes and within 2 hours following hydrocortisone therapy (1 mg) in 25- to 26-week gestation infants with vasopressor-resistant hypotension.[83] Gaissmaier and Pohlandt noted improvement in vasopressor-resistant hypotension within 4–8 hours following a single injection of dexamethasone.[128] Seri et al.[30] and Noori et al.[129] reported an increase in blood pressure within 2 hours of hydrocortisone and low-dose dexamethasone (0.1 mg/kg) administration, respectively. Mizobuchi found a similar response after a single dose of 2 mg/kg dose of hydrocortisone.[141] Ng et al. found more infants were weaned off vasopressor-inotropes by 72 hours after receiving hydrocortisone vs placebo (79% vs. 33%, $P = 0.001$).[142] In 15 newborn infants Noori et al. studied the hemodynamics following hydrocortisone (2 mg/kg, followed by 1 mg/kg q 12 hours) and showed an increase in blood pressure at 6 hours, a parallel increase in systemic vascular resistance, and a decrease in dopamine dosage without initial changes in stroke volume or left ventricular output.[135] In seven term ill newborn infants given dexamethasone at 0.2 mg/kg/day, an increase in blood pressure was noted by 4 hours after initial dosing, with a concomitant decrease in heart rate and vasopressor dosage.[55] Vasopressors were discontinued in

all infants within 72 hours of initiating dexamethasone. In a larger study of ill late preterm and term neonates there was a significant change in blood pressure over the first 24 hours after hydrocortisone and an overall decrease in vasopressor dose and heart rate within 12 hours.[44] In 12 term infants given hydrocortisone for low cardiac output syndrome after cardiac surgery, the blood pressure increased 3 hours after hydrocortisone.[130] Baker et al. also found an increase in blood pressure, starting 2 hours after the first dose of hydrocortisone, and a decrease in the total vasopressor-inotrope requirement at 6 hours in a study of 117 critically ill term and preterm newborns.[114] In summary, most newborn infants respond with improved blood pressure within 2–4 hours of initiation of corticosteroids and weaning from inotropes as early as 6 hours after initiation and most by 72 hours.

## DURATION OF ADRENAL INSUFFICIENCY

In most infants with possible adrenal insufficiency-associated hypotension, blood pressure recovers in less than a few days after corticosteroid initiation, with few preterm infants requiring longer treatment. This is similar to what is found in acutely ill adults where *the reversal of shock*, as measured by the timing of withdrawal of vasopressors, occurs earlier after receiving hydrocortisone versus placebo (3.3 vs. 5.8 median days).[42] In a group of adults with sepsis and higher illness severity, the median time to vasopressor withdrawal with corticosteroids versus placebo also favored the treated group (7 vs. 9 days, respectively).[42]

In preterm infants, Colasurdo et al. found that in nine sick infants of 26 weeks' gestation with clinical symptoms of relative adrenal insufficiency and low cortisol levels (mean $251 \pm 102$ nmol/L or $9.1 \pm 3.7$ mcg/dL), there was reversal of clinical signs within 2 days. Ng et al. reported that 79% of preterm infants <32 weeks' gestation with refractory hypotension receiving hydrocortisone for 5 days were successfully weaned from vasopressor support by 72 hours of age compared with only 33% who were receiving placebo.[54] Hochwald et al. also showed that a 2-day course of hydrocortisone compared with placebo decreased dopamine exposure by 34 hours versus 67 hours ($P = 0.04$).[143] Similarly, Efird et al. reported that prophylactic hydrocortisone therapy for 5 days (versus placebo) in ELBW infants reduced the use of vasopressors during the first 2 postnatal days.[144] On the other hand, in very premature baboons with relative adrenal insufficiency and vaso-pressor-resistant hypotension at a gestational age approximately equivalent to human gestation of 26 weeks, there was no decrease in urinary free cortisol levels over the first 2 postnatal weeks (the entire duration of the study).[87]

In term ill infants, Economou et al. found that, in 4 of 15 infants who were "low cortisol responders" relative to their illness, this state lasted until the fifth postnatal day.[97] In another study of critically ill newborn infants with refractory hypotension, Baker et al. used cortisol levels and the presence of hemodynamic instability to determine the duration of relative adrenal insufficiency and thereby the duration of hydrocortisone replacement therapy.[114] In total, 61 term infants received 3.5 median days of hydrocortisone therapy, whereas 37 extremely preterm infants enrolled in the study remained on hydrocortisone for a median of 15 days. In another study 1-day-old term and late preterm ill infants with random low cortisol values of less than 15 mcg/dL received longer courses of treatment with hydrocortisone for hypotension compared with those with higher cortisol values (5 vs. 2.5 median days).[44] Kamath et al. found a high incidence (67%) of cortisol values of less than 15 mcg/dL in hypotensive infants with congenital diaphragmatic hernia, all of whom received hydrocortisone for 10.9 ± 7.0 days.[98]

The duration of relative adrenal insufficiency varies with age, disease severity, etiology, and response to treatment. In general, relative adrenal insufficiency seems to last less than a week in term infants and no longer than 2 weeks in very preterm infants, irrespective of whether it is defined by cortisol values or by the short-term cardiovascular response to corticosteroid replacement therapy. However, exposure to corticosteroids should be limited as much as possible and most infants appear to have significantly less inotrope exposure after 72 hours.

## Outcomes

While corticosteroids have continued to show positive effects on stabilizing cardiovascular insufficiency, there remains caution because of the limited data on safety due to the lack of RCTs. It is well known that high-dose corticosteroids in all populations have associated adverse effects. High-dose corticosteroids have been shown to increase mortality and infection rates in septic and ill adults and increase rates of neurodevelopmental delays (i.e., cerebral palsy) in preterm infants.[53,145] It is not clear that lower dose hydrocortisone is without potential risk long term. In a recent small study of preterm infants with septic shock, hydrocortisone improved blood pressure, urine output, and oxygen requirement. There was, however, a decrease in 1-year survival in those who received hydrocortisone, suggesting more information is needed.[146] In addition, there may be particular populations of infants more at risk of complications due to hydrocortisone such as found in the study by Peeple et al.[136] In hypotensive infants on inotropes who received hydrocortisone, those with cortisol values >15 mcg/dL showed less improvement in vasoactive burden, increased hyperglycemia (P = 0.015), and increased death independent of the hydrocortisone dose (OR 26.3, range 3.5–198.3, P = 0.002), suggesting that hydrocortisone therapy should be avoided in infants who are not cortisol deficient.

Shorter-term outcomes in newborn infants have shown that both low- and high-dose corticosteroids have been associated with hyperglycemia, hypertension, and hypertrophic cardiomyopathy.[147-149] In addition, there have been reports of spontaneous ileal perforations when preterm infants are co-exposed to hydrocortisone or dexamethasone and cyclooxygenase inhibitors (i.e., indomethacin).

Despite these potential complications, the data from RCTs on hydrocortisone treatment for the prevention of BPD in preterm infants are reassuring. Hydrocortisone use in preterm infants for the prevention of BPD has shown either positive long-term outcomes (neurodevelopment or mortality) or at least no difference versus placebo.[145,148,150,151]

Given the pros and cons of using corticosteroids, they should, at the minimum, be considered for patients with fulminant manifestations of critical illness, especially those with volume and vasopressor-resistant hypotension, as there is equipoise to indicate that they may improve outcome with acceptable risks when used at the lowest effective dose and shortest course possible.

## Summary

Clinical, biochemical, and physiologic evidence indicates that adrenal insufficiency and vasopressor-resistant hypotension are serious conditions in sick preterm and term infants and that these conditions respond to corticosteroid therapy, with improvements in cardiovascular status. Adequate HPA axis and adrenal function are vital to postnatal adaptation in extremely premature infants and critically ill late preterm and term newborns. Yet, recent findings provide important insights into adrenal insufficiency and vasopressor-resistant hypotension and stimulate consideration of mechanisms for adrenal insufficiency and vasopressor-resistant hypotension. Management of the critically ill hypotensive infant remains challenging and requires a better understanding of the pathophysiology of neonatal shock and improvements in our ability to monitor cardiac output, organ blood flow, and tissue perfusion in real time at the bedside.

In addition, we still need to improve our understanding of the pathogenesis and epidemiology of adrenal insufficiency and vasopressor-resistant hypotension, especially in terms of the determinants, mechanisms, and characteristics of these conditions, and their relationship with each other and with acute and long-term morbidity/mortality. Ultimately, we need to provide evidence that our interventions also improve clinically meaningful outcomes. Another challenge is to improve the diagnostic methods to assess adrenal function and vasopressor-resistant hypotension and define the criteria for treatment. We need to be able to determine which patient needs therapy, at what dose and for how long, and what evaluations provide the most reliable information early in the course of the disease, such as the use of echocardiograms and cortisol values. Are serum cortisol values the optimal measure of adrenal function? Can one improve diagnostic accuracy and prognosis by combining the findings of different tests in conjunction with the status of the patient? Will simultaneous measurements of inflammatory mediators improve our understanding and guide therapy? By improving our ability to establish accurate and timely diagnosis of adrenal insufficiency, will we be able to target high-risk patients for investigational and clinical interventions and avoid unnecessary exposure of lower-risk infants to corticosteroid therapy?

More comprehensive issues to be addressed include identifying the factors that influence the choice of corticosteroid treatment and establishing the dosage, duration, and response to therapy of the individual patient.[152] We also need to find out whether corticosteroid regimens need to be adjusted according to disease severity or the response to treatment to maximize effectiveness and minimize harm. Scientifically and ethically sound research and carefully designed studies will resolve these questions but answers may also require a different approach than only applying rigorous RCTs. Any approach should include framework for recognition, treatment strategy, and implementation and performance assessment of feasibility, adherence, effectiveness, and outcomes.

## REFERENCES

1. Fernandez E, Watterberg KL, Faix RG, et al. Incidence, management, and outcomes of cardiovascular insufficiency in critically ill term and late preterm newborn infants. *Am J Perinatol.* 2014;31(11):947-956. doi:10.1055/s-0034-1368089.
2. Rios DR, Moffett BS, Kaiser JR. Trends in pharmacotherapy for neonatal hypotension. *J Pediatr.* 2014;165(4):697-701.e1. doi:10.1016/j.jpeds.2014.06.009.
3. Sehgal A, Osborn D, McNamara PJ. Cardiovascular support in preterm infants: a survey of practices in Australia and New Zealand. *J Paediatr Child Health.* 2012;48(4):317-323. doi:10.1111/j.1440-1754.2011.02246.x.
4. Ng PC, Wong SP, Chan IH, Lam HS, Lee CH, Lam CW. A prospective longitudinal study to estimate the "adjusted cortisol percentile" in preterm infants. *Pediatr Res.* 2011;69(6):511-516. doi:10.1203/PDR.0b013e31821764b1.
5. Aleem S, Robbins C, Murphy B, et al. The use of supplemental hydrocortisone in the management of persistent pulmonary hypertension of the newborn. *J Perinatol.* 2021;41(4):794-800. doi:10.1038/s41372-021-00943-9.
6. Davis AL, Carcillo JA, Aneja RK, et al. American college of critical care medicine clinical practice parameters for hemodynamic support of pediatric and neonatal septic shock. *Crit Care Med.* 2017;45(6):1061-1093. doi:10.1097/CCM.0000000000002425.
7. Annane D, Pastores SM, Rochwerg B, et al. Guidelines for the diagnosis and management of critical illness-related corticosteroid insufficiency (CIRCI) in critically ill patients (Part 1): Society of Critical Care Medicine (SCCM) and European Society of Intensive Care Medicine (ESICM) 2017. *Intensive Care Med.* 2017;43(12):1751-1763. doi:10.1007/s00134-017-4919-5.
8. Kohn Loncarica G, Fustinana A, Jabornisky R. Recomendaciones para el manejo del shock septico en ninos durante la primera hora (segunda parte) [Recommendations for the management of pediatric septic shock in the first hour (part two)]. *Arch Argent Pediatr.* 2019;117(1):e24-e33. doi:10.5546/aap.2019.eng.e24.

9. Goldsmith JP, Keels E. Recognition and management of cardio-vascular insufficiency in the very low birth weight newborn. *Pediatrics.* 2022;149(3):e2021056051. doi:10.1542/peds.2021-056051.

10. Ibrahim H, Sinha IP, Subhedar NV. Corticosteroids for treating hypotension in preterm infants. *Cochrane Database Syst Rev.* 2011;(12):CD003662. doi:10.1002/14651858.CD003662.pub4.

11. Watterberg KL. Hydrocortisone dosing for hypotension in new-born infants: less is more. *J Pediatr.* 2016;174:23-26.e1. doi:10.1016/j.jpeds.2016.04.005.

12. Schwarz CE, Dempsey EM. Management of neonatal hypoten-sion and shock. *Semin Fetal Neonatal Med.* 2020;25(5):101121. doi:10.1016/j.siny.2020.101121.

13. Giesinger RE, McNamara PJ. Hemodynamic instability in the critically ill neonate: an approach to cardiovascular support based on disease pathophysiology. *Semin Perinatol.* 2016;40(3):174-188. doi:10.1053/j.semperi.2015.12.005.

14. Ng PC. Adrenocortical insufficiency and refractory hypoten-sion in preterm infants. *Arch Dis Child Fetal Neonatal Ed.* 2016;101(6):F571-F576. doi:10.1136/archdischild-2016-311289.

15. Batton BJ, Li L, Newman NS, et al. Feasibility study of early blood pressure management in extremely preterm infants. *J Pediatr.* 2012;161(1):65-69.e1. doi:10.1016/j.jpeds.2012.01.014.

16. Watterberg KL, Fernandez E, Walsh MC, et al. Barriers to en-rollment in a randomized controlled trial of hydrocortisone for cardiovascular insufficiency in term and late preterm newborn infants. *J Perinatol.* 2017;37(11):1220-1223. doi:10.1038/jp.2017.131.

17. Menon K, McNally D, O'Hearn K, et al. A randomized con-trolled trial of corticosteroids in pediatric septic shock: a pilot feasibility study. *Pediatr Crit Care Med.* 2017;18(6):505-512. doi:10.1097/PCC.0000000000001121.

18. Bhayat SI, Gowda HM, Eisenhut M. Should dopamine be the first line inotrope in the treatment of neonatal hypotension? Review of the evidence. *World J Clin Pediatr.* 2016;5(2):212-222. doi:10.5409/wjcp.v5.i2.212.

19. Nisticò D, Bossini B, Benvenuto S, Pellegrin MC, Tornese G. Pediatric adrenal insufficiency: challenges and solutions. *Ther Clin Risk Manag.* 2022;18:47-60. doi:10.2147/tcrm.S294065.

20. Buonocore F, McGlacken-Byrne SM, Del Valle I, Achermann JC. Current insights into adrenal insufficiency in the newborn and young infant. *Front Pediatr.* 2020;8:619041. doi:10.3389/fped.2020.619041.

21. Cohen J, Venkatesh B. Relative adrenal insufficiency in the in-tensive care population; background and critical appraisal of the evidence. *Anaesth Intensive Care.* 2010;38(3):425-436.

22. Cooper MS, Stewart PM. Adrenal insufficiency in critical ill-ness. *J Intensive Care Med.* 2007;22(6):348-362. doi:10.1177/0885066607307832.

23. Marik PE. Critical illness-related corticosteroid insufficiency. *Chest.* 2009;135(1):181-193. doi:10.1378/chest.08-1149.

24. Fernandez EF, Watterberg KL. Relative adrenal insufficiency in the preterm and term infant. *J Perinatol.* 2009;29(suppl 2):S44-S49. doi:10.1038/jp.2009.24.

25. de Jong FH, Mallios C, Jansen C, Scheck PA, Lamberts SW. Etomidate suppresses adrenocortical function by inhibition of 11 beta-hydroxylation. *J Clin Endocrinol Metab.* 1984;59(6):1143-1147.

26. Schneider AJ, Voerman HJ. Abrupt hemodynamic improve-ment in late septic shock with physiological doses of glucocor-ticoids. *Intensive Care Med.* 1991;17(7):436-437.

27. Colasurdo MA, Hanna CE, Gilhooly JT, Reynolds JW. Hydrocortisone replacement in extremely premature infants with cortisol insufficiency. *Clin Res.* 1989;37:180A.

28. Ward RM, Kimura RE, Rich Denson C. Addisonian crisis in extremely premature neonates. *Clin Res.* 1991;39:11A.

29. Hanna CE, Keith LD, Colasurdo MA, et al. Hypothalamic pitu-itary adrenal function in the extremely low birth weight infant. *J Clin Endocrinol Metab.* 1993;76(2):384-387.

30. Seri I, Tan R, Evans J. Cardiovascular effects of hydrocortisone in preterm infants with pressor-resistant hypotension. *Pediatrics.* 2001;107(5):1070-1074.

31. Briegel J, Forst H, Kellermann W, Haller M, Peter K. Haemody-namic improvement in refractory septic shock with cortisol replacement therapy. *Intensive Care Med.* 1992;18(5):318.

32. Caplan RH, Wickus GG, Reynertson RH, Kisken WA. Occult hy-poadrenalism in critically ill patients. *Arch Surg.* 1994;129(4):456.

33. Fauser A, Pohlandt F, Bartmann P, Gortner L. Rapid increase of blood pressure in extremely low birth weight infants after a single dose of dexamethasone. *Eur J Pediatr.* 1993;152(4):354-356.

34. Reynolds JW, Hanna CE. Glucocorticoid-responsive hypoten-sion in extremely low birth weight newborns. *Pediatrics.* 1994;94(1):135-136.

35. Scott SM, Watterberg KL. Effect of gestational age, postnatal age, and illness on plasma cortisol concentrations in premature infants. *Pediatr Res.* 1995;37(1):112-116.

36. Watterberg KL, Scott SM. Evidence of early adrenal insuffi-ciency in babies who develop bronchopulmonary dysplasia. *Pediatrics.* 1995;95(1):120-125.

37. Bourchier D, Weston PJ. Randomised trial of dopamine com-pared with hydrocortisone for the treatment of hypotensive very low birthweight infants. *Arch Dis Child Fetal Neonatal Ed.* 1997;76(3):F174-F178.

38. Hanna CE, Jett PL, Laird MR, Mandel SH, LaFranchi SH, Reyn-olds JW. Corticosteroid binding globulin, total serum cortisol, and stress in extremely low-birth-weight infants. *Am J Perinatol.* 1997;14(4):201-204. doi:10.1055/s-2007-994127.

39. Ng PC, Lam CW, Fok TF, et al. Refractory hypotension in pre-term infants with adrenocortical insufficiency. *Arch Dis Child Fetal Neonatal Ed.* 2001;84(2):F122-F124.

40. Korte C, Styne D, Merritt TA, Mayes D, Wertz A, Helbock HJ. Adrenocortical function in the very low birth weight infant: improved testing sensitivity and association with neonatal out-come. *J Pediatr.* 1996;128(2):257-263. doi:10.1016/s0022-3476(96)70404-3.

41. Cooper MS, Stewart PM. Corticosteroid insufficiency in acutely ill patients. *N Engl J Med.* 2003;348(8):727-734. doi:10.1056/NEJMra020529.

42. Annane D, Sebille V, Charpentier C, et al. Effect of treatment with low doses of hydrocortisone and fludrocortisone on mortality in patients with septic shock. *JAMA.* 2002;288(7):862-871. doi:10.1001/jama.288.7.862.

43. Menon K, Ward RE, Lawson ML, et al. A prospective multi-center study of adrenal function in critically ill children. *Am J Respir Crit Care Med.* 2010;182(2):246-251. doi:10.1164/rccm.200911-1738OC.

44. Fernandez E, Schrader R, Watterberg K. Prevalence of low cortisol values in term and near-term infants with vasopressor-resistant hypotension. *J Perinatol.* 2005;25(2):114-118. doi:10.1038/sj.jp.7211211.

45. Soliman AT, Taman KH, Rizk MM, Nasr IS, Alrimawy H, Hamido MS. Circulating adrenocorticotropic hormone (ACTH)

and cortisol concentrations in normal, appropriate-for-gestational-age newborns versus those with sepsis and respiratory distress: cortisol response to low-dose and standard-dose ACTH tests. *Metabolism.* 2004;53(2):209-214. doi:10.1016/j.metabol.2003.09.005.

46. Ho JT, Al-Musalhi H, Chapman MJ, et al. Septic shock and sepsis: a comparison of total and free plasma cortisol levels. *J Clin Endocrinol Metab.* 2006;91(1):105-114. doi:10.1210/jc.2005-0265.

47. Guttentag SH, Rubin LP, Douglas R, Ringer SA, Berg G, Liley H. The glucocorticoid pathway in ill and well extremely low birth-weight infants. *Pediatric Res.* 1991;29:77A.

48. Scott SM, Alverson DC, Backstrom C, Bessman S. Positive effect of cortisol on cardiac output in the preterm infant. *Pediatric Res.* 1995;236A.

49. Rezai M, Fullwood C, Hird B, et al. Cortisol levels during acute illnesses in children and adolescents: a systematic review. *JAMA Netw Open.* 2022;5(6):e2217812. doi:10.1001/jamanetworkopen.2022.17812.

50. Bhat V, Saini SS, Sachdeva N, Walia R, Sundaram V, Dutta S. Adrenocortical dysfunctions in neonatal septic shock. *Indian J Pediatr.* 2022;89(7):714-716. doi:10.1007/s12098-021-03955-7.

51. Khashana A, Ahmed H, Ahmed A, et al. Cortisol precursors in neonates with vasopressor-resistant hypotension in relationship to demographic characteristics. *J Matern Fetal Neonatal Med.* 2018;31(18):2473-2477. doi:10.1080/14767058.2017.1344966.

52. Annane D. Glucocorticoids in the treatment of severe sepsis and septic shock. *Curr Opin Crit Care.* 2005;11(5):449-453. doi:10.1097/01.ccx.0000176691.95562.43.

53. Annane D, Pastores SM, Arlt W, et al. Critical illness-related corticosteroid insufficiency (CIRCI): a narrative review from a Multispecialty Task Force of the Society of Critical Care Medicine (SCCM) and the European Society of Intensive Care Medicine (ESICM). *Intensive Care Med.* 2017;43(12):1781-1792. doi:10.1007/s00134-017-4914-x.

54. Langer M, Modi BP, Agus M. Adrenal insufficiency in the critically ill neonate and child. *Curr Opin Pediatr.* 2006;18(4):448-453. doi:10.1097/01.mop.0000236397.79580.85.

55. Tantivit P, Subramanian N, Garg M, Ramanathan R, deLemos RA. Low serum cortisol in term newborns with refractory hypotension. *J Perinatol.* 1999;19(5):352-357.

56. Fernandez EF, Montman R, Watterberg KL. ACTH and cortisol response to critical illness in term and late preterm newborns. *J Perinatol.* 2008;28(12):797-802. doi:10.1038/jp.2008.190.

57. Rivers EP, Gaspari M, Saad GA, et al. Adrenal insufficiency in high-risk surgical ICU patients. *Chest.* 2001;119(3):889-896.

58. Dimopoulou I, Tsagarakis S, Kouyialis AT, et al. Hypothalamic-pituitary-adrenal axis dysfunction in critically ill patients with traumatic brain injury: incidence, pathophysiology, and relationship to vasopressor dependence and peripheral interleukin-6 levels. *Crit Care Med.* 2004;32(2):404-408. doi:10.1097/01.CCM.0000108885.37811.CA.

59. Hoen S, Asehnoune K, Brailly-Tabard S, et al. Cortisol response to corticotropin stimulation in trauma patients: influence of hemorrhagic shock. *Anesthesiology.* 2002;97(4):807-813. doi:10.1097/00000542-200210000-00010.

60. Watterberg KL, Shaffer ML, Garland JS, et al. Effect of dose on response to adrenocorticotropin in extremely low birth weight infants. *J Clin Endocrinol Metab.* 2005;90(12):6380-6385. doi:10.1210/jc.2005-0734.

61. Dickstein G, Shechner C, Nicholson WE, et al. Adrenocorticotropin stimulation test: effects of basal cortisol level, time of day, and suggested new sensitive low dose test. *J Clin Endocrinol Metab.* 1991;72(4):773-778.

62. Annane D. Time for a consensus definition of corticosteroid insufficiency in critically ill patients. *Crit Care Med.* 2003;31(6):1868-1869. doi:10.1097/01.CCM.0000066445.91548.20.

63. Arnold J, Leslie G, Bowen J, Watters S, Kreutzmann D, Silink M. Longitudinal study of plasma cortisol and 17-hydroxyprogesterone in very-low-birth-weight infants during the first 16 weeks of life. *Biol Neonate.* 1997;72(3):148-155.

64. Agus M. One step forward: an advance in understanding of adrenal insufficiency in the pediatric critically ill. *Crit Care Med.* 2005;33(4):911-912. doi:10.1097/01.ccm.0000159724.29534.cf.

65. Contreras LN, Arregger AL, Persi GG, Gonzalez NS, Cardoso EM. A new less-invasive and more informative low-dose ACTH test: salivary steroids in response to intramuscular corticotrophin. *Clin Endocrinol (Oxf).* 2004;61(6):675-682. doi:10.1111/j.1365-2265.2004.02144.x.

66. Hoen S, Mazoit JX, Asehnoune K, et al. Hydrocortisone increases the sensitivity to alpha1-adrenoceptor stimulation in humans following hemorrhagic shock. *Crit Care Med.* 2005;33(12):2737-2743. doi:10.1097/01.ccm.0000189743.55352.0e.

67. Marik PE, Zaloga GP. Adrenal insufficiency during septic shock. *Crit Care Med.* 2003;31(1):141-145. doi:10.1097/01.CCM.0000044483.98297.89.

68. Brierley J, Carcillo JA, Choong K, et al. Clinical practice parameters for hemodynamic support of pediatric and neonatal septic shock: 2007 update from the American College of Critical Care Medicine. *Crit Care Med.* 2009;37(2):666-688. doi:10.1097/CCM.0b013e31819323c6.

69. Masumoto K, Kusuda S, Aoyagi H, et al. Comparison of serum cortisol concentrations in preterm infants with or without late-onset circulatory collapse due to adrenal insufficiency of prematurity. *Pediatr Res.* 2008;63(6):686-690. doi:10.1203/PDR.0b013e31816c8fcc.

70. Iijima S. Late-onset glucocorticoid-responsive circulatory collapse in premature infants. *Pediatr Neonatol.* 2019;60(6):603-610. doi:10.1016/j.pedneo.2019.09.005.

71. Lamberts SW, Bruining HA, de Jong FH. Corticosteroid therapy in severe illness. *N Engl J Med.* 1997;337(18):1285-1292. doi:10.1056/NEJM199710303371807.

72. Annane D, Briegel J, Sprung CL. Corticosteroid insufficiency in acutely ill patients. *N Engl J Med.* 2003;348(21):2157-2159. doi:10.1056/NEJM200305223482123.

73. Joosten KF, de Kleijn ED, Westerterp M, et al. Endocrine and metabolic responses in children with meningococcal sepsis: striking differences between survivors and nonsurvivors. *J Clin Endocrinol Metab.* 2000;85(10):3746-3753.

74. Chrousos GP. The hypothalamic-pituitary-adrenal axis and immune-mediated inflammation. *N Engl J Med.* 1995;332(20):1351-1362. doi:10.1056/NEJM199505183322008.

75. Meduri GU, Muthiah MP, Carratu P, Eltorky M, Chrousos GP. Nuclear factor-kappaB- and glucocorticoid receptor alpha- mediated mechanisms in the regulation of systemic and pulmonary inflammation during sepsis and acute respiratory distress syndrome. Evidence for inflammation-induced target tissue resistance to glucocorticoids. *Neuroimmunomodulation.* 2005;12(6):321-338. doi:10.1159/000091126.

76. Briegel J, Jochum M, Gippner-Steppert C, Thiel M. Immunomodulation in septic shock: hydrocortisone differentially regulates cytokine responses. *J Am Soc Nephrol.* 2001;12(suppl 17):S70-S74.

77. Tsuneyoshi I, Kanmura Y, Yoshimura N. Methylprednisolone inhibits endotoxin-induced depression of contractile function in human arteries in vitro. *Br J Anaesth.* 1996;76(2):251-257.

78. Annane D, Bellissant E, Sebille V, et al. Impaired pressor sensitivity to noradrenaline in septic shock patients with and without impaired adrenal function reserve. *Br J Clin Pharmacol.* 1998;46(6):589-597.

79. Liggins GC. The role of cortisol in preparing the fetus for birth. *Reprod Fertil Dev.* 1994;6(2):141-150.

80. McLean M, Smith R. Corticotrophin-releasing hormone and human parturition. *Reproduction.* 2001;121(4):493-501.

81. Ng PC, Lee CH, Lam CW, et al. Transient adrenocortical insufficiency of prematurity and systemic hypotension in very low birthweight infants. *Arch Dis Child Fetal Neonatal Ed.* 2004;89(2):F119-F126.

82. Huysman MW, Hokken-Koelega AC, De Ridder MA, Sauer PJ. Adrenal function in sick very preterm infants. *Pediatr Res.* 2000;48(5):629-633.

83. Helbock HJ, Insoft RM, Conte FA. Glucocorticoid-responsive hypotension in extremely low birth weight newborns. *Pediatrics.* 1993;92(5):715-717.

84. Hingre RV, Gross SJ, Hingre KS, Mayes DM, Richman RA. Adrenal steroidogenesis in very low birth weight preterm infants. *J Clin Endocrinol Metab.* 1994;78(2):266-270.

85. Lee MM, Rajagopalan L, Berg GJ, Moshang Jr T. Serum adrenal steroid concentrations in premature infants. *J Clin Endocrinol Metab.* 1989;69(6):1133-1136.

86. Heckmann M, Wudy SA, Haack D, Pohlandt F. Reference range for serum cortisol in well preterm infants. *Arch Dis Child Fetal Neonatal Ed.* 1999;81(3):F171-F174.

87. Yoder B, Martin H, McCurnin DC, Coalson JJ. Impaired urinary cortisol excretion and early cardiopulmonary dysfunction in immature baboons. *Pediatr Res.* 2002;51(4):426-432.

88. Coalson JJ, Winter VT, Siler-Khodr T, Yoder BA. Neonatal chronic lung disease in extremely immature baboons. *Am J Respir Crit Care Med.* 1999;160(4):1333-1346.

89. Thomas S, Murphy JF, Dyas J, Ryalls M, Hughes IA. Response to ACTH in the newborn. *Arch Dis Child.* 1986;61(1):57-60.

90. al Saedi S, Dean H, Dent W, Cronin C. Reference ranges for serum cortisol and 17-hydroxyprogesterone levels in preterm infants. *J Pediatr.* 1995;126(6):985-987. doi:10.1016/s0022-3476(95)70229-6.

91. Watterberg KL, Gerdes JS, Cook KL. Impaired glucocorticoid synthesis in premature infants developing chronic lung disease. *Pediatr Res.* 2001;50(2):190-195.

92. Ng PC, Lam CW, Lee CH, et al. Reference ranges and factors affecting the human corticotropin-releasing hormone test in preterm, very low birth weight infants. *J Clin Endocrinol Metab.* 2002;87(10):4621-4628.

93. Bolt RJ, van Weissenbruch MM, Cranendonk A, Lafeber HN, Delemarre-Van De Waal HA. The corticotrophin-releasing hormone test in preterm infants. *Clin Endocrinol (Oxf).* 2002;56(2):207-213. doi:10.1046/j.0300-0664.2001.01467.x.

94. Arnold JD, Bonacruz G, Leslie GI, Veldhuis JD, Milmlow D, Silink M. Antenatal glucocorticoids modulate the amplitude of pulsatile cortisol secretion in premature neonates. *Pediatr Res.* 1998;44(6):876-881.

95. Palta M, Gabbert D, Weinstein MR, Peters ME. Multivariate assessment of traditional risk factors for chronic lung disease in very low birth weight neonates. The Newborn Lung Project. *J Pediatr.* 1991;119(2):285-292.

96. Linder N, Davidovitch N, Kogan A, et al. Longitudinal measurements of 17alpha-hydroxyprogesterone in premature infants during the first three months of life. *Arch Dis Child Fetal Neonatal Ed.* 1999;81(3):F175-F178.

97. Economou G, Andronikou S, Challa A, Cholevas V, Lapatsanis PD. Cortisol secretion in stressed babies during the neonatal period. *Horm Res.* 1993;40(5-6):217-221.

98. Kamath BD, Fashaw L, Kinsella JP. Adrenal insufficiency in newborns with congenital diaphragmatic hernia. *J Pediatr.* 2010;156(3):495-497.e1. doi:10.1016/j.jpeds.2009.10.044.

99. Pittinger TP, Sawin RS. Adrenocortical insufficiency in infants with congenital diaphragmatic hernia: a pilot study. *J Pediatr Surg.* 2000;35(2):223-225; discussion 225-226. doi:10.1016/s0022-3468(00)90013-7.

100. Gutai J, George R, Koeff S, Bacon GE. Adrenal response to physical stress and the effect of adrenocorticotropic hormone in newborn infants. *J Pediatr.* 1972;81(4):719-725.

101. Khashana A, Saarela T, Ramet M, Hallman M. Cortisol intermediates and hydrocortisone responsiveness in critical neonatal disease. *J Matern Fetal Neonatal Med.* 2017;30(14):1721-1725. doi:10.1080/14767058.2016.1223032.

102. Perez M, Wedgwood S, Lakshminrusimha S, Farrow KN, Steinhorn RH. Hydrocortisone normalizes phosphodiesterase-5 activity in pulmonary artery smooth muscle cells from lambs with persistent pulmonary hypertension of the newborn. *Pulm Circ.* 2014;4(1):71-81. doi:10.1086/674903.

103. Alsaleem M, Malik A, Lakshminrusimha S, Kumar VH. Hydrocortisone improves oxygenation index and systolic blood pressure in term infants with persistent pulmonary hypertension. *Clin Med Insights Pediatr.* 2019;13:1179556519888918. doi:10.1177/1179556519888918.

104. Mokra D, Mokry J, Tonhajzerova I. Anti-inflammatory treatment of meconium aspiration syndrome: benefits and risks. *Respir Physiol Neurobiol.* 2013;187(1):52-57. doi:10.1016/j.resp.2013.02.025.

105. Prasanth K, Kamat M, Khilfeh M, Davis V. Adrenocorticotropic hormone and cortisol levels in term infants born with meconium-stained amniotic fluid. Comparative study observational study. *J Perinat Med.* 2014;42(6):699-703. doi:10.1515/jpm-2014-0244.

106. Kovacs K, Szakmar E, Meder U, et al. A randomized controlled study of low-dose hydrocortisone versus placebo in dopamine-treated hypotensive neonates undergoing hypothermia treatment for hypoxic-ischemic encephalopathy. *J Pediatr.* 2019;211:13-19.e3. doi:10.1016/j.jpeds.2019.04.008.

107. Khashana A, Ahmed E. Hyperdehydroepiandrosterone in neonates with hypoxic ischemic encephalopathy and circulatory collapse. *Pediatr Neonatol.* 2017;58(6):504-508. doi:10.1016/j.pedneo.2016.09.010.

108. Khashana A, Ojaniemi M, Leskinen M, Saarela T, Hallman M. Term neonates with infection and shock display high cortisol precursors despite low levels of normal cortisol. *Acta Paediatr.* 2016;105(2):154-158. doi:10.1111/apa.13257.

109. Robertson JO, Criss CN, Hsieh LB, et al. Steroid use for refractory hypotension in congenital diaphragmatic hernia. *Pediatr Surg Int.* 2017;33(9):981-987. doi:10.1007/s00383-017-4122-3.

110. Marik PE, Pastores SM, Annane D, et al. Recommendations for the diagnosis and management of corticosteroid insufficiency in critically ill adult patients: consensus statements from an international task force by the American College of Critical Care Medicine. *Crit Care Med.* 2008;36(6):1937-1949. doi:10.1097/CCM.0b013e31817603ba.

111. Aucott SW. The challenge of defining relative adrenal insufficiency. *J Perinatol.* 2012;32(6):397-398. doi:10.1038/jp.2012.21.
112. Venkatesh B, Mortimer RH, Couchman B, Hall J. Evaluation of random plasma cortisol and the low dose corticotropin test as indicators of adrenal secretory capacity in critically ill patients: a prospective study. *Anaesth Intensive Care.* 2005;33(2):201-209.
113. Metzger DL, Wright NM, Veldhuis JD, Rogol AD, Kerrigan JR. Characterization of pulsatile secretion and clearance of plasma cortisol in premature and term neonates using deconvolution analysis. *J Clin Endocrinol Metab.* 1993;77(2):458-463.
114. Baker CF, Barks JD, Engmann C, et al. Hydrocortisone administration for the treatment of refractory hypotension in critically ill newborns. *J Perinatol.* 2008;28(6):412-419. doi:10.1038/jp.2008.16.
115. Kline GA, Buse J, Krause RD. Clinical implications for biochemical diagnostic thresholds of adrenal sufficiency using a highly specific cortisol immunoassay. *Clin Biochem.* 2017;50(9):475-480. doi:10.1016/j.clinbiochem.2017.02.008.
116. Ng PC, Wong GW, Lam CW, et al. The pituitary-adrenal responses to exogenous human corticotropin-releasing hormone in preterm, very low birth weight infants. *J Clin Endocrinol Metab.* 1997;82(3):797-799.
117. Karlsson R, Kallio J, Irjala K, Ekblad S, Toppari J, Kero P. Adrenocorticotropin and corticotropin-releasing hormone tests in preterm infants. *J Clin Endocrinol Metab.* 2000;85(12):4592-4595.
118. Karlsson R, Kallio J, Toppari J, Kero P. Timing of peak serum cortisol values in preterm infants in low-dose and the standard ACTH tests. *Pediatr Res.* 1999;45(3):367-369.
119. Watterberg KL, Gerdes JS, Gifford KL, Lin HM. Prophylaxis against early adrenal insufficiency to prevent chronic lung disease in premature infants. *Pediatrics.* 1999;104(6):1258-1263.
120. Watterberg KL, Gerdes JS, Cole CH, et al. Prophylaxis of early adrenal insufficiency to prevent bronchopulmonary dysplasia: a multicenter trial. *Pediatrics.* 2004;114(6):1649-1657. doi:10.1542/peds.2004-1159.
121. Hochwald O, Holsti L, Osiovich H. The use of an early ACTH test to identify hypoadrenalism-related hypotension in low birth weight infants. *J Perinatol.* 2012;32(6):412-417. doi:10.1038/jp.2012.16.
122. Gill H, Barrowman N, Webster R, Ahmet A. Evaluating the low-dose ACTH stimulation test in children: ideal times for cortisol measurement. *J Clin Endocrinol Metab.* 2019;104(10):4587-4593. doi:10.1210/jc.2019-00295.
123. LeDrew R, Bariciak E, Webster R, Barrowman N, Ahmet A. Evaluating the low-dose ACTH stimulation test in neonates: ideal times for cortisol measurement. *J Clin Endocrinol Metab.* 2020;105(12):dgaa635. doi:10.1210/clinem/dgaa635.
124. Trainer PJ, McHardy KC, Harvey RD, Reid IW. Urinary free cortisol in the assessment of hydrocortisone replacement therapy. *Horm Metab Res.* 1993;25(2):117-120. doi:10.1055/s-2007-1002056.
125. Vezina HE, Ng CM, Vazquez DM, Barks JD, Bhatt-Mehta V. Population pharmacokinetics of unbound hydrocortisone in critically ill neonates and infants with vasopressor-resistant hypotension. *Pediatr Crit Care Med.* 2014;15(6):546-553. doi:10.1097/PCC.0000000000000152.
126. Menon K, McNally D, Acharya A, et al. Random serum free cortisol and total cortisol measurements in pediatric septic shock. *J Pediatr Endocrinol Metab.* 2018;31(7):757-762. doi:10.1515/jpem-2018-0027.
127. Sweeney DA, Natanson C, Banks SM, Solomon SB, Behrend EN. Defining normal adrenal function testing in the intensive care unit setting: a canine study. *Crit Care Med.* 2010;38(2):553-561. doi:10.1097/CCM.0b013e3181cb0a25.
128. Gaissmaier RE, Pohlandt F. Single-dose dexamethasone treatment of hypotension in preterm infants. *J Pediatr.* 1999;134(6):701-705. doi:10.1016/s0022-3476(99)70284-2.
129. Noori S, Siassi B, Durand M, Acherman R, Sardesai S, Ramanathan R. Cardiovascular effects of low-dose dexamethasone in very low birth weight neonates with refractory hypotension. *Biol Neonate.* 2006;89(2):82-87. doi:10.1159/000088289.
130. Suominen PK, Dickerson HA, Moffett BS, et al. Hemodynamic effects of rescue protocol hydrocortisone in neonates with low cardiac output syndrome after cardiac surgery. *Pediatr Crit Care Med.* 2005;6(6):655-659. doi:10.1097/01.pcc.0000185487.69215.29.
131. Paquette L, Friedlich P, Ramanathan R, Seri I. Concurrent use of indomethacin and dexamethasone increases the risk of spontaneous intestinal perforation in very low birth weight neonates. *J Perinatol.* 2006;26(8):486-492. doi:10.1038/sj.jp.7211548.
132. Hassan AH, von Rosenstiel P, Patchev VK, Holsboer F, Almeida OF. Exacerbation of apoptosis in the dentate gyrus of the aged rat by dexamethasone and the protective role of corticosterone. *Exp Neurol.* 1996;140(1):43-52. doi:10.1006/exnr.1996.0113.
133. Shinwell ES, Karplus M, Reich D, et al. Early postnatal dexamethasone treatment and increased incidence of cerebral palsy. *Arch Dis Child Fetal Neonatal Ed.* 2000;83(3):F177-F181.
134. Higgins S, Friedlich P, Seri I. Hydrocortisone for hypotension and vasopressor dependence in preterm neonates: a meta-analysis. *J Perinatol.* 2010;30(6):373-378. doi:10.1038/jp.2009.126.
135. Noori S, Friedlich P, Wong P, Ebrahimi M, Siassi B, Seri I. Hemodynamic changes after low-dosage hydrocortisone administration in vasopressor-treated preterm and term neonates. *Pediatrics.* 2006;118(4):1456-1466. doi:10.1542/peds.2006-0661.
136. Peeples ES. An evaluation of hydrocortisone dosing for neonatal refractory hypotension. *J Perinatol.* 2017;37(8):943-946. doi:10.1038/jp.2017.68.
137. Sushko K, Al-Rawahi N, Watterberg K, et al. Efficacy and safety of low-dose versus high-dose hydrocortisone to treat hypotension in neonates: a protocol for a systematic review and meta-analysis. *BMJ Paediatr Open.* 2021;5(1):e001200. doi:10.1136/bmjpo-2021-001200.
138. Czock D, Keller F, Rasche FM, Haussler U. Pharmacokinetics and pharmacodynamics of systemically administered glucocorticoids. *Clin Pharmacokinet.* 2005;44(1):61-98. doi:10.2165/00003088-200544010-00003.
139. Perogamvros I, Aarons L, Miller AG, Trainer PJ, Ray DW. Corticosteroid-binding globulin regulates cortisol pharmacokinetics. *Clin Endocrinol (Oxf).* 2011;74(1):30-36. doi:10.1111/j.1365-2265.2010.03897.x.
140. Reynolds JW, Colle E, Ulstrom RA. Adrenocortical steroid metabolism in newborn infants. V. Physiologic disposition of exogenous cortisol loads in the early neonatal period. *J Clin Endocrinol Metab.* 1962;22:245-254.
141. Mizobuchi M, Iwatani S, Sakai H, Yoshimoto S, Nakao H. Effect of hydrocortisone therapy on severe leaky lung syndrome in ventilated preterm infants. *Pediatr Int.* 2012;54(5):639-645. doi:10.1111/j.1442-200X.2012.03636.x.
142. Ng PC, Lee CH, Bnur FL, et al. A double-blind, randomized, controlled study of a "stress dose" of hydrocortisone for rescue treatment of refractory hypotension in preterm infants. *Pediatrics.* 2006;117(2):367-375. doi:10.1542/peds.2005-0869.

143. Hochwald O, Pelligra G, Osiovich H. Adding hydrocortisone as 1st line of inotropic treatment for hypotension in very low birth weight infants: authors' reply. *Indian J Pediatr.* 2014;81(9):988. doi:10.1007/s12098-013-1276-4.

144. Efird MM, Heerens AT, Gordon PV, Bose CL, Young DA. A randomized-controlled trial of prophylactic hydrocortisone supplementation for the prevention of hypotension in extremely low birth weight infants. *J Perinatol.* 2005;25(2):119-124. doi:10.1038/sj.jp.7211193.

145. Doyle LW, Cheong JL, Hay S, Manley BJ, Halliday HL. Early (< 7 days) systemic postnatal corticosteroids for prevention of bronchopulmonary dysplasia in preterm infants. *Cochrane Database Syst Rev.* 2021;10(10):CD001146. doi:10.1002/14651858.CD001146.pub6.

146. Altit G, Vigny-Pau M, Barrington K, Dorval VG, Lapointe A. Corticosteroid therapy in neonatal septic shock-do we prevent death? *Am J Perinatol.* 2018;35(2):146-151. doi:10.1055/s-0037-1606188.

147. Mhanna C, Pinto M, Koechley H, et al. Postnatal glucocorticoid use impacts renal function in VLBW neonates. *Pediatr Res.* 2022;91(7):1821-1826. doi:10.1038/s41390-021-01624-1.

148. Watterberg KL, Walsh MC, Li L, et al. Hydrocortisone to improve survival without bronchopulmonary dysplasia. *N Engl J Med.* 2022;386(12):1121-1131. doi:10.1056/NEJMoa2114897.

149. Jiang J, Zhang J, Kang M, Yang J. Transient hypertrophic cardiomyopathy and hypertension associated with hydrocortisone in preterm infant: a case report. *Medicine (Baltimore).* 2019;98(33):e16838. doi:10.1097/MD.0000000000016838.

150. Baud O, Trousson C, Biran V, Leroy E, Mohamed D, Alberti C. Two-year neurodevelopmental outcomes of extremely preterm infants treated with early hydrocortisone: treatment effect according to gestational age at birth. *Arch Dis Child Fetal Neonatal Ed.* 2019;104(1):F30-F35. doi:10.1136/archdischild-2017-313756.

151. Peltoniemi O, Kari MA, Heinonen K, et al. Pretreatment cortisol values may predict responses to hydrocortisone administration for the prevention of bronchopulmonary dysplasia in high-risk infants. *J Pediatr.* 2005;146(5):632-637. doi:10.1016/j.jpeds.2004.12.040.

152. Aucott SW. Hypotension in the newborn: who needs hydrocortisone? *J Perinatol.* 2005;25(2):77-78. doi:10.1038/sj.jp.7211225.

# Chapter 24

# Hemodynamically Based Management of Circulatory Compromise in the Newborn

Nicholas Evans

## Key Points

- There is little outcome-based evidence to guide circulatory support in the newborn.
- In clinical situations of high risk for circulatory compromise, there are a range of hemodynamics.
- A "one size fits all" approach to neonatal circulatory support is neither logical nor likely to be successful.
- It is logical to define the individual hemodynamic in a baby and apply therapy on the basis of those individual findings.

## Introduction

Shock refers to a circulatory state where the delivery of oxygen to the organs and tissues of the body is inadequate to meet demand. In neonatology, the terms hypotension and shock have tended to be used synonymously. This is erroneous, and while many shocked babies will be hypotensive, not all hypotensive babies are shocked and not all shocked babies are hypotensive. While true shock is uncommon in neonatology, borderline states of circulatory incompetence are common in sick and very premature babies.

## Pathophysiology

Circulatory competence depends on adequate systemic blood flow, which is dependent on cardiac output. Cardiac output is the product of ventricular stroke volume and heart rate. Ventricular stroke volume is determined by preload (positively), myocardial performance (positively), and afterload (negatively, above an individually variable threshold). Thus cardiac output can be increased by

increasing stroke volume, heart rate, or both. Blood pressure is the product of cardiac output and systemic vascular resistance (SVR) (related to afterload), so blood pressure can be improved by increasing cardiac output or SVR, or both.

Neonatal circulatory compromise can result from four basic mechanisms: reduced intravascular volume (low preload), intrinsic or extrinsic compromise of myocardial performance, obstruction in the circulation (high afterload), and loss of vascular tone or distributive disorders of the peripheral circulation. In the first three processes the main hemodynamic feature is low systemic blood flow, which results in tissue hypo-perfusion and hypoxia. In contrast, in vasodilatory shock, as long as myocardial performance keeps up with the increased workload, there is a normal or high systemic blood flow. In vasodilatory shock abnormal distribution of the circulation or microcirculatory alterations may play an important role in the development of tissue hypoxia. Microcirculatory shock is the condition in which the microcirculation fails to support tissue oxygenation in the face of normal systemic hemodynamics.[1]

This complexity is magnified many times in the newborn because we are dealing with a circulation in transition. The fetal channels may not close, leading to blood either bypassing the lungs by shunting right to left or recirculating through them by shunting left to right. This depends on the pressure differentials in the pulmonary and systemic circulation. If the fetal channels do close (as they often do in near-term or term babies) and the pulmonary vascular resistance remains high, then the circulation may be compromised because the blood cannot get through the lungs to reach the systemic circulation.

Hemodynamics may vary between different clinical situations and even between babies in the same clinical situation, so to determine the logical approach to managing shock in an individual baby, there is a need to understand the mechanism of circulatory compromise in that baby and to apply therapy logically on the basis of our understanding of the actions of the pharmacological agents that are available.

This is not an area where a "one size fits all" evidence-based approach is likely to be effective. There is too much variation between babies and in the same baby with time. In this chapter, the author will summarize the important information needed to derive an individual hemodynamic, list the common patterns of abnormal hemodynamics and examine the evidence in relation to available circulatory support interventions in the newborn. Then a logical approach to utilizing these interventions based on hemodynamic scenarios that are commonly found in the newborn in clinical situations of high circulatory risk is suggested.

## Relevant Hemodynamic Information

How to best define an individual hemodynamic is controversial. Many neonatologists still use vital signs, mainly blood pressure, and this will reflect the reality for many with limited access to technologies such as Doppler ultrasound and/or NIRS. But, to define a hemodynamic, one really needs both a measure of pressure and a measure of flow so that resistance can be estimated. From that, it is possible to derive whether it is flow or resistance or both that you need to increase to support pressure.

How best to define flow is also controversial, particularly whether that should be a measure of total systemic flow or a marker of individual organ blood flow, usually the brain. Both are clearly important, and the ideal situation would be to be able to measure systemic and organ blood flow as well as blood pressure. Indeed, the future may be comprehensive, real-time hemodynamic monitoring, as described in Chapter 14. One would also need a measure of preload or volume status, but this marker remains elusive except in cases of extreme hypovolemia. The author would argue that it is difficult to define an individualized approach to the circulation without any information about what is happening in the organ that drives the circulation and, indeed, the organ

you are trying to manipulate with your interventions, the heart. Without this knowledge, you are flying blind.

Cardiac ultrasound assessment of an individual hemodynamic is complex, and the measurements will be covered in more detail in the relevant chapters of this book. It is clearly important to document structural normality, fetal channel shunts, volume status, myocardial function, and estimated pulmonary pressure but the essentials for circulatory support are a measure of blood pressure, a measure of systemic blood flow, and in some babies an estimate of pulmonary blood flow. The author uses superior vena cava flow and/or right ventricular output as markers of systemic blood flow and left pulmonary artery velocity as an estimate of pulmonary blood flow. Ideally, in addition, information on blood flow distribution to the organs needs to be available to fully understand the cardiovascular status of the neonate.

## Patterns of Abnormal Neonatal Hemodynamics

Neonatal hemodynamics exist on a continuum, not in the discrete categories that are described in the following sections. Notwithstanding this, there are several patterns of abnormal hemodynamics seen in the newborn, and it is the author's opinion that it is helpful to model your thinking around these categories. While these will be discussed separately below, it must be highlighted that there will be overlap between these hemodynamic patterns in individual babies. It is also important to emphasize the importance of integrating the cardiac ultrasound findings with the clinical history, respiratory/ventilatory status, and vital signs to define the likely diagnosis and individual therapeutic needs. There are essentially five patterns of abnormal hemodynamics found in the newborn. These are summarized in Table 24.1. These patterns are given as follows:

### HYPOVOLEMIC HEMODYNAMIC (SEE ALSO CHAPTER 21)

Absolute hypovolemia is rare in the newborn, but it is seen in the immediate postnatal period in babies that have suffered intrapartum fetal blood loss and, postnatally, with subgaleal hemorrhage and post-surgical blood loss. Such babies may have a perinatal or clinical

**TABLE 24.1  Diagnosis and Management of Common Neonatal Hemodynamics. Note That These Hemodynamics Are Not Mutually Exclusive and Babies May Have Features of More Than One Hemodynamic. Criteria in Italics Indicate the Key Feature of Each Hemodynamic**

| Hemodynamic | Clinical Situations | Vital Signs | Cardiac US Flow Measures | Other Cardiac US Findings | Management |
|---|---|---|---|---|---|
| Hypovolemic hemodynamic | • Perinatal fetal blood loss<br>• Subgaleal hemorrhage<br>• Abdominal emergencies | • Pallor<br>• Tachycardia<br>• Low BP | • Low or low normal SBF depending on degree of volume loss. | • *Biventricular poor filling.* | • Give 20 mL/kg isotonic saline IV over 5–10 minutes depending on severity.<br>• If acute blood loss, follow with 20 mL/kg of uncrossmatched O-negative blood (cross-match only if time) over 10-30 minutes depending on severity.<br>• Monitor impact with full blood count, coagulation, vital signs, and cardiac ultrasound.<br>• Further volume expansion/blood as indicated, consider implementing massive transfusion protocol if ongoing blood loss exceeds 40 mL/kg.[57] |
| Low systemic flow hemodynamic | • Very preterm <12 h<br>• Any baby with a high ventilation/oxygen need<br>• Asphyxia | • Variable, BP low or normal | • *Low SBF* | • Poor myocardial function may be apparent. | • Give 10 mL/kg isotonic saline over 30 minutes.<br>• At the same time, commence dobutamine infusion at 10 mcg/kg/min. Monitor response with cardiac US and/or heart rate.<br>• If systemic blood flow not improving, increase dobutamine to 20 mcg/kg/min<br>• If blood pressure remains low, add dopamine 5 mcg/kg/min and titrate to minimal acceptable blood pressure.<br>• Review cardiac ultrasound at 24 h, particularly in very preterm babies, and wean dobutamine over 4-6 hours if flow measures have normalized (which they usually will). |
| Vasodilatory hemodynamic | • Sepsis<br>• Preterm baby after 24 h, sometimes earlier<br>• Recovery from shock or asphyxia | • *BP low*<br>• Other vital signs variable | • Normal or high SBF | • Good myocardial function<br>• Well filled ventricles | • If early postnatal in a preterm baby, it may be reasonable to observe, depending on BP and other vital signs. Spontaneous improvement is common.<br>• Otherwise give 10 mL/kg isotonic saline over 30 minutes. Consider more in probable septic shock. At the same time, commence dopamine at 5 mcg/kg/min. Monitor impact with BP.<br>• If not improving, increase dopamine in 2 mcg/kg/min increments to a maximum of 15 mcg/kg/min in order to achieve a minimally acceptable MBP.<br>• Reduce dopamine if MBP goes significantly above the minimally acceptable MBP.<br>• If BP does not improve, consider:<br>• **In septic shock:** Refer to Chapter 21.<br>• **In late preterm hypotension:** if refractory to dopamine, consider hydrocortisone 1 mg/kg 8- to 12-hourly |

*Continued on following page*

**TABLE 24.1** Diagnosis and Management of Common Neonatal Hemodynamics. Note That These Hemodynamics Are Not Mutually Exclusive and Babies May Have Features of More Than One Hemodynamic. Criteria in Italics Indicate the Key Feature of Each Hemodynamic (Continued)

| Hemodynamic | Clinical Situations | Vital Signs | Cardiac US Flow Measures | Other Cardiac US Findings | Management |
|---|---|---|---|---|---|
| Low pulmonary blood flow PPHN | • High FiO$_2$ with relatively normal lungs (clinically and on CXR) | • Poor oxygenation<br>• BP normal or low<br>• Variable | • Normal or low SBF<br>• *Low mean velocity in LPA* | • Exclude CHD<br>• Dilated poorly contracting RV<br>• Poorly filled LV<br>• *High PAP*<br>• Dominant R-to-L bidirectional shunt through ductus and/or FO | • Commence iNO 5–10 ppm. Monitor response with oxygenation and cardiac ultrasound; both will usually improve.<br>• If low systemic blood flow persists, start milrinone 0.2–0.5 mcg/kg/min (or dobutamine) and consider isotonic saline.<br>• If low blood pressure persists, particularly if oxygenation varying with MBP, consider norepinephrine starting at 0.05 mcg/kg/min and increasing to 1.0 mcg/kg/min or epinephrine starting at 0.05 mcg/kg/min and increasing to 1.0 mcg/kg/min depending on BP response. |
| Normal pulmonary blood flow PPHN | • High FiO$_2$ with abnormal signs (clinically and on CXR) | • BP normal or low<br>• Other vital signs variable | • Often low SBF on day 1<br>• *Normal mean velocity in LPA* | • Exclude CHD<br>• Usually normal contractility<br>• *Moderate to high PAP*<br>• Bidirectional shunt through ductus and/or FO | • Optimize respiratory management, surfactant (repeat surfactant even if there is no apparent response), ventilation, etc.<br>• Consider iNO depending on oxygenation and pulmonary artery pressure.<br>• Monitor response with oxygenation and cardiac ultrasound. The effect of iNO is more variable.<br>• If low systemic blood flow, consider starting milrinone (or dobutamine, depending on myocardial function) and consider isotonic saline.<br>• If low blood pressure, particularly if oxygenation varying with MBP, consider norepinephrine starting at 0.05 mcg/kg/min and increasing to 1.0 mcg/kg/min or epinephrine starting at 0.05 mcg/kg/min and increasing to 1.0 mcg/kg/min depending on BP response. |

**Definitions:**

**Low systemic blood flow (SBF):** RV output <150 mL/kg/min and/or SVC flow <50 mL/kg/min.

**Low pulmonary blood flow (PBF):** Left pulmonary artery (LPA) mean velocity <20 cm/s.

**Minimally acceptable blood pressure:** Controversial, MBP use above gestational age suggested.

*BP*, blood pressure; *CHD*, congenital heart disease; *FBC*, full blood count; *FO*, foramen ovale; *iNO*, inhaled nitric oxide; *LPA*, left pulmonary artery; *LV*, left ventricle, *MBP*, mean blood pressure; *PAP*, pulmonary artery pressure; *PPHN*, persistent pulmonary hypertension of the newborn; *RV*, right ventricle; *SBF*, systemic blood flow.

history consistent with blood loss and, on examination, will be pale and invariably tachycardic. If they have progressed beyond the compensatory phase, they will have low blood pressure. The main cardiac ultrasound finding is dramatic poor biventricular filling, so the chambers look small and often have an appearance of poor contractility, reflecting low preload. The walls of the left ventricle may appear to touch each other in systole. The systemic veins will also be poorly filled and measures of systemic blood flow will be low or low normal depending on the degree of hypovolemia.

Hemoglobin falls quickly after blood loss and evidence of a low hemoglobin as measured on a hematocrit or emergency full blood count may assist in diagnosis. Also, most blood gas machines include a hemoglobin measurement, so look for that on your cord gas if one has been performed.

### Case History 1

Preterm rupture of membranes at 34 weeks progressed to preterm labor at 36 weeks. Maternal group B streptococcus positive and given intrapartum antibiotics. Ventouse delivery for failure to progress and maternal temperature. No nuchal cord, no intrapartum hemorrhage. Apgars 2 at one minute, 6 at 5 minutes, and 8 at 10 minutes, still pale and unwell looking at 10 minutes.

Cord arterial gas was as follows: pH 7.28, base excess (BE) −7, and lactate 4 mmol/L. On examination, heart rate 190, mean BP 28 mmHg, and respiratory rate 40. Scalp was boggy on examination, with possible small subgaleal hemorrhage. Venous gas at 50 minutes: pH 7.02, BE −15, lactate 8.3 mmol/L, and hemoglobin 90 g/L. Given 20 mL/kg normal saline and cardiac ultrasound performed.

Neonatologist-performed cardiac ultrasound showed poor filling of both ventricles. Figure 24.1 shows the end-systolic frame with the walls of the left ventricle touching each other.

Interpretation: Diagnosis consistent with severe hypovolemia. Given 20 mL/kg of uncrossmatched O-negative blood over 20 minutes with marked clinical improvement. Cardiac ultrasound repeated, and Figure 24.2 shows the improved ventricular filling with the LV walls no longer touching in end-systole. A further 20 mL/kg of blood was given over an hour.

Outcome: Maternal Kleihauer test result consistent with 90 mL of fetal blood in the maternal circulation.

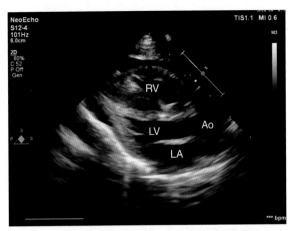

**Fig. 24.1 Low parasternal long-axis view at end-systole in this severely hypovolemic baby.** The poor filling of the left ventricle is shown by the touching of the walls. The right ventricle is also small.

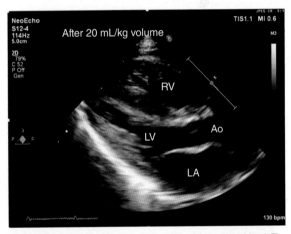

**Fig. 24.2 Same view after giving 20 mL/kg of O-negative blood.** The end-systolic separation of the LV walls is now apparent. Upon assessment, this baby was still hypovolemic and a further 20 mL/kg of blood was given.

Diagnosis of acute hypovolemia from combined effect of an acute fetomaternal hemorrhage and a subgaleal hemorrhage. Cardiac ultrasound and cord arterial gas allowed quick confirmation of diagnosis from the main differential, which would be perinatal asphyxia.

### VASODILATORY HEMODYNAMIC

This loss of vascular resistance pattern is invariable in hypotensive preterm babies who are more than 24 hours old and can be seen during the first 24 hours, sometimes in combination with low systemic blood flow (see below). It is also seen on recovery from shock or severe asphyxia and is the invariable hemodynamic in late-onset sepsis (see Chapter 21).[2] These babies will either be very preterm or have a clinical history consistent with sepsis or asphyxia. They will be hypotensive, often tachycardic, and the impact on other clinical signs and markers of shock such as lactate will depend on severity. The cardiac ultrasound findings will show well-filled ventricles with a good, sometimes hyperdynamic, appearance to the myocardial function, and measures of systemic blood flow will be high normal or high, reflecting the loss of resistance. If treatment is delayed, myocardial function will deteriorate as, after a certain period, myocardial oxygen delivery starts failing to meet tissue oxygen demand.

### Case History 2

Preterm baby born at 29 weeks with good initial course, but sudden deterioration on day 7 with clinical sepsis. Full septic screen and commenced on vancomycin and gentamicin. Baby had pale shocked appearance with tachycardia, mean blood pressure of 18 mmHg, and a rising blood lactate. Hypotension, not responsive to both dobutamine and dopamine at 20 mcg/kg/min, was noted. Neonatologist-performed cardiac ultrasound done for investigation of unresponsive hypotension.

Cardiac ultrasound showed a hyperdynamic heart with a closed ductus arteriosus. LV output was very high at 600 mL/kg/min (Normal range [NR] 150–300 mL/kg/min). This can be seen in Figure 24.3, with high velocities in the ascending aorta (left) and middle cerebral artery (right). The normal average maximum velocities are shown by the *dotted lines.*

Interpretation: LV output is systemic blood flow when the ductus is closed. High systemic blood flow with low blood pressure is consistent with vasodilatory shock. The therapy was focused on pressors, so dobutamine was ceased. Norepinephrine and then vasopressin were commenced.

Outcome: Blood cultures grew *Pseudomonas aeruginosa.* The blood pressure was non-responsive to the added pressor therapy and the lactate continued to rise. The baby passed about 24 hours later with ischemic increased echogenicity changes evolving on the cerebral ultrasound. The case highlights that tissue ischemia can occur in the presence of normal or high systemic blood flow, pointing to the role of distributive or micro-circulatory shock.

## LOW SYSTEMIC BLOOD FLOW HEMODYNAMIC

This pattern usually reflects absolute or relative myocardial dysfunction with relative myocardial dysfunction, meaning that a myocardium is struggling against increased afterload or, in the case of the preterm myocardium, afterload for which it is not adapted. This is

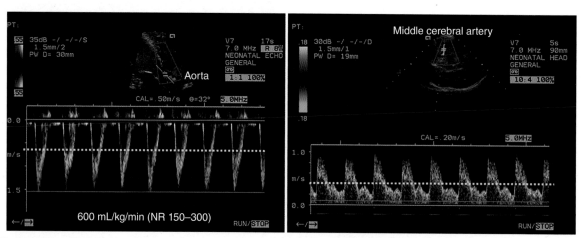

**Fig. 24.3** High velocities in the ascending aorta (*left*) and middle cerebral artery (*right*), with the normal maximum velocities shown by the *dotted line.* The high LV output in this severely hypotensive baby is characteristic of vasodilatory shock.

the most common pattern of abnormal hemodynamic seen in the very preterm baby in the first 12 hours after delivery (Chapter 20). It probably reflects maladaptation of the immature myocardium to the higher afterloads of extra-uterine life, possibly compounded by the negative circulatory effects of positive pressure ventilation as well as shunts out of the systemic circulation through the fetal channels.[3] It is unusual to find this pattern in preterm babies after the first 24 hours, where the abnormal hemodynamic is invariably vasodilatory.[2,3] Low systemic blood flow due to afterload compromise is the usual pathophysiology of the cardiorespiratory compromise seen after PDA ligation,[4] and recipients of twin-twin transfusion syndrome seem particularly vulnerable to developing this hemodynamic. Low systemic blood flow is found in more mature babies with high ventilator and oxygen requirements, where primary myocardial dysfunction merges with the PPHN hemodynamic discussed below.[5] Low systemic blood flow is also found in clinical situations associated with an injured myocardium, most commonly in the asphyxiated newborn but also in viral myocarditis or congenital cardiomyopathies. It is also important to remember that myocardial compromise can be external to the heart, as in cardiac tamponade.

The impact of low systemic blood flow on vital signs is variable, particularly in the preterm baby, where blood pressure may be normal. Because of this, recognition of low systemic blood flow often depends on proactive use of cardiac ultrasound in the high-risk clinical situations mentioned above. The findings on cardiac ultrasound will be low SVC flow (<50 mL/kg/min) and/or low RV output (<150 mL/kg/min) and, particularly in the more mature baby, poor myocardial function may well be subjectively apparent as well assessed by myocardial function measures. Cardiac tamponade will show as an echolucent surrounding to the myocardium compressing the chambers and impairing contractility.

## Case History 3

Spontaneous onset of preterm labor in a 27-week monozygotic twin pregnancy. On delivery, undiagnosed twin polycythemia anemia sequence apparent. Twin 2 was the recipient twin with hemoglobin 257 g/L and hematocrit 72%. Intubated, ventilated, and given surfactant. Mean blood pressure at 4 hours was in the range of 45–50 mmHg. Neonatologist-performed cardiac ultrasound performed because of high-risk hemodynamic situation.

Cardiac ultrasound showed mild myocardial hypertrophy with a 2.0 mm PDA shunting left to right. Figure 24.4 shows the pulsed Doppler traces from which RV output and SVC flow were derived. Both show low velocities suggesting low systemic blood flow. RV output was 145 mL/kg/min (NR 150–300 mL/kg/min) and SVC flow was 41 mL/kg/min (NR 50–100 mL/kg/min).

Interpretation: Low systemic blood flow in context of raised blood pressure is consistent with afterload compromise. Recipient twins are at high risk for developing afterload compromise, so the pre-emptive focus was on using interventions that would reduce cardiac work. Dobutamine was commenced at 20 mcg/kg/h and a 30 mL/kg dilutional plasma exchange performed.

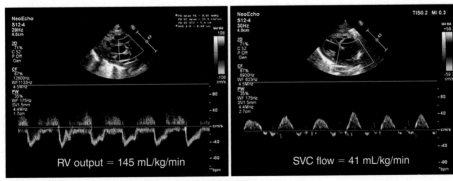

**Fig. 24.4 Low velocities in the main pulmonary artery (*left*) and superior vena cava (*right*), consistent with a baby in low systemic blood flow.** In the presence of normal or high blood pressure this likely reflects afterload compromise.

Outcome: Baby remained stable and RV output improved to 180 mL/kg/min at 24 hours and 240 mL/kg/min at 36 hours. Full recovery occurred with a normal head ultrasound.

## PERSISTENT PULMONARY HYPERTENSION HEMODYNAMICS (SEE ALSO CHAPTERS 25 AND 27)

The plural is pointedly used in the title of this subsection because the hemodynamics are as varied as the causes of the high ventilation and oxygen requirements that often lead neonatologists to consider PPHN as a diagnosis. It is important to remember that pressure in the pulmonary arterial system is determined by the same factors as in the systemic circulation, that is, flow and resistance. So, just like the systemic circulation, pulmonary arterial pressure can be high because flow is high or resistance is high, or because both are high.

In fact, the hemodynamics here represent a continuum with, at one end, the classic concept of PPHN with high resistance, low pulmonary blood flow, and right-to-left shunts across the fetal channels and, at the other end, normal pulmonary blood flow with a varying degree of increased pulmonary vascular resistance and pressure as well as variable fetal channel shunts. There is a parallel in these hemodynamics with the classic categorization of PPHN into primary (with relatively normal lungs) and secondary (with parenchymal lung disease), with primary PPHN more likely to have a low pulmonary blood flow hemodynamic and secondary PPHN more likely to have a normal pulmonary blood flow hemodynamic.[5] Discussing these two hemodynamics in turn.

### Low Pulmonary Blood Flow PPHN

This hemodynamic is commonly seen in term or late preterm babies with idiopathic primary PPHN. Clinically these babies will have increased oxygen requirements that are out of keeping with any parenchymal lung disease and often will have relatively normal chest x-rays and may have relatively mild increased work of breathing. This hemodynamic is also found in babies with hypoplastic lungs from conditions such as diaphragmatic hernia, renal anomalies associated with decreased fetal urine production, or premature prolonged rupture of the membranes. It is uncommon in very preterm babies except those born after prolonged

oligohydramnios, where it is the hemodynamic that is invariably found. This was traditionally explained as due to pulmonary hypoplasia; however, the responsiveness to inhaled nitric oxide suggests a significant reversible component to the pulmonary hypertension in these babies (see Case History 4 in Chapter 9).[6,7]

Congenital heart disease must be excluded in these babies as soon as possible. Assuming the heart is structurally normal, cardiac ultrasound usually shows evidence of supra-systemic pulmonary pressure with predominantly right-to-left shunting through the ductus (if patent) and bidirectional shunting through the foramen ovale. There will be low-velocity flow in the left pulmonary artery (mean velocity < 0.2 m/s), a finding which predicts responsiveness to iNO.[8] Measures of systemic blood flow may be normal, particularly if the flow through the fetal channels is not restricted. If the flow through the fetal channels is restricted, then systemic blood flow may be low, with the likely pathophysiology being low pulmonary blood flow restricting systemic blood flow. The left ventricle can only pump on what it receives from the right ventricle.

### Normal Pulmonary Blood Flow PPHN

This hemodynamic is most commonly seen in babies with severe acquired lung disease, such as meconium aspiration, pneumonia, or hyaline membrane disease. The main clinical feature is a history and chest x-ray changes that are consistent with one of these diagnoses. The babies will usually have presented with severe respiratory distress and, when ventilated, will have high oxygen and pressure requirements. These babies must also have congenital heart disease excluded as soon as possible. If the heart is structurally normal, then pulmonary pressures in these babies will be variable and many of these babies will have sub-systemic pulmonary artery pressures. Within this group of babies, there is a positive relationship between oxygenation index and pulmonary artery pressure, with the most severe babies usually having peri- or supra-systemic pulmonary artery pressures.[5] Like the pulmonary artery pressures, shunts will be variable but will often be more left-to-right than right-to-left in the pattern. The ductus arteriosus often constricts early and closes by the second postnatal day. There is a high incidence of low systemic blood flow on the first day with improvement with time, much as seen in very preterm babies.[5]

## Circulatory Support Interventions

In a 2014 European-based survey of neonatal circulatory support,[9] the most common first-line interventions were volume expansion (85%), dopamine (62%), dobutamine (18%), dopamine and dobutamine used together (18%), epinephrine (2%), and norepinephrine (1%). The same interventions were used in varying frequency as second-line interventions but steroids (10%) and milrinone (1%) were also used as second-line interventions. The pharmacology of these agents is covered in Chapter 5, but is there any evidence that they provide benefit?

### VOLUME EXPANSION

Volume expansion is probably one of the most widely used circulatory support interventions despite evidence that true hypovolemia is rare. We have little understanding of the effects of volume expansion in a normovolemic infant. Volume expansion will increase preload on the heart. This will be life-saving in a truly hypovolemic baby, but in a normovolemic infant there may well be an immediate increase in cardiac output; however, maintenance of this will depend on how long the extra volume stays in the circulation. If volume expansion keeps being pushed, the distribution of extra volume out of the intravascular compartment may well create interstitial edema in the lungs and other organs of the body. Excessive volume expansion in preterm babies may be associated with higher mortality.[10]

Studies have shown that volume expansion in hypotensive preterm babies has little effect on blood pressure.[11] One study in preterm babies with low systemic blood flow showed an immediate increase in systemic blood flow but the researchers did not follow for how long this increase was maintained.[11] Cerebral blood flow, whether studied using Xenon extraction[12] or near-infrared spectroscopy,[13,14] does not seem to be consistently increased by volume in hypotensive preterm infants. Clinical trials of routine early volume expansion in preterm babies with fresh frozen plasma, plasma substitutes, or isotonic saline have shown no improvement in outcomes when compared to no intervention.[15] Delayed umbilical cord clamping probably provides

benefit, in part, optimizing blood, volume at birth with an extra 10–20 mL/kg of blood, and there is evidence that this intervention does improve outcomes. The Cochrane review of delayed cord clamping shows probably improved survival and better neurodevelopmental outcomes.[16] Delayed cord clamping should be standard of care in preterm babies whenever possible.

The evidence to guide what type of fluid to use in volume expansion is not consistent. Two small trials in preterm babies showed no difference between isotonic saline and 5% albumin in improving blood pressure,[17,18] and one slightly larger trial showed that hypotensive preterm babies given 5% albumin were more likely to achieve normal blood pressure and less likely to be given vasopressors than those randomized to saline.[19]

Because relative hypovolemia in the context of a mechanically ventilated baby is difficult to exclude, there is merit in including some volume expansion in a circulatory support protocol but volumes in excess of 20 mL/kg should be used with caution unless there is a clear diagnosis of hypovolemia as in case history 1.

### DOPAMINE

The clinical trial evidence around dopamine is largely related to its effect on blood pressure. There is consistent data that it is more effective than volume and dobutamine at increasing blood pressure[20,21] and similarly efficacious to epinephrine,[22] steroids,[23] and vasopressin.[24] Much of this effect on blood pressure seems to be due to the vasopressor effect, and the evidence around effects on systemic and cerebral blood flow is less consistent.[25] Dopamine at doses between 4 and 10 mcg/kg/min increased cardiac output in a cohort of late preterm and term infants, most of whom were asphyxiated.[25,26] In hypotensive preterm babies, Zhang et al showed no significant effect on cardiac output.[27] Roze et al showed a reduction in left ventricular output with a dose of dopamine sufficient to normalize BP,[28] and Osborn et al showed no change in superior vena cava flow, with dopamine despite achieving a significant increase in BP.[11] The latter study showed a rise in LV wall stress (a marker of afterload) on increasing the dose of dopamine from 10 to 20 mcg/kg/min, consistent with an α-adrenergic effect at high doses.[29] There is no evidence that this vasoconstriction significantly limits cerebral blood flow.

Studies of changes in cerebral blood flow after dopamine, mainly in hypotensive preterm babies and using NIRS surrogate markers of CBF, tend to show either increases or no change.

With reference to effects of dopamine on the pulmonary vasculature, the study is limited to preterm babies with PDA. Liet et al.[30] showed variable effects on the ratio of systemic to pulmonary pressure, but overall, no change in that ratio. Bouissou et al.[31] showed an increase in pulmonary artery pressure in response to 8 mcg/kg/min of dopamine. They also showed an increase in SVC flow, which they suggest may relate to a reduction in PDA shunt.

So, in summary, dopamine will reliably increase blood pressure, and it probably does this more by increasing systemic vascular resistance than systemic blood flow. The weight of evidence is that dopamine likely increases cerebral blood flow, but higher doses should be used with caution as high afterload in either the systemic or pulmonary circulation could result in compromise. In addition, dopamine has a broader spectrum of effects on other organs including the inhibition of TSH production in the pituitary gland, with special clinical relevance for the newborn. There is no evidence of the impact of dopamine on clinical outcomes.

## DOBUTAMINE

Dobutamine is a synthetic catecholamine that was modified from isoprenaline to reduce some of the chronotropic effects. The vasodilatory effect of dobutamine is likely why clinical trials have consistently shown dobutamine is not as good as dopamine at improving blood pressure in hypotensive preterm babies,[20] but, in the few studies which have measured it, dobutamine seems better than dopamine at improving systemic blood flow.[11,28] There was no difference in neurodevelopment at 3 years in the only trial to report this, though the trial was not powered for this outcome.[32] One small randomized trial has compared dobutamine to placebo in babies with low systemic blood flow and showed that systemic blood flow improved in both groups, but other markers of perfusion were significantly better in babies treated with dobutamine.[33] This study was unable to show any differences or changes in NIRS markers of cerebral blood flow with either dobutamine or placebo. Other observational studies have shown an impact on Doppler markers of organ blood flow including cerebral blood flow,[34] but the placebo effect in the Bravo et al study[33] reminds us that most blood flow parameters will improve spontaneously after about 12 hours of age in very preterm babies.

In summary, dobutamine has dose-related central inotropic and chronotropic effects with peripheral vasodilation. It is likely to be most effective where there is myocardial dysfunction and/or increased afterload, leading to low systemic blood flow. It is unlikely to be effective when hypotension is due to vasodilatation.

## EPINEPHRINE (ADRENALINE)

Epinephrine has very similar dose-related effects to dopamine. There has been limited study of the cardiovascular effects of epinephrine in the newborn. The previously cited randomized trial of dopamine and epinephrine in hypotensive preterm babies showed similar effects in improving blood pressure and cerebral oxygenation index, though the epinephrine group had significantly higher lactate and more hyperglycemia than those randomized to dopamine.[22] This was one of the few neonatal cardiovascular support trials that have assessed neurodevelopmental outcome, and they showed no difference between the two groups at 2–3 years of age.[35]

In summary, the vasoconstrictive effects of epinephrine make it best suited to management of vasodilatory shock. Like dopamine, caution should be applied when using higher doses because of the risk of afterload compromise.

## NOREPINEPHRINE (NORADRENALINE)

There is no clinical trial evidence on the use of norepinephrine in the newborn and not much observational data. A retrospective study of norepinephrine use in 48 babies born before 33 weeks showed that normotension could be achieved in all but one baby at a median dose of 0.5 mcg/kg/min. Apart from tachycardia (in 31%), no immediate side effects were observed.[36] One small cohort study showed improved blood pressure in term babies with septic shock refractory to dopamine and dobutamine.[37] An observational study in term babies with pulmonary hypertension suggested that norepinephrine has a beneficial effect on both systemic and pulmonary hemodynamics by causing systemic vasoconstriction and pulmonary vasodilatation.[38] There is no long-term safety data on the use of norepinephrine but it may have a role in refractory vasodilatory shock and in babies with PPHN and low blood pressure.

## VASOPRESSIN

There has been one small randomized trial ($n = 20$) that compared vasopressin with dopamine in hypotensive preterm infants.[39] Outcomes were limited to physiological parameters and both agents had similar effects in increasing blood pressure, while vasopressin had less tachycardic effect. Otherwise, there are small case series of improvement in blood pressure in preterm babies with inotrope refractory hypotension.[40,41] There is some evidence from animal studies that vasopressin has a vasodilatory effect on the pulmonary vasculature.[41] This would be consistent with the observational report of the use of vasopressin in 10 babies with PPHN refractory to inhaled nitric oxide.[42] A vasopressin infusion improved blood pressure, reduced oxygenation index, and improved urine output. There is not enough safety data to recommend routine use of vasopressin but it may have a role in vasodilatory shock refractory to vasopressor-inotropes.

## MILRINONE

The role of milrinone is best established in preventing and treating low cardiac output syndrome (LCOS) after cardiac bypass surgery, where a large RCT has shown that milrinone significantly reduced the incidence of LCOS in a neonatal and pediatric population.[43] The similarities between LCOS and the postnatal drop in systemic blood flow seen in some preterm babies led to a trial of milrinone to prevent low systemic blood flow in preterm babies.[44] This trial showed no difference in the incidence of low systemic blood flow between milrinone and placebo, though milrinone did increase the need for vasopressor-inotropes to support blood pressure and seemed to slow the constriction of the ductus arteriosus. The afterload-reducing properties of milrinone led to an observational study that suggested that milrinone may prevent the afterload compromise that can follow PDA ligation in preterm babies.[45] The pulmonary vasodilatory properties may also explain the observation

of improvement in oxygenation and hemodynamics in babies with PPHN refractory to inhaled nitric oxide.[46] There is also one small case series of milrinone being used in conjunction with inhaled nitric oxide in seven preterm babies with pulmonary hypertension with improvement in oxygenation index, right ventricle myocardial function, and pulmonary pressure.[47] Milrinone may have a role in the management of hemodynamics associated with systemic or pulmonary vasoconstriction but there is not enough safety data to recommend routine use. It should be used with caution in very preterm babies because of the long half-life and risk of hypotension.[48]

## HYDROCORTISONE

In a recent review of circulatory support measures in a US pediatric health information system,[49] hydrocortisone was second to dopamine as the most commonly used drug in extremely-low-birth-weight infants (dopamine 83% vs. hydrocortisone 33%). This is surprising as we don't know much about the hemodynamic impact of hydrocortisone, apart from the effect on blood pressure. Bourchier et al.[50] randomized hypotensive preterm babies to hydrocortisone or dopamine and showed both had similar effects on blood pressure. Ng et al.[51] randomized preterm babies needing more than 10 mcg/kg/min of dopamine to hydrocortisone or placebo and showed faster weaning of inotropes in those treated with hydrocortisone. Efird et al.[52] randomized preterm babies to hydrocortisone or placebo and confirmed vasopressor use was reduced. To the best of the author's knowledge, just one study has looked at the hemodynamic effects of hydrocortisone. In a cohort of 15 preterm and 5 term babies with hypotension requiring high-dose dopamine, Noori et al.[53] showed that the immediate effect of hydrocortisone on blood pressure was mediated via an increase in systemic vascular resistance without change in cardiac output or stroke volume; however, later, with weaning of dopamine, there were increases in stroke volume and cardiac output.

None of these studies looked at longer-term outcomes and the current Cochrane review on corticosteroids to treat hypotension in preterm babies urges caution, concluding with, "With long term benefit or safety data lacking, steroids cannot be recommended routinely for the treatment of hypotension in preterm infants".[54] This review is now over 10 years old, and although not addressing the circulatory support use of hydrocortisone, some reassurance about risk of long-term harm from hydrocortisone can be drawn from the follow-up of two RCTs of hydrocortisone to prevent chronic lung disease, the PREMILOC trial[55] and the NICHD trial,[56] neither of which showed any difference in disability at 2–3 years compared to placebo.

There is some observational evidence of an increased risk of GI perforation, particularly when hydrocortisone is used in conjunction with indomethacin. It is prudent to avoid using these two drugs together.

In summary, we know a lot about how our interventions affect blood pressure, less about how they affect hemodynamics, and almost nothing about how they affect outcomes. In light of this, it is the author's view that the logical way to approach circulatory support in the newborn is to use an individual or "precision based" approach. That is, one should try to define the individual hemodynamic as accurately as possible and apply logical treatment based on what we know about the effects of the interventions on physiology.

## Targeting Treatment to the Defined Individual Hemodynamic

Considering, in turn, the logical approach to managing each of the abnormal hemodynamics discussed above.

### MANAGEMENT OF HYPOVOLEMIA

A demonstrably hypovolemic baby needs immediate volume replacement with isotonic saline and/or blood as soon as available. The latter may need to be un-crossmatched O-negative blood if the urgency of the situation demands it. Babies with ongoing blood loss of more than 40 mL/kg are vulnerable to developing transfusion-related coagulopathy and should be managed according to the principles of a massive transfusion protocol where platelets and clotting factors are replaced proactively according to a defined schedule (see Chapter 21).[57]

### MANAGEMENT OF VASODILATORY SHOCK

The suggested management of septic shock is covered in detail in Chapter 21 and there are overlaps between the management of septic shock and that of post-asphyxial vasodilatory shock.

In preterm neonates with vasodilatory hypotension, the first question is whether it needs to be treated. If the hypotension is borderline and there are no changes in the markers of perfusion such as lactate and/or urine output, then an expectant approach may be reasonable. The decision in these cases also depends on the etiology of the vasodilatory shock as, for instance, in preterm neonates with suspected sepsis, there should be a lower threshold to initiate cardiovascular support. In babies with blood pressure well below the normal range and/or with other markers of poor tissue perfusion, intervention is indicated.

The logical intervention for a vasodilatory hemodynamic is a vasopressor. Some volume expansion may help to fill the additional vascular space created by the vasodilation. It is suggested to start some volume expansion (up to 20 mL/kg) as well as dopamine (because there is most experience with this vasopressor) at 5 mcg/kg/min and titrate the infusion rate up in small, perhaps 2 mcg/kg/min, dosage increments to achieve a minimal acceptable blood pressure. As long as the drug infusion is likely beyond the dead space of the giving set, one doesn't need to wait for a response longer than approximately 5 minutes to find out if the given dose needs to be increased again. It's unusual to need more than 10 mcg/kg/min, but if the blood pressure remains low at higher doses of dopamine (20 mcg/kg/min), then consideration could be given to adding another pressor because the hypotension may well be resistant to dopamine.

Different neonatologists will recommend different second-line vasopressors in this situation, including epinephrine, norepinephrine, and vasopressin as well as hydrocortisone. There is no evidence to guide the choice. Our preference would be to add hydrocortisone at 1 mg/kg 8-hourly in that we know a bit more about its hemodynamic effects (e.g., it probably acts as a vasopressor by potentiating catecholamine receptors) and it covers the risk of relative or absolute adrenocortical insufficiency. Due to hydrocortisone's prolonged half-life in preterm neonates <34 weeks' gestation, 12-hourly dosing has recently been recommended for this patient population as a starting dosage interval with the option to shorten the dosage interval if the increase in BP is not sustained for the 12 hours.[58] After that, we would consider norepinephrine or vasopressin, with a preference for the former because there is more reported experience.[36]

## MANAGEMENT OF LOW SYSTEMIC BLOOD FLOW

Most of these babies are not hypovolemic, but borderline volume status is difficult to exclude and there is some evidence of short-term improvement in systemic blood flow in preterm babies with low systemic blood flow in response to volume,[11] so we would suggest some volume expansion in these babies with 10 mL/kg of isotonic saline. The pathophysiology here would indicate the need for augmentation of myocardial function and, particularly if the blood pressure is normal, with an agent that will tend to reduce afterload. At the same time as the volume, we would suggest starting dobutamine at 10 mcg/kg/min. One practical difficulty in this situation is how to monitor the effect of Dobutamine which may or may not increase blood pressure even though systemic blood flow has improved. Ideally, repeat the cardiac ultrasound for markers of systemic blood flow about an hour after starting the infusion, but experientially, if that option is not available, then titrate up the dose until some chronotropic effect is seen, as this will make it likely that inotropy has been achieved. Dobutamine has a good dose-response relationship and, unless there is severe tachycardia, doses of up to 20 mcg/kg/min are unlikely to do harm.[11] The more mature baby with low systemic blood flow is often quite responsive to dobutamine, but low systemic blood flow in the preterm baby may be refractory to the intervention.[11] If the blood pressure is low, then that suggests combined low flow and vasodilation, and it is suggested to add in dopamine at 5 mcg/kg/min and titrate up to a minimally acceptable blood pressure. The concept of titrating to a minimally acceptable blood pressure becomes more important during this early postnatal period because of the risk of afterload compromise. There tends to be an assumption that more is better when it comes to blood pressure, so people are quick to start vasopressor-inotropes if the blood pressure is low but slow to reduce them if the blood pressure gets pushed well into the normal range or high.

It is also important to consider the optimal time for weaning inotropes. The natural history of systemic blood flow in preterm and term babies is for flow to improve between 12 and 24 hours of age. There is often a reluctance to wean the vasopressor-inotropes or inotropes and the theoretical risk this creates is that

continuing treatment may drive reperfusion in a system that is in spontaneous recovery. We would suggest repeat cardiac ultrasound at 24 hours of age to confirm normal systemic blood flow and then an aggressive wean of the cardiovascular medications over about 4–6 hours. If one doesn't have access to cardiac ultrasound, then it's reasonable to wean the inotropes anyway, as long as vital signs and other perfusion markers are normal.

The situation in the very preterm baby may be confounded by the presence of large left-to-right ductal shunting even at this early time. This moves blood out of the systemic circulation back to the pulmonary circulation and this may be a factor contributing to low systemic blood flow. Management of the patent ductus arteriosus is outside the scope of this chapter (see Chapters 16–19) but early medical closure of the poorly constricted ductus arteriosus with a large left to right shunt could be considered.

## MANAGEMENT OF LOW PULMONARY BLOOD FLOW PPHN (SEE CHAPTER 27 FOR DETAILS)

The primary problem in this hemodynamic is high pulmonary vascular resistance due to pulmonary vasoconstriction, so therapy needs to be aimed at dilating the pulmonary arterioles. Inhaled nitric oxide would be the first choice for this and, when this hemodynamic is associated with otherwise normal lungs, there is usually a brisk response to iNO and a normalization of the hemodynamic.

In babies who are not responsive to iNO, consideration should be given to adding milrinone if the systemic blood pressure is normal or, if the baby has hypotension, norepinephrine. Care is needed using milrinone in the setting of a wide-open PDA with bidirectional shunt, and borderline systemic blood pressure, to avoid dropping the SBP, which may worsen right-to-left shunt and therefore oxygenation. In iNO unresponsive babies, where the ductus arteriosus is constricting, there is some logic to consider opening the ductus arteriosus with prostaglandin E2. This will serve to decompress the right heart and improve systemic blood flow, albeit with relatively poorly oxygenated blood. In neonates not responding or not having a sustained response to iNO, addition of sildenafil can be considered the next step in the management.

## MANAGEMENT OF NORMAL PULMONARY BLOOD FLOW PPHN

The primary problem in these babies is pulmonary. The cardiac and pulmonary vascular effects are secondary to that pulmonary disease. With respect to high-pressure ventilation, it is important to remember that inappropriately high positive intrathoracic pressures will have a negative effect on cardiac output and pulmonary artery pressure will have to be higher to drive the blood through the lungs. The primary focus in these babies should be on optimizing respiratory and conventional ventilator management with surfactant, optimizing ventilator settings, or using other modes of ventilation (as indicated). If oxygenation is still poor despite optimized respiratory management, then consider iNO depending on the estimated pulmonary artery pressure and the patient's oxygenation status.

The effect of iNO in this hemodynamic is more variable. If systemic blood flow is low, consider dobutamine or milrinone as above and, if blood pressure is low, particularly if oxygenation varies with the blood pressure changes, consider norepinephrine or epinephrine titrating to the blood pressure response.

## Conclusions

In the absence of outcome-based evidence to guide circulatory support in the newborn, it is the author's view that the logical approach is one that uses individual or precision-based therapy. That is, one should try to diagnose the individual hemodynamic as accurately as possible and apply treatment logically to that hemodynamic based on what we know about the effects of the pharmacological interventions on cardiovascular physiology. Like all approaches to circulatory support in the newborn, there is no evidence that this improves outcomes.

## REFERENCES

1. Kanoore Edul VS, Ince C, Dubin A. What is microcirculatory shock? *Curr Opin Crit Care.* 2015;21(3):245-252.
2. de Waal KA, Evans N. Hemodynamics in preterm infants with late-onset sepsis. *J Pediatr.* 2010;156(6):918-922.
3. Kluckow M, Evans N. Low superior vena cava flow and intraventricular haemorrhage in preterm infants. *Arch Dis Child Fetal Neonatal Ed.* 2000;82:188-194.
4. El-Khuffash AF, Jain A, Dragulescu A, McNamara PJ, Mertens L. Acute changes in myocardial systolic function in preterm infants undergoing patent ductus arteriosus ligation: a tissue Doppler and myocardial deformation study. *J Am Soc Echocardiogr.* 2012;25(10):1058-1067.
5. Evans N, Kluckow M, Currie A. Range of echocardiographic findings in term neonates with high oxygen requirements. *Arch Dis Child Fetal Neonatal Ed.* 1998;78(2):F105-F111.
6. Semberova J, O'Donnell SM, Franta J, Miletin J. Inhaled nitric oxide in preterm infants with prolonged preterm rupture of the membranes: a case series. *J Perinatol.* 2015;35(4):304-306.
7. Shah DM, Kluckow M. Early functional echocardiogram and inhaled nitric oxide: usefulness in managing neonates born following extreme preterm premature rupture of membranes (PPROM). *J Paediatr Child Health.* 2011;47(6):340-345.
8. Roze JC, Storme L, Zupan V, Morville P, Dinh-Xuan AT, Mercier JC. Echocardiographic investigation of inhaled nitric oxide in newborn babies with severe hypoxaemia. *Lancet.* 1994; 344(8918):303-305.
9. Stranak Z, Semberova J, Barrington K, et al. International survey on diagnosis and management of hypotension in extremely preterm babies. *Eur J Pediatr.* 2014;173(6):793-798.
10. Ewer AK, Tyler W, Francis A, Drinkall D, Gardosi JO. Excessive volume expansion and neonatal death in preterm infants born at 27–28 weeks gestation. *Paediatr Perinat Epidemiol.* 2003; 17(2):180-186.
11. Osborn D, Evans N, Kluckow M. Randomized trial of dobutamine versus dopamine in preterm infants with low systemic blood flow. *J Pediatr.* 2002;140(2):183-191.
12. Lundstrom K, Pryds O, Greisen G. The haemodynamic effects of dopamine and volume expansion in sick preterm infants. *Early Hum Dev.* 2000;57(2):157-163.
13. Kooi EM, van der Laan ME, Verhagen EA, Van Braeckel KN, Bos AF. Volume expansion does not alter cerebral tissue oxygen extraction in preterm infants with clinical signs of poor perfusion. *Neonatology.* 2013;103(4):308-314.
14. Bonestroo HJ, Lemmers PM, Baerts W, van Bel F. Effect of antihypotensive treatment on cerebral oxygenation of preterm infants without PDA. *Pediatrics.* 2011;128(6):e1502-e1510.
15. Osborn DA, Evans N. Early volume expansion for prevention of morbidity and mortality in very preterm infants. *Cochrane Database Syst Rev.* 2004;2004(2):CD002055.
16. Rabe H, Gyte GML, Díaz Rossello JL, Duley L. Effect of timing of umbilical cord clamping and other strategies to influence placental transfusion at preterm birth on maternal and infant outcomes. *Cochrane Database of Syst Rev.* 2019;(9):CD003248. doi:10.1002/14651858.CD003248.pub4.10.
17. Oca MJ, Nelson M, Donn SM. Randomized trial of normal saline versus 5% albumin for the treatment of neonatal hypotension. *J Perinatol.* 2003;23(6):473-476.
18. So KW, Fok TF, Ng PC, Wong WW, Cheung KL. Randomised controlled trial of colloid or crystalloid in hypotensive preterm infants. *Arch Dis Child Fetal Neonatal Ed.* 1997;76(1):F43-F46.
19. Lynch SK, Mullett MD, Graeber JE, Polak MJ. A comparison of albumin-bolus therapy versus normal saline-bolus therapy for hypotension in neonates. *J Perinatol.* 2008;28(1):29-33.
20. Subhedar NV, Shaw NJ. Dopamine versus dobutamine for hypotensive preterm infants. *Cochrane Database Syst Rev.* 2003; (3):CD001242.
21. Osborn DA, Evans N. Early volume expansion versus inotrope for prevention of morbidity and mortality in very preterm infants. *Cochrane Database Syst Rev.* 2001;(2):CD002056.

22. Pellicer A, Valverde E, Elorza MD, et al. Cardiovascular support for low birth weight infants and cerebral hemodynamics: a randomized, blinded, clinical trial. *Pediatrics*. 2005;115(6):1501-1512.

23. Ibrahim H, Sinha IP, Subhedar NV. Corticosteroids for treating hypotension in preterm infants. *Cochrane Database Syst Rev*. 2011;(12):CD003662.

24. Rios DR, Kaiser JR. Vasopressin versus dopamine for treatment of hypotension in extremely low birth weight infants: a randomized, blinded pilot study. *J Pediatr*. 2015;166(4):850-855.

25. Walther FJ, Siassi B, Ramadan NA, Wu PY. Cardiac output in newborn infants with transient myocardial dysfunction. *J Pediatr*. 1985;107:781-785.

26. Padbury JF, Agata Y, Baylen BG, et al. Dopamine pharmacokinetics in critically ill newborn infants. *J Pediatr*. 1987; 110(2):293-298.

27. Zhang J, Penny DJ, Kim NS, Yu VY, Smolich JJ. Mechanisms of blood pressure increase induced by dopamine in hypotensive preterm neonates. *Arch Dis Child Fetal Neonatal Ed*. 1999; 81(2):F99-F104.

28. Roze JC, Tohier C, Maingueneau C, Lefevre M, Mouzard A. Response to dobutamine and dopamine in the hypotensive very preterm infant. *Arch Dis Child*. 1993;69:59-63.

29. Osborn DA, Evans N, Kluckow M. Left ventricular contractility in extremely premature infants in the first day and response to inotropes. *Pediatr Res*. 2007;61(3):335-340.

30. Liet JM, Boscher C, Gras-Leguen C, Gournay V, Debillon T, Roze JC. Dopamine effects on pulmonary artery pressure in hypotensive preterm infants with patent ductus arteriosus. *J Pediatr*. 2002;140(3):373-375.

31. Bouissou A, Rakza T, Klosowski S, et al. Hypotension in preterm infants with significant patent ductus arteriosus: effects of dopamine. *J Pediatr*. 2008;153(6):790-794.

32. Osborn DA, Evans N, Kluckow M, Bowen JR, Rieger I. Low superior vena cava flow and effect of inotropes on neurodevelopment to 3 years in preterm infants. *Pediatrics*. 2007;120(2): 372-380.

33. Bravo MC, Lopez-Ortego P, Sanchez L, et al. Randomized, placebo-controlled trial of dobutamine for low superior vena cava flow in infants. *J Pediatr*. 2015;167(3):572-578.e1-e2.

34. Robel-Tillig E, Knupfer M, Pulzer F, et al. Cardiovascular impact of dobutamine in neonates with myocardial dysfunction. *Early Hum Dev*. 2007;83(5):307-312.

35. Pellicer A, Bravo MC, Madero R, et al. Early systemic hypotension and vasopressor support in low birth weight infants: impact on neurodevelopment. *Pediatrics*. 2009;123(5):1369-1376.

36. Rowcliff K, de Waal K, Mohamed AL, Chaudhari T. Noradrenaline in preterm infants with cardiovascular compromise. *Eur J Pediatr*. 2016;175(12):1967-1973.

37. Tourneux P, Rakza T, Abazine A, Krim G, Storme L. Noradrenaline for management of septic shock refractory to fluid loading and dopamine or dobutamine in full-term newborn infants. *Acta Paediatr*. 2008;97(2):177-180.

38. Tourneux P, Rakza T, Bouissou A, Krim G, Storme L. Pulmonary circulatory effects of norepinephrine in newborn infants with persistent pulmonary hypertension. *J Pediatr*. 2008;153(3): 345-349.

39. Bidegain M, Greenberg R, Simmons C, et al. Vasopressin for refractory hypotension in extremely low birth weight infants. *J Pediatr*. 2010;157(3):502-504.

40. Meyer S, Loffler G, Polcher T, et al. Vasopressin in catecholamine-resistant septic and cardiogenic shock in very-low-birthweight infants. *Acta Paediatr*. 2006;95(10):1309-1312.

41. Walker BR, Haynes Jr J, Wang HL, Voelkel NF. Vasopressin-induced pulmonary vasodilation in rats. *Am J Physiol*. 1989;257 (2 Pt 2):H415-H422.

42. Mohamed A, Nasef N, Shah V, McNamara PJ. Vasopressin as a rescue therapy for refractory pulmonary hypertension in neonates: case series. *Pediatr Crit Care Med*. 2014;15(2):148-154.

43. Hoffman TM, Wernovsky G, Atz AM, et al. Efficacy and safety of milrinone in preventing low cardiac output syndrome in infants and children after corrective surgery for congenital heart disease. *Circulation*. 2003;107(7):996-1002.

44. Paradisis M, Evans N, Kluckow M, et al. Randomized trial of milrinone versus placebo for prevention of low systemic blood flow in very preterm infants. *J Pediatr*. 2009;154(2): 189-195.

45. El-Khuffash AF, Jain A, Weisz D, Mertens L, McNamara PJ. Assessment and treatment of post patent ductus arteriosus ligation syndrome. *J Pediatr*. 2014;165(1):46-52.e1.

46. McNamara PJ, Shivananda SP, Sahni M, Freeman D, Taddio A. Pharmacology of milrinone in neonates with persistent pulmonary hypertension of the newborn and suboptimal response to inhaled nitric oxide. *Pediatr Crit Care Med*. 2013;14(1):74-84.

47. James AT, Bee C, Corcoran JD, McNamara PJ, Franklin O, El-Khuffash AF. Treatment of premature infants with pulmonary hypertension and right ventricular dysfunction with milrinone: a case series. *J Perinatol*. 2015;35(4):268-273.

48. Paradise's M, Jiang X, McLachlan AJ, Evans N, Kluckow M, Osborn D. Population pharmacokinetics and dosing regimen design of milrinone in preterm infants. *Arch Dis Child Fetal Neonatal Ed*. 2007;92(3):F204-F209.

49. Rios DR, Moffett BS, Kaiser JR. Trends in pharmacotherapy for neonatal hypotension. *J Pediatr*. 2014;165(4):697-701.e1.

50. Bourchier D, Weston PJ. Randomised trial of dopamine compared with hydrocortisone for the treatment of hypotensive very low birthweight infants. *Arch Dis Child Fetal Neonatal Ed*. 1997;76(3):F174-F178.

51. Ng PC, Lee CH, Bnur FL, et al. A double-blind, randomized, controlled study of a "stress dose" of hydrocortisone for rescue treatment of refractory hypotension in preterm infants. *Pediatrics*. 2006;117(2):367-375.

52. Efird MM, Heerens AT, Gordon PV, Bose CL, Young DA. A randomized-controlled trial of prophylactic hydrocortisone supplementation for the prevention of hypotension in extremely low birth weight infants. *J Perinatol*. 2005;25(2):119-124.

53. Noori S, Friedlich P, Wong P, Ebrahimi M, Siassi B, Seri I. Hemodynamic changes after low-dosage hydrocortisone administration in vasopressor-treated preterm and term neonates. *Pediatrics*. 2006;118(4):1456-1466.

54. Ibrahim H, Sinha IP, Subhedar NV. Corticosteroids for treating hypotension in preterm infants. *Cochrane Database of Syst Rev*. 2011;2011(12):CD003662. doi:10.1002/14651858.CD003662. pub4. Accessed 31 March 2022.

55. Baud O, Trousson C, Biran V, et al. Association between early low-dose hydrocortisone therapy in extremely preterm neonates and neurodevelopmental outcomes at 2 years of age. *JAMA*. 2017;317(13):1329-1337.

56. Watterberg KL, Walsh MC, Lei L, et al. Hydrocortisone to improve survival without bronchopulmonary dysplasia. *NEJM*. 2022;386:1121-1131.

57. Diab YA, Wong EC, Luban NL. Massive transfusion in children and neonates. *Br J Haematol*. 2013;161(1):15-26.

58. Watterberg KL. Hydrocortisone dosing for hypotension in newborn infants: less is more. *J Pediatr*. 2016;174:23-26.e1.

# PATHOPHYSIOLOGY AND TREATMENT OF PULMONARY HYPERTENSION OF THE NEWBORN

# Chapter 25

# Pathophysiology and Assessment of Acute Pulmonary Hypertension of the Newborn

Yogen Singh and Satyan Lakshminrusimha

## Introduction

Acute pulmonary hypertension (aPH) in the neonatal period is common in sick newborn infants being treated in the neonatal intensive care unit (NICU). The causes and underlying pathophysiology are multifactorial. Acute pulmonary hypertension in the newborn is secondary to impaired or delayed relaxation of the pulmonary vasculature associated with a diverse group of cardiopulmonary pathologies such as meconium aspiration syndrome (MAS), congenital diaphragmatic hernia (CDH), sepsis, respiratory distress syndrome (RDS), prolonged premature rupture of membranes (PPROM), persistent hypoxia, hypoxic-ischemic encephalopathy (HIE), congenital heart disease CHD), heart failure, and alveolar capillary dysplasia, or without a known cause (idiopathic).[1,2] Whatever the cause, most infants with aPH present soon after birth. Hence often this clinical presentation is termed persistent pulmonary hypertension of the newborn (PPHN), previously referred to as persistent fetal circulation (PFC).[3]

Acute pulmonary hypertension (PH) is the phenotypical presentation of various underlying conditions – it is a syndrome of impaired circulatory adaptation at birth.[4] The hallmark of aPH physiology is a sustained elevation of pulmonary vascular resistance (PVR) and labile hypoxemia after birth.[5] Despite advances in understanding of perinatal pathophysiology and neonatal management strategies, its prevalence (2 per 1000 live births) has not changed significantly.[1,6] Most infants with aPH are born at term or late preterm, although around 2% of cases are born prematurely.[7] Acute PH remains one of the leading causes of critical illness in the NICU, with a mortality rate of 5–10%, and this has

not changed significantly despite advances in management and better understanding of pathophysiology.[1] It is critical to understand the etiopathogenesis, altered physiology, and impact of treatment interventions on the underlying pathophysiology, allowing adoption of a physiology-based approach which may help in decreasing morbidity and mortality.

This chapter is primarily focused on pathophysiology and evaluation of aPH, including the role of advanced hemodynamic evaluation in assessing severity and management of aPH and controversies / clinical dilemmas around cardio-centric management. The pharmacological treatment of aPH (Chapter 5), chronic pulmonary hypertension, and PH associated with bronchopulmonary dysplasia (BPD) in premature infants (Chapter 26) and CDH in term infants (Chapter 29) have been described in other chapters.

## Classification of aPH

During the sixth World Symposium of Pulmonary Arterial Hypertension (PAH) held in 2018 in Nice, France, the classification of PAH was updated.[8,9] Due to its particular anatomic and physiologic nature, aPH in the neonatal period has been moved to a separate subcategory – "Persistent PH of the newborn syndrome". However, in our opinion controversy persists in its nomenclature and classification because aPH is neither "persistent" nor present from birth in all infants. It develops secondary to high PVR (which may fail to drop or worsen from an underlying condition) and right and left ventricular dysfunction leading to circulatory failure, associated with acute hypoxia.

While the sixth World Symposium of PAH classification of pediatric pulmonary hypertension is useful, a more commonly used classification of aPH based

**481**

upon etiology, primary (idiopathic) and secondary PPHN, would be more useful to the clinician (Figure 25.1).

Compared to pediatric pulmonary hypertension, only around 10–20% of cases of aPH are idiopathic; most cases (80–90%) occur from abnormally constricted pulmonary vasculature due to MAS, sepsis, CDH, RDS, pneumonia, HIE / perinatal hypoxia, or CDH – this is referred to as secondary aPH. Recent data from California suggest that infection (30%), MAS (24%), idiopathic (20%), RDS (7%), and CDH (6%) are the five leading causes of aPH in newborns.[1] In these cases it can be difficult to separate chronic intrauterine remodeling from acute pulmonary vasoconstriction due to parenchymal lung disease. Primary or idiopathic aPH refers to the absence of parenchymal lung disease/other neonatal disease to explain elevated pulmonary arterial pressure and implies intrauterine

pulmonary vascular remodeling. In neonates this accounts for only 10–20% of cases. Some cases of idiopathic aPH may potentially have a genetic basis.

## Pathophysiology of Acute Pulmonary Hypertension in the Newborn

The PVR during the fetal period is high due to mechanical (fluid-filled alveoli, prominent endothelium), biochemical (high levels of endothelin and serotonin and low levels of nitric oxide and prostacyclin – see Figure 25.2), and alveolar hypoxia.[10,11] Chronic intrauterine hypoxia, exposure to non-steroidal anti-inflammatory drugs (NSAIDs),[12,13] and serotonin-reuptake inhibitors (SSRI) have been associated with vascular remodeling and aPH. However, the association between NSAID use during pregnancy and aPH has been questioned.[14] The imbalance of vasodilator

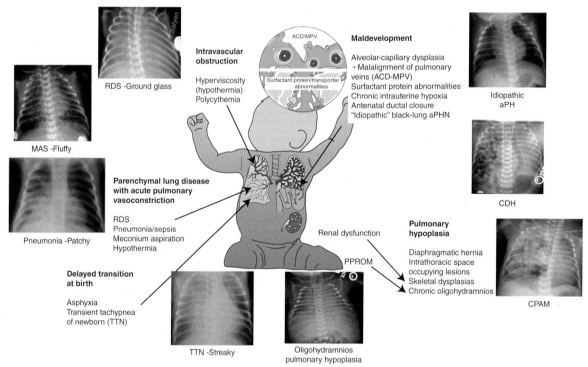

**Fig. 25.1 Pathophysiological classification of acute pulmonary hypertension (*aPH*) with some representative radiological images. *CDH*,** congenital diaphragmatic hernia; *CPAM*, congenital pulmonary adenomatoid malformation; *MAS*, meconium aspiration syndrome with hyperexpansion and fluffy infiltrates; *Pneumonia*, with patchy infiltrates, although occasionally may resemble RDS; *PPROM*, preterm, prolonged rupture of membranes; *RDS*, respiratory distress syndrome with ground glass appearance and air bronchograms; *TTN*, transient tachypnea of the newborn with streaky infiltrates and fluid in the minor fissure. (Copyright Satyan Lakshminrusimha.)

and vasoconstrictor mediators leads to inadequate pulmonary vasodilation at birth, leading to pulmonary hypertension.

Sepsis, specifically group B streptococcal infection, is associated with aPH.[15] Sepsis and pneumonia result in acidosis, hypoxia, and release of pulmonary vasoconstrictor mediators such as thromboxane.[16] In addition, systemic hypotension and shock secondary to sepsis decreases systemic vascular resistance (SVR), leading to right-to-left shunt and hypoxemia.

Perinatal asphyxia, meconium aspiration, hypoxic-ischemic encephalopathy, and therapeutic hypothermia are commonly associated with aPH[17-19] and are discussed in Chapter 22.

## Mechanisms of Pulmonary Vascular Remodeling

Current strategies in the treatment of aPH focus solely on pulmonary vasodilation; effective therapies to reverse pulmonary vascular remodeling and restore angiogenesis do not receive adequate focus (Figures 25.2 and 25.3).[20] In addition to pulmonary vasoconstriction, vascular remodeling and vascular hypoplasia are important contributors to the pathophysiology of aPH. Conditions such as CDH, MAS with intrauterine onset, BPD with aPH, and idiopathic (black lung) aPH demonstrate reduced blood vessel density with remodeling with hypertrophy and hyperplasia of tunica media and adventitial thickening contributing to increased PVR. This vascular remodeling is promoted by factors such as hypoxia-inducible factor-1α (HIF-1α), endothelin-1, reactive oxygen species (ROS), and PPAR-γ. In contrast, therapies that increase cAMP and cGMP in the pulmonary arterial smooth muscle cells tend to be anti-proliferative (Figure 25.2).

HIF-1α is a master transcriptional regulator of developmental and cellular response to hypoxia. Among various factors, HIF-1α upregulates transcription of vascular endothelial growth factor (VEGF) and erythropoietin. Elevated HIF-1α protein has been reported in experimental models of aPH, including pulmonary arterial endothelial cells derived from lambs, with aPH induced by antenatal ductal ligation.[21] The expression of hexokinase-II, a target gene of HIF-1α, is also elevated in aPH pulmonary arterial endothelial cells.

Increased ROS production and oxidative stress contributes to pathophysiology of aPH and vascular remodeling.[22-26] Increased ROS can inhibit prolyl hydroxylases that target HIF-1α for degradation.[27-29] Reduced VEGF leads to decreased angiogenesis and vascular hypoplasia and also leads to reduced nitric oxide (NO). Reduced NO levels lead to decreased cGMP and protein kinase-G levels and are associated with decreased mitochondrial transcription factor levels, electron transport chain protein levels, vascular tube formation, and cell migration.[20,30] These changes were reversed by cinaciguat (a soluble guanyl cyclase activator), 8-bromo-cGMP, and sildenafil (a phosphodiesterase-5 inhibitor).[20]

Reduced AMP kinase (AMPK) activity contributes to impaired mitochondrial function, reduced eNOS, and decreased branching and vessel formation in lambs with aPH induced by antenatal ductal ligation.[31] In utero treatment of these lambs with metformin stimulates AMPK and restores vessel density in the lungs of these lambs.[31]

Rho kinase (ROCK) signaling is a complex pathway responsible for smooth muscle contraction, cellular proliferation, migration, differentiation, and gene expression in various vascular beds, including the neonatal pulmonary circulation.[32-34] In experimental models of aPH increased ROCK activity increases calcium sensitization and vascular tone and contributes to hypertensive remodeling mediated through endothelin-1 and peroxisome proliferator-activated receptor-γ (PPAR-γ) pathway.[32,33] PPAR-γ is a member of the nuclear receptor superfamily, decreases pulmonary arterial smooth muscle cell (PASMC) proliferation, and is abundantly expressed in vascular smooth muscle cells and endothelial cells in the lung.[35] Agonists of PPAR-γ decrease ROCK activity and reduce proliferation of PASMC.[32]

The cellular mechanisms responsible for vascular hypoplasia and remodeling are shown in Figure 25.3. Agents that increase cGMP (sildenafil, cinaciguat and NO),[36,37] those that decrease ROS (antioxidants),[25,38] ROCK inhibitors (Y-27632, fasudil),[34] AMPK stimulators (metformin),[31] endothelin receptor blockers (bosentan),[33] and PPAR-γ agonists (rosiglitazone)[32] have the potential to promote pulmonary vasodilation and reverse vascular modeling in aPH and are being currently used or investigated as potential therapeutic agents.

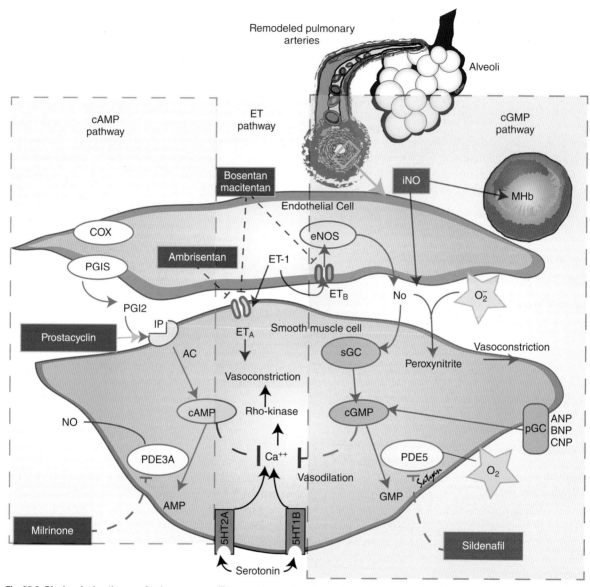

**Fig. 25.2 Biochemical pathways of pulmonary vasodilators and vasoconstrictors.** Therapeutic agents acting through these pathways are shown in *black boxes. 5HT,* serotonin; *AC,* adenylate cyclase; *ANP,* atrial natriuretic peptide; *BNP,* brain natriuretic peptide; *CNP,* C-type natriuretic peptide; *COX,* cyclooxygenase enzyme; *ET,* endothelin; *ET$_A$ and ET$_B$,* endothelin receptors A and B; *IP,* prostacyclin receptor; *MHb,* methemoglobin; *NO,* nitric oxide; *PDE,* phosphodiesterase; *pGC,* particulate guanylate cyclase; *PGI$_2$,* prostacyclin; *PGIS,* prostacyclin synthase enzyme; *sGC,* soluble guanylate cyclase. (Copyright Satyan Lakshminrusimha.)

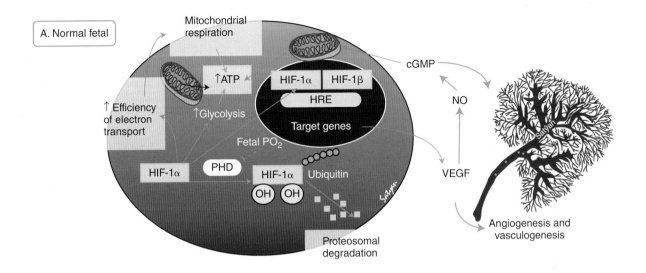

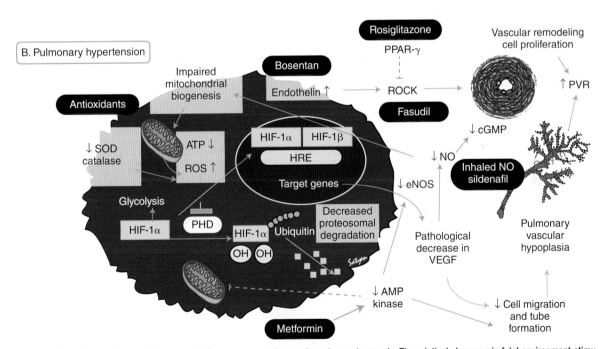

**Fig. 25.3** (A) Pathways involved in in-utero fetal pulmonary angiogenesis and vasculogenesis. The relatively hypoxemic fetal environment stimulates the hypoxia-inducible factor (*HIF*) to stimulate glucose metabolism and vascular endothelial growth factor (*VEGF*) synthesis, leading to nitric oxide (*NO*) production. Cyclic GMP (*cGMP*) stimulates vascular growth. (B) In animal models of pulmonary hypertension breakdown of HIF-1α is inhibited, leading to high levels, but there is a pathological decrease in VEGF and AMP kinase resulting in decreased cell migration and tube formation leading to pulmonary vascular hypoplasia. Increased endothelin and Rho kinase (*ROCK*) pathways, along with deficiency of NO, cGMP, and peroxisome proliferator-activated receptor-γ (*PPAR-γ*), result in vascular modeling and proliferation. Therapeutic agents (shown in *black boxes*) are currently being investigated to reverse vascular remodeling in aPH. (Copyright Satyan Lakshminrusimha [with input from Dr. Ganesh G. Konduri].)

# Clinical Presentation and Diagnosis of Acute Pulmonary Hypertension in the Newborn

Acute hypoxemic respiratory failure with persistent hypoxemia is a hallmark feature of aPH and differentiating cyanotic CHD from acute PH is critical in a hypoxemic cyanosed infant. The initial evaluation should include a thorough history of risk factors for aPH, a meticulous physical examination, simultaneous measurement of pre-ductal (right upper limb) and post-ductal (lower limb) oxygen saturation to check the difference between them, chest radiography, and arterial blood gas analysis. Pre- and post-ductal oxygen saturation and $PaO_2$ measurements can help in differentiating aPH from cyanotic CHD. Pre-/post-ductal saturation differences of greater than 5–10% or $PaO_2$ differences of 10–20 mmHg between right upper limb and lower limbs, with pre-ductal levels being higher than post-ductal levels, are considered significant. The lack of a pre-/post-ductal saturation difference does not exclude a diagnosis of aPH, as the ductus arteriosus must be patent for this feature to be noted. Hypoxemia is often labile and variable in aPH, unlike the fixed hypoxemia seen in cyanotic CHD.[4,39]

The chest X-ray is particularly helpful in diagnosing respiratory pathology. It may help in differentiating the etiology of aPH (such as MAS, pneumonia, RDS, CDH, etc.) and may also help in differentiating types of CHD.[40,41] Hypoxemia disproportionate to the severity of parenchymal disease on chest radiography suggests idiopathic PH or underlying cyanotic heart disease (Figure 25.1). *Pulmonary oligemia* is seen in tetralogy of Fallot (TOF), Ebstein anomaly, critical pulmonary stenosis, and pulmonary atresia due to decreased pulmonary flow. *Pulmonary plethora* is seen in transposition of great arteries (TGA) with intact interventricular septum, truncus arteriosus, tricuspid atresia, total anomalous pulmonary venous connection (TAPVC), and single ventricle.[41] From a pulmonary management perspective, aPH secondary to parenchymal lung disease needs optimal PEEP or mean airway pressure to expand the lung to FRC and to prevent expiratory airflow obstruction in TTN and MAS. In contrast, aPH secondary to pulmonary hypoplasia associated with CDH or oligohydramnios may benefit from lung protective ventilation (with relatively low PEEP).[42] Finally, infants with idiopathic

aPH may benefit more from early use of pulmonary vasodilators.[4]

The hyperoxia test may be useful in differentiating the cardiac causes from respiratory causes in cyanotic newborns. On confirmation of central cyanosis by measuring the arterial partial pressure of oxygen ($PaO_2$), response of $PaO_2$ to 100% oxygen inhalation is tested (hyperoxia test). Oxygen should be administered through a plastic hood for at least 10 minutes in order to fill the alveolar spaces completely with oxygen. In a cyanotic CHD the rise in $PaO_2$ is usually no more than 10–30 mmHg and hardly ever exceeds 100 mmHg. With pulmonary diseases, $PaO_2$ often rises greater than 100 mmHg. However, infants with massive intra-pulmonary shunt from severe respiratory disease may not show a rise in $PaO_2$ to 100 mmHg. Conversely, some infants with cyanotic defects with a large pulmonary blood flow, such as TAPVC, may demonstrate a rise in $PaO_2$ of 100 mmHg or higher. A hyperoxia test should be interpreted in the context of the clinical picture and the degree of pulmonary pathology seen on x-ray.[41,43] With the availability of bedside echocardiography, the hyperoxia test is rarely performed but it is still a very helpful bedside test when echocardiography is not available.

# Echocardiographic Evaluation of Acute Pulmonary Hypertension of Newborn

Echocardiography remains the gold-standard bedside test to confirm the diagnosis of acute PH, monitor the response to the therapeutic interventions, and rule out underlying cyanotic or critical CHD. It can help in confirming the diagnosis of acute pulmonary hypertension and to assess its severity. In the absence of right ventricular (RV) outflow obstruction, pulmonary artery systolic pressure (PASP) can be estimated using tricuspid regurgitation velocity or ductus arteriosus shunt when present.

The pulmonary artery systolic pressure (PASP) can be estimated using echocardiography in the presence of tricuspid regurgitation (TR), as demonstrated (Figure 25.4). The pressure gradient between the RV and right atrium (RA) is calculated by using the modified Bernoulli's principle.[44,45] PASP is estimated by adding RA pressure, which is usually about 5 mmHg, to the peak pressure gradient between RV and RA obtained on continuous wave (CW) Doppler, when there is no RV outflow tract obstruction (Figures 25.4 and 25.5).

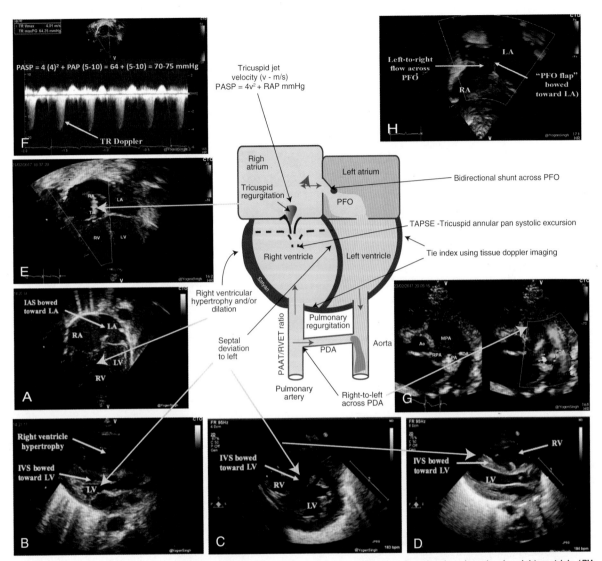

**Fig. 25.4 Echocardiography images showing features of aPH on 2D images.** Image (A) Apical four-chamber view showing right ventricle (*RV*) hypertrophy, interventricular septum (*IVS*) bowing toward left ventricle (*LV*), and inter-atrial septum bowing toward left atrium (*LA*). Image (B) Parasternal long-axis view showing RV and IVS hypertrophy with bowing of IVS toward LV. Image (C) Parasternal short-axis view showing significant bowing of IVS toward LV due to supra-systemic pulmonary artery pressure. Image (D) Parasternal long-axis view showing RV dilatation and hypertrophy with paradoxical septal movements in an infant with PPHN and RV failure. Echocardiography images showing estimation of pulmonary artery systolic pressure (*PASP*) and shunts in PPHN are shown in images E–H. (E) Apical four-chamber showing tricuspid regurgitation (*TR*) jet on color flow mapping, (F) Doppler assessment of TR velocity (Vmax 4 m/s), which equates to an estimated PASP of around 70–75 mmHg, (G) right-to-left shunt across patent ductus arteriosus (PDA) suggesting supra-systemic PASP, (H) Subcostal view showing bidirectional transatrial shunt across patent foramen ovale (PFO) – left-to-right blood flow direction seen on frozen image and "flap of PFO" bowed toward left atrium. TAPSE – tricuspid annular plane systolic excursion – can be used to assess right ventricular function. Tei index using tissue Doppler imaging can be used to assess both right and left ventricular function. *PAAT*, pulmonary arterial acceleration time; *RVET*, right ventricular ejection time. (Copyright Yogen Singh and Satyan Lakshminrusimha 2021. Modified from Ref. 5.)

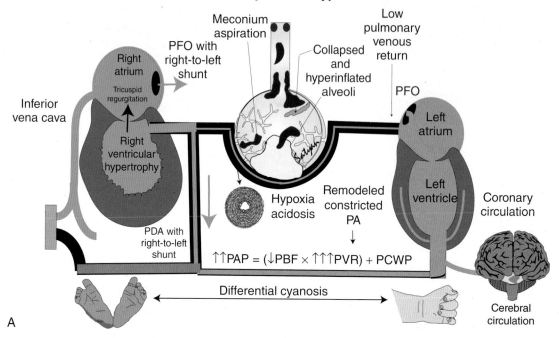

## Pulmonary arterial hypertension

$$\uparrow\uparrow PAP = (\downarrow PBF \times \uparrow\uparrow\uparrow PVR) + PCWP$$

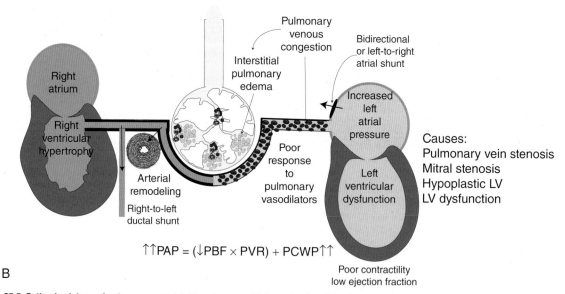

## Pulmonary venous hypertension

Causes:
Pulmonary vein stenosis
Mitral stenosis
Hypoplastic LV
LV dysfunction

$$\uparrow\uparrow PAP = (\downarrow PBF \times PVR) + PCWP\uparrow\uparrow$$

**Fig. 25.5 Pathophysiology of pulmonary arterial (A) and venous (B) hypertension.** (A) Pulmonary arterial hypertension is characterized by right ventricular hypertrophy, tricuspid regurgitation, right-to-left or bidirectional shunt across the PDA and PFO, and differential cyanosis. *PAP*, pulmonary arterial pressure; *PBF*, pulmonary blood flow; *PCWP*, pulmonary capillary wedge pressure; *PVR*, pulmonary vascular resistance. (B) Pulmonary venous (or postcapillary) hypertension can be secondary to various causes but left ventricular dysfunction can be commonly associated with aPH and can cause pulmonary edema that is worsened by inhaled nitric oxide. (Copyright Satyan Lakshminrusimha.)

However, pulmonary pressures may be underestimated if there is impaired RV contractility, and TR may be absent in up to one-third of infants with aPH.

$$\text{Pulmonary artery systolic pressure} = 4 \times (\text{TR velocity})^2 + \text{RA pressure (5 mmHg)}$$

The severity of pulmonary hypertension can be qualitatively estimated by appraising interventricular septum (IVS) and LV shape in the parasternal short-axis view, although the reliability of this method is questionable. Normally, the left ventricle (LV) is circular in shape as the interventricular septum is dependent on the interventricular pressure gradient. With rising PAP, the IVS will flatten, and paradoxical septal movements may be seen in severe PH with suprasystemic pulmonary artery pressures. These effects are also known as ventriculo-ventricular interaction. End-systolic and maximal eccentricity indices are quantitative measures of LV circularity. An eccentricity index of > 1.3 is suggestive of pulmonary arterial hypertension. The severity of pulmonary hypertension can also be estimated by the direction and velocity of shunt across a patent ductus arteriosus (PDA) but may be limited because of the long and tortuous nature of the duct that renders the Bernoulli equation less reliable. A pure right-to-left shunt across a PDA suggests suprasystemic pulmonary artery pressure (PAP), while a bidirectional transductal shunt suggests isosystemic pulmonary artery pressure. PASP can also be estimated by measuring the shunt velocity across the ductus arteriosus.

Pulmonary regurgitation is not common in neonates, but when present, it can help in estimating mean and end-diastolic pulmonary artery pressure. Detailed description of echocardiographic techniques used for assessment of aPH is beyond the scope of this article. A summary of echocardiography parameters commonly used in clinical practice is shown in Figure 25.4 and Table 25.1.

Serial echocardiography assessment can help in understanding evolving pathophysiology and response to the therapeutic intervention. Echocardiography assessment and hemodynamic evaluation can help in targeting specific intervention and they can guide the choice of appropriate pulmonary vasodilator and vasoactive therapy (see Chapter 27).[45,46]

## Role of Advanced Hemodynamic Evaluation in Management of Acute Pulmonary Hypertension

Infants with aPH often have hemodynamic instability and need cardioactive medications. Some infants with hypovolemia may need fluid therapy, while infants with severe cardiac function without hypovolemia may be harmed by excessive fluid therapy. Similarly, some infants may need pure vasopressor therapy, while others would benefit from inotropic or lusitropic therapy. Echocardiography can be used to evaluate hemodynamics at the bedside and to target specific interventions. Preload (cardiac filling), afterload (pulmonary vascular resistance and systemic vascular resistance), and cardiac contractility can be evaluated at the bedside. Comprehensive evaluation of pulmonary hemodynamics should include characterization of pulmonary artery pressure, RV function, and the impact on left and right ventricular output. Every first echocardiography evaluation should be comprehensive and include the necessary imaging and sweeps to confirm normal cardiac anatomy and exclude anatomic heart disease. This assessment may be performed by a neonatologist with training in targeted neonatal echocardiography but should be reviewed in a timely manner by a pediatric cardiologist. In addition, echocardiography can be used to study the trend and response to therapy by serial assessments. We recommend that this detailed assessment should be a routine and standard of care in infants with aPH associated with hemodynamic instability, and serial echocardiography assessment should be performed to monitor the disease progress, changing pathophysiology, and response to treatment.[45,46]

## Controversies and Clinical Dilemmas and Physiology-Based Management of Acute Pulmonary Hypertension in the Newborn

### LUNG RECRUITMENT

Lung expansion to functional residual capacity (FRC) results in low PVR. Lung overexpansion (above FRC) decreases venous return and compresses the alveolar vessels in the lung, increasing PVR. In contrast, lung

| TABLE 25.1 | Echocardiographic Parameters Used for Assessment of aPH |
|---|---|
| | **Echocardiographic Parameter** |

**A.) Diagnosis of pulmonary hypertension and its severity – evaluation of pulmonary hemodynamics**

| Conventional echo parameters | 1. Disproportionately large right side of the heart with right ventricle (RV) hypertrophy and/or RV dilatation on visual inspection – use multiple views to assess cardiac asymmetry |
|---|---|
| | 2. Estimation of pulmonary artery systolic pressure (PASP) – by measuring tricuspid regurgitation gradient (when present) or ductal shunt using Doppler assessment |
| | 3. Direction of blood flow across patent ductus arteriosus (PDA) – **Right-to-left shunt:** supra-systemic PAP; **Left-to-right shunt:** sub-systemic PAP; and **Bidirectional shunt:** PAP equal to systemic blood pressure |
| | 4. Direction of blood flow across patent foramen ovale (PFO) – usually bidirectional in aPHN and seldom purely right to left |
| | 5. Flattening of interventricular septum – helps in estimating severity of aPHN in absence of TR or PDA; can be categorized as mild, moderate, and severe flattening |
| | 6. Pulmonary artery Doppler – shape (normal spectral or with dicrotic notch), pulmonary artery acceleration time (PAAT), PAAT:RVET (RV ejection time) ratio |
| | 7. End-systolic LV eccentricity index (EI) |

**B.) Assessment of right ventricle function**

| Conventional echo parameters for RV function assessment | 1. Qualitative assessment on visual inspection in multiple echo views – subjective and prone to inaccuracy; useful in emergency situations |
|---|---|
| | 2. Tricuspid annular plane systolic excursion (TAPSE) |
| | 3. RV fractional area change (FAC) |
| | 4. RV output measurement |
| Advanced echo parameters for research only | 1. Assessment of RV systolic and diastolic function on tissue Doppler imaging (TDI) |
| | 2. Speckle tracking/strain rate |

**C.) Assessment of left ventricle function**

| Conventional echo parameters for LV function assessment | 1. Qualitative assessment on visual inspection in multiple echo views – subjective and prone to inaccuracy; useful in emergency situations |
|---|---|
| | 2. Fraction shortening (%FS) |
| | 3. Ejection fraction (%EF) |
| | *(Note: fraction shortening may be unreliable in presence of RV hypertrophy and dysfunction)* |
| | 4. LV output measurement |
| | 5. Myocardial performance index or Tei index using tissue Doppler Imaging (TDI) |
| Advanced echo parameters for research only | 1. Assessment of LV systolic and diastolic function on tissue Doppler imaging (TDI) |
| | 2. Myocardial performance index or Tei index using TDI |
| | 3. Speckle tracking/strain rate |

collapse increases the resistance in extra-alveolar pulmonary vessels and increases PVR.[47] In infants with normal lung volumes achieving an 8 to 9 rib expansion on a chest x-ray is ideal. However, in infants with hypoplastic lungs (such as CDH), FRC might be achieved with only a 6–7 rib expansion on the contralateral side. Lung point-of-care ultrasound (POCUS) may help in assessing and optimizing lung expansion. It has been recommended by the European Society of Pediatric and Neonatal Intensive Care Society

(ESPNIC) international guideline on use of POCUS in neonates and children.[48] Attempts to overexpand the lung to achieve 8 to 9 rib expansion with high PEEP or mean airway pressure in CDH can increase the risk of volutrauma, air leak, and increased PVR. Hence low PEEP (3–5 cm $H_2O$) and limiting PIP to 25 cm $H_2O$ is optimal for initial conventional ventilation in CDH.[49] Neonates with parenchymal lung disease such as RDS, MAS, or pneumonia may require much higher pressures to recruit the lung. Initiating iNO without optimal lung recruitment is a common cause of lack of sustained response to iNO.[50] For iNO to be effective, it needs to reach the alveoli and pulmonary vasculature (i.e., PASMC, the target cell) with alveoli expanded to FRC.[51]

## SURFACTANT

In aPH secondary to neonatal parenchymal lung disease recruitment of the lung with adequate pressure and use of surfactant if $FiO_2$ >0.4 is often needed to maintain preductal $SpO_2$ >90%. Additionally, it may enhance the response to iNO and reduce the need for ECMO.[52,53] In the absence of surfactant asymmetric lung expansion results in collapsed and hyperexpanded alveoli, increasing ventilation-perfusion mismatch and PVR. With the use of surfactant and optimal lung recruitment, uniform expansion of alveoli results in lower PVR and enhances the ability for iNO to reach the alveoli and pulmonary vasculature.[54]

## OXYGENATION

Both oxygen and iNO are potent and specific pulmonary vasodilators. However, when high concentrations of inspired oxygen are used (~$FiO_2$ = 1.0), there is increased formation of ROS such as superoxide anions in the lung leading to induction of PDE5 activity reducing the effectiveness of iNO.[55-58] Use of iNO in combination with $FiO_2$ ~1.0 results in increased formation of peroxynitrite in the pulmonary vasculature.[38] Based on these results, it is important to wean $FiO_2$ from 1.0 to <0.6 if possible after initiation of iNO in aPH.[59]

The American Thoracic Society (ATS)/American Heart Association (AHA) guidelines recommend oxygen therapy for infants with $SpO_2$ <92%, especially for those with pulmonary hypertension associated with respiratory disease. They also add that $FiO_2$ >0.6 may be ineffective in pulmonary hypertension, owing to extrapulmonary shunting, and may aggravate lung injury.[60] The European Pulmonary Vascular Disease Network recommends a preductal $SpO_2$ of 91–95% when aPH is suspected or established.[61] There are no clinical trials evaluating the optimal $FiO_2$ or $SpO_2$ in aPH. Animal studies using ductal ligation and meconium aspiration models of aPH suggest that targeting a preductal $SpO_2$ in the 90–97% range results in low PVR.[62-64] Based on these results, setting lower $SpO_2$ alarm limit

at 89% and upper alarm limit at 98–99% appears prudent during management of aPH. Each infant with aPH should be carefully evaluated to optimally balance oxidative stress associated with high $FiO_2$ and pulmonary vasoconstriction secondary to hypoxia.

## SYSTEMIC BLOOD PRESSURE AND VASOPRESSORS IN APH

Systemic hypotension leading to aggravation of right-to-left shunt and hypoxemia is commonly seen in aPH.[65] A common practice is to RVSP by echocardiography and use dopamine to increase systemic systolic pressure above the RVSP. While this practice might temporarily decrease right-to-left shunting and transiently improve oxygenation, it has the following negative consequences: (i) vasopressor agents, especially dopamine, are non-specific and increase both systemic and pulmonary arterial pressure, especially at doses >10–15 mcg/kg/min[66]; (ii) the right-to-left shunt across the PDA often serves as a pop-off valve limiting excessive right ventricular afterload and failure; limiting this shunt by increasing systemic blood pressure to supraphysiological levels will hasten right ventricular failure; and (iii) many cases of aPH associated with systemic hypotension have a component of left ventricular dysfunction with low cardiac output. Intense systemic vasoconstriction increases afterload to the already preload-compromised left ventricle. In these cases the right-to-left ductal shunt maintains systemic circulation. Increasing systemic vascular resistance with non-specific vasopressors will limit right-to-left shunt and lead to systemic ischemia, causing oliguria, lactic acidosis, and renal failure. Hence from a systemic hemodynamic perspective, "blue blood is better than no blood".[66] For these reasons, we recommend avoiding non-specific vasopressors such as dopamine and recommend the use of norepinephrine[67] or vasopressin[68] to increase blood pressure to physiological levels (normal range for gestational age). Care must be exercised while using vasopressin to avoid oliguria and hyponatremia by closely monitoring urine output and serum electrolytes.[68]

## LEFT VENTRICULAR DYSFUNCTION (FIGURE 25.5B)

Infants with aPH secondary to left CDH, sepsis, and asphyxia are likely to have LV dysfunction. Infants with LV dysfunction demonstrate poor contractility, low ejection fraction, and left atrial dilation. Despite elevated pulmonary arterial pressures and a right-to-left ductal shunt, these patients may present with a bidirectional (mostly left-to-right) or exclusively left-to-right shunt at the atrial level due to high left atrial pressure, pulmonary venous hypertension, and pulmonary edema. Inhaled NO can worsen pulmonary edema, leading to respiratory deterioration. Non-responders to iNO with CDH had a higher likelihood of LV systolic dysfunction and ECMO compared to responders.[69] It is prudent to use an inotrope such as milrinone to enhance left ventricular function instead of iNO in patients with left ventricular dysfunction. In patients with asphyxia and HIE undergoing therapeutic hypothermia, milrinone should be used cautiously in the presence of renal dysfunction, as systemic hypotension can occur due to impaired clearance of milrinone.[70]

## Conclusions

Acute pulmonary hypertension is common in infants being treated in the neonatal intensive care and continues to have high mortality and co-morbidities. Early diagnosis and targeted intervention based on the altered pathophysiology is crucial in the management of acute pulmonary hypertension. Although the diagnosis of acute pulmonary hypertension can be made clinically, echocardiography remains the gold-standard bedside investigation to establish diagnosis of acute pulmonary hypertension, assess its severity, and provide hemodynamic data to support specific interventions and monitor response to treatment. While standard echocardiography to assess for CHD is important, evaluation of hemodynamics using echocardiography can further help in understanding and managing the pathophysiology.

## REFERENCES

1. Steurer MA, Jelliffe-Pawlowski LL, Baer RJ, Partridge JC, Rogers EE, Keller RL. Persistent pulmonary hypertension of the newborn in late preterm and term infants in California. *Pediatrics*. 2017;139(1):e20161165.
2. Martinho S, Adao R, Leite-Moreira AF, Bras-Silva C. Persistent pulmonary hypertension of the newborn: pathophysiological mechanisms and novel therapeutic approaches. *Front Pediatr*. 2020;8:342.
3. Spitzer AR, Davis J, Clarke WT, Bernbaum J, Fox WW. Pulmonary hypertension and persistent fetal circulation in the newborn. *Clin Perinatol*. 1988;15(2):389-413.
4. Lakshminrusimha S, Keszler M. Persistent pulmonary hypertension of the newborn. *Neoreviews*. 2015;16(12):e680-e692.
5. Singh Y, Lakshminrusimha S. Pathophysiology and management of persistent pulmonary hypertension of the newborn. *Clin Perinatol*. 2021;48(3):595-618.
6. Walsh-Sukys MC, Tyson JE, Wright LL, et al. Persistent pulmonary hypertension of the newborn in the era before nitric oxide: practice variation and outcomes. *Pediatrics*. 2000;105 (1 Pt 1):14-20.
7. Kumar VH, Hutchison AA, Lakshminrusimha S, Morin FC III, Wynn RJ, Ryan RM. Characteristics of pulmonary hypertension in preterm neonates. *J Perinatol*. 2007;27(4):214-219.
8. Rosenzweig EB, Abman SH, Adatia I, et al. Paediatric pulmonary arterial hypertension: updates on definition, classification, diagnostics and management. *Eur Respir J*. 2019;53(1):1801916.
9. Simonneau G, Montani D, Celermajer DS, et al. Haemodynamic definitions and updated clinical classification of pulmonary hypertension. *Eur Respir J*. 2019;53(1):1801913.
10. Lakshminrusimha S, Steinhorn RH. Pulmonary vascular biology during neonatal transition. *Clin Perinatol*. 1999;26(3):601-619.
11. Delaney C, Gien J, Grover TR, Roe G, Abman SH. Pulmonary vascular effects of serotonin and selective serotonin reuptake inhibitors in the late-gestation ovine fetus. *Am J Physiol Lung Cell Mol Physiol*. 2011;301(6):L937-L944.
12. Talati AJ, Salim MA, Korones SB. Persistent pulmonary hypertension after maternal naproxen ingestion in a term newborn: a case report. *Am J Perinatol*. 2000;17(2):69-71.
13. Alano MA, Ngougmna E, Ostrea Jr EM, Konduri GG. Analysis of nonsteroidal antiinflammatory drugs in meconium and its relation to persistent pulmonary hypertension of the newborn. *Pediatrics*. 2001;107(3):519-523.
14. Van Marter LJ, Hernandez-Diaz S, Werler MM, Louik C, Mitchell AA. Nonsteroidal antiinflammatory drugs in late pregnancy and persistent pulmonary hypertension of the newborn. *Pediatrics*. 2013;131(1):79-87.
15. Shankaran S, Farooki ZQ, Desai R. β-Hemolytic streptococcal infection appearing as persistent fetal circulation. *Am J Dis Child*. 1982;136(8):725-727.
16. Schweer H, Seyberth HW, Kuhl PG, Meese CO. Unusual metabolism of prostacyclin in infants with persistent septic pulmonary hypertension. *Eicosanoids*. 1990;3(4):237-242.
17. Lapointe A, Barrington KJ. Pulmonary hypertension and the asphyxiated newborn. *J Pediatr*. 2011;158(suppl 2):e19-e24.
18. Lakshminrusimha S, Shankaran S, Laptook A, et al. Pulmonary hypertension associated with hypoxic-ischemic encephalopathy-antecedent characteristics and comorbidities. *J Pediatr*. 2018;196:45-51.e3.
19. Rios DR, Lapointe A, Schmolzer GM, et al. Hemodynamic optimization for neonates with neonatal encephalopathy caused by a hypoxic ischemic event: physiological and therapeutic considerations. *Semin Fetal Neonatal Med*. 2021:26:101277.
20. Sharma M, Rana U, Joshi C, et al. Decreased cyclic guanosine monophosphate-protein kinase G signaling impairs angiogenesis in a lamb model of persistent pulmonary hypertension of the newborn. *Am J Respir Cell Mol Biol*. 2021;65(5):555-567.
21. Makker K, Afolayan AJ, Teng RJ, Konduri GG. Altered hypoxia-inducible factor-1alpha (HIF-1alpha) signaling contributes to impaired angiogenesis in fetal lambs with persistent pulmonary hypertension of the newborn (PPHN). *Physiol Rep*. 2019;7(3):e13986.

22. Wedgwood S, Steinhorn RH, Lakshminrusimha S. Optimal oxygenation and role of free radicals in PPHN. *Free Radic Biol Med.* 2019;142:97-106.

23. Wedgwood S, Steinhorn RH, Bunderson M, et al. Increased hydrogen peroxide downregulates soluble guanylate cyclase in the lungs of lambs with persistent pulmonary hypertension of the newborn. *Am J Physiol Lung Cell Mol Physiol.* 2005;289(4): L660-L666.

24. Wedgwood S, Lakshminrusimha S, Fukai T, Russell JA, Schumacker PT, Steinhorn RH. Hydrogen peroxide regulates extracellular superoxide dismutase activity and expression in neonatal pulmonary hypertension. *Antioxid Redox Signal.* 2011;15:1497-1506.

25. Wedgwood S, Lakshminrusimha S, Farrow KN, et al. Apocynin improves oxygenation and increases eNOS in persistent pulmonary hypertension of the newborn. *Am J Physiol Lung Cell Mol Physiol.* 2012;302(6):L616-L626.

26. Wedgwood S, Lakshminrusimha S, Czech L, Schumacker PT, Steinhorn RH. Increased p22[phox]/Nox4 expression is involved in remodeling through hydrogen peroxide signaling in experimental persistent pulmonary hypertension of the newborn. *Antioxid Redox Signal.* 2013;18(14):1765-1776.

27. Scortegagna M, Ding K, Oktay Y, et al. Multiple organ pathology, metabolic abnormalities and impaired homeostasis of reactive oxygen species in Epas1-/- mice. *Nat Genet.* 2003;35(4): 331-340.

28. Semenza GL. Involvement of hypoxia-inducible factor 1 in pulmonary pathophysiology. *Chest.* 2005;128(suppl 6): 592S-594S.

29. Semenza GL. Pulmonary vascular responses to chronic hypoxia mediated by hypoxia-inducible factor 1. *Proc Am Thorac Soc.* 2005;2(1):68-70.

30. Afolayan AJ, Eis A, Alexander M, et al. Decreased endothelial nitric oxide synthase expression and function contribute to impaired mitochondrial biogenesis and oxidative stress in fetal lambs with persistent pulmonary hypertension. *Am J Physiol Lung Cell Mol Physiol.* 2016;310(1):L40-L49.

31. Rana U, Callan E, Entringer B, et al. AMP-kinase dysfunction alters notch ligands to impair angiogenesis in neonatal pulmonary hypertension. *Am J Respir Cell Mol Biol.* 2020; 62(6):719-731.

32. Gien J, Tseng N, Seedorf G, Roe G, Abman SH. Peroxisome proliferator activated receptor-gamma-Rho-kinase interactions contribute to vascular remodeling after chronic intrauterine pulmonary hypertension. *Am J Physiol Lung Cell Mol Physiol.* 2014;306(3):L299-L308.

33. Gien J, Tseng N, Seedorf G, Roe G, Abman SH. Endothelin-1 impairs angiogenesis in vitro through Rho-kinase activation after chronic intrauterine pulmonary hypertension in fetal sheep. *Pediatr Res.* 2013;73(3):252-262.

34. McNamara PJ, Murthy P, Kantores C, et al. Acute vasodilator effects of Rho-kinase inhibitors in neonatal rats with pulmonary hypertension unresponsive to nitric oxide. *Am J Physiol Lung Cell Mol Physiol.* 2008;294(2):L205-L213.

35. Abbott BD, Wood CR, Watkins AM, Das KP, Lau CS. Peroxisome proliferator-activated receptors alpha, Beta, and gamma mRNA and protein expression in human fetal tissues. *PPAR Res.* 2010;2010:690907.

36. Huang W, Liu N, Tong X, Du Y. Sildenafil protects against pulmonary hypertension induced by hypoxia in neonatal rats via activation of PPARgammamediated downregulation of TRPC. *Int J Mol Med.* 2022;49(2):19.

37. Roberts Jr JD, Chiche JD, Weimann J, Steudel W, Zapol WM, Bloch KD. Nitric oxide inhalation decreases pulmonary artery remodeling in the injured lungs of rat pups. *Circ Res.* 2000; 87(2):140-145.

38. Lakshminrusimha S, Russell JA, Wedgwood S, et al. Superoxide dismutase improves oxygenation and reduces oxidation in neonatal pulmonary hypertension. *Am J Respir Crit Care Med.* 2006;174(12):1370-1377.

39. Lesneski A, Hardie M, Ferrier W, Lakshminrusimha S, Vali P. Bidirectional ductal shunting and preductal to postductal oxygenation gradient in persistent pulmonary hypertension of the newborn. *Children (Basel).* 2020;7(9):137.

40. Minocha P, Agarwal A, Jivani N, Swaminathan S. Evaluation of neonates with suspected congenital heart disease: a new cost-effective algorithm. *Clin Pediatr.* 2018;57(13):1541-1548.

41. Singh Y, Lakshminrusimha S. Perinatal cardiovascular physiology and recognition of critical congenital heart defects. *Clin Perinatol.* 2021;48(3):573-594.

42. Guevorkian D, Mur S, Cavatorta E, Pognon L, Rakza T, Storme L. Lower distending pressure improves respiratory mechanics in congenital diaphragmatic hernia complicated by persistent pulmonary hypertension. *J Pediatr.* 2018;200:38-43.

43. Singh Y, Chee YH, Gahlaut R. Evaluation of suspected congenital heart disease. *Paediatr Child Health.* 2015;25(1):7-12.

44. Singh Y. Echocardiographic evaluation of hemodynamics in neonates and children. *Front Pediatr.* 2017;5:201.

45. de Boode WP, Singh Y, Molnar Z, et al. Application of neonatologist performed echocardiography in the assessment and management of persistent pulmonary hypertension of the newborn. *Pediatr Res.* 2018;84(suppl 1):68-77.

46. Tissot C, Singh Y. Neonatal functional echocardiography. *Curr Opin Pediatr.* 2020;32(2):235-244.

47. Simmons DH, Linde LM, Miller JH, O'Reilly RJ. Relation between lung volume and pulmonary vascular resistance. *Circ Res.* 1961;9(2):465-471.

48. Singh Y, Tissot C, Fraga MV, et al. International evidence-based guidelines on Point of Care Ultrasound (POCUS) for critically ill neonates and children issued by the POCUS Working Group of the European Society of Paediatric and Neonatal Intensive Care (ESPNIC). *Crit Care.* 2020;24(1):65.

49. Snoek KG, Reiss IK, Greenough A, et al. Standardized postnatal management of infants with congenital diaphragmatic hernia in Europe: The CDH EURO consortium consensus – 2015 update. *Neonatology.* 2016;110(1):66-74.

50. Dadiz R, Nair J, D'Angio CT, Ryan RM, Lakshminrusimha S. Methemoglobin and the response to inhaled nitric oxide in persistent pulmonary hypertension of the newborn. *J Neonatal Perinatal Med.* 2020;13(2):175-182.

51. Pabalan MJ, Nayak SP, Ryan RM, Kumar VH, Lakshminrusimha S. Methemoglobin to cumulative nitric oxide ratio and response to inhaled nitric oxide in PPHN. *J Perinatol.* 2009; 29:698-701.

52. Konduri GG, Lakshminrusimha S. Surf early to higher tides: surfactant therapy to optimize tidal volume, lung recruitment, and iNO response. *J Perinatol.* 2021;41(1):1-3.

53. Konduri GG, Sokol GM, Van Meurs KP, et al. Impact of early surfactant and inhaled nitric oxide therapies on outcomes in term/late preterm neonates with moderate hypoxic respiratory failure. *J Perinatol.* 2013;33(12):944-949.

54. Gonzalez A, Bancalari A, Osorio W, et al. Early use of combined exogenous surfactant and inhaled nitric oxide reduces treat-

ment failure in persistent pulmonary hypertension of the newborn: a randomized controlled trial. *J Perinatol.* 2021;41:32-38.

55. Brennan LA, Steinhorn RH, Wedgwood S, et al. Increased superoxide generation is associated with pulmonary hypertension in fetal lambs: a role for NADPH oxidase. *Circ Res.* 2003; 92(6):683-691.

56. Farrow KN, Wedgwood S, Lee KJ, et al. Mitochondrial oxidant stress increases PDE5 activity in persistent pulmonary hypertension of the newborn. *Respir Physiol Neurobiol.* 2010; 174(3):272-281.

57. Farrow KN, Lee KJ, Perez M, et al. Brief hyperoxia increases mitochondrial oxidation and increases Pde5 activity in fetal pulmonary artery smooth muscle cells. *Antioxid Redox Signal.* 2012;17(3):460-470.

58. Farrow KN, Lakshminrusimha S, Czech L, et al. Superoxide dismutase and inhaled nitric oxide normalize phosphodiesterase 5 expression and activity in neonatal lambs with persistent pulmonary hypertension. *Am J Physiol Lung Cell Mol Physiol.* 2010;299:L109-L116.

59. Sharma V, Berkelhamer SK, Lakshminrusimha S. Persistent pulmonary hypertension of the newborn. *Maternal Health, Neonatol Perinatol.* 2015;1:14.

60. Abman SH, Hansmann G, Archer SL, et al. Pediatric pulmonary hypertension: guidelines from the American heart association and American thoracic society. *Circulation.* 2015;132:2037-2099.

61. Hansmann G, Koestenberger M, Alastalo TP, et al. 2019 updated consensus statement on the diagnosis and treatment of pediatric pulmonary hypertension: The European Pediatric Pulmonary Vascular Disease Network (EPPVDN), endorsed by AEPC, ESPR and ISHLT. *J Heart Lung Transplant.* 2019;38(9):879-901.

62. Rawat M, Chandrasekharan P, Gugino SF, et al. Optimal oxygen targets in term lambs with meconium aspiration syndrome and pulmonary hypertension. *Am J Respir Cell Mol Biol.* 2020; 63:510-518.

63. Lakshminrusimha S, Konduri GG, Steinhorn RH. Considerations in the management of hypoxemic respiratory failure and persistent pulmonary hypertension in term and late preterm neonates. *J Perinatol.* 2016;36(suppl 2):S12-S19.

64. Lakshminrusimha S, Swartz DD, Gugino SF, et al. Oxygen concentration and pulmonary hemodynamics in newborn lambs with pulmonary hypertension. *Pediatr Res.* 2009; 66(5):539-544.

65. Siefkes HM, Lakshminrusimha S. Management of systemic hypotension in term infants with persistent pulmonary hypertension of the newborn: an illustrated review. *Arch Dis Child Fetal Neonatal Ed.* 2021;106:446-455.

66. McNamara PJ, Giesinger RE, Lakshminrusimha S. Dopamine and neonatal pulmonary hypertension-pressing need for a better pressor? *J Pediatr.* 2022;246:242-250.

67. Tourneux P, Rakza T, Bouissou A, Krim G, Storme L. Pulmonary circulatory effects of norepinephrine in newborn infants with persistent pulmonary hypertension. *J Pediatr.* 2008;153(3): 345-349.

68. Acker SN, Kinsella JP, Abman SH, Gien J. Vasopressin improves hemodynamic status in infants with congenital diaphragmatic hernia. *J Pediatr.* 2014;165(1):53-58.e1.

69. Lawrence KM, Monos S, Adams S, et al. Inhaled nitric oxide is associated with improved oxygenation in a subpopulation of infants with congenital diaphragmatic hernia and pulmonary hypertension. *J Pediatr.* 2020;219:167-172.

70. Bischoff AR, Habib S, McNamara PJ, Giesinger RE. Hemodynamic response to milrinone for refractory hypoxemia during therapeutic hypothermia for neonatal hypoxic ischemic encephalopathy. *J Perinatol.* 2021;41(9):2345-2354.

# Chapter 26

# Chronic Pulmonary Hypertension

Philip T. Levy and Amish Jain

## Key Points

- Chronic pulmonary hypertension (cPH), a severe form of pulmonary vascular disease, is characterized by a sustained and progressive elevation of pulmonary vascular resistance, pulmonary artery pressures, and resultant exposure of the right ventricle to high afterload.
- cPH most commonly affects extreme preterm infants with bronchopulmonary dysplasia (BPD) but has also been identified in preterm infants without overt lung disease.
- Comprehensive assessment should aim to delineate the specific hemodynamic profiles associated with cPH, with a thorough clinical exam and conventional and emerging quantitative echocardiography measures to help guide therapeutic interventions.
- Infants with established BPD should be screened for cPH with echocardiography.
- The indications to consider evaluation by cardiac catheterization are to determine severity of PH, identify contributing cardiovascular co-morbidities, and elucidate poor responders to PH-targeted therapy.
- The management of established cPH focuses on the following principles: (i) supportive cardiorespiratory care (optimizing ventilatory support, diuretics, calorie intake) (ii) pharmacotherapy to induce pulmonary vasodilation, and (iii) monitoring right ventricular function.

## Introduction

Chronic pulmonary hypertension (cPH) in neonates is a heterogeneous disease process characterized by an elevation of pulmonary artery pressures (PAP) and prolonged exposure of the right ventricle (RV) to high afterload that collectively contribute to higher morbidity and mortality.[1-4] The diagnosis and management of the hemodynamic status of preterm infants with cPH can be challenging, owing to the multitude of etiologies and the unique characteristics of the pulmonary circulatory system. The causes of neonatal cPH may be described based on endotype of the pulmonary vasculature.[1,2,5] These include conditions associated with maladaptive pulmonary vasculature (e.g., chronic lung disease [CLD], pulmonary hypoplasia and genetic conditions like trisomy 21), those associated with maldeveloped pulmonary vasculature, and those associated with congested pulmonary vasculature caused by high pulmonary blood flow (PBF), or by raised pulmonary capillary wedge pressure (PCWP). However, physiologically, the spectrum of neonatal cPH can be understood from the direct relationship between mean PAP (mPAP) and pulmonary vascular resistance (PVR), PBF, and PWCP, defined by the following equation: $mPAP = (PVR \times PBF) + PCWP$.[1] Traditionally, cPH has been thought to originate from a secondary progressive rise in PVR beyond the first month of age (often with initial successful postnatal transition) and is seen most frequently as a secondary complication with CLD. High mPAP from exposure to high PBF, most commonly in the context of atrial-level left to right shunt, or a combination of high PBF and PVR, is not uncommon. Less frequent and currently not fully understood, high PCWP conditions may also contribute to cPH in this patient population. Chronically elevated mPAP increases afterload on the immature right ventricle (RV), which may lead to ventricular remodeling, RV congestion (dilatation), and in severe cases RV systolic dysfunction and poor cardiac output.

A comprehensive clinical and echocardiography assessment focused on evaluating the major determinants of mPAP, possibly combined with echocardiography measures of myocardial performance and cardiac biomarkers, and with judicious use of invasive diagnostic modalities, can help define underlying etiologies. This approach will provide hemodynamic profiles of the disease in patients, allowing clinicians to adopt a physiology-driven individualized management plan.[1,2] This is important as recent pilot data also indicates an association between neonatal cPH and impaired growth and neurodevelopment during early childhood in preterm infants, after accounting for CLD severity.[6] This chapter discusses the risk factors, underlying etiopathologies, and hemodynamic assessment of cPH in neonates and provides a physiology-based approach for the diagnosis of the variability of the presenting phenotypes of neonatal cPH with special considerations based on new recommendations and emerging diagnostic methods.

## Epidemiology and Risk Factors

Although term-born infants can also develop cPH in association with chronic lung disease, congenital heart disease (CHD), and structural and genetic abnormalities of the airways, pulmonary vasculature, or parenchyma,[1] the focus of this chapter is cPH in preterm neonates. That population accounts for the greatest proportion of patients seen in pediatric pulmonary hypertension clinics. Pulmonary hypertension can present in premature infants at different stages of initial hospital stay with varying hemodynamic signatures, including acute and early (e.g., delayed perinatal transition with persistent elevation of PVR), acute and late (associated with acute complications such as sepsis and pulmonary hemorrhage), and chronic and late (i.e., cPH), which is typically sustained well beyond the initial hospital stay.[7] The chronic and late form of pulmonary hypertension commonly lasts into infancy and early childhood and may have pulmonary vascular ramifications across the lifespan. Extremely premature neonates, born <28 weeks' gestational age, are particularly vulnerable to developing cPH and have been the focus of the majority of research to date. In preterm infants cPH is intricately linked, though not always, to the occurrence and severity of CLD.[8-15] While the overall incidence of cPH in this patient population is ~20%, the reported range is 14–44%, depending on the severity of underlying CLD.[4,16-18] Interestingly, even infants with mild or no CLD have some risk for pulmonary vascular disease and overt cPH.[8-12,19] Recent evidence indicates that 2–20% of infants born less than 30 weeks' gestation without

BPD may develop evidence of pulmonary hypertension during the neonatal period.[3] However, clinical observations suggest that this disease, at least in the short term, may not be as aggressive and pathological as overt cPH associated with moderate to severe CLD. Several prospective and retrospective cohort studies have now confirmed that, compared to CLD without cPH, infants with cPH are at much higher risk of in-hospital and post-discharge mortality as well as respiratory morbidities, such as duration off mechanical ventilation and home oxygen therapy.[3,9,11,13,15,20-22] Among preterm neonates with cPH diagnosed at 36 weeks postmenstrual age (PMA), the rate of reported associated mortality ranged from 20 to 50% and was linked closely with the severity of cPH.[18,23] Among infants with evidence of supra-systemic pulmonary pressures at 36 weeks PMA, the mortality rate may be as high as 60–70%, with most occurring within the first 6–8 months after diagnosis.[18,23] Among survivors though, the natural history of cPH appears to follow the pattern of CLD itself, where the disease commonly resolves with growth over 36 to 42 months.[23] However, physiologically, echocardiographic evidence of subclinical relative pulmonary vascular disease persists in neonates with CLD well into late childhood and beyond.[24-26] Further, the burden of cPH may extend beyond the neonatal period and is associated with respiratory diseases during early childhood,[21] poor growth,[27] and sub-optimal neurodevelopment.[3,21]

Maternal and fetal risk factors can affect the development of pulmonary vasculature and how it adapts to extra-uterine life. Physiologically, reduced vascular branching, altered pattern of vascular distribution, disruption of vascular signaling pathways, endothelial injury, and abnormal smooth muscle proliferation are some of the underlying mechanisms of the progressive increase in PVR.[28] Exacerbating factors include air trapping induced abnormal stretch of small pulmonary arteries, atelectasis leading to constraining pulmonary vessels, and acute episodes of hypoxia and hypercarbia, all of which can induce pulmonary artery vasoconstriction and altered vessel morphology in premature neonates.[15] These can lead to injury of the lung parenchyma and affect the molecular pathways responsible for increased pulmonary vasomotor tone, leading to cPH.[29,30] Epidemiologically, the known risk factors contributing to development of cPH in preterm neonates may be seen as demographic variables, which are unlikely to be amenable to interventions, and postnatal acquired variables, which clinicians may have an opportunity to alter (Figure 26.1).[31,32] The degree of prematurity remains the most consequential risk factor for developing cPH in preterm neonates.[33] Other demographic factors include poor intrauterine growth, pulmonary hypoplasia–related conditions such as prolonged oligohydramnios, and factors promoting in utero pulmonary vascular remodeling, such as maternal hypertension and diabetes, antenatal closure of ductus arteriosus, twin-to-twin transfusion syndrome, chylothorax, and hydrops fetalis. Acquired postnatal factors may include known risk factors for severity of CLD, such as hyperoxia, duration of mechanical ventilation, inflammatory conditions like sepsis, necrotizing enterocolitis and ventilation-associated pneumonia, chronic aspiration, chronic exposure to shunts resulting in high pulmonary blood flow (large patent ductus arteriosus, atrial, or ventricular septal defects), and cumulative burden of hypoxemia by virtue of

activation of hypoxic pulmonary vasoconstriction. Further, occurrence of pulmonary edema is *both* a contributory factor to worsening of cPH and a consequence of cPH itself, as fluid leaks into the lung interstitial space due to high intravascular pressure. The subsequent rise in interstitial pressure causes further obliteration of pulmonary microvasculature and redistribution of blood to even smaller vascular compartments, raising intravascular pressure.

In addition, early echocardiographic evidence of pulmonary vascular disease has been identified as a risk factor for subsequent development of cPH by 36 weeks PMA.[8,9,11,21,34] Levy et al.,[9] utilizing deformation imaging, demonstrated that changes in ventricular septal strain patterns in the first postnatal week were associated with a higher risk of cPH (RR 2.15; 95% CI 1.18–4.33). Mourani et al.,[8,21] in a large prospective cohort, observed that ventricular septal wall flattening at 7 days of age was associated with increased risk of the subsequent diagnosis of cPH at 36 weeks PMA (RR 2.85; 95% CI 1.28–6.33). However, the sensitivity and specificity of early

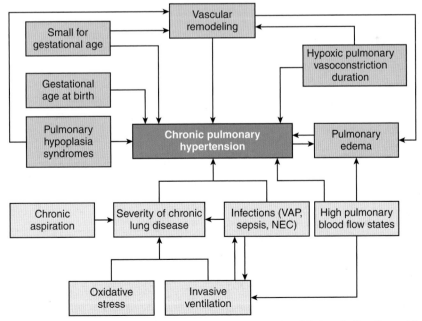

**Fig. 26.1** Risk factors for chronic pulmonary hypertension (*cPH*) in preterm neonates: for clinical application, the contributing factors may be considered as demographics that are not amenable to change (*shown in blue color*) or acquired during initial hospital stay that may be altered by quality improvement initiatives (*shown in orange color*). *NEC*, necrotizing enterocolitis; *VAP*, ventilation-associated pneumonia.

changes was only 62% and 61%, respectively, to identify subsequent cPH cases. In several infants with early echocardiographic signs the pulmonary vascular changes resolved without cPH diagnosis at 36 weeks PMA and in some infants without any early vascular changes, cPH resulted. The optimal timing and diagnostic criteria to identify preterm neonates with significant pulmonary vascular disease, early in the disease course, are still being investigated.[35]

Preterm infants with BPD are at risk for dysregulation of pulmonary vasculature, characterized by vascular growth arrest. This delicate pulmonary vascular system is further impacted by states of hyperoxia, alveolar hypoxia, and hemodynamic perturbations, which all play a role in proliferation of the smooth muscle and integration of myofibroblasts and fibroblasts into the vessel walls. These vascular changes ultimately lead to elevation of the pulmonary vascular resistance with decreased compliance and vascular narrowing, and ultimately cPH, RV strain, and RV failure. In addition, systemic arterial stiffness will lead to increased afterload, LV hypertrophy and dysfunction, and possibly pulmonary edema.

## Neonatal Right Ventricle in cPH: Main Determinant of Symptoms and Outcome

cPH is a disease of altered RV-pulmonary vasculature interactions where the main determinant of the clinical symptoms and prognosis is the progressive response of the RV to pressure loading (Figure 26.2). The challenge for the neonatal RV in cPH is to remain hemodynamically coupled to the pulmonary circulation.[36] Initially, the RV adapts to the increasing vascular load by enhancing contractility to maintain PBF, by virtue of the myocardium's inherent contractile reserve. Ongoing exposure to altered loading conditions then leads to RV remodeling and adaptive responses. An important adaptive mechanism that enhances the contractile capabilities of the RV is muscle hypertrophy with increased wall thickness, referred to as homeotropic adaptation. This is a relatively beneficial adaptation, as it allows the RV to maintain output while keeping its wall stress and oxygen demand low (wall stress is directly related to chamber diameter and inversely to the wall thickness). Sustained and progressive pressure-volume loading of the RV, however, may lead

to maladaptive ventricular remodeling in which the RV dilates, referred to as heterotropic adaptation. While a dilated RV can maintain normal cardiac output by virtue of higher end-diastolic volume despite lower ejection fraction, through the Frank-Starling principle, it comes at the expense of significant rise in wall stress and oxygen consumption. At this stage, the end-diastolic pressures in the RV increase, which can then transmit upstream, raising the central venous pressure, clinically resulting in systemic and pulmonary edema (RV congestion or congestive heart failure). The dilated RV also pushes the interventricular septum leftwards, distorting the normal left ventricular geometry,[37] which reduces the ability of the left ventricular contraction to support RV output by trans-septal pressure conduction (left ventricular contraction can support up to 40% of RV output), placing further contractile load on the failing RV. As the sarcomeres reach the maximal length corresponding to the plateau of the Frank-Starling curve, further dilation only causes rise in wall stress without any corresponding increase in the cardiac output. This may precipitate progression to end-stage overt RV failure, characterized by severely reduced contractility, uncoupling of RV from the high afterload, critically reduced RV output, and clinically, profound oxygenation failure and shock. In clinical practice most patients demonstrate a combination of homeotropic and heterotropic adaptive response, the relative extent of which may vary between individuals, producing patient-to-patient variability in the clinical phenotype despite similar afterload exposure.

Among preterm neonates with cPH, heterotropic adaptation with RV dilatation appears to be the predominant response as the preterm myocardium is often incapable of rapid increase in wall thickness, making them highly vulnerable to the adverse outcome of progressive RV dilatation and failure.[38] Furthermore, since the preterm myocardium is composed of underdeveloped contractile mechanisms with disorganized myofibrils, an immature calcium handling system, and inadequately compliant collagen, it has inherently reduced diastolic properties and compliance, making it highly sensitive to pressure/volume loading conditions.[39] Further, preterm neonates have a relatively low total pulmonary vascular capacity (less total number of alveoli-capillary units), which is further reduced in the presence of parenchymal disease

**Upstream impact of cPH on the right ventricle**

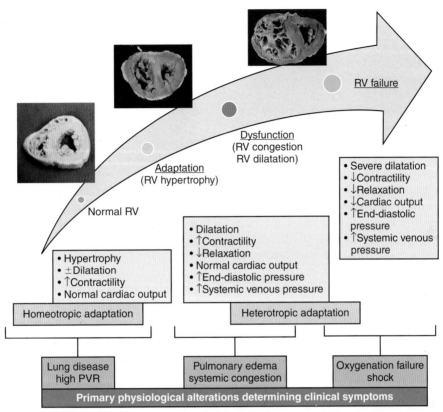

Fig. 26.2 **Pathophysiological impact of sustained progressive rise of pulmonary vascular resistance (*PVR*) on the right ventricle (*RV*).** The RV may remodel by hypertrophy (homeotropic adaptation), which increases the contractility, maintains cardiac output, and also keeps the wall stress (afterload felt by the myocardial walls) low, and/or by dilatation (heterotropic adaptation), which maintains cardiac output by increasing preload (Frank-Starling curve) but at the cost of high wall stress (wall stress is directly related to chamber diameter and inversely to wall thickness). Beyond a certain point, further increase in dilatation does not lead to any increase in cardiac output, leading to overt severe RV failure.

like CLD, making preterm pulmonary vasculature less tolerant to volume overload and susceptible to getting congested and developing cPH, in the setting of relatively smaller left-to-right shunts than term-born neonates might tolerate.

## Clinical Symptoms and Signs

The phenotypic presentation of cPH is governed by slow, sustained exposure to elevated PAP and RV adaptation to it, which is in stark contrast to the typical severe acute hypoxic respiratory failure and hemodynamic lability associated with an acute pulmonary hypertensive crisis, until late stage of RV failure

ensues.[4,36] Preterm neonates with cPH typically present with more subtle respiratory symptoms such as dependence on respiratory support and oxygen therapy rather than overt oxygenation and respiratory failure. Given the major overlap in clinical symptoms and respiratory course, cPH may be difficult to distinguish clinically from the underlying lung disease (CLD) itself, particularly early in the disease course.[4,36] Therefore clinicians are required to be proactive and have a high index of suspicion. Any neonate with chronic parenchymal lung disease where the respiratory course deviates from the expected, such as unexpected and unexplained worsening of oxygenation status late in the hospital course or lack of expected improvement, should be considered for evaluation of cPH. Ongoing pressure-volume overload often leads to RV dilatation and raised central venous pressure, manifesting through a varying combination of signs of pulmonary heart disease i.e., cardiac symptoms and signs occurring secondary to a primary pulmonary pathology. In the context of cPH it indicates occurrence of upstream congestive right heart failure, producing signs such as excessive weight gain, systemic dependent edema, hepatomegaly, pulmonary edema, and/or inability to establish oral feeding due to dyspnea.[36] In the late stages overt RV failure will present as progression to profound and refractory hypoxic respiratory failure and systemic shock from severe low RV output. Another possible manifestation and complication of neonatal cPH is an out-of-proportion hypoxemia and acute pulmonary hypertension precipitated by intercurrent illnesses such as sepsis, viral infections, or even urinary tract infections (acute on chronic pulmonary hypertension). It is thus important for clinicians to counsel parents of neonates with cPH before discharge from the hospital about risk of PH crises due to viral illnesses and the need for early evaluation by the pediatric care provider. It is important to communicate the disease course with primary care providers (especially the increased risk of an acute deterioration after a viral illness) and ensure robust follow-up.

## Diagnostic Assessment for cPH in Preterm Neonates

As described above, optimal diagnosis and monitoring of cPH in preterm neonates requires heightened clinician's awareness of the problem and a high index of suspicion, liberal usage of noninvasive imaging, along with judicious use of invasive and advanced assessments (Table 26.1).[38,40] The gold-standard investigation for confirming diagnosis, pathophysiology, and vasoreactivity of cPH is cardiac catheterization; however, its invasive nature and associated risk for complications makes it an undesirable option for the majority of preterm neonates.[41] Given these pragmatic considerations, echocardiography is the most commonly employed modality and is considered the standard of care to screen, establish diagnosis and disease severity, and provide longitudinal follow-up to monitor disease progression and response to interventions,[4,42,43] as recommended in current practice guidelines[44] and expert opinions.[4,36,45-47]

### ROLE OF COMPREHENSIVE ECHOCARDIOGRAPHY IN CPH ASSESSMENT IN NEONATES

Using a comprehensive approach, bedside echocardiography provides relevant hemodynamic information, which, when integrated with the phenotypic

**TABLE 26.1   Recommended Diagnostic Approach for Chronic Pulmonary Hypertension (cPH) in Neonates**

| Diagnostic Approach | Pulmonary Hypertension Assessment |
|---|---|
| I. Echocardiography | Clinical standard investigation for screening of patients with CLD, Establish initial diagnosis and severity of cPH. Utilize for longitudinal monitoring to detect disease progression and response to interventions. |
| II. Cardiac catheterization | Although gold-standard investigation, clinical utilization highly limited by risk of complications owing to patient size and stability. Currently, its use is reserved for select circumstances, such as (a) severity and underlying pathophysiology of PH not clear on echocardiography, (b) need to identify contributing cardiovascular co-morbidities and role of cardiac shunts, and (c) need to elucidate underlying pathophysiology and confirm vasoreactivity in cases of poor response or worsening with PH-targeted therapy. |
| III. Cardiac magnetic resonance | Provides a noninvasive option to assess right and left heart size and function, along with pulmonary and systemic flow mechanics and shunt fraction (phase contrast MRI), especially useful in patients that are not candidates for cardiac catheterization. Currently, availability is limited to specialized centers and often is cumbersome to organize and can only be used for sporadic assessment, even when available. |
| IV. Computerized tomography | Is particularly used as an aid for the evaluation of chronic lung disease, airway disease, pulmonary artery size, and identification of pulmonary vein stenosis. |

clinical presentation, offers a pathway for which to develop a scientifically-based diagnostic impression, determine a pathophysiologically appropriate management strategy, and evaluate response to therapeutic interventions.[38] Using a systematic approach, echocardiography-derived measurements may be considered under three broad categories (Table 26.2): (1) qualitative, semi-quantitative, and quantitative assessment of pulmonary pressures (RV afterload assessment); (2) evaluation of right and left ventricular size and pump performance; and (3) appraisal of shunts.[2]

### RV Afterload Assessment and Pulmonary Hemodynamics

Although several surrogate quantitative echocardiography methods are available to evaluate and monitor RV afterload, it is usually desirable, whenever feasible, to indirectly calculate pulmonary arterial pressures. This may be achieved by interrogation of regurgitation jets across tricuspid or pulmonary valves or flow across a PDA or VSD, as available. Among these, by far the most commonly employed method in clinical practice is estimation of RV systolic pressure from the tricuspid regurgitation jet velocity (TRJV) using the modified Bernoulli equation (RVSP = 4 × [TRJV]$^2$ + right atrial pressure).[48] In addition, PVR can be assessed with the TRJV interrogation based on its relationship to velocity time integral along the RV outflow tract (TRJV:VTI),[49] as well as dynamic compliance,[50] and pulmonary artery capacitance.[51] While these may add value to our understanding of the disease and degree of pulmonary bed vasoreactivity, their use in preterm neonates with cPH needs validation. A complete tricuspid regurgitation jet, however, is only present in ~30% of cPH cases at 36 weeks PMA, limiting the clinical applicability of this measure. A complete pulmonary valve regurgitation jet is even less often

| TABLE 26.2 Comprehensive Assessment of Neonatal Chronic Pulmonary Hypertension by Echocardiography | |
|---|---|
| **Categories** | **Characteristics** |
| **Severity of PH (RV Afterload)[1]** | |
| Septal wall configuration[2] | Septal wall flattening in end-systole estimates RVSP in response to changes in RV afterload (qualitative estimate of RVSP < or ≥ systolic blood pressure) |
| Eccentricity Index (EI)[3] | Ratio of the LV dimensions parallel and perpendicular to the septum in systole and diastole, a quantitative measure for degree of septal flattening |
| Doppler integration of the tricuspid valve (TRJV) | Quantitative estimate of RVSP by the modified Bernoulli equation |
| Doppler integration of the pulmonary valve (PAAT, PAAT/RVET) | Provides reliable noninvasive semi-quantitative surrogate of mPAP, PVR, and compliance[4] |
| **RV Performance[5]** | |
| Morphology | Four-chamber view of outflow tracts and linear dimensions of cavity, wall thickness, end-systolic and end-diastolic areas |
| Fractional area of change (FAC) | Change in cavity dimensions (estimate of RV ejection fraction) |
| Tricuspid annular plane systolic excursion (TAPSE) | Provides an estimate of longitudinal myocardial shortening and RV systolic performance |
| Tissue Doppler imaging (DI) | Provides quantitative measures of RV systolic (S') and diastolic (E' and A') function |
| Strain and strain rate | Assessment of RV systolic function (strain), diastolic function (diastolic strain rate), and contractility (systolic strain rate) |
| RV velocity time integral (VTI) and RV output | Estimate of RV stroke volume and, in the absence of a PDA, pulmonary blood flow |
| RV-PA coupling (TAPSE/PAAT and strain/PAAT) | Reliable estimate of invasive coupling hemodynamics (not validated in preterm neonates with cPH) |

*Continued on following page*

**TABLE 26.2** **Comprehensive Assessment of Neonatal Chronic Pulmonary Hypertension by Echocardiography (Continued)**

| Categories | Characteristics |
| --- | --- |
| **LV Performance[6]** | |
| Morphology | Four-chamber view of outflow tracts and linear dimensions of cavity, wall thickness, end-systolic, and end-diastolic areas |
| Ejection fraction / shortening fraction | Assess LV systolic function |
| Mitral annular plane systolic excursion (MAPSE) | Provides an estimate of longitudinal myocardial shortening and LV systolic performance |
| Tissue Doppler imaging (DI) | Provides quantitative measures of RV systolic (S′) and diastolic (E′ and A′) function |
| Strain and strain rate | Assessment of LV systolic function (strain), diastolic function (diastolic strain rate), and contractility (systolic strain rate) |
| LV velocity time integral (VTI) and LV output | Estimate of LV stroke volume and, in the absence of PDA, systemic blood flow |
| Pulmonary vein Doppler | Qualitative assessment of net pulmonary blood flow |
| **Appraisal of Shunt** | |
| Patent ductus arteriosus | Quantitative and qualitative estimate of PASP and mPAP using relationship with systemic blood pressure |
| Atrial level shunt (PFO/ASD) | Qualitative estimation of RA to LA pressure relationship (right-to-left shunt indicates supra-systemic PASP) |
| Ventricular septal defect (VSD) | Quantitative and qualitative estimate of RVSP using relationship with systemic systolic blood pressure |

*FAC*, fractional area change; *PAAT*, pulmonary artery acceleration time; *PADP*, pulmonary artery diastolic pressure; *PASP*, pulmonary artery systolic pressure; *RVET*, RV ejection time; *RVSP*, RV systolic pressure; *TRJV*, tricuspid regurgitant jet velocity.
[1]Cardiac catheterization is used for the assessment of severe PH. Specific indications listed in Table 26.2.
[2]The degree of septal wall flattening in end-systole provides an estimate of RV systolic pressure (RVSP).
[3]Diastolic LV EI is a reflective marker of RV volume overload and systolic EI reflects RV pressure overload. A pressure-loaded RV in cPH will deviate the septum in systole and reduce the perpendicular dimension, resulting in an end-systolic LV EI $\geq$ 1.0.
[4]Visual inspection of the Doppler flow envelope across the RV outflow tract has been shown to be a sensitive predictor of altered pulmonary hemodynamics in neonates with PH. The characteristic mid-systolic notch (the "flying W") and its different patterns integrate all the indicators of pulmonary vascular load and RV function and have been used to detect a fall in the RV afterload during the early transitional period in healthy term infants.
[5]RV peformance FAC, TAPSE, tissue Doppler imaging, and deformation have all been validated in term and preterm infants with emerging reference patterns in health and disease states.
[6]LV perfomance systolic disease is pretty rare in this setting – diastolic failure appears to be the primary contributor.

available, but when present, it may be used to measure both mPAP and end-diastolic pulmonary pressure by peak regurgitant velocity and end-diastolic regurgitant velocity, respectively.[52] Using TRJV to estimate RVSP, pulmonary artery diastolic pressure may also be estimated by the following equation: PADP = 0.49 × RVSP.[53] Though, its utility in cPH in preterm neonates is unknown.

Qualitatively, visual inspection of the intraventricular septal wall configuration, particularly degree of flattening in end-systole (parasternal short axis view) obtained at the level of papillary muscles, is used for assessment of presence and, semi-quantitatively, severity of cPH. This measure is the most frequently employed index in neonatal cPH studies to date, as it is easy and available in almost all patients, including sequential assessments. A flat interventricular septum at end-systole ("D-shaped" left ventricle) indicates RVSP to be between 50 and 100% of systolic blood pressure, while the septum being concave toward the left side (paradoxical septum motion) indicates RVSP to be greater than systolic blood pressure.[54] While a perfectly round septum ("O-shaped" left ventricle) most certainly rules out cPH, and inter-rater reliability of this measure is very good at either extreme of disease, it remains a qualitative index with inferior reliability in moderate disease.[55] The eccentricity index (EI) is a measure that quantifies the degree of septal flattening by calculation of the ratio between left ventricular anteroposterior and septolateral linear dimensions; a ratio >1.0 indicates raised RV pressures at the corresponding time in the cardiac cycle.[56] While raised EI at end-diastole suggests RV volume overload (from ASD/PFO shunt), end-systolic EI reflects RV pressure loading.[57] While exact diagnostic thresholds for cPH in neonates have not been well established, pilot studies indicate that an end-systolic EI $\geq 1.3$ may reflect RVSP more than half-systemic and diminished RV systolic performance.[58] However, EI may be a useful marker for longitudinal evaluation of disease severity and response to treatments. Qualitative presence of RV hypertrophy and dilation is also a strong indicator of cPH.[56,59] Finally, it should be noted that in cases of severe hypertension, systolic EI may not be reliable.

Pulse wave Doppler interrogation of the RV outflow tract and flow in the main pulmonary artery also provides supplementary indices, which are easy to obtain in the majority of patients and can be very useful for screening for pulmonary vascular disease and estimation of change over time or response to therapies.[60] The presence of a mid- or late-systolic notch in the Doppler trace of RV outflow tract is indicative of raised PVR, validated against invasive measurement in adult patients.[61] With regards to time periods on the Doppler trace of the main pulmonary artery, the pre-ejection period, referring to the time between the onset of ventricular depolarization and onset of ejection of blood across the pulmonary valve, is directly proportional to PAP.[62] RV ejection time (RVET) is relative to stroke volume and has an inverse relationship to pulmonary artery compliance. Pulmonary artery acceleration time (PAAT), considered to be the most useful time-dependent index in cPH, is the time interval from the onset to the peak velocity of Doppler trace and is inversely related to PVR and systolic PAP.[41] PAAT and its ratio with RVET have been validated against cardiac

catheterization measures of PVR and cPH in children and adults,[41] and changing patterns over time have been established for term and preterm infants.[34,63,64] Although PAAT <70 ms at 36 weeks PMA in preterm neonates is suggested to reflect raised pulmonary arterial pressure,[65] specific validated diagnostic thresholds for cPH, which correspond to risk of adverse outcomes, are not known. We find PAAT and its ratio to RVET to be highly useful in clinical practice and recommend sequential evaluations for preterm neonates being scanned for cPH and related follow-up.

### Assessment of RV Performance

The intricate cardiopulmonary interactions and myocardial remodeling seen in cPH may result in varying degrees of systolic and diastolic RV dysfunction in the context of alterations in afterload. Morphological measures of RV performance provide diagnostic clues as to how the structure of the RV responds to increases in afterload. Assessment of RV performance may be characterized by three separate techniques (Figure 26.3): (i) change in cavity dimensions (e.g., RV fractional area change [FAC]); (ii) displacement and velocity of single point along the myocardial wall (e.g., tricuspid annular plane systolic excursion [TAPSE], tissue Doppler imaging, tissue Doppler velocities); and (iii) deformation of a segment of the wall (e.g., strain analysis).[66] RV FAC reflects a change in cavity size and is a surrogate of RV ejection fraction.[67] Although typically measured from the apical four-chamber view, evidence suggests that capturing the FAC from the apical three-chamber view accurately reflects the longitudinal shortening in systole from the RV infundibulum and is less influenced by interventricular septal motion.[68] Recent studies of BPD-associated cPH reported lower values of FAC at 36 weeks PMA compared to asymptomatic preterm infants.[67,69] Although RV FAC linearly increases with gestational age at birth and weight, normal values are considered to be >35% by 1 month of age.[67,70] TAPSE measures the longitudinal distance (displacement) that the tricuspid valve annulus moves during systole and provides an estimate of longitudinal myocardial shortening and RV systolic performance. Although it is an easily reproducible measure that is not influenced by heart rate,[71] TAPSE only reflects the displacement of the tricuspid annulus at a single point and does not account for the tethering

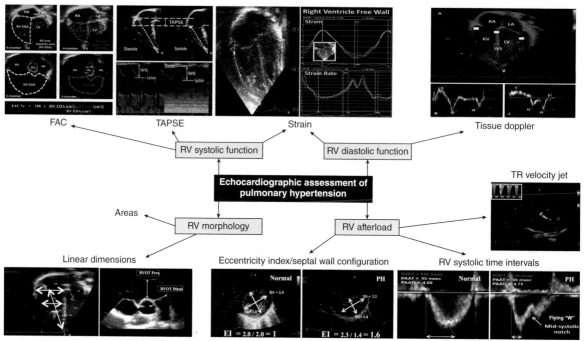

**Fig. 26.3 Echocardiographic assessment of pulmonary hypertension.** A comprehensive assessment is highly recommended and should include qualitative and quantitative measures of pulmonary hemodynamics (RV afterload) as well as its impact on the right ventricle morphology and function. A simultaneous, using similar methods, interrogation of the left ventricle is also carried out.

effect of regional wall motion abnormalities and segmental RV dysfunction.[72] Similar to FAC, TAPSE is a load-dependent measure,[73] with established normative data at birth in preterm infants.[72] Low TAPSE < 4 mm predicts the need for ECMO or death in term infants with acute PH.[74] TAPSE increases linearly from early gestation to term equivalency; therefore these cut-off values cannot be extrapolated to preterm infants with cPH. In a prospective multicenter study TAPSE was decreased in preterm infants with cPH as early as 1 month of age compared to term infants and preterm infants without BPD or evidence of cPH.[26] Emerging evidence suggests that TAPSE is decreased in some preterm infants with cPH at 36 weeks PMA,[19,75] although specific values that predict adverse outcomes are not known.

Tissue Doppler imaging is a quantitative echocardiography modality that measures the velocity of muscle movement at a single point along the myocardial wall; it can be performed in pulsed-wave and color Doppler modes.[76] Although pulse wave tissue Doppler imaging has higher temporal resolution,

color tissue Doppler imaging increases spatial resolution and provides visualization of multiple segments of the RV from one single view.[76] Longitudinal myocardial motion velocity of the RV free wall from base to apex in systole and the reverse in diastole, evaluated at the level of attachment of the anterior leaflet of the tricuspid valve, measures the peak systolic (s′), early diastolic (e′), and late diastolic (a′) velocities.[68] Normative reference values for preterm infants according to gestational age and birth weight are available, and the measure has been validated as an index of RV longitudinal function in older populations.[77-80] There is some evidence that tissue Doppler imaging is associated with early respiratory course in term neonates with PH secondary to congenital diaphragmatic hernia,[81] but data in preterm neonates are lacking.[76,80] Speckle-tracking echocardiography, on the other hand, assesses myocardial deformation, which is defined by the systolic change in the shape of a segment of the myocardium.[76,82] Characterization of RV performance with strain and strain rate analysis may be utilized to assess loading conditions and ventricular contractility in preterm infants[66]; normative values are now available.[9,76] In some neonatal diseases deformation imaging may be more sensitive than conventional measures for identifying ventricular dysfunction.[9,74,76,83,84] The day-to-day clinical utility of these measures in neonatal practice is still a subject of investigation.

### Right Ventricular Pulmonary Arterial Coupling

The RV and pulmonary arterial circulation function as one unit, commonly referred to as the RV-PA axis.[37] In cPH the increased vascular load combined with the inherent susceptibility of the preterm myocardium to afterload may cause the RV to uncouple from its load, predisposing preterm neonates to progress more quickly to decreased RV performance and overt RV failure. Recent evidence suggests that an index of ventriculo-arterial coupling may serve as a measure of RV pump function associated with outcome in PH patients.[85] For instance, the relationship of TAPSE to PAAT is suggested to be a surrogate of RV-PA coupling[86] and associated with PH[87] in older infants but warrants future investigation in premature infants with cPH.

### Left Ventricular Systolic and Diastolic Function and Systemic Hemodynamics

Although cPH is a type of pulmonary heart disease that primarily impacts RV performance, later in the disease course, simultaneous left ventricular assessment to fully characterize the disease phenotype, understand the stage at diagnosis, and monitor progression is highly recommended. Left ventricular diastolic dysfunction (along with pulmonary vein stenosis) can often masquerade as cPH. The assessment of left ventricular systolic and diastolic function follows a similar approach as RV characterization, including assessment of left atrial inflow (pulmonary vein velocities, indicating pulmonary blood flow), left ventricular filling (mitral valve inflow), preload (end-diastolic volumes), morphology (distorted shape by septal bulge), function (systolic and diastolic measures), and flow (stroke volume and left ventricular output). Left ventricular systolic and diastolic function can be characterized by ejection fraction, shortening fraction, mitral annular plane systolic excursion (MAPSE, similar method to TAPSE), tissue Doppler imaging, and deformation.[76,82]

LV systolic disease is rare in cPH and diastolic failure appears to be the primary contributor. As such, LV dysfunction is extremely important in the assessment of cPH and specific techniques are described in Chapter 10.

### Appraisal of Shunts

The complete assessment of intra- (e.g., patent foramen ovale and VSD, when present) and extra-cardiac shunts (e.g., PDA) is critical, as they not only provide easy and reliable measures for estimation of PAP but also may explain the primary pathology causing cPH (excessive PBF resulting in volume overload and raised pulmonary arterial pressure versus high PVR or combination). This is critical to guide management decisions regarding use of pulmonary vasodilator therapies. The presence of an exclusive right-to-left ductal shunt is always abnormal and indicates suprasystemic PASP, while a bidirectional shunt indicates near-systemic PASP.

### Assessment of Pulmonary Veins

Pulmonary vein flow patterns and gradients must be evaluated at each echocardiogram performed for cPH, especially when there is direct or indirect evidence of pulmonary vascular disease.[4] However, pulmonary vein evaluation is not universally included in the evaluation of infants with cPH.[88] There is increasing recognition of the potential contribution of pulmonary venous stenosis in PVD and cPH in preterm neonates with severe CLD, specifically those with a past history of necrotizing enterocolitis.[4,89,90] In this patient population pulmonary vein stenosis is an acquired illness, which develops over time, and is thought to be secondary to exposure to inflammatory mediators.[91] Importantly, although echocardiography may be able to identify pulmonary venous stenosis, cardiac catheterization, CT angiography, or cardiac MRI is required for a detailed characterization of vessel involvement. A recent case series of preterm infants with pulmonary vein stenosis showed that only 56% of patients were diagnosed correctly solely by echocardiography.[92] Another report showed that of 26 preterm infants studied via cardiac catheterization to characterize cPH, pulmonary vein stenosis was identified in 7 (27%), of which only 3 had been suspected by echocardiography.[93] Evaluation for pulmonary vein stenosis must be considered in cases where cPH is worsening despite optimization of cardiopulmonary support and vasodilator therapies.

## ROLE OF INVASIVE AND ADVANCED NONINVASIVE INVESTIGATIONS

### Cardiac Catheterization

Echocardiography may not always be able to accurately identify cPH, estimate disease severity, or differentiate underlying contributing etiopathologies. Cardiac catheterization is the gold standard investigation for pulmonary hypertensive disorders and has the fidelity to not only confirm diagnosis but also provide a thorough hemodynamic understanding; specifically, estimates of right atrial pressure, RV performance, direct measurement of mPAP, flow, and PCWP (allowing for calculation of PVR) may be obtained. Further, it also provides an opportunity to directly test the vasoreactivity of the pulmonary vasculature to guide subsequent clinical management. In this specific patient population, owing to small patient size and inherent clinical instability, the specific goals of cardiac catheterization and the diagnostic, prognostic, and therapeutic benefits must be weighed against the risk of complications (e.g., need for general anesthesia, cardiac arrhythmia, vascular and cardiac injury, thrombosis).[94] In addition, the physiologic data is acquired in a sedated and muscle-relaxed state, which may not be accurately representative of the patients' normal ambient circumstances. Recent expert consensus opinions and guidelines have incorporated the consideration for cardiac catheterization in the framework for management of cPH in preterm neonates, however, with some differences.[4,44,46,95,96] Earlier guidelines suggested deploying cardiac catheterization in the preterm neonate with cPH with the same approach as for older children, specifically after exhausting ventilatory supportive measures and before initiating targeted pulmonary vasodilator therapies.[44] However, this approach was not practical in small, acutely ill infants. Therefore the guidelines have been revised to incorporate a more selective use of cardiac catheterization, restricted to special circumstances, especially when etiology is unclear or there is lack of response to one or two trials of pulmonary vasodilator therapies.[95,96] Cardiac catheterization may also be helpful when echocardiography is

normal but the clinical picture suggests incipient cPH, such as in the setting of recurrent pulmonary edema requiring high diuretic use.

### Cardiac MRI and CT

Additional advanced noninvasive imaging techniques, such as cardiac magnetic resonance imaging (MRI) and computerized tomography (CT), may offer complementary tools to examine cardiac function, morphology, and hemodynamics; in particular, these modalities may be helpful for patients who are not good candidates to undergo catheterization but where echocardiography alone is deemed insufficient.[4,97] Cardiac MRI provides both morphological and functional indices, including right and left ventricular mass, shape, systolic function, and estimates of pulmonary and systemic blood flow and shunt fraction, when applicable. Although it has been shown to predict outcomes for adults with pulmonary hypertension,[98] the reliability and clinical utility in children is still under investigation. Further, for preterm neonates with cPH, its availability is mostly limited to specialized centers, and even it is often too cumbersome to organize for sequential assessments.[99,100] Movement artifacts and duration of examination are additional challenges in this patient population. Nevertheless, it offers a noninvasive tool for intermittent use and against which echocardiography markers may be fine-tuned to enhance their clinical applications. Cardiac magnetic resonance–augmented cardiac catheterization may offer a novel approach in future to validate some of the qualitative estimates (e.g., septal wall configuration) against invasive hemodynamics (e.g., PVR and mPAP).[101]

Cardiac CT has been particularly utilized to diagnose or rule out additional contributing etiologies such as pulmonary vein stenosis.[97] CT angiography can be employed to characterize the presence, size, and significance of bronchial or systemic collateral arteries, as well as that of pulmonary venous anatomy, prompting a call from some authors to use it as the initial investigation of choice prior to cardiac catheterization.[89] While CT may be a useful adjunct for evaluation of the vascular anatomy and the extent of chronic lung diseases and airway disease, until protocols are developed to minimize radiation exposure, its use will remain highly selective in the preterm population.

## ROLE FOR CARDIAC BIOMARKERS

Several recent studies have attempted to identify early biomarkers (e.g., B-type natriuretic peptide [BNP],[102,103] N-terminal pro-B-type natriuretic peptide [NT-pBNP],[104] circulating microRNAs,[105] oxidant stress and nitric oxide precursor metabolites[106]) that may be associated with or predictive of cPH in neonates. However, only BNP and NT-pBNP have been suggested as clinical parameters of interest for measuring at diagnosis and follow-up to aid in cPH management. Neither has been shown to correlate with alteration in pulmonary hemodynamics in neonates with acute pulmonary hypertension,[102] despite their promise in older children with acute pulmonary hypertension.[107] It is worth noting that there appears to be a wide range of normal data and no established cut-off exists to aid diagnosis of significant cPH/congestive heart failure in neonates. Further, these peptides are non-specific for cPH and may also be elevated with right or left heart volume loading, such as with PFO or PDA, confounding their interpretation. Nevertheless, there is a consensus that these biomarkers, when combined with echocardiography on a sequential basis, can help clinicians assess disease progression and response to therapies. Circulating microRNAs represent another class of interesting biomarkers that have been explored in CLD and PH in infants and children,[105,108] but more evidence is needed to understand their specific role for estimation of vascular function in preterm infants with cPH.

## SCREENING GUIDELINES FOR CPH IN PRETERM NEONATES

There are several guidelines and consensus statements published over the last decade by multi-disciplinary panels of experts with the intention to provide a practical framework for diagnosis and management of preterm infants with cPH.[4,44,65,109] A consistent recommendation across panels is to perform echocardiographic screening for cPH in all infants with established CLD, at 36 weeks PMA. However, at the time of CLD diagnosis, there is already a high prevalence of cPH, which limits the scope of subsequent management in ameliorating clinical burden of disease, particularly with regard to respiratory morbidities during the initial hospital stay. The optimal time to screen for cPH and diagnostic criteria and the merits of early-targeted intervention remain key knowledge gaps in neonatology. Some consensus-based guidelines indicate that in the presence of specific risk factors (e.g., birth <28 weeks' gestation, small for gestational age, history of oligohydramnios, and/or prolonged mechanical ventilation), earlier screening for cPH prior to 36 weeks PMA may be beneficial. We recommend that an earlier screening for cPH in neonates with chronic lung disease may be considered if the clinical respiratory course is deemed to be deviating from expected, even if it is before 36 weeks PMA. After initial screening, frequency of follow-up evaluations will largely be individualized, dictated by the degree and severity of the disease phenotype. Among infants with a negative screen, it is suggested to repeat evaluation every 1–2 months if symptoms persist, such as persistent oxygen requirement, impaired growth, or feeding difficulties.

## Management of cPH in Preterm Neonates

Although several observational studies have now established the association of cPH in preterm neonates with adverse outcomes and identified several risk factors, the evidence with regard to treatment remains sparse, with no treatment trials available to guide clinical practice. Therefore, while we wait for more evidence, the current clinical management of cPH in CLD neonates is largely based upon vigilance, individualized care plans, common sense approach based on physiological principles, and expert consensus.[95,96] This management strategy revolves around ensuring prompt diagnosis, defining clinical signs that may be driven by cPH on top of pre-existing CLD, considering possible contributing factors, and deciding which future investigations or therapies are needed. Once the diagnosis of cPH secondary to CLD has been established, the clinical management focuses on the following principles:

(i) *Supportive respiratory care:* Like the management of severe CLD itself, provision of supportive and adequate ventilatory support and considering (and treating) potential contribution of other respiratory co-morbidities are the key first steps in management of cPH occurring secondary to CLD. A significant under-recruitment of the alveoli, by activating hypoxic pulmonary vasoconstriction, an adaptive response in the lungs to maintain ventilation-perfusion matching through vaso-constriction of the adjoining pre-capillary arterioles to reduce the blood passing through the hypoxic alveoli, will not only contribute to an increase in overall PVR but also promote adverse remodeling of pulmonary vasculature.[110] On the other hand, overdistended alveoli will compress the capillaries and increase the total PVR by increasing its alveolar component (total PVR = alveolar PVR + extra-alveolar PVR). An ideal ventilatory strategy will be to maintain lungs at functional residual capacity where PVR related to lung volume is at its lowest.[111] This goal may be tricky to achieve in a heterogenous condition like CLD, where the same ventilation pressure may cause overdistention of some parts but remain inadequate to recruit others. One suggestion will be to use ventilation pressures where no further improvement in oxygenation (or hypoxic episodes) is observed, but a reduction in pressures causes worsening (i.e., minimal effective mean airway pressure). The other important goals of ventilation strategy should be a) to maintain as normal as feasible minute ventilation to avoid hypercarbia and respiratory acidosis, which otherwise may contribute by inducing pulmonary vasoconstriction (avoiding hypocarbia as it results in cerebral vasoconstriction), and b) to minimize the cumulative burden of hypoxemic episodes. If the latter is not achieved by optimizing ventilatory pressures, clinicians may consider providing supplemental oxygen and set targets for peripheral oxygen saturation ($SpO_2$) slightly higher, between 93% and 97%, to avoid both hypoxemia and hyperoxia. Lastly, all cases of cPH should be carefully evaluated and considered for relevant investigations of contributing respiratory co-morbid factors such as reflux, silent aspiration, and airway disease.

(ii) *Supportive cardiopulmonary care:* Unlike acute pulmonary hypertensive disorders where symptoms are secondary to sudden ventilation-perfusion mismatch, symptoms of cPH are insidious and governed by a slow sustained increase in hydrostatic pressure in the pulmonary vascular bed, almost always mediated through interstitial and alveolar pulmonary edema and, subsequently, RV congestive heart failure. Clinically this may be recognized by the presence of significant peripheral edema, lung imaging (x-ray or ultrasound), or RV dilatation on echocardiography. Early recognition and treatment with an optimal dose of diuretics (Chapter 5), reducing fluid intake, and readjusting calorie intake accordingly may not only provide symptomatic improvement but also improve pulmonary pressures by removing the secondary contribution of interstitial edema on rising PVR. Although the ideal diuretic agent and dosing is not established for neonatal cPH, the optimal nature of provided therapy should be adjudicated by demonstration of induced diuresis and weight (excessive volume) loss. A dilated RV is already in preload excess, so extreme caution should be practiced in prescribing extra volume (e.g., boluses).

(iii) *Pharmacotherapy to induce pulmonary vasodilation:* Symptomatic patients who fail to improve or continue to worsen despite taking the measures presented previously should be considered for targeted pulmonary vasodilator therapy. Consideration should be given to the clinical need to rule out the contribution of shunts and collaterals (flow-driven cPH) and post-capillary causes (pulmonary vein stenosis, left ventricular dysfunction) before commencement of vasodilator therapy. If needed, additional specific investigations may be undertaken, as highlighted above. Otherwise, reserving advanced investigations for unresponsive patients is considered an acceptable course of action. There are many pulmonary vasodilator agents available, targeting different cellular pathways to induce pulmonary vasodilation (Table 26.3). See Chapter 5 for detailed pharmacological information. However, for most, there is little data available for neonates with cPH. Among available agents, sildenafil and bosentan have been described the most in published literature and appear to be safe and effective, though evidence is restricted to uncontrolled case reports and case series. In cPH the reduction in pulmonary pressures with these agents is expected to be modest in the

**TABLE 26.3 Options and Mechanism of Action for Potentially Feasible Pharmacotherapies for cPH**

| Drug | Mechanism | Neonatal |
|------|-----------|----------|
| **Nitric Oxide-cGMP Pathway** | | |
| Sildenafil | PDE5 inhibitor | Most widely used first-line agent for CLD-cPH. |
| Tadalafil | PDE5 inhibitor | Alternative to sildenafil with less frequent dosing. No published study data on use in neonatal cPH. |
| Riociguat | Stimulator of soluble guanylate cyclase (sGC) | "Dual" mode of action (sGC activator and stimulator), no published study data on use in neonatal cPH. |
| **Prostacyclin Analogue** | | |
| Iloprost | PCA | No published study data in BPD-PH. |
| Epoprostenol | PCA | No published study data in BPD-PH. |
| Treprostinil | PCA | No published study data in BPD-PH. |
| Selexipag | "PCA" (IP receptor agonist) | No published study data in BPD-PH. |
| **Endothelial Receptor Agonists** | | |
| Bosentan | ERA | $ET_{1A}$- and $ET_{1B}$-receptor antagonist. In published literature, appears to be the second most used agent in clinical practice for preterm neonates with cPH. It may, however, increase liver transaminases and lowers plasma sildenafil levels when used in combination. |
| Macitentan | ERA | $ET_{1A}$- und $ET_{1B}$-receptor antagonist. No reported liver toxicity and does not appear to affect plasma sildenafil level. Only limited reported experience in neonatal cPH. |
| Ambrisentan | ERA | Selective $ET_{1A}$-receptor inhibition. May increase liver transaminases but does not affect plasma sildenafil levels. No published clinical experience in neonatal cPH. |

*cGMP*, Cyclic guanosine monophosphate; *ERA*, endothelin receptor antagonist; *ET*, endothelin; *IP*, prostacyclin receptor; *PAH*, pulmonary arterial hypertension;

short term, and symptoms may take some time to show improvement, unlike use of pulmonary vasodilators in acute pulmonary hypertension. Hence treatment effectiveness should be evaluated over weeks and not days, provided no significant worsening is observed.

(iv) *Involvement of multidisciplinary care teams and follow-up services:* cPH is a complex heart-lung disorder, which requires longitudinal care spanning both in-patient and out-patient services to ensure optimal clinical outcomes. Given the wide array of potential contributing factors and potential need for advanced investigations, a multi-disciplinary team approach is highly recommended. While the exact nature of the team and services involved may vary depending upon local factors, typically,

it is expected to include some combination of neonatologists, pediatric cardiologists, and pulmonologists with special expertise in pulmonary hypertension and CLD, pediatric dieticians, nurse practitioners, occupational therapists, and developmental pediatricians. All patients diagnosed with cPH needing treatment, even if responsive and appearing to resolve during initial hospital stay, must be provided follow-up evaluations after discharge, ideally with pediatric pulmonary hypertension clinics.

## Conclusion

Neonatal cPH is a pathophysiologic disorder characterized by elevated PAP and impaired RV performance with high morbidity and mortality. The diagnosis and management of cPH requires clinical awareness of risk factors; high index of suspicion; and knowledge of specific symptoms, signs, and hemodynamic phenotypes; as well as an understanding of the pros and cons of the different investigational modalities available. Longitudinal assessment can offer valuable physiological insights into disease progression and response to therapies. Finally, interdisciplinary approaches that include teams of neonatologists, cardiologists, and pulmonologists are essential for the comprehensive care and optimizing outcomes of infants with cPH.

## REFERENCES

1. Jain A, McNamara PJ. Persistent pulmonary hypertension of the newborn: advances in diagnosis and treatment. *Semin Fetal Neonatal Med.* 2015;20(4):262-271.
2. Bhattacharya S, Sen S, Levy PT, Rios DR. Comprehensive evaluation of right heart performance and pulmonary hemodynamics in neonatal pulmonary hypertension. *Curr Treat Options Cardiovasc Med.* 2019;21(2):10.
3. Arjaans S, Zwart EAH, Ploegstra MJ, et al. Identification of gaps in the current knowledge on pulmonary hypertension in extremely preterm infants: a systematic review and meta-analysis. *Paediatr Perinat Epidemiol.* 2018;32:258-267.
4. Krishnan U, Feinstein JA, Adatia I, et al. Evaluation and management of pulmonary hypertension in children with bronchopulmonary dysplasia. *J Pediatr.* 2017;188:24-34.
5. Giesinger RE, More K, Odame J, Jain A, Jankov RP, McNamara PJ. Controversies in the identification and management of acute pulmonary hypertension in preterm neonates. *Pediatr Res.* 2017;82:901-914.
6. Choi EK, Shin SH, Kim EK, Kim HS. Developmental outcomes of preterm infants with bronchopulmonary dysplasia-associated pulmonary hypertension at 18–24 months of corrected age. *BMC Pediatrics.* 2019;19(1):26-33.
7. Jain A, McNamara PJ. Persistent pulmonary hypertension of the newborn: advances in diagnosis and treatment. *Semin Fetal Neonatal Med.* 2015;20:262-271.
8. Mourani PM, Sontag MK, Younoszai A, et al. Early pulmonary vascular disease in preterm infants at risk for bronchopulmonary dysplasia. *Am J Respir Crit Care Med.* 2015;191:87-95.
9. Levy PT, El-Khuffash A, Patel M, et al. Maturational patterns of systolic ventricular deformation mechanics by two-dimensional speckle tracking echocardiography in preterm infants over the first year of age. *J Am Soc Echocardiogr.* 2017;30:685-698.
10. Weismann CG, Asnes JD, Bazzy-Asaad A, Tolomeo C, Ehrenkranz RA, Bizzarro MJ. Pulmonary hypertension in preterm infants: results of a prospective screening program. *J Perinatol.* 2017;37:572-577.
11. Bhat R, Salas AA, Foster C, Carlo WA, Ambalavanan N. Prospective analysis of pulmonary hypertension in extremely low birth weight infants. *Pediatrics.* 2012;129(3):e682-e689.
12. Mehler K, Udink Ten Cate FE, Keller T, Bangen U, Kribs A, Oberthuer A. An echocardiographic screening program helps to identify pulmonary hypertension in extremely low birthweight
13. Mirza H, Ziegler J, Ford S, Padbury J, Tucker R, Laptook A. Pulmonary hypertension in preterm infants: prevalence and association with bronchopulmonary dysplasia. *J Pediatr.* 2014;165:909-914.e1.
14. Steinhorn R, Davis JM, Göpel W, et al. Chronic pulmonary insufficiency of prematurity: developing optimal endpoints for drug development. *J Pediatr.* 2017;191:15-21.e11.
15. Mourani PM, Abman SH. Pulmonary hypertension and vascular abnormalities in bronchopulmonary dysplasia. *Clin Perinatol.* 2015;42:839-855.
16. Berenz A, Vergales JE, Swanson JR, Sinkin RA. Evidence of early pulmonary hypertension is associated with increased mortality in very low birth weight infants. *Am J Perinatol.* 2017;34:801-807.
17. Murthy K, Dykes FD, Padula MA, et al. The children's hospitals neonatal database: an overview of patient complexity, outcomes and variation in care. *J Perinatol.* 2014;34(8):582-586.
18. Khemani E, McElhinney DB, Rhein L, et al. Pulmonary artery hypertension in formerly premature infants with bronchopulmonary dysplasia: clinical features and outcomes in the surfactant era. *Pediatrics.* 2007;120:1260-1269.
19. Vayalthrikkovil S, Vorhies E, Stritzke A, et al. Prospective study of pulmonary hypertension in preterm infants with bronchopulmonary dysplasia. *Pediatr Pulmonol.* 2018;14:358.
20. Levy PT, Jain A, Nawaytou H, et al. Risk assessment and monitoring of chronic pulmonary hypertension in premature infants. *J Pediatr.* 2020;217:199-209.
21. Mourani PM. Early pulmonary vascular disease in preterm infants is associated with late respiratory outcomes in childhood. *Am J Respir Crit Care Med.* 2019;199:1020-1027.
22. Northway WJ, Rosan RC, Porter DY. Pulmonary disease following respirator therapy of hyaline-membrane disease. Bronchopulmonary dysplasia. *N Engl J Med.* 1967;276:357-368.
23. Arjaans S, Haarman MG, Roofthooft MTR, et al. Fate of pulmonary hypertension associated with bronchopulmonary dysplasia beyond 36 weeks postmenstrual age. *Arch Dis Child Fetal Neonatal Ed.* 2021;106:45-50.
24. Naumburg E, Söderström L, Huber D, Axelsson I. Risk factors for pulmonary arterial hypertension in children and young adults. *Pediatr Pulmonol.* 2016;52:636-641.
25. Levy PT, Patel MD, Choudhry S, Hamvas A, Singh GK. Evidence of echocardiographic markers of pulmonary vascular disease in asymptomatic preterm infants at one year of age. *J Pediatr.* 2018;197:48-56.
26. Erickson CT, Patel MD, Choudhry S, et al. Persistence of right ventricular dysfunction and altered morphometry in asymptomatic preterm Infants through one year of age: cardiac phenotype of prematurity. *Cardiol Young.* 2019;29:945-953.
27. Nakanishi H, Uchiyama A, Kusuda S. Impact of pulmonary hypertension on neurodevelopmental outcome in preterm infants with bronchopulmonary dysplasia: a cohort study. *J Perinatol.* 2016;36:890-896.
28. De Paepe ME, Mao Q, Powell J, et al. Growth of pulmonary microvasculature in ventilated preterm infants. *Am J Respir Crit Care Med.* 2006;173(2):204-211.
29. Pearson DL, Dawling S, Walsh WF, et al. Neonatal pulmonary hypertension – urea-cycle intermediates, nitric oxide production, and carbamoyl-phosphate synthetase function. *N Engl J Med.* 2001;344(24):1832-1838.
30. Fletcher K, Chapman R, Keene S. An overview of medical ECMO for neonates. *Semin Perinatol.* 2018;42(2):68-79.

31. Aikio O, Metsola J, Vuolteenaho R, Perhomaa M, Hallman M. Transient defect in nitric oxide generation after rupture of fetal membranes and responsiveness to inhaled nitric oxide in very preterm infants with hypoxic respiratory failure. *J Pediatr*. 2012;161:397-403.e1.

32. Bendapudi P, Rao GG, Greenough A. Diagnosis and management of persistent pulmonary hypertension of the newborn. *Paediatr Respir Rev*. 2015;16:157-161.

33. Higgins RD, Jobe AH, Koso-Thomas M, et al. Bronchopulmonary dysplasia: executive summary of a workshop. *J Pediatr*. 2018;197:300-308.

34. Patel M, Breatnach CR, James AT, et al. Echocardiographic assessment of right ventricle afterload in preterm infants: maturational patterns of pulmonary artery acceleration time over the first year of age and implications for pulmonary hypertension. *J Am Soc Echocardiogr*. 2019;32:884-894.

35. Thomas L, Baczynski M, Deshpande P, et al. Multicentre prospective observational study exploring the predictive value of functional echocardiographic indices for early identification of preterm neonates at risk of developing chronic pulmonary hypertension secondary to chronic neonatal lung disease. *BMJ Open*. 2021;11(3):e044924.

36. Neary E, Jain A. Right ventricular congestion in preterm neonates with chronic pulmonary hypertension. *J Perinatol*. 2018;38:1708-1710.

37. Vonk Noordegraaf A, Westerhof BE, Westerhof N. The relationship between the right ventricle and its load in pulmonary hypertension. *J Am Coll Cardiol*. 2017;69:236-243.

38. El-Khuffash A, McNamara PJ. Hemodynamic assessment and monitoring of premature infants. *Clin Perinatol*. 2017;44:377-393.

39. Bussmann N, Breatnach C, Levy PT, McCallion N, Franklin O, El-Khuffash A. Early diastolic dysfunction and respiratory morbidity in premature infants: an observational study. *J Perinatol*. 2018;38:1205-1211.

40. Keller RL. Pulmonary hypertension and pulmonary vasodilators. *Clin Perinatol*. 2016;43:187-202.

41. Levy PT, Patel MD, Groh G, et al. Pulmonary artery acceleration time provides a reliable estimate of invasive pulmonary hemodynamics in children. *J Am Soc Echocardiogr*. 2016;29:1056-1065.

42. EL-Khuffash AF, McNamara PJ. Neonatologist-performed functional echocardiography in the neonatal intensive care unit. *Semin Fetal Neonatal Med*. 2011;16:50-60.

43. Evans N, Gournay V, Cabanas F, et al. Point-of-care ultrasound in the neonatal intensive care unit: international perspectives. *Semin Fetal Neonatal Med*. 2011;16:61-68.

44. Abman SH, Hansmann G, Archer SL, et al. Pediatric pulmonary hypertension: guidelines from the American heart association and American Thoracic Society. *Circulation*. 2015;132(21):2037-2099.

45. Tracy MC, Cornfield DN. The evolution of disease. *Curr Opin Pediatr*. 2017;29:320-325.

46. Hilgendorff A, Apitz C, Bonnet D, Hansmann G. Pulmonary hypertension associated with acute or chronic lung diseases in the preterm and term neonate and infant. The European Paediatric Pulmonary Vascular Disease Network, endorsed by ISHLT and DGPK. *Heart*. 2016;102:ii49-ii56.

47. Katz SL, Luu TM, Nuyt AM, et al. Long-term follow-up of cardiorespiratory outcomes in children born extremely preterm: recommendations from a Canadian consensus workshop. *Paediatr Child Health*. 2017;22:75-79.

48. Yock PG, Popp RL. Noninvasive estimation of right ventricular systolic pressure by Doppler ultrasound in patients with tricuspid regurgitation. *Circulation*. 1984;70:657-662.

49. Abbas AE, Fortuin FD, Schiller NB, Appleton CP, Moreno CA, Lester SJ. A simple method for noninvasive estimation of pulmonary vascular resistance. *J Am Coll Cardiol*. 2003;41:1021-1027.

50. Dyer K, Lanning C, Das B, et al. Noninvasive Doppler tissue measurement of pulmonary artery compliance in children with pulmonary hypertension. *J Am Soc Echocardiogr*. 2006;19:403-412.

51. Friedberg MK, Feinstein JA, Rosenthal DN. Noninvasive assessment of pulmonary arterial capacitance by echocardiography. *J Am Soc Echocardiogr*. 2007;20:186-190.

52. Abbas AE, Fortuin FD, Schiller NB, Appleton CP, Moreno CA, Lester SJ. Echocardiographic determination of mean pulmonary artery pressure. *Am J Cardiol*. 2003;92:1373-1376.

53. Friedberg MK, Feinstein JA, Rosenthal DN. A novel echocardiographic Doppler method for estimation of pulmonary arterial pressures. *J Am Soc Echocardiogr*. 2006;19:559-562.

54. Kim GB. Pulmonary hypertension in infants with bronchopulmonary dysplasia. *Korean J Pediatr*. 2010;53:688.

55. Smith A, Purna JR, Castaldo MP, et al. Accuracy and reliability of qualitative echocardiography assessment of right ventricular size and function in neonates. *Echocardiography*. 2019;36:1346-1352.

56. Ehrmann DE, Mourani PM, Abman SH, et al. Echocardiographic measurements of right ventricular mechanics in infants with bronchopulmonary dysplasia at 36 weeks postmenstrual age. *J Pediatr*. 2018;203:210-217.e1.

57. de Boode WP, Singh Y, Molnar Z, et al. Application of neonatologist performed echocardiography in the assessment and management of persistent pulmonary hypertension of the newborn. *Pediatr Res*. 2018;84(suppl 1):68-77.

58. Abraham S, Weismann CG. Left ventricular end-systolic eccentricity index for assessment of pulmonary hypertension in infants. *Echocardiography*. 2016;33(6):910-915.

59. Berenz A, Vergales JE, Swanson JR, Sinkin RA. Evidence of early pulmonary hypertension is associated with increased mortality in very low birth weight infants. *Am J Perinatol*. 2017;34:801-807.

60. Nagiub M, Lee S, Guglani L. Echocardiographic assessment of pulmonary hypertension in infants with bronchopulmonary dysplasia: systematic review of literature and a proposed algorithm for assessment. *Echocardiography*. 2015;32:819-833.

61. Arkles JS, Opotowsky AR, Ojeda J, et al. Shape of the right ventricular Doppler envelope predicts hemodynamics and right heart function in pulmonary hypertension. *Am J Respir Crit Care Med*. 2011;183(2):268-276.

62. Hsieh KS, Sanders SP, Colan SD, MacPherson D, Holland C. Right ventricular systolic time intervals: comparison of echocardiographic and Doppler-derived values. *Am Heart J*. 1986;112:103-107.

63. Jain A, Mohamed A, Kavanagh B, et al. Cardiopulmonary adaptation during first day of life in human neonates. *J Pediatr*. 2018;200:50-57.

64. Jain A, Mohamed A, El-Khuffash A, et al. A comprehensive echocardiographic protocol for assessing neonatal right ventricular dimensions and function in the transitional period: normative data and z scores. *J Am Soc Echocardiogr*. 2014;27:1293-1304.

65. Hansmann G, Koestenberger M, Alastalo TP, et al. 2019 updated consensus statement on the diagnosis and treatment of pediatric pulmonary hypertension: the European Pediatric Pulmonary Vascular Disease Network (EPPVDN), endorsed by AEPC, ESPR and ISHLT. *J Heart Lung Transplant*. 2019;38(9):879-901.

66. Bussmann N, El-Khuffash A. Future perspectives on the use of deformation analysis to identify the underlying pathophysiological basis for cardiovascular compromise in neonates. *Pediatr Res.* 2019;85:591-595.

67. Levy PT, Dioneda B, Holland MR, et al. Right ventricular function in preterm and term neonates: reference values for right ventricle areas and fractional area of change. *J Am Soc Echocardiogr.* 2015;28:559-569.

68. Jain A, Mohamed A, El-Khuffash A, et al. A comprehensive echocardiographic protocol for assessing neonatal right ventricular dimensions and function in the transitional period: normative data and z scores. *J Am Soc Echocardiogr.* 2014;27(12):1293-1304.

69. Blanca AJ, Duijts L, van Mastrigt E, et al. Right ventricular function in infants with bronchopulmonary dysplasia and pulmonary hypertension: a pilot study. *Pulm Circ.* 2019;9:1-9.

70. James AT, Corcoran JD, Franklin O, EL-Khuffash AF. Clinical utility of right ventricular fractional area change in preterm infants. *Early Hum Dev.* 2016;92:19-23.

71. Arce OX, Knudson OA, Ellison MC, et al. Longitudinal motion of the atrioventricular annuli in children: reference values, growth related changes, and effects of right ventricular volume and pressure overload. *J Am Soc Echocardiogr.* 2002;15(9):906-916.

72. Koestenberger M, Nagel B, Ravekes W, et al. Systolic right ventricular function in preterm and term neonates: reference values of the tricuspid annular plane systolic excursion (TAPSE) in 258 patients and calculation of Z-score values. *Neonatology.* 2011;100(1):85-92.

73. Badano LP, Ginghina C, Easaw J, et al. Right ventricle in pulmonary arterial hypertension: haemodynamics, structural changes, imaging, and proposal of a study protocol aimed to assess remodelling and treatment effects. *Eur J Echocardiogr.* 2010;11(1):27-37.

74. Malowitz JR, Forsha DE, Smith PB, Cotten CM, Barker PC, Tatum GH. Right ventricular echocardiographic indices predict poor outcomes in infants with persistent pulmonary hypertension of the newborn. *Eur Heart J Cardiovasc Imaging.* 2015;16:1224-1231.

75. Seo YH, Choi HJ. Clinical utility of echocardiography for early and late pulmonary hypertension in preterm infants: relation with bronchopulmonary dysplasia. *J Cardiovasc Ultrasound.* 2017;25:124.

76. Breatnach CR, Levy PT, James AT, Franklin O, El-Khuffash A. Novel echocardiography methods in the functional assessment of the newborn heart. *Neonatology.* 2016;110:248-260.

77. Murase M, Morisawa T, Ishida A. Serial assessment of right ventricular function using tissue Doppler imaging in preterm infants within 7 days of life. *Early Hum Dev.* 2015;91:125-130.

78. Koestenberger M, Nagel B, Ravekes W, et al. Right ventricular performance in preterm and term neonates: reference values of the tricuspid annular peak systolic velocity measured by tissue Doppler imaging. *Neonatology.* 2013;103(4):281-286.

79. Breatnach CR, El-Khuffash A, James A, McCallion N, Franklin O. Serial measures of cardiac performance using tissue Doppler imaging velocity in preterm infants ,29weeks gestations. *Early Hum Dev.* 2017;108:33-39.

80. Di Maria MV, Younoszai AK, Sontag MK, et al. Maturational changes in diastolic longitudinal myocardial velocity in preterm infants. *J Am Soc Echocardiogr.* 2015;28:1045-1052.

81. Moenkemeyer F, Patel N. Right ventricular diastolic function measured by tissue Doppler imaging predicts early outcome in congenital diaphragmatic hernia. *Pediatr Crit Care Med.* 2014;15(1):49-55.

82. Breatnach CR, Levy PT, Franklin O, El Khuffash A. Strain rate and its positive force-frequency relationship: further evidence from a premature infant cohort. *J Am Soc Echocardiogr.* 2017;30:1045-1046.

83. Levy PT, Holland MR, Sekarski TJ, Hamvas A, Singh GK. Feasibility and reproducibility of systolic right ventricular strain measurement by speckle-tracking echocardiography in premature infants. *J Am Soc Echocardiogr.* 2013;26(10):1201-1213.

84. Cade WT, Levy PT, Tinius RA, et al. Markers of maternal and infant metabolism are associated with ventricular dysfunction in infants of obese women with type 2 diabetes. *Pediatr Res.* 2017;82:768-775.

85. Jone PN, Schafer M, Pan Z, Bremen C, Ivy DD. 3D echocardiographic evaluation of right ventricular function and strain: a prognostic study in paediatric pulmonary hypertension. *Eur Heart J Cardiovasc Imaging.* 2018;19:1026-1033.

86. Levy PT, El-Khuffash A, Woo KV, Hauck A, Hamvas A, Singh GK. A novel noninvasive index to characterize right ventricle pulmonary arterial vascular coupling in children. *JACC Cardiovasc Imaging.* 2019;12:761-763.

87. Levy PT, El Khuffash A, Woo KV, Singh GK. Right ventricular-pulmonary vascular interactions: an emerging role for pulmonary artery acceleration time by echocardiography in adults and children. *J Am Soc Echocardiogr.* 2018;31(8):962-964.

88. Baczynski M, Bell EF, Finan E, McNamara PJ, Jain A. Survey of practices in relation to chronic pulmonary hypertension in neonates in the Canadian Neonatal Network and the National Institute of Child Health and Human Development Neonatal Research Network. *Pulm Circ.* 2020;10(3):2045894020937126.

89. del Cerro MJ, Sabate Rotes A, Carton A, et al. Pulmonary hypertension in bronchopulmonary dysplasia: Clinical findings, cardiovascular anomalies and outcomes. *Pediatr Pulmonol.* 2013;49:49-59.

90. del Cerro MJ, Moledina S, Haworth SG, et al. Cardiac catheterization in children with pulmonary hypertensive vascular disease: consensus statement from the Pulmonary Vascular Research Institute, Pediatric and Congenital Heart Disease Task Forces. *Pulm Circ.* 2016;6:118-125.

91. Swier NL, Richards B, Cua CL, et al. Pulmonary vein stenosis in neonates with severe bronchopulmonary dysplasia. *Am J Perinatol.* 2016;33:671-677.

92. Mahgoub L, Kaddoura T, Kameny AR, et al. Pulmonary vein stenosis of ex-premature infants with pulmonary hypertension and bronchopulmonary dysplasia, epidemiology, and survival from a multicenter cohort. *Pediatr Pulmonol.* 2017;52:1063-1070.

93. Frank BS, Schäfer M, Grenolds A, Ivy DD, Abman SH, Darst JR. Acute vasoreactivity testing during cardiac catheterization of neonates with bronchopulmonary dysplasia-associated pulmonary hypertension. *J Pediatr.* 2019;208:127-133.

94. O'Byrne ML, Kennedy KF, Kanter JP, Berger JT, Glatz AC. Risk factors for major early adverse events related to cardiac catheterization in children and young adults with pulmonary hypertension: an analysis of data from the IMPACT (Improving Adult and Congenital Treatment) Registry. *J Am Heart Assoc.* 2018;7:1-12.

95. Rosenzweig EB, Abman SH, Adatia I, et al. Paediatric pulmonary arterial hypertension: updates on definition, classification, diagnostics and management. *Eur Respir J.* 2019;53:1-18.

96. Hansmann G, Sallmon H, Roehr CC, et al. Pulmonary hypertension in bronchopulmonary dysplasia. *Pediatr Res.* 2021;89(3):446-455.

97. Latus H, Kuehne T, Beerbaum P, et al. Cardiac MR and CT imaging in children with suspected or confirmed pulmonary hypertension/pulmonary hypertensive vascular disease. Expert consensus statement on the diagnosis and treatment of paediatric pulmonary hypertension. The European Paediatric Pulmonary Vascular Disease Network, endorsed by ISHLT and DGPK. *Heart.* 2016;102(suppl 2):ii30-ii35.

98. van Wolferen SA, Marcus JT, Boonstra A, et al. Prognostic value of right ventricular mass, volume, and function in idiopathic pulmonary arterial hypertension. *Eur Heart J.* 2007; 28:1250-1257.

99. Blalock S, Chan F, Rosenthal D, Ogawa M, Maxey D, Feinstein J. Magnetic resonance imaging of the right ventricle in pediatric pulmonary arterial hypertension. *Pulm Circ.* 2013;3: 350-355.

100. Moledina S, Pandya B, Bartsota M, et al. Prognostic significance of cardiac magnetic resonance imaging in children with pulmonary hypertension. *Circ Cardiovasc Imaging.* 2013; 6:407-414.

101. Pandya B, Quail MA, Steeden JA, et al. Real-time magnetic resonance assessment of septal curvature accurately tracks acute hemodynamic changes in pediatric pulmonary hypertension. *Circ Cardiovasc Imaging.* 2014;7:706-713.

102. König K, Guy KJ, Walsh G, Drew SM, Barfield CP. Association of BNP, NTproBNP, and early postnatal pulmonary hypertension in very preterm infants. *Pediatr Pulmonol.* 2016;51:820-824.

103. Cuna A, Kandasamy J, Sims B. B-type natriuretic peptide and mortality in extremely low birth weight infants with pulmonary hypertension: a retrospective cohort analysis. *BMC Pediatr.* 2014;14:68-73.

104. Dasgupta S, Aly AM, Malloy MH, Okorodudu AO, Jain SK. NTproBNP as a surrogate biomarker for early screening of pulmonary hypertension in preterm infants with bronchopulmonary dysplasia. *J Perinatol.* 2018;38:1252-1257.

105. Lal CV, Olave N, Travers C, et al. Exosomal microRNA predicts and protects against severe bronchopulmonary dysplasia in extremely premature infants. *JCI Insight.* 2018;3:30.

106. Montgomery AM, Bazzy-Asaad A, Asnes JD, Bizzarro MJ, Ehrenkranz RA, Weismann CG. Biochemical screening for pulmonary hypertension in preterm infants with bronchopulmonary dysplasia. *Neonatology.* 2016;109:190-194.

107. Warwick G, Thomas PS, Yates DH. Biomarkers in pulmonary hypertension. *Eur Respir J.* 2008;32:503-512.

108. Kheyfets VO, Sucharov CC, Truong U, et al. Circulating miRNAs in pediatric pulmonary hypertension show promise as biomarkers of vascular function. *Oxid Med Cell Longev.* 2017;2017:1-11.

109. Abman SH, Collaco JM, Shepherd EG, et al. Interdisciplinary care of children with severe bronchopulmonary dysplasia. *J Pediatr.* 2017;181:12-28.e11.

110. Dunham-Snary KJ, Wu D, Sykes EA, et al. Hypoxic pulmonary vasoconstriction: from molecular mechanisms to medicine. *Chest.* 2017;151(1):181-192.

111. Simmons DH, Linde LM, Miller JH, O'Reilly RJ. Relation between lung volume and pulmonary vascular resistance. *Circ Res.* 1961;9(2):465-471.

# Chapter 27

# Pathophysiologically Based Management of Pulmonary Hypertension of the Newborn

Stephanie M. Boyd, Trassanee Chatmethakul, and Patrick J. McNamara

## Key Points

- Acute pulmonary hypertension (aPH), classically referred to as persistent pulmonary hypertension of the newborn (PPHN) when occurring during the perinatal transition period, is characterized by failure of the normal postnatal decline in pulmonary vascular resistance (PVR). Elevated pulmonary arterial pressure (PAP) may also occur via alternative mechanisms, including left ventricular diastolic heart failure and excessive pulmonary blood flow.

- Hypoxemia, with or without accompanying systemic hypoperfusion, is the clinical manifestation of several different underlying pathophysiological phenotypes of PH. Right ventricular (RV) myocardial hypoxia and ischemia play an important role in the pathophysiology of circulatory impairment.

- Treatment strategies for PH should consider the underlying hemodynamic disturbance(s) and be targeted toward individual pathophysiology. Targeted neonatal echocardiography (TnECHO) is an important assessment tool that enables adjudication of the underlying physiology, targeting of treatment, documentation of response to treatment, and identification of when to wean therapy.

- The approach to management should include optimization of respiratory support, care of the underlying condition, and specific hemodynamic therapy with cardiotropic agents and/or pulmonary vasodilators in accordance with the underlying phenotypic presentation of PH.

## Introduction

Neonatal pulmonary hypertension is a heterogenous condition affecting both term and preterm neonates with a range of underlying disease processes, the hallmark of which is elevated pulmonary arterial pressure (PAP). Mean PAP (mPAP) is dependent upon pulmonary vascular resistance (PVR), cardiac output (CO) (and shunts), and left atrial pressure. Calculation of mPAP is possible, using pulmonary capillary wedge pressure (PCWP) as a proxy for left atrial pressure:

$$mPAP = [PVR \times CO] + PCWP$$

The primary pathophysiologic event in aPH occurring during the perinatal transition period, classically referred to as persistent pulmonary hypertension of the newborn (PPHN), is interruption to or failure of the normal postnatal decline in pulmonary vascular resistance (PVR). This may be due to maladaptation (e.g., perinatal asphyxia, meconium aspiration syndrome), maldevelopment of the pulmonary vasculature (e.g., in utero closure of the ductus arteriosus), or pulmonary underdevelopment or hypoplasia in the setting of e.g., congenital diaphragmatic hernia or oligohydramnios. Whatever the underlying etiology, there is associated dysregulation of the pulmonary vascular bed and changes in cardiac loading conditions, with significant hemodynamic consequences. Although PPHN is a commonly used descriptor, aPH may be a more appropriate term for the constellation of features that include hypoxemia and right ventricular dysfunction, due to the protracted time taken for physiological decline in PVR after birth in healthy newborn infants. Persistent elevations in PAP after birth are essentially ubiquitous, and for healthy infants, not pathological. In the setting of aPH, the resultant low oxygen saturation is poorly tolerated after birth and affected neonates may develop multi-organ dysfunction/failure because of hypoxemia and inadequate tissue perfusion. The hemodynamic consequences of aPH (Chapter 25) may include right ventricular dysfunction, dilation and hypertrophy due to increased

afterload, and impairments in pulmonary blood flow. Adverse systemic effects include hypoxemia, abnormal left ventricular (LV) mechanics, and low cardiac output. Although generally considered to be a primary disorder of elevated PVR, it is evident from the "mPAP equation" that elevations in cardiac output and/or left atrial pressure may also result in raised pulmonary pressure, with implications for management. Accurate delineation of the pathology requires comprehensive hemodynamic assessment and a detailed understanding of the interplay of the neonatal cardiovascular system with the various underlying disease processes (Table 27.1).

**TABLE 27.1 Biological Phenotypes Contributing to Elevated Pulmonary Arterial Pressure, Associated Echocardiography Findings, and Suggested Treatment Approaches**

| PH Phenotype | Pathophysiology | Echocardiography Features | Suggested Treatment Approach |
|---|---|---|---|
| **Acute PH** | | | |
| Arterial (classic) | Hypoxic pulmonary vasoconstriction, V/Q mismatch | Dilated and hypertrophied RV, septal flattening in systole, predominantly R→L PDA and atrial shunts, ↑PAAT:RVET, PA Doppler notching, ↓LVO | Optimize lung recruitment and supportive care, offload RV with pulmonary vasodilators, support systemic arterial pressure with vasoconstrictors which do not ↑PVR |
| Flow-mediated | High volume of blood in a circuit with limited capacitance, endothelial dysfunction, oxidative stress | Dilated RV and/or LV, discordant ventricular outputs with either ↑RVO, ↑LVO, or both, septal flattening in diastole if ASD/VSD | Shunt management; maintain ↑PVR, avoid selective pulmonary vasodilators |
| Left heart dysfunction | Poor LV compliance and high LVEDP, resulting in impaired flow through pulmonary circuit | Dilated LV, LV systolic and diastolic dysfunction [↓MVE, ↑IVRT↓PV velocities], MR and/or AI, ↓LVO | LV afterload reduction, inotropy, maintain R→L ductal shunt if ↓SBF, maintain ↑PVR, diuretics for pulmonary edema |
| **Chronic PH** | | | |
| Arterial (classic), e.g., associated with BPD | Pulmonary vascular remodeling, impaired angiogenesis, alveolar hypoxia/hyperoxia | Dilated, hypertrophied RV, septal flattening in systole, predominantly R→L PDA and atrial shunts, ↑PAAT:RVET, PA Doppler notching, ↓ LVO | Optimize lung recruitment and supportive care, offload RV with pulmonary vasodilators, consider diuretics if RV dilation |
| Flow-mediated | High volume of blood in a circuit with limited capacitance, interstitial edema, pulmonary vascular remodeling | Dilated RV or LV, discordant ventricular outputs with either ↑RVO, ↑LVO, or both, septal flattening in diastole if ASD/VSD | Shunt management; maintain ↑PVR, avoid selective pulmonary vasodilators |
| Systemic hypertension | High LV afterload causing ↑LVEDP, LA hypertension, pulmonary venous congestion | Dilated LV, LV diastolic dysfunction (↓MVE, ↑IVRT, ↓PV velocities), MR and/or AI | Antihypertensive therapy; role for ACE inhibitors/ARBs; avoid pulmonary vasodilators |

*ACE*, angiotensin-converting enzyme; *AI*, aortic insufficiency; *ARB*, angiotensin II receptor blocker; *ASD*, atrial septal defect; *BPD*, bronchopulmonary dysplasia; *IVRT*, isovolumetric relaxation time; *L*, left; *LA*, left atrium; *LV*, left ventricle; *LVEDP*, left ventricular end-diastolic pressure; *LVO*, left ventricular output; *MR*, mitral regurgitation; *MVE*, mitral valve early wave; *PA*, pulmonary artery; *PAAT*, pulmonary artery acceleration time; *PDA*, patent ductus arteriosus; *PV*, pulmonary vein; *PVR*, pulmonary vascular resistance; *R*, right; *RV*, right ventricle; *RVET*, right ventricular ejection time; *RVO*, right ventricular output; *SBF*, systemic blood flow; *V/Q*, ventilation/perfusion; *VSD*, ventricular septal defect.
Adapted from Giesinger R, Kinsella JP, Abman SH, McNamara PJ. Pulmonary hypertension phenotypes in the newborn. In: Dakshinamurti S, ed. *Hypoxic respiratory failure in the newborn: from origins to clinical management.* Boca Raton: Taylor & Francis Group; 2021.

## Clinical Presentation

The clinical manifestations of aPH depend on the degree of elevation of PAP; the presence, direction, and magnitude of shunting through the patent ductus arteriosus (PDA) and/or patent foramen ovale (PFO); right and left ventricular performance and ability to adapt to changes in cardiac loading conditions; and the presence of associated morbidities. The severity of aPH can run the full clinical spectrum, from mild hypoxemia with varying degrees of respiratory distress to severe hypoxemia and cardiopulmonary instability necessitating advanced intensive care support. Hypoxemia in the newborn may result from lung parenchymal and/or cardiovascular pathology, and differentiating the contributors to poor oxygenation clinically can be challenging. Multiple lung and vascular pathologies may also coexist in the same patient. For example, in the setting of aPH secondary to meconium aspiration, atelectasis, intrapulmonary shunting, alveolar edema, and hyperinflation may all be present together with pulmonary vascular remodeling, hypoxic vasoconstriction, and myocardial dysfunction due to perinatal hypoxia-ischemia. Hypoxemia out of proportion to the degree of underlying lung disease and lability in oxygenation are both characteristic of aPH, and presence of either of these clinical features should raise suspicion of a cardiopulmonary vascular component to the infant's presentation. Approaches to treatment vary according to the severity of the pathophysiology, the underlying cause(s), and the hemodynamic phenotype. Consequently, an in-depth understanding of the pathophysiology (Figure 27.1) is essential to allow individualization of therapy and appropriate targeting of treatment modalities.

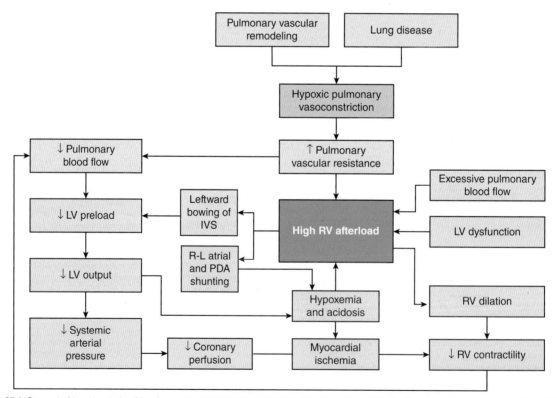

**Fig. 27.1 Suggested treatment algorithm for acute pulmonary hypertension.** *D/C*, discontinue; *FiO₂*, fraction of inspired oxygen; *iNO*, inhaled nitric oxide; *LV*, left ventricle; *PGE*, prostaglandin E₁; *PVR*, pulmonary vascular resistance; *RV*, right ventricle; *TH*, therapeutic hypothermia; *TnECHO*, targeted neonatal echocardiography.

## Pathophysiology

### ACUTE PULMONARY HYPERTENSION OF ARTERIAL (CLASSIC) ORIGIN

Due to the complexity of interactions between PVR, lung aeration, and myocardial adaptation, perinatal transition is a time of heightened vulnerability for the newborn cardiovascular system. Perturbations in this physiological framework due to any combination of perinatal hypoxia-ischemia, infection, and/or pulmonary parenchymal disease may interfere with the normal physiological decline in PVR and result in development of aPH. As a result of the elevated PVR in arterial (classic) aPH, hypoxic vasoconstriction ensues, which is an adaptive response to optimize ventilation-perfusion (V/Q) matching.[1] Poor lung recruitment and overdistension from positive pressure ventilation can worsen hypoxic vasoconstriction, due to both increases in PVR and impaired carbon dioxide clearance, resulting in acidosis. It is important to realize that PVR is lowest at optimal lung recruitment, that is, at or near FRC.[2] With excessive lung volume, some pulmonary capillaries undergo narrowing and stretching, whereas reduced lung volume can lead to capillary tortuosity or kinking, both of which increase PVR.[2] Careful titration of positive pressure ventilation based on clinical, blood gas, and radiological assessment is therefore necessary. Particular care should be taken to avoid lung overinflation in the setting of hypoxic-ischemic encephalopathy, where lung compliance and FRC may be normal and hypoxemia instead a manifestation of altered pulmonary vascular reactivity. Overly aggressive attempts at lung recruitment in this context may be complicated by further impairments in PBF,[3] as well as systemic compromise from reductions in LV stroke volume and LV end-diastolic volume (LVEDV).[4] Over-distension also has the potential to compromise pulmonary venous flow, which may be difficult to distinguish clinically from progression of aPH driven by high PVR.[5] Additional non-pulmonary factors related to either the underlying disease process, such as sepsis, perinatal asphyxia, and hypovolemia, or iatrogenesis, such as treatment with vasopressors that can cause pulmonary vasoconstriction (e.g., high-dose dopamine), may further drive increases in PVR. Elevated PVR leads to increased RV afterload[6] and bidirectional or right-to-left shunting through the PFO and PDA. Right-to-left atrial

shunting contributes to a reduction in RV preload.[7] Right-to-left ductal shunting, though contributing to hypoxemia and reduced PBF, may provide a pop-off mechanism for the RV exposed to high afterload and an additional source of post-ductal perfusion where there is significant LV impairment.

Elevated pulmonary pressure results in a reduction in the pressure gradient between the RV cavity and the pulmonary vascular bed. The initial increase in RV afterload results in compensatory RV hypertrophy and increased contractility (referred to as "coupling" or homeometric adaptation).[8] Increased contractility is mediated by changes in the sarcomere length-tension relationship and cardiomyocyte force-frequency relationship and increased calcium sensitivity.[9] The force-frequency relationship describes the adaptive response of the neonatal myocardium to tachycardia, leading to improved force generation with increasing heart rate.[10] To maintain cardiac output in the face of increased afterload, the RV dilates and heart rate increases. These changes preserve stroke volume initially by way of the increase in stroke volume associated with increased preload – via the Frank-Starling mechanism, with a larger ventricle emptying proportionally less blood – and an intact force-frequency response. This process is referred to as heterotopic adaptation.[11] Unable to generate sufficient pressure for complete ejection of blood with each cardiac beat, RV emptying becomes progressively inadequate, leading to an increase in RV end-systolic pressure and, because less blood is ejected during systole, an increase in RV end-diastolic pressure.[11] In addition, the force-frequency response is blunted as cardiac dysfunction develops. Progressive dilatation increases wall stress and myocardial oxygen consumption and eventually leads to a reduction in stroke volume.[8] RV dilatation also changes the configuration of the cardiac chamber into one that is more spherical, which is associated with functional regurgitation across the tricuspid valve and increased right atrial pressure.[12] Where elevation of PVR is excessive and sustained, ischemia, hypoxemia, and myocardial stretching lead to progressive RV dysfunction and uncoupling.[8,13] This is associated with leftward bowing of the interventricular septum (IVS), which is caused by prolonged contraction of the RV free wall when compared with the septum or LV free wall, impairing diastolic LV filling.[14] Together with RV dilation, this leads to further impairment of RV function and decreased PBF.[15] Through ventricular interdependence, the leftward shift in septal configuration also reduces LVEDV, LV stroke volume,[9] and RV systolic contractile force,[16,17] resulting in systemic hypoperfusion, acidosis, and further reductions in PBF. In some infants a cycle of reduced PBF, worsening acidosis, hypoxemia, ventilation-perfusion mismatch, and cardiac dysfunction may develop, with a clinical phenotype of hypoxemic respiratory failure and cardiocirculatory impairment.

## ACUTE PULMONARY HYPERTENSION RELATED TO EXCESSIVE PULMONARY BLOOD FLOW

Increased pulmonary blood flow, such as that observed in left-to-right shunt lesions, may result in elevations in pulmonary arterial pressure. The most obvious mechanism for this is an increase in pressure driven by increased flow through a circuit with a finite capacity to expand to accommodate the additional circulating volume. Muscular hypertrophy of the pulmonary vasculature, with secondary elevation in PVR, also occurs in response to a sustained increase in PBF.[18,19] An additional contributor is a disturbance of endothelial function resulting in altered pulmonary vasoreactivity; specifically, selective impairment of endothelium-dependent pulmonary vasodilation. Based on animal models, this may be attributable to both high basal activity of nitric oxide (NO) that is not readily increased[20] and dysregulation of endothelial NO synthase,[21] induced by increased pulmonary blood flow and pulmonary hypertension. This attenuates the fetal endothelial release of NO in response to sheer stress[22] such as that generated by excessive pulmonary blood flow and may contribute to elevated mPAP in this setting.

Newborns with large preductal systemic to venous connections resulting in high-volume shunts are particularly at risk of complications from right heart pressure and volume loading. For example, the vein of Galen aneurysmal malformation (VGAM) is a rare cerebral arteriovenous malformation (AVM) with major hemodynamic implications. In utero, the low resistance of a cerebral AVM is balanced by the low-resistance placental circuit. With removal of the placenta and transition to the high afterload systemic neonatal circulation, up to 70% of the cardiac output is directed toward the cerebral vasculature.[23] Superior

vena caval flow may be up to 10 times normal, reflecting high flow through the AVM.[24] This may result in a profound reduction in lower body perfusion, with lactic acidosis and post-ductal arterial hypotension. The ventricles receive increased preload, which in the case of the RV must be ejected against increased afterload, predisposing to RV dysfunction and failure. Supra-systemic pulmonary hypertension occurs,[24] which is associated with right to left shunting at atrial and ductal levels.[23,24] This perpetuates hypoxemia, which further compromises ventricular performance. Chronic volume and pressure loading leads to RV dilation, which increases susceptibility to afterload-mediated dysfunction[25] as adaptive mechanisms fail.[17] RV coronary perfusion normally occurs throughout systole and diastole and is characterized by a lower flow and oxygen extraction when compared with the LV.[17] The maladaptive, dilated, and hypertrophied RV has a higher oxygen requirement and inefficient oxygen utilization,[17] with coronary perfusion limited to diastole by the increased RV pressure.[26] Elevations in RV end-diastolic pressure, leading to increased right atrial and central venous pressure, and therefore reduced diastolic coronary flow to the RV constitute a potential additional source of impaired perfusion in the setting of PH.[11] Intracranial vascular "steal" through the AVM, which is associated with retrograde diastolic descending aortic flow, may further compromise tenuous coronary perfusion via low coronary root pressure, creating a "pseudocoarctation" physiology.[27] This effect is additive with the increased ventricular pressure in reducing subendocardial perfusion, contributing to myocardial ischemia and RV dysfunction.[23] Non-judicious use of pulmonary vasodilators may exacerbate these effects, particularly in the setting of an open ductus. Despite the increase in PVR, the shunt in VGAM is obligatory, such that pulmonary vasoconstriction does not offset the high-output cardiac failure, as might occur in congenital cardiac disease. This is postulated as a contributor to the severity of cardiac failure in infants with VGAM.[28]

## ACUTE PULMONARY HYPERTENSION SECONDARY TO LEFT VENTRICULAR DYSFUNCTION

Poor function of the left ventricle results in inefficient ejection of end-diastolic volume, which results in a progressive increase in left ventricular end-diastolic pressure (LVEDP). This leads to pulmonary venous congestion, increased pulmonary capillary pressure, and a hydrostatic gradient across the interstitium, resulting in fluid transudation to alveolar spaces, i.e., pulmonary edema. Similar to left-to-right shunt lesions, endothelial dysfunction is also implicated as contributory to elevated pulmonary pressure in obstructive pulmonary venous hypertension.[29] Left and right ventricular dysfunction may coexist in transitional aPH, although there are subgroups in whom LV disease may occur independently. Fetal and neonatal echocardiographic studies of infants with congenital diaphragmatic hernia (CDH) support disturbances of fetal LV development and postnatal LV dysfunction as part of the pathogenesis of hypoxemia in affected infants.[30-33] Early LV systolic function correlates with markers of clinical disease severity in CDH and may be a primary determinant of illness severity rather than a secondary consequence of cardiovascular instability.[30] These findings have implications for treatment, and use of pulmonary vasodilators, since increasing pulmonary blood flow and LV preload may risk exacerbating existing LV diastolic dysfunction and pulmonary venous hypertension.[34,35] Flash pulmonary edema has been observed with pulmonary vasodilator therapy in pulmonary venous disease.[36] Conversely, improvements in RV performance by afterload reduction may indirectly augment LV performance through ventricular interdependence.[30] A multicenter randomized trial of sildenafil and inhaled NO in CDH (CoDiNOS trial) utilizing cardiac function assessment may provide additional guidance on use of pulmonary vasodilators in this setting.[37] In general, pulmonary vasodilators should be used with caution in infants with LV dysfunction and are likely to be harmful where LV impairment is severe.

## Chronic Pulmonary Hypertension (cPH)

The pathophysiology of cPH (Chapter 26) is influenced by the development of the pulmonary vasculature and the status of the lung parenchyma.[15] Maldeveloped pulmonary vasculature with abnormal lung parenchyma and elevated PVR is typical of BPD and pulmonary hypoplasia. Maldeveloped pulmonary vasculature is less commonly encountered and is observed in, for example, alveolar capillary dysplasia

(ACD) and primary surfactant deficiencies. ACD with misaligned pulmonary veins may, however, account for a greater proportion of unexplained PH in infants than previously thought.[38] Chronic PH secondary to pulmonary venous congestion may be due to either increased PBF (e.g., left-to-right shunts), or increased pulmonary capillary wedge pressure).[15] Elevated PCWP, or left atrial pressure, in the newborn most commonly occurs due to LV dysfunction or acquired pulmonary vein stenosis, although left-sided cardiac lesions may also produce this cPH phenotype.

## CHRONIC PULMONARY HYPERTENSION SECONDARY TO BPD

Chronic PH associated with BPD (BPD-cPH) is characterized by abnormal remodeling and growth arrest of the pulmonary vasculature,[39,40] and impaired angiogenesis and alveolarization,[39,41] resulting in abnormal pulmonary vascular function with increased PVR, high RV afterload, and RV dysfunction. Abnormal pulmonary vascular remodeling is triggered by postnatal hypoxia/hyperoxia.[39] Additive insults, such as endothelial dysfunction, and inflammatory stimuli, such as infection and ventilator-induced lung injury, are thought to perpetuate alveolar hypoxia[39,40,42] in at-risk infants. Antenatal factors, including inflammation, intrauterine growth restriction, and the lung microbiome,[43] are also implicated in the pathogenesis. There is evidence that echocardiographic evidence of PH within the first 7–14 days after birth may predict subsequent moderate-severe BPD or death at 36 weeks postmenstrual age,[44,45] underscoring the importance of abnormal pulmonary vascular development in the development of BPD. Conversely, a very low risk of late PH has been observed in the absence of PH at 7 days of age.[45] The approach to management includes lung optimization alongside treatment with pulmonary vasodilators (e.g., sildenafil). Both clinical improvement and reductions in pulmonary artery pressure have been documented with sildenafil therapy.[46] In the presence of RV dilatation, diuretics may also be considered for optimizing RV configuration.[5] Although long-term benefits of diuretics have not been demonstrated in infants with BPD, improvements in both oxygenation and pulmonary mechanics have been observed.[47] In addition, a retrospective study demonstrated high rates of symptomatic improvement in BPD-cPH, with diuretic treatment where RV dilatation was used as the treatment threshold.[48]

## CHRONIC PULMONARY HYPERTENSION SECONDARY TO EXCESSIVE PULMONARY BLOOD FLOW

Sustained left to right shunt and resultant pulmonary over-circulation may occur in particular at atrial level (e.g., PFO or atrial septal defect [ASD]) or at ductal level,[5] where a PDA persists over an extended period of time. Chronic over-circulation results in pulmonary vascular remodeling, which is also a potential driver of eventual PDA closure.[49] Elevations in pulmonary arterial pressure are initially due to increased PBF and, with chronicity, result in changes to pulmonary vascular architecture and reactivity.[50,51] Both shear stress injury and endothelial dysfunction are implicated in the pathogenesis,[52] as in acute flow-driven PH. In high-volume shunts leading to unrestrictive pulmonary artery flow, increases in PVR may eventually be sufficient to lead to PDA shunt reversal in some patients.[50,51] Infants with coexistent ASD and PDA, or other multi-level shunts, are at greatest risk of abnormal pulmonary physiology due to dual sources of over-circulation.[5] This is highlighted by the 2.44-fold increase in PH among preterm infants with an ASD in an echocardiographic study of 334 infants born at <32 weeks' gestation.[53] Pulmonary vasodilator use in this setting may be harmful both due to the drop in PVR resulting in an increased SVR:PVR ratio and the risk of contributing to oxidative stress.[5] Adequate shunt management in the mainstay of therapy. In the case of PDA this may include pharmacological or interventional (surgical or transcatheter) closure. Although diuretics are often used for symptomatic management, historical studies of furosemide have noted prostaglandin-mediated dilatation of ductus arteriosus vessels in an animal model[54] and an increased incidence of PDA.[55] While judicious fluid management is sensible, aggressive fluid restriction has been associated with a greater risk of acute kidney injury[56] as well as concerns regarding nutritional intake. In addition, reducing overall circulating fluid volume without any effect on the proportion of cardiac output directed toward the lungs poses a risk of exacerbating existing post-ductal hypoperfusion from PDA run-off.[57] Conversely, diuretics are a key aspect of management for patients with ASD, with device closure performed successfully in infants as small as 2–2.5 kg.[58]

## CHRONIC PULMONARY HYPERTENSION SECONDARY TO LV DYSFUNCTION

While cPH and right ventricular function are the usual focus of cardiovascular sequelae of BPD, there is increasing interest in the contribution of LV disease to BPD-related symptomatology.[59-62] Clinical identification of preterm born infants with respiratory morbidity and comorbid LV pathology is challenging, since features of post-capillary pulmonary venous hypertension closely mimic those of BPD with primary parenchymal pathology. Persistence of pulmonary edema despite diuresis and worsening of pulmonary edema in response to pulmonary vasodilator therapy are "red flags" for underlying LV disease.[61]

In association with LV mal-compliance, high rates of systemic hypertension have been observed among infants with BPD.[63-65] The increased afterload imposed by aortic stiffness associated with systemic hypertension (loss of Windkessel effect) is postulated to produce sufficient back pressure over time to result in disturbances of left heart function and pulmonary venous hypertension.[61] Additionally, polymorphisms in angiotensin-converting (AT-converting) enzyme genes have been identified in infants with CDH and features of PH[66] and alterations in the AT-II receptor pathway have been shown to reduce hyperoxia-mediated heart and lung injury in a neonatal rat model.[67] The role of AT-II in modulating blood pressure via both increasing SVR and stimulating release of norepinephrine and vasopressin highlights the potential for a neurohormonal contribution to neonatal hypertension and BPD.[5] Furthermore, the effectiveness of an endothelin receptor antagonist in reducing PH and RV hypertrophy in a neonatal rat model provides additional translational data as to the importance of the endothelium in the pathogenesis of PH in newborns.[68] There is preliminary evidence that improvement of cardiorespiratory indices, and diastolic function in particular, may be achieved by treatment with ACE inhibitors.[69] RV output has been shown to be increased, accompanied by a significant lowering of PVR with ACE inhibition in a small case series of infants with severe BPD unresponsive to conventional therapies.[69] Additionally, improvement in LV diastolic function indices with ACE inhibitor treatment has been observed in neonates with systemic hypertension and LV diastolic dysfunction.[70] Anti-hypertensive therapy with ACE inhibitors is suggested as a treatment option for LV disease in this patient group, with appropriate monitoring of renal function and caution with co-administration of diuretics.[5] Due to the risk of precipitation of pulmonary edema and worsening of pulmonary venous hypertension, pulmonary vasodilator therapy is best avoided in preterm born infants with chronic PH of this nature, although in some patients true pulmonary arterial and venous hypertension may coexist, requiring combination therapy.

## Delineation of PH Phenotype

Assessment of underlying pathophysiology in PH may be challenging clinically as labile hypoxemia and co-morbid pulmonary disease are common to several hemodynamic phenotypes. The final common pathway is high RV afterload leading to RV dysfunction, with or without systemic effects from disturbances in LV morphology and function. Delineating flow-driven PH from that caused by primary elevations in PVR or mal-compliance of the LV is important for instituting disease-specific management. For example, pulmonary vasodilator therapy may be harmful in the context of pulmonary venous hypertension from LV disease. Targeted neonatal echocardiography (TnECHO) may aid in adjudication of the underlying cause(s) of PH, as well as titrating treatment against clinical response.[71,72]

## Echocardiography-Based Assessment in aPH

The approach to a newborn with suspected PH includes confirmation of the elevation in mPAP; assessment of PVR and right ventricular performance; exclusion of major structural congenital cardiac disease that can mimic primary PH; and evaluation of LV function, systemic blood flow, and the magnitude and directionality of intracardiac shunts. Qualitative measures of RV size and function, even by trained evaluators, are unreliable,[73] and biventricular cardiac dysfunction is common.[74] Comprehensive appraisal of both RV and LV performance is recommended.

A number of congenital cardiac defects, including total anomalous pulmonary venous drainage (TAPVD) and transposition of the great arteries (TGA), may present with severe hypoxemia and mimic aPH. Presence of labile hypoxemia and/or systemic hypotension makes aPH more likely[75]; however, this is not absolute and distinguishing between aPH and congenital cardiac lesions on clinical grounds can be challenging. Initiation of prostaglandin E$_1$ while awaiting definitive anatomical assessment may be appropriate depending on the clinical presentation. Specialist advice should be sought early, and cardiac structural evaluation should occur as part of the first echocardiogram, or at the earliest opportunity.[76] This is important so as not to delay specialist cardiology input and care in a cardiac surgical center, as well as because some treatments for aPH, such as pulmonary vasodilator therapy, can worsen hemodynamics in subgroups of infants with congenital cardiac disease.

Typical findings in resistance-mediated aPH include RV systolic and diastolic failure due to increased afterload, decreased RV stroke volume and filling, decreased PBF with V/Q mismatch, RV dilatation resulting in a D-shaped left ventricle with a decrease in LV preload and stroke volume, and right-to-left ductal shunting through the PDA and/or PFO.[76] TnECHO, also referred to as clinician-performed ultrasound, is a useful adjunct to clinical assessment. It may be utilized to confirm the diagnosis of aPH and disease severity, delineate the underlying pathophysiology to guide treatment selection and therapeutic target(s), monitor response to therapy, and wean supportive treatment as the infant's condition improves. Echocardiographic measurements commonly employed in assessment of aPH are outlined in Table 27.2.

### EVALUATION OF PULMONARY ARTERY PRESSURE AND PULMONARY VASCULAR RESISTANCE

Pulmonary artery pressure may be estimated by several different methods. These are discussed in detail in Chapters 9 and 10 and include tricuspid valve regurgitation (TR) peak velocity, PDA right-to-left flow peak velocity, interventricular septum (IVS) configuration, and LV systolic eccentricity index (LV-sEI).[76] For estimation of PAP using the TR jet, the angle of insonation should

**TABLE 27.2   Echocardiographic Assessment of Acute Pulmonary Hypertension**

| Hemodynamic Parameter | Clinical Application | Advantages | Limitations |
|---|---|---|---|
| **Assessment of Pulmonary Arterial Pressure** | | | |
| RVSP using TR jet (mmHg) | Direct measure of RV systolic pressure | Moderate correlation with invasive measures of RVSP[77] | • Angle dependent and requires complete envelope<br>• TR jet may not be present despite significant PH |
| Septal curvature – subjective assessment<br>Eccentricity index | Assessment of RV versus LV pressure<br>Assessment of RV versus LV pressure | Easily measured and universally present<br>Reproducible, validated in newborns | • Subjective measure<br>• Low interobserver reliability<br>• Pressure relative to LVSP; may underestimate RVSP in systemic hypertension |
| PAAT<br>PAAT:RVET (ms)<br>Mid-systolic notching of PA Doppler waveform | Serial assessment to monitor PVR over time or with treatment | Easily measured | • PAAT affected by HR<br>• Underestimated by RV dysfunction<br>• Unreliable in presence of shunts<br>• Limited evidence in neonates<br>• Single time-point measures |
| **Assessment of Right Heart Function** | | | |
| RVO (mL/kg/min) | Marker of pulmonary blood flow and RV function | • Well studied in neonates across a range of physiological and disease states<br>• Serial evaluations useful for following disease progression and treatment response | • Accuracy dependent on Doppler angle and precise measurement<br>• May be overestimated where RVOT dilated<br>• Affected by atrial shunt |
| TAPSE (mm) | Measure of RV function | • Normative data exist for newborns[78]<br>• Provides information about longitudinal RV contractility; good correlation with estimations of RV global function<br>• Independent of HR and shunts<br>• Easily measured | • Angle and load dependent<br>• Exaggerated by severe TR<br>• May overestimate global function if regional wall dysfunction (rare in the neonatal population) |
| RV FAC | Measure of global RV function | Normative data exist for newborns[79] | • Requires high-quality imaging<br>• Affected by septal motion in apical four-chamber view |
| TDI of IVS and RV free wall | Assessment of systolic and diastolic function | May be useful for monitoring response to treatment | • Requires high-quality imaging<br>• Dependent on angle of insonation |
| **Assessment of Systemic Blood Flow** | | | |
| LVO (mL/kg/min) | Marker of systemic blood flow and LV function | • Well-studied in neonates across a range of physiological and disease states<br>• Serial evaluations useful for following disease progression and treatment response | • Accuracy dependent on Doppler angle and precise measurement<br>• Affected by PDA shunt |

### TABLE 27.2  Echocardiographic Assessment of Acute Pulmonary Hypertension (Continued)

| Hemodynamic Parameter | Clinical Application | Advantages | Limitations |
|---|---|---|---|
| **Assessment of Shunts** | | | |
| PDA: ratio of pulmonary artery to aortic pressure (PAP:AOP) based on shunt direction: Uses Doppler of ductus arteriosus | Direct comparison of pulmonary to systemic arterial pressure | Useful for qualifying RVSP as subsystemic, systemic, or supra-systemic | • PDA may not be present<br>• May be unreliable depending on PDA morphology (e.g., tortuous, restrictive, or S-shaped)<br>• Dynamic – varies with ambient conditions (e.g., pH, $SpO_2$) |
| Atrial communication: shunt direction | • Predominantly R-L shunt suggestive of ↑RVSP; pure R-L shunt requires exclusion of TAPVD<br>• L-R shunt in setting of other features of ↑PAP requires assessment for ↑LA pressure, pulmonary venous hypertension, and LV dysfunction | • Important in understanding drivers of flow-mediated PH (PDA, ASD)<br>• May provide clues as to etiology of ↑PAP | • Atrial communication not always present |

*AOP*, aortic pressure; *ASD*, atrial septal defect; *HR*, heart rate; *L*, left; *LA*, left atrial; *LV*, left ventricle; *LVSP*, left ventricular systolic pressure; *PA*, pulmonary artery; *PAAT*, pulmonary artery acceleration time; *PAP*, pulmonary artery pressure; *PDA*, patent ductus arteriosus; *PH*, pulmonary hypertension; *PVR*, pulmonary vascular resistance; *R*, right; *RV*, right ventricle; *RVET*, right ventricular ejection time; *RVO*, right ventricular output; *RVOT*, right ventricular outflow tract; *RVSP*, right ventricular systolic pressure; *TAPSE*, tricuspid annular plane systolic excursion; *TAPVD*, total anomalous pulmonary venous drainage; *TR*, tricuspid regurgitant/regurgitation.

Adapted from Jain A, Giesinger RE, Dakshinamurti S, et al. Care of the critically ill neonate with hypoxemic respiratory failure and acute pulmonary hypertension: framework for practice based on consensus opinion of neonatal hemodynamics working group. *J Perinatol.* 2022;42:3–13.

be less than 20° to avoid underestimation of systolic pulmonary artery pressure. The modified Bernoulli equation is used and right atrial pressure, though not measured, is assumed to be 3–5 mmHg.[76] Assessment of the TR jet in multiple views is advantageous in this regard. The measurement is generally reliable if accurate measurement is taken using a full Doppler spectral envelope, with moderate correlation observed with catheter laboratory measures of PAP.[77] Tricuspid regurgitation is present in approximately 70% of infants with aPH.[80] Absence of a measurable TR velocity does not imply absence of PH,[81] and evaluation of PAP using this method is not reliable in the presence of right ventricular outflow tract obstruction or RV failure.[76] Pulmonary regurgitation peak velocity can also be used to estimate PAP using the modified Bernoulli equation, with RV diastolic pressure assumed to be 2–5 mmHg. Although

PAP may be estimated using transductal right-to-left flow peak velocity if right-to-left shunting occurs for ≥30% of the cardiac cycle, this is often not reliable,[76] and assessment of direction of the ductal shunt is probably more useful.

Configuration of the IVS, either qualitatively or using the LV-sEI, can also be used to estimate PAP. Normal ventricular geometry consists of an O-shaped LV, with an RV systolic pressure (RVSP) of <50% of LV pressure (LVP). With increased pulmonary pressure, flattening of the IVS occurs, resulting in a loss of circularity and D-shaped LV (estimated RVSP of 50–100% of LVP). With further increases in RV afterload, the RV eventually curves into the LV, producing a crescent-shaped LV and an estimated RVSP that is systemic or supra-systemic (≥100% of LVP).[76,82] Changes in IVS configuration relative to the cardiac cycle can provide some insight as to the likely under-lying pathophysiology. In resistance-driven aPH due to elevated PVR, bowing of the IVS occurs due to prolonged contraction of the RV free wall (against the increased afterload) when compared with the septum or LV free wall.[14] This results in predominant flatten-ing or bowing of the IVS during systole and impair-ment of LV diastolic filling.[14] Conversely, in the set-ting of flow-driven PH secondary to a left-to-right shunt lesion, the RV pressure relative to the LV is higher in diastole, due to increased filling from left-to-right shunt. The LV-sEI provides an objective estimate of IVS flattening/bowing[76] and uses the end-systolic ratio of the anterior-inferior and septal-posterolateral LV cavity dimensions, respectively. Interobserver agreement is higher for LV-sEI than for subjective assessment of septal configuration[83] and values of ≥1.3 show strong correlation with catheterization laboratory measurements with good sensitivity and specificity.[84] The normal value is 1, and more than half-systemic RV pressure has been demonstrated at values of ≥1.3 in an echocardiographic study of 216 newborns at risk of PH.[83]

Right ventricular systolic time intervals have been validated for estimation of PVR,[85] including in newborns.[86] A pulmonary artery acceleration time (PAAT), also referred to as time to peak velocity (TPV), of <90 ms identifies PH with a sensitivity of 97% and specificity of 95%.[85] A PAAT to RV ejection time (RVET) ratio of <0.31 also reliably detects PH, with a value of <0.23 suggestive of marked elevation of PAP.[85] Additional measures of PVR, such as the tricuspid regurgitation velocity to RV outflow time-velocity integral (TRV/VTI[RVOT]) and pulmonary ar-tery compliance, may also be used; however, these are outside the scope of this chapter. Impaired myo-cardial performance results in dilatation of right heart structures, and this is visible qualitatively during echocardiographic assessment. Although accuracy is marginally greater in the hands of expert assessors, reliability of qualitative RV evaluation in newborns has not been established[73] and should not be used in isolation.

## ASSESSMENT OF RIGHT VENTRICULAR FUNCTION

Appraisal of RV function is a crucial aspect of hemo-dynamic assessment in aPH. Reductions in several RV function measures have been associated with

poor outcome in infants with aPH, including tricus-pid annular plane systolic excursion (TAPSE) and RV global longitudinal peak strain.[87] A TAPSE of <4 mm has been shown to be predictive of ECMO or death,[87] and in a retrospective study TAPSE and LV systolic velocity were lower in patients who subsequently died or required ECMO.[74] Neonatal normative values have been published for TAPSE,[78] although limitations include angle and load depen-dency.[76] In infants with comorbid HIE undergoing therapeutic hypothermia, lower RV and LV systolic and RV diastolic performance have been demon-strated,[74] and cerebral function and oxygenation are correlated with RV function.[88] Importantly, impaired RV performance in this population has been associ-ated with adverse outcomes,[89] including an indepen-dent association between TAPSE <6 mm and a composite outcome of death, diagnosis of cerebral palsy, or low developmental assessment scores.[90] In addition, early echocardiography evidence of aPH and RV dysfunction have been associated with death and adverse outcomes, including requirement for ECMO, in infants with CDH.[91] RV fractional area change (FAC) is a quantitative measure for which normative values in term and preterm newborns (25–45%) have been published.[92] Values of 19% have been associated with death or a requirement for ECMO.[87] Detailed RV function assessment is reviewed in Chapters 10 and 11.

Newer measures, such as RV longitudinal strain using speckle tracking echocardiography (STE), show greater correlation with cardiac magnetic resonance (MR) RV ejection fraction and may be more sensitive in detection of myocardial dysfunction at earlier stages of disease[93] – these techniques are discussed in detail in Chapter 11. A reduction in both RV and LV global longitudinal strain have been observed in neonatal aPH[74] and RV function in response to iNO treatment has been monitored longi-tudinally using STE.[94] In term infants with PPHN who were iNO non-responders, RV strain and strain rates improved over a 24-period following administration of milrinone,[95] highlighting their utility in identifying and monitoring cardiac dysfunction in aPH. Diastolic func-tion may be studied using tissue Doppler by measuring the tricuspid inflow velocities (Early [E], Late [A] and ratio [E:A]) during diastole, performed from the apical four-chamber view using PW Doppler. Peak systolic (s′), early diastolic (e′), and late diastolic (a′) myocardial velocities can be measured using TDI, as well as the systolic to diastolic (S/D) ratio and isovolumic relaxation time (IVRT). Both systolic and diastolic velocities using TDI have been shown to be reduced in aPH, including the subgroup of infants with CDH.[96]

## ASSESSMENT OF LEFT VENTRICULAR FUNCTION

Left ventricular dysfunction in aPH may be the primary pathology in the setting of post-capillary aPH. More commonly, LV dysfunction is secondary to a combination of RV impairment, due to ventricular interdependence and/or altered ventricular-ventricular interactions, reduced PBF with decreased LV preload, and myocardial ischemia with low coronary perfusion pressure. Decreased LV performance may contribute to the pathophysiology and clinical features of aPH. Decreased LV size and output have been shown to correlate with a requirement for advanced therapies in aPH, such as ECMO and prolonged mechanical ventilation.[97] A low LV output (LVO) and diminished LV stroke volume with a normal or mildly reduced LV-EF due to right-to-left shunting (reduced preload) and changes in septal configuration are common findings in term and late preterm infants with resistance-driven aPH.[76] The role of the LV in the pathophysiology of cardiorespiratory compromise in CDH is increasingly recognized,[98,99] and early LV dysfunction and severe aPH are independent predictors of adverse outcome in "low risk" infants with the condition.[100] LV dysfunction in CDH may result in post-capillary aPH secondary to pulmonary venous hypertension coexisting with classical, resistance-driven aPH. Afterload reduction with selective pulmonary vasodilators (e.g., iNO) in this context may worsen LV diastolic dysfunction and perpetuate hypoxemia. Determining the relative contribution of LV disease to symptomatology is important for guiding therapy, with inotropic (and lusitropic) support likely to be advantageous where LV impairment is significant, particularly where there is existing diastolic dysfunction. Prolongation of IVRT, reduction in the ratio of passive to active transmitral flow (E:A ratio; due to reliance of the stiff LV on the atrial "kick" for filling), and elevation in LV e:e′ and LV dilatation are suggestive of LV diastolic impairment.

Echocardiography assessment of LV function is reviewed in detail in Chapters 9–11. LV output (LVO ) measurement is suggested as a surrogate marker of systemic perfusion and LV function in

aPH.[1] The myocardial performance index (MPI) is generally used to estimate global LV function, although RV function in neonates may also be assessed using MPI[72,76] and neonatal normative values have been published.[79] Ventricular dysfunction leads to elevated MPI though increased isovolumic contraction and relaxation times, though, like many echocardiography measures, the MPI is load dependent. Both RV and LV MPI have been shown to be elevated in infants with aPH.[101] Additional measures, such as ejection fraction and TDI of the IVS and LV free wall or STE, are also recommended for comprehensive appraisal of LV function.[76]

## ASSESSMENT OF EXTRAPULMONARY SHUNTS

Assessment of extrapulmonary shunts is important for understanding PH hemodynamics and clinical decision-making. Right-to-left shunting at ductal and atrial level have been associated with adverse outcomes in heterogeneous groups of neonates with PH.[87,102] It is important to recognize that the magnitude of the pulmonary-systemic shunt is a marker of disease severity rather than the cause of adverse outcomes and, in many patients, plays a beneficial role. For example, right-to-left ductal shunting both augments systemic perfusion and provides a pop-off mechanism for the RV exposed to high afterload. Although right-to-left atrial shunting is a hallmark of aPH due to high PVR, exclusive right-to-left shunting should prompt cardiac anatomical assessment to exclude total anomalous pulmonary venous drainage, in which there is an obligate right-to-left atrial shunt. Left-to-right flow via the atrial communication in the setting of markers of raised mPAP should raise concern regarding LV function and the presence of pulmonary venous hypertension and elevated left atrial pressure. It is in this subset of patients that pulmonary vasodilation is likely to be deleterious. Infants with congenital diaphragmatic hernia, where LV maldevelopment and dysfunction occur in conjunction with abnormalities of the pulmonary vascular bed, may present with this phenotype. With respect to ductal shunt, right-to-left flow for ≥30% of the cardiac cycle is consistent with raised mPAP, and right-to-left flow for >60% of systole has been associated with suprasystemic level PAP in term neonates with aPH.[103] The neonatal RV myocardium is highly sensitive to increases in afterload, more so even than the LV.[25] Right-to-left ductal shunting may offload the failing RV and support systemic perfusion, but at the expense of post-ductal oxygenation.[15] Nonetheless, maintaining patency of the ductus with a low-dose prostaglandin infusion represents a therapeutic option in infants with severe aPH, impaired RV performance, and a restrictive PDA with the classic arterial aPH phenotype or in association with congenital diaphragmatic hernia. This effect may be magnified in patients with a large preductal systemic to venous connections, where post-ductal perfusion may be severely compromised; therefore maintaining patency of the ductus may be necessary to avert critical post-ductal hypoperfusion.

## Treatment Principles

Therapeutic approaches to aPH should be based upon a clear understanding of the physiologic concepts underpinning neonatal cardiovascular care and a detailed assessment of individual hemodynamics. Treatment goals include reduction of PVR, augmentation of RV performance as required, restoration of adequate systemic blood flow, ensuring adequate RV perfusion pressure, supportive care of the underlying condition, and correction of associated metabolic and hematologic derangements. A suggested algorithm for cardiovascular management in aPH is outlined in Figure 27.2.

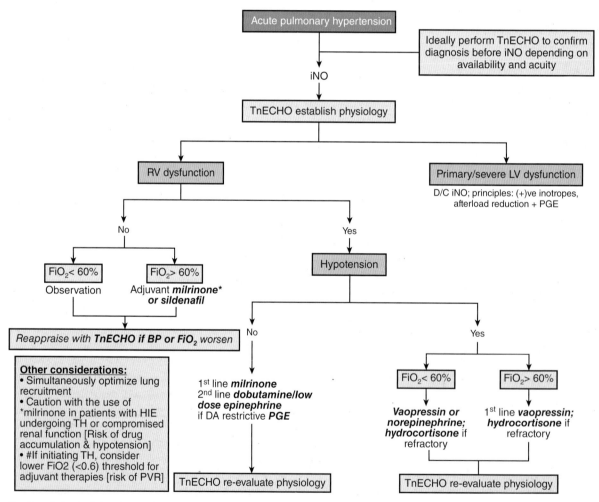

**Fig. 27.2 Pathophysiological contributors to acute pulmonary hypertension.**[11] *IVS*, interventricular septum; *L*, left; *LV*, left ventricle; *PDA*, patent ductus arteriosus; *R*, right; *RV*, right ventricle.

Optimizing lung recruitment guided by the pathophysiology of aPH and clinical, biochemical, and radiological response to treatment is important in terms of both supportive care for the underlying disease process, and for providing an optimal milieu for lowering PVR. *Oxygen* is a potent and selective pulmonary vasodilator; thus increased oxygen tension results in a reduction of PVR. Ideal oxygen saturation and/or arterial $PO_2$ targets in PH are not completely clear, however, and there is wide practice variation.[104] Pulmonary vasoconstriction occurs in response to both alveolar hypoxia and hypoxemia,[105] though hyperoxia is also harmful[106] and may blunt the vasodilatory response to iNO.[107] A steep inverse relationship has been demonstrated between PAP and $PaO_2$ in animal models between 20 and 40 mmHg.[108] A plateau observed at 50 mmHg suggests that additional benefit in reduction of PVR is unlikely to be achieved with further increases in $PaO_2$, and hyperoxia brings with it risks of free radical accumulation[106] and an adverse effect on PVR.[109] In general, oxygen saturations of 91–95% and $PaO_2$ values between 50 and 80 mmHg are recommended.[110] The optimal post-ductal $PaO_2$, which is influenced by right-to-left ductal shunt, is unclear, however, and caution should be applied in placing strong emphasis on $PaO_2$ values obtained from an umbilical arterial catheter in this setting.

*Carbon dioxide*-related changes to pulmonary vascular tone differ between the normal and injured lung, and they also vary depending on pulmonary pressures and the presence of endogenous NO. Of importance, the effect of hypoxia on the pulmonary vasculature is more pronounced than any effect of pH and/or $CO_2$.[111] It is also important to consider the acid-base status in the context of $O_2$ administration and its effect on pulmonary vessels. Animal studies have shown that hypercapnia and lower pH exaggerate hypoxic pulmonary vasoconstriction,[112] which is an adaptive response to promote V/Q matching. Therefore avoiding acidosis offers some protection against pulmonary vasoconstriction in response to hypoxia.[113] Normal values of $pCO_2$ (35–45 mmHg) are generally desirable, with a pH of 7.3–7.45. Oxygenation and ventilation targets may differ for congenital diaphragmatic hernia due to the importance of minimizing injury to vulnerable, hypoplastic lungs and evidence of benefit for "gentle" respiratory support strategies; this is discussed in detail in Chapter 29. *Sedation*, usually with opioids and

benzodiazepines, is widely used in aPH to minimize fluctuation in oxygenation and to facilitate ventilation; however, use is not without side-effects. In addition to the potential for the development of systemic hypotension, generalized edema, reduced cerebral blood flow, and deterioration of lung function with the prolonged use of sedation, the usefulness of sedative agents in the setting of aPH has not been subjected to well-designed studies. Judicious but adequate analgesia and sedation is recommended, though muscle relaxation is best avoided where possible due to an association with increased mortality.[114]

*Targeted PH therapy* should be considered after supportive treatment for underlying cardiorespiratory disturbances has been optimized. Before consideration of *pulmonary vasodilator therapy*, care should be taken to exclude primary or severe LV dysfunction and pulmonary venous hypertension, for which treatment principles include positive inotropy and LV afterload reduction. Where needed, *prostaglandin* may also be used in this setting to augment systemic blood flow by maintaining a right-left PDA shunt. Treatment for high PVR, in addition to provision of adequate supplemental oxygen, is often with iNO in the first instance. *Inhaled NO* is preferentially distributed to the ventilated segments of the lungs, underscoring the importance of optimal lung recruitment prior to the initiation of specific pulmonary vasodilator therapy. Administration of iNO results in an improved ventilation/perfusion ratio, decreased intra-alveolar shunting, and improved oxygenation. Infants who have evidence of raised PVR with decreased pulmonary blood flow and an open PDA with predominantly right-to-left shunting are most likely to have a dramatic response to iNO. If a patient responds, oxygenation generally improves within 30–60 minutes after commencing therapy. Depending on the underlying physiology, non-specific pulmonary vasodilators may be useful adjuvant therapy for aPH; for example, milrinone, prostaglandin, or sildenafil (see Chapter 5 for detailed pharmacology). It is important to be cognizant, however, of the fact that use of non-specific pulmonary vasodilators will be accompanied by systemic vasodilation and thereby a reduction in SVR. As such, in the setting of comorbid systemic arterial hypotension, restoration of sufficient systemic arterial pressure to maintain RV perfusion pressure is advisable prior to commencement. *Milrinone,* a phosphodiesterase-3 inhibitor that is both an inodilator and lusitrope, has been associated with improvements in both oxygenation[115] and cardiac function[116] in newborns with PH. Synergistic activity when combined with iNO has also been demonstrated in adult animal models.[117] Importantly, the drug is not associated with the tachycardia and increased myocardial oxygen consumption observed with sympathomimetic inotropes such as dobutamine. Caution is advised in the use of milrinone in infants with hypoxic-ischemic encephalopathy (HIE) undergoing therapeutic hypothermia, however, in whom delayed renal clearance poses a risk of toxic drug accumulation and a more marked systemic hypotensive response.[118]

With preserved LV function and a coupled RV, pulmonary vasodilatation using iNO may produce a sufficient reduction in PVR and thereby PAP[119] to improve RV performance and result in recovery of PBF.[11,120] *Adequate circulating volume* should be ensured, and volume expansion may be advantageous where RV function is impaired, and the pressure passive pulmonary circulation is therefore aided by higher central venous pressure.[11] In the absence of hypovolemia or specific disease states where maintaining adequate preload for cardiac output is of particular concern (e.g., hypertrophic obstructive cardiomyopathy), multiple fluid boluses beyond 10–20 mL/kg (of 0.9% saline or Ringer's lactate) are infrequently required. In the absence of RV dysfunction either milrinone or sildenafil represent good treatment options for reduction in PVR. *Sildenafil*, a phosphodiesterase-5 inhibitor, has shown efficacy for aPH treatment in low-resource settings,[121,122] where the cost of iNO can be prohibitive. A multicenter randomized controlled trial conducted in the United States, UK, and Europe, however, did not demonstrate benefit of sildenafil above iNO in infants with PPHN or hypoxic respiratory failure at risk of PPHN.[123] Animal studies suggest that sildenafil may be effective in infants with aPH and prolonged exposure to hyperoxic ventilation.[107,124]

Where there is evidence of cardiac dysfunction and/or low systolic arterial pressure, *inotropic support* should be considered. In the absence of systemic hypotension, milrinone is a good first-line agent. Evidence for efficacy of *milrinone* in newborns with PH is currently limited to case series,[115,116] although randomized trials are in progress.[37,125] Where milrinone

may be less desirable (e.g., HIE with therapeutic hypothermia, significant prematurity), *dobutamine and low-dose epinephrine* (e.g., 0.03–0.05 mcg/kg/min) represent suitable second-line options. There is limited evidence for the use of dobutamine; however, evidence exists for increases in systemic blood flow in preterm newborns in the perinatal transition period.[126] The drug is more chronotropic than epinephrine, even at low doses,[127] of which clinicians should be particularly mindful when considering use in infants who are already tachycardic. Dobutamine is not associated with increases in PVR. Epinephrine increases PVR; however, there is a proportionate increase in SVR.[128] In an animal model of perinatal asphyxia with poor cardiac function, epinephrine, dobutamine, and milrinone all demonstrated efficacy in improving cardiac output and carotid and intestinal perfusion, without adverse effects on the pulmonary vasculature.[129] Further research on inotropic support in aPH tailored to individual pathophysiology is required.

Although arbitrary systemic blood pressure targeting with the goal of producing left-to-right flow across extrapulmonary shunts is widely practiced, this is not a physiologically nor evidence-based approach to aPH management and is not advocated.[11] Low systemic arterial pressure (SAP) in aPH may require *vasopressor therapy* once treatment for high RV afterload and support of RV performance has been optimized. Achieving adequate SAP is important for augmenting coronary perfusion pressure and thereby minimizing RV ischemia, which contributes to the cascade of circulatory impairment in aPH. Dopamine, though commonly used, produces non-specific pulmonary and systemic vasoconstriction and may have an adverse effect on aPH physiology.[11] Animal models suggest that in the presence of aPH, dopamine produces marked elevation of PAP without improving oxygenation; therefore it is not recommended.[130,131] *Vasopressin* is a systemic vasoconstrictor that acts via V1 receptors on vascular smooth muscle cells, with a mechanism of action that differs according to tissue-specific distribution of V1 receptors. Vasodilation has been demonstrated in the pulmonary vascular bed in an animal model,[132] mediated via endothelial cell V1 receptor-driven release of NO.[132] For this reason, vasopressin may be preferred for support of systemic blood pressure in aPH where oxygen requirement remains high despite pulmonary vasodilator therapy. There is evidence for benefit of vasopressin on hemodynamic indices in various shock states in children and adults,[133,134] and case series demonstrating improvements in oxygenation,[135,136] and SAP,[135,137] in aPH. Careful attention to salt and water balance is necessary with use of vasopressin, including frequent serum electrolyte assessment and early supplementation with sodium, due to multifactorial disturbances in serum sodium levels including potent natriuresis in some patients.

*Norepinephrine* represents an additional vasopressor option in aPH; however, there is limited neonatal evidence for use. Lakshminrusimha et al. demonstrated an increase in PVR with norepinephrine in an animal model,[138] particularly with coadministration of a high concentration of inspired oxygen, which may be poorly tolerated by patients with significant RV dysfunction and/or significant labile hypoxemia. Norepinephrine has also been shown to increase PVR in adult human studies.[139,140] An observational study in term newborns with aPH of moderate severity did demonstrate increased LV output, SAP, and minor improvement in oxygenation[141]; however, further evidence for safety and efficacy of norepinephrine in neonatal aPH is awaited. *Corticosteroids* such as hydrocortisone potentiate vasoactive responses to catecholamines[142] and may be considered adjunctive therapy for refractory hypotension in aPH. In addition, in an ovine ductal ligation model of PPHN, hydrocortisone decreased hyperoxia-induced changes in soluble guanylate cyclase and phosphodiesterase 5, thereby increasing cGMP and improving oxygenation.[143] Further cardiovascular pharmacology information is available in Chapter 5.

## Cardiovascular Management in Specific Disease States Associated With aPH

Special circumstances that require a more nuanced, disease process-specific approach to newborn cardiovascular care are discussed in detail in Chapter 29. These conditions include arteriovenous malformation, hypertrophic cardiomyopathy in infants of diabetic mothers, congenital diaphragmatic hernia, and preterm aPH. A summary of management considerations for the first two pathologies, as they relate to the included case studies, is included as follows:

## LARGE PREDUCTAL SYSTEMIC TO VENOUS CONNECTIONS

Cardiovascular management in VGAM and other large preductal systemic to venous connections can be challenging. Treatment with pulmonary vasodilators can be detrimental in some patients as this may prompt development of left-to-right ductal shunting, which can compromise post-ductal perfusion reliant on a large volume transductal right-to-left shunt. The resulting post-ductal hypoperfusion may be severe enough to result in "pseudocoarctation" physiology.[27] Conversely, pulmonary vasodilation may be highly desirable in select patients with severe aPH and RV decompensation due to elevated PVR, particularly in the event of pulmonary hypertensive crisis.[27] Hemodynamic management in VGAM requires careful appraisal of the complex pathophysiology and balancing of mPAP to avoid RV failure without further compromising the fragile systemic circulation. Treatment principles include achieving adequate shunt control, which is often via interventional neurosurgical means in the setting of VGAM, maintenance of ductal patency to preserve lower body perfusion, and judicious use of pulmonary vasodilators (based on the dominant physiology).

## HYPERTROPHIC OBSTRUCTIVE CARDIOMYOPATHY (HOCM)

Acute pulmonary hypertension may be a presenting feature in infants with hypertrophic obstructive cardiomyopathy (HOCM) related to maternal diabetes. Attention should be paid to lung recruitment to optimize PVR; however, consideration should be given to conventional ventilation strategies rather than high-frequency oscillation, where possible. The latter results in a sustained elevation of mean airway pressure and can have a negative effect on PBF. Pulmonary vasodilators, such as iNO, are appropriate where there is echocardiography evidence of raised pulmonary pressure. Maintenance of adequate circulating volume is important for preservation of left atrial filling pressure and augmentation of cardiac preload, where inadequate preload risks exacerbating functional LV outflow tract (LVOT) obstruction.[144] Increases in heart rate are undesirable due to the diastolic dysfunction characteristic of HOCM; coronary perfusion and stroke volume are critically reliant on lower hearts for adequate diastolic filling time.[137] For this reason, sympathomimetic cardiotropes should generally be avoided. Vasopressin is a suitable vasopressor for maintaining systemic arterial pressure in patients with HOCM physiology, without the negative effect of chronotropy, and there may also be advantages in terms of a favorable effect on PVR.[136] Additionally, vasopressin augments aortic root pressure through systemic vasoconstriction, producing a beneficial effect on left heart filling and mitigating LVOT obstruction. Close attention should be paid to salt and water balance, as transient disturbances in serum sodium are observed with vasopressin therapy.[137]

## Chronic Pulmonary Hypertension

The approach to treatment of chronic PH is discussed in detail in Chapter 26. Consensus guidelines suggest actively screening for cPH in at-risk infants,[145-147] including those with established chronic lung disease (CLD) of prematurity (or bronchopulmonary dysplasia [BPD]) and congenital diaphragmatic hernia. In addition to estimation of mPAP using the tricuspid regurgitant jet, the ratio of PAAT to RVET can be used in assessment of PVR in cPH, including as a means of assessing response to pulmonary vasodilators over time.[5] A ratio of <0.31 is considered low and consistent with raised pulmonary pressure.[148] TAPSE < z-score −3 and RV:LV end-systolic ratio >1.5 are also suggested as echocardiography markers of risk for cPH in BPD.[39] Biomarkers, namely brain natriuretic peptide and its N-terminal cleavage product (NT-proBNP), have been investigated for use in diagnosis and management of BPD.[149,150] NT-proBNP concentrations are significantly higher in infants with BPD and correlate with clinical respiratory disease severity.[149] Absolute values of NT-proBNP may be less useful in diagnosis of BPD or assessment of disease severity, though together with echocardiography can be helpful in evaluation of disease progression and response to therapy.[39] Cardiac catheterization should be strongly considered when assessment of PH severity is not possible using echocardiography, as well as where responsiveness to therapy for PH is poor, and to quantify disease severity, evaluate the contribution of shunts, and exclude other causes of pulmonary

vascular disease.[15] Of particular concern is pulmonary vein stenosis (PVS), the diagnosis of which is often delayed and associated with poor survival.[151] PVS can be the cause of cPH in infants with chronic lung disease of prematurity,[152] in whom multiple risk factors for abnormal pulmonary hemodynamics coexist. Initial echocardiography may be normal, and PVS is a progressive disease, making diagnosis challenging.[152] This highlights the importance of echocardiography for clarification of cardiac anatomy in addition to functional assessment in infants suspected to have PH, as well as the need to accurately delineate underlying pathophysiology.

Limited data exist to guide management of cPH in preterm born infants with BPD.[48] Treatment goals include reduction in PVR, support and offloading of the RV, avoidance of coronary ischemia and cardiac failure, and improvement in cardiorespiratory symptoms and signs, thus avoiding aggravation of PH.[39] Optimization of non-invasive respiratory support to avoid V/Q mismatch and localized hypoxic vasoconstriction from atelectasis is advised.[39] Sildenafil is generally considered as first-line therapy for augmenting pulmonary vasodilation in BPD-cPH, particularly in patients who are iNO responders. Endothelin receptor antagonists such as bosentan, inhaled epoprostenol, or intravenous treprostinil represent second-line options, although evidence of efficacy is limited. The need to introduce a second PH-targeted medication or worsening of symptoms using dual pharmacotherapy should prompt assessment with cardiac catheterization.[39] In addition, a standardized management approach using diuretics for patients with echocardiography evidence of RV dilatation may result in symptomatic improvement.[48] Infants with severe BPD are more likely to experience growth failure,[153] and adequate attention to caloric intake is important for growth in the setting of higher metabolic requirements. There is a risk of PH crisis with stressful procedures in infants with BPD-cPH,[39] such as with endotracheal intubation for treatment of retinopathy of prematurity. Adequate sedation and analgesia should be ensured for procedures, which should incorporate senior clinician oversight. The role of postcapillary pathology, that is, LV diastolic dysfunction causing high LA pressure and pulmonary venous congestion, in driving respiratory morbidity in infants with BPD is increasingly being recognized.[61] Diastolic function assessment in this setting may include myocardial performance index,[59,61] as well as transmitral E:A ratio and IVRT.[61] LV afterload reduction with ACE inhibition for infants with severe BPD and evidence of LV diastolic dysfunction and systemic hypertension is an emerging strategy into which further investigation is warranted.[69,70]

Chronic shunts produce cardiac dilatation and alterations in cardiac output, with the latter being measurable using LVO and RVO. Atrial level shunts will result in RA/RV dilation and an increase in RVO relative to LVO, whereas chronic PDA shunts result in LA/LV dilation and an increase in LVO (generally >300 mL/kg/min). Increased transductal flow also eventually tends to lead to stretching of the atrial communication, which results in an increase in both ventricular outputs.[5] In addition to assessment of left heart volume loading, IVRT and mitral valve E:A ratio may provide some insight into left heart pressure loading. Large left-to-right ductal shunt increases venous return and thereby left atrial pressure. This results in earlier mitral valve opening and increased early passive filling, which causes the IVRT to be shortened (<40 ms) and results in "pseudonormalization" of the E:A ratio to >1. Both elevated PVR and chronic excessive PBF may contribute to cPH in the setting of longstanding PDA. With flow-mediated PH, most patients continue to have evidence of left heart volume loading, including high pulmonary vein and mitral valve flow velocities, short IVRT, and dilated left heart structures.[5,154] While ductal closure may ameliorate pulmonary overcirculation and improve respiratory status in shunt-driven cPH, once progression to PVR-mediated cPH occurs, PDA closure should be avoided due to risks of precipitating pulmonary hypertensive crisis and significant RV dysfunction.[5] A staged approach for infants with a large PDA shunt and severe PH has been proposed, incorporating serial assessment with both echocardiography and cardiac catheterization, including evaluation of pulmonary pressure during test PDA occlusion.[155]

## Case Studies

The following case studies provide examples of some of the distinct PH phenotypes, and illustrate how comprehensive hemodynamic assessment and in-depth understanding of physiological drivers of disease may be used to provide individually tailored newborn cardiovascular care.

## CASE STUDY 1: SEVERE ACUTE PULMONARY HYPERTENSION OF ARTERIAL (CLASSIC) ORIGIN

A term female infant was born to a diabetic mother (gestational diabetes; diet controlled). The infant was delivered by elective cesarean section (C-section) secondary to a history of maternal previous C-section and meconium-stained amniotic fluid. Apgar scores were 4, 6, and 8 at 1, 5, and 10 minutes, respectively. After birth, the infant developed progressive hypoxemia and respiratory acidosis, prompting endotracheal intubation. Despite administration of surfactant (CUROSURF® [poractant alfa]), the infant remained profoundly hypoxemic, requiring fractional inspired oxygen ($FiO_2$) 1.0. In addition, the patient developed systemic hypotension (mean BP = 20 mmHg) based on noninvasive (cuff) blood pressure. The chest radiograph (CXR) showed increased cardiothoracic ratio with relatively clear lung fields. The infant was treated with 20 ppm inhaled nitric oxide (iNO) and fluid resuscitation with 10 mL/kg of normal saline bolus. In addition, an intravenous infusion of dopamine infusion was initiated and titrated to 6 mcg/kg/min, which led to normalization of the mean blood pressure. Despite this, the infant remained hypoxemic with an oxygen saturation ($SpO_2$) of 90% in $FiO_2$ 1.0. There was also persistent lactic acidosis (capillary blood gas pH 7.21, $PCO_2$ 44, BE −10, lactic acid 12 mmol/L) and poor perfusion; therefore the infant was transferred to a tertiary care center for consideration of extracorporeal membrane oxygenation (ECMO) support. Upon arrival, the patient was reviewed by the neonatal hemodynamics team and TnECHO was performed.

*Overall Interpretation*: The echocardiogram showed severe (suprasystemic) pulmonary hypertension with RV dilation and reduced RV systolic dysfunction in the presence of a small, restrictive patent ductus arteriosus (PDA) with predominantly right-to-left shunt (Table 27.3 and Figure 27.3). There was normal LV systolic performance but low cardiac output.

*Discussion*: The primary goal of care was to administer cardiopulmonary medications which lower pulmonary vascular resistance, enhance RV systolic performance, and achieve a systemic to pulmonary

## TABLE 27.3    Echocardiographic Findings for Case Study 1

**Assessment of Pulmonary Hypertension**

| Test | Result | Normal Range |
|---|---|---|
| RVSP by TR | 80 mmHg | <35 mmHg[156,157] |
| sEI | 4 | 1 ± 0.06[159] |
| Ductal shunt | Right to left | |
| Atrial level shunt | Right to left | |
| PAAT | 37 ms | 55 ± 7 ms[158] |
| RVET | 163 ms | 216 ± 16 ms[158] |
| RVET:PAAT | 4.4 | 4 ± 0.5[158] |

**Assessment of Right Heart Function**

| Test | Result | Normal Range |
|---|---|---|
| RVO | 64 mL/min/kg | 250 ± 78 mL/kg/min[158] |
| TAPSE | 5 mm | 9 ± 1 mm[160] |
| RV FAC | 0.33 | 38 ± 6%[160] |
| RV S' (TDI) | 5.2 cm/s | 6.8 ± 2.1 cm/s[165] |

**Assessment of Left Heart Function**

| Test | Result | Normal Range |
|---|---|---|
| LVO | 86 mL/min/kg | 143 ± 43 mL/kg/min[158] |
| EF by Simpson biplane | 80% | 53 ± 6%[161-164] |
| Septum S' (TDI) | 2.4 cm/s | 3.5 ± 0.5 cm/s[161] |
| Septum e/E' (TDI) | 17 | |
| LV S' (TDI) | 4.7 cm/s | 4.6 ± 0.6 cm/s[161] |
| LV e/E' (TDI) | 14 | |
| Mitral E/A | 1.04 | 1 ± 0.3[166] |
| IVRT | 36 ms | 52 ± 10 ms[161] |

*EF*, ejection fraction; *LVO*, left ventricular output; *PAAT*, pulmonary artery acceleration time; *RV FAC*, right ventricular fractional area change; *RVET*, right ventricular ejection time; *RVO*, right ventricular output; *RVSP by TR*, right ventricular systolic pressure by tricuspid regurgitation; *sEI*, systolic eccentricity index; *TAPSE*, tricuspid annular plane systolic excursion; *TDI*, tissue Doppler imaging.

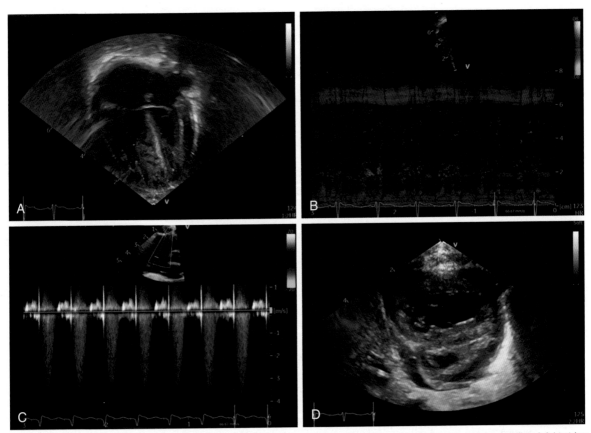

**Fig. 27.3** (A) Qualitative assessment from apical four-chamber view demonstrating prominence of the right heart with severely dilated right atrium (*RA*) and right ventricle (*RV*); (B) Quantitative assessment of right ventricular systolic function in apical four-chamber view with M-mode of tissue Doppler imaging showing moderate to severe RV systolic dysfunction (tricuspid annular plane systolic excursion [*TAPSE*] = 5 mm); (C) Continuous Doppler wave interrogation of tricuspid regurgitation (*TR*) jet from parasternal short-axis view showing tricuspid regurgitation (*TR*) maximal pressure gradient ~80 mmHg (Right ventricular systolic pressure [*RVSP*] estimates pulmonary pressures of at least 80 mmHg + right atrial pressure [*RAP*]). (D) Assessment of ventricular wall motion in parasternal short-axis view showing paradoxical interventricular septal (*IVS*) motion with the IVS bowing into the LV and an elevated eccentricity index in end-systole (sEI = 4).

pressure gradient across the PDA, thereby improving pulmonary blood flow and the efficacy of oxygenation and carbon dioxide clearance.[1] The infant was immediately transitioned from intravenous dopamine to intravenous vasopressin over a period of 1 hour with maximal dose of vasopressin of 0.8 mU/kg/min to maintain systemic blood pressure, minimize pulmonary vasoconstriction, and optimize the transductal pressure gradient.[11] There was concern regarding acute kidney injury at the time of admission, with anuria and elevated creatinine. An intravenous dobutamine infusion of 10 mcg/kg/min was commenced and was selected over milrinone due to concerns about milrinone metabolism and clearance in the setting of renal dysfunction.[118] Repeat echocardiography evaluation showed moderately reduced RV systolic function (TAPSE 6 mm, RV FAC 0.34); therefore an intravenous infusion of prostaglandin (PGE-1) was started at 0.03 mcg/kg/min to offload right ventricular afterload. TnECHO evaluation 24 hours later showed normalized biventricular systolic function, interval improvement of pulmonary hypertension, and a large PDA with an unrestrictive bidirectional shunt. At this stage, the infusion of PGE was discontinued. This case illustrates the importance of maintaining a high clinical suspicion of acute PH in an infant with severe hypoxemia out of proportion of the degree of paren-chymal lung disease, merits of vasopressor selection with more favorable profile on PVR, and the important modulator role of PGE-1 in optimizing RV function.

## CASE STUDY 2: ACUTE PULMONARY HYPERTENSION RELATED TO EXCESSIVE PULMONARY BLOOD FLOW

A 36-week male infant (birth weight of 2708 g), with an in utero diagnosis of cerebral arteriovenous malfor-mation with cutaneous extension, was born by emer-gency cesarean section secondary to prolonged fetal deceleration. The infant was vigorous at birth with normal spontaneous breathing and heart rate above 100 bpm. The preductal $SpO_2$ remained below 50% despite receipt of CPAP via facemask and $FiO_2$ 1.0. Endotracheal intubation was performed, and the infant was transported to the NICU. iNO at 20 ppm was started for a clinical diagnosis of hypoxemic respiratory failure but the patient remained hypoxemic with respi-ratory acidosis (arterial blood gas: pH 7.02, $PCO_2$ 73, $PO_2$ 42, BE $-12$) and elevated lactic acid (8.8 mmol/L). Blood pressure and heart rate on admission were 53/34 mmHg and 168 bpm, respectively. TnECHO evalu-ation was performed at 4 postnatal hours to assess heart function and pulmonary hemodynamics, due to the magnitude of illness severity.

*Overall Interpretation*: Echocardiogram showed su-prasystemic pulmonary hypertension with increased RV output (flow-driven) secondary to a large cerebral arteriovenous malformation (low resistance shunt) (Table 27.4 and Figure 27.4).

*Discussion:* As the nature of PH was related to in-creased pulmonary blood flow [pressure = flow × resistance + left atrial pressure], iNO was weaned off to optimize systemic blood flow. To limit excessive pulmonary blood flow, specific targets for permissive hypercapnia ($pCO_2$ 50–60) and $SpO_2$ (85–90%) were set. An intravenous infusion of PGE-1 was rec-ommended to maintain ductal patency and ensure continual right-to-left ductal shunt to supply the post-ductal systemic circulation. This was followed by weaning of $FiO_2$ and improvement in respiratory and lactic acidosis (lactic acid 5.3 mmol/L). Neuro-surgery consultation was arranged for consideration of surgical intervention of the arteriovenous malfor-mation. Magnetic resonance imaging showed a large intracranial vascular malformation, pial arteriovenous

fistulas, dural arteriovenous fistulas, and neoangio-genesis (Figure 27.5). The infant successfully under-went embolization of bilateral middle meningeal and left occipital arteries with reduction in intracranial arteriovenous shunting by 50–70%. There was im-provement in systemic perfusion, heart rate, and blood pressures (HR 140 bpm, BP 65/45 mmHg) and resolution of lactic acidosis (lactic acid 1.5 mmol/L). In summary, patients with a large preductal systemic to venous connection may present with a dilated pressure and volume loaded right heart and right-to-left ductal shunt. Due to the magnitude of pre-ductal systemic steal, a right-to-left ductal shunt is essential to support post-ductal organ perfusion. This case il-lustrates that, according to the Darcy law of fluid dynamics, elevated pulmonary arterial pressure may relate to increased pulmonary blood flow; therefore pulmonary vasodilators should be avoided in this situation. In the presence of ductal patency further reductions in PVR may reduce the magnitude of right to left ductal shunt, further compromising post-ductal perfusion.

## CASE STUDY 3: ACUTE PULMONARY HYPERTENSION WITH HYPERTROPHIC CARDIOMYOPATHY

A 9-day-old term female infant of a diabetic mother (diabetes mellitus type II, poorly controlled with insu-lin with maternal $HbA_{1C}$ of 11%) was born by cesar-ean section secondary to fetal macrosomia with ceph-alopelvic disproportion at a community hospital. The resuscitation was uneventful, with Apgar scores of 8 and 9 at 1 and 5 minutes, respectively. The infant was admitted to NICU at the community hospital on post-natal day 2 with severe hypoxemia [$SpO_2$ 60% (pre-ductal) and 39% (post-ductal)]. Due to a presumptive diagnosis of acute PH and systemic hypertension, iNO (20 ppm), an intravenous infusion of milrinone at 0.5 mcg/kg/min, and PRN bolus of calcium channel blocker were commenced. Due to the refractory nature of the illness, the patient was referred for hemodynamics consultation and consideration of ECMO. Upon arrival at the tertiary academic center, the infant was on conven-tional mechanical ventilation (pressure-regulated volume control [PRVC] tidal volume [TV] 6 mL/kg, PEEP 10, rate 45, inspiratory time [iT] 0.4) and was receiving $FiO_2$ 1.0. The patient was noted to be tachycardic (180–190 bpm) with systemic hypertension (BP 130/110 mmHg)

## TABLE 27.4  Echocardiographic Findings for Case Study 2

### Assessment of Pulmonary Hypertension

| Test | Result | Normal Range |
| --- | --- | --- |
| RVSp by TR | 85 mmHg | <35 mmHg[156,157] |
| sEI | 1.6 | 1 ± 0.06[159] |
| Ductal shunt | Right to left | |
| Atrial level shunt | Right to left | |
| PAAT | N/A | 55 ± 7 ms[158] |
| RVET | N/A | 216 ± 16 ms[158] |
| RVET:PAAT | N/A | 4 ± 0.5[158] |

### Assessment of Right Heart Function

| Test | Result | Normal Range |
| --- | --- | --- |
| RVO | 196 mL/min/kg | 250 ± 78 mL/kg/min[158] |
| TAPSE | 9.3 mm | 9 ± 1 mm[160] |
| RV FAC | 0.42 | 38 ± 6%[160] |
| RV S' (TDI) | N/A | 6.8 ± 2.1 cm/s[165] |

### Assessment of Left Heart Function

| Test | Result | Normal Range |
| --- | --- | --- |
| LVO | 303 mL/min/ kg | 143 ± 43 mL/kg/min[158] |
| EF by Simpson biplane | 60% | 53 ± 6%[161-164] |
| Septum S' (TDI) | N/A | 3.5 ± 0.5 cm/s[161] |
| Septum e/E' (TDI) | N/A | |
| LV S' (TDI) | N/A | 4.6 ± 0.6 cm/s[161] |
| LV e/E' (TDI) | N/A | |
| Mitral E/A | 1.28 | 1 ± 0.3[166] |
| IVRT | 70 ms | 52 ± 10 ms[161] |

EF, ejection fraction; LVO, left ventricular output; PAAT, pulmonary artery acceleration time; RV FAC, right ventricular fractional area change; RVET, right ventricular ejection time; RVO, right ventricular output; RVSP by TR, right ventricular systolic pressure by tricuspid regurgitation; sEI, systolic eccentricity index; TAPSE, tricuspid annular plane systolic excursion; TDI, tissue Doppler imaging.

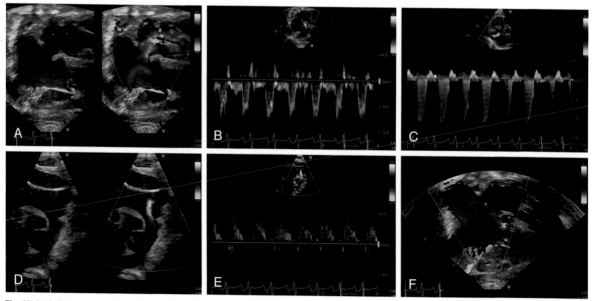

**Fig. 27.4** (A, B) Assessment of atrial level shunt from subcostal view revealing a large atrial level communication with exclusive right to left shunt. (C) Continuous Doppler wave interrogation of tricuspid regurgitation (*TR*) jet from parasternal short-axis view showing TR maximal pressure gradient ~85 mmHg (right ventricular systolic pressure [*RVSP*] estimates pulmonary pressures of at least 85 mmHg + right atrial pressure [*RAP*]). (D, E) Assessment of post-ductal descending aorta with pulsed wave Doppler at supra-sternal arch view revealed the presence of post-ductal holo-diastolic flow reversal including reversal into the proximal arch and preductal vessels. (F) Assessment via subcostal view demonstrated a dilated superior vena cava (*SVC*).

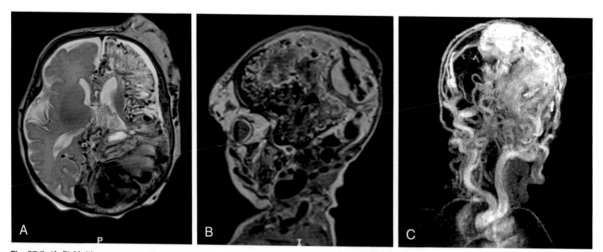

**Fig. 27.5** (A, B) Multisequence, multiplanar MRI of the brain with Gadavist IV contrast axial T1 and parasagittal T1 showing numerous dilated arteries and veins, most prominently on the left, but with some seen on the right. There is abnormal signal and enhancement in the left parietal calvarium. (C) Multisequence, multiplanar MRA of the head with Gadavist IV contrast showing the intra- and extracranial arteries, veins, and dural venous sinuses are diffusely dilated, concerning for diffuse pial AV fistula.

and clinical features of a low cardiac output state (decreased urine output, pale, mottled skin, and elevated lactic acid [4 mmol/L]). Shortly after arrival, there was an acute decompensation with desaturation to $SpO_2$ ~60s% and extreme tachycardia (heart rate ranges 200–230 bpm). The pre- to post-ductal oxygen saturation difference was more than 40%. A fall in arterial blood pressure (cuff BP showed abrupt decrease in BP by 70 mmHg in both SBP and DBP) was noted. The arterial blood gas revealed pH 7.21, $pCO_2$ 65, $pO_2$ 34, and base excess (BE) −2, with lactic acid 4.2 mmol/L. Chest radiograph showed under-recruited lungs and an increased cardiothoracic ratio. TnECHO was obtained to assess heart function and pulmonary hemodynamics.

*Overall Interpretation*: Echocardiography showed severe interventricular septal hypertrophy, without left ventricular outflow tract obstruction, and a hyperdynamic LV. There was normal biventricular systolic function but with severely decreased cardiac output. Severe pulmonary hypertension was also present in the setting of a widely patent ductus arteriosus (3.5 mm) with bidirectional shunt, mainly right to left (Table 27.5 and Figure 27.6).

*Discussion*: This large-for-gestational-age infant, born to a mother with diabetes, presented with echocardiography features of acute pulmonary hypertension and LV/septal hypertrophy, resulting in low biventricular cardiac outputs. The principles of management include optimization of left heart preload by lowering PVR (pulmonary vasodilators), maintaining high LV afterload (systemic vasoconstrictors), maintaining ductal patency in patients with LV outflow tract obstruction, and avoidance of tachycardia.[137,167] The approach to hemodynamic care was as follows (see Chapter 29):

1. Optimization of lung recruitment but maintaining the patient on conventional ventilation to allow for brief periods between inspirations of lower intrathoracic pressure to mitigate the negative impact of sustained elevation in mean airway pressure on pulmonary blood flow seen in high-frequency oscillation.[168]
2. To maximize pulmonary vasodilation and pulmonary venous return, the patient was continued on iNO (20 ppm) and intravenous PGE-1 at dose 0.05 mcg/kg/min was commenced.
3. Prevention of hypovolemia including liberal infusion of fluids (normal saline boluses, for instance) to maintain adequate preload to LV.
4. An intravenous infusion of vasopressin at titrated dose of 0.6 mU/kg/min was administered as the preferrable vasopressor due to favorable effects on PVR and lack of chronotropy.[137,167] In addition, by maintaining high aortic root pressure, it prevents the LV from completely emptying at the end of systole, which positively impacts left heart filling and mitigates the risk of LV outflow tract obstruction.
5. Additional strategies to lower heart rate and metabolic demands included use of intravenous sedation, avoidance of high body temperature, and avoidance of cardiovascular medications (e.g., dopamine, dobutamine, epinephrine, norepinephrine) with positive chronotropic and/or inotropic effects that may exacerbate the impairment in LV filling.
6. Use of short-acting beta-blockers [e.g., intravenous esmolol] for rate was avoided in this phase of the illness due to the severity of concurrent pulmonary hypertension.

Over the next 12 hours, the infant made good clinical progress. The heart rate decreased to 120's bpm with blood pressure improving to ~110/60 mmHg. $FiO_2$ was able to be weaned to 0.25–0.3. Follow-up TnECHO showed improvement in pulmonary arterial pressure and normalization of cardiac output.

## CASE STUDY 4: CPH RELATED TO LEFT VENTRICULAR DIASTOLIC DYSFUNCTION

The index case was a male infant born at 25 weeks' gestational age with a weight of 710 g. The initial care was provided at a community neonatal intensive care unit and complicated by RDS with evolving BPD, neonatal sepsis, and resolved acute kidney injury. He was diagnosed with congenital pulmonary valve stenosis on postnatal day 41 and was referred for balloon valvuloplasty, which was performed on postnatal day 71. The infant's oxygenation and ventilation both initially improved following the procedure, and he was able to be extubated to nasal continuous positive airway pressure at PEEP 7 $cmH_2O$ with $FiO_2$ 0.5. Repeat TnECHO evaluation 1 week following the procedure (at 36 weeks postmenstrual age [PMA]) showed moderate tricuspid regurgitation, which estimated right ventricular systolic pressure (RVSP) of at least 44 mmHg + right atrial pressure (RAP). This was initially speculated to be secondary to instrumentation during his percutaneous

## TABLE 27.5 Echocardiographic Findings for Case Study 3

### Assessment of Pulmonary Hypertension

| Test | Result | Normal Range |
|---|---|---|
| RVSp by TR | 115 mmHg | <35 mmHg[156,157] |
| sEI | 2.97 | 1 ± 0.06[159] |
| Ductal shunt | Bidirectional | |
| Atrial level shunt | Bidirectional | |
| PAAT | N/A | 55 ± 7 ms[158] |
| RVET | N/A | 216 ± 16 ms[158] |
| RVET:PAAT | N/A | 4 ± 0.5[158] |

### Assessment of Right Heart Function

| Test | Result | Normal Range |
|---|---|---|
| RVO | 57 mL/min/kg | 250 ± 78 mL/kg/min[158] |
| TAPSE | 10.5 mm | 9 ± 1 mm[160] |
| RV FAC | 0.37 | 38 ± 6%[160] |
| RV S′ (TDI) | 7 cm/s | 6.8 ± 2.1 cm/s[165] |

### Assessment of Left Heart Function

| Test | Result | Normal Range |
|---|---|---|
| LVO | 66 mL/min/ kg | 143 ± 43 mL/kg/min[158] |
| EF by Simpson biplane | 86% | 53 ± 6%[161–164] |
| Septum S′ (TDI) | 5.4 cm/s | 3.5 ± 0.5 cm/s[161] |
| Septum e/E′ (TDI) | 19 | |
| LV S′ (TDI) | 6 cm/s | 4.6 ± 0.6 cm/s[161] |
| LV e/E′ (TDI) | 18 | |
| Mitral E/A | 0.76 | 1 ± 0.3[166] |
| IVRT | 60 ms | 52 ± 10 ms[161] |

*EF*, ejection fraction; *LVO*, left ventricular output; *PAAT*, pulmonary artery acceleration time; *RV FAC*, right ventricular fractional area change; *RVET*, right ventricular ejection time; *RVO*, right ventricular output; *RVSP by TR*, right ventricular systolic pressure by tricuspid regurgitation; *sEI*, systolic eccentricity index; *TAPSE*, tricuspid annular plane systolic excursion; *TDI*, tissue Doppler imaging.

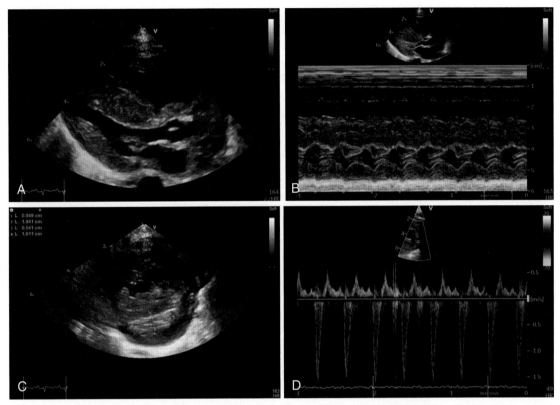

**Fig. 27.6** (A, B) Assessment of the interventricular septum and septal wall thickness with 2-dimensional and M-mode evaluation from parasternal long-axis view demonstrating severe interventricular septal hypertrophy (interventricular septal wall thickness at end-diastole [*IVSd*] z-score = 1) and LV hypertrophy (LV posterior wall thickness at end-diastole [*LVPWd*] z-score = 5) but without LV outflow tract obstruction. (C) Assessment of ventricular wall motion in parasternal short-axis view showing flattening of the interventricular septum (*IVS*) with elevated eccentricity index (*EI*) in both end-systole (*sEI* = 2.97) and end-diastole (*dEI* = 2.04). (D) Assessment of ductal-level shunt with supra-sternal arch view demonstrating a large patent ductus arteriosus (3.5 mm) with bidirectional (72% R-L by VTI and 55% R-L by time) shunt.

pulmonary balloon valvuloplasty, and conservative management was recommended based on the expectation that this would likely improve over time. In the following 2 weeks the infant gradually developed progressive hypoxemia and respiratory acidosis, which required escalation in respiratory support to nasal continuous positive airway pressure at PEEP 9 cmH$_2$O with FiO$_2$ 0.55. Additional treatment with diuretics (short 3 day course of furosemide and maintenance chlorothiazide) was provided. The respiratory deterioration coincided with progressive development of systemic hypertension, as defined by systolic blood pressures greater than 95th percentile (average BP over 24 hours was 98/65 mmHg). A work-up for systemic hypertension showed normal serum creatinine and no evidence of renal artery

stenosis or renal vein thrombosis on renal Doppler ultrasound. TnECHO was performed to assess pulmonary hemodynamics and left ventricular diastolic function.

*Overall Interpretation*: The echocardiogram showed moderate pulmonary hypertension with mildly dilated RV with normal RV systolic function. Neither RVO nor PVRi was calculated, due to presence of pulmonary valve stenosis and pulmonic insufficiency that limit the reliability of these measurements. There was, however, evidence of LV diastolic dysfunction, characterized by prolongation of isovolumic relaxation time, reduction in passive:active transmitral flow (E:A ratio), and elevation in LV e:e′ and left heart dilation with elevated left atrial to aortic (LA:Ao) diameter (Table 27.6 and Figure 27.7).

**TABLE 27.6    Echocardiographic Findings for Case Study 4**

| Assessment of Pulmonary Hypertension | | | Assessment of Right Heart Function | | | Assessment of Left Heart Function | | |
| --- | --- | --- | --- | --- | --- | --- | --- | --- |
| Test | Result | Normal Range | Test | Result | Normal Range | Test | Result | Normal Range |
| RVSP by TR | 53 mmHg | <35 mmHg[156,157] | RVO | N/A due to PS, PI | 250 ± 78 mL/kg/min[158] | LVO | 197 mL/min/kg | 143 ± 43 mL/kg/min[158] |
| sEI | 1.23 | 1 ± 0.06[159] | TAPSE | 10.3 mm | 9 ± 1 mm[160] | EF by Simpson biplane | 64% | 53 ± 6%[161-164] |
| Ductal shunt | None | | RV FAC | 0.43 | 38 ± 6%[160] | Septum S' (TDI) | 4.17 cm/s | 3.5 ± 0.5 cm/s[161] |
| Atrial level shunt | Left to right | | RV S' (TDI) | 8 cm/s | 6.8 ± 2.1 cm/s[165] | Septum e/E' (TDI) | 18.79 | |
| PAAT | N/A due to PS, PI | 55 ± 7 ms[158] | | | | LV S' (TDI) | 4.25 cm/s | 4.6 ± 0.6 cm/s[161] |
| RVET | N/A due to PS, PI | 216 ± 16 ms[158] | | | | LV e/E' (TDI) | 17.9 | |
| RVET:PAAT | N/A due to PS, PI | 4 ± 0.5[158] | | | | Mitral E/A | 0.69 | 1 ± 0.3[166] |
| | | | | | | IVRT | 60 ms | 52 ± 10 ms[161] |

*EF*, ejection fraction; *LVO*, left ventricular output; *PAAT*, pulmonary artery acceleration time; *RV FAC*, right ventricular fractional area change; *RVET*, right ventricular ejection time; *RVO*, right ventricular output; *RVSP by TR*, right ventricular systolic pressure by tricuspid regurgitation; *sEI*, systolic eccentricity index; *TAPSE*, tricuspid annular plane systolic excursion; *TDI*, tissue Doppler imaging.

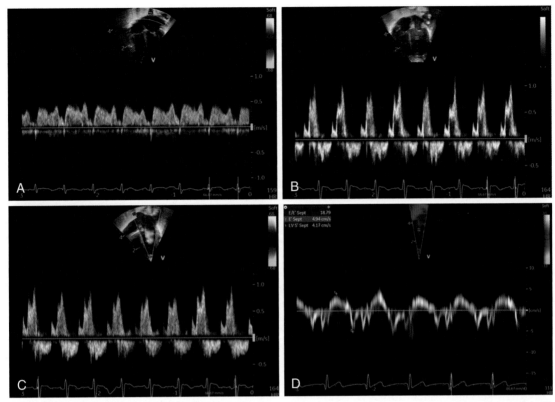

**Fig. 27.7** (A) Assessment of pulmonary vein flow with pulsed wave Doppler from apical four-chamber view demonstrating atrial reversal of flow in diastole of pulmonary vein Doppler (A wave) suggestive of elevated left atrial (*LA*) pressure. (B) Assessment of mitral valve inflow with pulsed wave Doppler from apical four-chamber view showing mitral valve transmitral Doppler E:A ratio = 0.69. (E:A < 1, which is typical of preterm infants with inherent diastolic dysfunction, and is indicative of LV diastolic dysfunction in this term corrected age infant who would be expected to have an E:A ratio ~ 1). (C) Assessment of isovolumic relaxation time (*IVRT*), which is the period of diastole between aortic valve closure and mitral valve opening during which the heart is relaxing but blood is neither entering nor exiting. Prolonged IVRT in this patient is an additional feature consistent with LV diastolic dysfunction. (D) Assessment of left ventricular diastolic function with tissue Doppler imaging from apical four-chamber view demonstrating elevated E/e', also suggestive of LV diastolic dysfunction.

*Discussion:* The clinical trajectory was unexpected and did not follow the natural course after pulmonary valvuloplasty. Rather, there was a progressive increase in right ventricular pressure that was temporally related to worsening of respiratory status, systemic hypertension, and echocardiography evidence of LV diastolic dysfunction. Comprehensive TnECHO evaluation suggested that the nature of chronic PH was consistent with postcapillary pulmonary venous hypertension secondary to left-sided heart disease. Antihypertensive treatment with enalapril, an angiotensin-converting enzyme (ACE) inhibitor, was commenced with positive response and normalization of blood pressure. Follow-up TnECHO evaluation 2 weeks following initiation of enalapril (in a normotensive state) showed PH resolution (estimated RVSP ~25 mmHg [+ RAP]) with normalization of indices of LV diastolic function (E:A ratio 0.95, IVRT 45, LV E:e' 12 [septal] and 11 [lateral] walls, respectively). Respiratory support was weaned to nasal continuous positive airway pressure at PEEP 7 cmH$_2$O secondary to improvement in hypoxia and hypercarbia. This case highlights the variance in chronic PH phenotypes in neonates born extremely preterm and the importance of consideration of LV diastolic dysfunction and impaired ventricular compliance. In addition, this case demonstrates the potential merits of ACE inhibitors for LV function and respiratory health.[70] Inhaled pulmonary vasodilators should be avoided in patients with LV diastolic dysfunction due to risk of worsening pulmonary edema.

## Conclusion

Pulmonary hypertension of the newborn represents a heterogeneous group of pathophysiological scenarios, any of which may present as hypoxic respiratory failure. It is crucial to understand the underlying pathophysiology in order to guide appropriate clinical management and avoid selection of therapy likely to worsen individual hemodynamics. Although the pivotal pathophysiological feature in classical arterial aPH is raised PVR, there are several additional important factors that will influence the clinical presentation and therapeutic decision-making. These factors include parenchymal lung abnormalities with significant V/Q mismatch, ischemic insult to the myocardium and other organs, the presence of an open ductus arteriosus and patent foramen ovale, the volume status of the circulation, interdependence between the two cardiac ventricles at multiple levels, and the ability of the neonatal myocardium to respond to changes in loading conditions. Assessment of underlying pathophysiology in PH may be challenging using clinical criteria alone. Labile hypoxemia and pulmonary parenchymal pathology are common to several hemodynamic phenotypes of PH. The ultimate pathophysiological driver of disease is increased RV afterload, leading to RV dysfunction, with or without systemic complications from altered LV morphology and function. Delineating flow-driven PH from resistance-driven PH or mal-compliance of the LV is essential for treating the primary cause(s) of elevated pulmonary pressure. Establishing the most appropriate treatment strategy for the individual infant may be guided by use of TnECHO to adjudicate hemodynamics and assess responses to intensive care therapies. This individualization of treatment approach is increasingly common in all areas of medicine and is particularly suited to the hemodynamic scenarios presenting as neonatal PH.

## REFERENCES

1. Jain A, Giesinger RE, Dakshinamurti S, et al. Care of the critically ill neonate with hypoxemic respiratory failure and acute pulmonary hypertension: framework for practice based on consensus opinion of neonatal hemodynamics working group. *J Perinatol.* 2022;42:3-13.
2. Lumb A, Horncastle E. Pulmonary physiology. In: Hemmings Jr H, Egan TD, eds. *Pharmacology and Physiology for Anesthesia: Foundations and Clinical Application.* 2nd ed. Philadelphia, PA: Elsevier; 2019:586-612.
3. Polglase G, Morley CJ, Crossley KJ, et al. Positive end-expiratory pressure differentially alters pulmonary hemodynamics and oxygenation in ventilated, very premature lambs. *J Appl Physiol.* 2005;99:1453-1461.
4. Reller M, Donovan EF, Kotagal UR. Influence of airway pressure waveform on cardiac output during positive pressure ventilation of healthy newborn dogs. *Pediatr Res.* 1985;19:337-341.
5. Giesinger R, Kinsella JP, Abman SH, McNamara PJ. Pulmonary hypertension phenotypes in the newborn. In: Dakshinamurti S, ed. *Hypoxic Respiratory Failure in the Newborn: From Origins to Clinical Management.* Boca Raton, FL: Taylor & Francis Group; 2021.
6. Gentles T. The right ventricle and persistent pulmonary hypertension of the newborn commentary on Patel N et al. Assessment of right ventricular function using tissue Doppler imaging in infants with pulmonary hypertension. *Neonatology.* 2009; 96:200-202.
7. Siefkes H, Lakshminrusimha S. Management of systemic hypotension in term infants with persistent pulmonary hypertension of the newborn (PPHN) – an illustrated review. *Arch Dis Child Fetal Neonatal Ed.* 2021;106(4):446-455.
8. Noordegraaf A, Westerhof BE, Westerhof N. The relationship between the right ventricle and its load in pulmonary hypertension. *J Am Coll Cardiol.* 2017;69(2):236-243.
9. Oishi P, Fineman JR. Pulmonary hypertension. *Pediatr Crit Care Med.* 2016;17:S140-S145.
10. Schmidt M, White PA, Khambadkone S, et al. The neonatal but not the mature heart adapts to acute tachycardia by beneficial modification of the force-frequency relationship. *Pediatr Cardiol.* 2011;32:562-567.
11. McNamara P, Giesinger RE, Lakshminrusimha S. Dopamine and neonatal pulmonary hypertension – pressing need for a better pressor? *J Pediatr.* 2022;246:242-250.
12. Rosenkranz S, Gibbs JS, Wachter R, De Marco T, Vonk-Noordegraaf A, Vachiéry JL. Left ventricular heart failure and pulmonary hypertension. *Eur Heart J.* 2016;37(12):942-954.
13. Arrigo M, Huber LC, Winnik S, et al. Right ventricular failure: pathophysiology, diagnosis and treatment. *Card Fail Rev.* 2019; 5(3):140-146.
14. Sanz J, Sánchez-Quintana D, Bossone E, Bogaard HJ, Naeije R. Anatomy, function, and dysfunction of the right ventricle: JACC state-of-the-art review. *Cardiol.* 2019;73(12):1463-1482.
15. Ruoss J, Rios DR, Levy PT. Updates on management for acute and chronic phenotypes of neonatal pulmonary hypertension. *Clin Perinatol.* 2020;47:593-615.
16. Bronicki R, Anas NG. Cardiopulmonary interaction. *Pediatr Crit Care Med.* 2009;10:313-322.
17. Ren X, Johns RA, Gao WD. Right heart in pulmonary hypertension: from adaptation to failure. *Pulm Circ.* 2019;9(3):1-20.
18. Dahdah N, Alesseh H, Dahms B, Saker F. Severe pulmonary hypertensive vascular disease in two newborns with aneurysmal vein of Galen. *Pediatr Cardiol.* 2001;22(6):538-541.

19. Reddy V, Meyrick B, Wong J, Khoor A, Liddicoat JR, Hanley FL. In utero placement of aortopulmonary shunts. A model of postnatal pulmonary hypertension with increased pulmonary blood flow in lambs. *Circulation.* 1995;92(3):606-613.

20. Reddy V, Wong J, Liddicoat JR, Johengen M, Chang R, Fineman JR. Altered endothelium-dependent responses in lambs with pulmonary hypertension and increased pulmonary blood flow. *Am J Physiol.* 1996;271:H562-H570.

21. Black S, Fineman JR, Steinhorn RH, Bristow J, Soifer SJ. Increased endothelial NOS in lambs with increased pulmonary blood flow and pulmonary hypertension. *Am J Physiol.* 1998;275(5):H1643-H1651.

22. Rairigh R, Storme L, Parker TA, et al. Inducible NO synthase inhibition attenuates shear stress-induced pulmonary vasodilation in the ovine fetus. *Am J Physiol.* 1999;276(3):L513-L521.

23. Frawley G, Dargaville PA, Mitchell PJ, Tress BM, Loughnan P. Clinical course and medical management of neonates with severe cardiac failure related to vein of Galen malformation. *Arch Dis Child Fetal Neonatal Ed.* 2002;87:F144-F149.

24. Patel N, Mills JF, Cheung MMH, Loughnan PM. Systemic haemodynamics in infants with vein of Galen malformation: assessment and basis for therapy. *J Perinatol.* 2007;27:460-463.

25. Reller M, Morton MJ, Reid DL, Thornburg KL. Fetal lamb ventricles respond differently to filling and arterial pressures and to in utero ventilation. *Pediatr Res.* 1987;22(6):621-626.

26. Van Wolferen S, Marcus JT, Westerhof N, et al. Right coronary artery flow impairment in patients with pulmonary hypertension. *Eur Heart J.* 2008;29:120-127.

27. Giesinger R, Elsayed YN, Castaldo MP, McNamara PJ. Targeted neonatal echocardiography-guided therapy in vein of Galen aneurysmal malformation: a report of two cases with a review of physiology and approach to management. *AJP Rep.* 2019;9(2):e172-e176.

28. Jedeikin R, Rowe RD, Freedom RM, Olley PM, Gillan JE. Cerebral arteriovenous malformation in neonates. The role of myocardial ischemia. *Pediatr Cardiol.* 1983;4(1):29-35.

29. Serraf A, Hervé P, Labat C, et al. Endothelial dysfunction in venous pulmonary hypertension in the neonatal piglet. *Ann Thorac Surg.* 1995;59(5):1155-1161.

30. Patel N, Massolo AC, Kipfmueller F. Congenital diaphragmatic hernia-associated cardiac dysfunction. *Semin Perinatol.* 2020;44:151168.

31. Altit G, Bhombal S, Van Meurs K, Tacy TA. Diminished cardiac performance and left ventricular dimensions in neonates with congenital diaphragmatic hernia. *Pediatr Cardiol.* 2018;39(5):993-1000.

32. Kinsella J, Steinhorn RH, Mullen MP, et al. The left ventricle in congenital diaphragmatic hernia: Implications for the management of pulmonary hypertension. *J Pediatr.* 2018;197:17-22.

33. Massolo A, Paria A, Hunter L, Finlay E, Davis CF, Patel N. Ventricular dysfunction, interdependence, and mechanical dispersion in newborn infants with congenital diaphragmatic hernia. *Neonatology.* 2019;116(1):68-75.

34. Loh E, Stamler JS, Hare JM, Loscalzo J, Colucci WS. Cardiovascular effects of inhaled nitric oxide in patients with left ventricular dysfunction. *Circulation.* 1994;90:2780-2785.

35. Gien J, Kinsella JP. Management of pulmonary hypertension in infants with congenital diaphragmatic hernia. *J Perinatol.* 2016;36:S28-S31.

36. Von Schnakenburg C, Peuster M, Norozi K, et al. Acute pulmonary edema caused by epoprostenol infusion in a child with scimitar syndrome and pulmonary hypertension. *Pediatr Crit Care Med.* 2003;4(1):111-114.

37. Cochius-den Otter S, Schaible T, Greenough A, et al. The CoDiNOS trial protocol: an international randomised controlled trial of intravenous sildenafil versus inhaled nitric oxide for the treatment of pulmonary hypertension in neonates with congenital diaphragmatic hernia. *BMJ Open.* 2019;9(11):e032122.

38. Onda T, Akimoto T, Hayasaka I, et al. Incidence of alveolar capillary dysplasia with misalignment of pulmonary veins in infants with unexplained severe pulmonary hypertension: The roles of clinical, pathological, and genetic testing. *Early Hum Dev.* 2021;155:105323.

39. Hansmann G, Sallmon H, Roehr CC, Kourembanas S, Austin ED, Koestenberger M, for the European Pediatric Pulmonary Vascular Disease Network (EPPVDN). Pulmonary hypertension in bronchopulmonary dysplasia. *Pediatr Res.* 2020;89:446-455.

40. Lignelli E, Palumbo F, Myti D, Morty RE. Recent advances in our understanding of the mechanisms of lung alveolarization and bronchopulmonary dysplasia. *Am J Physiol Lung Cell Mol Physiol.* 2019;317:L832-L887.

41. De Paepe M, Hanley LC, Lacourse Z, Pasquariello TA, Mao Q. Pulmonary dendritic cells in lungs of preterm infants: neglected participants in bronchopulmonary dysplasia? *Pediatr Dev Pathol.* 2011;14(1):20-27.

42. Thébaud B, Goss KN, Laughon M, et al. Bronchopulmonary dysplasia. *Nat Rev Dis Primers.* 2019;5(1):78.

43. Hwang J, Rehan VK. Recent advances in bronchopulmonary dysplasia: pathophysiology, prevention, and treatment. *Lung.* 2018;196(2):129-138.

44. Mirza H, Ziegler J, Ford S, Padbury J, Tucker R, Laptook A. Pulmonary hypertension in preterm infants: prevalence and association with bronchopulmonary dysplasia. *J Pediatr.* 2014;165(5):909-914.e1.

45. Mourani P, Sontag MK, Younoszai A, et al. Early pulmonary vascular disease in preterm infants at risk for bronchopulmonary dysplasia. *Am J Respir Crit Care Med.* 2015;191(1):87-95.

46. Cohen J, Nees SN, Valencia GA, Rosenzweig EB, Krishnan US. Sildenafil use in children with pulmonary hypertension. *J Pediatr.* 2019;205:29-34.e1.

47. Stewart A, Brion LP. Intravenous or enteral loop diuretics for preterm infants with (or developing) chronic lung disease. *Cochrane Database Syst Rev.* 2011;9:CD001453.

48. Baczynski M, Kelly E, McNamara PJ, Shah PS, Jain A. Short and long-term outcomes of chronic pulmonary hypertension in preterm infants managed using a standardized algorithm. *Pediatr Pulmonol.* 2020;56:1155-1164.

49. Rahde Bischoff A, Cavallaro Moronta S, McNamara PJ. Going home with a patent ductus arteriosus: is it benign? *J Pediatr.* 2021;240:10-13.

50. Philip R, Nathaniel Johnson J, Naik R, et al. Effect of patent ductus arteriosus on pulmonary vascular disease. *Congenit Heart Dis.* 2019;14:37-41.

51. Philip R, Lamba V, Talati A, Sathanandam S. Pulmonary hypertension with prolonged patency of the ductus arteriosus in preterm infants. *Children (Basel).* 2020;7:139.

52. Hamrick S, Sallmon H, Rose AT, et al. Patent ductus arteriosus of the preterm infant. *Pediatrics.* 2020;146(5):e20201209.

53. Vyas-Read S, Guglani L, Shankar P, Travers C, Kanaan U. Atrial septal defects accelerate pulmonary hypertension diagnoses in premature infants. *Front Pediatr.* 2018;6:342.

54. Toyoshima K, Momma K, Nakanishi T. In vivo dilatation of the ductus arteriosus induced by furosemide in the rat. *Pediatr Res.* 2010;67:173-176.

55. Green T, Thompson TR, Johnson DE, Lock JE. Furosemide promotes patent ductus arteriosus in premature infants with the respiratory distress syndrome. *N Engl J Med.* 1983;308:743-748.

56. Sung S, Lee MH, Ahn Sy, Chang YS, Park WS. Effect of nonintervention vs oral ibuprofen in patent ductus arteriosus in preterm infants: a randomized clinical trial. *JAMA Pediatr.* 2020;174(8):755-763.

57. De Buyst J, Rakza T, Pennaforte T, Johansson AB, Storme L. Hemodynamic effects of fluid restriction in preterm infants with significant patent ductus arteriosus. *J Pediatr.* 2012;161(3):404-408.

58. Bishnoi R, Everett AD, Ringel RE, et al. Device closure of secundum atrial septal defects in infants weighing less than 8 kg. *Pediatr Cardiol.* 2014;35(7):1124-1131.

59. Yates A, Welty SE, Gest AL, Cua CL. Changes in patients with bronchopulmonary dysplasia. *J Pediatr.* 2008;152:766-770.

60. Mourani P, Ivy DD, Rosenberg AA, Fagan TE, Abman SH. Left ventricular diastolic dysfunction in bronchopulmonary dysplasia. *J Pediatr.* 2008;152:291-293.

61. Seghal A, Malikiwi A, Paul E, Tan K, Menahem S. A new look at bronchopulmonary dysplasia: postcapillary pathophysiology and cardiac dysfunction. *Pulm Circ.* 2016;6(4):508-515.

62. Bokiniec R, Właskienko P, Borszewska-Kornacka M, Szymkiewicz-Dangel J. Evaluation of left ventricular function in preterm infants with bronchopulmonary dysplasia using various echocardiographic techniques. *Echocardiography.* 2017;34(4):567-576.

63. Abman S, Warady BA, Lum GM, Koops BL. Systemic hypertension in infants with bronchopulmonary dysplasia. *J Pediatr.* 1984;104:928-931.

64. Anderson A, Warady BA, Daily DK, Johnson JA, Thomas MK. Systemic hypertension in infants with severe bronchopulmonary dysplasia: associated clinical factors. *Am J Perinatol.* 1993;10:190-193.

65. Alagappan A, Malloy MH. Systemic hypertension in very low birth weight infants with bronchopulmonary dysplasia: incidence and risk factors. *Am J Perinatol.* 1998;15:3-8.

66. Solari V, Puri P. Genetic polymorphisms of angiotensin system genes in congenital diaphragmatic hernia associated with persistent pulmonary hypertension. *J Pediatr Surg.* 2004;39(3):302-306.

67. Wagenaar N, Sengers RMA, Laghmani EH, et al. Angiotensin II type 2 receptor ligand PD123319 attenuates hyperoxia–induced lung and heart injury at a low dose in newborn rats. *Am J Physiol Lung Cell Mol Physiol.* 2014;307(3):L261-L272.

68. Wagenaar G, Laghmani EH, de Visser YP, et al. Ambrisentan reduces pulmonary arterial hypertension but does not stimulate alveolar and vascular development in neonatal rats with hyperoxic lung injury. *Am J Physiol Lung Cell Mol Physiol.* 2013;304(4):L264-L275.

69. Seghal A, Krishnamurthy MB, Clark M, Menahem S. ACE inhibition for severe bronchopulmonary dysplasia – an approach based on physiology. *Physiol Rep.* 2018;6(17):e13821.

70. Stanford A, Reyes M, Rios DR, et al. Safety, feasibility, and impact of enalapril on cardiorespiratory physiology and health in preterm infants with systemic hypertension and left ventricular diastolic dysfunction. *J Clin Med.* 2021;10:4519.

71. Hébert A, Lavoie PM, Giesinger RE, et al. Evolution of training guidelines for echocardiography performed by the neonatologist: toward hemodynamic consultation. *J Am Soc Echocardiogr.* 2019; 32(6):785-790.

72. Mertens L, Seri I, Marek J, et al. Targeted neonatal echocardiography in the neonatal intensive care unit: practice guidelines and recommendations for training. *Eur J Echocardiogr.* 2011; 12(10):715-736.

73. Smith A, Purna JR, Castaldo MP, et al. Accuracy and reliability of qualitative echocardiography assessment of right ventricular size and function in neonates. *Echocardiography.* 2019;36(7): 1346-1352.

74. Jain A, El-Khuffash AF, van Herpen CH, et al. Cardiac function and ventricular interactions in persistent pulmonary hypertension of the newborn. *Pediatr Crit Care Med.* 2021;22(2):e145-e157.

75. Gupta N, Kamlin CO, Cheung M, Stewart M, Patel N. Improving diagnostic accuracy in the transport of infants with suspected duct-dependent congenital heart disease. *J Paediatr Child Health.* 2014;50:64-70.

76. De Boode W, Singh Y, Molnar Z, et al. Application of neonatologist performed echocardiography in the assessment and management of persistent pulmonary hypertension of the newborn. *Pediatr Res.* 2018;84:68-77.

77. D'Alto M, Romeo E, Argiento P, et al. Accuracy and precision of echocardiography versus right heart catheterization for the assessment of pulmonary hypertension. *Cardiology.* 2017; 168:4058-4062.

78. Skinner J, Hunter S, Hey EN. Haemodynamic features at presentation in persistent pulmonary hypertension of the newborn and outcome. *Arch Dis Child Fetal Neonatal Ed.* 1996;74:F26-F32.

79. O'Leary M, Assad TR, Xu M, et al. Lack of a tricuspid regurgitation Doppler signal and pulmonary hypertension by invasive measurement. *J Am Heart Assoc.* 2018;7:e009362.

80. Bendapudi P, Rao GG, Greenough A. Diagnosis and management of persistent pulmonary hypertension of the newborn. *Pediatr Respir Rev.* 2015;16:157-161.

81. Abraham S, Weismann CG. Left ventricular end-systolic eccentricity index for assessment of pulmonary hypertension in infants. *Echocardiography.* 2016;33(6):910-915.

82. Burkett D, Patel SS, Mertens L, Friedberg MK, Ivy DD. Relationship between left ventricular geometry and invasive hemodynamics in pediatric pulmonary hypertension. *Circ Cardiovasc Imaging.* 2020;13(5):e009825.

83. Levy P, Patel MD, Groh G, et al. Pulmonary artery acceration time provides a reliable estimate of invasive pulmonary hemodynamics in children. *J Am Soc Echocardiogr.* 2016;29(11): 1056-1065.

84. Patel M, Breatnach CR, James AT, et al. Echocardiographic assessment of right ventricular afterload in preterm infants: maturational patterns of pulmonary artery acceleration time over the first year of age and implications for pulmonary hypertension. *J Am Soc Echocardiogr.* 2019;32(7):884-894.e4.

85. Malowitz J, Forsha DE, Smith PB, Cotten CM, Barker PC, Tatum GH. Right ventricular echocardiographic indices predict poor outcomes in infants with persistent pulmonary hypertension of the newborn. *Eur Heart J.* 2015;16:1224-1231.

86. Koestenberger M, Nagel B, Ravekes W, et al. Systolic right ventricular function in preterm and term neonates: reference values of the tricuspid annular plane systolic excursion (TAPSE) in 258 patients and calculation of Z-score values. *Neonatology.* 2011;100(1):85-92.

87. Rodriguez M, Coredera A, Martinez-Orgado J, Arruza L. Cerebral blood flow velocity and oxygenation correlate predominantly with right ventricular function in cooled neonates with moderate-severe hypoxic-ischemic encephalopathy. *Eur J Pediatr.* 2020; 179(10):1609-1618.

88. Giesinger R, El Shahed AI, Castaldo MP, et al. Impaired right ventricular performance is associated with adverse outcome after hypoxic ischemic encephalopathy. *Am J Respir Crit Care Med.* 2019;200(10):1294-1305.

89. Giesinger R, Elsayed YN, Castaldo MP, et al. Neurodevelopmental outcome following hypoxic ischaemic encephalopathy and therapeutic hypothermia is related to right ventricular performance at 24-hour postnatal age. *Arch Dis Child Fetal Neonatal Ed.* 2022;107(1):70-75.

90. Aggarwal S, Shanti C, Lelli J, Natarajan G. Prognostic utility of noninvasive estimates of pulmonary vascular compliance in neonates with congenital diaphragmatic hernia. *J Pediatr Surg.* 2019;54(3):439-444.

91. Levy P, Dioneda B, Holland MR, et al. Right ventricular function in preterm and term neonates: reference values for right ventricle areas and fractional area of change. *J Am Soc Echocardiogr.* 2015;28(5):559-569.

92. Smolarek D, Gruchala M, Sobiczewski W. Echocardiographic evaluation of right ventricular systolic function: The traditional and innovative approach. *Cardiol J.* 2018;24(5):563-572.

93. Sehgal A, Ibrahim M, Tan K. Cardiac function and its evolution with pulmonary vasodilator therapy: a myocardial deformation study. *Echocardiography.* 2014;31:E185-E188.

94. James A, Corcoran JD, McNamara PJ, Franklin O, El-Khuffash AF. The effect of milrinone on right and left ventricular function when used as a rescue therapy for term infants with pulmonary hypertension. *Cardiol Young.* 2015;26:1-10.

95. Patel N, Mills JF, Cheung MMH. Assessment of right ventricular function using tissue Doppler imaging in infants with pulmonary hypertension. *Neonatology.* 2009;96(3):193-199.

96. Peterson A, Deatsman S, Frommelt MA, Mussatto K, Frommelt PC. Correlation of echocardiographic markers and therapy in persistent pulmonary hypertension of the newborn. *Pediatr Cardiol.* 2009;30(2):160-165.

97. Tingay D, Kinsella JP. Heart of the matter? Early ventricular dysfunction in congenital diaphragmatic hernia. *Am J Respir Crit Care Med.* 2019;200(12):1462-1464.

98. Patel N, Lally PA, Kipfmueller F, et al. Ventricular dysfunction is a critical determinant of mortality in congenital diaphragmatic hernia. *Am J Respir Crit Care Med.* 2019;200(12):1522-1530.

99. Dao D, Patel N, Harting MT, Lally KP, Lally PA, Buchmiller TL. Early left ventricular dysfunction and severe pulmonary hypertension predict adverse outcomes in "low-risk" congenital diaphragmatic hernia. *Pediatr Crit Care Med.* 2020;21(7):637-646.

100. Jain A, Mohamed A, El-Khuffash A, et al. A comprehensive echocardiographic protocol for assessing neonatal right ventricular dimensions and function in the transitional period: normative data and z scores. *J Am Soc Echocardiogr.* 2014;27(12):1293-1304.

101. Aggarwal S, Natarajan G. Echocardiographic correlates of persistent pulmonary hypertension of the newborn. *Early Hum Dev.* 2015;91:285-289.

102. Breinig S, Dicky O, Ehlinger V, Dulac Y, Marcoux MO, Arnaud C. Echocardiographic parameters predictive of poor outcome in persistent pulmonary hypertension of the newborn (PPHN): preliminary results. *Pediatr Cardiol.* 2021;42(8):1848-1853.

103. Musewe N, Poppe D, Smallhorn JF, et al. Doppler echocardiographic measurement of pulmonary artery pressure from ductal Doppler velocities in the newborn. *J Am Coll Cardiol.* 1990;15(2):446-456.

104. Alapati D, Jassar R, Shaffer TH. Management of supplemental oxygen for infants with persistent pulmonary hypertension of newborn: a survey. *Am J Perinatol.* 2017;34:276-282.

105. Hauge A. Hypoxia and pulmonary vascular resistance. The relative effects of pulmonary arterial and alveolar PO2. *Acta Physiol Scand.* 1969;76:121-130.

106. Rawat M, Lakshminrusimha S, Vento M. Pulmonary hypertension and oxidative stress: where is the link? *Semin Fetal Neonatal Med.* 2022;27:101347.

107. Farrow K, Groh BS, Schumacker PT, et al. Hyperoxia increases phosphodiesterase 5 expression and activity in ovine fetal pulmonary artery smooth muscle cells. *Circ Res.* 2008;102(2):226-233.

108. Rudolph A, Yuan S. Response of the pulmonary vasculature to hypoxia and H+ ion concentration changes. *J Clin Invest.* 1966;45:399-411.

109. Belik J, Jankov RP, Pan J, Tanswell AK. Peroxynitrite inhibits relaxation and induces pulmonary artery muscle contraction in the newborn rat. *Free Radic Biol Med.* 2004;37:1384-1392.

110. Chandrasekharan P, Rawat M, Lakshminrusimha S. How do we monitor oxygenation during the management of PPHN? Alveolar, arterial, mixed venous oxygen tension or peripheral saturation? *Children (Basel).* 2020;7(10):180.

111. Kregenow DA, Swenson ER. The lung and carbon dioxide: implications for permissive and therapeutic hypercapnia. *Eur Respir J.* 2002;20(1):6-11.

112. Ketabchi F, Ghofrani HA, Schermuly RT, et al. Effects of hypercapnia and NO synthase inhibition in sustained hypoxic pulmonary vasoconstriction. *Respir Res.* 2012;13(1):7.

113. Afolayan AJ, Eis A, Alexander M, et al. Decreased endothelial nitric oxide synthase expression and function contribute to impaired mitochondrial biogenesis and oxidative stress in fetal lambs with persistent pulmonary hypertension. *Am J Physiol Lung Cell Mol Physiol.* 2016;310(1):L40-L49.

114. Walsh-Sukys M, Tyson JE, Wright LL, et al. Persistent pulmonary hypertension of the newborn in the era before nitric oxide: practice variation and outcomes. *Pediatrics.* 2000;105:14-20.

115. McNamara P, Laique F, Muang-In S, Whyte HE. Milrinone improves oxygenation in neonates with severe persistent pulmonary hypertension of the newborn. *J Crit Care.* 2006;21:217-222.

116. James A, Corcoran JD, McNamara PJ, Franklin O, El-Khuffash AF. The effect of milrinone on right and left ventricular function when used as a rescue therapy for term infants with pulmonary hypertension. *Cardiol Young.* 2016;26:90-99.

117. Deb B, Bradford K, Pearl RG. Additive effects of inhaled nitric oxide and intravenous milrinone in experimental pulmonary hypertension. *Crit Care Med.* 2000;28:795-799.

118. Bischoff A, Habib S, McNamara PJ, Giesinger RE. Hemodynamic response to milrinone for refractory hypoxemia during therapeutic hypothermia for neonatal hypoxic ischemic encephalopathy. *J Perinatol.* 2021;41:2345-2354.

119. Tworetzky W, Bristow J, Moore P, et al. Inhaled nitric oxide in neonates with persistent pulmonary hypertension. *Lancet.* 2001;357:118-120.

120. Creagh-Brown B, Griffiths MJD, Evans TW. Bench-to-bedside review: inhaled nitric oxide therapy in adults. *Crit Care.* 2009;13(3):221.

121. Kelly L, Ohlsson A, Shah PS. Sildenafil for pulmonary hypertension in neonates. *Cochrane Database Syst Rev.* 2017;8:CD005494.

122. El-Ghandour M, Hammad B, Ghanem M, Antonios MAM. Efficacy of milrinone plus sildenafil in the treatment of neonates with persistent pulmonary hypertension in resource-limited settings: results of a randomized, double-blind trial. *Paediatr Drugs.* 2020;22:685-693.

123. Pierce C, Zhang MH, Jonsson B, et al. Efficacy and safety of IV sildenafil in the treatment of newborn infants with, or at risk of, persistent pulmonary hypertension of the newborn (PPHN): a multicenter, randomized, placebo-controlled trial. *J Pediatr.* 2021;237:154-161.e3.

124. Farrow K, Wedgwood S, Lee KJ, et al. Mitochondrial oxidant stress increases PDE5 activity in persistent pulmonary hypertension of the newborn. *Respir Physiol Neurobiol.* 2010;174(3):272-281.

125. El-Khuffash A, McNamara PJ, Breatnach C, et al. The use of milrinone in neonates with persistent pulmonary hypertension of the newborn – a randomised controlled trial pilot study (MINT 1): study protocol and review of literature. *Matern Health Neonatal Perinatol.* 2018;4:24.

126. Osborn D, Evans N, Kluckow M. Randomized trial of dobutamine versus dopamine in preterm infants with low systemic blood flow. *J Pediatr.* 2002;140(2):183-191.

127. Butterworth JI, Prielipp RC, Royster RL, et al. Dobutamine increases heart rate more than epinephrine in patients recovering from aortocoronary bypass surgery. *J Cardiothorac Vasc Anesth.* 1992;6:535-541.

128. Barrington K, Finer NN, Chan WK. A blind, randomized comparison of the circulatory effects of dopamine and epinephrine infusions in the newborn piglet during normoxia and hypoxia. *Crit Care Med.* 1995;23(23):740-748.

129. Joynt C, Bigam DL, Charrois G, Jewell LD, Korbutt G, Cheung PY. Milrinone, dobutamine or epinephrine use in asphyxiated newborn pigs resuscitated with 100% oxygen. *Intensive Care Med.* 2010;36(6):1058-1066.

130. Cheung PY, Barrington KJ, Pearson RJ, Bigam DL, Finer NN, Van Aerde JE. Systemic, pulmonary and mesenteric perfusion and oxygenation effects of dopamine and epinephrine. *Am J Respir Crit Care Med.* 1997;155:32-37.

131. Cheung PY, Barrington KJ. The effects of dopamine and epinephrine on hemodynamics and oxygen metabolism in hypoxic anesthetized piglets. *Crit Care.* 2001;5:158-166.

132. Evora P, Pearson PJ, Schaff HV. Arginine vasopressin induces endothelium-dependent vasodilatation of the pulmonary artery. V1-receptor-mediated production of nitric oxide. *Chest.* 1993;103(4):1241-1245.

133. Rosenzweig E, Starc TH, Chen JM, et al. Intravenous arginine-vasopressin in children with vasodilatory shock after cardiac surgery. *Circulation.* 1999;100:II182-II186.

134. Patel B, Chittock DR, Russell JA, Walley KR. Beneficial effects of short-term vasopressin infusion during severe septic shock. *Anesthesiology.* 2002;96:576-582.

135. Mohamed A, Nasef N, Shah V, McNamara PJ. Vasopressin as a rescue therapy for pulmonary hypertension in neonates: case series. *Pediatr Crit Care Med.* 2014;15(2):148-154.

136. Mohamed A, Louis D, Surak A, Weisz DE, McNamara PJ, Jain A. Vasopressin for refractory persistent pulmonary hypertension of the newborn in preterm neonates – a case series. *J Matern Fetal Neonatal Med.* 2022;35(8):1475-1483.

137. Boyd S, Riley KL, Giesinger RE, McNamara PJ. Use of vasopressin in neonatal hypertrophic cardiomyopathy: case series. *J Perinatol.* 2021;41:126-133.

138. Lakshminrusimha S, Russell JA, Wedgwood S, et al. Superoxide dismutase improves oxygenation and reduces oxidation in neonatal pulmonary hypertension. *Am J Respir Crit Care Med.* 2006;174:1370-1377.

139. Jeon Y, Ryu JH, Lim YJ, et al. Comparative hemodynamic effects of vasopressin and norepinephrine after milrinone-induced hypotension in off-pump coronary artery bypass surgical patients. *Eur J Cardiothorac Surg.* 2006;29(6):952-956.

140. Abdelazziz M, Abdelhamid HM. Terlipressin versus norepinephrine to prevent milrinone-induced systemic vascular hypotension in cardiac surgery patient with pulmonary hypertension. *Ann Cardiac Anaesth.* 2019;22:136-142.

141. Tourneux P, Rakza T, Bouissou A, Krim G, Storme L. Pulmonary circulatory effects of norepinephrine in newborn infants with persistent pulmonary hypertension. *J Pediatr.* 2008;153:345-349.

142. Yang S, Zhang L. Glucocorticoids and vascular reactivity. *Curr Vasc Pharmacol.* 2004;2(1):1-12.

143. Perez M, Lakshminrusimha S, Wedgwood S, et al. Hydrocortisone normalizes oxygenation and cGMP regulation in lambs with persistent pulmonary hypertension of the newborn. *Am J Physiol Lung Cell Mol Physiol.* 2012;302(6):L595-L603.

144. Robinson B, Eshaghpour E, Ewing S, Baumgart S. Hypertrophic obstructive cardiomyopathy, in an infant of a diabetic mother: support by extracorporeal membrane oxygenation and treatment with β-adrenergic blockade and increased intravenous fluid administration. *ASAIO J.* 1998;44(6):845-847.

145. Abman S, Hansmann G, Archer SL, et al. Pediatric pulmonary hypertension: guidelines from the American heart association and American thoracic society. *Circulation.* 2015;132(21):2037-2099.

146. Krishnan U, Feinstein JA, Adatia I, et al. Evaluation and management of pulmonary hypertension in children with bronchopulmonary dysplasia. *J Pediatr.* 2017;188:24-34.e1.

147. Hansmann G, Koestenberger M, Alastalo TP, et al. 2019 updated consensus statement on the diagnosis and treatment of pediatric pulmonary hypertension: the European Pediatric Pulmonary Vascular Disease Network (EPPVDN), endorsed by AEPC, ESPR and ISHLT. *J Heart Lung Transplant.* 2019;38(9):879-901.

148. Fitzgerald D, Evans N, Van Asperen P, Henderson-Smart D. Subclinical persisting pulmonary hypertension in chronic neonatal lung disease. *Arch Dis Child Fetal Neonatal Ed.* 1994;70:F118-F122.

149. Joseph L, Nir A, Hammerman C, Goldberg S, Shalom EB, Picard E. N-terminal pro-B-type natriuretic peptide as a marker of bronchopulmonary dysplasia in premature infants. *Am J Perinatol.* 2010;27(5):381-386.

150. Rodríguez-Blanco S, Oulego-Erroz I, Alonso-Quintela P, Terroba-Seara S, Jiménez-González A, Palau-Benavides M. N-terminal-probrain natriuretic peptide as a biomarker of moderate to severe bronchopulmonary dysplasia in preterm infants: a prospective observational study. *Pediatr Pulmonol.* 2018;53:1073-1081.

151. Mahgoub L, Kaddoura T, Kameny AR, et al. Pulmonary vein stenosis of ex-premature infants with pulmonary hypertension and bronchopulmonary dysplasia, epidemiology, and survival from a multicenter cohort. *Pediatr Pulmonol.* 2017;52(8):1063-1070.

152. Laux D, Rocchisani MA, Boudjemline Y, Gouton M, Bonnet D, Ovaert C. Pulmonary hypertension in the preterm infant with chronic lung disease can be caused by pulmonary vein stenosis: a must-know entity. *Pediatr Cardiol.* 2016;37(2):313-321.

153. Wang LY, Luo HJ, Hsieh WS, et al. Severity of bronchopulmonary dysplasia and increased risk of feeding desaturation and growth delay in very low birth weight preterm infants. *Pediatr Pulmonol.* 2010;45(2):165-173.

154. de Freitas Martins F, Ibarra Rios D, Helena F Resende M, et al. Relationship of patent ductus arteriosus size to echocardiographic markers of shunt volume. *J Pediatr.* 2018;202: 50-55.e3.

155. Niu M, Mallory GB, Justino H, Ruiz FE, Petit CJ. Treatment of severe pulmonary hypertension in the setting of the large patent ductus arteriosus. *Pediatrics.* 2013;131(5):e1643-e1649.

156. Giesinger RE, Boyd SM, Rios DR, McNamara PJ. Towards optimization of cardiovascular stability in neonates with hypertrophic cardiomyopathy: uniqueness of the neonatal cardiovascular system. *J Perinatol.* 2021;41(4):907-908.

157. Shekerdemian LS, Shore DF, Lincoln C, Bush A, Redington AN. Negative-pressure ventilation improves cardiac output after right heart surgery. *Circulation.* 1996;94(suppl 9): II49-II55.

158. Galiè N, Torbicki A, Barst R, et al. Guidelines on diagnosis and treatment of pulmonary arterial hypertension. The task force on diagnosis and treatment of pulmonary arterial hypertension of the European Society of Cardiology. *Eur Heart J.* 2004;25(24):2243-2278.

159. Shiraishi H, Yanagisawa M. Pulsed Doppler echocardiographic evaluation of neonatal circulatory changes. *Br Heart J.* 1987;57(2):161-167.

160. Jain A, Mohamed A, Kavanagh B, et al. Cardiopulmonary adaptation during first day of life in human neonates. *J Pediatr.* 2018;200:50-57.e2.

161. Burkett DA, Patel SS, Mertens L, Friedberg MK, Ivy DD. Relationship between left ventricular geometry and invasive hemodynamics in pediatric pulmonary hypertension. *Circ Cardiovasc Imaging.* 2020;13(5):e009825.

162. Koestenberger M, Ravekes W, Everett AD, et al. Right ventricular function in infants, children and adolescents: reference values of the tricuspid annular plane systolic excursion (TAPSE) in 640 healthy patients and calculation of z score values. *J Am Soc Echocardiogr.* 2009;22(6):715-719.

163. Jain A, El-Khuffash AF, Kuipers BCW, et al. Left ventricular function in healthy term neonates during the transitional period. *J Pediatr.* 2017;182:197-203.e2.

164. Zecca E, Romagnoli C, Vento G, De Carolis MP, De Rosa G, Tortorolo G. Left ventricle dimensions in preterm infants during the first month of life. *Eur J Pediatr.* 2001;160(4):227-230.

165. Skelton R, Gill AB, Parsons JM. Reference ranges for cardiac dimensions and blood flow velocity in preterm infants. *Heart.* 1998;80(3):281-285.

166. Nagasawa H. Novel regression equations of left ventricular dimensions in infants less than 1 year of age and premature neonates obtained from echocardiographic examination. *Cardiol Young.* 2010;20(5):526-531.

167. Koestenberger M, Nagel B, Ravekes W, et al. Right ventricular performance in preterm and term neonates: reference values of the tricuspid annular peak systolic velocity measured by tissue Doppler imaging. *Neonatology.* 2013;103(4):281-286.

168. Rios DR, Martins FF, El-Khuffash A, Weisz DE, Giesinger RE, McNamara PJ. Early role of the atrial-level communication in premature infants with patent ductus arteriosus. *J Am Soc Echocardiogr.* 2021;34(4):423-432.e1.

# PATHOPHYSIOLOGY AND TREATMENT IN OTHER HEMODYNAMIC SITUATIONS

# Chapter 28

# Hemodynamic Management in Resource-Challenged Countries

Rema S. Nagpal, Pradeep Suryawanshi, and Mohit Sahni

## Key Points

- Low- and middle-income countries contribute to a major portion of the global neonatal disease burden, accounting for >90% of neonatal mortality.
- Perinatal asphyxia, gram-negative sepsis, and prematurity are major contributors to the neonatal disease burden in LMIC countries.
- Understanding the pathophysiology of the underlying disease process is crucial to appropriate hemodynamic management.
- Hemodynamic management should include an integrated evaluation of the clinical/laboratory parameters, with a comprehensive echocardiographic assessment. This will assist in identifying the pathophysiology of disease and aid in judicious use of vasoactive medication.

## Introduction

Low- and middle-income countries account for 92% of the global disease burden.[1] There is tremendous health "inequality" between high-income countries (HIC) and low- and middle-income countries (LMIC) in the provision and availability of health care services, particularly neonatal health care. These inequalities exist due to differences in health financing, availability and training of the health workforce, health infrastructure in the NICUs, and the establishment of safety protocols. An estimated 2.5 million neonatal deaths occur each year, with South Asia and Sub-Saharan Africa contributing to 36% and 43% of these deaths, respectively. HIC countries contribute to <1% of neonatal deaths, highlighting the vast inequalities in the provision of neonatal care.[2] Neonatal mortality rates (NMRs) are 25 and 27 per 1,000 live births in South Asia and Sub-Saharan Africa, respectively, while rates are as low as 2–4 per 1,000 live births in many HICs.[2] To survive major illnesses, these infants often need highly technical and expensive newborn intensive care, which may not be available in LMIC countries.

## Hemodynamic Monitoring in Neonates

Hemodynamics encompasses the interaction between heart function, cardiac loading conditions, and the dynamics of systemic and pulmonary blood flow and is controlled by homeostatic mechanisms. The goal of hemodynamic (HD) "monitoring" is to track cardiovascular health over time and aid understanding of the underlying pathophysiology of the disease process, timely detection of hemodynamic compromise, rapid initiation of targeted therapy, and the monitoring of treatment effect. Since the predominant disease processes in LMIC countries include perinatal asphyxia, sepsis (particularly gram-negative sepsis), and prematurity itself, this chapter will concentrate on monitoring the hemodynamic changes in these disease processes.

## Approach to Clinical Diagnosis in Neonates Requiring Hemodynamic Monitoring

### PERINATAL HISTORY

A detailed history is invaluable in providing clues to determine the reasons for clinical deterioration in neonates. Relevant areas include poor antenatal care, signs compatible with intraamniotic infection and preterm premature rupture of membranes leading to early onset of sepsis, delivery before hospital admission/home delivery predisposing to asphyxia and hypothermia, maternal diseases like diabetes which predispose to RDS and congenital heart disease, severe pre-eclampsia/eclampsia predisposing to chronic intrauterine hypoxia and intrauterine growth restriction, and drug intake such as nonsteroidal anti-inflammatory drugs (NSAIDs).

## Hemodynamic Assessment Tools in Resource-Challenged Settings

A comprehensive clinical examination should be performed including heart rate, respiratory rate and pattern, presence of tachypnea, grunting, blood pressure (BP) measurements and their interpretation, peripheral pulses (to rule out coarctation), pulse volume (as indicators for PDA and warm shock), presence of cyanosis, pulse oximetry, and a pre-post ductal difference in saturations. Indirect clinical assessments like capillary fill time and perfusion index are also helpful. Laboratory assessments using arterial blood gases and lactate levels are useful in the hemodynamic

assessment of a sick neonate. However, these clinical parameters are inadequate when used in isolation (Figure 28.1).

The objective markers, which are surrogate evidence of the state of cardiovascular stability in neonates, can be divided as follows: "Central" or major markers derived from echocardiography, which assess blood flow and estimated pressure in the central part of the circulatory system (heart, pulmonary artery, vena cava, and aorta), and "Peripheral" parameters, which provide a regional assessment of oxygen delivery, including amplitude-integrated electroencephalogram (aEEG) and near-infrared spectroscopy (NIRS). In resource-limited countries, where echocardiography, aEEG, and NIRS are frequently not available, the clinical parameters have a greater utility and need to be carefully evaluated and interpreted.

### CLINICAL PARAMETERS – UTILITY IN HEMODYNAMIC ASSESSMENT

The commonly used clinical bedside signs of perfusion adequacy in neonates include heart rate, blood pressure, and an assessment of capillary perfusion. However, these markers alone are inadequate in providing accurate information regarding the magnitude

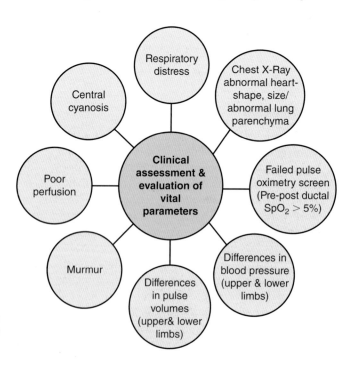

**Fig. 28.1 Suggested hemodynamic assessment algorithm using clinical parameters to determine need for further evaluation using echocardiography.**

of hemodynamic compromise or underlying pathophysiology. Monitoring tools that aid physicians in these countries include:

## Heart Rate

Heart rate is an accurate and routinely monitored parameter in the NICU. Alterations in heart rate (bradycardia <80/min, or tachycardia >180/min) may suggest cardiovascular compromise. Neonates have limitations in their ability to increase the stroke volume; therefore heart rate may increase to compensate for a drop in cardiac output (CO). Since there are multiple other causes for bradycardia/tachycardia in neonates, they are not good indicators of cardiovascular compromise.

## Blood Pressure (BP)

Routine BP measurement is commonly used as a surrogate for cardiovascular wellbeing, even in HIC countries.[3-5] The BP is determined by CO and systemic vascular resistance (SVR). However, an "adequate" mean BP may not equate to an "adequate" CO (see Chapter 3); for example, neonates with high BP due to elevated SVR may actually have a reduced CO. Therefore ideally, CO and BP will need to be monitored simultaneously to determine tissue perfusion. Interpreting BP values, without an objective assessment of cardiac output (using echocardiography), as is followed in many LMICs, may be detrimental in neonates who are critically unwell. In the absence of echocardiography combining parameters like mean BP <30 mmHg and capillary refill time ≥3 seconds increases the sensitivity for detecting measures of low CO such as low superior vena cava (SVC).[6] Hypotension, which occurs in one-third of preterm neonates,[7] needs vigilant monitoring, due to its effect on the cerebral blood flow auto-regulation, particularly if the mean blood pressure falls to <30 mmHg.[8,9] Invasive BP monitoring, which may not always be possible in LMICs, needs adequate staff training, while non-invasive measurements need appropriate cuff sizes[10] and tend to overestimate invasive BP values, particularly in immature hypotensive preterm infants.[11,12]

## Oxygen Saturation Index (OSI)

The oxygenation index (OI) and the OSI are measures that reflect the severity of hypoxic respiratory failure (HRF) in a neonate and are used to trend the degree of oxygen impairment (Table 28.1). The OI is utilized in some centers to determine the need to initiate iNO and is part of the criteria for commencing ECMO.[13] Limitations of the OI are that it is invasive, it requires an indwelling arterial catheter, and it is only intermittently performed. OSI is useful in settings where arterial catheter insertion and monitoring are difficult to perform, utilizes the saturation by pulse oximetry ($SpO_2$), and allows for continuous assessment of the severity of the HRF. In studies comparing OI and OSI in ventilated neonates the correlation coefficient compared strongly (0.89–0.95)[14,15] and was good in the $SpO_2$ range of 85–95% ($r = 0.94$). For ranges >95% or <65%, the correlation was poor ($r = 0.75$).[16] OSI correlated more strongly with HRF in preterm infants <34 weeks (<28 weeks, $r = 0.93$; 28–33 weeks, $r = 0.93$) compared with late preterm ($r = 0.86$) and term ($r = 0.70$) infants.[16] OSI can be used to predict various levels of OI,[14] making it a potentially useful, noninvasive tool. The regression equation from the derived data showed strong linear association of OSI with OI. A simple relationship between the two measures is that OI values can be derived or predicted from OSI values based on the equation OI $= 2 \times$ OSI.[14] The strong correlation between OI and OSI makes OSI a useful tool to predict OI in babies with HRF in an LMIC setting. There are, however, some caveats; specifically, $SpO_2$ and $PaO_2$ only correlate linearly when $SpO_2$ ranges between 80% and 97%, but not in the extremes, where OSI may be unreliable.

| TABLE 28.1 Oxygenation Index and Oxygen Saturation Index | |
| --- | --- |
| **Oxygenation Index** | **Oxygen Saturation Index** |
| OI = MAP × $FiO_2$ × 100/$PaO_2$ mmHg (MAP is measured in cm $H_2O$) | OSI = MAP × $FiO_2$ × 100/$SpO_2$ (MAP is measured in cm $H_2O$) |
| Interpretation[13]: Moderate HRF: 16–25 Severe HRF: 26–40 Very severe HRF: >40 | Interpretation: Mild hypoxemia: 1–4.9 Moderate hypoxemia: 5–7.5 Severe hypoxemia: 7.6–15 Critical hypoxemia: >15 |

## d. Assessment Of Capillary Perfusion[17]

### CapillaryRefill Time (CRT)

CRT is a commonly used, but unreliable, clinical parameter, which is affected by ambient temperature variations, pressure application, maturity of the neonatal skin, and drugs. A CRT >3 seconds in isolation has a 55% sensitivity and 81% specificity for the prediction of low systemic blood flow, and therefore it is not a good indicator of cardiovascular compromise.[6,18]

### Perfusion Index (PI)

PI is a continuous noninvasive parameter, measured by a pulse oximeter, and calculates the ratio of the pulsatile infrared signal (arterial blood flow) to the non-pulsatile infrared signal (static flow of skin) in the peripheral tissue. It correlates with peripheral perfusion, cardiac output, and stroke volume.[19] It reflects the amplitude of the pulse oximeter waveform and is expressed as a percentage (0.02–20%). It is an objective measure of neonatal illness, and the lowest PI is documented at postnatal 12–18 hours.[20] Values <1.24 have been identified as an indicator of severe illness in neonates.[21] Regional cerebral saturation of oxygenation ($rScO_2$) and cerebral fractional tissue oxygen extraction (cFTOE) also correlate with PI at 24–72 hours.[20] PI could be a useful tool in LMIC countries as a measure of perfusion and is already available from the pulse oximeter.

### Plethysmography Variability Index (PVI)

(Figure 28.2) A useful, noninvasive parameter, also measured by pulse oximetry, is plethysmography variability index (PVI), which is a dynamic index (from 0 to 100) measuring the relative variability of the plethysmography waveform. Higher variability of the plethysmography waveform indicates preload dependence and the need for fluid administration. PVI is calculated as follows: $((PI_{max} - PI_{min})/PI_{max}) \times 100$. It may be affected by clinical deterioration, hypotension, volume insufficiency, or other parameters such as ventilation.[22,23]

In an Indian study[24] that evaluated the changes in PVI in preterm neonates with sepsis and associated hypovolemia, the mean PVI was 28% ± 5 and decreased by 11% ± 5 on resolution of shock. In neonates with associated hypovolemic shock, the average PVI at the onset of shock (31% ± 3) decreased in these infants on the management of hypovolemia by 14% ± 2. PVI correlated positively with the collapsibility of the inferior vena cava (IVC), which suggested need for fluids, though the correlation was weak. Multiple studies[25-27] indicate that PVI may be used as a marker of hypovolemia in hemodynamically unstable neonates, particularly in neonates with no access to cardiac ultrasound.

### Serum Lactate

Serum lactate is a good indicator of tissue perfusion and tissue ischemia; specifically, plasma levels >2.5 mmol/L might indicate low cardiac output and impaired tissue perfusion.[28] Levels may rise before clinical deterioration and worsening serial lactate levels suggest severe disease status and likely higher mortality. The common causes of high lactates include hemodynamic causes of hypoxemia, sepsis, necrotizing enterocolitis, multiple organ dysfunction, and drugs like adrenaline (which increases glycogenolysis and glycolysis in the liver).[29] Lactate levels should be used along with other clinical indicators of poor tissue perfusion and not in isolation.[30]

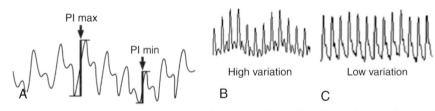

**Fig. 28.2 Plethysmography variability index (PVI).** A) Plethysmography waveform in a pulse oximeter. *Arrows* indicate maximum and minimum pulsatility index (PI). (B) High variation in the waveform between maximum and minimum PI suggests there is scope to give fluids. (C) Low variation in the waveform suggests an unlikely response to fluids.

## CENTRAL HEMODYNAMIC MONITORING

An important aspect of central hemodynamic monitoring is measurement of cardiac output, which is determined by the heart rate (HR) and stroke volume (SV). An assessment of stroke volume is further determined by the assessment of the preload, cardiac contractility (assessed by echocardiography), and afterload (assessed by systemic blood pressures).

### Preload Assessment

Preload assessment in neonates, using jugular venous pressure, is not possible due to the presence of a short neck. Cardiac ultrasound is a useful modality for fluid assessment and responsiveness but may have limited availability in LMIC. Some useful parameters in the echocardiographic assessment include (i) IVC diameter (Figure 28.3) and collapsibility index[31]; (ii) eyeballing of the left ventricle (LV) with "kissing ventricles" suggesting an underfilled LV[31]; (iii) reduced ejection fraction by the Simpson biplane method which uses LV end-diastolic areas[32]; and (iv) variation in the velocity time integral (VTI) at the LV outflow tract (LVOT). A value of >15% predicts need for fluids with a sensitivity/specificity of >90%.[33,34] Low bedside BP measurement is a good, albeit late, indicator of volume status. As mentioned above, the plethysmography variability index is a new tool that could be used as an indicator of fluid status in resource-challenged settings.

### Measurement of Cardiac Output and Contractility

Measurement of LV output equals the systemic blood flow, but only in the absence of a ductal shunt. Measurement of right ventricular (RV) output is reflective of the systemic venous return (in the absence of any atrial shunting). Flow measured in the SVC is normally between 30% and 50% of the total systemic blood flow.[35] Echocardiographic assessment of CO,[36] if available, is the only available modality in resource-restricted settings to measure CO. Although the intra-observer variability of the measurement is high, and inter-observer variability is even higher, it still remains a helpful noninvasive mode of measuring cardiac output.[37-40]

Cardiac ultrasound may be used for comprehensive assessment of chamber dilatation, ventricular systolic function (fractional shortening, ejection fraction) (Figures 28.4 and 28.5) and diastolic function, the presence and direction of flow through transitional shunts (ductus arteriosus, foramen ovale), pulmonary artery pressures, cardiac outputs, and fluid status. It is helpful for enhanced characterization of the hemodynamics in neonates with a significant PDA, pulmonary hypertension, perinatal asphyxia and sepsis, and guiding escalation of inotropic/vasopressor or lusitropic support. There is, however, need for a close collaboration with a pediatric cardiology team to rule out undiagnosed structural heart disease.[41,42] More detailed description of echocardiographic parameters may be found in Chapters 9 and 10.

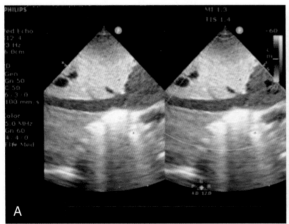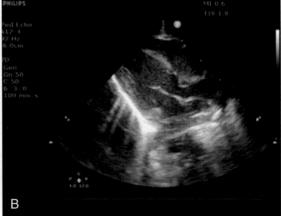

**Fig. 28.3** (A) Subcostal view shows a prominent inferior vena cava and no indication of fluid boluses. (B) Well-filled ventricles in parasternal long-axis view.

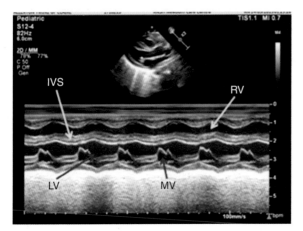

**Fig. 28.4** Fractional shortening is estimated by placing the M-mode through the tips of the mitral leaflets in the parasternal long-axis view and measuring the LV end-diastolic (*LVEDD*) and end-systolic diameter (*LVESD*). The ejection fraction is calculated as (LVEDD − LVESD)/LVEDD. It is a measure of LV systolic function. *IVS*, Interventricular septum; *LV*, left ventricle; *MV*, mitral valve; *RV*, right ventricle.

## Afterload Assessment

Afterload is the force against which the heart has to contract in order to eject its stroke volume and depends on the BP, systemic vascular resistance (SVR), and vascular compliance. High afterload situations are seen in the transitional phase on postnatal day 1 (particularly in ELBW neonates) due to clamping the umbilical cord, "cold" shock in sepsis (peripheral vasoconstriction), and at a later time point following PDA ligation. Low afterload is seen in "warm" shock in sepsis and with a patent ductus arteriosus. Measured LV output provides insights regarding the afterload status, as infants with "warm shock" due to sepsis may have high cardiac output. LV afterload or SVR is a derived value from the mean arterial pressure (MAP), CO, and central venous pressure according to the following equation: SVR = MAP/CO (mmHg/L/kg/min) (normal = 150–200 mmHg/L/kg/min). The diastolic BP may also be considered an indirect measure of the afterload status.

## PERIPHERAL HEMODYNAMIC MONITORING AND ASSESSMENT[43]

The adequacy of $O_2$ delivery depends on BP, SVR, and cardiac output. Therefore assessment of the microcirculation is more complex and affected by multiple factors. The assessment of adequate end-organ function may be supported by the following biomarkers: brain function (cerebral dopplers using ultrasound), regional cerebral oxygen saturation ($rCsO_2$) using near-infrared spectroscopy, and amplitude-integrated electroencephalogram, lung function (from respiratory rate, pattern of breathing), renal function (urine output, urea and creatinine), and liver function (using liver enzymes, clotting factors).[44,45] The available hemodynamic assessment tools available in NICUs of many LMICs are shown in Figure 28.6.

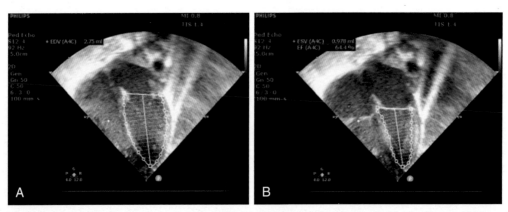

**Fig. 28.5** Apical four-chamber view for measurement of left ventricle ejection fraction which is calculated by the Simpson biplane method from (A) LV end-diastolic volume (*LV EDV*) and (B) LV end-systolic volume (*LV ESV*). LV EDV − LV ESV/LV EDV × 100 = 64.4% (normal value is >55%).

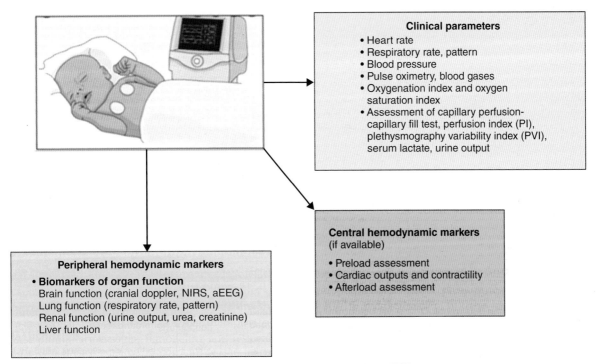

**Clinical parameters**
- Heart rate
- Respiratory rate, pattern
- Blood pressure
- Pulse oximetry, blood gases
- Oxygenation index and oxygen saturation index
- Assessment of capillary perfusion-capillary fill test, perfusion index (PI), plethysmography variability index (PVI), serum lactate, urine output

**Central hemodynamic markers**
(if available)
- Preload assessment
- Cardiac outputs and contractility
- Afterload assessment

**Peripheral hemodynamic markers**
- **Biomarkers of organ function**
  Brain function (cranial doppler, NIRS, aEEG)
  Lung function (respiratory rate, pattern)
  Renal function (urine output, urea, creatinine)
  Liver function

Fig. 28.6 Hemodynamic assessment tools in the NICU.

## Hemodynamic Management of a Critically Ill Neonate With Hypoxic Respiratory Failure and Acute Pulmonary Hypertension in LMIC Countries

Hypoxic respiratory failure (HRF) with/without pulmonary hypertension (PH) is a complex illness, with rapidly changing hemodynamics, requiring skilled diagnostic ability and resource-intensive management. It is a frequent cause of mortality in LMIC countries. The standard approach to clinical diagnosis and monitoring includes historical clues, comprehensive newborn examination, chest radiography and its interpretation, pulse oximetry for oxygen saturation, and a comprehensive echocardiography assessment.[46] Management strategies include optimizing oxygenation, ventilation, and hemodynamics and judicious use of pulmonary vasodilators and inotropes/vasopressors.

The consensus opinion of the Neonatal Hemodynamics Working Group (2022)[46] suggests that clinicians should adopt a low threshold for comprehensive echocardiography assessment. There is a great deal of heterogeneity in management among NICUs, both in HIC and LMIC countries. Use of inhaled nitric oxide (iNO), high-frequency ventilation (HFV), and extracorporeal membrane oxygenation (ECMO) has greatly revolutionized management and improved survival, but these modalities are expensive and require training, which are not easily available in a resource-limited setting.

In a survey done in Canada, Australia, and New Zealand (2008)[47] severity of the disease was assessed by echocardiography (86%), arterial blood gas measurements (83%), oxygenation index (78%), and $FiO_2$ (74%). In a subsequent survey (2015)[48] the use of echocardiography had increased (95%), and most (77%) used iNO as the first-line pulmonary vasodilator; the estimated mortality was 8.3%. In Indian studies,[49,50] in whom the diagnosis of acute PH was confirmed by echocardiography (neonatologist performed or cardiologist performed) but iNO was not available, overall mortality was 29.6%.[49] The mortality figures are similar to other data from Asia (20.6%),[51] Pakistan (26.6%),[52] Egypt (25%),[53] and Portugal (32%).[54]

There are diagnostic and management variations between LMIC and HIC countries. A comprehensive approach to management of neonates with HRF ± acute PH in the NICU includes hemodynamic assessment by integration of the clinical parameters like BP, oxygen saturation, blood gases, lactate (Table 28.2), and comprehensive echocardiography to ascertain the underlying pathophysiology (vasoconstrictor, vasodilator physiology, or mixed picture) (Table 28.3).

## ECHOCARDIOGRAPHIC ASSESSMENT FOR NEONATES WITH HYPOXIC RESPIRATORY FAILURE AND ACUTE PULMONARY HYPERTENSION

Echocardiography remains the gold standard for the diagnosis of PH. In a survey among 148 Indian NICUs[55] 72% of respondents had neonatologist-performed point-of-care ultrasound (NP-POCUS) services (predominantly cardiac US), while the remaining units had either pediatric (64%) or adult cardiology (33%) services.[55] In an Indian study of 187 neonates[56] suspected PDA (50%), hemodynamic instability (12.4%), suspected PH (6.6%), and hypotension (13.5%) were the commonest reasons for assessment. The investigators reported that following

| TABLE 28.2 | Integrated Evaluation of Hypoxic Respiratory Failure in Neonates in Resource Limited Settings | |
|---|---|---|
| CLINICAL EVALUATION | Signs of Systemic Circulatory compromise | Oliguria, tachycardia, Increased CRT, low BP |
| | Signs of Pulmonary Circulatory compromise | Increasing $FiO_2$, ventilation requirements |
| | Markers of organ dysfunction | Gut: Bloody stools (ischemic gut) |
| | | CNS: Apneas, Seizures |
| | | Renal: Oliguria, creatinine deranged |
| | | Liver: Liver function tests deranged |
| | | Lung: Hypoxic respiratory failure |
| | | Suprarenal: Cortisol, ACTH deranged |
| NONINVASIVE MONITORING (Monitor trends) | Diastolic BP | Reflects Systemic vascular resistance, Intravascular volume |
| | Mean BP | Maintains tissue perfusion |
| | Pulse Pressure | Reflects systolic function of heart (Stroke Volume and Myocardial performance) |
| | Systolic pressure | Normal Pulse pressure =15–20 mmHg |
| | | (Low < 10 mmHg) |
| | | Increases with Gestational Age |
| | Look at heart rate trends | |
| | Perfusion Index | |
| | Plethysmography Variability Index | |
| OXYGEN INDICES | Oxygenation Index | OI > 15 |
| | Oxygen Saturation Index | OSI > 7.5 is severe hypoxemia |
| CARDIAC ULTRASOUND (Rule out CHD) | Assessment of: | Ventricular outputs |
| | | Ventricular systolic & diastolic performance |
| | Preload | Shunt evaluation- direction, velocity |
| | Cardiac contractility | Severity of Pulmonary hypertension |
| | Afterload | Calculate SVR |
| | | (Normal SVR = 150–200 mmHg/L/kg/min) |
| DETERMINE DISEASE PATHOPHYSIOLOGY | Vasoconstrictor physiology OR Vasodilator physiology | |
| | **MAKE A PHYSIOLOGY BASED MEDICAL RECOMMENDATION FOR MANAGEMENT** | |

**TABLE 28.3 Pathophysiology-Based Approach to Hemodynamic Management of a Sick Neonate**

| | | Vasoconstrictor Physiology | Vasodilator Physiology | PDA Physiology |
|---|---|---|---|---|
| Clinical Assessment | Assess perfusion lactates Urine output | Who Is at Risk? ELBW – failure to adapt postnatally Pulmonary hypertension Perinatal asphyxia | Who Is at Risk? Gram-negative Sepsis (warm shock) Suprarenal dysfunction Medication – anesthetic agents, morphine | Who Is at Risk? Extreme premature neonates |
| | | Cold shock in sepsis | | |
| BP Assessment | Systolic BP Diastolic BP Mean BP Pulse Pressure | Low or normal Normal or high Normal Narrow | Normal or low Low Low Normal | Normal or high Low Low Wide |
| ECHO Findings | Ventricular outputs Systolic performance Diastolic performance Shunts Pulmonary pressures Systemic vascular resistance (SVR) | Low cardiac outputs Impaired systolic performance Impaired diastolic performance Shunts ± Normal or high pulmonary pressures SVR High | High cardiac outputs Normal systolic performance Impaired or Normal diastolic performance Shunts ± Normal or high pulmonary pressures Low SVR | LV output high RV output normal High pulmonary flows Ductal "steal" |
| Management | | Inotrope (with vasodilatation) | Vasopressors | NSAIDs |
| Inotropes | | 1st Line: Dobutamine Milrinone | 1st line: Norepinephrine Vasopressin | |
| Others – Management | | Cautious fluids Steroids | Avoid dopamine if pulmonary pressures high | |

the echocardiographic assessment, treatment was modified in 42.5% of cases; specifically, addition and/or change in the treatment or avoidance of unnecessary intervention were noted. An increasing number of units from LMIC countries are now adopting clinician-performed ultrasound as a useful hemodynamic assessment tool. The components of the initial clinician-performed ultrasound in neonates with HRF and/or PH are as follows:

  i. Anatomic assessment to rule out structural cardiac disease. The clinical mimics of PH including restrictive pulmonary blood flow disorders (e.g., critical pulmonary stenosis/atresia, obstructed total anomalous pulmonary venous connections), left heart obstructive lesions (e.g., coarctation of aorta), and flow-driven PH (e.g., cerebral arteriovenous malformations) (Figure 28.7) should be ruled out.

 ii. Systematic evaluation of pulmonary artery pressure (PAP) and/or pulmonary vascular resistance,[31,57] RV/LV systolic performance,[36,57] and quantification of pulmonary and systemic blood flow.

iii. Echocardiography information should be interpreted in the context of the given clinical scenario to enable a phenotype-based approach to selection of pulmonary vasodilators or inotropes/vasopressors. Multiple evaluations may be needed over the next 12–24 hours[46] until clinical stability is attained.

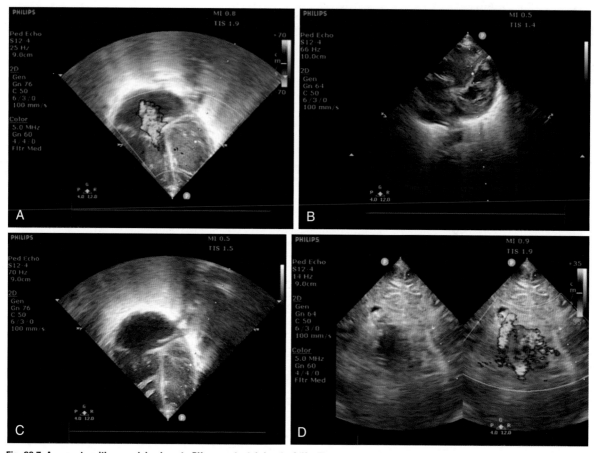

**Fig. 28.7 A neonate with unexplained acute PH on postnatal day 1 of life.** The patient had (A) significant tricuspid regurgitant jet with raised pulmonary artery pressures, (B) crescentic intraventricular septum, (C) dilated right atrium and right ventricle, and (D) cranial ultrasound revealed an arterio-venous malformation.

## PRACTICAL CHALLENGES IN MANAGEMENT OF NEONATES WITH HRF/PH IN RESOURCE-CONSTRAINED SETTINGS

Adequate oxygenation to maintain target saturations, adequate ventilation, and provision of hemodynamic support are the keys to management.

### Oxygen Therapy

Oxygen is a powerful pulmonary vasodilator. It helps to avoid hypoxic pulmonary vasoconstriction; however, hyperoxia should be avoided since it can generate reactive oxygen species, worsen pulmonary vasoconstriction, and render other pulmonary vasodilators like iNO ineffective.[58] LMIC countries face multiple challenges in the provision and availability of oxygen itself,[59] availability of $O_2$ flow monitors, provision of humidity, patient interface devices, and important monitoring equipment like pulse oximeters, which are unavailable or insufficient in some units.

In a survey to evaluate practice variations among neonatologists in oxygen management in term neonates with pulmonary hypertension,[60] there were wide variations in target oxygen saturations; specifically, more than 70% of physicians targeted SpO$_2$ >95–98%[60] and 37% targeted PaO$_2$ 60–100 mmHg, whereas 11% targeted PaO$_2$ >120 mmHg. The weaning strategies revealed variation between clinician practices.[60] Target oxygen saturations of 90-95% are recommended in acute PH to achieve $PaO_2$ 60–90 mmHg.[46,61,62]

Useful oxygen monitoring tools for LMICs include pulse oximetry and oxygenation indices such as OI, OSI, $SpO_2$, and $PaO_2$. Evidence-based clinical practice guidelines with standardized oxygen targets, which will reduce oxygen fluctuations, practice variation, and improve outcomes, are recommended. Early transfer of a critically sick neonate to a tertiary care center, after stabilization, where better therapies and monitoring facilities are likely to be available, would be prudent.

### Inhaled Nitric Oxide (iNO)

iNO is the only FDA-approved pulmonary vasodilator in developed countries.[46,61] The major considerations in usage of iNO in LMIC countries are its cost and availability. The recommended medical-grade iNO, with impurities by other oxides of nitrogen <1%, is very expensive in India ($125/h, £80/h, or 1–1.5 lakh Indian rupees/day) and not easily available.[63] A study from India[63] has highlighted the beneficial role of industrial grade iNO (impurities of <2%) for treatment of neonates with HRF, which is much less costly. The current daily costs of treating a neonate with (industrial-grade) iNO in India is the equivalent of $320–350 (Rs. 25,000) per day, which is prohibitive in LMIC countries. In the same Indian study[63] of 25 neonates with HRF treated with iNO, 70% of neonates showed a successful response. The overall survival rate was 42% (100% iNO non-responders and 39% iNO responders did not survive). The response was superior if the etiology of HRF were secondary to MAS, RDS, and perinatal asphyxias, as compared to sepsis. In total, 30% of neonates with HRF are non-responders and need other pulmonary vasodilators.[46,61,64] This intervention, which has the potential to rapidly improve the clinical condition, however, remains unaffordable to most neonates with HRF in resource-constrained settings mainly due to the prohibitive costs of its usage.

### Pharmacological Strategies Other Than Nitric Oxide in LMIC Countries

### PDE-5 Inhibitors (Sildenafil)

Endogenous NO activates soluble guanylate cyclase (sGC), resulting in an increase in cyclic guanosine monophosphate (cGMP), which leads to pulmonary smooth muscle relaxation. Oxidative stress causes an increase in phosphodiesterase-5 (PDE-5) and phosphodiesterase-3 (PDE-3), which inactivate cGMP and cyclic adenosine monophosphate (cAMP), respectively, thereby promoting pulmonary vasoconstriction. Therefore sildenafil (selective inhibitor of endogenous PDE-5) and milrinone (selective inhibitor of PDE-3) promote vasodilatation. Sildenafil may be the ideal first-line drug in LMIC countries where iNO is not feasible. In <30% of neonates[46,61,64] who are iNO non-responders, sildenafil was shown to be a useful adjunctive therapy. Sildenafil has also been shown to reduce mortality in PH when compared to placebo (RR 0.20; 95% CI 0.07 to 0.56).[64] A pilot RCT of oral sildenafil (1–2 mg/kg every 6 hours) conducted in Colombia[65] showed improved oxygenation in neonates with severe PH compared with placebo-treated infants. The physiological parameters of OI and $PaO_2$ showed steady improvement 6–12 hours after the first dose of sildenafil. It may not be as useful in cases of PH secondary to sepsis, where the pathophysiology consists of overproduction of nitric oxide, leading to systemic vasodilation.[64] The commonest side effect of sildenafil is systemic hypotension, but in most cases treatment is usually well tolerated.

Oral sildenafil, used as the primary therapy for PH in LMIC countries in the absence of iNO, is effective and safe. Studies of IV sildenafil have shown similar benefits.[66,67] The potential benefits of sildenafil have been shown in LMICs.[68-70] In an Indian study[71] of neonates with PH, conducted over an 8-year period ($n$ = 187), oral sildenafil led to a reduction in the pulmonary pressure and improvement in $PaO_2$, $A-aDO_2$, and a/A. There is a surprising paucity of RCTs of Sildenafil in LMIC; therefore large multicenter trials are needed to determine the impact of treatment as it is a very affordable drug and currently is the first-line choice, in the absence of iNO.

### PDE-3 Inhibitors (Milrinone)

PDE 3 inhibitors, like milrinone, inhibit the breakdown of cAMP, leading to pulmonary vasodilatation. It is also an inotropic agent, with lusitropic effects, which improves ventricular function.[62] The initiation of milrinone in PH leads to an improvement in $PaO_2$ ($P$ = 0.002), a sustained reduction in $FiO_2$ ($P$ < 0.001), improvement in oxygenation index ($P < 0.001$), mean airway pressure ($P = 0.03$), and reduction in inhaled nitric oxide dose ($P < 0.001$).[72] In a three-arm RCT, sildenafil combined with milrinone was more effective in cases of PH than either drug alone in reducing PH and improving survival.[73] This study suggests that the use of milrinone in combination with sildenafil, in a resource-limited setting, has a beneficial synergistic effect with better outcomes, especially in severe PH.

## Magnesium Sulfate

Magnesium antagonizes calcium ion entry into smooth muscle cells and thus promotes vasodilatation.[74] There are published case reports and case series,[75,76] but no RCTs determining its effectiveness in newborns. With the advent of nitric oxide as a selective pulmonary vasodilator, the use of magnesium sulfate has become minimal. In preterm/term neonates with aPH ($n = 28$), administration of $MgSO_4$ led to an improvement in alveolar-arterial oxygen gradient (A-aDO$_2$) by >40%, and an increase in post-ductal $SpO_2$ by >10%.[75] Overall, 71% of neonates demonstrated a good clinical response, with 50% of patients responding within 1 hour and 35% within 1–4 hours. This study suggests that $MgSO_4$, which is a non-selective pulmonary vasodilator, may have a good clinical response in hypoxemic patients where inhaled nitric oxide is not available. Systemic hypotension (in 75% of cases) may be a limiting factor for usage.[75] This cheap and readily available drug makes it a potentially useful adjunct in LMIC countries, but more research is needed.

## Use of Surfactant therapy

In neonates with parenchymal lung disease (e.g., respiratory distress syndrome [RDS], meconium aspiration syndrome [MAS] and congenital pneumonias/sepsis) and acute PH, lung recruitment strategies and surfactant administration should be considered prior to pulmonary vasodilator therapy. While the role of surfactant in RDS is well studied, patients with MAS may also benefit from surfactant.[77,78] The use of bolus surfactant did not reduce mortality in established MAS; however, it reduced duration of hospital stay by 2–4 days (95% CI −7.11 to −2.24)[78] and reduced days of mechanical ventilation (−9.76 to −1.03).[78] This greatly impacts the cost of neonatal care in LMIC

countries and may be beneficial. However, the average weight of a late preterm/term neonate with MAS is greater; therefore the cost implications of surfactant administration in LMIC countries will need to be weighed against the benefits.

The role of surfactant administration in bacterial pneumonias remains debatable.[79] Pneumonia is known to cause secondary surfactant deficiency, through reduced surfactant production, surfactant dysfunction, inactivation, or peroxidation,[79] providing a strong rationale for its use. In a cohort of patients with early-onset pneumonia,[80] in OI (11.15-3.7, $P < 0.05$) and arterial/alveolar PO$_2$ (0.09–0.3, $P < 0.01$) there was improvement by 1 hour, whereas mean airway pressure (MAP) and FiO$_2$ (0.82–0.52) ($P < 0.01$) improved by 12 hours after surfactant. This is a simple but expensive intervention, available in LMIC settings. A cost-benefit analysis would be useful for physicians in LMIC countries.

## SUGGESTED MANAGEMENT ALGORITHM IN HRF

The choice of inotropes is determined by the pathophysiology noted on echocardiography. We suggest an integrated evaluation for neonates with HRF (Table 28.2) and a management algorithm (Table 28.4) for these neonates in the absence of inhaled nitric oxide.

## Hemodynamic Management of Perinatal Asphyxia in LMIC Countries

In HIC countries intrapartum-related injuries are rare, with a reported incidence of 1.6 cases per 1000 live births.[81] In contrast, many LMIC countries have a high burden of asphyxia, due to obstetric demand challenges (poor antenatal visit coverage, inadequate access to health care facility, and low literacy levels), obstetric supply challenges (absence of skilled birth care, poor intrapartum care), and inability to access NICU care.[81] The neonatal mortality rate is 20- to 50-fold higher than in HIC countries. Overall, 46%[82,83] of global neonatal asphyxia mortality burden is from the Sub-Saharan region. In India one of the leading causes of mortality is intrapartum-related events including perinatal asphyxia.[84]

The initial assessment in asphyxiated neonates includes integration of clinical information as done in any neonate with HRF. The likely pathophysiological mechanisms are then ascertained, to determine whether the baby has HRF due to primary lung pathology (e.g., MAS, congenital pneumonias), likely cardiac pathology, or signs of compromise to the pulmonary and systemic circulation. In a study (2018–2019) of neonates with perinatal asphyxia conducted by the Indian Neonatal Collaborative (INC), which is a network of 28 tertiary care neonatal units including public and private hospitals,[85] variation in management was noted. The incidence of hemodynamic instability can vary from 33% to 77% in asphyxiated neonates receiving therapeutic hypothermia to 25–83% in asphyxiated neonates not being cooled.[86]

## Hemodynamic Management of Gram-Negative Sepsis in LMIC Countries

The global incidence and mortality attributable to neonatal sepsis is high, particularly in LMIC countries.[87,88] In an Indian study looking at the incidence and profile of sepsis among neonates born in tertiary care NICUs,[89] 14.3% (95% CI 13.8–14.9) of neonates had a clinical illness consistent with sepsis, and 6.2% had culture-positive sepsis (95% CI 5.8–6.6). Nearly two-thirds of cases were early-onset sepsis, and 64% of the isolates were gram-negative infections (*Acinetobacter* [22%], *Klebsiella* [17%], and *Escherichia coli* [14%]).[89] Sepsis (both culture-proven and suspected sepsis) was the underlying cause of death in 24%; of note, mortality (48%) was higher if the sepsis was culture-positive.[89] In a similar study of mortality among preterm neonates <33 weeks' gestation, based on three hospital-based datasets in India,[90] 25.4% of deaths were attributed to sepsis. These data indicate the high incidence and mortality of sepsis in a country like India, where most infections are of gram-negative origin. The contributors to mortality include lack of adequate monitoring tools and multidrug resistance, which was as high as 82% in *Acinetobacter*, 54% in *Klebsiella*, and 38% in *E. coli*.[89] The findings of the Indian studies are in sharp contrast to studies from HIC countries, where late-onset sepsis was more common,[91,92] gram-positive organisms were the causative agent,[91,92] and antimicrobial resistances were comparatively low.[91,92]

## PATHOPHYSIOLOGY-BASED APPROACH TO MANAGEMENT IN NEONATAL SEPSIS

The clinical patterns of sepsis are "warm shock" and "cold shock" presentations which have been well described.[93] While "warm shock" relates to a vasodilatory state (low SVR, hypotension, bounding pulses, brisk CRT, high cardiac outputs), "cold shock" represents a vasoconstrictive state (mottled appearance, weak peripheral pulses and delayed CRT). The BP initially may be normal-high with narrow pulse pressures but the cardiac output is diminished. Clinical assessment with parameters like heart rate, CRT, urine output, and lactate, while being surrogate markers for cardiovascular wellbeing, are insufficient to determine the pathophysiological presentation of neonates with suspected sepsis. Isolated BP measurements are poor indicators of cardiac output. Therefore echocardiography, if available, has a useful role in determining the pathophysiological status of the septic neonate.

In an Indian study comparing 52 preterm infants with septic shock (the majority had warm shock) versus controls, LV output was higher in infants with sepsis versus controls (305 mL/kg/min [IQR 204, 393] vs 233 mL/kg/min [IQR 204, 302]; $P < 0.001$), ejection fraction was comparable (indicating a hyperdynamic circulation), and 60% had evidence of PDA.[94] This suggested that vasoregulatory failure (or vasodilator physiology) was the predominant pathophysiological state. Ductal patency occurs because infection promotes cyclooxygenase expression and increases prostaglandin levels.[95] Tomerak et al.[96] noted that septic preterm neonates also had evidence of some diastolic dysfunction. In another study on late-onset sepsis,[97] indices of blood flow were high (RVO 555 [133], LVO 441 [164], and SVC flow 104 [39] mL/kg/min, mean [SD]), suggesting "vasodilatation" as the primary pathophysiology. Survivors showed an increase in MBP in the first 12 hours. Pulmonary hypertension has also been reported in almost 50% of culture-proven septic neonates.[98]

The key to successful management of septic shock in neonates, besides early institution of antibiotics, is understanding the underlying pathophysiology and integrating it into the management decisions regarding choice of vasopressors and inotropes. This can be

**TABLE 28.4 Management Algorithm for Neonates Admitted With Hypoxemic Respiratory Failure in LMIC Countries**

| **Step 1: Stabilization, Lung Recruitment, Establish Diagnosis** | |
|---|---|
| Identify risk factors | Birth asphyxia<br>Meconium-stained amniotic fluid<br>Diaphragmatic hernia<br>Pulmonary hypoplasia<br>Maternal drug intake (NSAIDs, SSRIs)<br>RDS, hypothermia, acidosis of unexplained origin |
| Suspect acute pulmonary hypertension if[46]:<br>FiO$_2$ > 0.35 despite appropriate respiratory support<br>Pre-/post-ductal difference in SpO$_2$ >5% (pulse oximetry or arterial blood gases)<br>More than two unexplained desaturations (SpO$_2$ <85%) in 12 h period<br>Unexplained hypotension or poor perfusion in a patient at high risk for acute PH (e.g., perinatal asphyxia,<br>   meconium-stained liquor) | |
| Oxygen<br>Monitoring vitals<br>Lung recruitment maneuvers<br>Early surfactant administration<br>(RDS, MAS, pneumonia?)<br>Antibiotics as necessary<br>Keep Hb >12 g/dL<br>Maintain systolic BP >5th centile<br>Echocardiography<br>Early initiation of nitric oxide<br>(If OI > 15)<br>Miscellaneous | Keep SpO$_2$ 90–95%, PaO$_2$ 60–90 mmHg, PaCO$_2$ 35–45 mmHg<br>Check difference in pre-post ductal saturations (>5%) (suggests<br>   presence of a duct)<br>Chest X-ray<br>Temperature, blood sugar monitoring<br>Gentle ventilation<br>BP monitoring (keep >5th centile)<br><br><br><br>Use as 1st line if available<br><br>Central lines, cluster care<br>Sedation, as needed |
| **Step 2: Pulmonary Vasodilation, Inotropes** | |
| Oral or intravenous sildenafil<br>Consider magnesium sulfate | 1st line –if nitric oxide not available) |
| Miscellaneous | Quiet environment, minimal handling<br>Fluids, vasopressors with minimal pulmonary vasoconstriction<br>   (norepinephrine, vasopressin)<br>Avoid dopamine/high-dose epinephrine<br>Steroids if fluid and catecholamine resistant |
| **Step 3: Pathophysiology-Based Approach** | |
| Determine need for inotropes/vasopressors<br>based on pathophysiology of disease process | Vasoconstrictor physiology – dobutamine, milrinone<br>Fluids, steroids if no response<br>Vasodilator physiology – vasopressors, inotropes |
| **Step 4: Longitudinal Re-Evaluation** | |
| Repeat Echocardiography every 12–24 h | |

achieved with cardiac ultrasound performed early in the disease process, to determine whether the clinical presentation is a vasodilatory or vasoconstrictor physiology (Table 28.3). LMIC countries, where gram-negative sepsis is a major concern in NICUs, will need to generate further literature on echocardiographic variations between early versus late-onset sepsis, between gram-negative and gram-positive sepsis, and responses to the initial fluid management and vasoactive drugs.

## Case 1: Neonate With Perinatal Asphyxia With Hypoxic Respiratory Failure

A term male infant was born at a peripheral district-level hospital at 39 + 4 weeks, by emergency cesarean section, following fetal bradycardia, and meconium-stained liquor. The Apgar scores were 3, 5, and 9 at 1, 5, and 10 minutes, respectively, the cord pH was 6.9, base deficit was −16, and plasma lactate was 8 mmol/L. The baby was intubated at birth and positive pressure ventilation (PIP 22/PEEP 6 cm $H_2O$) was initiated with an $FiO_2$ of 0.9. iNO was not available and therapeutic hypothermia (TH) was not offered. The baby was transferred to a tertiary hospital and arrived by 4 hours of life.

### CLINICAL ASSESSMENT

The baby was lethargic, and hypotonic, on NICU admission. The $FiO_2$ requirements were high in order to maintain an $SpO_2$ of 90–94%. The infant developed seizures 2 hours after admission. The chest X-ray revealed features of MAS. Systolic (SBP), diastolic (DBP), mean (MBP), and pulse pressures (PP) were 36 mmHg, 28 mmHg, 30 mmHg, and 8 mmHg, respectively. The baby had labile oxygenation on handling, and there was a pre-post ductal difference in saturation of 10%. At the tertiary hospital, iNO was not available, and TH was not offered.

### CARDIAC ULTRASOUND

Cardiac ultrasound revealed the following (Figure 28.8):
  i. Preload – No IVC collapsibility (subcostal view)
  ii. Pulmonary hypertension and RV dysfunction: RV output 150 mL/kg/min (low); right ventricular systolic pressure was estimated at 50 mmHg via the tricuspid regurgitant jet peak velocity jet. Tricuspid annular plane systolic excursion (TAPSE) was consistent with impaired RV performance
  iii. Low LV output 140 mL/kg/min and impaired LV systolic performance (fractional shortening of 15.5%)
  iv. Evidence of RV and LV diastolic dysfunction was seen
  v. Shunt appraisal: Ductus arteriosus flow – predominantly right to left, PFO flow was left to right with a small shunt volume

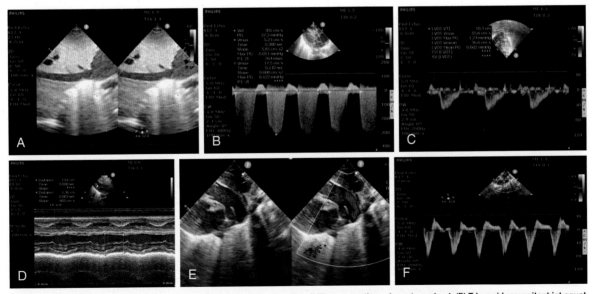

**Fig. 28.8** (A) Prominent inferior vena cava in subcostal view, with no collapsibility, suggesting adequate preload. (B) Tricuspid regurgitant jet equating to pulmonary systolic pressure of 50 mmHg. (C) LV velocity time integral (VTI) is 10.3 cm, suggesting low left ventricular output (LVO – 140 mL/kg/min). (D) Reduced fractional shortening (15.5%) suggesting LV systolic dysfunction. (E) Right-to-left ductal shunting indicating that pulmonary pressures are supra-systemic (F) Duct Doppler shows predominantly right-to-left duct suggesting high pulmonary pressures.

## ANALYSIS

This is a term infant with HRF and MAS and evidence of hypoxic-ischemic encephalopathy (HIE). The baby had systemic hypotension (<3rd centile), with supra-systemic pulmonary hypertension and biventricular dysfunction. The high lactate suggested poor tissue perfusion. The calculated systemic vascular resistance is high, indicating a *vasoconstrictor* physiology.

## THERAPEUTIC GOALS/MANAGEMENT

- Ventilation was optimized in view of parenchymal lung disease with the infant switched to high-frequency oscillatory ventilation.
- Fluid boluses were avoided, since myocardial contractility was poor, and the inferior vena cava appeared full on echocardiography.
- In view of the hypotension and myocardial dysfunction, a drug with inotropic and vaso-pressor effect was chosen (low dose epinephrine upto a maximum of 0.1 mcg/kg/min) to minimize pulmonary vasoconstriction. Dopamine was avoided because of its potential pulmonary vasoconstricting effects at higher doses (at least in animal models). Milrinone was not considered, specifically due to concerns about impaired liver metabolism and renal excretion in babies with HIE, particularly if cooling was offered.[99]
- As the ultrasound findings were consistent with LV impairment from ventricular interdependance rather than primary LV dysfunction, sildenafil was added to decrease PVR and improve pulmonary blood flow since iNO was not available.

## TRENDS AND OUTCOME

There was a slow improvement in BP and lactate levels normalized within 36 hours, so epinephrine and sildenafil were tapered and ceased. The ventilator settings were reduced and the infant was stabilized. The baby was discharged by postnatal day 20.

## Case 2: Preterm Neonate With Sepsis

A preterm male neonate, born at 28 + 4 weeks, weighing 800 g at birth, developed apnea on postnatal day 21 and was noticed to be lethargic, tachypneic, and tachycardic (HR 180 bpm) and needed mechanical ventilation. The arterial gases revealed a metabolic acidosis. There was a central venous line in situ, since the baby had multiple episodes of feeding intolerance and had not reached full feeds.

## CLINICAL ASSESSMENT

The baby had bounding pulses and adequate perfusion. There was no murmur. SBP, DBP, MBP, and pulse pressure were 40 mmHg, 19 mmHg, 25 mmHg, and 21 mmHg, respectively. The baby was commenced on antibiotics after taking appropriate cultures. The lumbar puncture was diagnostic of meningitis.

## CARDIAC ULTRASOUND

The initial cardiac ultrasound revealed (Figure 28.9):
  i. Pericardial effusion was ruled out and preload assessment appeared unremarkable.
  ii. Ventricular function: LV output was high (420 mL/kg/day). Subjective assessment of the LV function suggested hyperdynamic performance. RV output was normal.
  iii. Pulmonary arterial pressure as estimated by the peak velocity of the tricuspid regurgitation jet was raised (40 mmHg) and TAPSE was suggestive of normal RV systolic performance for gestational age.
  iv. Shunt appraisal: The ductus arteriosus was closed, and the PFO showed a small left-to-right shunt.

## ANALYSIS

This preterm baby showed a sudden clinical deterioration with widened pulse pressures. The LV output was high, suggesting *vasodilator* physiology. The ductus arteriosus was closed, and there were features of raised pulmonary pressures, possibly as a result of sepsis.

## THERAPEUTIC GOALS/MANAGEMENT

- 20 mL/kg normal saline was given as a bolus in view of the low SVR state.
- Antibiotics were commenced after all the appropriate cultures were taken and ventilation was optimized.
- In view of the diastolic hypotension, vasopressor support was started (noradrenaline). Dopamine was avoided in view of its potential pulmonary vasoconstricting effects at higher doses.
- Sequential BP monitoring was done and the baby was frequently assessed for signs of shock.

## TRENDS AND OUTCOME

The baby's condition continued to deteriorate; he developed oliguria, delayed perfusion, hypotension, and worsening acidosis, suggesting progression to septic shock. Serial echocardiograms revealed fall in the LV outputs, worsening diastolic dysfunction, and worsening TAPSE. The baby was started on inotropes (epinephrine) in addition to the norepinephrine. The blood culture showed growth of gram-negative bacillus *Acinetobacter*. The baby died 3 days after commencement of management.

## Training and Accreditation for Clinician-Performed Ultrasound or Echocardiography in LMIC Countries

Clinician-performed ultrasound (CPU) is increasingly being recognized as an important bedside hemodynamic monitoring tool for the neonate and is gaining wide acceptance. While there are established training programs in HIC countries,[100-102] access to training in LMIC countries has been limited so far.[103] In a survey conducted by the authors[55] only 25% of the neonatologists performing ultrasounds had undergone a structured and certified training course. Only 9 units of the 148 respondents completed a formal training program (ranging from <1 month (22%) to 6–12 months (33%). So far, India, with its vast pool of qualified neonatologists, does not have an accredited program with a formal curriculum for either CPU or neonatal hemodynamics. In contrast, the benefits of having a structured training program were noted in a Canadian center[104] performing targeted neonatal echocardiography (TnECHO), where 48% of echocardiograms were followed by a change in clinical management within 6 hours. An appropriately

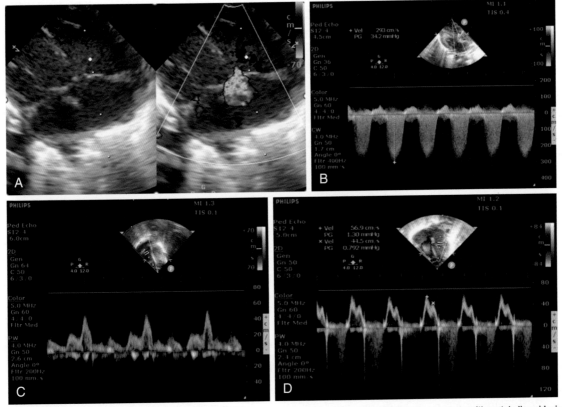

**Fig. 28.9** (A, B) Presence of tricuspid regurgitant jet with high pulmonary pressures on Day of life (DOL) 21 in a neonate with metabolic acidosis raised suspicion of sepsis. (C) Tricuspid valve showed a low E:A ratio (0.5:1), which suggested mild diastolic dysfunction. (D) A simultaneous mitral valve E:A ratio (1.27) also suggested impaired diastolic function.

*Continued on following page*

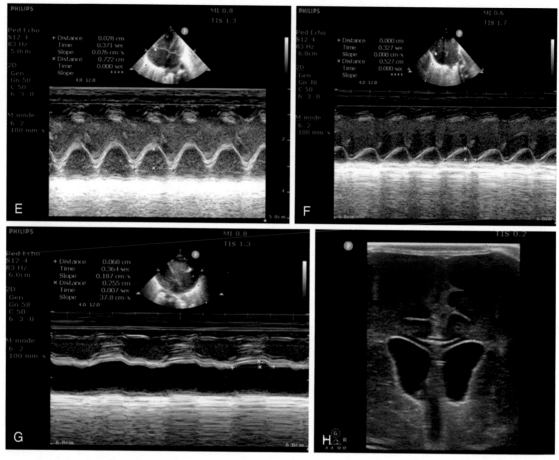

**Fig. 28.9, cont'd** (E) Tricuspid annular plane systolic excursion (TAPSE) was initially normal (F, G) TAPSE progressively worsened over the next 48–72 hours (from 7.2 mm [*Panel E*] to 2.7 mm [*Panels F and G*]). (H) Cranial ultrasound showed ventriculitis and ventriculomegaly. The baby died on day 24 of life due to *Acinetobacter* sepsis with meningitis.

structured training program is necessary for clinicians, in order to ensure that the measurements and data collection are robust, accurate, and reliable. With the otherwise limited available resources for hemodynamic monitoring and monitoring tools in LMIC countries, the benefits of POCUS and potential value to patient outcomes are immense. The requirements for formal training are discussed further in Chapter 9.

While image acquisition and optimization are the initial steps of the hemodynamics evaluation, physiologic information must be thoughtfully integrated within the clinical context to formulate a

diagnostic impression and medical recommendations to enhance patient outcomes. Comprehensive, advanced hemodynamics programs (Table 28.5) have been successfully implemented in North America[104] and Australia and serve as a role model for LMIC countries (Table 28.5).

## Status of Pediatric Cardiac Care in LMIC Countries[105-107]

The status of pediatric cardiac care in an LMIC country like India has been compared with a HIC country like the United States. There is a staggering shortfall of

**TABLE 28.5 Comparison of Training Programs for Neonatal Clinician-Performed Ultrasound**

| | India (Proposed Model) | Australia | North America |
|---|---|---|---|
| Course Name | FNPU<br>Fellowship in Neonatologist Performed Ultrasound | CCPU<br>Certificate in Clinician Performed Ultrasound | TnECHO<br>Targeted Neonatal Echocardiography |
| Duration | 6 months | 1–3 years | 1 year |
| Number of imaging Assessments | 100 | 75 | 300 |
| Pediatric Cardiologist as Team Member | Essential | Preferred | Preferred |
| No. of Supervisors | 2 + 1 | 1 | 1 |
| Site of Training | On and off site | On and off site | On site |
| Maintenance of Certification | NIL | 25 cases each year for 5 years | NIL |
| Log Book | Mandatory | Mandatory | Mandatory |

pediatric cardiology services that impact neonatal cardiac care and serves as an endorsement for neonatal hemodynamics training in LMICs to aid improvement in clinical outcomes.

## Conclusion

LMIC countries face enormous challenges in the delivery of neonatal care, and some of the significant treatment modalities are unavailable. Clinical parameters alone are inadequate to assess the hemodynamic status of a critically sick neonate, and more objective tools like cardiac ultrasound are useful. Structured training programs in cardiac ultrasound would be a strong addition to the armamentarium of the clinician in resource-restricted countries. Clinicians need to undertake an integrated evaluation of the clinical status, and cardiac ultrasound, to determine the disease pathophysiology, which aids in management decisions.

## REFERENCES

1. Franzen SRP, Chandler C, Lang T. Health research capacity development in low-and-middle income countries: reality or rhetoric? A systematic meta-narrative review of the qualitative literature. *BMJ Open.* 2017;7(1):e012332. doi:10.1136/bmjopen-2016-012332.
2. United Nations Children's Fund. *The State of the World's Children 2021: On My Mind-Promoting, protecting and caring for children's mental health.* New York: UNICEF; October 2021.
3. Stranak Z, Semberova J, Barrington K, et al. International survey on diagnosis and management of hypotension in extremely preterm babies. *Eur J Pediatr.* 2014;173(6):793-798. doi:10.1007/s00431-013-2251-9.
4. Dempsey EM, Barrington KJ. Diagnostic criteria and therapeutic interventions for the hypotensive very low birth weight infant. *J Perinatol.* 2006;26(11):677-681. doi:10.1038/sj.jp.7211579.
5. Sehgal A, Osborn D, McNamara PJ. Cardiovascular support in preterm infants: a survey of practices in Australia and New Zealand. *J Paediatr Child Health.* 2012;48(4):317-323. doi:10.1111/j.1440-1754.2011.02246.x.
6. Osborn DA, Evans N, Kluckow M. Clinical detection of low upper body blood flow in very premature infants using blood pressure, capillary refill time, and central-peripheral temperature difference. *Arch Dis Child Fetal Neonatal Ed.* 2004;89(2):168F-F173. doi:10.1136/adc.2002.023796.
7. Subhedar N. Treatment of hypotension in newborns. *Semin Neonatol.* 2003;8(6):413-423. doi:10.1016/S1084-2756(03)00117-9.
8. Munro MJ, Walker AM, Barfield CP. Hypotensive extremely low birth weight infants have reduced cerebral blood flow. *Pediatrics.* 2004;114(6):1591-1596. doi:10.1542/peds.2004-1073.
9. Børch K, Lou HC, Greisen G. Cerebral white matter blood flow and arterial blood pressure in preterm infants. *Acta Paediatr.* 2010;99(10):1489-1492. doi:10.1111/j.1651-2227.2010.01856.x.
10. Pickering TG, Hall JE, Appel LJ, et al. Recommendations for blood pressure measurement in humans: an AHA scientific statement from the council on high blood pressure research professional and public education subcommittee. *J Clin Hypertens.* 2005;7(2):102-109. doi:10.1111/j.1524-6175.2005.04377.x.
11. Dempsey E, Seri I. Definition of normal blood pressure range: the elusive target. In: Elsevier, ed. *Hemodynamics and Cardiology: Neonatology Questions and Controversies.* 3rd ed. Philadelphia: Elsevier; 2019:47.

12. Dasnadi S, Aliaga S, Laughon M, Warner D, Price W. Factors influencing the accuracy of noninvasive blood pressure measurements in NICU infants. *Am J Perinatol.* 2014;32(7): 639-644. doi:10.1055/s-0034-1390345.

13. Golombek SG, Young JN. Efficacy of inhaled nitric oxide for hypoxic respiratory failure in term and late preterm infants by baseline severity of illness: a pooled analysis of three clinical trials. *Clin Ther.* 2010;32(5):939-948. doi:10.1016/j.clinthera.2010.04.023.

14. Rawat M, Chandrasekharan PK, Williams A, et al. Oxygen saturation index and severity of hypoxic respiratory failure. *Neonatology.* 2015;107(3):161-166. doi:10.1159/000369774.

15. Doreswamy SM, Chakkarapani AA, Murthy P. Oxygen saturation index, a noninvasive tool for monitoring hypoxemic respiratory failure in newborns. *Indian Pediatr.* 2016;53(5): 432-433.

16. Muniraman HK, Song AY, Ramanathan R, et al. Evaluation of oxygen saturation index compared with oxygenation index in neonates with hypoxemic respiratory failure. *JAMA Netw Open.* 2019;2(3):e191179. doi:10.1001/jamanetworkopen.2019.1179.

17. Gupta S, Donn SM. Assessment of neonatal perfusion. *Semin Fetal Neonatal Med.* 2020;25(5):101144. doi:10.1016/j.siny.2020.101144.

18. Leflore JL, Engle WD. Capillary refill time is an unreliable indicator of cardiovascular status in term neonates. *Adv Neonatal Care.* 2005;5(3):147-154. doi:10.1016/j.adnc.2005.02.008.

19. Pinto Lima A, Beelen P, Bakker J. Use of a peripheral perfusion index derived from the pulse oximetry signal as a noninvasive indicator of perfusion. *Crit Care Med.* 2002;30(6):1210-1213. doi:10.1097/00003246-200206000-00006.

20. Alderliesten T, Lemmers PMA, Baerts W, Groenendaal F, van Bel F. Perfusion Index in preterm infants during the first 3 days of life: reference values and relation with clinical variables. *Neonatology.* 2015;107(4):258-265. doi:10.1159/000370192.

21. de Felice C, Latini G, Vacca P, Kopotic RJ. The pulse oximeter perfusion index as a predictor for high illness severity in neonates. *Eur J Pediatr.* 2002;161(10):561-562. doi:10.1007/s00431-002-1042-5.

22. McGrath SP, Ryan KL, Wendelken SM, Rickards CA, Convertino VA. Pulse oximeter plethysmographic waveform changes in awake, spontaneously breathing, hypovolemic volunteers. *Anesth Analg.* 2011;112(2):368-374. doi:10.1213/ANE.0b013e3181cb3f4a.

23. Partridge BL. Use of pulse oximetry as a noninvasive indicator of intravascular volume status. *J Clin Monit.* 1987;3(4):263-268.

24. Pawale D, Murki S, Kulkarni D, et al. Plethysmography variability index (PVI) changes in preterm neonates with shock – an observational study. *Eur J Pediatr.* 2021;180(2):379-385. doi:10.1007/s00431-020-03749-7.

25. Vidal M, Ferragu F, Durand S, Baleine J, Batista-Novais AR, Cambonie G. Perfusion index and its dynamic changes in preterm neonates with patent ductus arteriosus. *Acta Paediatr.* 2013;102(4):373-378. doi:10.1111/apa.12130.

26. Raja DJA, Balasankar DS, Mathiarasan DrK. Perfusion index and Plethysmographic variability index values in spontaneously breathing clinically stable term neonates in room air in the first 10 days of life. *Pediatric Rev Int J Pediatric Res.* 2017;4(8):531-536. doi:10.17511/ijpr.2017.i08.06.

27. Latini G, Dipaola L, de Felice C. First day of life reference values for pleth variability index in spontaneously breathing term newborns. *Neonatology.* 2012;101(3):179-182. doi:10.1159/000331774.

28. Deshpande SA, Platt MPW. Association between blood lactate and acid-base status and mortality in ventilated babies. *Arch Dis Child Fetal Neonatal Ed.* 1997;76(1):F15-F20. doi:10.1136/fn.76.1.F15.

29. Rodríguez-Balderrama I, Ostia-Garza PJ, Villarreal-Parra RD, Tijerina-Guajardo M. Risk factors and the relation of lactic acid to neonatal mortality in the first week of life. *Medicina Universitaria.* 2016;18(70):3-9. doi:10.1016/j.rmu.2015.12.001.

30. Singh Y, Villaescusa JU, da Cruz EM, et al. Recommendations for hemodynamic monitoring for critically ill children – expert consensus statement issued by the cardiovascular dynamics section of the European Society of Paediatric and Neonatal Intensive Care (ESPNIC). *Crit Care.* 2020;24(1):620. doi:10.1186/s13054-020-03326-2.

31. Singh Y. Echocardiographic evaluation of hemodynamics in neonates and children. *Front Pediatr.* 2017;5:201. doi:10.3389/fped.2017.00201.

32. Lang RM, Bierig M, Devereux RB, et al. Recommendations for chamber quantification: a report from the American Society of Echocardiography's Guidelines and Standards Committee and the Chamber Quantification Writing Group, developed in Conjunction with the European Association of Echocardiography, a Branch of the European Society of Cardiology. *J Am Soc Echocardiogr.* 2005;18(12):1440-1463. doi:10.1016/j.echo.2005.10.005.

33. Slama M, Masson H, Teboul JL, et al. Respiratory variations of aortic VTI: a new index of hypovolemia and fluid responsiveness. *Am J Physiol Heart Circ Physiol.* 2002;283(4): H1729-H1733. doi:10.1152/ajpheart.00308.2002.

34. Feissel M, Mangin I, Ruyer O, Faller JP, Michard F, Teboul JL. Respiratory changes in aortic blood velocity as an indicator of fluid responsiveness in ventilated patients with septic shock. *Chest.* 2001;119(3):867-873. doi:10.1378/chest.119.3.867.

35. Kluckow M. Use of ultrasound in the haemodynamic assessment of the sick neonate. *Arch Dis Child Fetal Neonatal Ed.* 2014;99(4):F332-F337. doi:10.1136/archdischild-2013-304926.

36. Tissot C, Singh Y, Sekarski N. Echocardiographic evaluation of ventricular function – for the neonatologist and pediatric intensivist. *Front Pediatr.* 2018;6:79. doi:10.3389/fped.2018.00079.

37. Groves AM, Kuschel CA, Knight DB, Skinner JR. Echocardiographic assessment of blood flow volume in the superior vena cava and descending aorta in the newborn infant. *Arch Dis Child Fetal Neonatal Ed.* 2008;93(1):F24-F28. doi:10.1136/adc.2006.109512.

38. Lee A, Liestol K, Nestaas E, Brunvand L, Lindemann R, Fugelseth D. Superior vena cava flow: feasibility and reliability of the off-line analyses. *Arch Dis Child Fetal Neonatal Ed.* 2010; 95(2):F121-F125. doi:10.1136/adc.2009.176883.

39. de Boode WP, van der Lee R, Horsberg Eriksen B, et al. The role of neonatologist performed echocardiography in the assessment and management of neonatal shock. *Pediatr Res.* 2018; 84(suppl 1):57-67. doi:10.1038/s41390-018-0081-1.

40. El-Khuffash AF, McNamara PJ. Neonatologist-performed functional echocardiography in the neonatal intensive care unit. *Semin Fetal Neonatal Med.* 2011;16(1):50-60. doi:10.1016/j.siny.2010.05.001.

41. Singh Y, Gupta S, Groves AM, et al. Expert consensus statement "Neonatologist-performed Echocardiography (NoPE)" – training and accreditation in UK. *Eur J Pediatr.* 2016;175(2): 281-287. doi:10.1007/s00431-015-2633-2.

42. Kluckow M, Seri I, Evans N. Echocardiography and the Neonatologist. *Pediatr Cardiol.* 2008;29(6):1043-1047. doi:10.1007/s00246-008-9275-3.

43. Weindling M, Paize F. Peripheral haemodynamics in newborns: best practice guidelines. *Early Hum Dev.* 2010;86(3):159-165. doi:10.1016/j.earlhumdev.2010.01.033.

44. Azhibekov T, Noori S, Soleymani S, Seri I. Transitional cardiovascular physiology and comprehensive hemodynamic monitoring in the neonate: relevance to research and clinical care. *Semin Fetal Neonatal Med.* 2014;19(1):45-53. doi:10.1016/j.siny.2013.09.009.

45. Noori S, McCoy M, Anderson MP, Ramji F, Seri I. Changes in cardiac function and cerebral blood flow in relation to peri/intraventricular hemorrhage in extremely preterm infants. *J Pediatr.* 2014;164(2):264-270.e3. doi:10.1016/j.jpeds.2013.09.045.

46. Jain A, Giesinger RE, Dakshinamurti S, et al. Care of the critically ill neonate with hypoxemic respiratory failure and acute pulmonary hypertension: framework for practice based on consensus opinion of neonatal hemodynamics working group. *J Perinatol.* 2022;42(1):3-13. doi:10.1038/s41372-021-01296-z.

47. Shivananda S, Ahliwahlia L, Kluckow M, Luc J, Jankov R, McNamara P. Variation in the management of persistent pulmonary hypertension of the newborn: a survey of physicians in Canada, Australia, and New Zealand. *Am J Perinatol.* 2012;29(7):519-526. doi:10.1055/s-0032-1310523.

48. Nakwan N. The practical challenges of diagnosis and treatment options in persistent pulmonary hypertension of the newborn: a developing country's perspective. *Am J Perinatol.* 2018; 35(14):1366-1375. doi:10.1055/s-0038-1660462.

49. Sardar S, Pal S, Mishra R. A retrospective study on the profile of persistent pulmonary hypertension of newborn in a tertiary care unit of Eastern India. *J Clin Neonatol.* 2020;9(1):18. doi:10.4103/jcn.JCN_68_19.

50. Panda SK, Mohakud NK, Rath S, Panda SS, Nayak MK. Clinical outcomes of neonates with persistent pulmonary hypertension in a teaching hospital, Eastern India. *Sri Lanka J Child Health.* 2021;50(2):272-279.

51. Nakwan N, Jain S, Kumar K, et al. An Asian multicenter retrospective study on persistent pulmonary hypertension of the newborn: incidence, etiology, diagnosis, treatment and outcome. *J Matern Fetal Neonatal Med.* 2020;33(12):2032-2037. doi:10.1080/14767058.2018.1536740.

52. Razzaq A, Quddusi AI, Nizami N. Risk factors and mortality among newborns with persistent pulmonary hypertension. *Pak J Med Sci.* 2013;29(5):1099-1104. doi:10.12669/pjms.295.3728.

53. Mohsen AA, Amin A. Risk factors and outcomes of persistent pulmonary hypertension of the newborn in neonatal intensive care unit of Al-Minya University Hospital in Egypt. *J Clin Neonatol.* 2013;2(2):78. doi:10.4103/2249-4847.116406.

54. Rocha G, Baptista MJ, Guimarães H. Persistent pulmonary hypertension of non cardiac cause in a neonatal intensive care unit. *Pulm Med.* 2012;2012:818971. doi:10.1155/2012/818971.

55. Deshpande S, Suryawanshi P, Sharma N, et al. Survey of point-of-care ultrasound uptake in Indian neonatal intensive care units: results and recommendations. *J Neonatol.* 2019;33(1–4): 13-21. doi:10.1177/0973217919897855.

56. Khamkar AM, Suryawanshi PB, Maheshwari R, et al. Functional neonatal echocardiography: Indian experience. *J Clin Diagnostic Res.* 2015;9(12):SC11-SC14. doi:10.7860/JCDR/2015/14440.6971.

57. de Boode WP, Singh Y, Molnar Z, et al. Application of neonatologist performed echocardiography in the assessment and management of persistent pulmonary hypertension of the newborn. *Pediatr Res.* 2018;84(suppl 1):68-77. doi:10.1038/s41390-018-0082-0.

58. Lakshminrusimha S, Swartz DD, Gugino SF, et al. Oxygen concentration and pulmonary hemodynamics in newborn lambs with pulmonary hypertension. *Pediatr Res.* 2009; 66(5):539-544. doi:10.1203/PDR.0b013e3181bab0c7.

59. Zelasko J, Omotayo MO, Berkelhamer SK, et al. Neonatal oxygen therapy in low- and middle-income countries: a pragmatic review. *J Glob Health Rep.* 2020;4:1-4. doi:10.29392/001c.12346.

60. Alapati D, Jassar R, Shaffer T. Management of supplemental oxygen for infants with persistent pulmonary hypertension of newborn: a survey. *Am J Perinatol.* 2016;34(3):276-282. doi:10.1055/s-0036-1586754.

61. Sharma M, Callan E, Konduri GG. Pulmonary vasodilator therapy in persistent pulmonary hypertension of the newborn. *Clin Perinatol.* 2022;49(1):103-125. doi:10.1016/j.clp.2021.11.010.

62. Rath C, Kluckow M. Pathophysiologically based management of persistent pulmonary hypertension of the newborn. In: Seri I, Kluckow M, eds. *Hemodynamics and Cardiology: Neonatology Questions and Controversies.* 3rd ed. Philadelphia: Elsevier; 2019:155-176.

63. Razak A, Nagesh NK, Venkatesh HA, Snehal D. Inhaled nitric oxide in neonates with severe hypoxic respiratory failure-early Indian experience. *J Neonatol.* 2013;27(2):1-3. doi:10.1177/0973217920130201.

64. Kelly LE, Ohlsson A, Shah PS. Sildenafil for pulmonary hypertension in neonates. *Cochrane Database Syst Rev.* 2017;8(8):CD005494. doi:10.1002/14651858.CD005494.pub4.

65. Baquero H, Soliz A, Neira F, Venegas ME, Sola A. Oral sildenafil in infants with persistent pulmonary hypertension of the newborn: a pilot randomized blinded study. *Pediatrics.* 2006;117(4): 1077-1083. doi:10.1542/peds.2005-0523.

66. Steinhorn RH, Kinsella JP, Pierce C, et al. Intravenous sildenafil in the treatment of neonates with persistent pulmonary hypertension. *J Pediatr.* 2009;155(6):841-847.e1. doi:10.1016/j.jpeds.2009.06.012.

67. Lakshminrusimha S, Mathew B, Leach CL. Pharmacologic strategies in neonatal pulmonary hypertension other than nitric oxide. *Semin Perinatol.* 2016;40(3):160-173. doi:10.1053/j.semperi.2015.12.004.

68. Daga S, Verma B, Valvi C. Sildenafil for pulmonary hypertension in non-ventilated preterm babies. *Internet J Pediatr Neonatol.* 2007;8(1):1-4.

69. Thandaveshwara D, Krishnegowda S, Hosur D, Doreswamy SM. Effect of sildenafil on mortality in term neonates with hypoxemic respiratory failure due to persistent pulmonary hypertension (SIPHON) – a randomised control trial. *J Nepal Paediatr Soc.* 2021;41(2):177-183. doi:10.3126/jnps.v41i2.32403.

70. Singh P, Upadhyay J, Digal KC, Shrivastava Y, Basu S. Oral sildenafil therapy for the management of mild persistent pulmonary hypertension of the newborn in term neonates. *Indian J Child Health (Bhopal).* 2020;7(10):415-417. doi:10.32677/IJCH.2020.v07.i10.005.

71. Prithviraj D, Reddy B, Abhijit D, Reddy R. Oral sildenafil in persistent pulmonary hypertension of the newborn in invasive and non-invasive ventilated babies-its effect on oxygenation indices. *Int J Sci Study.* 2016;4(2):203-209.

72. McNamara PJ, Shivananda SP, Sahni M, Freeman D, Taddio A. Pharmacology of milrinone in neonates with persistent pulmonary hypertension of the newborn and suboptimal response to inhaled nitric oxide. *Pediatr Criti Care Med.* 2013;14(1):74-84. doi:10.1097/PCC.0b013e31824ea2cd.

73. El-Ghandour M, Hammad B, Ghanem M, Antonios MAM. Efficacy of milrinone plus sildenafil in the treatment of neonates with persistent pulmonary hypertension in resource-limited settings: results of a randomized, double-blind trial. *Pediatr Drugs.* 2020;22(6):685-693. doi:10.1007/s40272-020-00412-4.

74. Patole SK, Finer NN. Experimental and clinical effects of magnesium infusion in the treatment of neonatal pulmonary hypertension. *Magnes Res.* 1995;8(4):373-388.

75. Rajadurai VS, Ngiam N, Agarwal P, Tan TH. Magnesium sulphate infusion for the treatment of persistent pulmonary hypertension of the newborn. *Pediatr Res.* 1999;45(4, Part 2 of 2):316A. doi:10.1203/00006450-199904020-01882.

76. Abdelkreem E, Mahmoud SM, Aboelez MO, Abd El Aal M. Nebulized magnesium sulfate for treatment of persistent pulmonary hypertension of newborn: a pilot randomized controlled trial. *Indian J Pediatr.* 2021;88(8):771-777. doi:10.1007/s12098-020-03643-y.

77. el Shahed AI, Dargaville PA, Ohlsson A, Soll R. Surfactant for meconium aspiration syndrome in term and late preterm infants. *Cochrane Database Syst Rev.* 2014;(12):CD002054. doi:10.1002/14651858.CD002054.pub3.

78. Natarajan CK, Sankar MJ, Jain K, Agarwal R, Paul VK. Surfactant therapy and antibiotics in neonates with meconium aspiration syndrome: a systematic review and meta-analysis. *J Perinatol.* 2016;36(suppl 1):S49-S54. doi:10.1038/jp.2016.32.

79. Tan K, Lai NM, Sharma A. Surfactant for bacterial pneumonia in late preterm and term infants. *Cochrane Database Syst Rev.* 2012;(2):CD008155. doi:10.1002/14651858.CD008155.pub2.

80. Deshpande S, Suryawanshi P, Ahya K, Maheshwari R, Gupta S. Surfactant therapy for early onset pneumonia in late preterm and term neonates needing mechanical ventilation. *J Clin Diagnostic Res.* 2017;11(8):SC09-SC12. doi:10.7860/JCDR/2017/28523.10520.

81. Lee AC, Kozuki N, Blencowe H, et al. Intrapartum-related neonatal encephalopathy incidence and impairment at regional and global levels for 2010 with trends from 1990. *Pediatr Res.* 2013;74(suppl 1):50-72. doi:10.1038/pr.2013.206.

82. Ahmed I, Ali SM, Amenga-Etego S, et al. Population-based rates, timing, and causes of maternal deaths, stillbirths, and neonatal deaths in South Asia and Sub-Saharan Africa: a multi-country prospective cohort study. *Lancet Glob Health.* 2018;6(12):e1297-e1308. doi:10.1016/S2214-109X(18)30385-1.

83. Usman F, Imam A, Farouk ZL, Dayyabu AL. Newborn mortality in Sub-Saharan Africa: why is perinatal asphyxia still a major cause? *Ann Glob Health.* 2019;85(1):112. doi:10.5334/aogh.2541.

84. Liu L, Chu Y, Oza S, et al. National, regional, and state-level all-cause and cause-specific under-5 mortality in India in 2000–15: a systematic analysis with implications for the sustainable development goals. *Lancet Global Health.* 2019;7(6):e721-e724.

85. Kumar C, Peruri G, Plakkal N, Oleti TP, Aradhya AS, Tandur B. Short-term outcome and predictors of survival among neonates with moderate or severe hypoxic ischemic encephalopathy: data from the Indian neonatal collaborative. *Indian Pediatr.* 2022;59(1):21-24.

86. Giesinger RE, Bailey LJ, Deshpande P, McNamara PJ. Hypoxic-ischemic encephalopathy and therapeutic hypothermia: the hemodynamic perspective. *J Pediatr.* 2017;180:22-30.e2. doi:10.1016/j.jpeds.2016.09.009.

87. Zaidi AK, Huskins WC, Thaver D, Bhutta ZA, Abbas Z, Goldmann DA. Hospital-acquired neonatal infections in developing countries. *Lancet.* 2005;365(9465):1175-1188. doi:10.1016/S0140-6736(05)71881-X.

88. Popescu CR, Cavanagh MMM, Tembo B, et al. Neonatal sepsis in low-income countries: epidemiology, diagnosis and prevention. *Expert Rev Anti Infect Ther.* 2020;18(5):443-452. doi:10.1080/14787210.2020.1732818.

89. Investigators of the Delhi Neonatal Infection Study (DeNIS) Collaboration. Characterisation and antimicrobial resistance of sepsis pathogens in neonates born in tertiary care centres in Delhi, India: a cohort study. *Lancet Glob Health.* 2016;4(10):e752-e760. doi:10.1016/S2214-109X(16)30148-6.

90. Jain K, Sankar MJ, Nangia S, et al. Causes of death in preterm neonates (<33 weeks) born in tertiary care hospitals in India: analysis of three large prospective multicentric cohorts. *J Perinatol.* 2019;39(suppl 1):13-19. doi:10.1038/s41372-019-0471-1.

91. Vergnano S, Menson E, Kennea N, et al. Neonatal infections in England: the NeonIN surveillance network. *Arch Dis Child Fetal Neonatal Ed.* 2011;96(1):F9-F14. doi:10.1136/adc.2009.178798.

92. Stoll BJ, Hansen N, Fanaroff AA, et al. Late-onset sepsis in very low birth weight neonates: the experience of the NICHD neonatal research network. *Pediatrics.* 2002;110(2):285-291. doi:10.1542/peds.110.2.285.

93. Kharrat A, Jain A. Hemodynamic dysfunction in neonatal sepsis. *Pediatr Res.* 2022;91(2):413-424. doi:10.1038/s41390-021-01855-2.

94. Saini SS, Kumar P, Kumar RM. Hemodynamic changes in preterm neonates with septic shock. *Pediatr Crit Care Med.* 2014;15(5):443-450. doi:10.1097/PCC.0000000000000115.

95. Kim ES, Kim EK, Choi CW, et al. Intrauterine inflammation as a risk factor for persistent ductus arteriosus patency after cyclooxygenase inhibition in extremely low birth weight infants. *J Pediatr.* 2010;157(5):745-750.e1. doi:10.1016/j.jpeds.2010.05.020.

96. Tomerak RH, El-Badawy AA, Hussein G, Kamel NRM, Razak ARA. Echocardiogram done early in neonatal sepsis. *J Investig Med.* 2012;60(4):680-684. doi:10.2310/JIM.0b013e318249fc95.

97. de Waal K, Evans N. Hemodynamics in preterm infants with late-onset sepsis. *J Pediatr.* 2010;156(6):918-922.e1. doi:10.1016/j.jpeds.2009.12.026.

98. Deshpande S, Suryawanshi P, Holkar S, et al. Pulmonary hypertension in late onset neonatal sepsis using functional echocardiography: a prospective study. *J Ultrasound.* 2022;25(2):233-239. doi:10.1007/s40477-021-00590-y.

99. Bischoff AR, Habib S, McNamara PJ, Giesinger RE. Hemodynamic response to milrinone for refractory hypoxemia during therapeutic hypothermia for neonatal hypoxic ischemic encephalopathy. *J Perinatol.* 2021;41(9):2345-2354. doi:10.1038/s41372-021-01049-y.

100. Australasian Society for Ultrasound in Medicine. *Certificate in Clinician Performed Ultrasound.* Available at: https://www.asum.com.au/education/ccpu-course/neonatal-ccpu-course.

101. Mertens L, Seri I, Marek J, et al. Targeted neonatal echocardiography in the neonatal intensive care unit: practice guidelines and recommendations for training: writing group of the American Society of Echocardiography (ASE) in collaboration with the European Association of Echocardiography (EAE) and the Association for European Pediatric Cardiologists (AEPC). *Eur J Echocardiogr.* 2011;12(10):715-736. doi:10.1093/ejechocard/jer181.

102. de Boode WP, Singh Y, Gupta S, et al. Recommendations for neonatologist performed echocardiography in Europe:

consensus statement endorsed by European Society for Paediatric Research (ESPR) and European Society for Neonatology (ESN). *Pediatr Res*. 2016;80(4):465-471. doi:10.1038/pr.2016.126.

103. Muhame RM, Dragulescu A, Nadimpalli A, et al. Cardiac point of care ultrasound in resource limited settings to manage children with congenital and acquired heart disease. *Cardiol Young*. 2021;31(10):1651-1657. doi:10.1017/S1047951121000834.

104. Papadhima I, Louis D, Purna J, et al. Targeted neonatal echocardiography (TNE) consult service in a large tertiary perinatal center in Canada. *J Perinatol*. 2018;38(8):1039-1045. doi:10.1038/s41372-018-0130-y.

105. Saxena A. Congenital heart disease in India: a status report. *Indian Pediatr*. 2018;55(12):1075-1082.

106. Hoffman JIE. The global burden of congenital heart disease : review article. *Cardiovasc J Afr*. 2013;24(4):141-145. doi:10.5830/CVJA-2013-028.

107. Saxena A. Status of pediatric cardiac care in developing countries. *Children*. 2019;6(2):34. doi:10.3390/children6020034.

# Chapter 29

# Hemodynamic Management in Special Circumstances

Elaine Neary, TJ Boly, and Regan Giesinger (E)[†]

## Key Points

1. Neonates with hypertrophic cardiomyopathy due to diabetes who have cardiovascular instability benefit from a strategy that avoids positive inotropy and high peak end-expiratory pressure and prioritizes left heart volume loading and increased left ventricular afterload.

2. Neonates with pre-ductal arteriovenous malformations may have flow-mediated pulmonary hypertension and pseudocoarctation physiology if left-to-right ductal shunt (either due to natural decline in systemic vascular resistance or secondary to inhaled nitric oxide therapy) is added to the large intracranial shunt. Treatment for pulmonary arterial hypertension (e.g., inhaled nitric oxide) should only be considered for neonates who also have hypoxemic respiratory failure.

3. Pulmonary arterial hypertension is more common in the transitional period for preterm infants. The frequency response to nitric oxide is comparable to term infants with acute pulmonary hypertension in the transitional period. The optimal starting dose, duration, and weaning schedule require further study.

4. Neonates with congenital diaphragmatic hernia may have either a right heart (e.g., pulmonary arterial hypertension) or left heart (e.g., pulmonary venous hypertension) phenotype. The clinical manifestations may be similar. Echocardiography demonstration of the direction of atrial shunt prior to nitric oxide therapy may be advantageous.

5. Twin-to-twin transfusion syndrome, particularly if not treated with in utero laser photocoagulation of affected vessels, may manifest as hypertrophic cardiomyopathy in the recipient twin and both twins may benefit from early echocardiography-based phenotypic delineation.

## Introduction

There are several biological conditions that highlight important physiological concepts and require special attention when caring for an infant faced with cardiovascular compromise. As neonatologists, we generally treat a population of patients with structurally normal hearts but abnormal cardiovascular physiology. That is crucial because that makes up the bulk of clinical practice for each licensed independent practitioner every day; however, it is also important to consider how these principles may need to be adapted to other unique situations. In this chapter we will focus on the application of physiological principles to the management of the infant of a diabetic mother with hypertrophic cardiomyopathy, pre-ductal arteriovenous malformation, preterm arterial pulmonary hypertension (PH), congenital diaphragmatic hernia (CDH), and twin-to-twin transfusion.

## Infants of Diabetic Mothers and Hemodynamic Management

### BACKGROUND

Diabetes mellitus is a common maternal morbidity, associated with higher body mass index, higher maternal age, and sedentary lifestyle, affecting 9–25% of pregnancies.[1-4] The term "infant of a diabetic mother (IDM)" refers to neonates born to a woman with persistently elevated blood sugar during pregnancy.[5] Infants of diabetic mothers, even with good glycemic control, are at five times increased risk of both morphological and functional cardiac changes because of characteristic fetal metabolic abnormalities such as hyperglycemia and hyperinsulinemia.[5-7]. Fetal exposure to these conditions often contributes to neonatal morbidity, which may be transient or permanent and predispose to cardiovascular disease in adulthood.[1,8] Even asymptomatic infants may have subclinical functional impairment.[5]

## IDM AND MORPHOLOGICAL CHANGES

Congenital heart disease, including septal defects, transposition of the great arteries, persistent truncus arteriosus, and patent ductus arteriosus (PDA), is associated with maternal diabetes.[1] Cardiomyopathy including hypertrophic obstructive cardiomyopathy, is identified in 13–44% of cases, with the greatest risk associated with maternal type 1 diabetes.[9,10] Hypertrophic cardiomyopathy is described as a combination of asymmetric septal hypertrophy and diastolic dysfunction.[9,11] These cardiac structural changes may be due to hyperglycemia, activating a cascade of cellular events and changes in gene expression.[1] They have also been found to be associated with hyperinsulinemia and IGF-1, which promotes hypertrophy in cardiomyocytes, leading to decreased myocardial compliance.[1] Asymmetric septal hypertrophy is typically due to a greater density of insulin receptors in this region as compared to other areas of the cardiac muscle. This may lead to left ventricular outflow tract (LVOT) obstruction and systolic anterior mitral valve displacement.[10] Although good maternal glycemic control may improve heart development and mitigate the risk of increased ventricular thickness compared to infants of poorly controlled diabetic mothers,[5] it does not eliminate the risk of septal hypertrophy.[12]

Echocardiography can be utilized to demonstrate structural and functional changes commonly found in IDMs; specifically, it is useful to examine the interventricular septum and posterior wall thickness and measure left ventricular (LV) systolic and diastolic function.[13,14] Biomarkers such as cardiac-specific troponin I (cTnI) and N-terminal pro-brain natriuretic peptide (NT-pro BNP) may also be used to predict HOCM and LV dysfunction. cTnI is an inhibitory protein involved in cardiac muscle relaxation released in settings of myocardial injury. Serum levels are correlated with the degree of septal hypertrophy, which may be due to suboptimal coronary artery oxygen delivery to compensate for high myocardial oxygen demand.[15]

## IDM, TRANSITION, AND FUNCTIONAL IMPAIRMENT

IDM are at increased risk of respiratory distress syndrome because fetal hyperinsulinemia impairs surfactant production.[16,17] Lung disease may lead to secondary acute pulmonary hypertension (PH); however, animal studies have also shown increased muscularization of pulmonary arteries and fewer pulmonary vessels at birth, suggesting that a predisposition to pulmonary vascular disease may exist in the absence of lung disease. Maternal diabetes is also associated with chronic fetal hypoxia and polycythemia, which are risk factors for PAH at birth.[18,19] Katheria et al. demonstrated that even following well-controlled DM during pregnancy, the IDM is at risk of abnormal transitional hemodynamics. This was supported by lower right ventricular output compared to controls.[8] These data are also consistent with the report by Seppänen et al., who showed that the closure of the ductus arteriosus and postnatal decrease in pulmonary artery pressure are delayed in IDMs when compared with control infants during the first postnatal days.[6] The consequences of hypertrophic cardiomyopathy may include impaired systemic blood flow and hyperdynamic LV systolic function, which is often observed to coexist with diastolic dysfunction.[8] However, even in the absence of hypertrophic cardiomyopathy, functional cardiac changes may be evident. As compared to well-controlled DM pregnancies and healthy controls, IDMs following poor control during pregnancy showed a significant reduction in LV global strain and strain rate. This suggests glycemic control influences the degree of impairment in myocardial systolic function, which persists at least through 6 months postnatal age. Additionally, persistence of the ductus arteriosus may be more prevalent among IDMs following poor glycemic control,[5] which may have important implications for preterm IDMs. Interestingly, early functional impairment itself has been suggested to induce cardiac hypertrophy.[1]

## IDM AND ADULT LIFE

The potential benefit of evaluating fetal cardiac function may lie in its prognostic value for long-term cardiovascular health. Fetal studies have shown that in utero reprogramming of genes involved in metabolic processes can occur secondary to maternal diabetes, especially when associated with a high-fat diet.[20] Several biochemical markers associated with adult cardiovascular disease have been identified as higher among IDMs than control infants. These include increased cellular adhesion molecules, markers of endothelial damage, and dysfunctional endothelial colony-forming cells. Elevated levels of angiotensin II, which potentiates stronger vasoconstriction in the presence of endothelin 1, and apoptosis of umbilical venous endothelial cells have been demonstrated in human IDMs.[12] While limited longitudinal data specific to the heart is available, these findings may provide biological support to epidemiological studies suggesting a greater burden of cardiovascular disease among IDMs later in life.

## Hemodynamic Management of IDM With Obstructive Hypertrophic Cardiomyopathy

In most instances infants with hypertrophic cardiomyopathy are asymptomatic and the hypertrophy resolves within months of birth as the stimulus for the insulin production disappears.[9,11] A subset of cases, however, develop cardiogenic pulmonary edema and/or shock with severe hypotension due to either LVOT obstruction and/or low LV preload resulting in a low cardiac output. Low cardiac output in these patients is associated with lower cerebral resistance to compensate for low flow through the carotid arteries.[21,22] Medication choices involve understanding of the physiology of hypertrophic cardiomyopathy. The most fundamental consideration is that hypertrophic muscle contracts well with often supra-normal systolic function but doesn't relax well (impaired compliance), resulting in diastolic dysfunction. Practically, this translates into a problem of keeping the LV filled and a need for high LA pressure. During systole, the LV has the capacity to eject and may completely empty before the cavity pressure declines below aortic root pressure. Thus maintenance of high aortic root pressure is one strategy to maintain LV volume. The pattern of deterioration among patients with hypertrophic cardiomyopathy is predictable and should inform the urgency of treatment. The LV becomes underfilled and compensatory tachycardia reduces diastolic duration and further compromises stroke volume. The gradient to flow in the coronary arteries, from the hypotensive aortic root to the hypertensive coronary sinus, is not compatible with coronary blood flow, and the hypertrophic cardiac muscle has a high tissue

oxygen demand. The result may be death from cardiac ischemia if prompt management is not instituted to correct the critically low coronary perfusion pressure and either restore LV filling or maintain right to left ductal shunting to support cardiac output. Once a patient becomes significantly hypotensive, emergent intervention should be instituted.

- *Pharmacologic Treatment of hypotension:* The physiologic goal of treatment is to maintain a high filling pressure, optimize intracardiac volume loading, and avoid tachycardia. Therefore a liberal approach to use of crystalloid therapy is recommended.[23] Intravenous vasopressin has been proposed as beneficial in the setting of hypertrophic obstructive cardiomyopathy physiology. Vasopressin has the potential to augment both cardiac preload and afterload due to effects on both free water absorption and systemic vasoconstriction while simultaneously avoiding tachycardia and excessive positive inotropy.[11] The rationale behind this may be threefold; *first*, increased systemic vascular resistance (SVR) may increase a left-to-right ductal shunt, which may be beneficial in this population because the resultant increase in pulmonary blood flow may augment left atrial filling and improve cardiac output. In addition, enhanced left heart volume loading may prevent the premature and complete emptying of the left ventricle; *second*, higher afterload because of increased SVR results in reduced velocity of fiber shortening, limiting ejection time. As a result of incomplete emptying of the LV, there is greater end-systolic volume, which adds to preload to improve cardiac output; *third*, the anti-diuretic effect of vasopressin may increase circulating volume, and this may be beneficial in the acute phases of treatment. In a retrospective case series by Boyd et al, six infants with hypertrophic obstructive cardiomyopathy (five of whom were IDMs) were treated with vasopressin resulting in clinical and biochemical improvement, which warrants further investigation with a prospective randomized trial.[11] Norepinephrine, although primarily an α-agonist, has some β1 activity and is not recommended due to the prevalence of tachycardia with NE use. Phenylephrine is used in adults and in anesthetic practice for treatment of shock due to obstructive cardiomyopathy, though there is limited experience with this agent in most neonatal intensive care units.

## GENERAL CARDIOVASCULAR CARE FOR PATIENTS WITH HOCM

The management of acute PH and/ or shock in the infant of a diabetic mother requires modification from routine neonatal intensive care strategies if significant septal hypertrophy is identified, particularly in the presence of LVOT obstruction. The most appropriate approach depends on the degree of obstruction to left heart outflow. *If the dominant clinical concern is hypoxia* and LVOT obstruction is mild or absent, treatment of PH with strategies that reduce pulmonary vascular resistance (PVR) such as inhaled nitric oxide (iNO) is the most appropriate. Conditions in which the left heart is preload compromised result in closer approximation of the septum and the mitral valve and therefore may exacerbate obstruction. This includes excessive mean airway pressure, particularly in the setting of high-frequency ventilation, where diastolic filling time may be limited. In addition, vasodilator drugs, such as milrinone, should be avoided. Positive inotropes (epinephrine, dobutamine, and dopamine) are contraindicated as more forceful contraction may worsen obstruction and, by inducing tachycardia, may reduce diastolic time, hence further limiting filling. *For neonates with hypotension and moderate or severe LVOT obstruction,* in whom adequate augmentation of LV filling is not possible, a strategy in which the PVR is kept elevated, and the right heart (via right-to-left ductal shunt) is temporarily used to supply systemic circulation may be the only way to accomplish adequate systemic blood flow. In this case prostaglandin E1 (PGE-1) to maintain ductal patency and avoidance of pulmonary vasodilators is warranted. Veno-arterial extracorporeal membrane oxygenation may be an alternative for neonates with refractory shock, though there is limited published evidence.[24,25] In the short term therapeutic hypothermia, which is associated with reduced HR, may be advantageous for these patients; however, this requires prospective study. The changes in heart rate, upon rewarming, in the setting of hypoxic-ischemic encephalopathy and therapeutic hypothermia, may negatively impact the physiology of these patients.

## CHRONIC THERAPY FOR PATIENTS WITH HYPERTROPHIC OBSTRUCTIVE CARDIOMYOPATHY

Long-term management may be required, though hypertrophic cardiomyopathy in infants of diabetic mothers is transient and typically resolves over 3–6 months. Beta-blockers may improve left heart filling based on their ability to reduce heart rate and for their negative inotropic properties.[9] In the acute phase, however, beta-blockers can precipitate symptomatic PH crisis, which may adversely affect LA filling; therefore caution should be exercised. Calcium channel blockers (e.g., verapamil, diltiazem) may also be used to reduce myocardial stiffness. Drugs that reduce systemic afterload (e.g., nitrates, angiotensin-converting enzyme inhibitors, milrinone) should be avoided in this population as they may worsen LVOT obstruction. Diuretics should be used with caution when hypertrophic cardiomyopathy is severe enough to cause pulmonary edema as dehydration may compromise LV filling.

## SUMMARY

There is evidence of a strong association between maternal diabetes and impaired fetal cardiac function in IDMs. Studies directly demonstrating the relationship between fetal cardiac diastolic dysfunction on ultrasound and future cardiovascular health are lacking. There is a need for further longitudinal studies aimed at demonstrating the plausible association between maternal diabetes and fetal cardiac function in utero, in relation to clinical outcomes and offspring development.[1] Cardiovascular management is focused on maintenance of LV filling by liberal use of volume boluses and judicious use of vasopressin as the first-line agent for systemic hypotension. In the situation where filling is refractory to fluid and vasopressin, maintenance of ductal shunt to support pulmonary blood flow (and indirectly load the LA) or systemic blood flow (if maintained right-to-left in the setting of severe LVOT obstruction) may be warranted.

# Pre-ductal Arteriovenous Malformation and Hemodynamic Management

## BACKGROUND

Arteriovenous malformations are vascular connections that can lead to alterations in the flow of blood to cerebral, pulmonary, and hepatic locations. A vein of

Galen malformation (VGAM) is a congenital arterio-venous fistula in the brain that develops in the early embryonic stage resulting in a high-volume pre-ductal left-to-right shunt. Clinical features vary from the differential effects of altered blood flow to the systemic versus pulmonary vascular beds, which can present at different time-points from the early newborn period to late childhood and are associated with increased morbidity and mortality. Infants with VGAM can be asymptomatic initially; however, as the normal postnatal transition occurs, with changing systemic and PVR, infants may become clinically symptomatic with features of poor tissue oxygen delivery.

## SYSTEMIC CONSEQUENCES OF VGAM PHYSIOLOGY

In utero, severe decompensation is rare because the low resistance of the cerebral VGAM is balanced by the low resistance of the placenta, which ensures perfusion of the peripheral organs. With loss of the placenta at birth, up to 80% of cardiac output is directed to the cerebral circulation due to high blood flow through the low-resistance fistula.[26-28] Therefore the volume overload caused by VGAM worsens after birth. Patel et al showed superior vena caval flow in this condition may be 10 times higher than that of normal values in their description of three infants with VGAM.[26] Higher cardiac output has been associated with higher mortality in the fetus with this condition and may be a useful prognostic indicator in the postnatal period. The right ventricle (RV) suffers from both volume and pressure overload; however, "high-output cardiac failure" is a biological misnomer for the clinical presentation with end-organ dysfunction of patients with VGAM. A more accurate term may be *pseudocoarctation* because the high flow to the brain acts functionally like an anatomic juxta-ductal obstruction. The high blood flow through the low-resistance fistula can reduce blood flow to the remainder of the body and may result in progressive hypotension, which may be profound secondary to *pseudocoarctation* physiology.[29] *Pseudocoarctation* physiology is a result of intracranial steal with low coronary root pressure and retrograde transverse and descending aortic arch flow. This means blood flow to the remainder of the body is reduced and can lead to multiorgan ischemia-mediated failure and death. Moreover, myocardial ischemia and infarction have been previously described in these infants. The ischemic myocardial damage stems from a decrease in right coronary blood flow and contributes to the cardiac decompensation.

## PULMONARY CONSEQUENCES OF VGAM PHYSIOLOGY

In utero, the fetal vascular bed of infants with VGAM physiology is exposed to substantially more flow than is typical as soon as the capacity of the ductus to shunt blood away from the lung is overcome. This leads to maldevelopment of the pulmonary vascular bed as characterized by pulmonary vascular muscularization and vascular hyperreactivity, which manifests as *resistance-mediated pulmonary arterial hypertension (PAH)*. Intrinsically, patients with VGAM may also present with *flow-mediated PAH*, given that a substantial volume of blood may fill vessels accustomed to a much smaller volume of flow every minute. It is important to be able to clinically distinguish between these two phenotypes because the principles of management are dichotomous. The former presents with oxygenation failure and typical echocardiographic findings of PAH, while the latter, however, is characterized by a baby who appears generally stable on low (or no) supplemental oxygen but has exclusively or predominantly right-to-left ductal shunt. The lack of compromise to oxygenation relates to the fact these patients have a normal to high right ventricular output (typically low in resistance-mediated PAH), which may be used to distinguish both conditions echocardiographically. A third, *mixed phenotype* may occur because high pulmonary blood flow over a sustained period can lead to RV dilation and subsequent RV dysfunction due to increased energy demand. This contributes to adverse effects on LV diastolic performance due to abnormal septal configuration and may contribute to left heart–mediated pulmonary edema. The combination of these three cardiovascular phenotypes may lead to multifactorial oxygenation failure after birth. The presence of supra-systemic PAH may be an indicator of poor prognosis[26]; however, the relevance of each of these physiologies to a broad population of patients requires further study using comprehensive echocardiography.

## Hemodynamic Management of Infants with Pre-ductal AVM

The physiological contributors to cardiovascular disease among patients with pre-ductal AVMs are highly complex and dynamic. Therapy should be guided by detailed physiological assessment performed serially and a high index of suspicion for changes in ambient conditions. A further consideration is that these neonates are highly vulnerable to brain injury based on abnormal blood flow, vascular distension and compression, and venous congestion. As such, they are at high risk of seizures which could present with subtle physiological deviations, including oxygen desaturation, hyper- or hypotension, etc. Neurological electrical monitoring and empiric phenobarbital use in the setting of sudden decompensation should be considered. Given the bio-physiologic complexity, infants with VGAM should preferentially be admitted to a specialized center with the capacity for both comprehensive longitudinal echocardiography hemodynamic care and for staged endo-vascular embolization.

The goals of management are to (i) maintain a balance of systemic and pulmonary blood flow while providing adequate but not excessive oxygen supplementation, (ii) ensure adequate RV performance, and (iii) assess brain integrity in terms of candidacy for staged embolization. With careful cardiovascular management, emergency embolization should be a rare, if ever, event. This is particularly important because undergoing embolization, with its dramatic changes in loading conditions and physiology, may create an additional risk of poor patient outcomes. The approach to management is dependent on phenotypic characterization of patients with flow-driven PH and resistance-driven PH as treatments such as iNO, which may help the latter, may be harmful to the former. Patients who present with low (or no) supplemental oxygen requirement to maintain pre-ductal $SpO_2$ >85–88% but who have echocardiographic findings which suggest acute PAH (e.g., RV dilation, septal flattening, significant right-to-left component of ductal shunt), are likely to have *flow-mediated PAH*. In these patients the goal of care is to avoid excessive reduction in PVR, thereby promoting right-to-left ductal flow to direct sufficient blood flow toward the systemic circulation to avoid *pseudocoarctation physiology*. In addition, iNO is not indicated and may precipitate lactic acidosis and renal failure.[29]

On the contrary, the initial management of patients with hypoxemic respiratory failure *and* VGAM should align with the usual approach to *resistance-mediated PH* with or without RV dysfunction (see Chapter 27). Judicious use of iNO, $CO_2$ targets, and oxygen with optimization of ventilation and sedation are essential components of cardiorespiratory care. In patients without significant lung disease these measures may be very successful in lowering PVR and caution must

be exercised to avoid reversal of the (from right to left to left to right) ductal shunt. Weaning to the lowest tolerated dose of oxygen and iNO are important. The aim is to lower pulmonary pressures, to a level that reduces the risk of RV dysfunction by promoting left-to-right flow through the ductus arteriosus, but not at the expense of exacerbating systemic steal and the risk of "pseudocoarctation physiology". Documentation of normal RV function and treatment of dysfunction with a positive inotrope like dobutamine or low-dose epinephrine is suggested. An intravenous infusion of PGE-1 may also be useful in reducing RV afterload, when RV function is compromised.

Hypotension in *pseudocoarctation physiology* may be due to a closing/restrictive PDA, excessive left-to-right ductal shunt, or RV dysfunction; therefore care should be guided by longitudinal echocardiography. Empiric choices of therapy may include positive inotropy, PGE-1, and shunt modulation strategies such as more liberal $CO_2$ goals, lower target oxygen saturation, and weaning/discontinuation of iNO if applicable. In patients with resistance-mediated PH, low cardiac output is the most likely pathophysiology, and empiric treatment could be either directed toward RV dysfunction or systemic vasoconstriction with agents such as vasopressin or norepinephrine. Caution is advised using norepinephrine concurrently with 100% oxygen and iNO due to its vasoconstrictive effects demonstrated in large animal models.[30] Due to the dynamic nature of the physiology, longitudinal targeted neonatal echocardiography (TnECHO) is recommended to guide therapy. The post-embolization period, when multiple feeding vessels are ablated, may be followed by dramatic increases in LV afterload that may lead to impaired LV function. Early post-interventional echocardiography and judicious use of intravenous milrinone may be of value.

## SUMMARY

Infants with VGAM need to be carefully evaluated for signs of PH and systemic hypoperfusion and managed accordingly. Therapeutic goals are to balance systemic and pulmonary blood flow, maintain RV performance, and monitor for neurological abnormalities. Although embolization is the definitive therapy for flow-mediated PH, correction of other ambient conditions is often necessary to achieve optimal operative stability. An algorithm has been published with this in mind by Giesinger et al, as illustrated in Figure 29.1.[29]

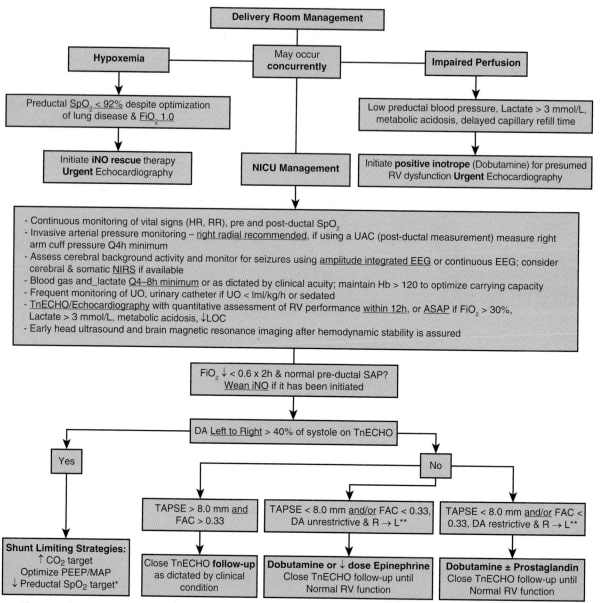

**Fig. 29.1 Suggested management algorithm for the cardiovascular stabilization of neonates with vein of Galen aneurysmal malformation.** *CO₂*, Carbon dioxide; *DA*, ductus arteriosus; *EEG*, electroencephalogram; *FAC*, fractional area change; *FiO₂*, fraction of inspired oxygen; *HR*, heart rate; *iNO*, inhaled nitric oxide; *L*, left; *LOC*, level of consciousness; *MAP*, mean airway pressure; *NIRS*, near-infrared spectroscopy; *PEEP*, positive end expiratory pressure; *R*, right; *RR*, respiratory rate; *RV*, right ventricle; *SpO₂*, oxygen saturation; *TAPSE*, tricuspid annulus plane systolic excursion; *TnECHO*, targeted neonatal echocardiography; *UO*, urinary output.[29]

## Preterm Acute PH and Hemodynamic Management

Acute PH occurs in 1.9/1000 live births, with mortality ranging from 4% to 33%.[31] The fact that preterm infants, particularly extreme preterms <27 weeks' gestation, also experience acute PH is increasingly recognized. A recent Japanese cohort study suggests an incidence as high as 18.5% of infants born at 22 weeks' gestation, with a gradual reduction by maturity thereafter.[32] As such, understanding the biological contributors to this disease, the maturity of the physiologic mechanisms required during normal postnatal adaptation, and the impact on both the cardiovascular system and neonate more broadly are important (Figure 29.2). Sections on term acute PH (Chapters 25 and 27) and chronic PH (Chapter 26) may be referenced for more detail.

### EMBRYOLOGY OF THE PULMONARY VASCULATURE

The development of the pulmonary vasculature is a process that occurs concurrently with development of the lung parenchyma. The proximal pulmonary arteries and veins arise from proliferation of endothelial cells from existing vessels in the developing heart.[34] The most distal pulmonary vessels develop from pluripotent mesenchymal cells from blood islands which differentiate into endothelial cells.[35] The proximal and distal vessels are joined together between 5 and 17 weeks of gestation, during the pseudoglandular stage of lung development.[36] As the lungs continue to develop, pulmonary vessels grow alongside each acinus.[34] After 20 weeks of gestation, pulmonary arteries and arterioles have completed development of wall musculature.[34] The developing pulmonary arterial system has approximately twice the thickness of musculature as compared to those in adults, and the smallest arterioles have more pronounced musculature[36]; however, there is animal evidence to suggest that arterial smooth muscle controlling vascular tone is mature in later gestation. Studies in the fetal lamb have suggested that the pulmonary vascular bed does not receive increased cardiac output in response to

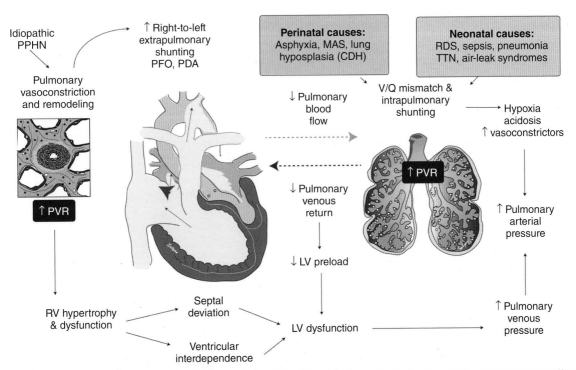

**Fig. 29.2 Pathophysiology of extrapulmonary shunts, ventricular dysfunction, and interventricular function interdependence in acute pulmonary hypertension.** *CDH,* Congenital diaphragmatic hernia; *LV,* left ventricle; *MAS,* meconium aspiration syndrome; *PVR,* pulmonary vascular resistance; *RV,* right ventricle; *TTN,* transient tachypnea of newborn. (With permission.[33])

maternal hyperoxygenation at 20 weeks, suggesting the immature pulmonary vasculature does not vasodilate in response to oxygen.[37] As gestation progresses to 30 weeks, however, the vasculature does become responsive to maternal hyperoxygenation, suggesting maturation of the vasoreactivity of these vessels later in gestation.[34,37-39] Importantly, endothelial nitric oxide synthase (eNOS) is present throughout gestation, suggesting that, if stimulated, it would respond to vasodilatory mediators.

## PRE- AND POSTNATAL FACTORS THAT CONTRIBUTE TO PH

Despite the inherent elevated vascular resistance of the fetal pulmonary vessels, several in utero factors may affect the normal development of these vessels and result in a delayed transition or PH following delivery (Figure 29.3). Prolonged premature rupture of membranes and oligohydramnios results in abnormal development of the lungs and alveoli, which in turn leads to poor growth of the pulmonary vasculature with thickened smooth muscle layers.[40] Abnormal placentation and intrauterine growth restriction lead to decreased alveolarization, pulmonary vessel density, and endogenous nitric oxide production.[41] Maternal factors, including obesity; diabetes mellitus; and use of tobacco, nonsteroidal anti-inflammatory drugs, or selective serotonin reuptake inhibitors, can affect the development of the pulmonary vasculature and its reactivity to endogenous pulmonary vasodilators.[42-45]

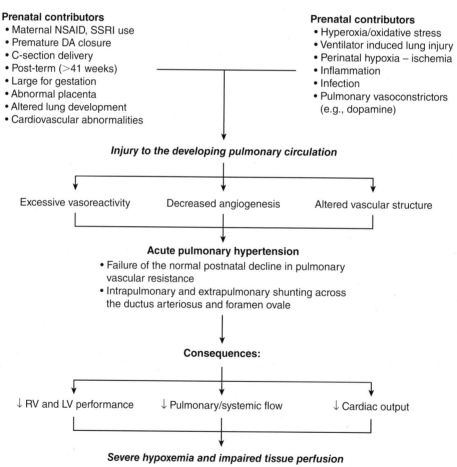

**Fig. 29.3 Pathogenesis of acute pulmonary hypertension.** *DA,* Ductus arteriosus; *LV,* left ventricle; *NSAID,* nonsteroidal anti-inflammatory drug; *PFO,* patent foramen ovale; *PVR,* pulmonary vascular resistance; *RV,* right ventricle; *SSRI,* selective serotonin reuptake inhibitor. Adapted from Ref. 37 with permission.

Finally, factors around the time of delivery, including fetal distress and cesarean delivery (both emergent and elective), can contribute to delayed transition to a neonatal cardiopulmonary physiology.[38,45]

Following delivery, multiple conditions can result in persistence of elevated pulmonary vascular resistance (Figure 29.4), of which preterm infants are particularly at risk. Lung disease due to respiratory distress syndrome (RDS) is intrinsically more common among preterm infants, affecting nearly all preterm infants born <24 weeks' gestational age.[46] Similarly, the immature myocardium may be at increased vulnerability to sudden the increase in afterload generated by the loss of the low-resistance placental circulation.[47,48] Left heart disease may predispose neonates to pulmonary venous hypertension, which may be difficult to distinguish from parenchymal lung disease and pulmonary arterial hypertension. However, relatively fewer, disorganized myofibrils,[49] a preponderance of non-contractile tissue,[50] and immature calcium handling systems[51] may predispose immature neonates to hypoxic respiratory

failure due to pulmonary edema. Although uncommon, congenital heart disease should always remain in the differential diagnosis, including for preterm infants.

## TREATMENT OF ACUTE PH

The general approach to acute PH in preterm should be consistent with the recommended approach in term infants (see Chapter 27). The focus of care should be on the following principles: *first*, pharmacologic and non-pharmacologic strategies that lower PVR; *second*, use of positive inotropes to support RV systolic function; and *third*, use of vasopressors that do not vasoconstrict the pulmonary vascular bed (Figure 29.5). Additional important factors in preterm infants are the initial steps of determining and attaining optimal functional residual capacity, which may include optimizing lung recruitment through mechanical ventilation or surfactant therapy for RDS while avoiding overexpansion of the airspaces.[38] Supplemental oxygen should be provided to maintain pre-ductal saturations from 90% to 95%[52]; however,

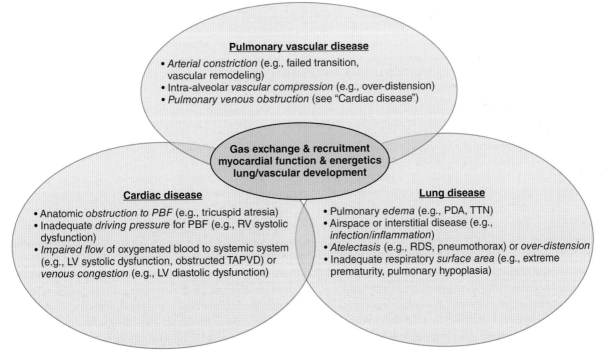

**Fig. 29.4 Possible contributors to hypoxic respiratory failure in preterm infants.** Complex pathophysiology may exist when multiple overlapping disease processes occur concurrently. There is considerable interdependency intrinsic in cardiorespiratory interactions. *LV,* Left ventricle; *PDA,* patent ductus arteriosus; *RDS,* respiratory distress syndrome; *RV,* right ventricle; *TAPVD,* total anomalous pulmonary venous drainage; *TTN,* transient tachypnea of the newborn.[52]

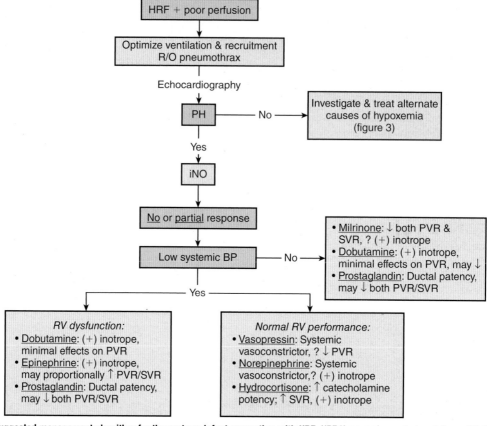

**Fig. 29.5 Suggested management algorithm for the preterm infant presenting with HRF.** *HRF,* Hypoxemic respiratory failure; *iNO,* inhaled nitric oxide; *PDA,* patent ductus arteriosus; *PH,* pulmonary hypertension; *PVR,* pulmonary vascular resistance; *R/O,* rule out; *RV,* right ventricle; *SVR,* systemic vascular resistance.[52]

immature patients may respond differently to postnatal oxygen supplementation. Responsiveness to oxygen increases throughout gestation, with the greatest change in the third trimester[53]; however, when exposed to hyperbaric oxygen, the increase in pulmonary blood flow is significantly blunted compared to infants born at term. It is important to remember that the provision of high inspired oxygen concentrations may be detrimental. Exposure to 24 hours of hyperoxia is associated with lung injury and inflammation[54] and the antioxidant defense systems of preterm animals demonstrate significant maturation toward term.[55,56] This suggests that extremely preterm infants have a greater vulnerability to reactive oxygen species as compared to term infants. It may be prudent to consider target pre-ductal $SpO_2$ in the 90–93% range

to avoid these extremes, but this recommendation is not evidence based.

iNO is currently recommended for use in late preterm and term infants with acute PH.[38] Its use in premature infants remains controversial as randomized controlled trials involving iNO use in this population have failed to show a significant benefit on the outcome of bronchopulmonary dysplasia.[52] It is necessary to note, however, that these studies enrolled infants on the basis of respiratory illness and not according to their underlying physiology; specifically, patients were not enrolled based on an echocardiography diagnosis of PH[52] (Table 29.1). Several studies have found that extremely premature infants *do respond* to iNO for hypoxic respiratory failure, especially in the first 72 hours of life, during the transition period of the pulmonary

**TABLE 29.1 Characteristics of Randomized Controlled Trials of Nitric Oxide for Early Rescue Therapy of Hypoxic Respiratory Failure in Preterm Infants[59]**

| Identifier | GA/wt, n | Inclusion Criteria | Intervention/Duration | Primary Outcome | PH on Echo (n, %) |
|---|---|---|---|---|---|
| The Franco-Belgium Collaborative NO Trial Group.[60] | <33/40, n = 85 | • OI 12.5–30<br>• ≤7 days of life | • 10–20 ppm (based on OI)<br>• Duration unclear | Reduction in OI after 2 h | Not reported |
| Srisuparp, et al., 2002[61] | < 2 kg, n = 34 | • Clinical RDS, surfactant<br>• OI varied by BW (min 4, max 12)<br>• ≤72 h of life | • 20 ppm<br>• Max of 7 days | Effects of iNO on oxygenation | Not reported |
| Su et al., 2008[62] | ≤31/40 gestation & ≤1.5 kg, n = 65 | • OI ≥ 25 | • 5–20 ppm<br>• ↓ by 1 ppm q 6 h as dictated by $FiO_2$ | Effects of iNO on oxygenation | Not reported |
| Wei et al., 2014[63] | ≤34/40, n = 60 | • MV, 2 h after surfactant<br>• OI ≥ 11<br>• <7 days of life | • 5 ppm starting<br>• At least 7 days or when extubated | OI before and during treatment | Not reported |

*OI*, oxygenation Index; ppm, *parts per million; RDS*, respiratory distress syndrome; *BW*, birth weight; *iNO*, inhaled nitric oxide; *MV*, mechanical ventilation.

vasculature.[57,58] Ahmed et al. demonstrated a response rate comparable to term infants during transition among patients with echocardiography confirmed PH.[58] iNO diffuses through the alveoli into capillary smooth muscle cells and results in selective pulmonary vasodilation with minimal systemic effects, improving perfusion to the well-aerated portion of the lungs.[38,33] The lungs must be appropriately aerated and expanded for iNO to be effective[38] (Figure 29.6). Infants that respond to iNO may have a rapid improvement in oxygenation, with higher oxygen saturations and lower supplemental oxygen requirements. In a subset of infants there may be worsening of their clinical status after initiation of iNO. If this occurs, the clinician should consider alternate diagnoses including congenital heart disease and diminished LV function.[38] The evidence for a specific starting dose of iNO among preterm infants is weak. Extrapolating from term data, it is typical to start at 20 ppm; however, it is possible that a similar therapeutic effect would be achieved at a lower starting dose, and some practitioners may start at a dose of 5 ppm. There is also little evidence to guide weaning of iNO in the preterm infant. Theoretically, the preterm infant with an open ductus is at risk of escalating left to right shunt as PVR falls. Initiation of iNO is typically associated with a pre-existing low-flow state and the subsequent escalation in pre-ductal cardiac output from increasing PDA flow may predispose to ischemia-reperfusion hemorrhage of the germinal matrix. Use of the minimum tolerated dose of NO with an aggressive approach to early weaning may be beneficial.

Dobutamine may be used for infants with ventricular dysfunction to improve systolic function and increase pulmonary or systemic flow. It has been shown to increase cardiac output among preterm infants, and this effect is mediated by an increase in contractility.[64] Vasopressin is an effective and biologically plausible vasopressor for preterms with PH and systemic hypotension.[65] Vasopressin binds to the V1 receptor on the systemic vascular smooth muscle cell causing systemic vasoconstriction and increased blood pressure; in the pulmonary vasculature the V1 receptor is primarily on the endothelial cell and, when bound, causes intracellular release of NO and vasodilation of the adjacent vascular smooth muscle cell.[66] Among preterm infants with iNO refractory PH, adjuvant vasopressin has been associated with improved oxygenation and improved metrics of systemic hemodynamics, including higher urine output.[65] Serum electrolytes need to be closely monitored during vasopressin administration due to both its anti-diuretic hormone effect and its potency as a natriuretic. Sodium supplementation is advisable

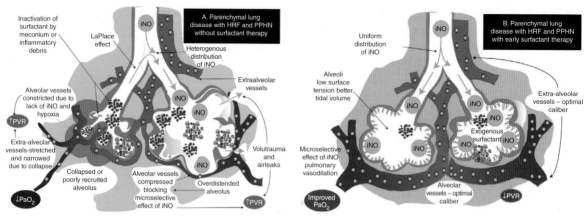

**Fig. 29.6 Effect of lung inflation, surfactant, and iNO on PVR.** In conditions such as MAS and pneumonia heterogeneous lung disease with surfactant deficiency leads to collapsed and overdistended alveoli (A). Underinflation or collapse compresses extra-alveolar pulmonary vessels and prevents their access to oxygen and iNO, causing high PVR (left-sided alveolus in [A]). Overdistended alveoli compress alveolar pulmonary vessels and prevent them from dilating in response to iNO and oxygen; overdistension increases the risk of air leak (right-sided alveolus in [A]). Following optimal lung recruitment and surfactant use, uniform distension of alveoli and optimal recruitment will allow oxygen and iNO to reach pulmonary vessels decreasing PVR and improving PaO$_2$. *HRF,* Hypoxemic respiratory failure; *iNO,* inhaled nitric oxide; *PaO$_2$,* partial pressure of oxygen; *PPHN,* persistent pulmonary hypertension of the newborn; *PVR,* pulmonary vascular resistance. (With permission.[33])

when values approach the lower limit of a normal range. Milrinone can be used to treat multiple underlying physiologies which contribute to PAH. Milrinone induces systemic and pulmonary vasodilation through inhibition of phosphodiesterase III, which can improve pulmonary blood flow, but it must be used with caution in infants with systemic hypotension.[38,33] Among preterm infants, milrinone has been associated with reduction in oxygenation index and iNO requirement in addition to improved indices of myocardial performance.[67] The specific inotropic properties of milrinone, independent of afterload reduction, have yet to be conclusively proven. The immature myocyte has a paucity of sarcolemma, which is milrinone's site of action. Afterload reduction to both the left and right ventricle alone, however, may be sufficient to achieve a clinical response.

Infants with acute PH can have varied presentations due to many underlying pathologies. By performing frequent, TnECHO assessments, the underlying physiology can be better understood, and therapies can be targeted to treat the abnormal physiology. Hemodynamic assessment of these infants can provide insight into the most appropriate cardioactive medication to begin and can rapidly assess the cardiopulmonary response to these therapies. In addition, infants who are more likely to respond positively to iNO, based on

the underlying physiology, can be better determined using hemodynamic assessment and thus can avoid potentially worsening the respiratory component of the disease if inappropriate treatments are used. By using targeted, physiology-driven information and treatment recommendations, disturbances in neonatal hemodynamics can be more precisely treated.

## Congenital Diaphragmatic Hernia and Hemodynamic Management

### BACKGROUND

CDH occurs in 1 in every 3000 live births, though the incidence may be higher due to early death among those with severe disease. The defect in the diaphragm forms between the 8th and 10th week of gestation, allowing herniation of the abdominal contents into the thorax and limiting growth and development of the thoracic organs. The postnatal consequences of this developmental aberrancy can be severe and require prompt assessment and intervention. In this section the use of a targeted hemodynamic approach to management of infants with CDH will be explored.

### HEART AND LUNG DEVELOPMENT IN INFANTS WITH CDH

Infants with CDH are known to have abnormal lung and pulmonary vasculature development. While most early research focused on the compressive effects of the abdominal contents on the developing lungs, more recent research has found that there may be genetic changes that impair the growth of the heart, lungs, and pulmonary vasculature. Genetic mutations can be observed in approximately 30–50% of all CDH cases.[68,69] Most CDHs develop due to spontaneous mutations, which cause impaired closure of the diaphragm during development.[70] Large chromosomal defects are found in 10-35% of infants with CDH.[71] Derangements in two individual genes, GATA4 and NR2F2, have been found to lead to CDH in multiple studies.[71,72] GATA4 is a transcription factor that is required for normal lung and diaphragm development, and GATA4 knockout mice are used as an animal model of CDH.[73] NR2F2 is a nuclear receptor activated by retinoic acid, and loss of this receptor has been shown to lead to CDH.[74] Some cases of CDH are due to syndromic mutations. These include autosomal recessive (LRP2, STRA6), autosomal dominant (WT1, GATA4), and X-linked (GPC3) mutations with CDH occurrence in 10–50% of the infants affected by these syndromes.[71]

While these genetic changes have been shown to directly affect diaphragm development, they also influence the development of the lungs and the pulmonary vessels. Mutations in GATA4 and ZFPM2 result in poor lung growth, decreased bronchial branching, and abnormal mesenchyme and epithelial differentiation.[71,72] The lungs of infants with CDH demonstrate reduced alveolarization and decreased collagen deposition in the interstitium, leading to decreased pulmonary compliance.[72] Genetic changes are less understood in the development of abnormal pulmonary vasculature in CDH; however, with transcriptional changes in other growth factors, there may be changes in vascular endothelial growth factor, endothelial adhesion molecules, and thromboxane B2 which affect growth of the vessels and response to vasodilatory agents. It is known that the pulmonary vasculature in infants with CDH demonstrates increased smooth muscle with variable response to pulmonary vasodilators.[35]

The herniated abdominal contents further limit the growth of the alveoli and pulmonary vessels. The amount of compressive inhibition of growth depends on the size of the diaphragmatic defect, the location of the defect, and the degree of abdominal contents in the thorax. Larger defects, right-sided hernias, and herniation of the stomach and liver have been associated with a more significant degree of pulmonary hypoplasia.[75] As pulmonary vasculature development follows that of alveolar growth, there is an overall reduction in pulmonary vessels. These vessels also develop abnormally, with increased smooth muscle thickness and decreased response to pulmonary vasodilators.[35,72]

In addition to the stunted growth of the lung, there is increased risk of associated congenital heart defects (Figure 29.7). Approximately 10% of infants with CDH have an associated heart defect, with the most common being a ventricular and/or atrial septal defect.[76] More significant cardiac lesions, including hypoplastic left heart syndrome, total anomalous pulmonary venous return, and transposition of the great arteries, are associated with increased mortality rates in infants with CDH.[76] In addition, just as with the lung, the abdominal contents can have a compressive effect on the aorta and the left-sided structures, leading to aortic or LV hypoplasia. This effect can be observed as early as 24 weeks of gestation and continues through term.[77]

## FETAL PREDICTION OF CDH SEVERITY

There are several measures that can be used in utero to assess the severity of the CDH. The lung-to-head ratio (LHR) is a measure obtained using prenatal ultrasound. This ratio is indicative of the degree of pulmonary hypoplasia during gestation, with a ratio of less than 1 indicative of severe hypoplasia.[79] In 2007 Jani et al published a modified LHR, comparing the observed to an expected ratio for gestational age. The observed to expected LHR (O/E LHR) corrects for growth that occurs with gestation. An O/E LHR of less than 25% is predictive of severe disease[80] (Figure 29.8). To further assess the degree of pulmonary hypoplasia, fetal MRI can be performed to measure total fetal lung volume, with lower estimated volumes associated with significant growth impairment.[81] Pulmonary artery hypoplasia can be indexed by the modified McGoon index using prenatal ultrasound. The sum of the diameters of the left and right pulmonary arteries is compared to the diameter of the descending aorta at the level of the diaphragm. A ratio less than 1.3 is predictive of severe pulmonary artery hypoplasia.[82] These measurements can be used to guide the initial therapy in infants who require treatment at the time of delivery.

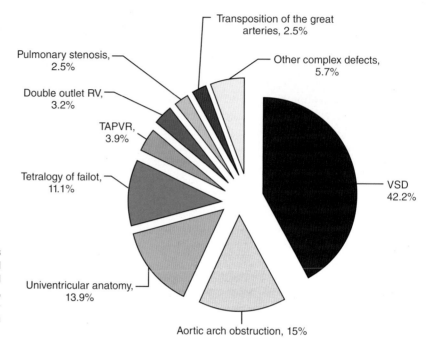

**Fig. 29.7 Types of cardiac defects observed in patients with congenital diaphragmatic hernia and congenital heart disease.** *RV*, right ventricle; *TAPVR*, total anomalous pulmonary venous drainage; *VSD*, ventricular septal defect. (With permission.[78])

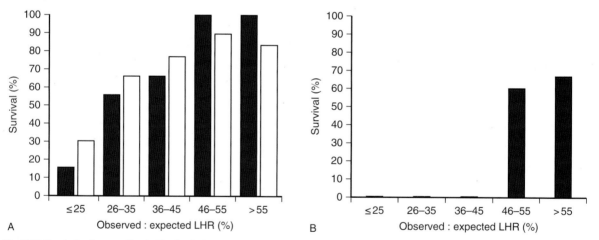

**Fig. 29.8 Survival rate according to the fetal observed to expected lung area to head circumference ratio (*LHR*) in fetuses with isolated left-sided (A) and right-sided (B) diaphragmatic hernia.** The *filled bars* represent fetuses with intrathoracic herniation of the liver and the *open bars* represent those without herniation. (With permission.[80])

## POSTNATAL HEMODYNAMIC ASSESSMENT OF INFANTS WITH CDH

Early comprehensive echocardiography assessment of the infant's hemodynamic status following birth, preferably prior to initiation of a trial of iNO, is imperative to guide therapy. Ideally, this first evaluation should include a comprehensive screen for anatomy as well as delineating the underlying physiology including distinguishing between **pulmonary arterial (PAH)** and **pulmonary venous (PVH)** hypertensive phenotypes. PAH is due to the disrupted growth and development of the pulmonary arteries and arterioles, leading to high RV afterload, RV maladaptation, and low pulmonary blood flow. In turn, this contributes to LV preload compromise, abnormal LV conformation, and impaired cardiac output. Clinically, this leads to hypoxemia, hypercarbia, and acidosis, which further promotes pulmonary vasoconstriction, leading to worsening PAH[33] (Figure 29.9). PVH may be seen in a subset of patients due to LV diastolic dysfunction. In this phenotype high LV and hence LA end-diastolic pressure leads to pulmonary venous congestion and pulmonary edema, which may mimic the respiratory course of PAH.[83] It is very important to distinguish between these two phenotypes, as treatment is considerably different, and potentially harmful if incorrectly applied. For example, non-judicious use of pulmonary vasodilators, primarily indicated for infants with PAH, to an infant with PVH may cause clinical deterioration and worsening of the underlying physiology, as it will reduce the gradient of flow into the LA and may worsen pulmonary edema. The main clue to the difference between these two phenotypes is the directionality of the atrial level shunt. Whereas an exclusive or predominant right-to-left atrial level shunt is pathognomonic of PAH, an exclusive or predominant left-to-right atrial shunt suggests high LA pressure and is consistent with PVH. If possible, early echocardiography (prior to initiation of iNO) to appraise the underlying hemodynamics, severity of PH and/or RV dysfunction and ascertainment of atrial shunt direction should be considered.

Even if not possible prior to iNO, a comprehensive echocardiogram should be performed as soon as feasible, particularly for infants requiring >50% oxygen or with concerns for systemic perfusion/blood pressure.[85]

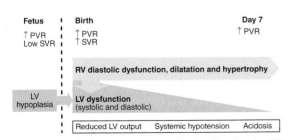

**Fig. 29.9 Pathophysiology of early cardiac dysfunction in CDH.** *LV,* left ventricle; *PVR,* pulmonary vascular resistance; *RV,* right ventricle; *SVR* systemic vascular resistance. (With permission.[84])

It has been shown that approximately 50% of these infants develop cardiac dysfunction within the first 48 postnatal hours.[84] Cardiac dysfunction may arise due to physiologic derangements, including poor oxygen delivery to the myocardium or worsening acidosis, increased stress due to higher afterload, or congenital structural malformations of the myocardium.[84,86] A variety of methods for assessing PAH have been extensively discussed in Chapter 27 and are applicable among patients with CDH.[84] Finally, an early echocardiographic examination is needed to identify possible congenital heart defects. As discussed previously, there is an increased risk of structural heart disease in infants with CDH. It is important to identify these changes early so appropriate treatment may be provided to ensure adequate pulmonary or systemic blood flow.

## Hemodynamic Stabilization and Treatment in CDH

Initial stabilization of infants with CDH begins at delivery. Infants should be intubated after delivery to adequately ventilate the lung on the unaffected side, as well as limit the amount of air swallowed by the infant during respiration, which will cause gaseous distension of the stomach and intestine and further impair pulmonary parenchymal and vascular compliance.[87] Transition to mechanical ventilation with judicious use of mean airway pressure while achieving adequate $CO_2$ clearance aids with the management of PAH in these infants.[87,88] In addition, continuous decompression of the stomach is needed to limit the intestinal compression on the lung.[87]

Following initial respiratory stabilization, an echocardiogram can be obtained, and therapies can be targeted to each infant's cardiovascular physiology. Pulmonary arterial hypertension can be treated with pulmonary vasodilators, such as iNO, PGE-1, and milrinone.[88] A negative response to iNO should prompt early echocardiography to exclude a primary left heart phenotype and weaning of treatment. PGE-1 may be favored in infants with evidence of structural heart disease to maintain ductal patency. Milrinone should be used cautiously in infants with evidence of perinatal hypoxic or ischemic injury, as concurrent renal injury limits milrinone excretion and can lead to significant systemic hypotension, particularly when combined with hypothermia.[89] For infants with evidence of ventricular dysfunction, intravenous dobutamine, low-dose epinephrine, or milrinone can be used.[84] Preliminary trials examining the use of additional pulmonary vasodilators, such as epoprostenol and treprostinil, have shown that these medications can effectively manage PAH in this cohort.[90] In patients with systemic hypotension, judicious use of vasopressors with a favorable pulmonary vascular profile (e.g., vasopressin, norepinephrine) is warranted (see Chapter 27). There is no evidence of benefit of intravenous dopamine and animal experimental data suggest potentially harmful pulmonary vasoconstriction; therefore, dopamine should be avoided in either of the CDH phenotypes. For infants with refractory PH, difficult ventilation requiring excessive airway pressure, or worsening oxygenation despite medical therapy, cannulation to extracorporeal membrane oxygenation (ECMO) should be considered. In infants with CDH the relative indications and contraindications for ECMO cannulation are shown in Table 29.2.[87] The use of ECMO allows time to modulate PAH and allow the normal postnatal decline in PVR to occur to whatever degree it is going to do so prior to surgical intervention and in some centers as a bridge to "on ECMO" surgical repair. Patients with an irreversible cause of ventilation/oxygenation failure may not be considered strong candidates for ECMO based on medical futility. Weight <2 kg or gestational age <34 weeks are relative contraindications due to technical limitations of vascular access and complications of prematurity combined with risks of ECMO.[91]

Longitudinal TnECHO and hemodynamic consultation may aid the assessment of infants with CDH and ease the transition to postnatal physiology where available. By determining the severity of the cardiovascular component, and frequently reassessing it with clinical changes, therapies can be directed to adequately treat the degree of PAH present. Hemodynamic assessments can also aid in management of pre- or post-ECMO cannulation and can continue to work at optimization of the pulmonary vascular bed to reduce overall morbidity and mortality in this population.

## Twin-to-Twin Transfusion Syndrome

Twin-to-twin transfusion syndrome (TTTS) affects 10–15% of monochorionic-diamniotic pregnancies and contributes significantly to both perinatal morbidity and mortality.[92] The donor twin experiences chronic hypovolemia and intrauterine growth restriction. In contrast, the recipient experiences chronic volume overload, afterload exposure, and hydrops.[93,94] If left untreated, mortality rate may approach 100% for either or both fetuses and survivors may experience adverse neurodevelopmental outcomes and other severe morbidities.[95] Prevention of TTTS-related cardiovascular morbidity may be accomplished with in utero selective laser photocoagulation of the communicating placental vessels, which improves survival and mitigates the abnormal circulatory and loading conditions.[96,97]

**TABLE 29.2    Indications and Relative Contraindications for ECMO Among CDH Patients[91]**

| CDH ELSO/EURO Indications | Relative Contraindications |
|---|---|
| **Oxygenation:** OI > 40 for 4 h or $PaO_2$ < 40 for 2 h; pre-ductal $SpO_2$ < 80–85% persistently | **Malformations:** lethal chromosomal disease or malformation |
| **Acidosis:** Lactate > 5 mmol/L; pH < 7.15–7.2 (metabolic or respiratory); $PCO_2$ > 70 mmHg | **Cardiac:** Major structural heart disease |
| **Systemic blood flow:** Refractory poor perfusion or hypotension; UO < 0.5 mL/kg/h | **Intracranial hemorrhage:** Grade III/IV IVH |
| **Lung protective:** If requiring PIP > 26–28 cm $H_2O$ or MAP 14–17 (HFO) to attain $CO_2$ < 70 | **Prolonged mechanical ventilation** with high pressures (irreversible lung disease) |

*OI,* oxygenation index; *PaO₂,* partial pressure of oxygen; *SpO₂,* oxygen saturation; *PCO₂,* partial pressure of carbon dioxide; *UO,* urinary output; *PIP,* peek inspiratory pressure; *MAP,* mean airway pressure; *HFO,* high frequency oscillation; *IVH,* interventricular haemhorrage

## CARDIOVASCULAR CONSEQUENCES OF TTTS

TTTS results in concentric hypertrophic cardiomyopathy, particularly for the recipient twin, if not treated in utero. This manifests as marked ventricular dysfunction with echocardiography evidence of abnormal strain, strain rate, and tissue Doppler–derived measures of diastolic dysfunction in the first postnatal week. The pathogenesis is incompletely understood; however, the pattern of abnormalities is consistent with a combination of abnormal loading conditions and impaired contractility.[98] Placentally derived renin-angiotensin system effectors and imbalances in endothelin may be important contributors to diastolic dysfunction, which may precede systolic dysfunction in the untreated fetus and may continue to contribute to postnatal disease.[99,100] Finally, anatomic heart disease, specifically valvular disease, is more common among affected fetuses, predominantly in the recipient twin.[101] The most affected is the pulmonary valve; however, tricuspid and mitral disease may occur.[101]

## Hemodynamic Stabilization and Treatment in TTTS

Early echocardiography may be beneficial for both the donor and the recipient twin. Both structural and functional heart disease are common and should be anticipated. Choice of treatment for ventricular systolic dysfunction depends on arterial pressure levels. For patients with cardiac dysfunction and normal or high blood pressure, intravenous milrinone and dobutamine are good first-line therapies. In contrast, for patients with cardiac dysfunction and low blood pressure, a more potent inotrope with vasopressor activity such as epinephrine or combination therapy with an inotrope and vasopressor (e.g., vasopressin) may be more appropriate. The role of partial exchange in patients with polycythemia, which may further increase ventricular afterload, should be considered in patients with refractory heart dysfunction.

## Conclusion

Neonates with adverse in utero environment or genetic/developmental abnormalities may represent patients with special vulnerabilities and unique physiology. All the pathophysiology described in this chapter may result in a need to modify screening and/or therapy to attain optimal outcome. The ability to identify these deviations and physiologic nuances early may result in earlier stabilization or improved outcomes and comprehensive echocardiography may be an important modulator of approach.

## REFERENCES

1. Depla AL, De Wit L, Steenhuis TJ, et al. Effect of maternal diabetes on fetal heart function on echocardiography: systematic review and meta-analysis. *Ultrasound Obstet Gynecol.* 2021; 57(4):539-550. doi:10.1002/uog.22163.
2. Ferrara A. Increasing prevalence of gestational diabetes mellitus: a public health perspective. *Diabetes Care.* 2007;30(suppl 2): S141-S146. doi:10.2337/dc07-s206.
3. Sacks DA, Hadden DR, Maresh M, et al. Frequency of gestational diabetes mellitus at collaborating centers based on IADPSG consensus panel-recommended criteria: the Hyperglycemia and Adverse Pregnancy Outcome (HAPO) Study. *Diabetes Care.* 2012;35(3):526-528. doi:10.2337/dc11-1641.
4. Alapati D, Jassar R, Shaffer TH. Management of supplemental oxygen for infants with persistent pulmonary hypertension of newborn: a survey. *Am J Perinatol.* 2017;34(3):276-282. doi: 10.1055/s-0036-1586754.
5. Samanth J, Padmakumar R, Vasudeva A, Lewis L, Nayak K, Nayak V. Persistent subclinical myocardial dysfunction among infants of diabetic mothers. *J Diabetes* Complications. 2022; 36(1):108079. doi:10.1016/j.jdiacomp.2021.108079.
6. Seppänen MP, Ojanperä OS, Kääpä PO, Kero PO. Delayed postnatal adaptation of pulmonary hemodynamics in infants of diabetic mothers. *J Pediatr.* 1997;131(4):545-548. doi:10.1016/s0022-3476(97)70059-3.
7. Vela-Huerta M, Aguilera-López A, Alarcón-Santos S, Amador N, Aldana-Valenzuela C, Heredia A. Cardiopulmonary adaptation in large for gestational age infants of diabetic and nondiabetic mothers. *Acta Paediatr (Oslo, Norway: 1992).* 2007;96(9): 1303-1307. doi:10.1111/j.1651-2227.2007.00414.x.
8. Katheria A, Leone T. Altered transitional circulation in infants of diabetic mothers with strict antenatal obstetric management: a functional echocardiography study. *J Perinatol.* 2012;32(7): 508-513. doi:10.1038/jp.2011.135.
9. Paauw ND, Stegeman R, de Vroede M, Termote JUM, Freund MW, Breur J. Neonatal cardiac hypertrophy: the role of hyperinsulinism-a review of literature. *Eur J Pediatr.* 2020;179(1): 39-50. doi:10.1007/s00431-019-03521-6.
10. Mehta A, Hussain K. Transient hyperinsulinism associated with macrosomia, hypertrophic obstructive cardiomyopathy, hepatomegaly, and nephromegaly. *Arch Dis Child.* 2003;88(9):822-824.
11. Boyd SM, Riley KL, Giesinger RE, McNamara PJ. Use of vasopressin in neonatal hypertrophic obstructive cardiomyopathy: case series. *J Perinatol.* 2021;41(1):126-133. doi:10.1038/s41372-020-00824-7.
12. Mitanchez D, Yzydorczyk C, Siddeek B, Boubred F, Benahmed M, Simeoni U. The offspring of the diabetic mother – short- and long-term implications. *Best Pract Res Clin Obstet Gynaecol.* 2015;29(2):256-269. doi:10.1016/j.bpobgyn.2014.08.004.
13. Cimen D, Karaaslan S. Evaluation of cardiac functions of infants of diabetic mothers using tissue Doppler echocardiography. *Turk Pediatri Ars.* 2014;49(1):25-29. doi:10.5152/tpa.2014.843.

14. Kozak-Barany A, Jokinen E, Kero P, Tuominen J, Ronnemaa T, Valimaki I. Impaired left ventricular diastolic function in newborn infants of mothers with pregestational or gestational diabetes with good glycemic control. *Early Hum Dev.* 2004;77(1–2):13-22. doi:10.1016/j.earlhumdev.2003.11.006.

15. Korraa A, Ezzat MH, Bastawy M, Aly H, El-Mazary AA, Abd El-Aziz L. Cardiac troponin I levels and its relation to echocardiographic findings in infants of diabetic mothers. *Ital J Pediatr.* 2012;38:39. doi:10.1186/1824-7288-38-39.

16. Gewolb IH, O'Brien J. Surfactant secretion by type II pneumocytes is inhibited by high glucose concentrations. *Exp Lung Res.* 1997;23(3):245-255.

17. Morriss Jr FH. Infants of diabetic mothers. Fetal and neonatal pathophysiology. *Perspect Pediatr Pathol.* 1984;8(3):223-234.

18. Colpaert C, Hogan J, Stark AR, et al. Increased muscularization of small pulmonary arteries in preterm infants of diabetic mothers: a morphometric study in noninflated, noninjected, routinely fixed lungs. *Pediatr Pathol Lab Med.* 1995;15(5):689-705.

19. Baack ML, Forred BJ, Larsen TD, et al. Consequences of a maternal high-fat diet and late gestation diabetes on the developing rat lung. *PLoS One.* 2016;11(8):e0160818. doi:10.1371/journal.pone.0160818.

20. Upadhyaya B, Larsen T, Barwari S, Louwagie EJ, Baack ML, Dey M. Prenatal exposure to a maternal high-fat diet affects histone modification of cardiometabolic genes in newborn rats. *Nutrients.* 2017;9(4):407. doi:10.3390/nu9040407.

21. Kojo M, Ogawa T, Yamada K, Sonoda H, Saito K. Multivariate autoregressive analysis of carotid artery blood flow waveform in an infant of a diabetic mother with cardiomyopathy. *Acta Paediatr Jpn.* 1995;37(5):588-593.

22. Van Bel F, Van de Bor M, Walther FJ. Cerebral blood flow velocity and cardiac output in infants of insulin-dependent diabetic mothers. *Acta Paediatr Scand.* 1991;80(10):905-910.

23. Balan C, Wong AV. Sudden cardiac arrest in hypertrophic cardiomyopathy with dynamic cavity obstruction: the case for a decatecholaminisation strategy. *J Intensive Care Soc.* 2018;19(1):69-75. doi:10.1177/1751143717732729.

24. Goldberg JF, Mery CM, Griffiths PS, et al. Extracorporeal membrane oxygenation support in severe hypertrophic obstructive cardiomyopathy associated with persistent pulmonary hypertension in an infant of a diabetic mother. *Circulation.* 2014;130(21):1923-1925. doi:10.1161/circulationaha.114.010678.

25. Arzuaga BH, Groner A. Utilization of extracorporeal membrane oxygenation in congenital hypertrophic cardiomyopathy caused by maternal diabetes. *J Neonatal Perinatal Med.* 2013;6(4):345-348. doi:10.3233/npm-1372913.

26. Patel N, Mills JF, Cheung MM, Loughnan PM. Systemic haemodynamics in infants with vein of Galen malformation: assessment and basis for therapy. *J Perinatol.* 2007;27(7):460-463. doi:10.1038/sj.jp.7211752.

27. Patton DJ, Fouron JC. Cerebral arteriovenous malformation: prenatal and postnatal central blood flow dynamics. *Pediatr Cardiol.* 1995;16(3):141-144. doi:10.1007/bf00801914.

28. Mendez A, Codsi E, Gonzalez Barlatay F, Lapointe A, Raboisson MJ. Pulmonary hypertension associated with vein of Galen malformation. Fetal cardiac hemodynamic findings and physiological considerations. *J Perinatol.* 2022;42(1):143-148. doi:10.1038/s41372-021-01297-y.

29. Giesinger RE, Elsayed YN, Castaldo MP, McNamara PJ. Targeted neonatal echocardiography-guided therapy in vein of Galen aneurysmal malformation: a report of two cases with a review of physiology and approach to management. *AJP Rep.* 2019;9(2):e172-e176. doi:10.1055/s-0039-1688765.

30. Lakshminrusimha S, Russell JA, Wedgwood S, et al. Superoxide dismutase improves oxygenation and reduces oxidation in neonatal pulmonary hypertension. *Am J Respir Crit Care Med.* 2006;174(12):1370-1377. doi:10.1164/rccm.200605-676OC.

31. Lakshminrusimha S, Keszler M. Persistent pulmonary hypertension of the newborn. *Neoreviews.* 2015;16(12):e680-e692. doi:10.1542/neo.16-12-e680.

32. Nakanishi H, Suenaga H, Uchiyama A, Kusuda S. Persistent pulmonary hypertension of the newborn in extremely preterm infants: a Japanese cohort study. *Arch Dis Child Fetal Neonatal Ed.* 2018;103(6):F554-F561. doi:10.1136/archdischild-2017-313778.

33. Singh Y, Lakshminrusimha S. Pathophysiology and management of persistent pulmonary hypertension of the newborn. *Clin Perinatol.* 2021;48(3):595-618. doi:10.1016/j.clp.2021.05.009.

34. Gao Y, Raj JU. Regulation of the pulmonary circulation in the fetus and newborn. *Physiol Rev.* 2010;90(4):1291-1335. doi:10.1152/physrev.00032.2009.

35. Mous DS, Kool HM, Wijnen R, Tibboel D, Rottier RJ. Pulmonary vascular development in congenital diaphragmatic hernia. *Eur Respir Rev.* 2018;27(147):170104. doi:10.1183/16000617.0104-2017.

36. Hislop A, Reid L. Fetal and childhood development of the intrapulmonary veins in man – branching pattern and structure. *Thorax.* 1973;28(3):313-319. doi:10.1136/thx.28.3.313.

37. Rasanen J, Wood DC, Debbs RH, Cohen J, Weiner S, Huhta JC. Reactivity of the human fetal pulmonary circulation to maternal hyperoxygenation increases during the second half of pregnancy: a randomized study. *Circulation.* 1998;97(3):257-262. doi:10.1161/01.cir.97.3.257.

38. Mandell E, Kinsella JP, Abman SH. Persistent pulmonary hypertension of the newborn. *Pediatr Pulmonol.* 2021;56(3):661-669. doi:10.1002/ppul.25073.

39. Ghanayem NS, Gordon JB. Modulation of pulmonary vasomotor tone in the fetus and neonate. *Respir Res.* 2001;2(3):139-144. doi:10.1186/rr50.

40. Barth PJ, Rüschoff J. Morphometric study on pulmonary arterial thickness in pulmonary hypoplasia. *Pediatr Pathol.* 1992;12(5):653-663. doi:10.3109/15513819209024218.

41. Rozance PJ, Seedorf GJ, Brown A, et al. Intrauterine growth restriction decreases pulmonary alveolar and vessel growth and causes pulmonary artery endothelial cell dysfunction in vitro in fetal sheep. *Am J Physiol Lung Cell Mol Physiol.* 2011;301(6):L860-L871. doi:10.1152/ajplung.00197.2011.

42. Van Marter LJ, Leviton A, Allred EN, et al. Persistent pulmonary hypertension of the newborn and smoking and aspirin and nonsteroidal antiinflammatory drug consumption during pregnancy. *Pediatrics.* 1996;97(5):658-563.

43. Chambers CD, Hernandez-Diaz S, Van Marter LJ, et al. Selective serotonin-reuptake inhibitors and risk of persistent pulmonary hypertension of the newborn. *N Engl J Med.* 2006;354(6):579-587. doi:10.1056/NEJMoa052744.

44. Bearer C, Emerson RK, O'Riordan MA, Roitman E, Shackleton C. Maternal tobacco smoke exposure and persistent pulmonary hypertension of the newborn. *Environ Health Perspect.* 1997;105(2):202-206. doi:10.1289/ehp.97105202.

45. Hernandez-Diaz S, Van Marter LJ, Werler MM, Louik C, Mitchell AA. Risk factors for persistent pulmonary hypertension of the newborn. *Pediatrics.* 2007;120(2):e272-e282. doi:10.1542/peds.2006-3037.

46. da Cunha Durães MI, Flor-De-Lima F, Rocha G, Soares H, Guimarães H. Morbidity and mortality of preterm infants less than 26 weeks of gestational age. *Minerva Pediatr.* 2019; 71(1):12-20. doi:10.23736/s0026-4946.16.04609-0.

47. Toyono M, Harada K, Takahashi Y, Takada G. Maturational changes in left ventricular contractile state. *Int J Cardiol.* 1998;64(3):247-252.

48. Igarashi H, Shiraishi H, Endoh H, Yanagisawa M. Left ventricular contractile state in preterm infants: relation between wall stress and velocity of circumferential fiber shortening. *Am Heart J.* 1994;127(5):1336-1340.

49. Rudolph AM. Myocardial growth before and after birth: clinical implications. *Acta Paediatr.* 2000;89(2):129-133.

50. Friedman WF. The intrinsic physiologic properties of the developing heart. *Prog Cardiovasc Dis.* 1972;15(1):87-111.

51. Page E, Buecker JL. Development of dyadic junctional complexes between sarcoplasmic reticulum and plasmalemma in rabbit left ventricular myocardial cells. Morphometric analysis. *Circ Res.* 1981;48(4):519-522.

52. Giesinger RE, More K, Odame J, Jain A, Jankov RP, McNamara PJ. Controversies in the identification and management of acute pulmonary hypertension in preterm neonates. *Pediatr Res.* 2017;82(6):901-914. doi:10.1038/pr.2017.200.

53. Lewis AB, Heymann MA, Rudolph AM. Gestational changes in pulmonary vascular responses in fetal lambs in utero. *Circ Res.* 1976;39(4):536-541.

54. Patel A, Lakshminrusimha S, Ryan RM, et al. Exposure to supplemental oxygen downregulates antioxidant enzymes and increases pulmonary arterial contractility in premature lambs. *Neonatology.* 2009;96(3):182-192. doi:10.1159/000211667.

55. Walther FJ, Wade AB, Warburton D, Forman HJ. Ontogeny of antioxidant enzymes in the fetal lamb lung. *Exp Lung Res.* 1991;17(1):39-45.

56. Frank L, Sosenko IR. Prenatal development of lung antioxidant enzymes in four species. *J Pediatr.* 1987;110(1):106-110.

57. Baczynski M, Ginty S, Weisz DE, et al. Short-term and long-term outcomes of preterm neonates with acute severe pulmonary hypertension following rescue treatment with inhaled nitric oxide. *Arch Dis Child Fetal Neonatal Ed.* 2017;102(6):F508-F514. doi:10.1136/archdischild-2016-312409.

58. Ahmed MS, Giesinger RE, Ibrahim M, et al. Clinical and echocardiography predictors of response to inhaled nitric oxide in hypoxic preterm neonates. *J Paediatr Child Health.* 2019;55(7): 753-761. doi:10.1111/jpc.14286.

59. Giesinger RE, More K, Odame J, Jain A, Jankov RP, McNamara PJ. Controversies in the identification and management of acute pulmonary hypertension in preterm neonates. *Pediatr Res.* 2017;82(6):901-914. doi:10.1038/pr.2017.200.

60. The Franco-Belgium Collaborative NO Trial Group. Early compared with delayed inhaled nitric oxide in moderately hypoxaemic neonates with respiratory failure: a randomised controlled trial. The Franco-Belgium Collaborative NO Trial Group. *Lancet.* 1999;354:1066-1071.

61. Srisuparp P, Heitschmidt M, Schreiber MD. Inhaled nitric oxide therapy in premature infants with mild to moderate respiratory distress syndrome. *J Med Assoc Thai.* 2002;85(Suppl 2): S469-S478.

62. Su PH, Chen JY. Inhaled nitric oxide in the management of preterm infants with severe respiratory failure. *J Perinatol.* 2008;28:112-116.

63. Wei QF, Pan XN, Li Y, et al. [Efficacy of inhaled nitric oxide in premature infants with hypoxic respiratory failure]. Zhongguo Dang Dai Er Ke Za Zhi. *Chin J Contemp Pediatr.* 2014;16: 805-809.

64. Osborn D, Evans N, Kluckow M. Randomized trial of dobutamine versus dopamine in preterm infants with low systemic blood flow. *J Pediatr.* 2002;140(2):183-191. doi:10.1067/mpd.2002.120834.

65. Mohamed AA, Louis D, Surak A, Weisz DE, McNamara PJ, Jain A. Vasopressin for refractory persistent pulmonary hypertension of the newborn in preterm neonates – a case series. *J Matern Fetal Neonatal Med.* 2022;35(8):1475-1483. doi:10.1080/14767058.2020.1757642.

66. Eichinger MR, Walker BR. Enhanced pulmonary arterial dilation to arginine vasopressin in chronically hypoxic rats. *Am J Physiol.* 1994;267(6 Pt 2):H2413-H2419. doi:10.1152/ajpheart.1994.267.6.H2413.

67. James AT, Bee C, Corcoran JD, McNamara PJ, Franklin O, El-Khuffash AF. Treatment of premature infants with pulmonary hypertension and right ventricular dysfunction with milrinone: a case series. *J Perinatol.* 2015;35(4):268-273. doi:10.1038/jp.2014.208.

68. Russell MK, Longoni M, Wells J, et al. Congenital diaphragmatic hernia candidate genes derived from embryonic transcriptomes. *Proc Natl Acad Sci U S A.* 2012;109(8):2978-2983. doi:10.1073/pnas.1121621109.

69. Yu L, Sawle AD, Wynn J, et al. Increased burden of de novo predicted deleterious variants in complex congenital diaphragmatic hernia. *Hum Mol Genet.* 2015;24(16):4764-4773. doi:10.1093/hmg/ddv196.

70. Brady PD, Srisupundit K, Devriendt K, Fryns JP, Deprest JA, Vermeesch JR. Recent developments in the genetic factors underlying congenital diaphragmatic hernia. *Fetal Diagn Ther.* 2011;29(1):25-39. doi:10.1159/000322422.

71. Kardon G, Ackerman KG, McCulley DJ, et al. Congenital diaphragmatic hernias: from genes to mechanisms to therapies. *Dis Models Mech.* 2017;10(8):955-970. doi:10.1242/dmm.028365.

72. Ameis D, Khoshgoo N, Keijzer R. Abnormal lung development in congenital diaphragmatic hernia. *Semin Pediatr Surg.* 2017;26(3):123-128. doi:10.1053/j.sempedsurg.2017.04.011.

73. Ackerman KG, Wang J, Luo L, Fujiwara Y, Orkin SH, Beier DR. Gata4 is necessary for normal pulmonary lobar development. *Am J Respir Cell Mol Biol.* 2007;36(4):391-397. doi:10.1165/rcmb.2006-0211RC.

74. You LR, Takamoto N, Yu CT, et al. Mouse lacking COUP-TFII as an animal model of Bochdalek-type congenital diaphragmatic hernia. *Proc Natl Acad Sci U S A.* 2005;102(45): 16351-16356. doi:10.1073/pnas.0507832102.

75. Mann PC, Morriss Jr FH, Klein JM. Prediction of survival in infants with congenital diaphragmatic hernia based on stomach position, surgical timing, and oxygenation index. *Am J Perinatol.* 2012;29(5):383-390. doi:10.1055/s-0032-1304817.

76. Montalva L, Lauriti G, Zani A. Congenital heart disease associated with congenital diaphragmatic hernia: a systematic review on incidence, prenatal diagnosis, management, and outcome. *J Pediatr Surg.* 2019;54(5):909-919. doi:10.1016/j.jpedsurg.2019.01.018.

77. Massolo AC, Romiti A, Viggiano M, et al. Fetal cardiac dimensions in congenital diaphragmatic hernia: relationship with gestational age and postnatal outcomes. *J Perinatol.* 2021; 41(7):1651-1659. doi:10.1038/s41372-021-00986-y.

78. Graziano JN. Cardiac anomalies in patients with congenital diaphragmatic hernia and their prognosis: a report from the Congenital Diaphragmatic Hernia Study Group. *J Pediatr Surg.* 2005;40(6):1045-1050. doi:10.1016/j.jpedsurg.2005.03.025.

79. Metkus AP, Filly RA, Stringer MD, Harrison MR, Adzick NS. Sonographic predictors of survival in fetal diaphragmatic hernia. *J Pediatr Surg*. 1996;31(1):148-152. doi:10.1016/s0022-3468(96)90338-3.

80. Jani J, Nicolaides KH, Keller RL, et al. Observed to expected lung area to head circumference ratio in the prediction of survival in fetuses with isolated diaphragmatic hernia. *Ultrasound Obstet Gynecol*. 2007;30(1):67-71. doi:10.1002/uog.4052.

81. Khan AA, Furey EA, Bailey AA, et al. Fetal liver and lung volume index of neonatal survival with congenital diaphragmatic hernia. *Pediatr Radiol*. 2021;51(9):1637-1644. doi:10.1007/s00247-021-05049-0.

82. Suda K, Bigras JL, Bohn D, Hornberger LK, McCrindle BW. Echocardiographic predictors of outcome in newborns with congenital diaphragmatic hernia. *Pediatrics*. 2000;105(5):1106-1109. doi:10.1542/peds.105.5.1106.

83. Tonelli AR, Plana JC, Heresi GA, Dweik RA. Prevalence and prognostic value of left ventricular diastolic dysfunction in idiopathic and heritable pulmonary arterial hypertension. *Chest*. 2012;141(6):1457-1465. doi:10.1378/chest.11-1903.

84. Patel N, Kipfmueller F. Cardiac dysfunction in congenital diaphragmatic hernia: pathophysiology, clinical assessment, and management. *Semin Pediatr Surg*. 2017;26(3):154-158. doi:10.1053/j.sempedsurg.2017.04.001.

85. Gien J, Kinsella JP. Management of pulmonary hypertension in infants with congenital diaphragmatic hernia. *J Perinatol*. 2016;36(suppl 2):S28-S31. doi:10.1038/jp.2016.46.

86. Patel N, Lally PA, Kipfmueller F, et al. Ventricular dysfunction is a critical determinant of mortality in congenital diaphragmatic hernia. *Am J Respir Crit Care Med*. 2019;200(12):1522-1530. doi:10.1164/rccm.201904-0731OC.

87. Yu PT, Jen HC, Rice-Townsend S, Guner YS. The role of ECMO in the management of congenital diaphragmatic hernia. *Semin Perinatol*. 2020;44(1):151166. doi:10.1053/j.semperi.2019.07.005.

88. Puligandla PS, Grabowski J, Austin M, et al. Management of congenital diaphragmatic hernia: a systematic review from the APSA outcomes and evidence based practice committee. *J Pediatr Surg*. 2015;50(11):1958-1970. doi:10.1016/j.jpedsurg.2015.09.010.

89. Bischoff AR, Habib S, McNamara PJ, Giesinger RE. Hemodynamic response to milrinone for refractory hypoxemia during therapeutic hypothermia for neonatal hypoxic ischemic encephalopathy. *J Perinatol*. 2021;41(9):2345-2354. doi:10.1038/s41372-021-01049-y.

90. McIntyre CM, Hanna BD, Rintoul N, Ramsey EZ. Safety of epoprostenol and treprostinil in children less than 12 months of age. *Pulm Circ*. 2013;3(4):862-869. doi:10.1086/674762.

91. Rafat N, Schaible T. Extracorporeal membrane oxygenation in congenital diaphragmatic hernia. *Front Pediatr*. 2019;7:336. doi:10.3389/fped.2019.00336.

92. Moon-Grady AJ. Fetal echocardiography in twin-twin transfusion syndrome. *Am J Perinatol*. 2014;31(suppl 1):S31-S38. doi:10.1055/s-0034-1378146.

93. Manning N, Archer N. Cardiac manifestations of twin-to-twin transfusion syndrome. *Twin Res Hum Genet*. 2016;19(3):246-254. doi:10.1017/thg.2016.20. Available at: http://www.journals.cambridge.org/abstract_S1832427416000207.

94. Rychik J, Zeng S, Bebbington M, et al. Speckle tracking-derived myocardial tissue deformation imaging in twin-twin transfusion syndrome: differences in strain and strain rate between donor and recipient twins. *Fetal Diagn Ther*. 2012;32:131-137. Available at: http://eutils.ncbi.nlm.nih.gov/entrez/eutils/elink.fcgi?dbfrom=pubmed&id=22613884&retmode=ref&cmd=prlinks.

95. Harkness UF, Crombleholme TM. Twin-twin transfusion syndrome: where do we go from here? *Semin Perinatol*. 2005;29(5):296-304. Available at: http://linkinghub.elsevier.com/retrieve/pii/S0146000505000893.

96. Akkermans J, Peeters SH, Klumper FJ, Lopriore E, Middeldorp JM, Oepkes D. Twenty-five years of fetoscopic laser coagulation in twin-twin transfusion syndrome: a systematic review. *Fetal Diagn Ther*. 2015;38(4):241-253. Available at: https://www.karger.com/Article/FullText/437053.

97. Roberts D, Gates S, Kilby M, Neilson JP. Interventions for twin-twin transfusion syndrome: a Cochrane review. *Ultrasound Obstet Gynecol*. 2008;31(6):701-711. doi:10.1002/uog.5328.

98. Breatnach CR, Bussmann N, Levy PT, et al. Postnatal myocardial function in monochorionic diamniotic twins with twin-to-twin transfusion syndrome following selective laser photocoagulation of the communicating placental vessels. *J Am Soc Echocardiogr*. 2019;32(6):774-784.e1. doi:10.1016/j.echo.2019.02.004.

99. Raboisson MJ, Fouron JC, Lamoureux J, et al. Early intertwin differences in myocardial performance during the twin-to-twin transfusion syndrome. *Circulation*. 2004;110(19):3043-3048. Available at: http://circ.ahajournals.org/cgi/doi/10.1161/01.CIR.0000146896.20317.59.

100. Bensouda B, Fouron JC, Raboisson MJ, Lamoureux J, Lachance C, Leduc L. Relevance of measuring diastolic time intervals in the ductus venosus during the early stages of twin-twin transfusion syndrome. *Ultrasound Obstet Gynecol*. 2007;30(7):983-987. doi:10.1002/uog.5161.

101. Habli M, Lim FY, Crombleholme T. Twin-to-twin transfusion syndrome: a comprehensive update. *Clin Perinatol*. 2009;36(2):391-416. x. doi:10.1016/j.clp.2009.03.003.

# Chapter 30

# Critical Congenital Heart Disease: What Should the Neonatologist Know?

Shazia Bhombal, Ganga Krishnamurthy, Jay D. Pruetz, and Yogen Singh

## Introduction

The incidence of congenital heart disease (CHD) is estimated at approximately 8 per 1000 live births,[1] with up to 25–30% of CHD deemed critical congenital heart disease (CCHD). CCHD includes lesions that necessitate early interventions to avoid significant morbidity and mortality and require multidisciplinary subspecialty care from pediatric cardiologists, cardiothoracic surgeons, neonatologists, anesthesiologists, and pediatric cardiac intensivists. Detection of CCHD by prenatal ultrasound (fetal anomaly screening) or by newborn pulse oximetry screening can occur prior to decompensation resulting in decreased morbidity and mortality in this vulnerable population.[2-4] Although there have been remarkable advances in ultrasound technology and an increasing prenatal detection rate, a significant proportion of cases of CCHD are diagnosed postnatally.[5] In the United States prenatal detection of CCHD has gradually increased from 26% in 2006 to 43% in 2012, with improvements in ultrasound technology and improved screening guidelines that emphasized the outflow tract views.[6] As such, CCHD may be unknown at birth, and neonatologists or non-cardiologist acute care physicians may be the "first call" for a decompensating infant with CCHD. Congenital heart disease remains the leading cause of infant mortality at approximately 40% of all deaths resulting from birth defects; thus familiarity with signs and symptoms of CCHD is paramount in the care of a decompensating neonate.[7] This chapter focuses on understanding the presenting pathophysiology and outlines the initial management by neonatal providers for a patient with CCHD.

## Clinical Presentation of CCHD

Critical congenital heart disease traditionally refers to lesions deemed necessitating surgical or catheter-based procedures in the first year of life,[8] with the focus of this chapter on those requiring life-sustaining intervention within the first postnatal month. Neonates with CCHD can manifest with varying degrees of severity due to several different pathophysiologic states: (1) increasing cyanosis due to lack of mixing of systemic and pulmonary venous return or inadequate pulmonary arterial blood flow; (2) signs of hypoperfusion resulting from inadequate systemic blood flow due to obstruction of systemic blood flow or decreased systolic function; and (3) respiratory distress due to excessive pulmonary flow or pulmonary venous obstruction. Neonates may have features of more than one presentation type depending on the lesion type and postnatal age. Timing of presentation will depend on type of CHDs ([i] ductal-dependent lesions and timing of PDA closure, e.g., hypoplastic left heart syndrome [HLHS], [ii] patent foramen ovale [PFO]/central mixing dependent, e.g., transposition of the great arteries [TGA], and [iii] obstructed pulmonary venous return), the rate of drop in pulmonary vascular resistance (PVR), and associated heart lesions (see Table 30.1). In a study assessing time to significant hemodynamic compromise in the setting of undiagnosed CCHD, defined as severe metabolic acidosis, cardiac arrest, lab evidence of renal or hepatic insult, or seizure, most (83%) occurred after 12 postnatal hours. Aortic arch obstructive lesions comprised approximately 90% of cases with significant hemodynamic compromise that were potentially preventable.[9] In addition, early diagnosis of CCHD (antenatal or pre-discharge) had a higher survival

## TABLE 30.1 Timing of Presentation With CCHD

| Soon After Birth (Severe Cyanosis With Inadequate Mixing or Respiratory Compromise*) | Within First Days to 1–2 Weeks (PDA Dependent Perfusion) | Within First Month (PVR Decreases, CHF, Cyanosis, Hypoperfusion) |
|---|---|---|
| • TGA with restrictive/intact atrial septum<br>• HLHS with restrictive/intact atrial septum<br>• TAPVC with obstructed veins<br>• TOF with absent pulmonary valve* | • Pulmonary stenosis(PS)<br>• Pulmonary atresia<br>• TOF with severe PS<br>• VSD with PS<br>• Tricuspid atresia with PS<br>• Severe Ebstein's Anomaly<br>• Critical coarctation<br>• Interrupted aortic arch<br>• Critical aortic stenosis | • Truncus arteriosus<br>• Tricuspid atresia with VSD and no PS<br>• CAVC<br>• Pink TOF<br>• Unobstructed TAPVC |

Adapted from Desai et al.[69]
*Corresponds to respiratory compromise with TOF with absent pulmonary valve in column. *CAVC*, complete atrioventricular canal *CCHD*, critical congenital heart disease; *CHF*, congestive heart failure; *HLHS*, hypoplastic left heart syndrome; *PDA*, patent ductus arteriosus; *PS*, pulmonary stenosis; *PVR*, pulmonary vascular resistance; *TAPVC*, total anomalous pulmonary venous connection; *TGA*, transposition of the great arteries; *TOF*, tetralogy of Fallot; *VSD*, ventricular septal defect.

advantage versus late diagnosis following discharge from hospital (16% vs. 27%).[10]

## PHYSIOLOGY OF CCHD

Within CCHD, five categories of lesions prevail, with recognition that many lesions can fall into more than one category: (1) ductal-dependent pulmonary blood flow, (2) ductal-dependent systemic blood flow, (3) pulmonary venous obstruction, (4) mixing lesions, and (5) transposition of the great arteries (see Table 30.2). CCHD lesion types with inadequate

aortic or pulmonary outflow are termed "ductal-dependent", given the need for flow through the ductus arteriosus to provide or augment either pulmonary or systemic blood flow.

## Ductal-Dependent Pulmonary Circulation

In patients with ductal-dependent pulmonary circulation, prostaglandin E1/E2 is required to augment pulmonary blood flow. This obstruction can occur anywhere along the path through the right side of the

## TABLE 30.2 CCHD Categories

| DD Pulmonary Flow | DD Systemic Flow | Obstructive Lesions | Mixing Lesions | Parallel Circulation |
|---|---|---|---|---|
| • Pulmonary atresia with intact ventricular septum<br>• TOF with severe right outflow tract obstruction<br>• TOF with pulmonary atresia*<br>• Tricuspid atresia with severe PS+<br>• Severe Ebstein's Anomaly | • HLHS<br>• Interrupted aortic arch<br>• Critical aortic stenosis<br>• Coarctation of the aorta | • TAPVC with obstruction<br>• HLHS with RAS/IAS | • Tricuspid Atresia with VSD<br>• Truncus arteriosus<br>• Single ventricle variants | • Transposition of the great arteries# |

*CCHD*, critical congenital heart disease; *DD*, ductal dependent; *HLHS*, hypoplastic left heart syndrome; *PS*, pulmonary stenosis, *TAPVC*, total anomalous pulmonary venous connection, *TOF*, tetralogy of Fallot; *VSD*, ventricular septal defect.
*Pulmonary flow may be supplied by multiple aortopulmonary collaterals (MAPCAs) and not be DD.
+Most commonly normally related great vessels, with DD pulmonary flow; can be transposed great vessels and reliant on ductus to augment systemic flow.
#Parallel circulation requiring atrial level mixing.

heart, from the tricuspid valve (e.g., tricuspid atresia with normally related great vessels) to the right ventricular outflow tract (RVOT, e.g., pulmonary atresia with intact septum, and tetralogy of Fallot with severe pulmonary stenosis or Ebstein's anomaly with pulmonary obstruction) (see Figure 30.1). Flow through the ductus arteriosus in patients with ductal-depending pulmonary circulation will traverse from the aorta to the lungs, with increasing pulmonary flow (Qp) over time as the PVR decreases. In patients with ductal-dependent pulmonary circulation, decreased saturations could be a result of decreased Qp if pulmonary flow decreases, such as in the case of ductal closure or restriction, or due to decreased pulmonary venous saturation related to pulmonary edema in cases with increased Qp as PVR decreases. Chest radiograph can help differentiate between these conditions with oligemic lung fields as pulmonary flow decreases and plethoric lung fields in patients with increased Qp (see Figure 30.2).

## Ductal-Dependent Systemic Circulation

Lesions with ductal-dependent systemic flow include left-sided obstructive lesions that limit systemic blood flow without the presence of a patent ductus arteriosus

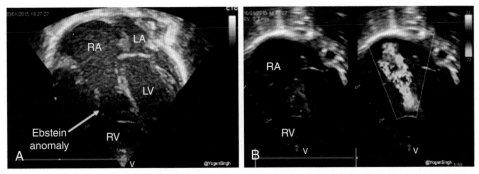

**Fig. 30.1** Ebstein's anomaly with failure of delamination of the septal leaflet of the tricuspid valve and obstruction to flow out the pulmonary artery. (A) 2D four-chamber apical view demonstrating atrialization of the right ventricle, (B) blue flow going away from the ventricle from the tricuspid valve into the atrialized right ventricle and right atrium.

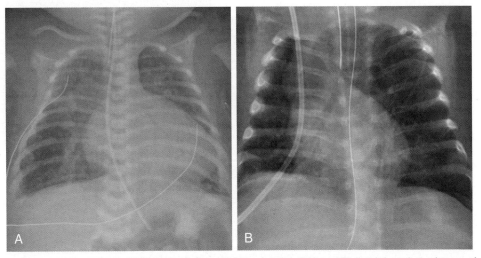

**Fig. 30.2** CXRs demonstrating (A) ductal-dependent systemic flow with hyperemic lung fields and (B) ductal-dependent pulmonary circulation with oligemic lung fields in setting of smaller ductal flow.

(PDA), such as interrupted aortic arch, severe coarctation, and hypoplastic left heart syndrome (HLHS) (see Table 30.1). As the ductus arteriosus (DA) restricts, patients may present in cardiogenic shock with hypoperfusion and acidosis and in extreme cases with death when the PDA closes. As the DA starts to constrict, pulses and perfusion can diminish, and if it continues to close completely, the patient may present in extremis with shock. Even once the DA is reopened successfully, the cardiac function may need time to recover as a result of the acidosis and the increased afterload on the left ventricle prior to surgical intervention. Early intervention may be necessary in patients with ductal-dependent systemic circulation. While most cases of HLHS can be stabilized by maintaining DA patency to provide adequate systemic flow, approximately 6–20% of HLHS cases have an intact or restrictive atrial septum, with pulmonary venous obstruction.[11-13] These infants present with early decompensation after birth, similar to d-TGA with restrictive atrial septum/intact atrial septum (RAS/IAS) though related to different pathophysiologic mechanism related to lack of egress from the left atrium and pulmonary vasculopathy. Infants with a restrictive or intact atrial septum present a time-critical emergency as they require immediate intervention for the creation of mixing at the atrial level despite successfully keeping the DA patent. Catheter-based or surgical intervention on the atrial septum is imperative to ensure adequate atrial mixing; nevertheless, even with intervention, mortality is still high.[13]

Catheter-based fetal septal interventions have been attempted in these infants, and while a recent analysis demonstrated procedural successes, this has not yet translated into improved survival when compared with a cohort of HLHS with patent atrial septum.[14]

## Non-Ductal-Dependent CCHD

Not all critical CHDs are necessarily ductal dependent, yet many still require intervention in the first postnatal month. CCHD with obstructed venous flow such as obstructive total anomalous pulmonary venous connection (TAPVC), mixing lesions such as truncus arteriosus, and transposition of the great arteries (TGA) are not ductal-dependent lesions by definition; however, patients with TGA may have some

benefit in use of PGE while obstructive TAPVC may either improve transiently or even worsen with its use. With TGA, the blood moves in parallel circuits, while not a traditional mixing lesion; specifically, systemic flow returns to the right heart and then is ejected out the aorta back to the body, while the pulmonary venous flow returns to the left heart and is ejected out the pulmonary artery back to the lungs. An atrial septal defect is required to allow oxygenated blood from the left atrium to the right atrium and out the aorta to the body (see Figure 30.3). In patients with

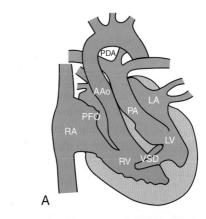

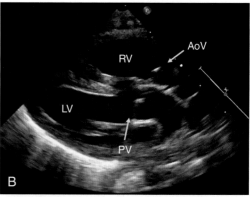

**Fig. 30.3** Transposition of the great arteries with parallel circulations that require an atrial septal defect for mixing from left to right atrium to allow flow across the aortic valve and to the body. Presence of a ventricular septal defect does not allow for adequate mixing – as PVR falls, blood flow will take the path of least resistance toward the pulmonary circulation from right to left ventricle and out to the pulmonary artery. (A) Diagram of TGA with a PDA and VSD present, (B) parasternal long-axis view of TGA with both great arteries seen in one plane due to failure to twist in utero. (Illustration courtesy of Satyan Lakshminrusimha.)

desaturation utilization of PGE will allow increased pulmonary flow to enter the left atrium and encourage further mixing at the atrial level. A common misconception is that utilization of PGE providing ductal patency provides mixing at the ductus level. In fact, what the DA often provides is effective pulmonary blood flow, such that deoxygenated systemic blood can get to the lungs and then return to the left atrium oxygenated and mix at the atrial level. It is important to remember that in patients with TGA, the expectation is for flow to traverse from the aorta with higher systemic vascular resistance across the PDA to the pulmonary arteries and lung as PVR falls. In some patients with a dysregulated postnatal transition, elevated PVR may further limit pulmonary blood flow and the efficacy of oxygenation, necessitating transient use of pulmonary vasodilators. A ventricular septal defect alone may not allow for adequate mixing as flow across the VSD is also dependent on the relative downstream resistances. Another physiologic consideration is the potential for reversed differential saturation in patients with d-TGA and pulmonary hypertension, with preductal saturations lower than post-ductal saturations. In these patients pulmonary venous flow enters the left atrium, into the left ventricle, and out the RVOT. In patients with elevated PVR in comparison to systemic vascular resistance (SVR), oxygenated blood will shunt right to left across the PDA and down the descending aorta, while systemic flow will enter the right atrium, with some mixing of oxygenated blood from the left to right atrium into the right ventricle, out the aorta.

Both patients with obstructive TAPVC and TGA with restrictive/intact atrial septum will present at or soon after birth with hypoxemia (decreased saturation) and will deteriorate regardless of ductal flow. In patients with obstructive TAPVC, which is most commonly infradiaphragmatic, PGE initiation may be detrimental as it may increase flow into a vascular bed with a downstream obstruction. In these cases, what is needed to prevent further morbidity and mortality is a rapid and definitive surgical repair to reconnect the pulmonary veins to the left atrium. TAPVC is particularly challenging to diagnose prenatally[15] and thus should be on the differential of a neonate with respiratory distress after delivery and similar CXR findings to meconium aspiration.

Finally, patients with truncus arteriosus have no protection of their pulmonary vascular bed, with only one valve separating intracardiac flow to systemic and pulmonary flow, with high risk of development of pulmonary vascular disease.[16] As PVR drops, increasing flow will steal from the systemic circulation to the pulmonary circulation, placing neonates with truncus arteriosus at high risk of end-organ hypoperfusion. In particular, these patients have a higher risk of developing necrotizing enterocolitis (NEC) from hypoperfusion to the gut.[17]

Although there are some situations where initiation of PGE may worsen a patient's condition, in most cases of CCHD (including TAPVC), PGE will either help or not significantly harm outcomes. Thus, from a neonatologist's perspective, *it is always reasonable to start prostaglandin when critical CHD is suspected until underlying anatomy is delineated by a pediatric cardiologist.*

## Clinical Presentation of CCHD

### CYANOSIS AND POSTNATAL PULSE OXIMETRY SCREENING

Cyanotic heart diseases, with hypoxemia as the primary presenting symptom, result from mixing of systemic flow (Qs) and pulmonary flow (Qp). Cyanosis occurs due to two mechanisms: (1) intracardiac shunting of deoxygenated blood from the right side of the heart to the left-side systemic circulation secondary to cyanotic CHD and (2) extrapulmonary right-to-left shunts at the levels of the PDA or PFO in acute pulmonary hypertension (PH). In the former, related to shunting of intracardiac mixing, the blood leaving the heart is already mixed, with both pre- and post-ductal saturations reflecting hypoxemia. The etiology includes both right-sided obstructive lesions (e.g., tricuspid atresia, tetralogy of Fallot, pulmonary atresia) and left-sided obstructed lesions (e.g., hypoplastic left heart syndrome), and mixing lesions without obstruction (e.g., truncus arteriosus, total anomalous pulmonary venous return, transposition of the great arteries). These seven cyanotic lesions with intracardiac shunting are the target of the postnatal CCHD pulse oximetry screen (see Table 30.3). Cyanosis due to extrapulmonary shunts for CCHD relates to cases of arch obstruction such as interrupted aortic arch with a PDA.

TABLE 30.3 **Targets of the CCHD Screen, 7 Primary Targets, 5 Secondary Targets Typically Associated With Some Hypoxemia[70]**

| Primary Targets of CCHD Screen | Secondary Targets of CCHD Screen |
|---|---|
| • Hypoplastic left heart syndrome<br>• Transposition of the great arteries<br>• Truncus arteriosus<br>• Total anomalous pulmonary venous connection<br>• Tricuspid atresia<br>• Pulmonary atresia with intact ventricular septum<br>• Tetralogy of Fallot | • Interrupted aortic arch<br>• Coarctation of the aorta<br>• Ebstein's anomaly<br>• Double outlet right ventricle<br>• Single ventricle |

Adapted from Oster et al.[70]

*CCHD*, critical congenital heart disease

In this situation measurement of preductal saturation (right arm) and post-ductal saturation (right leg) may show a significant difference between pre- and post-ductal $PaO_2$, indicating that the blood is shunted at the level of PDA from pulmonary to systemic circulation. Therefore it is important for neonatologists to recognize that an exclusive pre-/post-ductal saturation gradient is not pathognomonic of acute PH.

While hypoxemia is present in most neonates with CCHD, appreciation of cyanosis on clinical exam is challenging, with 4–5 g of deoxygenated Hb required to produce visible cyanosis. In a neonate with Hb 20 g/dL cyanosis would be noted clinically at an oxygen saturation of <80%, but at less than 60% in a neonate with a Hb of 10 g/dL[8]. Of note, neonates with CCHD and cyanosis often appear comfortable without respiratory distress, as opposed to patients with cyanosis and respiratory compromise leading to poor gas exchange and/or pulmonary hypertension with right to left ductal shunting.

With recognition that early diagnosis of CCHD improves outcomes, pulse oximetry screening was added to the US-recommended Uniform Screening Panel for newborns in 2011.[18] In a state review the estimated numbers of CCHD were 0.17% of the population (approximately 136 patients per year), 48 with a critical left heart lesion and 7 with missed critical left heart lesions. These numbers are more impressive when compared to the routine statewide screening program, which picked up 26 cases of galactosemia, 5 of phenylketonuria, and 0 of maple syrup urine disease. This reflects the importance of a screening program for critical CHD.[19] Prior to implementation of universal pulse oximetry screening, a state registry noted that CCHD was not diagnosed during initial hospitalization in approximately 23% of patients with CCHD. Patients born in level 1 or level 2 hospitals had later detection of CCHD than those born in a level 3 hospital, indicating that pulse oximetry screening may be particularly useful in level 1 and level 2 units.[20]

However, while addition of the pulse oximetry screening to the existing screening tools will help in detecting up to 80–92% of CCHD, some lesions remain under-detected, particularly left-sided heart obstruction. (Table 30.3).[9] Hence a neonatologist who is often the first point of contact for seeing these infants should have a low threshold for suspecting underlying CHD and initiating therapy such as prostaglandin E1 (PGE) and obtaining an echocardiogram. Echocardiography is the investigation of choice to diagnose CHD at bedside; however, pediatric cardiology services may not be readily available in all centers. Institutions with neonatal hemodynamic consult services where a neonatologist trained in targeted neonatal echocardiography or neonatologist-performed echocardiography (TNE or NPE, respectively) can utilize imaging to differentiate between varying pathologies. NPE-trained personnel have demonstrated the ability to identify structural heart disease when echocardiography was obtained prior to imaging by the cardiac service.[21] While the goal of NPE is not to diagnose congenital heart disease, in a decompensating patient, it may be life-saving and provide earlier access to pediatric cardiology in centers where these services are not routinely available.

Therefore all first echocardiograms must be comprehensive and, if not performed by a pediatric cardiologist, include all the necessary views/sweeps to enable exclusion of major forms of congenital heart disease. These images may be remotely reviewed by a pediatric cardiologist with imaging expertise. However, it is important to recognize that imaging may not be readily available for diagnosis of CHD and understanding the physiology and timing of presentation is integral to ensuring that CCHD is considered and managed in a neonate.

## HYPOPERFUSION

The initial presenting symptoms to a neonatologist may include limitation to systemic blood flow. Hypoperfusion may be observed in all categories of CCHD lesions. Hypoperfusion resulting from decreased systemic blood flow can manifest with lactic acidosis, end-organ dysfunction, cool extremities, and in severe cases circulatory collapse with shock. In a patient with ductal-dependent pulmonary blood flow (e.g., pulmonary atresia with intact ventricular septum), as PVR drops in the presence of a large PDA, increased flow left to right from the arch to the pulmonary vasculature can lead to decreased systemic flow, resulting in metabolic acidosis. This can be more pronounced in patients with mixing lesions without obstruction, such as truncus arteriosus. As PVR falls, increased ductal flow is shunted to the pulmonary vasculature unimpeded through systole and diastole, with patients with truncus arteriosus noted to have higher risk for development of NEC.[17] Finally, patients with CCHD with ductal-dependent systemic flow are at risk of systemic hypoperfusion; in particular, patients with HLHS are at higher risk for development of NEC compared with other congenital heart disease.[17,22]

## Postnatal Transition and Instability With CCHD

Transition at birth from fetal to postnatal circulation involves lung expansion and a drop in PVR with loss of the low-resistance placental circulation, resulting in increased systemic vascular resistance, diminishing contribution of fetal intracardiac shunts, and a shift to reliance on oxygen from the lungs rather than the placenta.[23,24] Most patients with CCHD remain relatively asymptomatic during the postnatal transition aside from lower oxygen saturation if a pulse oximeter is placed. Timing of presentation depends on the type of lesion and potential additional factors (Table 30.1). Lesions with severe obstruction to flow, limitation of cardiac output, or respiratory compromise resulting from CCHD present immediately after birth.

CCHD with instability during the immediate postnatal transition can be grouped into four categories: (1) inadequate pulmonary venous egress, such as in obstructed TAPVC and subtypes HLHS with intact or restrictive atrial septum; (2) inadequate intracardiac mixing of oxygenated blood to the systemic circulation in some cases of d-transposition of the great arteries (d-TGA) with restrictive atrial shunt; (3) associated airway anomalies which compromise the ability to ventilate such as severe cases of Ebstein's anomaly and tetralogy of Fallot (TOF) with absent pulmonary valve (APV); and (4) inadequate cardiac output in cases of severe fetal arrhythmias and/or decreased cardiac function.[25] Additionally, identification of the fetus with CCHD and hydrops may allow time for optimal delivery planning, weighing risks of early delivery with worsening hydrops. Patients with certain CCHD that can lead to an increase in central venous pressure may be at risk for fetal hydrops, such as lesions with significant atrioventricular (AV) valve regurgitation (e.g., AV septal defects, Ebstein's anomaly, tricuspid valve dysplasia). Two factors may contribute to development of hydrops: (1) the fetal myocardium is less compliant and does not tolerate small changes in preload well (due to diastolic stiffness) and (2) fetuses have increased capillary permeability, lower osmotic pressure, and reliance on lymphatics for drainage, contributing to increased extracellular fluid volume with small increases in CVP[26,27] Prenatal diagnosis and fetal hemodynamic monitoring of these critical forms of CHDs can allow for multidisciplinary planning for delivery and well-coordinated care during transition, as well as providing prenatal counseling to families.

## Perinatal Management Strategies to Optimize Postnatal Transition

Prenatal diagnosis of CCHD allows for adequate time to counsel families, create a perinatal transition plan, and prepare the multidisciplinary team for a well-coordinated delivery with postnatal care.[28] Delivery and transition plans must take into account the underlying cardiac anatomy, anticipated physiologic changes during transition from fetal to postnatal life, rate of risk of deterioration, the need for emergent neonatal intervention, and potential definitive surgical options. Risk stratification systems are designed according to the severity level of the CHD and include associated neonatal action plans. These stratification systems can designate the need for PGE, the mode of delivery (MOD), appropriate level of perinatal and neonatal care services available, and proximity to immediate access to cardiology and cardiothoracic surgery care.

Risk stratification and management systems using level of care (LOC) for neonates prenatally diagnosed with CHD have been shown to be highly accurate at predicting the postnatal care and need for emergent intervention at birth.[29,30] The four levels of care, with level 1 being lowest and level 4 being highest risk for compromise, are denoted based on the type of cardiac lesion and agreed on by the perinatal team, including obstetrics, neonatology, CT surgery, and cardiology, helping to guide the delivery and transition plan.[25,30] These classification strategies have been highly reproducible, with the exception of d-TGA, due to the difficulty in determining the risk for postnatal atrial level restriction. As a result, all d-TGA cases are automatically upgraded from LOC 3 to LOC 4 status.[30]

LOC 1 patients are low risk, not expected to necessitate support or intervention in the immediate newborn period, and include patients with atrial septal defects and ventricular septal defects. Level 2 denotes intermediate risk including patients with severe systemic or pulmonary outflow tract obstruction with ductal dependent flow. Patients with lesions in this category, such as HLHS, are typically stable in DR but require prostaglandin for ductal patency and transfer to cardiac center for intervention. Level 3, identifies patients at high risk for immediate postnatal catheter intervention or surgery such as HLHS with restrictive atrial septum or CHD with arrhythmia or decreased function. Finally, level 4 care indicates a high-risk population requiring immediate intervention postnatally, including HLHS with intact atrial septum, d-TGA with RAS/IAS, and severe Ebstein's with hydrops or incessant arrhythmia. Level 3 and 4 deliveries via planned cesarean section versus induction near term must be discussed with

the multidisciplinary team to assess ability for coordination of care and at a center with interventional/surgical services for rapid access.[25,30] If unable to deliver at a cardiac center and concern for rapid decompensation, particularly level 4 patients, transport team should be ready to transfer to a center with cardiac intervention services as soon as feasible (Table 30.4). Another institution implemented a slight variation to the LOC 1–4 risk stratification, separating CHD by need for emergent neonatal cardiac intervention (ENCI). In their model the classification system correctly stratified 90.4% of prenatally diagnosed CHD patients based on intervention need. No neonate with ENCI level 1 (low risk, e.g., ASD, VSD, mild PS) or level 2 (medium risk, not PGE dependent, e.g., complete AV canal, TOF/PS, truncus) needed neonatal emergent intervention.[29]

While some patients with CCHD can be delivered at centers without cardiac services, transportation of infants with CCHD to a higher-level cardiac care center for delivery and postnatal care has been shown to improve outcomes and is associated with lower overall health care costs.[31-33] Delivery planning includes timing as well as MOD. With recognition that preterm delivery and low birth weight have negative impact on outcomes, current recommendations endeavor to deliver these patients no earlier than 39 weeks of gestation.[34-37] It is notable that a prenatal diagnosis of CHD may alter the chosen MOD and has been shown to result in elevated rates of elective c-section for many forms of CHDs.[38,39] However, studies have asserted that vaginal birth is generally well-tolerated in CCHD neonates, with little evidence demonstrating that altering MOD improves outcomes in CHD infants.[39-41] Thus changes in delivery timing and MOD should only be considered in critical cases in order to provide rapid postnatal stabilization and intervention.

## Delivery Room Management

Most patients with CCHD are relatively stable in the DR; thus DR management begins by following the basic tenants of neonatal resuscitation to assess the infant's airway, breathing, and circulation. At delivery, cord clamping releases the low-resistance placenta from the fetal circuit, resulting in a sudden increase in left ventricular afterload. Simultaneously, respiratory effort aids in rapid decrease in PVR. Both of these

**TABLE 30.4   Risk-Stratification of Delivery Room Management of Neonates With CHD**

| Level of Care | Postnatal Expectation | CHD Examples | Delivery Recommendation | Cardiac DR Recommendation |
|---|---|---|---|---|
| 1 | No instability expected | ASD, VSD | Delivery at local hospital | Outpatient f/u |
| 2 | Stability in DR, but expected postnatal intervention | Ductal dependent lesions, e.g., HLHS, PA/IVS, severe TOF | Planned induction ≥39 weeks dependent on maternal care | Neonatologist in DR Transport to cardiac center |
| 3 | Instability requiring immediate care in DR | HLHS with RAS CHD or arrhythmia with decreased function | Planned induction at 38–39 weeks Plan for urgent intervention/transport as indicated | Neonatologist, cardiologist in DR, potential meds |
| 4 | Instability requiring immediate cath or surgical intervention | HLHS with IAS or TGA with RAS/IAS Arrhythmia with hydrops Severe Ebstein's anomaly or TOF/APV with hydrops | Mode and time of delivery planned with possible c-section at 38 weeks (possibly earlier if dysfunction or hydrops) | Specialty team in DR, potential for ECMO or side-by-side OR |

Adapted from Donofrio.[30,71,72]

*ASD*, atrial septal defect; *CHD*, congenital heart disease; *DR*, delivery room; *HLHS*, hypoplastic left heart syndrome; *ECMO*, extracorporeal membrane oxygenation; *IAS*, intact atrial septum; *OR*, operating room; *PA/IVS*, pulmonary atresia/intact ventricular septum; *RAS*, restrictive atrial septum; *TGA*, transposition of the great arteries; *TOF*, tetralogy of Fallot; *TOF/APV*, tetralogy of Fallot/absent pulmonary valve; VSD = ventricular septal defect.

postnatal factors lead to increased left atrial pressure, resulting in functional closure of the patent foramen ovale.[42,43] CCHD patients with an inability to traverse blood out of the left atrium, such as with HLHS with RAS/IAS, will present shortly after birth with respiratory distress and decreased cardiac output. However, most CCHD patients will tolerate transition well. In fact, delayed cord clamping has been noted to be safe in the CCHD population and is associated with a decrease in transfusions.[44] Elective intubation is not recommended and should be avoided when possible. The decision to intubate should be based on the assessment of the clinical respiratory and circulatory status, rather than the underlying cardiac diagnosis. Pulse oximetry should be initiated in the DR with the goal of judicious use of oxygen based on diagnosis. In patients with a known prenatal diagnosis of a CHD lesion associated with increased pulmonary blood flow such as HLHS, clinicians should avoid increased oxygen administration that will lower PVR and lead to over-circulation of blood to the lungs with risk of systemic steal. Ongoing circulatory assessment includes evaluation of heart rate (HR), color, pulses, and central capillary refill. For patients at risk of compromise in the DR requiring

surgical or ECMO capabilities, a multidisciplinary approach to planning side-by-side operating rooms, including the role of simulation, may provide an ability to streamline the process and enhance outcomes.[45]

## Postnatal Monitoring

Pre- and post-ductal oxygen saturation monitoring should be obtained depending on the diagnosis. Additional monitoring including line placement should be obtained in patients with CCHD for close assessment. Umbilical lines are preferred as they allow avoidance of vascular access points in patients with potential upcoming cardiac procedures including catheterizations. Use of point-of-care ultrasound (POCUS) at the bedside has been demonstrated to facilitate the success rate of umbilical line placement in cardiac patients.[46]

Prostaglandin E1/E2 should be initiated in infants with lesions requiring maintenance of the PDA, eventually needing surgical- or catheter-based intervention to provide a more stable source of pulmonary or systemic blood flow. Clinicians should be aware of potential side effects of a prostaglandin infusion, including early apnea and hypotension. The late side effect profile includes hyperostosis and gastric outlet obstruction, with one study noting occurrence of hyperostosis in 42% of patients with PGE1 infusion for <30 days and 100% when continued for >60 days.[47-49] Most infants with a CCHD and an open ductus arteriosus (such as those with a prenatal diagnosis or those who are diagnosed soon after birth) need a small dose of prostaglandin E1/E2 (0.01–0.02 mcg/kg/min) to keep the PDA open, while decompensated infants with a closed duct may initially require a larger dose (0.05–0.1 mcg/kg/min).[50] Most infants with a prostaglandin dose of under 0.025 mcg/kg/min are unlikely to have significant apnea or adverse effects, and they can be even transported safely without mechanical ventilation, while those on the higher dose (0.05–0.1 mcg/kg/min) are more likely to need mechanical ventilation.[50]

In patients with CCHD presenting postnatally with hypoxemia and concern for cardiovascular compromise, the clinical evaluation should include perfusion checks, laboratory tests such as lactate level, and monitoring of pre- and post-ductal saturations to determine the presence of right to left shunting through the PDA. However, echocardiography provides a definitive noninvasive bedside diagnostic tool for identifying underlying CHD and delineating the anatomy. It is suggested that any neonate that has a limited POCUS evaluation performed in the setting of cardiovascular or respiratory compromise should subsequently have a comprehensive echocardiogram performed to rule out CCHD.[51,52]

## Multidisciplinary Care of the Neonate with CCHD

With neonates comprising 25–30% of patients in cardiac intensive care units, neonatologists are involved in many institutions in the management of this complex and vulnerable population. In a survey of level 4 neonatal intensive care units (NICUs) prenatal consultation by a neonatologist for patients with CHDs occurred in 86%, and while most patients were admitted to the cardiac intensive care unit, 95% of hospitals had neonatologists involved in the management of neonates with congenital cardiac lesions.[53] Associated conditions, including multiple anomalies, genetic

associations, and prematurity, in particular, can benefit from multidisciplinary care. Epidemiologic studies suggest approximately 20–30% of CHD cases are associated with genetic or environmental causes, with gross chromosomal anomalies/aneuploidy comprising 8–10% of CHD cases. Determining underlying genetic associations can provide additional counseling opportunities for families, including testing family members, as well as directing clinicians to additional testing that may be needed.[54,55]

Prematurity with CHD adds more complexity to the neonatal care and is associated with increased mortality.[56-58] CHD has been associated with a twofold increased risk of spontaneous preterm birth.[59] In a single-center study, 18% of neonates admitted to the cardiac intensive care unit (CICU) were born prematurely with an overall hospital mortality rate of 21%, compared with 7% in patients born between 37 and 38 weeks' gestational age (GA), and 3% in those born between 39 and 40 weeks' GA, respectively. In addition, there was increased risk of 5-minute Apgar score ≤7, preintervention mechanical ventilation, and greater surgical complexity.[57] In a large international multicenter study of very preterm infants from 24 to 31 weeks' gestation, mortality was higher in the cohort with CHD compared to neonates without CHD at the same gestational age (18.6% vs. 8.9%, $P < 0.001$). It was also found that the preterm infant with CHD had a greater risk for the development of bronchopulmonary dysplasia; however, there were no differences seen in other co-morbidities, such as neonatal brain injury, necrotizing enterocolitis, or treated retinopathy of prematurity.[56] Another large cohort study of trends in 1-year morbidity and mortality in preterm infants with CHD 26–36 weeks' gestational age found that while the relative risk of death decreased by 10.6% each year, risk of morbidity increased 8.3% yearly. Interestingly, this study also noted significant increases in BPD risk over time, but no other major morbidities had a statistically significant increase in risk, such as NEC, interventricular hemorrhage, and periventricular leukomalacia, though risks did trend higher.[60] While it is clear that prematurity impacts outcomes, optimal timing of surgical intervention is less certain. Some centers have demonstrated success with delaying surgery,[61,62] with 2 kg being reported as a threshold for a change in mortality rate.[63] However, prolonged PGE1 and long-term total parenteral nutrition (TPN) are not without significant risks, such as infection, vascular injury, TPN cholestasis, and feeding intolerance. Some studies demonstrate worse outcomes with delayed surgery and advocate for early repair.[64,65] With a heterogenous complex population, combining expertise in management of prematurity with expertise in congenital heart disease through a multidisciplinary team approach is essential.

In cases of fetal diagnosis of CHD both prenatal and postnatal collaborative care allows for discussion of delivery room management and personnel and planning of postnatal care.[66] Currently there is a significant variation in the postnatal management of CCHD patients, with recognition that standardization of care may enhance care and prognosis.[67] In the setting of the cardiac ICU neonatologists with cardiovascular expertise may provide guidance on approach to mechanical ventilation, use of surfactant, feeding, neurocritical care, and vascular access.

## Summary

Prenatal detection of congenital heart disease has improved over the years, yet it is still diagnosed in only approximately half of patients, and this pick-up rate is only slightly better for cases of critical CHD at 50–75%.[68] Thus early recognition of the signs and symptoms of decompensation related to CCHD is paramount to providing high-quality neonatal care in this area. The postnatal transition represents a time of major physiologic adaptation during which the neonate with CCHD may be stressed by changes in PVR, cardiac loading conditions, and increased metabolic demands. This is particularly true in neonates with CHD that present with cyanosis, hypoperfusion, or inadequate mixing of the circulations. While many patients with CCHD can initially have stable hemodynamics at birth, an understanding of changing physiology surrounding patients with CHD is imperative to appropriate care in the delivery room and NICU. Multidisciplinary collaboration with well-developed risk stratification systems with planning of care strategies can enhance team communication and potentially improve outcomes in this complex population.

## REFERENCES

1. Montaña E, Khoury MJ, Cragan JD, Sharma S, Dhar P, Fyfe D. Trends and outcomes after prenatal diagnosis of congenital cardiac malformations by fetal echocardiography in a well defined birth population, Atlanta, Georgia, 1990-1994. *J Am Coll Cardiol.* 1996;28(7):1805-1809. doi:10.1016/S0735-1097(96)00381–6.
2. Tworetzky W, McElhinney DB, Reddy VM, Brook MM, Hanley FL, Silverman NH. Improved surgical outcome after fetal diagnosis of hypoplastic left heart syndrome. *Circulation.* 2001; 103(9):1269-1273. doi:10.1161/01.CIR.103.9.1269.
3. Holland BJ, Myers JA, Woods Jr CR. Prenatal diagnosis of critical congenital heart disease reduces risk of death from cardiovascular compromise prior to planned neonatal cardiac surgery: a meta-analysis. *Ultrasound Obstet Gynecol.* 2015;45(6):631-638. doi:10.1002/uog.14882.
4. Friedberg MK, Silverman NH, Moon-Grady AJ, et al. Prenatal detection of congenital heart disease. *J Pediatr.* 2009;155(1): 26-31.e1. doi:10.1016/j.jpeds.2009.01.050.
5. Escobar-Diaz MC, Freud LR, Bueno A, et al. Prenatal diagnosis of transposition of the great arteries over a 20-year period: improved but imperfect. *Ultrasound Obstet Gynecol.* 2015; 45(6):678-682. doi:10.1002/uog.14751.
6. Quartermain MD, Pasquali SK, Hill KD, et al. Variation in prenatal diagnosis of congenital heart disease in infants. *Pediatrics.* 2015;136(2):e378-e385. doi:10.1542/peds.2014-3783.
7. Gilboa SM, Salemi JL, Nembhard WN, Fixler DE, Correa A. Mortality resulting from congenital heart disease among children and adults in the United States, 1999 to 2006. *Circulation.* 2010;122(22):2254-2263. doi:10.1161/circulationaha. 110.947002.
8. Mahle WT, Newburger JW, Matherne GP, et al. Role of pulse oximetry in examining newborns for congenital heart disease. *Circulation.* 2009;120(5):447-458. doi:10.1161/circulationaha. 109.192576.
9. Schultz AH, Localio AR, Clark BJ, Ravishankar C, Videon N, Kimmel SE. Epidemiologic features of the presentation of critical congenital heart disease: implications for screening. *Pediatrics.* 2008;121(4):751-757. doi:10.1542/peds.2007-0421.
10. Eckersley L, Sadler L, Parry E, Finucane K, Gentles TL. Timing of diagnosis affects mortality in critical congenital heart disease. *Arch Dis Child.* 2016;101(6):516-520. doi:10.1136/archdischild-2014-307691.
11. Atz AM, Feinstein JA, Jonas RA, Perry SB, Wessel DL. Preoperative management of pulmonary venous hypertension in hypoplastic left heart syndrome with restrictive atrial septal defect. *Am J Cardiol.* 1999;83(8):1224-1228. doi:10.1016/s0002-9149(99)00087-9.
12. Rychik J, Rome JJ, Collins MH, DeCampli WM, Spray TL. The hypoplastic left heart syndrome with intact atrial septum: atrial morphology, pulmonary vascular histopathology and outcome. *J Am Coll Cardiol.* 1999;34(2):554-560. doi:10.1016/s0735-1097(99)00225-9.
13. Vlahos AP, Lock JE, McElhinney DB, Velde MEvd. Hypoplastic left heart syndrome with intact or highly restrictive atrial septum. *Circulation.* 2004;109(19):2326-2330. doi:10.1161/01. CIR.0000128690.35860.C5.
14. Jantzen DW, Moon-Grady AJ, Morris SA, et al. Hypoplastic left heart syndrome with intact or restrictive atrial septum. *Circulation.* 2017;136(14):1346-1349. doi:10.1161/CIRCULA-TIONAHA.116.025873.
15. Seale AN, Carvalho JS, Gardiner HM, et al. Total anomalous pulmonary venous connection: impact of prenatal diagnosis.

604 PART D  Common Hemodynamic Dilemmas in the Neonate

*Ultrasound Obstet Gynecol.* 2012;40(3):310-318. doi:10.1002/uog.11093.

16. Juaneda E, Haworth SG. Pulmonary vascular disease in children with truncus arteriosus. *Am J Cardiol.* 1984;54(10):1314-1320. doi:10.1016/S0002-9149(84)80089-2.

17. McElhinney DB, Hedrick HL, Bush DM, et al. Necrotizing enterocolitis in neonates with congenital heart disease: risk factors and outcomes. *Pediatrics.* 2000;106(5):1080-1087. doi:10.1542/peds.106.5.1080.

18. Mahle WT, Martin GR, Beekman RH, et al. Endorsement of health and human services recommendation for pulse oximetry screening for critical congenital heart disease. *Pediatrics.* 2012;129(1):190-192. doi:10.1542/peds.2011-3211.

19. Liske MR, Greeley CS, Law DJ, et al. Report of the tennessee task force on screening newborn infants for critical congenital heart disease. *Pediatrics.* 2006;118(4):e1250-e1256. doi:10.1542/peds.2005-3061.

20. Dawson AL, Cassell CH, Riehle-Colarusso T, et al. Factors associated with late detection of critical congenital heart disease in newborns. *Pediatrics.* 2013;132(3):e604-e611. doi:10.1542/peds.2013-1002.

21. Papadhima I, Louis D, Purna J, et al. Targeted neonatal echocardiography (TNE) consult service in a large tertiary perinatal center in Canada. *J Perinatol.* 2018;38(8):1039-1045. doi:10.1038/s41372-018-0130-y.

22. Lau PE, Cruz SM, Ocampo EC, et al. Necrotizing enterocolitis in patients with congenital heart disease: a single center experience. *J Pediatr Surg.* 2018;53(5):914-917. doi:10.1016/j.jpedsurg.2018.02.014.

23. Rudolph AM. *Congenital Diseases of the Heart: Clinical-Physiological Considerations.* 3rd ed. Chichester: Wiley-Blackwell; 2009.

24. Hooper SB, te Pas AB, Lang J, et al. Cardiovascular transition at birth: a physiological sequence. *Pediatr Res.* 2015;77(5):608-614. doi:10.1038/pr.2015.21.

25. Pruetz JD, Wang SS, Noori S. Delivery room emergencies in critical congenital heart diseases. *Semin Fetal Neonatal Med.* 2019;24(6):101034. doi:10.1016/j.siny.2019.101034.

26. Pruetz JD, Votava-Smith J, Miller DA. Clinical relevance of fetal hemodynamic monitoring: perinatal implications. *Semin Fetal Neonatal Med.* 2015;20(4):217-224. doi:10.1016/j.siny.2015.03.007.

27. Kiserud T. Physiology of the fetal circulation. *Semin Fetal Neonatal Med.* 2005;10(6):493-503. doi:10.1016/j.siny.2005.08.007.

28. Sanapo L, Pruetz JD, Słodki M, Goens MB, Moon-Grady AJ, Donofrio MT. Fetal echocardiography for planning perinatal and delivery room care of neonates with congenital heart disease. *Echocardiography.* 2017;34(12):1804-1821. doi:10.1111/echo.13672.

29. Harbison AL, Chen S, Shepherd JL, et al. Outcomes of implementing cardiac risk stratification and perinatal care recommendations for prenatally diagnosed congenital heart disease. *Prenat Cardiol.* 2020;(1):24-31. doi:10.5114/pcard.2020.99014.

30. Donofrio MT, Skurow-Todd K, Berger JT, et al. Risk-stratified postnatal care of newborns with congenital heart disease determined by fetal echocardiography. *J Am Soc Echocardiogr.* 2015;28(11):1339-1349. doi:10.1016/j.echo.2015.07.005.

31. Anagnostou K, Messenger L, Yates R, Kelsall W. Outcome of infants with prenatally diagnosed congenital heart disease delivered outside specialist paediatric cardiac centres. *Arch Dis Child Fetal Neonatal Ed.* 2013;98(3):F218-F221. doi:10.1136/archdischild-2011-300488.

32. Jegatheeswaran A, Oliveira C, Batsos C, et al. Costs of prenatal detection of congenital heart disease. *Am J Cardiol.* 2011;108(12):1808-1814. doi:10.1016/j.amjcard.2011.07.052.

33. Morris SA, Ethen MK, Penny DJ, et al. Prenatal diagnosis, birth location, surgical center, and neonatal mortality in infants with hypoplastic left heart syndrome. *Circulation.* 2014;129(3):285-292. doi:10.1161/CIRCULATIONAHA.113.003711.

34. Costello JM, Polito A, Brown DW, et al. Birth before 39 weeks' gestation is associated with worse outcomes in neonates with heart disease. *Pediatrics.* 2010;126(2):277-284. doi:10.1542/peds.2009-3640.

35. Cnota JF, Gupta R, Michelfelder EC, Ittenbach RF. Congenital heart disease infant death rates decrease as gestational age advances from 34 to 40 weeks. *J Pediatr.* 2011;159(5):761-765. doi:10.1016/j.jpeds.2011.04.020.

36. Wertaschnigg D, Manlhiot C, Jaeggi M, et al. Contemporary outcomes and factors associated with mortality after a fetal or neonatal diagnosis of ebstein anomaly and tricuspid valve disease. *Can J Cardiol.* 2016;32(12):1500-1506. doi:10.1016/j.cjca.2016.03.008.

37. Steurer MA, Baer RJ, Keller RL, et al. Gestational age and outcomes in critical congenital heart disease. *Pediatrics.* 2017;140(4):e20170999. doi:10.1542/peds.2017-0999.

38. Trento LU, Pruetz JD, Chang RK, Detterich J, Sklansky MS. Prenatal diagnosis of congenital heart disease: impact of mode of delivery on neonatal outcome. *Prenat Diagn.* 2012;32(13):1250-1255. doi:10.1002/pd.3991.

39. Peyvandi S, Nguyen TA, Almeida-Jones M, et al. Timing and mode of delivery in prenatally diagnosed congenital heart disease – an analysis of practices within the University of California Fetal Consortium (UCfC). *Pediatr Cardiol.* 2017;38(3):588-595. doi:10.1007/s00246-016-1552-y.

40. Reis PM, Punch MR, Bove EL, van de Ven CJM. Obstetric management of 219 infants with hypoplastic left heart syndrome. *Am J Obstet Gynecol.* 1998;179(5):1150-1154. doi:10.1016/S0002-9378(98)70123-1.

41. Walsh CA, MacTiernan A, Farrell S, et al. Mode of delivery in pregnancies complicated by major fetal congenital heart disease: a retrospective cohort study. *J Perinatol.* 2014;34(12):901-905. doi:10.1038/jp.2014.104.

42. Sanapo L, Moon-Grady AJ, Donofrio MT. Perinatal and delivery management of infants with congenital heart disease. *Clin Perinatol.* 2016;43(1):55-71. doi:10.1016/j.clp.2015.11.004.

43. Singh Y, Lakshminrusimha S. Perinatal cardiovascular physiology and recognition of critical congenital heart defects. *Clin Perinatol.* 2021;48(3):573-594. doi:10.1016/j.clp.2021.05.008.

44. Backes CH, Huang H, Cua CL, et al. Early versus delayed umbilical cord clamping in infants with congenital heart disease: a pilot, randomized, controlled trial. *J Perinatol.* 2015;35(10):826-831. doi:10.1038/jp.2015.89.

45. Yamada NK, Fuerch JH, Halamek LP. Simulation-based patient-specific multidisciplinary team training in preparation for the resuscitation and stabilization of conjoined twins. *Am J Perinatol.* 2017;34(6):621-626. doi:10.1055/s-0036-1593808.

46. Kozyak BW, Fraga MV, Juliano CE, et al. Real-time ultrasound guidance for umbilical venous cannulation in neonates with congenital heart disease. *Pediatr Crit Care Med.* 2022;23(5):e257-e266. doi:10.1097/pcc.0000000000002919.

47. Estes K, Nowicki M, Bishop P. Cortical hyperostosis secondary to prostaglandin E1 therapy. *J Pediatr.* 2007;151(4):441, 441.e1. doi:10.1016/j.jpeds.2007.02.066.

48. Woo K, Emery J, Peabody J. Cortical hyperostosis: a complication of prolonged prostaglandin infusion in infants awaiting cardiac transplantation. *Pediatrics*. 1994;93(3):417-420.

49. Akkinapally S, Hundalani SG, Kulkarni M, et al. Prostaglandin E1 for maintaining ductal patency in neonates with ductal-dependent cardiac lesions. *Cochrane Database Syst Rev*. 2018;2(2):Cd011417. doi:10.1002/14651858.CD011417.pub2.

50. Singh Y, Mikrou P. Use of prostaglandins in duct-dependent congenital heart conditions. *Arch Dis Child Educ Pract Ed*. 2018;103(3):137-140. doi:10.1136/archdischild-2017-313654.

51. Singh Y, Tissot C, Fraga MV, et al. International evidence-based guidelines on Point of Care Ultrasound (POCUS) for critically ill neonates and children issued by the POCUS Working Group of the European Society of Paediatric and Neonatal Intensive Care (ESPNIC). *Crit Care*. 2020;24(1):65. doi:10.1186/s13054-020-2787-9.

52. Singh Y, Bhombal S, Katheria A, Tissot C, Fraga MV. The evolution of cardiac point of care ultrasound for the neonatologist. *Eur J Pediatr*. 2021;180(12):3565-3575. doi:10.1007/s00431-021-04153-5.

53. Hamrick SEG, Ball MK, Rajgarhia A, Johnson BA, Digeronimo R, Levy PT. Integrated cardiac care models of neonates with congenital heart disease: the evolving role of the neonatologist. *J Perinatol*. 2021;41(7):1774-1776. doi:10.1038/s41372-021-01117-3.

54. Pierpont ME, Brueckner M, Chung WK, et al. Genetic basis for congenital heart disease: revisited: a scientific statement from the American Heart Association. *Circulation*. 2018;138(21):e653-e711. doi:10.1161/CIR.0000000000000606.

55. Cowan JR, Ware SM. Genetics and genetic testing in congenital heart disease. *Clin Perinatol*. 2015;42(2):373-393, ix. doi:10.1016/j.clp.2015.02.009.

56. Norman M, Håkansson S, Kusuda S, et al. Neonatal outcomes in very preterm infants with severe congenital heart defects: an international cohort study. *J Am Heart Assoc*. 2020;9(5):e015369. doi:10.1161/jaha.119.015369.

57. Cheng HH, Almodovar MC, Laussen PC, et al. Outcomes and risk factors for mortality in premature neonates with critical congenital heart disease. *Pediatr Cardiol*. 2011;32(8):1139-1146. doi:10.1007/s00246-011-0036-3.

58. Chu PY, Li JS, Kosinski AS, Hornik CP, Hill KD. Congenital heart disease in premature infants 25-32 weeks' gestational age. *J Pediatr*. 2017;181:37-41.e1. doi:10.1016/j.jpeds.2016.10.033.

59. Matthiesen NB, Østergaard JR, Hjortdal VE, Henriksen TB. Congenital heart defects and the risk of spontaneous preterm birth. *J Pediatr*. 2021;229:168-174.e5. doi:10.1016/j.jpeds.2020.09.059.

60. Steurer MA, Baer RJ, Chambers CD, et al. Mortality and major neonatal morbidity in preterm infants with serious congenital heart disease. *J Pediatr*. 2021;239:110-116.e3. doi:10.1016/j.jpeds.2021.08.039.

61. Shepard CW, Kochilas LK, Rosengart RM, et al. Repair of major congenital cardiac defects in low-birth-weight infants: is delay warranted? *J Thorac Cardiovasc Surg*. 2010;140(5):1104-1109. doi:10.1016/j.jtcvs.2010.08.013.

62. Jennings E, Cuadrado A, Maher KO, Kogon B, Kirshbom PM, Simsic JM. Short-term outcomes in premature neonates adhering to the philosophy of supportive care allowing for weight gain and organ maturation prior to cardiac surgery. *J Intensive Care Med*. 2012;27(1):32-36. doi:10.1177/0885066610393662.

63. Hickey EJ, Nosikova Y, Zhang H, et al. Very low-birth-weight infants with congenital cardiac lesions: is there merit in delaying intervention to permit growth and maturation? *J Thorac Cardiovasc Surg*. 2012;143(1):126-136.e1. doi:10.1016/j.jtcvs.2011.09.008.

64. Reddy VM, Hanley FL. Cardiac surgery in infants with very low birth weight. *Semin Pediatr Surg*. 2000;9(2):91-95. doi:10.1016/s1055-8586(00)70023-0.

65. Reddy VM, McElhinney DB, Sagrado T, Parry AJ, Teitel DF, Hanley FL. Results of 102 cases of complete repair of congenital heart defects in patients weighing 700 to 2500 grams. *J Thorac Cardiovasc Surg*. 1999;117(2):324-331. doi:10.1016/s0022-5223(99)70430-7.

66. Levy VY, Bhombal S, Villafane J, et al. Status of multidisciplinary collaboration in neonatal cardiac care in the United States. *Pediatr Cardiol*. 2021;42(5):1088-1101. doi:10.1007/s00246-021-02586-1.

67. Leon RL, Levy PT, Hu J, Yallpragada SG, Hamrick SEG, Ball MK. Practice variations for fetal and neonatal congenital heart disease within the Children's Hospitals Neonatal Consortium. *Pediatr Res*. 2022. doi:10.1038/s41390-022-02314-2.

68. Bakker MK, Bergman JEH, Krikov S, et al. Prenatal diagnosis and prevalence of critical congenital heart defects: an international retrospective cohort study. *BMJ Open*. 2019;9(7):e028139. doi:10.1136/bmjopen-2018-028139.

69. Desai K, Rabinowitz EJ, Epstein S. Physiologic diagnosis of congenital heart disease in cyanotic neonates. *Curr Opin Pediatr*. 2019;31(2):274-283. doi:10.1097/mop.0000000000000742.

70. Oster ME, Aucott SW, Glidewell J, et al. Lessons Learned From Newborn Screening for Critical Congenital Heart Defects. *Pediatrics*. 2016;137(5). doi:10.1542/peds.2015-4573.

71. Donofrio MT. Predicting the future: delivery room planning of congenital heart disease diagnosed by fetal echocardiography. *Am J Perinatol*. 2018;35(6):549-552. doi:10.1055/s-0038-1637764.

72. Donofrio MT, Levy RJ, Schuette JJ, et al. Specialized delivery room planning for fetuses with critical congenital heart disease. *Am J Cardiol*. 2013;111(5):737-747. doi:10.1016/j.amjcard.2012.11.029.

# Index

Note: Page numbers followed by "f" refer to illustrations; page numbers followed by "t" refer to tables; page numbers followed by "b" refer to boxes.

616 Index